NORTH TEXAS POISON CENTER
P.O. BOX 35926
DALLAS, TEXAS 75235

Handbook of Pesticide Toxicology

Handbook of Pesticide Toxicology

VOLUME 3
CLASSES OF PESTICIDES

EDITED BY

Wayland J. Hayes, Jr.
Vanderbilt University
School of Medicine
Nashville, Tennessee

Edward R. Laws, Jr.
Department of Neurological Surgery
George Washington University School of Medicine
Washington, D.C.

Academic Press, Inc.
Harcourt Brace Jovanovich, Publishers
San Diego   New York   Boston   London   Sydney   Tokyo   Toronto

Academic Press, Inc.
San Diego, California 92101

United Kingdom Edition published by
Academic Press Limited
24–28 Oval Road, London NW1 7DX

Library of Congress Cataloging-in-Publication Data

Handbook of pesticide toxicology / Wayland J. Hayes, Jr., Edward R.
  Laws, Jr., editors.
      p.   cm.
    Includes bibliographical references.
    Contents: v. 1. General principles -- v. 2-3. Classes of
pesticides.
    ISBN 0-12-334161-2   (v. 1 : alk. paper) -- ISBN 0-12-334162-0
(v. 2 : alk. paper) -- ISBN 0-12-334163-9   (v. 3 : alk. paper)
    1. Pesticides--Toxicology.   I. Hayes, Wayland J., Date.
  II. Laws, Edward R.
  RA1270.P4H36   1991
  615.9'02--dc20
                                                      90-313
                                                      CIP

Printed in the United States of America
90 91 92 93   9 8 7 6 5 4 3 2 1

To Philip Theophrastus Bombast von Hohenheim
called PARACELSUS who said

Was ist das nit gifft ist: alle ding sind
gifft/und nichts ohn gifft/Allein die dosis macht
das ein ding kein gift ist.

or in more familiar language
Dosage Alone Determines Poisoning

Contents of the Handbook

Contents of Volume 3

Carbamate Insecticides

Ronald L. Baron

Baron Associates

17.1 CLASSIFICATION OF CARBAMATES

Carbamate esters used as insecticides have this common structure:

$$R—O—C(O)—N(CH_3)—R'$$

where R is an alcohol, oxime, or phenol and R' is hydrogen or a methyl group (or, in the case of procarbamates, one of several N- or S-substituted moieties, as discussed in Section 17.2.4.1). These compounds, which inhibit acetylcholinesterase in both insects and mammals, are described in later sections of this chapter. Other carbamates do not inhibit acetylcholinesterase to any significant degree; they are described in Chapter 20 on herbicides and Chapter 21 on fungicides.

17.2 TOXICOLOGY OF ANTICHOLINESTERASE CARBAMATES

17.2.1 PHARMACOLOGICAL BASIS

Among both carbamates and organic phosphorus compounds are a few with a quaternary nitrogen at a suitable distance from the carbonyl carbon or from the phosphorus so that the nitrogen reacts with the anionic site of acetylcholinesterase. Some of these quaternary compounds are extremely active in mammals and inhibit insect acetylcholinesterase *in vitro,* but they are not effective insecticides. Much of what is known about the action of insecticidal carbamates in humans first was learned from study of one such compound, physostigmine, and its synthetic analogs. Physostigmine (Eserine) is an alkaloid extracted from the calabar bean, the seed of *Physostigma venenosum.* Along the Calabar River in West Africa, where the vine is found, slurries of the beans were used as ordeal poisons. Holmstedt (1972) records that the use of such poisons has not been abandoned.

17.2.1.1 Symptomatology

The signs and symptoms of acute toxicity are similar for all anticholinesterase carbamates and for all mammalian species. Onset and severity of symptoms are dose related. The first signs, usually occurring 15–30 min or less after oral administration, are excessive salivation and increased and irregular respiration, followed by lacrimation, urination, defecation, and muscular fasciculations and tremors. Constriction of pupils, exophthalmos, pallor, piloerection, anorexia, nausea, vomiting, ataxia, and bradycardia or tachycardia are often observed. In the most severe cases, these signs are followed by violent intestinal movements, associated with muscular weakness and spasms, progressing to convulsions. Either death or signs of recovery generally occur within one to several hours of exposure. The usual case of death is respiratory failure associated with bronchial constriction, excessive pulmonary secretions, and paralysis of the respiratory center or respiratory muscles. General agitation, lacrimation, salivation, constriction of pupils, poor coordination, and muscular twitching usually subside within 5–6 hr. In humans, spontaneous recovery from clinical signs and symptoms of peripheral or central nervous system disruption is complete 24 hr after acute overexposure.

17.2.1.2 Absorption, Distribution, Metabolism, and Excretion

The toxicity of carbamates is greatly influenced by the vehicle and route of exposure, and the importance of these factors varies among the insecticidal carbamates. Carbamates are readily absorbed during passage through the gastrointestinal tract, and absorption is in part related to the vehicle in which they are administered. Both vehicles and environmental conditions also influence the dermal absorption rate and thus the observed dermal toxicity. For example, in monkeys dermally exposed to methomyl, conditions of high temperature and relative humidity caused cholinergic symptoms to occur earlier, be more severe, and last longer than under normal conditions (du Pont, 1986). The most important human exposure route is dermal, and those most likely to be affected are those occupationally exposed, such as insecticide formulators and applicators and farm workers. The greatest risk to these individuals would be from working with carbamates under conditions of high temperature. Low-level exposure to residues in foods may occur wherever carbamates are used on edible commodities and where tolerances have been granted for such uses.

Whereas the anticholinesterase carbamates are subject to all the factors, including temperature, that influence toxicity and dermal absorption, as discussed in Section 3.2.2.5, the vapor pressure of certain of these compounds makes them particularly subject to the effects of temperature when they are sprayed on surfaces. For example, poisoning occurred when the experimental pesticide 3-isopropylphenyl-N-methylcarbamate was sprayed inside Nigerian houses to test its possible value for malaria control. In explanation, Hayes (1971) cited a report by Barlow and Flower noting that metal roofs exposed to tropical sunlight may reach temperatures of 70–90°C. Thus, chemicals sprayed on roofs at these temperatures would vaporize so rapidly that the sprayers would be exposed to a high concentration of vapor, in addition to the usual aerosol. It was noted that propoxur and promecarb, which were used with far less difficulty, were not only inherently less toxic but also less volatile at temperatures of 80°C or below.

Once absorbed, carbamates are rapidly distributed to the tissues and organs. Concentrations tend to be highest in organs and tissues involved in xenobiotic metabolism. Metabolism and elimination are relatively rapid; no evidence has been found for bioaccumulation of carbamates. A complete review of the biotransformation of any of the N-methyl or N,N-dimethyl carbamates is beyond the scope of this book. The mammalian metabolism of individual compounds is briefly reviewed in Section 17.3. Although the compounds show broad similarities in their metabolism, no two are identical. Furthermore, species differences in metabolism are more pronounced for some carbamates than for others.

Generally, the first step in carbamate metabolism is oxidation to provide a site that serves as the base for a conjugation reaction yielding water-soluble products for excretion. In a study of the oxidation of 33 methyl and dimethyl insecticides and related compounds by microsomal enzymes, examples of N-demethylation, aromatic ring hydroxylation, O-dealkylation, alkyl hydroxylation, sulfoxidation, conversion of N-methyl to N-formamide or N-hydroxymethyl groups, and formation of a dihydrodihydroxy derivative of an aromatic ring were encountered. Conjugates formed in mammals include O- and N-glucuronides, sulfates, and mercapturic acid derivatives. Changes of a carbamate insecticide that fail to separate the ester bond usually produce acetylcholinesterase inhibitors; some of these products are at least as potent as the parent compounds, contributing to the parent compounds' overall toxicity (Oonnithan and Casida, 1968). Hydrolysis of carbamates (enzymatic or spontaneous) yields an amine, carbon dioxide, and an alcohol, oxime, or phenol; the mechanism differs between methyl and dimethyl compounds. In the metabolism of carbamates to carbon dioxide, the carbon atoms involved may enter the normal carbon pool of the body, ultimately appearing in normal constituents of the tissues, milk, or excreta.

17.2.1.3 Mode of Action

Mechanisms of Action in the Nervous System In normal nervous system function, a burst of the neurotransmitter acetylcholine is released from a nerve cell terminal, diffuses across the synaptic cleft and transmits a nerve impulse to a specific cholinergic receptor. To end stimulation and restore the sensitivity of the receptor to new transmitter, acetylcholine at the receptor must continually be eliminated; this function is fulfilled by the enzyme acetylcholinesterase, which hydrolyzes acetylcholine to choline and acetic acid. By inhibiting acetylcholinesterase, anticholinesterase carbamates allow acetylcholine to accumulate at cholinergic junctions.

The cholinergic junctions may be classified into four categories on the basis of their differing sensitivity to the drugs nicotine, muscarine, atropine, and curare. One class of cholinergic junction contains only the skeletal neuromuscular junctions (of the somatic nervous system), where nerve and voluntary muscle meet. Such junctions are stimulated by nicotine and blocked by curare but not by atropine. Such stimulation produces what are referred to as *nicotinic effects*. When junctions are overstimulated, muscle fasciculation occurs. When the neuromuscular junctions are blocked, the muscle is paralyzed.

Another class of cholinergic junction includes the neuroeffector junctions of the parasympathetic systems. At these junctions, the parasympathetic nerves transmit impulses to the muscles and glands that are not voluntarily controlled, such as those of the intestine and the pupil. These junctions are not affected by nicotine or curare, but are stimulated by muscarine and blocked by atropine. Such parasympathetic stimulation of effectors produces *muscarinic effects*, which include slowing of the heart, constriction of the pupil, urination, lacrimation, and salivation. Many of the early symptoms of cholinergic poisoning are muscarinic and can be reversed or attenuated by atropine.

Of less importance to poisoning by carbamates are the cholinergic junctions of the sympathetic and parasympathetic autonomic ganglia. These comprise the intermediate synapses of the autonomic nerves, where impulses are relayed from neurons originating in the central nervous system (CNS) to neurons innervating the effectors. (Also in this category are the sympathetic nervous system junctions with the adrenal medulla and the sweat glands.) These junctions are stimulated by nicotine but not by muscarine, atropine, or curare, except at high concentrations. Sympathetic nerves innervate many smooth muscles of the eye, the bladder, the heart, and the salivary glands. Parasympathetic and sympathetic nerves often operate antagonistically; for example, the former slow the heart, constrict the pupil, and control the bladder muscles, while the latter accelerate the heart, dilate the pupil, and control the bladder's blood supply. The effects of autonomic ganglionic drugs are hard to predict because they often depend on whether the sympathetic or parasympathetic ganglion is the more affected.

The final group of cholinergic junctions important in carbamate poisoning are those of the CNS. The respiratory center of the brain is cholinergic; it controls respiration rate, and breathing stops if it is blocked. Convulsions also presumably are mediated via central neurons. At least some CNS junctions are stimulated by nicotine (such central effects are not, however, termed "nicotinic"). Other CNS junctions, particularly those of the respiratory center, are affected by atropine. Ionic compounds have virtually no effect on CNS junctions, and injected acetylcholine, muscarine, and curare have little effect.

Inhibition and Reactivation of Acetylcholinesterase Anticholinesterase carbamates react with, and are hydrolyzed by, esterases in a pattern analogous to the normal biological mechanism of acetylcholine–acetylcholinesterase activity. First, a reversible carbamate–acetylcholinesterase complex is formed; next follows a nonreversible carbamylation reaction with the enzyme; finally, decarbamylation frees the enzyme and reactivates the original acetylcholinesterase (Reiner and Aldridge, 1967; Aldridge and Reiner, 1972). The enzymatic process can be represented schematically as follows (Corbett *et al.*, 1984):

$$
\begin{array}{c}
\xrightarrow{\hspace{3.5cm}} \\
 K_i \downarrow \\
\text{EOH} + \text{AB} \underset{k_{-1}}{\overset{k_1}{\rightleftharpoons}} \text{EOH} \cdot \text{AB} \xrightarrow{\hspace{0.3cm} k_2 \hspace{0.3cm}} \underset{\substack{+ \\ \text{H} + \text{B}}}{\text{EOA}} \xrightarrow{\hspace{0.3cm} k_3 \hspace{0.3cm}} \underset{\substack{+ \\ \text{A} + \text{OH}}}{\text{EOH}}
\end{array}
$$

where AB stands for carbamate; EOH, acetylcholinesterase; EOA, carbamylated enzyme; B, alcohol, oxime, or phenol; and A, carbamate moiety.

Although the carbamylated form EOA is distinguished from the reversible form EOH·AB, EOA decarbamylates, by hydrolysis, to give rise to the original enzyme. Carbamylation therefore appears to be reversible from the point of view of the enzyme; however, it is not reversible from the point of view of the carbamate, which is cleaved and loses its anticholinesterase potency in the process.

For N-methylcarbamate esters in general, EOH·AB is formed almost instantly; kinetic values for the affinity constant K_a ($K_a = k^{-1}/k_1$) generally reflect this. Most N-methyl and N,N-dimethyl carbamates that have been studied *in vitro* inhibit acetylcholinesterase more readily than pseudocholinesterase; however, the degree of inhibition varies greatly among compounds. Furthermore, because carbamylated cholinesterases are unstable, the degree of inhibition at a steady state depends on the rate constants for both inhibition and spontaneous reactivation. N-carbamylated acetylcholinesterase undergoes spontaneous reactivation faster than does N-carbamylated pseudocholinesterase (Baron *et al.*, 1964). Therefore, *in vivo,* the plasma enzyme is sometimes inhibited for a longer period than the erythrocyte enzyme. For each of several compounds studied, rate constants for acetylcholinesterases from different animals were similar, as were rate constants for pseudocholinesterases (Simeon and Reiner, 1973). Species differences in carbamate toxicity are much less among mammals than among insects.

As discussed in Section 16.2.1.4 under Rate of Reaction, the phosphorylation of acetylcholinesterase by cholinergic organophosphate compounds corresponds to the electron-withdrawing power of their leaving (—X) groups. In contrast, the carbamylation of the enzyme by methylcarbamates depends on molecular complementarity and reactivity. Reactivity, in turn, depends on the nature of the leaving group; phenolic and oxime moieties are better leaving groups than benzyl alcohols (Hayes, 1982). Kuhr and Dorough (1976) and Corbett *et al.* (1984) review the kinetics of acetylcholinesterase inhibition in animals by insecticidal carbamates.

Duration of Action Although acetylcholinesterase inhibition by carbamates is rapidly and spontaneously reversible, some variation exists in the speed of spontaneous recovery. Following observations that the duration of inhibition of plasma acetylcholinesterase differed in workers exposed to propoxur and promecarb, Pleština and Svetličić (1973) investigated the matter in dogs. No qualitative difference in signs of poisoning was observed. Plasma acetylcholinesterase activity decreased rapidly in dogs injected with either compound. Plasma enzyme activity recovered promptly following the highest intramuscular dose of propoxur (20 mg/kg), but took 4 days to recover following an equitoxic dose of promecarb (60 mg/kg). When the two compounds were injected intravenously, the ratio of equitoxic dosages was reversed and the rate of recovery of enzyme activity was similar for the two compounds. These results indicate that both compounds were absorbed more slowly following intramuscular than intravenous injection, but the difference was much greater for promecarb. The continuing absorption of promecarb from its intramuscular deposit undoubtedly accounted for at least some of the continuing inhibition of enzyme. Whether promecarb also is less susceptible than propoxur to detoxication is unknown.

Methods of Measuring Acetylcholinesterase Activity The transience of acetylcholinesterase inhibition by carbamate esters makes it difficult to assay accurately. Vandekar (1980) has suggested that in human exposure the enzyme reactivates too rapidly for this measurement to be of any value in preventing occupational overexposure. In routine toxicological studies, previously exposed animals often are placed on a control diet 24 hr before terminal sacrifice, when an assay for several clinical chemistry parameters is to be made. By this procedure, acetylcholinesterase inhibition by carbamates cannot be detected because enzyme activity completely recovers within a few hours after exposure is stopped. This was demonstrated in experiments with rats fed aldoxycarb for 1 week or for 3 months and then assayed for acetylcholinesterase activity either immediately or after 24 hr. The immediate assay revealed acetylcholinesterase depression, and the delayed assay did not (Rhône-Poulenc, 1987).

Even with no delay between cessation of carbamate exposure and the assay, reversible acetylcholinesterase depression is difficult to detect by routine procedures. Spontaneous reversal of inhibition is rapid, and inhibition is reversed by simple dilution. Furthermore, because acetylcholine and the carbamate compete for the enzyme's active site, acetylcholinesterase inhibition is reduced by adding substrate (acetylcholine) to measure the reaction. (This effect also occurs naturally in the body and probably contributes to the spontaneous rapid recovery from cholinergic signs of poisoning following acetylcholinesterase inhibition.) Thus, the assay for acetylcholinesterase inhibition must be very rapid, taking less than 5 min, and must employ minimal dilutions and minimal amounts of substrate. Modifications of the colorimetric assay developed initially by Ellman *et al.* (1961) have been found to meet the demands for such a procedure, not only in the laboratory but also as a field screening procedure (Vandekar, 1980). In the case of subchronic or chronic exposure, such assays must be made immediately after exposure is ended. The common practice in laboratory toxicology studies of waiting 24 hr between the last exposure and the sacrifice is not acceptable with rapidly reversible acetylcholinesterase inhibitors like the carbamate pesticides.

17.2.2 CLINICAL CONSIDERATIONS

17.2.2.1 Comparison of Poisoning by Carbamates and by Organic Phosphorus Compounds

Poisoning by carbamates and by organic phosphorus compounds and the severity of its signs and symptoms depend not only on the degree of reduction of acetylcholinesterase activity in the nervous system but also on the rate of inhibition and the type of inhibitory action. Much of what is said in Section 16.2.2 applies to the carbamates also. The most striking differences between the clinical effects of the two groups are the much more rapid and spontaneous recovery from poisoning by carbamates and the relatively wide separation between the smallest dosage of any carbamate that will cause mild illness and the lethal dosage of the same compound. Both of these differences have their pharmacological basis in the relatively rapid and spontaneous reactivation of acetylcholinesterase inhibited by a carbamate (Vandekar *et al.*, 1965, 1971; Vandekar and Wilford, 1969). Another difference has the same basis; the ratio between the dosages producing the first signs of illness and causing death is constant for organic phosphorus compounds but depends on the rate of infusion for carbamates. Vandekar and Fajdetić (1966) showed, for a number of carbamates injected into the jugular vein of rats, that this ratio became larger as the rate of infusion was reduced; expressed as a quotient, it reached values around 50. In similar experiments with paraoxon, death occurred at dosage levels only about twice those producing the first signs of illness, regardless of infusion rate.

17.2.2.2 Treatment of Poisoning

Antidotal Studies with Animals   The muscarinic signs of carbamate insecticide poisoning are readily antagonized by atropine, which competitively blocks acetylcholine, but only at muscarinic receptors. Consequently, to the extent that carbamate poisoning involves action at muscarinic sites, atropine is an excellent antidote. Its effectiveness varies greatly with species; among mammals, atropine is extremely effective in humans and is least effective in mice. Species variations may be due to differences in the relative contribution of muscarinic effects to the poisoning process.

The nicotinic effects of anticholinesterase carbamates, involving the neuromuscular junction, have proved more difficult to control. In the case of aldicarb, decamethonium, a skeletal-

muscle relaxant, was not very effective, nor was tubocurare, although a combination of decamethonium and atropine was effective (Rhône-Poulenc, 1987).

Oximes, widely used in treatment of organophosphate poisoning, are frequently less effective or ineffective against carbamate poisoning. Several oximes were mildly antidotal to carbofuran and dioxacarb in mice (Bošković *et al.*, 1976). In other animal studies, 2-PAM was antidotal to aldicarb and to insecticide mixtures containing methomyl, both alone and with atropine; similar results were found for P2S and Toxogonin with aldicarb (Natoff and Reiff, 1973; Sterri *et al.*, 1979; Rhône-Poulenc, 1987; du Pont, 1986). However, atropine was in all these cases the more effective antidote. For mecarbam, tests with atropine were not reported, but 2-PAM was antidotal [Food Agriculture Organization/World Health Organization (FAO/WHO), 1981]. Although not an effective antidote to carbofuran, methiocarb, mexacarbate, thiodicarb, or trimethacarb, 2-PAM did not exacerbate the clinical signs of poisoning or interfere with the antidotal effectiveness of atropine (FAO/WHO, 1982; Dodd, 1987a,b; FMC, 1986a; Myers and Christopher, 1986). Similar results were found for Toxogonin with methiocarb and for P2S with pirimicarb, while other tests showed oximes to be markedly beneficial in the rat against isolan poisoning and slightly beneficial against dimetilan (Sanderson, 1961; FAO/WHO, 1977, 1982).

In contrast to results with all other carbamates, studies of carbaryl poisoning in laboratory animals showed oximes to be useless or actually harmful (Sanderson, 1961; Carpenter *et al.*, 1961; Aleksashina, 1969; Natoff and Reiff, 1973; Bošković *et al.*, 1976; Sterri *et al.*, 1979). This is the only instance in carbamate toxicology where such synergistic activity between a carbamate and an oxime has been noted, and it bears further investigation.

The abstract of a Soviet study (Kokshareva, 1982) reported that in rats, diethyxime (not further identified) at a dose of 20 mg/kg body weight was as effective as atropine in treating intoxication by several carbamate insecticides. The LD 50 was reduced about 3- to 9-fold for carbofuran, dioxacarb, ethiofencarb, and pirimicarb. Diethyxime therapy led to recovery of acetylcholinesterase activity both centrally and peripherally, including neuromuscular transmission, and the effects of coadministered diethyxime and atropine were additive.

Tetraethylammonium chloride was no more effective protection than atropine in rats given aminocarb, carbaryl, methiocarb, mexacarbate, propoxur, or four other *N*-methylcarbamates (Kimmerle, 1971). In monkeys, tetraethylammonium protected against a lethal dose of methomyl, though less effectively than atropine; results with hexamethonium were inconclusive (du Pont, 1986). Tetraethylammonium bromide was as effective as atropine in controlling the effects of carbofuran on mice and rats, but was less effective against mexacarbate and propoxur and much less so against aldicarb (Verschoyle and Barnes, 1969).

In summary, atropine is the recommended antidote, at a dosage of 2 mg/kg iv, repeated every 15–30 min or as necessary to maintain full atropinization. Diazepam is recommended in moderate or severe cases to relieve anxiety and because it may counteract some CNS-related symptoms not affected by atropine [World Health Organization (WHO), 1986]. Oximes should not be given unless organophosphate poisoning also is suspected. Other centrally acting drugs are not recommended.

Clinical Aspects of Poisoning Cases of accidental human overexposure to or suicide attempts with various carbamate insecticides (described in Section 17.3 under Accidental and Intentional Overexposure) have followed similar clinical courses characteristic of cholinergic poisoning as described in Section 17.2.1. Differences in severity, duration, and outcome have corresponded to differences in effective doses and in promptness and appropriateness of treatment. Spontaneous recovery without medical treatment has occurred generally within 4 hr of exposures producing symptoms of headache, lightheadedness or dizziness, weakness, excessive salivation, nausea, or vomiting. More severe symptoms have generally prompted medical treatment. Following treatment with sufficient atropine, individuals have recovered from poisoning that produced such symptoms as visual disturbances, profuse sweating, abdominal pain, incoordination, fasciculations, breathing difficulties, or changes in pulse rate. Recovery has been complete in some cases within 2 hr and in all cases within 1 day. Deaths have resulted in severe cases where treatment was delayed, insufficient atropine was administered, or other drugs were used. It is important to note, however, that treatment with atropine combined with general supportive treatment, such as artificial respiration and administration of fluids, has resulted in recovery even in cases where symptoms progressed to pulmonary edema or coma.

17.2.3 NONANTICHOLINESTERASE EFFECTS OF CARBAMATES

17.2.3.1 Delayed Neurotoxicity

The insecticidal carbamates have shown no evidence of an ability to induce a delayed neurotoxic syndrome similar to that seen with some organophosphorus compounds. In tests with 17 of the carbamates discussed in Section 17.3, following acute doses ranging from half to several times the LD 50, no behavioral evidence of neurotoxicity was observed during 22-day observation periods and no degeneration of the sciatic nerve was seen at autopsy (Carpenter *et al.*, 1961; Gaines, 1969; Kaplan and Sherman, 1976; FAO/WHO, 1977, 1978, 1980, 1981, 1982, 1983, 1986b; Dodd, 1987a,b; Union Carbide, 1984, 1985; Ciba-Geigy Limited, 1986; FMC, 1986b; Rhône-Poulenc, 1987). These observations are consistent with the mechanism by which delayed neuropathy is initiated. Neuropathy target esterase (NTE) must be organophosphorylated, followed by an "aging" reaction. Although some *N*-aryl carbamates can inhibit NTE, they do not permit an aging reaction; in fact, some carbamate NTE inhibitors were shown to protect hens against neuropathic effects of organophosphates (Johnson, 1970).

17.2.3.2 Mutagenicity

Considerable experimental evidence indicates that, as a class, methyl- and dimethylcarbamates are not mutagenic (e.g., WHO, 1986). Accounts of mutagenicity testing have been published for nearly all of the carbamates discussed in Section 17.3; selected references are provided here. Negative results have been obtained in the vast majority of assays for gene mutation, primary DNA damage, and chromosomal effects.

Gene mutation assays yielding negative results have included tests for forward or reverse mutation in the bacteria *Salmonella typhimurium*, *Escherichia coli*, and *Bacillus subtilis*, the yeast *Saccharomyces cerevisiae*, and rodent cells *in vitro*, as well as host-mediated assays and the *Drosophila* sex-linked recessive lethal assay. Assays for primary DNA damage in the above bacteria and yeast and in human and rodent cells *in vitro* have also given negative results, and negative results for chromosomal effects have been found in *Drosophila*, rodent cells *in vitro*, rodent somatic cells *in vivo*, and dominant lethal mutation assays with rodents (e.g., DeGiovanni-Donnelly *et al.*, 1968; Epstein *et al.*, 1972; Weil *et al.*, 1973; Guerzoni *et al.*, 1976; Simmon *et al.*, 1976, 1977; De Lorenzo *et al.*, 1978; FAO/WHO, 1977, 1978, 1980, 1981, 1982, 1983, 1985a,b; Jaszczuk and Syrowatka, 1980; Usha Rani *et al.*, 1980; Probst *et al.*, 1981; Quinto *et al.*, 1981; Valencia, 1981; Waters *et al.*, 1981; Gentile *et al.*, 1982; Wojciechowski *et al.*, 1982; Moriya *et al.*, 1983; Robertson *et al.*, 1983; Woodruff *et al.*, 1983; Jones *et al.*, 1984; Pilinskaya and Stepanova, 1984; Union Carbide, 1984, 1985; Ciba-Geigy Limited, 1986; du Pont, 1986; FMC, 1986a,b; Hodogaya Chemical Co., Ltd., 1986; Mitsubishi Chemical Industries Limited, 1986a,b; Otsuka, 1987; Rhône-Poulenc, 1987; Schering, 1987).

Weak mutagenicity has been reported for several of these carbamates, particularly at highly toxic dosages. However, the published studies reporting mutagenic effects tend to be methodologically flawed or provide insufficient information for meaningful evaluation of the results (e.g., as discussed by Vaughan-Dellarco, 1981, and Cranmer, 1986, in the case of carbaryl). Some have employed different protocols from those now accepted as standard. The reported positive assay results generally conflict with other published results or have not been replicated in subsequent studies.

For example, weak mutagenicity in *S. typhimurium* has been reported for aminocarb (Douglas *et al.*, 1982, 1983), carbaryl (Egert and Greim, 1976; Cook *et al.*, 1977; Rashid, 1978), carbofuran (Moriya *et al.*, 1983), and ethiofencarb (FAO/WHO, 1983). Guerzoni *et al.* (1976) reported positive results in a yeast reverse mutation assay with carbaryl, dioxacarb, methomyl, and propoxur. Weak mutagenicity in cultured rodent cells has been reported for aminocarb (Douglas *et al.*, 1983), carbaryl (Ahmed *et al.*, 1977b), carbofuran (Wojciechowski *et al.*, 1982; FMC, 1986a), formetanate HCl (Schering, 1987), and mecarbam (FAO/WHO, 1985a). Formetanate HCl was mutagenic in cultured human lymphocytes without, but not with, metabolic activation (Schering, 1987). Primary DNA damage was reported for aldicarb in *S. typhimurium* (Rashid and Mumma, 1986), for thiodicarb in *S. cerevisiae* (Union Carbide, 1984), and for carbaryl in human fibroblasts *in vitro* (Ahmed *et al.*, 1977a).

Carbaryl has been reported to be a spindle poison, tending to arrest mitosis in metaphase, especially at cytotoxic concentrations. The predominant mitotic abnormality reported was C-mitosis (Vasilos *et al.*, 1972; Önfelt, 1983), which could be counteracted by glutathione or rat liver S9. In cytotoxicity studies with mouse neuroblastoma cells, carbaryl was twice as toxic to undifferentiated cells as to differentiated cells (Shea, 1987). Carbaryl has been reported to cause chromosomal aberrations in studies with rodent and human cells *in vitro* (Kazarnoskaya and Vasilos, 1977; Ishidate and Odashima, 1977; Önfelt and Klasterska, 1983, 1984). *In vitro* induction of chromosomal aberrations in mammalian cells has also been reported for aldicarb (Debuyst and Van Larebeke, 1983; Gonzáles Cid and Matos, 1984), aminocarb (Douglas *et al.*, 1982, 1983), carbofuran (de Saint-Georges-Gridelet *et al.*, 1982; Pilinskaya and Stepanova, 1984; Georgian *et al.*, 1985), mexacarbate (Dodd, 1987), and pirimicarb (Pilinskaya, 1981a,b, 1982). Hoque (1972) reported chromosomal aberrations and phenotypic anomalies in the progeny of *Drosophila* fed carbaryl.

In *in vivo* cytogenetic studies, C-mitosis and other mitotic abnormalities in the intestinal epithelium were reported in rats given carbaryl (Vasilos *et al.*, 1975a,b). Although chromosomal aberrations in bone marrow cells were reported in mice given aldicarb (Sharaf *et al.*, 1982), this result could not be reproduced under identical conditions (Rhône-Poulenc, 1987). Propoxur gave positive results in a mouse dominant lethal test (Syrowatka *et al.*, 1971). Pirimicarb was reported to increase the frequency of chromosomal aberrations in human peripheral blood lymphocytes both in culture and in samples from workers exposed to pirimicarb vapors (Pilinskaya, 1981a,b, 1982). However, the effects were small and not dosage-related, and they were not confirmed in subsequent studies.

17.2.3.3 Carcinogenicity

No evidence has been found for carcinogenicity of the cholinergic methyl- and dimethylcarbamates. The results of chronic dietary studies with rodents are described for each compound in Section 17.3, under Effects on Organs and Tissues. The carcinogenicity of nitroso derivatives of carbamates is discussed in Section 17.2.4.3.

17.2.3.4 Immunology

The potential for specific immunotoxic effects has been investigated for relatively few carbamate insecticides; this testing is summarized for individual compounds in Section 17.3 under Effects on Organs and Tissues. Chronic dietary studies performed to meet registration requirements have generally revealed no histopathological or clinical chemical effects on endpoints related to immune function. Although some laboratory animals and *in vitro* systems have shown treatment-related changes in immunological parameters at nontoxic dosages of carbamates, such effects have generally been slight, inconsistent, or not clearly dose related. There is no convincing evidence that methyl- and dimethylcarbamates, as a class, have specific effects on the immune system.

17.2.3.5 Effects on Reproduction

Many carbamates have been tested for reproductive effects in a variety of mammalian species; this testing is summarized for each compound in Section 17.3 under Effects on Reproduction. Some reports (especially from Soviet researchers) have indicated effects on the endocrine system and on gametogenesis. The most common positive findings have been embryotoxicity at high (maternally toxic) doses. There is no evidence that the insecticidal carbamates in common use are teratogenic agents.

17.2.3.6 Behavioral Effects

Investigations of the neurobehavioral effects of carbamates have generally focused on behavioral effects following acute high-dosage administration, generally by injection. In tests of spontaneous activity, learning, or avoidance behaviors, acute exposures to carbamates have generally reduced animals' activity levels or response rates, but have not interfered with learning or memory *per se*. Reduced activity has generally been correlated with blood or brain acetylcholinesterase inhibition. Some longer-term exposures have been reported to increase spontaneous activity levels. In all cases, behavioral events were shown to be reversible, and recovery of most functions preceded complete recovery of acetylcholinesterase activity.

Transient dose-related decreases in spontaneous motor activity have been reported for rats and mice following acute sc or ip injection with BPMC, carbaryl, carbofuran, or propoxur at doses ranging from less than 1% to nearly 30% of the LD 50 (Iwami *et al.*, 1981; Gupta and Bagchi, 1982; Ruppert *et al.*, 1983; Kobayashi *et al.*, 1985). Single or repeated injection of mice with propoxur produced changes in rotarod performance and in open-field behavior (Kajita *et al.*, 1983). In 14-day studies with rats, carbaryl did not affect total daily running-wheel activity (Singh, 1973), but resulted in slightly increased open-field activity (Bracy *et al.*, 1979). Chronic dietary exposure to carbofuran did not affect locomotor activity of wild mice in a residential maze (Wolfe and Esher, 1980), but chronic dietary exposure to bendiocarb increased hyperactivity of rats in response to external stimuli (FAO/WHO, 1983). Subchronic inhalation exposure of cats to carbaryl caused a transient decrease in responsiveness in a classical conditioning experiment (Yakim, 1967). Carbaryl administered orally to mice on gestation days 8–12 at about half the LD 50 had no effect on locomotor activity of the young tested at weaning and at ages 2 months and 7 months (Gray *et al.*, 1986). Behavioral parameters unaffected by these carbamates in rodents included landing foot-spread (an indicator for peripheral neuropathies) (Ruppert *et al.*, 1983), handling/emotionality, muricide, and rearing (Bracy *et al.*, 1979).

In tests of rat learning and memory, rates of responding were decreased by acute or subchronic exposure to carbaryl or propoxur at low dosages, but memory *per se* was not affected

(Viter, 1978; Anger and Wilson, 1980; Pużyńska, 1980; Gordon *et al.*, 1981; Heise and Hudson, 1985a,b). Dési *et al.* (1974) reported a progressive decline in maze-running performance in rats fed carbaryl or propoxur, but not dioxacarb, over a 50-day exposure period. Anger and Setzer (1979) found that carbaryl increased monkeys' error rate and time per session in a repeated-chain acquisition task. In various studies with rats, carbaryl at low acute or subchronic dosages interfered with learned electric shock avoidance behavior, apparently via increased tolerance of shock. This interference was accentuated by pretreatment with the microsomal enzyme inhibitor SKF 525A and antagonized by atropine (Goldberg *et al.*, 1964, 1965; Sideroff and Santolucito, 1972; Tachibana *et al.*, 1973; Rhône-Poulenc, 1987).

Acute injection of mice with carbaryl affected electroretinogram (ERG) recordings of photopic and scotopic system responses (Carricaburu *et al.*, 1979). Slight changes in rat electroencephalogram (EEG) patterns were noted with subchronic dietary exposure to carbaryl, propoxur, and dioxacarb (Dési, 1983). Carbaryl at higher acute or subchronic dosages depressed cortical activity in rats but did not affect EEG recordings (Belonozhko and Kuchak, 1969). Chronic oral exposure of rhesus and squirrel monkeys to carbaryl at low dosages produced slight changes in EEG; the authors noted that testing under anesthesia could have influenced the results (Santolucito, 1970; Santolucito and Morrison, 1971). In human volunteers, carbaryl taken orally at up to 0.12 mg/kg per day for 6 weeks did not affect EEG recordings (Wills *et al.*, 1968).

17.2.4 CARBAMATE DERIVATIVES

17.2.4.1 Procarbamates

The structures of the simple anticholinesterase carbamates discussed in this chapter are shown in Table 17.1. Certain carbamate derivatives such as those shown in Fig. 17.1 exhibit insecticidal toxicity comparable to that of the parent carbamates, but lower mammalian toxicity. Such compounds are rapidly cleaved to release the parent carbamates; lower mammalian toxicities are due to preferential metabolism of the derivatives to nontoxic products. Fukuto and co-workers (e.g., Fukuto, 1983) demonstrated that substitution of the hydrogen on the carbamyl nitrogen atom of insecticidal methylcarbamate esters resulted in derivatives of lower mammalian toxicity, due to the slow conversion of the derivative to the original toxic methylcarbamate esters and the possibility for alternative metabolic routes in insects and mammals. Examples include two of the compounds discussed in Section 17.3: carbosulfan and thiodicarb are sulfide derivatives of carbofuran and methomyl, respectively. Other sulfide derivatives of carbofuran that have been developed commercially as insecticides include benfuracarb (2,3-dihydro-2,2-dimethyl-7-benzofuranyl *N*-{*N*-[2-(ethoxycarbonyl)ethyl]-*N*-isopropylsulfenamoyl}-*N*-methylcarbamate; Tanaka *et al.*, 1985) and furathiocarb [*O-n*-butyl *O'*-(2,2-dimethyl-2,3-dihydro-7-benzofuranyl)-*N,N'*-dimethyl *N,N'*-thiodicarbamate; Drabek and Bachmann, 1983].

Another line of procarbamate development has been to combine the insecticidal activity of carbamates with the superior acaricidal activity of formamidines. Eya and Fukuto (1986) described preparation and testing of a series of formamidine-*S*-carbamates incorporating the phenolic moiety of carbofuran or 3-isopropylphenyl methylcarbamate or the oxime of methomyl or oxamyl together with the formamidine demethylchlordimeform [*N'*-(4-chloro-2-methylphenyl)-*N*-methylmethanimidamide] or *N'*-(2,4-dimethylphenyl)-*N*-methylmethanimidamide. In many cases, these derivatives were more effective than the parent compounds against both insects and mites. Their favorable properties appear to be due to more rapid penetration into the pests and rapid release of the two parent pesticides.

17.2.4.2 Conjugates Formed by Plants

A potential route of human exposure to carbamate insecticides is ingestion of residues in treated crop plants. Because carbamate metabolism is rapid, such exposure is more likely to involve metabolites than the parent carbamates. Carbamate metabolism is generally similar in plants, animals, and microorganisms, differing primarily in relative rates for different pathways and in the nature of conjugates formed. Both oxidative and hydrolytic detoxification mechanisms are known to be important in plants. Although the intermediate plant metabolites are generally similar to those resulting from mammalian metabolism, the terminal metabolites in plants tend to be glucoside, phosphate, and amino acid conjugates. On consumption by mammals, such conjugates could potentially be further metabolized to liberate free carbamate metabolites. Carbamate metabolites exhibiting anticholinesterase activity usually are less toxic than the parent compounds. Although the mammalian toxicology of plant carbamate conjugates is generally not well known (Dorough, 1979; WHO, 1986), recent investigations indicate that the toxicological significance of these conjugates is slight.

Studies in which mammals were fed carbamate-treated plants or residues from such plants (e.g., Dorough and Wiggins, 1969; Knaak *et al.*, 1970; Marshall and Dorough, 1977; Rhône-Poulenc, 1987) have demonstrated rapid absorption of water-soluble glucoside metabolites and further metabolism of free or conjugated metabolites to glucuronide or sulfate products, which are rapidly excreted in the urine. Bound residues are generally eliminated in the feces.

17.2.4.3 Nitrosocarbamates

The nitroso derivatives of several carbamates have been synthesized and shown to be potent mutagens and carcinogens, in contrast to the parent compounds. Concern has been raised that nitrosation of carbamate pesticides either in the environment or under human stomach conditions could constitute a potential human health risk. Although endogenous formation of *N*-nitroso compounds has been demonstrated in humans following ingestion of a source of nitrite and an appropriate nitrosatable precursor, relatively high levels of the precursor and of nitrite were required (Oshima and Bartsch, 1981). Neither carbamate

Table 17.1
Structure of Carbamate Insecticides of the Form R—O—C(O)—N(CH₃)—R′

Compound	R	R′	Compound	R	R′
aldicarb	$CH_3-S-\underset{\underset{CH_3}{|}}{\overset{\overset{CH_3}{|}}{C}}-CH=N-$	—H	dioxycarb	(2-(1,3-dioxolan-2-yl)phenyl)	—H
aldoxycarb	$CH_3-\underset{\underset{O}{\|}}{\overset{\overset{O}{\|}}{S}}-\underset{\underset{CH_3}{|}}{\overset{\overset{CH_3}{|}}{C}}-CH=N-$	—H	primicarb	(dimethylaminopyrimidinyl)	—CH₃
aminocarb	(dimethylamino-methylphenyl)	—H	promecar	(methyl-isopropyl-phenyl)	—H
bendiocarb	(benzodioxol, 2,2-dimethyl)	—H	propoxur	(2-isopropoxyphenyl)	—H
4-benzothienyl-N-methyl carbamate	(4-benzothienyl)	—H	trimethacarb	(I) trimethylphenyl (II) trimethylphenyl	—H
bufencarb	(I) $\underset{C_3H_7\ \ CH_3}{CH}$-phenyl (II) $\underset{C_2H_5\ \ C_2H_5}{CH}$-phenyl	—H	XMC	(3,5-dimethylphenyl)	—H
carbaryl	(1-naphthyl)	—H	ethiofencarb	(2-(ethylthiomethyl)phenyl) CH_3-CH_2-S	—H
carbofuran	(2,3-dihydro-2,2-dimethylbenzofuran-7-yl)	—H			
dimetilan	$(CH_3)_2-N-\overset{}{C}-N\diagdown\underset{N}{\diagup}\ CH_3$	—CH₃			

(continued)

Table 17.1 (*Continued*)

Compound	R	R'	Compound	R	R'
fenobucar (BPMC)	(structure: 2-(1-methylpropyl)phenyl; CH with CH₃—CH₂ and CH₃)	—H	methiocarb	(structure: 3,5-dimethyl-4-(methylthio)phenyl; CH₃—S, CH₃, CH₃)	—H
formetanate hydrochloride	HCl · (CH₃)₂—N—CH=N— (phenyl)	—H	methomyl	CH₃—C=N—, CH₃—S	—H
isolan	(structure: pyrazole ring N—N, CH with CH₃ CH₃)	—H	mexacarbate	(structure: CH₃ CH₃ N, CH₃, CH₃ on dimethyl-methylamino phenyl)	—H
isoprocarb (MIPC)	(structure: CH₃ CH₃ CH phenyl)	—H	oxamyl	(structure: CH₃ N—C(=O)—C=N—, CH₃, S—CH₃)	—H
3-isopropylphenyl-*N*-methyl carbamate	(structure: CH₃ CH₃ CH phenyl)	—H	phencyclocarb	(structure: cyclopentyl phenyl)	—H

nor nitrate precursors occur at high levels under normal conditions.

Extrapolation of data from animal studies to predict potential human effects of nitrosocarbamates is complicated by the need to take into account the influence of pH, concentrations of reactants and other interacting chemicals, competing reactions, and the susceptibility of humans relative to that of animal models (WHO, 1986). In an attempt to simulate stomach conditions, Han (1975) incubated ^{14}C-labeled methomyl at pH 2 with macerated meat samples containing 16–20 ppm residual nitrite. Neither nitrosomethomyl nor its hydrolysis product *S*-methyl *N*-hydroxythioacetimidate was found. Beraud *et al.* (1979) found that nitrosocarbaryl formed rapidly in rat gastric juice incubated with sodium nitrite at 37°C. Rickard *et al.* (1982) demonstrated *in vitro* nitrosation of carbaryl and carbofuran at pH 1, but not at pH 2 or above; the nitrosocarbamates were most stable at pH 3–5. Nitroso derivatives of carbaryl and carbofuran were isolated from the stomach contents of guinea pigs given the carbamates orally with sodium nitrite; the yield was 0.5–2% of the carbamate doses, at a stomach pH between 1 and 2 (Rickard and

Dorough, 1984). Rat stomach contents (at pH 3.5–5.5) yielded only trace amounts of nitrosocarbamates.

Cummins (1982) reported experimental formation of a mutagenic nitroso derivative of propoxur in nitrogen dioxide atmospheres and in automotive exhaust. However, *N*-nitrosocarbamates are highly unstable, hygroscopic materials, and there is no indication that they are present in the environment. For example, environmental monitoring of water containing trace residues of aldicarb and nitrate has shown no indication of the presence of a nitroso derivative of aldicarb (Rhône-Poulenc, 1987).

Mutagenicity Nitroso derivatives of aldicarb, carbaryl, carbofuran, dioxacarb, ethiofencarb, formetanate HCl, methomyl, propoxur, and trimethacarb have been tested for mutagenicity. Various of these nitrosocarbamates caused gene mutation in bacteria; induced DNA damage in bacteria, *S. cerevisiae*, and human skin fibroblasts *in vitro;* and caused chromosomal aberrations in rodent cells *in vitro* (Elespuru *et al.*, 1974; Siebert and Eisenbrand, 1974; Uchiyama *et al.*, 1975; Marshall *et al.*, 1976;

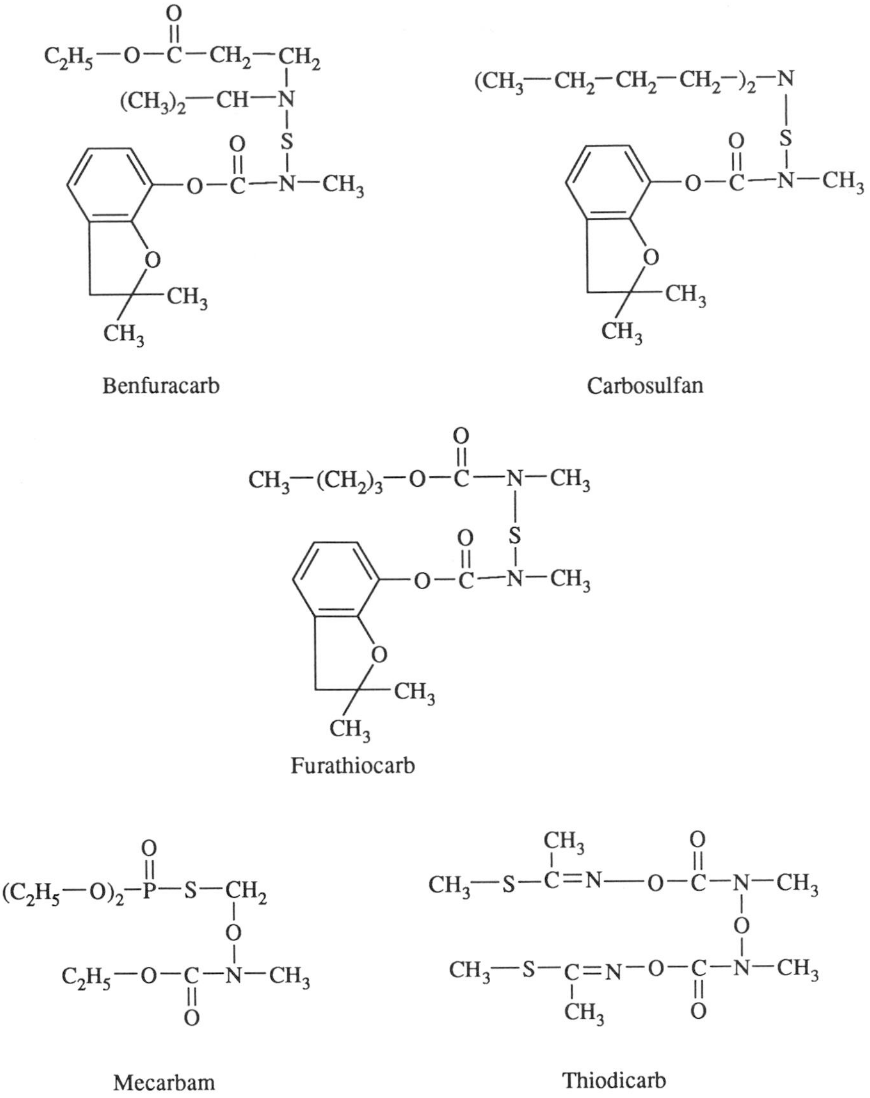

Figure 17.1 Some procarbamates.

Regan *et al.*, 1976; Blevins *et al.*, 1977a,b; Ishidate and Odashima, 1977; Seiler, 1977; Lijinsky and Andrews, 1979; Thust *et al.*, 1980; Ishidate *et al.*, 1981; Nelson *et al.*, 1981; Eto *et al.*, 1982; Rickard *et al.*, 1982). However, neither nitrosocarbaryl nor nitrosopropoxur caused chromosomal aberrations following administration orally to rats or ip to mice (Tyrkiel *et al.*, 1978). When parent carbamates were fed to mice with sodium nitrate, none caused chromosomal aberrations in bone marrow erythrocytes; compounds tested included carbaryl, carbofuran, ethiofencarb, formetanate HCl, and propoxur (Seiler, 1977).

Carcinogenicity Nitrosocarbamates have been shown to induce morphological transformation in a transplacental host-mediated hamster cell culture system (Quarles *et al.*, 1979a,b), to cause sarcomas in rats when injected sc (Eisenbrand *et al.*, 1975), to cause skin tumors in mice following acute or chronic application (Lijinsky and Winter, 1981; Deutsch-Wenzel *et al.*, 1985), and to cause stomach tumors in rats chronically exposed

by gavage (Lijinsky and Schmähl, 1978). However, when rats were given a combination of carbaryl and sodium nitrite, no excess of tumors was found in the treated adults or in the young of treated pregnant adults (Lijinsky and Taylor, 1977).

17.3 ANTICHOLINESTERASE CARBAMATES AND PROCARBAMATES

The anticholinesterase carbamates vary greatly in acute toxicity. They range from compounds that when formulated may be used with few precautions and even used for purposes that involve direct human exposure (as in the use of carbaryl against head lice) to compounds that must be formulated in special ways and used with care if injury is to be avoided. With few exceptions, the anticholinesterase carbamates are relatively safe for mammals. The balance of this chapter consists of individual descriptions of the toxicology of carbamate and procarbamate insecticides that have been studied in humans. The chemicals are discussed in alphabetical order, with emphasis on characteristics specific to the individual compounds rather than common to all insecticidal carbamates. The chemical structures of these compounds are shown in Table 17.1 (simple carbamates) and Fig. 17.1 (procarbamates), and their acute toxicity is summarized in Tables 17.2 through 17.4. Much information on the chemistry, biochemistry, and toxicology of the insecticidal carbamates may be found in a book by Kuhr and Dorough (1976). A more recent review of carbamate toxicology, emphasizing environmental aspects, is provided in the World Health Organization's Environmental Health Criteria series (WHO, 1986).

The author will supply information on the identity, properties, uses, and toxicity to laboratory animals for the following compounds for which no study in humans is available: aldoxycarb, aminocarb, benfuracarb, ethiofencarb, fenobucarb (BPMC), isoprocarb (MIPC), and XMC. The structural formulas of these compounds are shown in Table 17.1 and Fig. 17.1.

17.3.1 ALDICARB

17.3.1.1 Identity, Properties, and Uses

Chemical Name Aldicarb is 2-methyl-2(methylthio)-propionaldehyde O-(methylcarbamoyl)oxime. Its structure is shown in Table 17.1.

Synonyms The common name aldicarb (ANSI, BSI, ISO) is in general use. The trade name is Temik®. Code designations have included ENT 27093, OMS 771, NCI 08640, and UC 21149. The CAS registry number is 116-06-3.

Physical and Chemical Properties Aldicarb has the empirical formula $C_7H_{14}N_2O_2S$ and a molecular weight of 190.3. The pure material forms white crystals with a slightly sulfurous odor and a melting point of 100°C. The vapor pressure (mm Hg) is 1×10^{-5} at 0°C, 1×10^{-4} at 25°C, 7×10^{-4} at 50°C, and 4×10^{-3} at 75°C. The solubility of aldicarb at 20°C is 0.6% in water, 10% in toluene, 20% in isopropanol, 25% in ethanol, 35% in chloroform, and 40% in benzene. Aldicarb is stable under normal storage conditions and in acidic media but decomposes rapidly in alkaline media and at temperatures above 100°C.

History, Formulations, and Uses Aldicarb was introduced in the mid-1960s for systemic control of a wide variety of insects, mites, and nematodes on field crops, cotton, some vegetable and fruit crops, and ornamentals. Aldicarb is available in granular formulations and in combination with the fungicides PCNB and ethazol.

17.3.1.2 Toxicity to Laboratory Animals

Except as otherwise indicated, toxicological information is proprietary data developed by Union Carbide Agricultural Products Company, Inc. and is the property of Rhône-Poulenc (Baron and Merriam, 1988). An incomplete review of these data was published by the U.S. Environmental Protection Agency (EPA)

(Risher *et al.*, 1987). A complete review was provided by Baron and Merriam (1988).

Basic Findings The acute toxicity of aldicarb is summarized in Tables 17.2 and 17.3. Signs of acute toxicity were characteristic of acetylcholinesterase inhibition. Aldicarb was not irritating to the eyes or skin of rabbits and did not cause a skin sensitization reaction in guinea pigs.

Single oral doses of aldicarb caused transient depression of erythrocyte and plasma acetylcholinesterase activity at 0.011 mg/kg in rats and dogs and at 0.033 mg/kg in rabbits. Inhalation is not a significant route of exposure to aldicarb during manufacture or application. Cynomolgus monkeys fed bananas and watermelons containing aldicarb residues at 0.005 mg/kg body weight showed no evidence of acute cholinergic distress and no depression of erythrocyte acetylcholinesterase activity. Depression of plasma acetylcholinesterase activity was evident within 1–4 hr, reaching a maximum of 35%; recovery of enzyme activity was rapid.

In a 3-month study with rats, aldicarb in the diet at 0.5 mg/kg/day increased mortality and decreased food consumption. Organ weights were not affected by dosages of 0.02–0.5 mg/kg/day (Rhône-Poulenc, 1987). In mice, aldicarb in the diet at up to about 6.0 mg/kg/day for 13 weeks caused no significant somatic effects [National Cancer Institute (NCI), 1979]. In a 3-month study with dogs, aldicarb in the diet at 0.3 mg/kg/day had no effect on organ weights.

In a 14-day range-finding study with dogs, acetylcholinesterase inhibition was noted at dietary dosages exceeding 0.1 mg/kg/day. At the conclusion of a 1-year dietary study with dogs, aldicarb at up to 0.25 mg/kg/day had no effects other than inhibition of erythrocyte and plasma acetylcholinesterase activity. The no-effect level for acetylcholinesterase inhibition was 0.025 mg/kg/day for males and 0.05 mg/kg/day for females. Aldicarb in the diet of dogs at 0.1 mg/kg/day for 2 years had no effect on mortality, growth, hematologic values, or condition of organs and tissues. (Hamada, 1987a).

Aldicarb in the diet of rats for 2 years at up to 0.3 mg/kg/day did not affect mortality, growth, hematologic characteristics, or occurrence of histological abnormalities (Baron and Merriam, 1988).

Absorption, Distribution, Metabolism, and Excretion The basic metabolic pathway for aldicarb appears to be the same in all species studied. Aldicarb is rapidly oxidized to the relatively stable aldicarb sulfoxide; then, more slowly, a small portion of aldicarb sulfoxide is oxidized to aldicarb sulfone. Aldicarb, aldicarb sulfoxide, and aldicarb sulfone also are readily converted to the corresponding oximes and nitriles, which are, in turn, slowly degraded to the corresponding aldehydes, acids, and alcohols.

Aldicarb given orally to rats as a single acute dose was excreted primarily as aldicarb sulfoxide (40%) and sulfoxide oxime (30%); only trace amounts of aldicarb were found in the urine (Knaak *et al.*, 1966; Andrawes *et al.*, 1967). The major urinary metabolites in dogs and goats were the same as in rats

Table 17.2
Acute Oral Toxicity of Carbamate Insecticides (Technical)

Chemical	Species	Sex	LD 50 (mg/kg)	Vehicle	References
aldicarb	rat	both	0.46–1.23	(various)	Baron and Merriam (1988)
	mouse	both	0.38–1.50	oil	Baron and Merriam (1988)
	guinea pig		1.0	corn oil	Baron and Merriam (1988)
	rabbit		1.3	propylene glycol	Baron and Merriam (1988)
aldoxycarb	rat	M	20–32	corn oil	Union Carbide (1985)
	mouse	M	25	corn oil	FAO/WHO (1983); Union Carbide (1985)
	guinea pig	M	>50	corn oil	FAO/WHO (1983); Union Carbide (1985)
	rabbit	M	75	corn oil	FAO/WHO (1983); Union Carbide (1985)
aminocarb	rat	both	22–50		Gaines (1969); FAO/WHO (1980)
	guinea pig	M	60		FAO/WHO (1980)
bendiocarb	rat	both	34–156	(various)	FAO/WHO (1983); FBC (1986)
	mouse	both	28–45	(various)	FAO/WHO (1983); FBC (1986)
	hamster	F	141	water	FBC (1986)
	guinea pig	F	35	glycerol formal	FAO/WHO (1983)
	rabbit	both	35–40	glycerol formal	FAO/WHO (1983)
benfuracarb	rat	M	138		Otsuka (1987)
	mouse	M	175		Otsuka (1987)
	dog	both	ca. 300		Otsuka (1987)
BPMC	rat	both	350–657		Takahashi *et al.* (1983); Mitsubishi (1986a)
	mouse	both	173–380		Miyata and Saito (1981); Takahashi *et al.* (1983, 1984, 1987a); Miyaoka *et al.* (1984); Tsuda *et al.* (1984); Mitsubishi (1986a)
carbaryl	rat	both	233–850	(various)	Gaines (1960); Carpenter *et al.* (1961); Coulston (1968); Rybakova (1966); Yakim (1967); Metcalf (1971); Vandekar *et al.* (1971); Cranmer (1986)
	mouse	both	108–650	(various)	Bukin and Filatov (1965); Coulston (1968); Rybakova (1966); Yakim (1967); Cress and Strother (1974); Haley *et al.* (1974); Ahdaya *et al.* (1976)
	guinea pig		280		Carpenter *et al.* (1961)
	gerbil	F	491		Benson and Dorough (1984)
	rabbit		710		Carpenter *et al.* (1961)
	dog		250–795		Carpenter *et al.* (1961); Coulston (1968)
	cat		125–250		Carpenter *et al.* (1961); Yakim (1967)
	monkey		>1000		Coulston (1968)
	swine		1500–2000		Smalley *et al.* (1969)
carbofuran	rat	M	5.3–13.2	corn or peanut oil	FMC (1986a); Gaines and Linder (1986)

(continued)

Table 17.2 (*Continued*)

Chemical	Species	Sex	LD 50 (mg/kg)	Vehicle	References
	mouse		2.0		Fahmy *et al.* (1970)
	dog		19		Tobin (1970)
carbosulfan	rat	both	90–250	corn oil or none	FMC (1986b)
	mouse	both	33–124	corn oil	FMC (1986b)
	rabbit	both	37–53	corn oil or none	FMC (1986b)
dioxacarb	rat		53–80		Ciba-Geigy Limited (1986)
	mouse	both	48–130		Haley *et al.* (1974); Ciba-Geigy Limited (1986)
	Chinese hamster		843		Ciba-Geigy Limited (1986)
ethiofencarb	rat	both	308–500		FAO/WHO (1978); Karpenko *et al.* (1984)
	mouse	both	71–256		Christensen (1977); FAO/WHO (1978); Karpenko *et al.* (1984)
	guinea pig	F	113		Benson and Dorough (1984)
	gerbil	F	113		Benson and Dorough (1984)
	rabbit		118–225		FAO/WHO (1978); Karpenko *et al.* (1984)
	dog	F	>50		FAO/WHO (1978)
formetanate HCl	rat	both	15–26		Schering (1987)
	mouse	both	13–25		Haley *et al.* (1974); Schering (1987)
	dog	both	19		Schering (1987)
mecarbam	rat	both	25–53		FAO/WHO (1981)
	mouse	M	106		FAO/WHO (1981)
	guinea pig		65		FAO/WHO (1981)
	rabbit		60		FAO/WHO (1981)
	cat		<50		FAO/WHO (1981)
	sheep		20–25		FAO/WHO (1981)
methiocarb	rat	both	13–135	(various)	Zbinden and Flury-Roversi (1981); FAO/WHO (1982)
	guinea pig	both	14–100	(various)	FAO/WHO (1982)
	dog	both	10–25	(various)	Nelson and Lamb (1977); FAO/WHO (1982)
methomyl	rat	both	12–48	(various)	Dashiell and Kennedy (1984); Union Carbide (1984); du Pont (1986); Gaines and Linder (1986)
mexacarbate	rat	both	8.5–12.0		Gaines (1969); Dodd (1987b)
MIPC	rat	both	178–485		Mitsubishi (1986b); WHO (1986)
	mouse	both	128–512		Mitsubishi (1986b); WHO (1986)
	rabbit		ca. 500		WHO (1986)
oxamyl	rat	both	2.5–16		FAO/WHO (1981); Kennedy (1986)
	mouse	both	2.3–3.3		Kennedy (1986)
	guinea pig	M	7.1		Kennedy (1986)
pirimicarb	rat	F	68–221		FAO/WHO (1977)
	mouse	F	107		FAO/WHO (1977)
	dog	both	100–200		FAO/WHO (1977)
propoxur	rat	both	80–191		Gaines (1969); Vandekar *et al.* (1971); Dési (1983); Nelson *et al.* (1984); WHO (1986)
	mouse	both	37–109	(various)	Haley *et al.* (1974); Miyata and Saito (1981); WHO (1986)

(*continued*)

Table 17.2 (*Continued*)

Chemical	Species	Sex	LD 50 (mg/kg)	Vehicle	References
	guinea pig		40		WHO (1986)
thiodicarb	rat	both	39–136	(various)	Union Carbide (1984)
	mouse	both	226	corn oil	Union Carbide (1984)
	guinea pig	M	160	corn oil	Union Carbide (1984)
	rabbit	both	556	corn oil	Union Carbide (1984)
	monkey	both	467.2	capsule	Union Carbide (1984)
trimethacarb	rat	both	125–232		Gaines (1969); Dodd (1986)
	dog	M	225		Dodd (1987a)
XMC	rat	both	542–697		Hodogaya (1986)
	mouse	M	220–245		Takahashi *et al.* (1983, 1987b); Hodogaya (1986)
	rabbit	both	375–445		Hodogaya (1986)

(Baron and Merriam, 1988). The principal metabolites found in milk in the first 12 hr following acute administration of aldicarb to cows were aldicarb sulfone nitrile, sulfoxide nitrile, and sulfoxide oxime, with small amounts of aldicarb sulfoxide and aldicarb sulfone (Dorough and Ivie, 1968).

In rats administered single oral doses of [^{14}C]aldicarb, most of the aldicarb metabolites were excreted within 24 hr. After 4 days, more than 95% of the administered doses of *S*-methyl- and *tert*-butyl-labeled aldicarb had been excreted, and no residues were detected in body tissues. Of administered *N*-methyl label, 8–10% was found in body tissues after 11 days, by which time 72% of the dose had been excreted (including more than 20% exhaled as CO_2) (Knaak *et al.*, 1966). In another study with rats, 80% of a radiolabeled dose of aldicarb was eliminated in the urine and 4% in the feces within 24 hr after administration. Although residues were found at low levels in a variety of tissues during the first days after treatment, there was no indication that they accumulated in the body; by the fifth day, residues were no longer detected (Andrawes *et al.*, 1967). Following single oral doses of radiolabeled aldicarb to male rats with cannulated bile ducts, approximately 26% of the dose appeared in the bile in the first 24 hr, indicating that the biliary metabolites are largely reabsorbed and excreted in the urine (Marshall and Dorough, 1979).

When a lactating dairy cow received a single dose of [^{35}S]aldicarb, approximately 83% of the dose appeared in the urine within 24 hr. Traces of residues were noted in the feces and milk; the highest concentration in the milk was 0.062 ppm, 3 hr after administration (Dorough and Ivie, 1968). Subchronic dosing of cows and goats with aldicarb gave very similar patterns of excretion; trace levels of residues were found in body tissues following continuous treatment (Dorough *et al.*, 1970; Baron and Merriam, 1988).

To measure the excretion of aldicarb administered repeatedly, dogs were maintained on diets determining an intake of 0.75 mg/dog/day for 20 days before and 10 days after being given a single ^{14}C-labeled dose. Of the radioactivity recovered in the urine, 90% was found within 24 hr after administration of the radiolabeled aldicarb (Baron and Merriam, 1988).

Biochemical Effects   *In vitro*, aldicarb did not interfere with rat liver mitochondrial energy-linked functions at concentrations of up to 10^{-3} *M* (Abo-Khatwa and Hollingworth, 1974), and it did not inhibit rat brain monoamine oxidase (Kadir and Knowles, 1981).

Effects on Organs and Tissues   Results of mutagenicity tests with aldicarb are summarized in Section 17.2.3.2. In chronic dietary studies, aldicarb was not carcinogenic to rats at up to approximately 0.3 mg/kg/day or to mice at up to approximately 0.9 mg/kg/day (Namba *et al.*, 1971; Baron and Merriam, 1988). Aldicarb in acetone solution (up to 0.25%) applied to the shaved backs of mice for 28 months did not increase the incidence of tumors over that in controls.

Aldicarb administered to mice in the drinking water for 34 days at up to 0.364 mg/kg/day had no effect on body or organ weights, numbers or types of circulating white blood cells, or the microscopic pathology of the thymus, spleen, liver, kidneys, or lymph nodes. Also unaffected were the number of antibody-forming cells in the spleen and the amount of circulating antibody in the blood. Aldicarb had no effect on *in vivo* host resistance to infectious viral challenge, on the capacity of B and T lymphocytes to respond to nonspecific mitogens, or on the ability of T lymphocytes to recognize genetically different cell types in a mixed lymphocyte culture (Thomas *et al.*, 1987). The study failed to reproduce an alleged inverse dosage-related effect of aldicarb on these same parameters in mice (Olson *et al.*, 1986).

Effects on Reproduction   Aldicarb administered by gavage to pregnant rats on day 18 of gestation at 0.001, 0.01, or 0.10

Table 17.3
Acute Dermal Toxicity of Carbamate Insecticides (Technical)

Chemical	Species	Sex	LD 50 (mg/kg)	Vehicle	References
aldicarb	rat	both	3.2–>10	(various)	Baron and Merriam (1988)
	rabbit	M	5.0–20	(various)	Baron and Merriam (1988)
aldoxycarb	rat	M	1000	corn oil	Union Carbide (1985)
	rabbit	M	>20–200	water or oil	Union Carbide (1985)
aminocarb	rat	both	275–>1000		FAO/WHO (1980)
	mouse	F	31		Abdel-Wahab and Casida (1967)
bendiocarb	rat	both	566		FBC (1986)
benfuracarb	rat	M	>2000		Otsuka (1987)
BPMC	rat	both	>5000		Mitsubishi (1986a)
	mouse		4200		Kuhr and Dorough (1976)
carbaryl	rat	both	>5000		Cranmer (1986)
carbofuran	rat	both	>1000	acetone	Gaines and Linder (1986)
	rabbit	both	>2000		FMC (1986a)
carbosulfan	rabbit	both	>2000	undiluted	FMC (1986b)
dioxacarb	rat		ca. 3000		Ciba-Geigy Limited (1986)
	rabbit		1950–>10,000		Ciba-Geigy Limited (1986); WHO (1986)
ethiofencarb	rat	M	>1000–>1150		FAO/WHO (1978); WHO (1986)
	rabbit	both	>8000		FAO/WHO (1978)
formetanate HCl	rabbit	both	>10,200		Schering (1987)
mecarbam	rat	M	>1222		FAO/WHO (1981)
	guinea pig		>1222		FAO/WHO (1981)
	rabbit		229		FAO/WHO (1981)
methiocarb	rat	both	>300–>5000	(various)	FAO/WHO (1982)
	rabbit	both	>2000	saline	FAO/WHO (1982)
methomyl	rat	M	>1000–>2400	(various)	du Pont (1986); Gaines and Linder (1986)
	rabbit	both	556–>1500	(various)	Union Carbide (1984); du Pont (1986)
mexacarbate	rabbit	both	>2000		Dodd (1987)
MIPC	rat	both	>2000		Mitsubishi (1986b)
oxamyl	rat	M	>1200		Kennedy (1986)
	rabbit	M	740		Kennedy (1986)
pirimicarb	rat	F	>500		FAO/WHO (1977)
	rabbit		>500		FAO/WHO (1977)
propoxur	rat	both	1000–>2400		Gaines (1969); WHO (1986)
	rabbit	M	>500		Nelson et al. (1984)
thiodicarb	rat	M	2540		Union Carbide (1984)
	rabbit	both	>6310		Union Carbide (1984)
trimethacarb	rabbit	both	>2000–>2500		Dodd (1986)
XMC	rat	both	>5000		Hodogaya (1986)
	mouse	both	>5000		Hodogaya (1986)

mg/kg depressed acetylcholinesterase activity to a greater degree in the fetus than in the mother (Cambon et al., 1979), indicating that aldicarb crossed the placenta to the fetus and cleared the body more slowly than is normally observed in nonpregnant rats. The presence of an additional compartment, the fetus, probably had a major effect on the pharmacokinetics associated with distribution and excretion. Aldicarb also af-

fected the distribution of acetylcholinesterase isoenzymes differently in the fetus than in the mother (Cambon et al., 1980), again probably due to pharmacokinetic effects.

In three-generation studies with rats, aldicarb at up to 0.7 mg/kg/day did not affect mortality, histopathology, fertility, gestation, viability, or lactation. Aldicarb was not teratogenic when fed to rats at up to 1.0 mg/kg/day on the first 7 days of

Table 17.4
Acute Inhalation Toxicity of Carbamate Insecticides (Technical)

Chemical	Species	Sex	LD 50 (mg/kg)	Duration (hours)	References
aldoxycarb	rat	both	0.12–0.15	4	Fait *et al.* (1984); Union Carbide (1985)
aminocarb	rat	both	0.2	4	FAO/WHO (1980)
	rat	F	6	1	FAO/WHO (1980)
	mouse	F	4	1	FAO/WHO (1980)
BPMC	rat	both	>2.5		Mitsubishi (1986a)
carbaryl	rat		0.005–0.023	4	Cranmer (1986)
carbosulfan	rat	both	0.61–1.53		FMC (1986b)
dioxacarb	rat		0.17–0.20	6	Ciba-Geigy Limited (1986)
formetanate HCl	rat	both	0.29–2.8	4	Schering (1987)
mecarbam	rat		0.7	6	FAO/WHO (1981)
methiocarb	rat	both	>0.322	4	FAO/WHO (1985a)
methomyl	rat	M	0.45	4	du Pont (1986)
MIPC	rat	both	2.09		Mitsubishi (1986b)
oxamyl	rat	both	0.12–0.17	1	Kennedy (1986)
	rat	M	0.064	4	Kennedy (1986)
pirimicarb	rat		ca. 0.3		FAO/WHO (1977)
propoxur	rat	M	>1.44	1	Nelson *et al.* (1984)
thiodicarb	rat	both	0.1155–0.22	4	Union Carbide (1984)
	rat		>0.20	6	Union Carbide (1984)

gestation, from day 5 through day 15 of gestation, or from the start of pregnancy through weaning of the pups, or when administered to rabbits by gavage at up to 0.5 mg/kg/day on gestation days 7–27. No effects were observed on fertility, gestation, viability, or lactation.

Factors Influencing Toxicity No potentiation of toxicity to rats was observed when aldicarb was coadministered with carbaryl, 1-naphthol, or each of eight organophosphate esters. Similarly, the effects of aldicarb and methyl parathion coadministered to mice were additive.

17.3.1.3 Toxicity to Humans

The 1982 FAO/WHO Joint Meeting on Pesticide Residues estimated a human acceptable daily intake (ADI) for aldicarb of 0–0.005 mg/kg body weight (FAO/WHO, 1983). The EPA's acceptable daily intake is 0.001 mg/kg body weight.

Experimental Exposures Following two preliminary analyses of blood acetylcholinesterase activity, groups of four adult male volunteers were given aqueous solutions of aldicarb at acute oral doses of 0.025, 0.05, or 0.1 mg/kg body weight; in a repeated similar trial, two subjects were given doses of 0.05 or 0.26 mg/kg. A dose-related depression of whole-blood acetylcholinesterase from pretrial values was observed in all individuals, predominantly 1–2 hr after exposure. Acute cholinergic signs of overexposure were observed only in subjects

exposed to a dose of 0.1 mg/kg or higher. By 6 hr after administration, acetylcholinesterase activity had returned to normal and clinical cholinergic signs and symptoms had disappeared with no medical treatment. The subjects eliminated approximately 8% of the dose as carbamate ester within 8 hr, and an additional 2.4% was found in urine at the end of 24 hr. The balance of the dose was not accounted for by the analytical method used, which would not analyze noncarbamate metabolites.

The Safe Drinking Water Committee of the National Research Council (1986) used the data from this study in a statistical model to project the acetylcholinesterase response to low exposure levels. Calculations were based on each individual's highest pretrial values and maximum depression at either 1 or 2 hr after administration. The mean maximum inhibition was 73% at a dose of 0.1 mg/kg, 64% at 0.05 mg/kg, and 47% at 0.025 mg/kg. The Committee's model used probit and logit regression analyses of these data to project enzyme inhibitions of 30% at a dose of 0.01 mg/kg and 20% at 0.005 mg/kg. A primate study examining the acute effects of aldicarb residues on acetylcholinesterase depression confirmed the regression extrapolation, showing minimal inhibition of plasma acetylcholinesterase at 0.005 mg/kg (Baron and Merriam, 1988).

Accidental and Intentional Overexposure Through June 1986, in over 15 years of registered use of aldicarb products, 193 cases of alleged overexposure (primarily occupational) were reported to and thoroughly investigated by Rhône-Poulenc Ag Company (Baron and Merriam, 1988). (See also Peoples *et al.*, 1978, for cases reported to California physicians from 1974 through 1976.) The involvement of aldicarb was confirmed in 79 of these cases, by either clinical diagnosis or urinalysis for aldicarb and its acetylcholinesterase-inhibiting metabolites. In 65 cases, the involvement of aldicarb could not be confirmed; the pesticide played no role in the remaining 49.

Most cases of overexposure have occurred during loading or application; some have resulted from the improper handling of treated plants or soil. In the past some overexposures resulted from the use of application devices that tended to grind the granules, producing fine, inhalable particles. Labels for formulated aldicarb products now recommend against the use of such applicators. All of the confirmed cases of overexposure resulted from misuse of the product, by failure to follow label precautions. Approximately 40% of the confirmed overexposures have occurred in connection with use on ornamental plants; 18% of the confirmed cases were not use-related. No illnesses or deaths have resulted from the proper use of aldicarb products.

In cases of occupational overexposure to aldicarb, mild acute signs of poisoning have been recorded with depressions of blood acetylcholinesterase activity. Recovery has been rapid, and there have been no indications of any long-term sequelae in exposed workers. In some instances, recovery has been aided by hospitalization and atropine therapy. Nine deaths have been reported in the United States as allegedly the result of overexposure to aldicarb. The involvement of aldicarb was confirmed in only four cases; three of these were the result of ingestion of the product (intentional in two cases). In one published account, an agricultural worker who had been loading a granular aldicarb formulation without appropriate protective clothing or equipment and without having undergone baseline acetylcholinesterase testing (required in California) was run over by a tractor and killed. Although death was directly attributable to trauma, the body burden of aldicarb estimated from tissue analysis would have been sufficient to produce cholinergic symptoms (Lee and Ransdell, 1984). The authors suggested that incapacitation due to cholinergic symptoms could have been a contributing factor in this accidental death.

In 1966, when aldicarb was an experimental pesticide, the wife of an agricultural scientist treated the soil around a rose bush at her home with a 10% granular formulation. Twenty-four days later, she ate some leaves from a mint plant growing near the rose. About 30 min later, she developed typical cholinergic signs and symptoms, including nausea, vomiting, diarrhea, and involuntary urination. On hospitalization, she had pinpoint pupils, muscle fasciculations, weakness, and difficult respiration. Signs and symptoms were maximal 2 hr after onset. She was given atropine (5 mg total) and had recovered by 3.5 hr after onset. Samples of mint leaves from the treated area showed extraordinarily high aldicarb residue concentrations (186–318 ppm) (Hayes, 1982).

In another overexposure incident, a 7-month-old girl was given aldicarb powder intended for rose plants. Signs included pinpoint pupils, muscle twitching, excessive secretions, spontaneous evacuation of bladder and bowel, convulsions, and

cyanosis requiring assisted respiration. A total of 105.6 mg of atropine was administered; recovery was complete, and the child was discharged on the sixth day (Ramasamy, 1976).

Episodes of apparent aldicarb overexposure were reported from two Nebraska communities, where several people developed typical cholinergic signs and symptoms immediately after eating cucumbers grown hydroponically at the same greenhouse. All recovered without specific medical treatment. Aldicarb was detected in cucumbers from the greenhouse (at 6.6–10.7 ppm) and in the water (1.8 ppm) and gravel (0.6 ppm) of the hydroponic system. Aldicarb was not found in the well water supplying the greenhouse, and its means of introduction remained unknown (Aaronson *et al.*, 1980; Goes *et al.*, 1980). A similar, more recent overexposure case involving hydroponically grown cucumbers was reported from Canada. Transient illness developed when cucumbers containing high levels of aldicarb residues were consumed. This use of aldicarb products is neither registered nor recommended.

In a major misuse of aldicarb, watermelons treated in California were consumed in Oregon and other places. Rapid onset of gastrointestinal illness was seen in a number of individuals consuming watermelon. The incident was widely reported, even though there were no hospitalizations or fatalities. As the incident occurred early in the season, most of the illegally treated commodity was seized and destroyed in a significant detective program in California and Oregon [Morbidity and Mortality Weekly Reports (MMWR), 1986; Baron and Merriam, 1988].

In two epidemiological surveys conducted on Long Island, New York, for the U.S. EPA, cohorts were selected on the basis of aldicarb levels in their drinking water, and questionnaires to determine water and food consumption, symptoms experienced, and diagnosed illnesses were sent to 1035 residents of 462 households. Although the initial survey indicated a possible association between the incidence of diarrhea and levels of aldicarb in the water, the follow-up study, focusing on children, did not confirm this association. No relationship was detected between food consumption or water source and adverse health symptoms, and self-reported physician-diagnosed illnesses were not significantly related to levels of aldicarb in the water (Whitlock *et al.*, 1982).

Another survey attempted to relate self-reported symptoms suggestive of peripheral neuropathy to aldicarb levels in drinking water in Suffolk County, New York. The response rate was less than 20%. Responses were classified as "probably," "possibly," or "vaguely" suggestive of a neurologic syndrome. A significant correlation with aldicarb concentration was obtained only by combining all three categories of response, including reports of just one symptom or of symptoms not forming any cohesive syndrome. The authors concluded only that further study was needed (Sterman and Varma, 1983). However, controlled experiments with animals have shown no evidence of a neurotoxic syndrome following exposure to aldicarb or to any other carbamate insecticide.

A pilot epidemiological study by the Wisconsin Department of Health and Social Services (WDHSS) evaluated a wide range of clinical immunological parameters in 23 women exposed to aldicarb in their drinking water and in a nonexposed control group. All individuals in the study were healthy, showing no evidence of any pathological state. The groups did not differ in any immunological parameter except number of T8 lymphocytes; the number was elevated in five individuals in the exposed group and one control individual. Although elevated over the concurrent control values, the T8 values were still within the normal range for the laboratory performing the assay. Observation of an elevated stimulation assay response to one of a large number of antigens (*Candida*) was not considered immunologically significant, nor was it attributed to aldicarb exposure (Fiore *et al.*, 1986). This study was reviewed by U.S. and Canadian government agencies and an independent panel representing expertise in epidemiology, biostatistics, and clinical immunology. Reviewers concurred that the WDHSS study did not provide evidence for any immunotoxic effect of aldicarb, citing several serious limitations and flaws of the study.

Use Experience   Human exposure to aldicarb has been assessed under a variety of actual working conditions (field and greenhouse). Exposure, as determined by detection of blood acetylcholinesterase inhibition or of aldicarb residues in the urine, depends primarily on the means by which the formulated product is applied. Among workers applying a 10% granular aldicarb formulation to ornamental plants in greenhouses or in outdoor beds, either with or without protective clothing or equipment, no signs or symptoms of intoxication were observed. After application periods of up to 4 hr, levels of aldicarb residues in the workers' urine ranged from undetectable to a total of 0.3 mg.

Among workers applying 10 or 15% aldicarb formulations to crops by tractor in the United States and England, no signs or symptoms of intoxication were found. Low levels of aldicarb residues were occasionally detected in the workers' urine, especially when no protective clothing or equipment was worn. In studies conducted in India in which volunteers applied a 10% formulation to field crops by various manual methods, low levels of aldicarb residues were found in the workers' urine; excretion of aldicarb residues was complete within 48 hr after exposure. Although erythrocyte acetylcholinesterase activity was significantly depressed, no signs or symptoms of intoxication were observed. Furthermore, the potential for exposure was maximal in these studies, as the workers wore no protective clothing except gloves for hand broadcasting of the granules; they did not use masks, goggles, or respirators, and they did not wear shoes.

In a study conducted in Panama, 15 volunteers applied a 15% aldicarb formulation to banana plants for 3 days, using hand applicators under standard working conditions (temperatures of 24–32°C and relative humidities of 80–90%). Blood sampling after the work period showed slight acetylcholinesterase inhibition in two workers, both of whom spontaneously recovered in 1 day (Baron and Merriam, 1988). Similarly, tractor drivers and loaders applying aldicarb to cotton fields in the Sudan showed low levels of aldicarb residues in the urine at the end of a workday. By the following morning, residues had declined to undetectable

levels in most cases (Mann and Danauskas, 1984). No signs or symptoms of intoxication were seen in either of these studies.

In all of these studies, when overexposed workers were removed from the exposure situation, acetylcholinesterase activity always returned rapidly to normal and symptoms, if any, subsided; no lasting effects on the health of workers were noted.

17.3.2 BENDIOCARB

17.3.2.1 Identity, Properties, and Uses

Chemical Name   Bendiocarb is 2,2-dimethyl-1,3-benzodioxol-4-yl *N*-methylcarbamate. Its structure is shown in Table 17.1

Synonyms   The common name bendiocarb (ANSI, BSI, ISO, JMAF) is in general use. Trade names have included Dycarb®, Ficam®, Garvox®, Multamat®, Multimet®, Niomil®, Rotate®, Seedox®, Tattoo®, and Turcam®. Code designations have included ENT 27695, NC 6897, and OMS 1394. The CAS registry number is 22781-23-3.

Physical and Chemical Properties   Bendiocarb has the empirical formula $C_{11}H_{13}NO_4$ and a molecular weight of 223.2. It is an odorless white crystalline solid with a melting point of 128–130°C and a vapor pressure of 5×10^{-6} mm Hg at 25°C. Its solubility (grams per liter at 25°C) is 0.04 in water, 0.3 in kerosene, 0.35 in hexane, 10 in *o*-xylene and trichloroethylene, 40 in benzene and ethanol, 200 in acetone, chloroform, dichloromethane, and dioxane, 300 in glycerol and dimethyl sulfoxide, and 640 in dimethylformamide. Bendiocarb is stable at up to 100°C.

Formulations and Uses   Bendiocarb was developed for structural pest control in and around the home and is effective against a wide range of nuisance and disease vector pests. It is also used for insect control in corn and on turf and ornamentals and for adult mosquito as a residual treatment and as an adulticide in an ultralow-volume (ULV) spray. Formulations include wettable powders, a dust, granules, and a solution for ULV application.

17.3.2.2 Toxicity to Laboratory Animals

Basic Findings   The acute toxicity of bendiocarb is summarized in Tables 17.2 and 17.3. Signs of acute intoxication are typical of acetylcholinesterase inhibition. Tested in rabbits, bendiocarb was a mild skin and eye irritant.

In rats given oral 4-mg/kg doses of bendiocarb, inhibition of acetylcholinesterase activity in plasma and whole blood peaked at 65–80% at 10 min after administration. Recovery began within 30 min and was nearly complete in 3 days. In dogs ingesting bendiocarb for an acute dose of about 6–8.6 mg/kg, brain and whole-blood acetylcholinesterase activities were inhibited by more than 50% within 15 min after the feeding period. In whole blood, inhibition peaked at 2 hr and activity recovered within 3 hr, whereas in the brain, acetylcholinesterase activity remained fairly constant from 15 min to 3 hr after dosing. In dogs given bendiocarb orally at about 32.4 mg/kg, whole-blood acetylcholinesterase inhibition was 73% at 1 hr and 48% at 6 hr after administration, and cholinergic signs were seen within 24 min. Recovery was complete in 24–25 hr (FAO/WHO, 1983).

In a 21-day study with rats, dermal exposure to dosages of 200 mg/kg/day or higher produced cholinergic signs. Whole-blood acetylcholinesterase activity was inhibited more than 30% following one 200-mg/kg dose or 15 50-mg/kg/day doses. No pathological effects were observed (FAO/WHO, 1983).

In a 2-year study with dogs, bendiocarb in the diet at 500 ppm resulted in elevated serum cholesterol and depression of acetylcholinesterase activity by more than 20% in whole blood and brain. At dietary levels of 100 ppm or higher, serum calcium levels also were transiently decreased. There were no treatment-related changes in organ weights or histopathology of more than 30 tissues at these dosages, and no treatment-related effects were seen at a dietary level of 20 ppm. A no-effect level was 0.7 mg/kg/day (FAO/WHO, 1983, 1985).

In a 2-year study with rats, bendiocarb in the diet at 200 ppm decreased water consumption and blood and brain acetylcholinesterase activity; produced changes in several hematological, biochemical, and urinalysis parameters and in organ weights; and increased the incidence of lenticular opacities and stomach lesions. Incidence of the eye lesion appeared to be dose related, with a borderline no-effect level of 10 ppm. No other treatment-related histopathological effects were observed. A no-effect level was 0.38 mg/kg/day (FAO/WHO, 1983).

Absorption, Distribution, Metabolism, and Excretion   In rats given a 1-mg/kg oral dose of [^{14}C]bendiocarb, plasma levels of radioactivity peaked at 10 min after administration. Following a 2.5-mg/kg dose, radioactivity in the tissues 72 hr after administration ranged from 0.015 to 0.061 ppm (as bendiocarb). Six days after 10-day dietary administration of ring-labeled bendiocarb to rats ended, residues were detected in the fat, liver, kidneys, muscle, and brain, the levels being highest in fat tissue (Challis and Adcock, 1981; FAO/WHO, 1983).

In all species examined, bendiocarb was metabolized via cleavage of the carbamate ester group to yield the phenol (2,2-dimethyl-1,3-benzoxodiol-4-ol), which was excreted as sulfate and glucuronide conjugates. After acute oral administration of ring-labeled bendiocarb to rats, conjugates of the phenol accounted for more than 85% of the dose recovered in the urine within 24 hr, and remaining 15% comprised sulfate and glucuronide conjugates of at least seven minor metabolites, apparently including *N*-hydroxymethyl bendiocarb; no unchanged parent compound was found. The feces contained primarily the free phenol, with some unchanged bendiocarb. Metabolism was similar in rats given ring-labeled bendiocarb at 20 ppm in their diet for 10 days (Challis and Adcock, 1981; FAO/WHO, 1983). In mice, conjugates of the phenol accounted for 33–56% of an intubated ring-labeled dose; the only other metabolite was thought to be conjugated 6-hydroxybendiocarb. Bendiocarb metabolism and excretion were similar in hamsters and rabbits. In dogs given ring-labeled bendiocarb, the minor urinary metabolites were thought to be ring-hydroxylated derivatives; unchanged parent compound was not found in the urine but accounted for 80% of the radioactivity in the feces (FAO/WHO, 1983).

Within 2 days after oral administration of ring-labeled bendiocarb (at 0.125–10 mg/kg) to rats, 89–90% of the dose was eliminated in the urine, 2–6% in the expired air, and 2–6% in the feces (Challis and Adcock, 1981; FAO/WHO, 1983). In mice intubated with ring-labeled bendiocarb, more than 80% of the dose was excreted within 24 hr, primarily in the urine; less than 10% of the radioactivity was recovered in the feces (FAO/WHO, 1983).

Effects on Organs and Tissues   Results of mutagenicity testing with bendiocarb are summarized in Section 17.2.3.2. Bendiocarb was not carcinogenic to rats or mice in 2-year studies (FAO/WHO, 1983).

Bendiocarb inhibited platelet aggregation in human plasma *in vitro;* this effect was observed for lipophilic carbamates but not hydrophilic ones (Krug and Berndt, 1985).

Effects on Reproduction   In a three-generation reproduction study with rats, fertility and reproduction were not affected by bendiocarb at dietary levels of up to 250 ppm. Perinatal and postnatal administration of bendiocarb to dams at up to 800 ppm in the diet (a maternally toxic dosage) reduced pup weight gain and survival. No effects were seen at 400 ppm, the next-lowest dosage. When rats were intubated with bendiocarb at 4 mg/kg/day (a maternally toxic dosage) on days 6–15 of gestation, no teratogenic effects were observed. In rabbits, intubation with bendiocarb at up to 5 mg/kg/day on days 6–28 of gestation produced no evidence of adverse effects on embryonic or fetal development, although acetylcholinesterase activity was inhibited by up to 87% (at 5 mg/kg/day) (FBC, 1986).

17.3.2.3 Toxicity to Humans

The 1984 FAO/WHO Joint Meeting on Pesticide Residues estimated a human ADI for bendiocarb of 0–0.004 mg/kg body weight (FAO/WHO, 1985).

Experimental Exposure   In a series of experiments involving oral administrations of one to three oral doses of a 76% wettable powder formulation of bendiocarb to human subjects, dose levels ranged from 0.003 to 0.200 mg a.i./kg (a.i. = active ingredient). The threshold dose for mild cholinergic symptoms was between 0.15 and 0.20 mg/kg; the latter dosage was rapidly followed by mild vertigo, nausea, and sweating, with up to 40% inhibition of blood acetylcholinesterase activity. Recovery from these effects was notable 30 min after dosing and complete within 4 hr. The lowest dose depressing blood acetylcholinesterase activity without eliciting symptoms was 0.15 mg/kg, and the maximum no-effect level was at least 0.10 mg/kg, a dosage producing no detectable cumulative effect when ingested at 4-hr intervals (FBC, 1986).

Metabolism and excretion of an oral dose of [^{14}C]bendiocarb by a human subject was similar to the pattern observed in animals; more than 99% of the dose was eliminated in the urine in 22 hr, primarily as sulfate and glucuronide conjugates of the phenol, with minor amounts of conjugated bendiocarb and N-hydroxymethyl bendiocarb (Challis and Adcock, 1981).

Accidental and Intentional Overexposure   During evaluation of the safety of bendiocarb as a mosquito adulticide in Indonesia in 1981, one inexperienced sprayman showed cholinergic symptoms, characterized by excessive salivation, vomiting, and a pounding headache. His cholinesterase activity was found to be 63% of his baseline level. He recovered in less than 3 hr without any medical treatment, and his cholinesterase activity returned to normal by the following morning (FBC, 1986).

A second case of bendiocarb poisoning occurred when a spray-plane pilot was cleaning the interior of a plane that had been grossly contaminated with a 25% bendiocarb ULV formulation as a result of a pump malfunction. Working in extreme heat and humidity and without protective clothing, the pilot experienced severe chemical contamination; after about 2.5 hr of work, he stopped and lay down. He was uncoordinated and nauseated, vomited several times, and experienced pains in his arms, hands, and legs. Muscles in various parts of his body, especially the fingers, went into spasms, with uncontrolled twitching, and he experienced breathing difficulties. After decontamination and two injections of atropine, his hypotension recovered, with a complete return to normal within 2 hr. He was released from hospital after 8 hr and had recovered fully by the following day (FBC, 1986).

In a well-documented case of attempted suicide, a 34-year-old male was admitted to hospital within 30 min of ingesting 15 gm of an 80% wettable powder formulation of bendiocarb, along with 20 mg. of metoclopromide. On arrival, he was incoherent and verbal contact was impossible. He had pupillary constriction, the skin was flushed and sweating, and there was fasciculation of the eyelids and hand muscles. He was hypersecreting and hyperventilating, his pulse rate was 180 per minute, and his serum acetylcholinesterase activity was markedly depressed. Following prompt gastric lavage and the administration of charcoal suspension, atropine (1.5 mg) was given iv for a total dose of 12 mg in 8 hr. The patient became comatose and unconscious soon after admission. When respiratory difficulties arose, he was placed on a ventilator; a metabolic acidosis was corrected by sodium bicarbonate infusion, and hypokalemia was corrected by a potassium supplement. After 2 hr, he had recovered consciousness and the sweating had decreased, but muscle fasciculation and weakness continued and assisted ventilation was still needed. Four hours after admission, the patient could breathe unaided, and 9 hr postadmission, further treatment was not considered necessary. The following day, he had completely recovered (FBC, 1986).

Use Experience   No cases of bronchospasm due to inhalation of bendiocarb have been reported, nor have any other specific localized responses except miosis to bendiocarb contamination. There have been no confirmed cases of allergic response or hypersensitivity of any type due to bendiocarb during development, manufacture, and commercial use, other than reversible miosis following eye contact (FBC, 1986).

The safety of bendiocarb to spray operators and villagers when used as a residual mosquito adulticide was evaluated in two major studies, in Iran and Indonesia, conducted along the guidelines of a World Health Organization expanded Stage V evaluation program and involving a total of 26 spray operators. In Iran, during 232 person-days of exposure, sprayers apparently showed significant reversible inhibition of blood acetylcholinesterase, but only 16 reports of mild symptoms were noted. It is thought that the acetylcholinesterase inhibition observed was partly a consequence of contamination of the finger-prick blood samples with insecticide. Urine residue values were low, supporting this hypothesis. In the Indonesian study, during 192 sprayer-days, venous blood was sampled with a hypodermic needle to prevent sample contamination. Several spray operators had symptomless, slight to moderate inhibition of whole-blood acetylcholinesterase activity, with a mean of 87% of preexposure levels after 48 sprayer-days. Two spray operators reported transient adverse effects. In one case of significant toxicity, acetylcholinesterase activity was depressed by 38%; the sprayer recovered within 3 hr without medical treatment, and his acetylcholinesterase level was normal the next morning. The calculated mean dermal exposure to a spray operator for a full day of spraying (4.5 hr) was 26 mg, and mean urinary excretion among spray operators was 0.94 mg bendiocarb equivalents. Based on data from a total of 950 man days of monitoring, it was concluded that only about 6% of bendiocarb on the skin actually was absorbed. Bendiocarb was not detectable in the urine of most villagers; most of the exceptions were children. No complaints were made by villagers within 24 hr of reentering treated houses in either study (FBC, 1986).

17.3.3   4-BENZOTHIETHYL-N-METHYLCARBAMATE

This compound (see Table 17.1) was effective for control of human lice and caused no irritation or other side effects. However, some spraymen complained of skin irritation and other subjective symptoms that did not prevent continued work, and no rash or other signs were observed (Hayes, 1982).

17.3.4   BUFENCARB

Some sprayers involved in testing this compound (see Table 17.1) for malaria control showed typical signs of poisoning, especially vomiting, and a few villagers complained of itching (Hayes, 1982).

17.3.5   CARBARYL

17.3.5.1   Identity, Properties, and Uses

Chemical Name   Carbaryl is 1-naphthyl N-methylcarbamate. Its structure is shown in Table 17.1.

Synonyms The common name carbaryl (ANSI, BSI, ESA, ISO) is in general use except in Eastern Europe, where arylam may be used, and in the USSR, where the trade name Sevin® is used as a common name. Other trade names have included Atoxan®, Caprolin®, Carbacide®, Carbamine®, Carpolin®, Cekubaryl®, Denapon®, Denopton®, Devicarb®, Dicarbam®, Gamonil®, Hexavin®, Karbaspray®, Karbatox®, Karbosep®, Mervin®, NAC®, Panam®, Rayvon®, Septene®, Sevinox®, Sevidol®, Tercyl®, and Tricarnam®. Code designations have included ENT 23969, UC 7744, and OMS 29. The CAS registry number is 63-25-2.

Physical and Chemical Properties Carbaryl has the empirical formula $C_{12}H_{11}NO_2$ and a molecular weight of 201.20. The material is a white to light tan solid with a mild phenolic odor. It has a melting point of 142°C and a vapor pressure of less than 4×10^{-5} mm Hg at 26°C. The solubility of carbaryl in water is 40 ppm at 30°C. It is moderately soluble in most polar organic solvents, such as dimethylformamide, dimethyl sulfoxide, and acetone; slightly soluble in hexane, benzene, and methanol; and about 5% soluble in petroleum oils. Carbaryl is stable under normal storage conditions but is hydrolyzed rapidly at pH 10 or above.

History, Formulations, and Uses Carbaryl was first synthesized in 1953 and introduced in 1958 as a broad-spectrum contact insecticide with systemic properties. It is used for control of over 150 major pests on more than 120 crops, including field crops, forage, vegetables, fruit, nuts, shade trees, ornamentals, forests, lawns, turf, and rangeland, as well as control of pests of domestic animals. Carbaryl formulations include baits, dusts, wettable powders, granules, and oil, molasses, and aqueous dispersions and suspensions.

17.3.5.2 Toxicity to Laboratory Animals

Basic Findings The acute toxicity of carbaryl is summarized in Tables 17.2–17.4. The symptoms of acute intoxication are typical of acetylcholinesterase inhibition. In rabbits, carbaryl did not irritate the skin and produced only transient conjunctival irritation. Carbaryl did not cause a skin sensitization reaction in guinea pigs (Cranmer, 1986).

Although acute ip injection of mice with carbaryl lowered body temperature, an effect reduced by atropine, administration of a cholinergic organophosphate did so only slightly, suggesting that the effect was not due to acetylcholinesterase inhibition (Ahdaya et al., 1976). Acute oral, dermal, and inhalation exposure of rats and rabbits to carbaryl at doses ranging from 450 to 1500 mg/kg resulted in transient acetylcholinesterase inhibition in the brain, plasma, and erythrocytes ranging from 30% to greater than 65%. At the higher doses, other blood parameters also were affected (Yakim, 1967; Mount et al., 1981; Kossakowski and Lysek, 1982).

Histological examination of rats following inhalation exposure to carbaryl showed tracheal swelling and inflammation and ciliary detachment (Lee and Hong, 1985). Acute inhalation

exposure of cats to carbaryl at 82 mg/m³ caused signs of intoxication and inhibited blood acetylcholinesterase activity by 39–71%. No clinical signs were seen at 2 mg/m³ (Yakim, 1967). In a subchronic study with cats, cholinergic signs appeared during the first 2 hr of each 6-hr inhalation exposure to carbaryl at 63 mg/m³; at 40 mg/m³ blood acetylcholinesterase inhibition and behavioral effects were noted, but 4 months' exposure at 16 mg/m³ caused no toxic signs (Yakim, 1967).

When rats and gerbils were given carbaryl orally for 70 days at dosages that were increased weekly, all deaths occurred within 24 hr of the first administration of a given dosage. One of 12 rats died at a dosage of 120 mg/kg/day, and cumulative mortality was 7/12 at a dosage of 180 mg/kg/day; no further deaths occurred at dosages of up to 200 mg/kg/day. In gerbils, mortality was 2/12 at the initial dosage of 60 mg/kg/day, and the last animals died at a dosage of 100 mg/kg/day (Benson and Dorough, 1984). Two-month dietary exposure of rats to carbaryl at 100 ppm was reported to increase liver weight (Cecil et al., 1974). In a Soviet study, carbaryl inhibited acetylcholinesterase and caused changes in various liver function tests and in liver histology when administered to rats and rabbits by gavage at dosages as low as 0.38 mg/kg/day for 3 months (Kagan et al., 1970). Azizova (1976) reported histological CNS changes following 6-month exposure of rabbits to carbaryl at dosages of approximately 8–80 mg/kg/day. The effects were noted 45 days after dosing ended, and changes at the higher dosages were likened to the effects of meningoencephalitis. It is not clear to what extent effects noted in Soviet studies are due to impurities in carbaryl manufactured in the USSR.

In a 1-year study with dogs, carbaryl in the diet at 1250 ppm reduced body weight gain, increased liver weight, increased leukocyte and segmented neutrophil counts, decreased albumin levels, and inhibited acetylcholinesterase in the plasma, erythrocytes, and brain. Acetylcholinesterase inhibition was also observed at a dosage of 400 ppm, but not at 125 ppm. No other effects were observed on body or organ weights, food consumption, mortality, clinical signs, gross pathology, ophthalmology, clinical chemistry, or histopathology (Hamada, 1987b).

Carbaryl in the diet of rats for 2 years at 400 ppm (about 20 mg/kg/day) slightly depressed organ weights in males but did not affect mortality, hematology, or organ histopathology. No-effect levels were 9 mg/kg/day for males and 21 mg/kg/day for females. In shorter-term studies at higher dosages, liver and kidney effects were noted, which were transient and may have been secondary to stress (Carpenter et al., 1961).

Pigs receiving carbaryl in the diet at 150 mg/kg/day gradually developed myasthenia, incoordination, ataxia, tremor, and clonic muscular contractions terminating in paraplegia and prostration. Involvement was greater in the hindquarters. At 300 mg/kg/day, onset of effects was faster. Significant histopathology was confined to the CNS and the skeletal musculature; no consistent changes in peripheral nerves were observed. Atropine did not change the course of the chronic poisoning, but if carbaryl administration was stopped after the pigs had been paralyzed for a full day, most of them recovered slowly. Administration of hydrochlorothiazide (300 mg/day) led to recovery from paresis in 8 or 9 days even with continued exposure to carbaryl, but paralysis recurred 10 or more days after the treatment was stopped. The condition was fatal unless dosing was stopped or treatment was instituted soon after prostration occurred (Smalley *et al.*, 1969; Smalley, 1970). Whether the paralysis seen in pigs was caused by carbaryl or by a metabolite, perhaps peculiar to pigs, has not been explored. No pharmacological study seems to have been made to determine whether hydrochlorothiazide acts merely as a diuretic reducing the blood level of carbaryl or some critical metabolite or whether it changes the metabolism of carbaryl. These matters deserve investigation. Monkeys exposed to carbaryl did not develop prostration and tolerated a dosage of 600 mg/kg/day for 6 months (Serrone *et al.*, 1966). In other experiments, pigs made paraplegic by repeated administration of carbaryl at 125 mg/kg/day had decreased acetylcholinesterase activity in several parts of the brain and spinal cord. The paraplegic syndrome culminating in convulsions was also produced by an iv dose of 25 mg/kg (Michel *et al.*, 1971).

Absorption and Distribution   Penetration of carbaryl through rat skin depended on the solvent, being greater in acetone than in benzene or corn oil; rapid early penetration was by the parent compound (O'Brien and Dannelley, 1965). In a percutaneous absorption study with rats, about 57% of a continuously applied dose of [^{14}C]carbaryl (in acetone) penetrated the shaved skin in 168 hr. The absorption rate was 0.18 μg/cm^2/hr, and $t_{1/2}$ was 1.26 hr for absorption and 67 hr for elimination (Knaak *et al.*, 1984). In mice, $t_{1/2}$ for acute dermal penetration of [^{14}C]carbaryl in acetone was 12.8 min, and the label was detected in the blood, tissues, and excreta within 5–15 min after application. By 8 hr after application, 73.3% of the dose had appeared in the excreta, while 4.9% remained in the intestines and 2.6% in the liver; levels in other tissues and organs ranged from less than 0.1% to 0.6% (Shah *et al.*, 1981). In rabbits, dermal absorption of methyl-^{14}C-labeled carbaryl in acetone was nearly complete in 24 hr, and recovery of the dose in urine and feces was greatest in the first 24 hr (Shah and Guthrie, 1977).

Following intratracheal injection of a small volume of radioactive carbaryl as an aerosol, activity in the blood of rats peaked in 2–5 min. Within 3 days, 90% of the radioactivity was recovered in the urine and 2–5% in the feces (Nye and Dorough, 1976).

Based on disappearance rates, the half-life of carbaryl was 6.4 min in the empty small intestines and 2.6 min in the lungs of rats (Hwang and Schanker, 1974). Exhalation of ^{14}CO$_2$ by rats peaked 30–40 min after oral administration of carbonyl-labeled carbaryl (Casper and Pekas, 1971). In rats, carbaryl was absorbed more rapidly from the intestine than from the stomach. Absorption was most rapid when dimethyl sulfoxide (DMSO) was the vehicle and was more rapid with oil than with gum tragacanth or milk (Cambon *et al.*, 1981). In rats given [^{14}C]carbaryl by gastric intubation, 55% of the dose was present in the gastrointestinal tract after 1 hr and 32.5% after 5 hr (Tanaka *et al.*, 1981). In mice, about 69% of an intubated dose of carbaryl was absorbed within 60 min. The $t_{1/2}$ for absorption was 17 min, and blood levels peaked 35–40 min after admin-

istration. Within an hour, 16.9% of the dose appeared in the urine and 8.6% in exhaled CO$_2$ (Ahdaya *et al.*, 1981). Stomach absorption accounted for about 29% of total gastrointestinal absorption after 1 hr (Ahdaya and Guthrie, 1982).

Following gastric intubation of rats with [^{14}C]carbaryl, the percentage of the dose per gram of tissue ranged from less than 0.1% to nearly 0.4% after 1 hr; levels were highest in the liver, kidneys, and fat. After 5 hr, levels had significantly declined in liver and fat (Tanaka *et al.*, 1980). Following acute oral exposure of rats to carbaryl at 450–1500 mg/kg, residues were detected in tissues at 48 hr after dosing. In rats that died, minimum residue levels were 11.7 ppm in the liver, 5 ppm in the brain, and 3.6 ppm in the heart (Mount *et al.*, 1981).

Carbaryl showed considerable protein-binding ability in cultured human embryonic lung cells (Murakami and Fukami, 1982). In a protein-binding study with rats, carbaryl in the serum was found to bind primarily to albumin and partly to globulin and lipoprotein; in the cytosol fraction of the intestinal mucosa, it was bound to a low-molecular-weight component (Tanaka *et al.*, 1981).

Metabolism and Excretion   Animals metabolize carbaryl both by hydrolytic mechanisms—hydrolysis and hydroxylation to 1-naphthol and hydroxylated naphthylmethylcarbamates, which form glucuronide and sulfate conjugates—and by nonhydrolytic pathways. Biotransformation of carbaryl is basically similar in humans, rats, guinea pigs, monkeys, and sheep, the major different being the extent to which carbaryl was hydrolyzed to yield 1-naphthol. Much less hydrolysis occurs in monkeys or pigs than in humans, rats, or sheep (Knaak *et al.*, 1968; Sullivan *et al.*, 1972; Lin *et al.*, 1975).

Carbaryl has been shown to be metabolized *in vitro* by cells from both animal and plant sources. The main product was 1-naphthol; an array of other metabolites similar to those noted *in vivo* were also isolated (Dorough and Casida, 1964; Leeling and Casida, 1966; Baron and Locke, 1970; Mehendale and Dorough, 1971; Sullivan *et al.*, 1972; Wheeler and Strother, 1974a; Chin *et al.*, 1974, 1979; Lin *et al.*, 1975; Blase and Loomis, 1976).

In rats given radiolabeled carbaryl iv, 50% of a 0.1-mg dose was recovered from the bile within 6 hr. Of higher doses, progressively smaller percentages were recovered; at 1.0 mg, only 17% of the activity was recovered in the bile (Bend *et al.*, 1971). When rats with cannulated bile ducts were given an oral dose of ring-labeled carbaryl, within 48 hr they excreted 45.4% of the dose in the bile, 42.3% in the urine, and 1.4% in the feces (Marshall and Dorough, 1979). Following iv administration of [^{14}C]carbaryl to bile duct-cannulated rats, biliary excretion of a 1-mg dose was 15.5% in 30 min, leveling out at about 28% in less than 3 hr (Tanaka *et al.*, 1980).

Bend *et al.* (1971) presented evidence that water-soluble metabolites in the urine and bile of rats that had received iv or ip doses of ring- or carbonyl-labeled carbaryl were unidentified conjugates that could be hydrolyzed by acid, but not by enzymes, to thioethers, specifically *S*-(4-hydroxy-1-naphthyl)cysteine and *S*-(5-hydroxy-1-naphthyl)cysteine. Struble *et al.* (1983) identified biliary metabolites from bile-fistulated rats given oral doses of [^{14}C]carbaryl as 5,6-dihydro-5,6-

dihydroxycarbaryl glucuronide and conjugated carbaryl and hydroxycarbaryl isomers; these accounted for up to 32% of the dose secreted in the bile. Partial metabolism of carbaryl to CO_2 was demonstrated *in vitro* (Palut *et al.*, 1970). Both the methyl and the carbonyl carbon, but not ring carbon, were oxidized to carbon dioxide in rats, guinea pigs, and humans (Knaak *et al.*, 1965; Hassan *et al.*, 1966). Dogs excreted in their urine none of the metabolites found in rat urine (Knaak and Sullivan, 1967). A compound chromatographing similarly to naphthyl glucuronide was excreted by dogs, but it proved to be nonfluorescent, and its identity is unknown (Knaak *et al.*, 1965; Sullivan *et al.*, 1972). An early report that cows excreted unmetabolized carbaryl in the urine (Whitehurst *et al.*, 1963) has not been confirmed.

Small quantities of some intermediate metabolites of carbaryl were excreted in the milk of lactating cows (Dorough and Casida, 1964; Baron, 1968); at the low doses administered in these studies, 58–70% of the activity was recovered in the urine and 11–15% in the feces (Dorough, 1967).

Most mammals given naphthyl-labeled carbaryl excreted 68–74% of the dose in the urine and 2–11% in the feces within 24 hr of administration (Knaak *et al.*, 1965, 1968; Krishna and Casida, 1966; Dorough, 1967; Sullivan *et al.*, 1972). Dogs excreted only 30% of the dose in the urine and 15% in the feces (Knaak and Sullivan, 1967). Rats given N-methyl[^{14}C]carbaryl eliminated 12–24% of the dose in exhaled air and 53–54% in the urine within 48 hr (Hassan *et al.*, 1966; Krishna and Casida, 1966). Within 24 hr after administration of carbonyl-labeled carbaryl, rats eliminated 34–45% in the urine, 8% in the feces, and 30% as exhaled $^{14}CO_2$ (Knaak *et al.*, 1965; Hassan *et al.*, 1966). In a study comparing hydrolysis of carbaryl in four rodent species, 24-hr recoveries of a carbonyl-labeled dose as exhaled $^{14}CO_2$ were lower in rats and mice than in gerbils and guinea pigs; the reverse was found for urinary recoveries (Benson and Dorough, 1984).

Biochemical Effects   The Soviet literature reporting effects of carbaryl on hematologic parameters and blood and tissue levels of various enzymes and other biochemical constituents in laboratory animals is reviewed by Kuhr and Dorough (1976) and by Khaikina and Kuz'minskaia (1970). Despite extensive study, it remains unclear whether the changes reported are causes or effects and especially whether they are associated with carbaryl or with some impurity. Most observations have not been reproduced in laboratories outside of the USSR and Eastern Europe.

In rat tissues *in vitro*, the half-time for hydrolysis of carbaryl increased linearly with increasing dose, suggesting a toxic effect on the hydrolytic mechanism, which would indirectly increase carbamate toxicity (Hurst and Dorough, 1978). Miller *et al.* (1979) demonstrated that carbon derived from carbaryl binds to microsomal proteins and that the degree of binding is increased by pretreatment with phenobarbital and other inducers.

In isolated rat hepatocytes, carbaryl was reported to increase cytochrome P-450 level, reduce O_2 consumption and CO_2 production, inhibit gluconeogenesis, reduce lactate dehydrogenase and aspartate aminotransferase activities, and enhance glucose-6-phosphatase activity (Parafita and Fernandez Otero,

1983, 1984a,b). In another *in vitro* study, carbaryl decreased rat liver microsomal β-glucuronidase content (Lechner and Abdel-Rahman, 1985). Carbaryl inhibited rat brain monoamine oxidase *in vitro;* inhibition ranged from 27 to 81%, depending on the substrate (Kadir and Knowles, 1981). Carbaryl also inhibited synthesis of DNA, RNA, and protein in cultured rat and human embryonic lung cells (Lockard *et al.*, 1982; Murakami and Fukami, 1983).

Acute oral administration of carbaryl to rats at doses ranging from 50 to about 500 mg/kg affected blood and brain levels of a variety of enzymes, amino acids, neurotransmitters, and other substances. Effects reported included decreases in serum protein levels, blood free amino acid levels, and brain acetylcholinesterase concentrations and changes in free amino acid metabolism in the liver and brain. Increases were reported in serum levels of glucose, glutamic-oxaloacetic transaminase, and glutamic-pyruvic transaminase; adrenal and plasma corticosterone levels; tyrosine α-ketoglutarate transaminase activity in liver cytosol; norepinephrine turnover (but not steady-state concentration) in the heart; urinary excretion of catecholamine metabolites; and regional brain levels of monoamine oxidase, noradrenaline, 5-hydroxyindoleacetic acid, homovanillic acid, dopamine, and serotonin (Hassan, 1971; Szcepaniak *et al.*, 1980; Jayapragasam *et al.*, 1981; Ray and Poddar, 1983a,b, 1984, 1985b; Ray *et al.*, 1984; Jeleniewicz and Szczepaniak, 1985; Jeleniewicz *et al.*, 1984). Serotonin activity in rats was increased by a single 10-mg/kg dose of carbaryl (Mogilevchik *et al.*, 1970). Hassan and Santolucito (1971) suggested that increased brain levels of serotonin in the rat might be secondary to stress (via sympathoadrenergic stimulation). Ray and co-workers suggested possible involvement of a central cholinergic mechanism in enhancement of serotonin and catecholamine metabolism by carbaryl.

Acute ip injection of rats with carbaryl increased serum β-glucuronidase activity in a dose-related fashion but did not affect activities of other acid hydrolases in the serum (Kikuchi *et al.*, 1981). Acute iv administration of carbaryl to rats at 8–16 mg/kg depressed the activities of several liver serine esterases, including β-glucuronidase, but not lactate dehydrogenase (Pipy *et al.*, 1982). Intraperitoneal doses of carbaryl as low as 5 mg/kg produced a hyperglycemic response in intact or hypophysectomized rats, but not in adrenalectomized rats, and decreased brain acetylcholinesterase activity (Orzel and Weiss, 1966). Hyperglycemic responses have also been reported for rabbits and dogs (Weiss *et al.*, 1964, 1965). Wakakura *et al.* (1978) suggested that increased sympathoadrenergic activity was responsible for carbaryl's effects on hepatic glycogen metabolism.

Acute inhalation exposure of rats to carbaryl at 112–224 mg/m^3 prolonged pentobarbital sleeping time and decreased liver microsomal cytochrome P-450 content and NADPH-cytochrome *c* reductase activity. However, a 3-day exposure had the opposite effect on each of these parameters (Lee and Hong, 1985).

In rats, acute oral pretreatment with carbaryl at a high dose increased hexobarbital sleeping time, whereas subchronic exposure increased hexobarbital oxidation and aniline metabolism and decreased hexobarbital sleeping time (Stevens *et al.*, 1972a,b). In another study with rats, a single oral 500-mg/kg dose of carbaryl or seven doses of 71 mg/kg/day increased the activities of acid phosphatase, glutamic-oxaloacetic transaminase, and glutamic-pyruvic transaminase in the liver and kidney, but did not affect the activities of alkaline phosphatase, lactate dehydrogenase, or succinate dehydrogenase (Kiran *et al.*, 1985). A single 10-mg/kg dose of carbaryl or 21 daily doses to rats increased serum β-glucuronidase levels; the increase was 20-fold greater following the single administration. Carbaryl at 50 mg/kg/day for 21 days decreased liver β-glucuronidase and glutathione content (Abdel-Rahman *et al.*, 1985).

In mice, carbaryl by gavage at 100 mg/kg/day for 3 days did not affect liver cytochrome P-450 content, NADPH-dependent reductase activities, microsomal xenobiotic metabolism, or cytosolic glutathione-dependent enzyme activities (Robacker *et al.*, 1981). In mice given carbaryl for 2 weeks at 5000 ppm in the diet, cytochrome P-450 and cytochrome b_5 activity increased (Cress and Strother, 1974).

In a 90-day study with rats, carbaryl at 2000 ppm in the diet caused a decrease in NADPH-cytochrome c reductase activity and increases in cytochrome P-450 activity and liver weights (Neskovic, 1979). In rats given oral doses of carbaryl at 200 mg/kg/day 3 days a week for 90 days, acetylcholinesterase activities were decreased in the blood and brain, and ATPase and glucose-6-phosphatase activities were slightly increased (Dikshith *et al.*, 1976). Subchronic oral administration of carbaryl to rats at 95 mg/kg/day for 30 days slightly decreased erythrocyte alanine levels, but a 15-day exposure did not affect blood-free amino acid levels (Jeleniewicz and Szczepaniak, 1980). Kuz'minskaya *et al.* (1984) reported changes in brain serotonin and dopamine content in rats given carbaryl orally at moderate dosages for 10 days. Carbaryl given to rats for 3 months at a daily intragastric dose of 60 mg/kg/day decreased the levels of tryptophan and 2,3-diphosphoglycerate in the blood. The same treatment increased the brain concentration of γ-aminobutyric acid (GABA) and decreased that of glutathione, while not affecting levels of norepinephrine, serotonin, 5-hydroxyindoleacetic acid, or monoamine oxidase (Podolak-Majczak and Tyburczyk, 1984; Tyburczyk and Podolak-Majczak, 1984a,b).

Effects on Organs and Tissues   Results of mutagenicity testing with carbaryl and other carbamates are discussed in Section 17.2.3.2. Administration of the maximum tolerated dosage of carbaryl (either 4.64 mg/kg/day orally or 100 mg/kg/day via sc injection) to mice for about 18 months did not increase the incidence of tumors (Innes *et al.*, 1969). Carbaryl in the diet of rats at 400 ppm (about 19.6 mg/kg/day) for 2 years did not affect the incidence of tumors (Carpenter *et al.*, 1961), nor did carbaryl in the diet of mice at 40 ppm for 80 weeks (Weil and Carpenter, 1962). Results of a pulmonary tumor induction assay with mice were not statistically significant and were considered equivocal by the authors (Shimkin *et al.*, 1969). Triolo *et al.* (1982) reported that carbaryl at 1000 ppm in the diet of mice for 20 weeks did not cause tumors, but increased the ability of benzo[*a*]pyrene to induce lung tumors; this effect was associated with increased B[*a*]P hydroxylase activity in the lung (but not in the liver).

Marked vacuolation of the epithelium of the proximal tubules of rats and monkeys receiving very large doses of carbaryl were reported by Serrone *et al.* (1966). Rats given carbaryl at 250–500 mg/kg showed a dose-dependent reduction in absorption of radiolabeled zinc from the stomach (Kossakowski and Żuk, 1983). Oral administration of carbaryl at 56 mg/kg increased tension developed during complete tetanus of rat skeletal muscle 2 hr after dosing (Santolucito and Whitcomb, 1971).

Effects of carbaryl on thyroid function and morphology are probably stress-related. Single high intragastric doses of carbaryl to rabbits first decreased and then increased uptake of ^{125}I by thyroid (Kossakowski *et al.*, 1982), and subchronic ip injection of mice with carbaryl at 50 mg/kg/week caused functional and morphological thyroid changes (Rappoport, 1969, 1971). Intubation of rats with carbaryl at dosages of 0.7–15 mg/kg/day for 6 months exacerbated the development of endemic goiter in rats, an effect prevented by simultaneous administration of 7 μg of iodine per day as a supplement (Shtenberg and Khovaeva, 1970; Kusevitskiy *et al.*, 1970).

Carbaryl inhibited platelet aggregation in human plasma *in vitro* (Krug and Berndt, 1985). A 30-day exposure of rats to carbaryl at 10 ppm in their drinking water produced treatment-related liver histopathology and slight decreases in platelet count and activity of clotting factor VII; other parameters were not affected (Lox, 1984).

A number of studies related to the *in vitro* and *in vivo* effects of carbaryl on the immune system have been reported. *In vivo* toxic action of carbaryl can disrupt the immune system's ability to combat certain viral infections. Several authors have suggested that observed effects were due to subtle treatment-related stress. In animal studies, carbaryl administered at doses not causing overt clinical signs of poisoning has been reported to produce a variety of reversible and nonthreatening effects on the immune system. No such effects have been observed in humans.

In an *in vitro* screening assay, carbaryl suppressed the generation of a T cell-mediated cytolytic response in mouse splenocytes, whether or not the compound was preincubated with a rat liver mitochondrial preparation (Rodgers *et al.*, 1986).

In rats given acute iv injections of carbaryl at dosages of 3.8–30 mg/kg, all but the lowest dosage transiently reduced phagocytosis of carbon particles by the reticuloendothelial system. The suggested mechanism was selective macrophage impairment via inhibition of a cell-bound serine esterase (Pipy *et al.*, 1978, 1983; de Maroussem *et al.*, 1986). Carbaryl was reported to decrease phagocytic activity of leukocytes and antibody formation in rats and rabbits following repeated exposure at a dosage of 20 mg/kg/day (Perelygin *et al.*, 1971).

Near-lethal oral doses of carbaryl to mice for 5–28 days before parenteral administration of antigen impaired the humoral immune response (Wiltrout *et al.*, 1978). In the African rodent *Mastomys natalensis*, carbaryl in the diet at 150 ppm for 1 month had no significant effect on reaginic antibody production or type 1 hypersensitivity (André *et al.*, 1981). In a similar study with mice, production of systemic antibody (IgG$_1$) was increased; six other antibody classes were unaffected (André *et al.*, 1983). In rabbits given nontoxic dietary dosages of carbaryl (about 2–8 mg/kg/day) or carbofuran (about 0.5–1 mg/kg/day) for 4 weeks, Street and Sharma (1975) observed slight immunosuppressive effects (including effects on globulin production) that were not consistently dosage-related. The authors suggested that the effects might be due to nonspecific physiological stress, although they were not mediated by adrenal function.

In rats given carbaryl in their diet so that the dosage was 2–5 mg/kg/day for 30 days and then experimentally infected with *Erysipelothrix rhusiopathiae,* septicemia and mortality increased, survival time decreased, and the onset of bacteremia was hastened (Shabanov *et al.,* 1983b). Similar results were obtained for rats infected with *Staphylococcus* (Shabanov *et al.,* 1983a). In rabbits and guinea pigs, daily oral doses of carbaryl at 15 mg/kg/day for 42 days enhanced the autosensitizing effects of *S. typhimurium* vaccine. Exposure of guinea pigs to this dosage for 3 months resulted in a delayed hypersensitivity response (Akhundov *et al.,* 1981). Administration of carbaryl to rabbits at subtoxic dosages for 90 days resulted in increased hemolysin levels and spleen lymphatic tissue reaction (Roszkowski, 1978).

Dose-related changes were seen in serum complement-fixing activity, lysozyme level, and immunological function of the reticuloendothelial system, neutrophils, skin, and mucosa in rats given carbaryl daily at 0.8–4 mg/kg for 4.5 months (Olefir and Minster, 1977). Shtenberg *et al.* (1972) reported decreases in serum complement-fixing activity, hemagglutinin titers, and phagocytic activity of neutrophils in rats given carbaryl perorally at 2 mg/kg/day for 9 months.

Pretreatment with carbaryl was reported to enhance replication of varicella zoster virus, but not herpes simplex viruses type 1 or 2 or cytomegalovirus, in cultured human embryonic lung cells (Abrahamsen and Jerkofsky, 1981, 1983; Jerkofsky and Abrahamsen, 1983). However, Schmidt (1983) found that carbaryl delayed the early spread of varicella zoster virus and delta herpes virus in human embryonic lung cells without affecting the total numbers of infection centers. Schmidt suggested that apparent enhancement in other studies could have been due to timing of sampling. A scientific panel appointed by the government of New Brunswick, Canada, could find no evidence that spraying of New Brunswick forests with carbaryl for spruce budworm control was related to a reported increased incidence of Reye's syndrome (via viral enhancement) (Schneider *et al.,* 1976).

Effects on Reproduction The acute and subchronic effects of carbaryl on reproductive parameters has been studied in at least 12 mammalian species. Transplacental transfer of carbaryl in pregnant rats and mice is minimal. By 96 hr after oral administration of ^{14}C-labeled carbaryl on day 18 of gestation, 0.3% of the administered radioactivity was found in rat fetuses. Levels were highest in fetal liver (Declume and Derache, 1976, 1977; Declume and Benard, 1977, 1978). In pregnant mice and rats given single doses of [^{14}C]carbaryl, maternal tissue levels peaked 1–2 hr after administration and decreased steadily over the 24 hr after administration (Courtney *et al.,* 1983). Radioac-

tivity from carbaryl administered orally at parturition increased in the mammary gland and the neonates throughout the 48 hr after administration (Benard and Declume, 1979). Excretion of carbaryl differed qualitatively and quantitatively between pregnant and nonpregnant rats and mice, probably as a result of the pharmacodynamics of metabolism in another compartment (the fetus) following acute administration (Wheeler and Strother, 1974a; Strother and Wheeler, 1980).

Single oral doses of carbaryl to pregnant rats on day 18 of gestation inhibited fetal acetylcholinesterase in the blood at doses of 6.25 mg/kg or higher and in the brain at 50 mg/kg, 1 hr after administration. Carbaryl orally administered to rats on gestation days 11–22 decreased brain and liver acetylcholinesterase activity at a dosage of 50 mg/kg/day, but not at 5 mg/kg/day or lower. At 50 mg/kg/day, body weight was reduced in both dams and neonates (Declume *et al.,* 1979). Carbaryl affected acetylcholinesterase isoenzymes similarly in dams and fetuses (Cambon *et al.,* 1980).

Reviews of the reproductive effects of carbaryl (Weil *et al.,* 1972; Kuhr and Dorough, 1976; Cranmer, 1986) note frequent reports from the USSR of reproductive injury by even small doses of carbaryl. Many of these effects have not been verified in other laboratories. In these studies, rats were exposed to carbaryl by daily peroral intubation at dosages ranging from 2 to 30 mg/kg/day and for periods ranging from 1 to 12 months; one study assessed reproductive effects over five generations. Effects reported at dosages as low as 2 mg/kg/day (but more commonly at 5 mg/kg/day and higher) were functional and focal histological changes in the testes (including decreased spermatogenesis), changes in sperm function (including reduced motility and survival time), inhibition of oogenesis, and increased hypophyseal secretion of gonadotropic hormones. Increased duration of the estrous cycle was reported at dosages as low as 5 mg/kg/day (but more commonly higher than 50 mg/kg/day), and histological changes in the ovaries occurred at dosages of 7 mg/kg/day and higher. Reproductive effects reported for dosages as low as 2 mg/kg/day were decreased fertility in both sexes, increases in stillbirths and pup mortality, and delayed pup development (Vashakidze, 1965, 1967, 1975; Rybakova, 1966, 1967, 1968; Shtenberg and Rybakova, 1968; Orlova and Zhalbe, 1968; Shtenberg and Ozhovan, 1971). More recently, Trifonova (1984) reported reduced ovarian function at carbaryl dosages of 40–80 mg/kg/day but not at 20 mg/kg/day.

Teratogenic effects in rats have also been reported by Soviet investigators (e.g., Shtenberg and Torchinskiy, 1972). Vashakidze (1965) reported teratogenicity and decreased reproduction at subchronic intubated dosages of 100 mg/kg/day and higher, but not at 50 mg/kg/day. However, a single 50-mg/kg intubated dose on gestation day 9 or 10 was reported to cause terata. The terata reported by Orlova and Zhalbe (1968) at 5 mg/kg/day for 12 months were interpreted by Weil *et al.* (1972) to be the result of infection rather than carbaryl exposure. Explanation of the differences between Soviet and Western results in reproductive toxicity testing is complicated by differences in experimental procedures and lack of detail in published accounts. Reviewers (e.g., Weil *et al.,* 1973) have suggested that impurities may be responsible for reproductive effects found in Soviet studies, have questioned the appropriateness of the intubation exposure route, and have noted that the effects are not consistently dose related. Cranmer (1986) suggests "nonspecific stress due to treatment rather than carbaryl *per se*" as a means of interpreting Soviet data that were not reproducible in Western studies.

Male rats given carbaryl orally at 200 mg/kg/day on 3 days a week for 90 days reportedly showed no clinical signs, effects on fertility, or histopathologic changes in the testes, liver, kidney, or brain; sperm effects were not quantified (Dikshith *et al.*, 1976). Kitagawa *et al.* (1977) reported reduced numbers of spermatogonia and spermatozoa in rats given 3 mg of carbaryl per week orally for 1 year. Carbaryl given to mice at up to 34 mg/kg/day for 5 days did not affect either the weight of the testes and sex glands or the ability of the prostate to assimilate and metabolize testosterone (Thomas *et al.*, 1974; Dieringer and Thomas, 1974). In mice injected ip with 0.4 mg of carbaryl either once or daily for 1 week, the incidence of sperm abnormalities was reportedly increased, but no degenerative changes in the testes were seen (Degraeve *et al.*, 1976). However, carbaryl administered to mice ip for 5 days at up to 800 mg/kg/day or by gavage at 150 mg/kg every 2 days for up to 68 days did not affect testis weight or histology, sperm count, or frequency of sperm abnormalities (Martin, 1982; Osterloh *et al.*, 1983). Studies of men occupationally exposed to carbaryl (discussed in Section 17.3.5.3) revealed no effects on sperm count or morphology.

In three-generation reproduction studies with rats, carbaryl in the diet at 10,000 ppm (about 500 mg/kg/day, a maternally toxic dosage) reduced fertility. Dietary levels of 5000 ppm (about 250 mg/kg/day) or higher reduced viability, average litter size, and survival, and dietary levels of 2000 ppm (about 100 mg/kg/day) or more resulted in reduced weanling weights but no other change. Dietary carbaryl leading to a dosage of 10 mg/kg/day had no significant effect on fertility, gestation, lactation, or viability of pups. No gross abnormalities were seen in the pups at any dosage. Carbaryl at 100 mg/kg/day by peroral intubation (a maternally toxic dosage) increased mortality and reduced growth and fertility (Collins *et al.*, 1971; Weil *et al.*, 1972, 1973). Weil and co-workers concluded that no-effect levels for fetotoxicity in rats were 25 mg/kg/day for exposure by gavage and 100 mg/kg/day for dietary exposure.

In rats administered carbaryl in their diet for various periods during gestation, maternal weight gain was reduced at dosages of 100 mg/kg/day or higher, but the only reproductive effect was reduced postnatal survival of pups at 500 mg/kg/day. A no-effect level for fetotoxicity was 100 mg/kg/day (Weil *et al.*, 1972). In rats given dietary carbaryl on gestation days 6–15 and sacrificed on day 18, no effects were observed on fetal viability or development at levels of up to 7000 ppm (about 525 mg/kg/day) (Hart, 1971).

Carbaryl given to female mice in their diets at up to 200 ppm (30 mg/kg/day) on days 6–18 of gestation had no reproductive or teratologic effects (FAO/WHO, 1968). Similar results were reported for a two-generation test in which mice received carbaryl at dietary levels up to 2000 ppm (about 260 mg/kg/day) (De-

Norscia and Lodge, 1973). Carbaryl administered to mice by gavage at 100 mg/kg/day on gestation days 6–15 had no fetotoxic effects; dietary exposure at 5660 ppm (1166 mg/kg/day) resulted in decreased fetal size but no terata (Murray *et al.*, 1979). In a study in which mice were given carbaryl by sc injection on gestation days 6–14, observation of fetal anomalies at a dosage of 100 mg/kg/day could not be replicated; a no-effect level was 25 mg/kg/day. Dosages of 100 mg/kg/day or higher were maternally toxic (Kotin *et al.*, 1968).

Carbaryl administered to guinea pigs by gavage at 300 mg/kg/day (a toxic dosage) during organogenesis resulted in fetal skeletal anomalies; fetal mortality resulted from dosing on gestation days 11–21, but not from single doses during gestation (Robens, 1969). In another teratogenesis study with guinea pigs, carbaryl in the diet at up to 300 mg/kg/day for various periods during gestation had no effect on fertility, gestation, or teratogenic anomalies; a dosage of 300 mg/kg on gestation days 15–19 was fetotoxic. By peroral intubation, carbaryl at 200 mg/kg/day was toxic to dams, but not teratogenic or fetotoxic; an intubated dosage of 100 mg/kg had no significant effects (Weil *et al.*, 1972, 1973).

Carbaryl administered to rabbits by gavage at 200 mg/kg/day on gestation days 6–18 was maternally toxic and increased the incidence of terata; these effects were not seen at 150 mg/kg/day (Murray *et al.*, 1979). In another study with rabbits, no maternal, fetotoxic, or teratogenic effects resulted from dosages of up to 200 mg/kg/day on gestation days 5–15 (Robens, 1969).

In a three-generation study in which Mongolian gerbils were fed carbaryl at 1000–10,000 ppm, fertility, litter size, viability, and survival were reduced even at the lowest dosage, but only reduced survival was clearly dose related. No gross or histological abnormalities were observed in the young at any dosage (Collins *et al.*, 1971). In hamsters, single doses of up to 250 mg/kg by gavage on day 7 or 8 were fetotoxic but not teratogenic (Robens, 1969).

Carbaryl fed to pregnant dogs throughout gestation at dosages of 3.125–50 mg/kg/day resulted in increased stillbirths, difficult labor, and decreased litter size and postnatal viability and growth. An apparent contraceptive effect was seen at the highest dosage. Teratogenesis was observed at dosages of 6.25 mg/kg/day or higher; several of the pups exhibited multiple defects that were difficult to categorize (Smalley *et al.*, 1968). The reproductive and teratogenic effects were not consistently dosage related, and statistical analysis of the results was not reported. In dogs fed carbaryl at 2–12.5 mg/kg/day throughout gestation and weaning, postnatal survival was decreased at all dosages; at 5 mg/kg/day or higher, other reproductive parameters were also affected and terata were observed (Imming *et al.*, 1969).

In a teratogenicity study, cardiac anomalies were observed in lambs produced by sheep given carbaryl in the diet at 250 ppm, but not at 100 ppm, during breeding and gestation; however, the data were not statistically analyzed (Panciera, 1967). In two studies, miniature swine were given carbaryl starting at various times from 20 days before breeding to 7 days after breeding and continuing throughout gestation, at dosages of 4–32 mg/

kg/day. Observations of reduced fertility and increased still-births were not consistently dose related and were not tested for statistical significance. Terata were observed in one litter at a dosage of 16 mg/kg/day (Earl *et al.*, 1973).

No terata were found among the young of rhesus monkeys receiving carbaryl by gavage at up to 20 mg/kg/day throughout gestation; abortions were slightly but not significantly increased at these dosages (Dougherty *et al.*, 1971). In another study employing the same route and dosages on gestation days 20–38, no terata or signs of maternal or fetal toxicity were noted (Coulston *et al.*, 1974).

Factors Influencing Toxicity Mice pretreated with the liver microsomal enzyme inducer phenobarbital were less susceptible to carbaryl poisoning, and those pretreated with the microsomal enzyme inhibitor SKF 525A were more susceptible (Neskovic *et al.*, 1978). Toxicity of carbaryl was increased by pretreatment with the drugs reserpine and chlordiazepoxide and decreased by chlorpromazine and meprobamate (Weiss and Orzel, 1967). Carbaryl caused a threefold increase in the toxicity of coadministered niridazole to rats (Samaam *et al.*, 1984). Coadministration of lindane and carbaryl to rats produced a slight increase in their lethal effect (Lewerenz *et al.*, 1980). Carbaryl-induced tremors in rats were significantly reduced by pretreatment with L-dopa and exacerbated by haloperidol; these results were interpreted to suggest central cholaminergic–dopaminergic involvement (Ray and Poddar, 1985a).

In mice, 14-day dietary exposure to carbaryl at 5000 ppm was reported to double the LD 50 in subsequent oral administration. This subchronic exposure also decreased *in vivo* hydrolysis of another carbamate insecticide, mexacarbate (Cress and Strother, 1974). Oxidation of carbaryl *in vitro* by rat hepatic microsomes was increased by pretreatment of the animals with chlordane and decreased by pretreatment with methylmercury hydroxide. Both compounds accelerated urinary excretion of carbaryl (Lucier *et al.*, 1972).

Carbaryl was more toxic to rats whose dietary protein was based entirely on casein than to those given ordinary laboratory feed; the LD 50 values were 575 and 744 mg/kg, respectively. In rats given low-protein diets (0 or 3%), the LD 50 values were reduced to 67 and 89 mg/kg, respectively; in rats whose protein intake was 30% of normal, the LD 50 was 506 mg/kg (Boyd and Boulanger, 1968; Boyd and Krijnen, 1969). In another study with rats, tissue levels of ^{14}C-labeled carbaryl 1 hr after oral administration were generally higher in rats fed a low-protein diet than in rats fed a normal diet, suggesting more rapid carbaryl uptake under conditions of protein deficiency or starvation (Tanaka *et al.*, 1980, 1981). These observations take on added significance in areas of emerging economic development; however, the relationship of the LD 50 values to lower values obtained more recently in other laboratories casts some doubt on this whole area of investigation.

Carpenter *et al.* (1961) found no potentiation or antagonism when carbaryl was coadministered to rats with organophosphate or other noncarbamate pesticides. Coadministration of malathion and carbaryl to rats altered pharmacokinetic parameters

for both pesticides and delayed the elimination of [^{14}C]carbaryl from gastrointestinal tissues (Lechner and Abdel-Rahman, 1986). Diphenyl, *o*-phenylphenol, piperonyl butoxide, and thiabendazole potentiated the effects of carbaryl when administered in equitoxic acute oral doses to mice (Isshiki *et al.*, 1983).

17.3.5.3 Toxicity to Humans

The 1973 FAO/WHO Joint Meeting on Pesticide Residues estimated a human ADI for carbaryl of 0–0.01 mg/kg body weight (FAO/WHO, 1974).

Experimental Exposures The pI 50 (negative log of the *in vitro* I50 value) for carbaryl and human brain acetylcholinesterase is 5.59 (Patocka and Bajgar, 1971), suggesting that although carbaryl is an inhibitor of this enzyme, it is not as potent as many other cholinergic carbamates and organophosphates. Acute ingestion of carbaryl at up to 2.0 mg/kg by two men per dose level had no observable or reported effects. In another study, five men took carbaryl at 0.06 mg/kg/day and six men took from 0.12 to 0.13 mg/kg/day for 6 weeks. The following tests were run: BSP, EEG, plasma and erythrocyte acetylcholinesterase, complete blood count, blood chemistry, and urine analysis. No abnormality attributable to carbaryl was found at the lower dose; the only effect at the higher dose was a slight, reversible decrease in the ability of the proximal convoluted tubules to reabsorb amino acids. In addition, daily oral exposure of volunteers to carbaryl at up to 0.12 mg/kg/day for 6 weeks had no effect on EEG recordings (Wills *et al.*, 1968).

A scientist exploring the possible value of carbaryl as an anthelmintic attempted to test its safety to humans by ingesting 250 mg (approximately 2.8 mg/kg). After 20 min, he suddenly experienced violent epigastric pain, and a little later he began to sweat profusely. Although a 1-mg dose of atropine produced little improvement, he was able to continue work. He gradually developed great lassitude and vomited twice. One hour after taking the carbaryl, and after a total atropine dose of 3 mg, he felt better; after one more hour, he was completely recovered (Hayes, 1982).

Another similar incident involved a greater dose and more severe and protracted symptoms. A scientist ingested, on an empty stomach, a suspension containing about 420 mg of carbaryl (5.45 mg/kg). (He had previously taken larger doses about an hour after a meal without any resulting illness.) No symptoms appeared for 80 min. After 85 min, he noticed a slight change in vision lasting for 15–20 min. After 90 min, he began to feel nauseated and lightheaded; 2 mg of atropine helped, but the symptoms returned. By 17 min after the onset of symptoms, he had taken 4.8 mg of atropine, despite which he began to sweat very profusely. Hyperperistalsis developed (with little pain). Nausea persisted for about 2 hr, but without vomiting or diarrhea. He experienced a profound sense of weakness and preferred to remain perfectly still, but had no difficulty in breathing. The sensorium remained completely clear, and he was able to answer questions readily and correctly. Symptoms were maximal about 2 hr after their onset, at which time the pulse rate was 64 per minute (decreased from the subject's normal resting rate of 70), and the respiratory rate was 18 per minute. During the entire course of poisoning, no miosis, excess lacrimation or salivation, or rales were observed. Definite improvement, including some increase in strength, appeared a little less than 3 hr after the onset of symptoms, and recovery was nearly complete 4 hr after onset (Hayes, 1982).

When [^{14}C]carbaryl was applied to the forearms of volunteers, radioactivity in the urine increased until 8–12 hr after application and then gradually declined; radioactivity was still much greater in samples collected 96–120 hr after application than in those collected during the first 4 hr of exposure. Because preliminary studies showed that only 7.4% of an iv dose of [^{14}C]carbaryl was excreted in the urine, a large correction factor was applied in interpreting the small excretion that followed dermal application; by this interpretation, about 74% of the carbaryl applied to the skin was absorbed (Feldmann and Maibach, 1974).

Following single 2-mg/kg doses of carbaryl to two volunteers, recovery in the urine was 26–28% within 4 days. Metabolites identified by the fluorometric method included 4-(methylcarbamoyloxy)-1-naphthyl glucuronide (4–6%), 1-naphthyl glucuronide (10–15%), and 1-naphthyl sulfate (6–8%), and there was qualitative evidence of 1-naphthyl-methylimidocarbonate-O-glucuronide. One or more unidentified neutral compounds also were present. A slightly higher proportion of the dose from the same samples (37.8%) was recovered using a colorimetric method sensitive to total 1-naphthol (Knaak *et al.*, 1968). Only 1-naphthyl glucuronide (25 ppm) and 1-naphthyl sulfate (5 ppm) were measured in the urine of men who packaged carbaryl (Knaak *et al.*, 1965). Of single oral doses of carbaryl to nine volunteers, 41.5–52.7% was excreted in the urine by 49 hr after administration (Myers, 1977).

Two workers experimentally exposed to carbaryl in the air at 50 mg/m^3 for 2 workdays showed no signs of intoxication; their urinary 1-naphthol levels were 36–90 mg/liter on the first day and 23–24 mg/liter on the second [National Institute for Occupational Health and Safety (NIOSH), 1976].

Therapeutic Use Formulations of carbaryl have been used successfully to control human lice (Sussman *et al.*, 1969).

Accidental and Intentional Overexposure A drunken 39-year-old man swallowed approximately 500 ml of an 80% solution of carbaryl (estimated dosage of 5700 mg/kg). When he was hospitalized 90 min later, he was confused but still able to answer questions. Gastric lavage was performed, and drugs to stimulate circulation were administered; however, the patient became worse; he complained of disturbance of vision and developed pulmonary edema. Atropine was given intravenously and intramuscularly at half-hour intervals, for a total dose of 6 mg. A slight amelioration occurred, but there was no sign of full atropinization. Three hours after ingestion, 250 mg of 2-PAM was administered. Thereafter, pulmonary edema progressed rapidly, and the patient died 6 hr after the ingestion. Concentrations of carbaryl in the man's blood, liver, kidney, and urine were 14, 29, 25, and

31 ppm, respectively (Faragó, 1969). Although it has been suggested that death in this case may have been related to the use of 2-PAM (Kuhr and Dorough, 1976), no conclusion can be drawn. To date, this suicide is the only death unambiguously attributed to carbaryl (Cranmer, 1986).

A 19-month-old infant developed miosis, salivation, and muscular incoordination despite gastric lavage within 30 min after ingestion of an unknown amount of carbaryl. A single 0.3-mg dose of atropine sulfate was effective, and recovery apparently was complete in 12 hr (Henson, cited by Best and Murray, 1962).

When first introduced into Australia in 1961 and used without any particular care, carbaryl was responsible for a number of cases of poisoning, but no deaths. Illness involved abdominal pain, vomiting, headache, and blurred vision. Recovery was rapid except in one man who swallowed some formulation while cleaning a vat line. The other overexposed men had become soaked with spray and had not laundered their overalls (New South Wales, 1965). In another episode, men applied 85% water-wettable carbaryl powder as a dust, thinking that it was a 2% dust. They complained of burning and irritation of the skin, but recovered in a few hours without any treatment except bathing. Their blood acetylcholinesterase levels were slightly depressed (Hayes, 1982).

One day after accidental exposure to carbaryl dust and vapor, seven workers who reported symptoms of nausea, dizziness, and headache had an average urinary 1-naphthol concentration of 14.2 mg/liter (with a range of 2–31 mg/liter). Seven other exposed employees were asymptomatic, but showed higher urinary 1-naphthol levels, averaging 22.4 mg/liter (with a range of 10–42 mg/liter) (NIOSH, 1976).

In other cases of carbaryl poisoning described by the World Health Organization (WHO, 1967), spontaneous recovery was complete within several hours of exposure.

The poisoning of 41 of 72 workers by a mixture of carbaryl and the more poisonous compound propaphos is discussed in Section 16.8.1.3.

Use Experience Most use experience with carbaryl has been very favorable. Korean farmers given patch tests for contact dermatitis showed no hypersensitivity to carbaryl (Lee *et al.*, 1981). In a 19-month study of manufacturing workers exposed to carbaryl dust levels of usually 0.75 mg/m^3, but ranging from 0.23 to 40 mg/m^3 (requiring the use of personal dust masks), 1-naphthol levels exceeded 10 ppm in 40% of the urine samples (the normal range of 1.5–4.0 ppm). However, blood acetylcholinesterase levels were only occasionally depressed (by less than 30%), and no signs or symptoms of anticholinesterase action were noted (Best and Murray, 1962). Assuming that the concentration of 1-naphthol was fairly constant throughout the day and assuming a urinary output of 1.5 liters, 18.5 ppm would indicate an absorbed carbaryl dosage of about 38.7 mg/person/day or about 0.55 mg/kg/day. This dosage is considerably less than dosages causing moderate poisoning and was acquired during an entire workday, permitting detoxication during the course of absorption. The estimated maximum exposure value of 0.55 mg/kg/day is less than 0.7 mg/kg/day, a level considered safe for occupational intake based on the threshold limit value of 5 mg/m^3 (NIOSH, 1976).

Eight sprayers and two supervisors applied a 5% carbaryl spray at a rate of 2 gm/m^2 inside houses in a Nigerian village for 6 hr. The only clinical effect was a pronounced skin rash in a sprayer whose back was splashed with the insecticide. The sprayers showed a 15% average inhibition of plasma acetylcholinesterase the day after spraying, and levels returned to normal within 5 days. Samples of plasma from 63 villagers showed an average 8% decrease in acetylcholinesterase activity. Excretion of 1-naphthol was unchanged in the sprayers but increased significantly in the villagers, from 30.5 ppm before spraying to 50.3 ppm after (Vandekar, 1965).

In a study of agricultural workers in the Soviet Union, 3- to 4-day exposure to carbaryl at about 2 mg/m^3 resulted in inhibition of cholinesterase by 11–24%. Exposure to an average concentration of 4 mg/m^3 inhibited acetylcholinesterase by 13–30%, and exposure to 0.7 mg/m^3 had no effect. No toxic signs were observed in any subjects (Yakim, 1967).

In another study, potential exposures of carbaryl formulators and applicators were calculated to be 74 and 59 mg/hr, respectively, by the dermal route and about 1 mg/hr by respiration. Among formulators, urinary concentrations of 1-naphthol ranged from 0.2 to 65 ppm, with a mean of 8.9 ppm. The rate of excretion varied from 0.004 to 3.4 mg/hr, with a mean of 0.5 mg/hr, equivalent to excretion of carbaryl at 0.7 mg/hr and corresponding to absorption of 5.6 mg of carbaryl during the 8-hr day. The urinary 1-naphthol concentration increased gradually during work, peaked during late afternoon and early evening, and returned to a lower level by the next morning. The highest exposure level was calculated to represent 0.4% of a toxic dose per hour (Comer *et al.*, 1975). Excretion of norepinephrine, total metanephrines, and 3-methoxy-4-hydroxymandelic acid was not increased in workers exposed to carbaryl and other insecticides, and their excretion of epinephrine was significantly lower than that of controls (Richardson *et al.*, 1975); the difference most likely depended on dosage.

Among two groups of workers spraying trees with formulated carbaryl, mean dermal exposures were 128 and 59 mg/hr, and mean respiratory exposure was 0.1 mg/hr. Calculated maximum hourly doses were 0.12 and 0.02% of a toxic dose, and cholinesterase activity was not inhibited in these workers (Leavitt *et al.*, 1982). Among 38 urban volunteers making 50 applications of various carbaryl formulations by various methods (including home use on yards and pets), the maximum dermal exposure was 2.86 mg/kg/hr, and the maximum air concentration of carbaryl was 0.28 µg/liter. The estimated maximum exposure was 0.08% of a toxic dose per hour. Changes in erythrocyte acetylcholinesterase activity ranged from a decrease of about 23% to an increase of over 23%; the mean effect was a decrease of 1.4% (Gold *et al.*, 1982). Worst-case estimated exposure of the general population to carbaryl via spraying of Maine forests for spruce budworm control was 0.194% of the FAO/WHO ADI (Shehata *et al.*, 1984).

In a study comparing 101 nonexposed men with 49 men currently or previously employed in carbaryl production, no relationship was found between the intensity or duration of exposure and either sperm count or the fathering of children, and sex hormone levels were normal in the exposed workers (Whorton *et al.*, 1979). In reexamining the sperm samples from this study and comparing them against a new control group of 34 nonexposed workers in the same plant, Wyrobek *et al.* (1981) reported morphological abnormalities in the sperm from the exposed workers, not related to estimated exposure levels. Another evaluation of these same sperm samples showed no differences in sperm count or morphology between the exposed and control groups (MacLeod, 1982). The qualitative and quantitative evaluation of sperm abnormalities does not appear to reveal any adverse effects of occupational exposure.

Atypical Cases of Various Origins Overexposure to carbaryl resulting from treatment of a home for flea infestation produced flu-like symptoms, including headache, malaise, epigastric discomfort, and muscle spasms, in a 75-year-old man. His wife and son showed milder symptoms and recovered in about 1 month, but the man's symptoms worsened, as treatment of the house continued for a 5-month period. It is not known why the man's wife and son were not similarly affected or whether the carbaryl exposure was in any way related to the persistent symptoms. The authors noted that the man was taking cimetidine, a inhibitor of oxidative drug metabolism, during much of the exposure period (Branch and Jacqz, 1986).

17.3.6 CARBOFURAN

17.3.6.1 Identity, Properties, and Uses

Chemical Name Carbofuran is 2,3-dihydro-2,2-dimethyl-7-benzofuranyl *N*-methylcarbamate. Its structure is shown in Table 17.1.

Synonyms The common name carbofuran (ANSI, BSI, ISO) is in general use. Trade names have included Brifur®, Crisfuran®, Cristofuran®, Curaterr®, Furadan®, Pillarfuran®, and Yaltox®. Code designations have included BAY 70143, D 1221, ENT 27164, FMC 10242, NIA 10242, and OMS 864. The CAS registry number is 1563-66-2.

Physical and Chemical Properties Carbofuran has the empirical formula $C_{12}H_{15}NO_3$ and a molecular weight of 221.26. The pure material is a white, odorless crystalline solid with a melting point of 153–154°C. The technical material is a tan crystalline solid with a melting point of 150–152°C. Carbofuran has a vapor pressure (mm Hg) of 2×10^{-5} at 33°C and 1.1×10^{-4} at 50°C. The solubility of carbofuran (w/w at 25°C) is 0.07% in water, 4% in benzene or ethanol, 9% in cyclohexanone, 14% in acetonitrile, 15% in acetone, 25% in dimethyl sulfoxide, 27% in dimethylformamide, and 30% in *N*-methyl-2-pyrrolidone. Its solubility is less than 1% in xylene, petroleum ether, and kerosene. Carbofuran is unstable in alkaline media and degrades at temperatures above 130°C.

History, Formulations, and Uses   Carbofuran was developed in the 1960s and introduced in 1967 as a systemic and contact broad-spectrum, long-residual insecticide and nematicide for use on a variety of crops. Carbofuran is available as granules, a flowable formulation, a wettable powder, and a seed treater formulation.

17.3.6.2 Toxicity to Laboratory Animals

Basic Findings   The acute toxicity of carbofuran is summarized in Tables 17.2 and 17.3. Signs of acute intoxication are characteristic of acetylcholinesterase inhibition. Ocular exposure to carbofuran has caused death in rabbits. The physical nature of carbofuran and most commercial formulations makes inhalation exposure unlikely; however, carbofuran is highly toxic as a dust or aerosol when the particles are in the respirable range. Carbofuran was not irritating to the skin or eyes of rabbits and did not cause a skin sensitization reaction in guinea pigs (FMC, 1986a). Ferguson *et al.* (1984) calculated an *in vivo* molar I 50 of 1.2×10^{-8} for erythrocyte acetylcholinesterase activity in rats exposed to carbofuran.

Subchronic dermal exposure of rabbits to carbofuran at up to 1000 mg/kg/day did not cause any signs of toxicity (including depression of acetylcholinesterase activity). Dogs given carbofuran in their diet at 500 ppm for 1 year showed body weight losses (usually associated with a significant drop in food retention), emesis and loose stools, reduced brain and heart weights, testicular degeneration, inflammatory changes in the lungs, and depression of plasma acetylcholinesterase activity, hematocrit, hemoglobin, and erythrocyte count, with concurrent changes in electrolyte values. Depressed plasma acetylcholinesterase activity also was observed at a dietary level of 20 ppm; no treatment-related effects were seen at 10 ppm (FMC, 1986a).

Exposure of rats to carbofuran in the diet at 100 ppm for 2 years caused body weight depression and moderate reductions in plasma, erythrocyte, and brain acetylcholinesterase activity. In a similar study with mice, carbofuran in the diet at 500 ppm caused intermittent decreases in body weight; brain acetylcholinesterase activity was depressed at dietary levels of 125 ppm or higher. Carbofuran at 20 ppm in the diet had no effect in either rats or mice (FMC, 1986a). No-effect levels were considered to be 1.0 mg/kg/day for rats and 2.5 mg/kg/day for mice (FAO/WHO, 1981).

Absorption, Distribution, Metabolism, and Excretion   In dermal absorption studies with mice, penetration of ring-labeled [^{14}C]carbofuran in acetone was 72% in 15 min. By 8 hr after application, 73% of the dose was found in excretory products and 12% in the carcass; the stomach and intestines each accounted for about 3%, the liver for 1.0%, and the blood for 0.8% (Shah *et al.*, 1981).

In fasted mice, about 67% of an intubated ^{14}C-labeled dose of carbofuran was absorbed within 60 min; the $t_{1/2}$ for absorption was 10 min. Peak levels appeared in the blood within 35–40 min, and tissue levels of radioactivity indicated rapid distribution (Ahdaya *et al.*, 1981). A study in which ring-labeled carbofuran was intubated into fasted mice with stomachs ligated at the pylorus indicated significant stomach absorption (about 28% of total gastrointestinal absorption). Recovery of 2.6% of the dose from the intestine after 60 min indicated intestinal or liver secretion of carbofuran (Ahdaya and Guthrie, 1982). Following oral administration of radiolabeled carbofuran to rats, plasma levels peaked in less than 7 min, and radioactivity was evenly distributed among the tissues (Ferguson *et al.*, 1984). In other studies with rats and cows, radiolabel was detected in the blood very quickly, and blood levels peaked within 2 hr after administration (Dorough, 1968; Ivie and Dorough, 1968).

Inhalation exposure of rats to a radiolabeled aerosol of carbofuran resulted in more rapid absorption and greater acetylcholinesterase inhibition per unit dose than did oral exposure; the greater toxicity via inhalation was attributed to the prolonged availability of carbofuran not initially subject to a single 100% pass through the liver such as occurs after oral exposure (Ferguson *et al.*, 1982).

Metabolism of carbofuran is similar in the rat, mouse, and cow. Carbofuran is almost completely metabolized via oxidation at ring carbon number 3 (3-hydroxy carbofuran and 3-keto carbofuran) and hydrolytic cleavage of the ester linkage to yield the 7-hydroxy metabolites (3-hydroxy-7-phenol, 3-keto-7-phenol, and 7-phenol). A majority of these metabolites plus minor amounts of other related metabolites are excreted as glucuronide or sulfate conjugates. The *in vivo* rate of hydrolysis for carbofuran in rats calculated by Ferguson *et al.* (1984) was comparable to previously established values for mono-methylcarbamates. In studies with carbonyl-labeled [^{14}C]carbofuran, degradation of the carbonyl group resulted in the appearance of radiolabel in expired CO_2 and incorporation of $^{14}CO_2$ into normal body constituents. In the milk of a lactating cow, the major hydrolytic products were conjugated 3-keto-7-phenol and 3-hydroxy carbofuran; only 0.001% of the parent compound was found (Dorough, 1968; Ivie and Dorough, 1968; Metcalf *et al.*, 1968; Marshall and Dorough, 1979).

Within 24 hr after oral administration to rats, about 72% of a dose of ring-labeled carbofuran was excreted in the urine and about 2% in the feces. By 12 hr after oral administration of 0.4 mg/kg carbonyl-labeled carbofuran to rats, 40% of the radiolabel appeared in the expired CO_2 and 30% in the urine (Dorough, 1968). Of a lower oral dose (0.05 mg/kg), 41–47% appeared in expired $^{14}CO_2$ within 8 hr, although only 15% was found in the urine. By 8 hr after inhalation exposure of rats to a carbonyl-labeled carbofuran aerosol, 31–38% of the dose appeared in the expired CO_2, 9–12% in the urine, and 2–5% in the feces (Ferguson *et al.*, 1982). The ultimate fate of carbofuran in rats was independent of exposure route (intravenous vs. oral) (Krieger *et al.*, 1984).

Within 48 hr after administration of a ring-labeled dose of carbofuran, rats with cannulated bile ducts excreted 28.5% in the bile, 65.4% in the urine, and 0.4% in the feces. The radioactive material in the bile consisted of glucuronide conjugates; 60% was 3-hydroxy carbofuran. In the urine, 70% of the radioactivity was sulfate and glucuronide conjugates of hydrolytic products of carbofuran. The authors concluded that in the intact animal, the majority of biliary metabolites were reabsorbed from the intestine (enterohepatic circulation), further metabolized, and ultimately eliminated in the urine (Marshall and Dorough, 1979).

Within 60 min after intubation with ring-labeled carbofuran, fasted mice eliminated 24% of the radiolabel in the urine and 6% in the expired CO_2 (Ahdaya et al., 1981). Of an N-methyl-^{14}C-labeled dose to mice, less than 2% was expired as $^{14}CO_2$ (Metcalf et al., 1968).

After a cow was given a single oral dose of ring-labeled carbofuran, 94% of the dose appeared in the urine within 72 hr; 0.2% was found in the milk, and 0.7% in the feces. For carbonyl-labeled carbofuran, 72-hr recovery in the urine was 21%; this difference represented an estimated 73% hydrolysis of administered carbofuran, most of which occurred within 4 hr of administration (Ivie and Dorough, 1968).

Biochemical Effects   In addition to decreasing brain acetylcholinesterase activity, acute oral administration of carbofuran to rats at 10 mg/kg increased serum levels of sugar, glutamic-oxaloacetic transaminase, and glutamic-pyruvic transaminase, but did not affect serum proteins. Subchronic exposure at lower dosages did not influence these parameters (Jayapragasam et al., 1981).

Rotaru et al. (1981) reported a transient increase in serum lactate dehydrogenase activity in rats given carbofuran subchronically in their diet at 10 or 25 ppm; no significant histological changes in the liver were noted. Subchronic oral administration of carbofuran to rats at 5% of the LD 50, in addition to depressing acetylcholinesterase activity, resulted in increased brain serotonin metabolism and brain levels of dopamine, GABA, and glutathione; brain levels of noradrenaline, adrenaline, 3,4-dihydroxyphenylacetic acid, and glutamic acid were decreased (Tyburczyk, 1981). Following multiple 0.25-mg/kg intraperitoneal doses of carbofuran to mice, brain levels of GABA, epinephrine, norepinephrine, dopamine, and 5-hydroxytryptamine were increased, along with acetylcholine (Gupta et al., 1984). Changes in liver, kidney, brain, and serum lipid levels were reported in mice given multiple intraperitoneal doses of carbofuran at 0.125–0.5 mg/kg for 6 weeks (Gupta et al., 1986).

Effects on Organs and Tissues   Results of mutagenicity testing with carbofuran are summarized in Section 17.2.3.2. Carbofuran was not carcinogenic in chronic studies with mice (FMC, 1986a).

In an in vitro screening assay, carbofuran partially suppressed the generation of a T cell-mediated cytolytic response in mouse splenocytes, whether or not the compound was preincubated with a rat liver mitochondrial preparation (Rodgers et al., 1986).

Effects on Reproduction   Carbofuran stimulated the metabolism of [^{3}H]testosterone by rat and mouse prostate glands during short periods of incubation in vitro (Schein et al., 1976). Testicular degeneration, noted in a chronic toxicity study with dogs,

was not seen in similar studies with rats and mice, and no adverse effects were observed in reproduction studies (FMC, 1986a).

Carbofuran at dietary levels of up to 100 ppm did not cause reproductive toxicity in rats in a three-generation study. Reduced parental food consumption and body weights, with correspondingly reduced pup survival and body weights, were seen at a dose level of 100 ppm, but not at 20 ppm. Carbofuran at up to 50 ppm in the diet of male and female dogs did not affect their health or reproductive behavior and did not cause abnormalities in the pups (McCarthy et al., 1971; FMC, 1986a).

Carbofuran administered by gavage to pregnant rats on day 18 of gestation at 0.05 mg/kg produced a slight transient inhibition of blood acetylcholinesterase activity. Acetylcholinesterase depression was seen also in fetal livers at a dose of 0.25 mg/kg and in fetal brains at 2.50 mg/kg (Cambon et al., 1979). Carbofuran affected the distribution of acetylcholinesterase isoenzymes differently in fetuses than in dams (Cambon et al., 1980). This was most likely related to differing pharmacokinetics of carbofuran between fetuses and dams, rather than selectivity or sensitivity of the fetus.

Exposure of rats to carbofuran at up to 1.2 mg/kg/day by gavage on days 6–15 of gestation had no significant effects on dams or fetuses. Carbofuran at 60 ppm or more in the diet of rats on days 6–19 of gestation had no effect on pups other than reduced body weight related to maternal toxicity; no maternal toxicity was observed at 20 ppm. Other studies in which rats and mice received carbofuran by gavage daily during gestation revealed no teratogenic effects at maternally nonlethal doses (Courtney et al., 1985). In rabbits, carbofuran at up to 2.0 mg/kg/day (a maternally toxic dosage) on days 6–18 of gestation was not teratogenic (FMC, 1986a).

Offspring of mice receiving carbofuran in the diet daily throughout gestation showed changes in serum immunoglobin concentrations that were transient or not dosage related (Barnett et al., 1980). On review, previously reported findings of liver changes in the year-old offspring of mice given carbofuran at 0.05 of 0.10 mg/kg/day throughout gestation (Hoberman, 1978) were considered to have resulted from misinterpretation of normal histologic and cytologic variability (Willigan, 1980).

Factors Influencing Toxicity   No potentiation of toxicity was observed in rats when carbofuran was coadministered with other acetylcholinesterase inhibitors, including 13 organophosphates and 1 carbamate (FAO/WHO, 1977). In vitro hepatic microsomal oxidation of carbofuran was increased by pretreatment of rats with chlordane and decreased by pretreatment with methylmercury hydroxide. Both compounds accelerated urinary excretion of carbofuran, but did not affect cumulative excretion over 3 days (Lucier et al., 1972).

17.3.6.3 Toxicity to Humans

The 1980 FAO/WHO Joint Meeting on Pesticide Residues estimated a human ADI for carbofuran of 0–0.01 mg/kg body weight (FAO/WHO, 1981).

Experimental Exposures   *In vitro* human protein-binding studies indicated that of 73.6% bound carbofuran, 1.4 and 1.8% were partitioned in low-density and high-density lipoprotein, respectively, and 96.8% was distributed in albumin. In this study, various insecticide lipoprotein affinities were inversely related to water solubility (Maliwal and Guthrie, 1981). The major metabolite in the urine of human subjects following oral or dermal administration of carbofuran was the 7-phenol (FMC, 1986a).

Accidental and Intentional Overexposure   Case reports of occupational exposure given as examples by Tobin (1970) illustrate the fairly rapid onset of symptoms, mild illness, and corresponding rapid recovery (with or without atropine treatment) resulting from moderate carbofuran intoxication. In experiences with manufacturing, formulation, and application personnel, early symptoms of carbofuran poisoning included headache, lightheadedness, weakness, and nausea. Later signs and symptoms were miosis (sometimes preceded by a transient dilation), blurred vision, abdominal cramps, excessive salivation and perspiration, diarrhea, and vomiting. Symptomatology has not progressed beyond this point in use experience. The interval between exposure and onset of signs and symptoms was related to the size of the dose and varied from a few minutes to about an hour; duration of symptoms was likewise related to dosage. In mild cases, spontaneous recovery took from 1 to 4 hr (FMC, 1986a).

The morning following aerial misapplication of a flowable formulation of carbofuran to a corn field, approximately 150 high-school-age workers entered the treated field to detassel corn. Symptoms of nausea and dizziness began to appear, and 74 workers reported to the hospital, 45 of whom received medical attention; 29 were admitted, and 1 remained overnight. Treatment included atropine sulfate [U.S. Environmental Protection Agency (US EPA), 1978]. In a case from Bulgaria reported by Izmirova *et al.* (1981), a woman survived intoxication with 60 mg of carbofuran. Following inhibition to between 50 and 80% of normal, acetylcholinesterase activity recovered completely within 72 hr, by which time all symptoms had disappeared.

17.3.7 CARBOSULFAN

17.3.7.1 Identity, Properties, and Uses

Chemical Name   Carbosulfan is 2,3-dihydro-2,2-dimethyl-7-benzofuranyl[(dibutylamino)thio]   *N*-methylcarbamate. Its structure is shown in Fig. 17.1.

Synonyms   The common name carbosulfan (ANSI, BSI, ISO) is in general use. Trade names are Advantage® and Marshal®, a code designation is FMC 35001, and the CAS registry number is 55285-14-8.

Physical and Chemical Properties   Carbosulfan has the empirical formula $C_{20}H_{32}N_2O_3S$ and a molecular weight of 380.5.

The unstabilized technical material is a brown, viscous liquid. Carbosulfan has a vapor pressure of 0.31×10^{-6} mm Hg at 25°C. Its solubility in water is 0.3 ppm, but it is completely miscible in xylene, hexane, chloroform, methylene chloride, methanol, acetone, and other organic solvents. Technical carbosulfan is stable for 1 year at 22°C and for 30 months at 50°C, but decomposes at 80°C under 0.1 mm Hg.

History, Formulations, and Uses   Carbosulfan was first synthesized in the mid-1970s, developed in the late 1970s, and introduced internationally in the 1980s for control of soil and foliar insects on a variety of major vegetable, field, and orchard crops; U.S. registration is pending. Formulations are produced from a stabilized technical material containing 90% a.i. Carbosulfan is available in emulsifiable concentrates, granular formulations, wettable powders, and a dust.

17.3.7.2 Toxicity to Laboratory Animals

Basic Findings   The acute toxicity of carbosulfan is summarized in Tables 17.2–17.4. Signs of acute intoxication are typical of acetylcholinesterase inhibition. Carbosulfan was minimally irritating to the eyes of rabbits, producing conjunctivitis that subsided within 72 hr. Applied to the skin of rabbits, it produced slight erythema and edema lasting no longer than 6 days. Carbosulfan was determined to be a dermal sensitizer in the guinea pig patch test (FMC, 1986b).

Inhibition of erythrocyte acetylcholinesterase activity was maximal 1 min after iv administration of carbosulfan to rats; at doses of 0.086, 0.25, and 0.69 mg/kg, maximum inhibition was 62, 77, and 85%, respectively, and recovery occurred within 4 hr. After oral administration at 0.69 mg/kg, maximum erythrocyte acetylcholinesterase inhibition was 37% at 45 min, and recovery occurred within 5 hr. Acetylcholinesterase inhibition was better correlated with plasma levels of the metabolite carbofuran than with plasma levels of carbosulfan. Signs of toxicity were generally observed when acetylcholinesterase activity was inhibited by more than 35%, and tremors occurred at inhibition by more than 70% (Renzi and Kreiger, 1986).

In dogs given carbosulfan in their diet at 1000 ppm for 6 months, body weight gain and spleen weights were decreased and relative adrenal weights were increased. Changes in hematological and biochemical parameters (including acetylcholinesterase activity) and decreased relative spleen weight were seen at dosages of 500 ppm or higher. No treatment-related histopathological changes were observed, and survival was not affected. A dietary no-effect level for dogs was 50 ppm (FAO/WHO, 1985; FMC, 1986b).

Exposure of rats to carbosulfan at dietary levels of 500 ppm or higher for 2 years caused depression of body weight, food consumption, and acetylcholinesterase activity in the erythrocytes, plasma, and brain; iris atrophy was noted, but there was no loss of sight. A dosage of 2500 ppm also produced cholinergic symptoms, retinal degeneration, and changes in biochemical and hematological parameters (including elevated leukocyte counts). No treatment-related histopathological changes or reduction in survival were seen. A dietary no-effect level for rats was 20 ppm. In a similar study with mice, carbosulfan at 2500 ppm in the diet resulted in reduced body weight, increased relative brain weight, and slight hematological changes, but did not affect survival. Erythrocyte, plasma, and brain acetylcholinesterase activities and spleen weight were depressed at dosages of 500 ppm or higher, and sporadic decreases in body weight were observed at 500 and 20 ppm. A dietary no-effect level for mice was 10 ppm (DeProspo *et al.*, 1985; FAO/WHO, 1985; FMC, 1986b).

Absorption, Distribution, Metabolism, and Excretion Maximum plasma radioactivity was observed 4 min after iv administration and 30–240 min after oral administration of carbonyl-^{14}C-labeled carbosulfan to rats (Renzi and Krieger, 1986). Blood analysis of a female rat given a single oral dose of ring-labeled [^{14}C]carbosulfan revealed unchanged parent compound for 3 hr after administration. Approximately 72% of the radioactivity detected was attributed to parent compound (Marsden *et al.*, 1982). In the stomach contents of rats given carbonyl-labeled carbosulfan orally, approximately 50% of the radioactivity recovered 80 min after administration was parent compound (Umetsu and Fukuto, 1982).

In rats administered ring-, carbonyl-, and dibutylamine-(DBA-)labeled [^{14}C]carbosulfan in corn oil, tissue levels of radioactivity were low, varying with labeling position. Wholebody autoradiography and physiologic disposition studies with ring- and DBA-labeled carbosulfan demonstrated that absorption and distribution occurred within 30 min of oral administration. DBA-labeled carbosulfan was distributed more widely, reached higher tissue concentrations, and persisted longer than ring-labeled compound. Tissue concentrations of both labels peaked at 6 hr, and levels were highest in the blood, liver, kidneys, lungs, heart, and spleen (Marsden *et al.*, 1982; FAO/WHO, 1985; FMC, 1986b).

In studies on its metabolic fate in mammals, carbosulfan was rapidly cleaved at the N—S bond to yield carbofuran and dibutylamine. Carbofuran was either quickly transformed by oxidation at the benzylic carbon of the benzofuran ring or hydrolyzed at the carbamate linkage (see Section 17.2.1.2). Significant urinary metabolites were dibutylamine, 3-hydroxy carbofuran, and 3-keto-7-phenol, and minor products included carbofuran, *N*-hydroxymethyl carbofuran, *N*-desmethyl carbofuran, 3-keto-*N*-hydroxymethyl carbofuran, 3-keto-*N*-desmethyl carbofuran, and 3-hydroxy-*N*-desmethyl carbofuran. Oxidation at the sulfur atom of carbosulfan also yielded minor amounts of 3-keto carbosulfan, carbosulfan sulfone, 3-hydroxy carbosulfan, and 3-keto carbosulfan sulfone in the urine. The majority of the metabolites related to carbofuran were conjugated, but dibutylamine was excreted intact. Fecal metabolites were nonconjugated; carbosulfan, carbosulfan sulfone, carbofuran, and 3-hydroxy carbofuran were found in significant quantities. Other minor metabolic products included bis-carbosulfan disulfide, 3-keto carbosulfan, 3-hydroxy carbosulfan, 3-keto carbosulfan sulfone, 3-keto carbofuran, 3-hydroxy-*N*-hydroxymethyl carbofuran, 3-hydroxy-7-phenol, 3-keto-7-phenol, 7-phenol, and dibutylamine (Marsden *et al.*, 1982; FMC, 1986b).

Rats given [^{14}C]carbosulfan excreted 65–80% of the dose in respired air, urine, and feces within 24 hr; elimination was nearly quantitative after 4 days. In 96 hr, urinary excretion was about 90% for ring-labeled, 53% for DBA-labeled, and 35% for carbonyl-labeled carbosulfan. Of the carbonyl-labeled material, 38% was eliminated via expired CO_2; fecal elimination was about 17% for carbonyl-labeled and 28% for DBA-labeled material (Marsden *et al.*, 1982; FAO/WHO, 1985b; FMC, 1986b).

Goats given two daily oral doses of ring-labeled carbosulfan for 7 days eliminated 80% of the dose in the urine, 2–3% in the feces, about 2% as respired $^{14}CO_2$, and less than 1% in the milk. By 12 hr after the last administration, maximum tissue levels (as carbosulfan equivalents) were 0.05 ppm in animals dosed with 4.09 mg/day and 0.1 ppm at 10.9 mg/day. In another study, goats given two daily oral doses of DBA-labeled carbosulfan at 1061 mg/kg/day for 10 days eliminated 79% of the dose in the urine and 1–3% in the feces, milk, and expired gases. Maximum tissue residues were 0.61 ppm (FMC, 1986b).

Effects on Organs and Tissues Results of mutagenicity testing with carbosulfan are summarized in Section 17.2.3.2. Carbosulfan was not carcinogenic at dietary levels of up to 2500 ppm in 2-year studies with mice and rats (DeProspo *et al.*, 1985; FMC, 1986b).

Effects on Reproduction In a three-generation reproduction study with rats, carbosulfan at 250 ppm in the diet resulted in decreased adult and pup body weights, pup weight gains, and neonatal survival. Carbosulfan at levels up to 250 ppm had no effect on reproductive parameters and no histopathologic effects. Carbosulfan given to rats orally on days 6–19 of gestation at 20 mg/kg/day caused dose-related maternal toxicity, with decreased fetal body weight and increased incidence of developmental variations. Maternal and fetal body weight reductions were also observed at 10 mg/kg/day. In rabbits, carbosulfan given orally on days 6–28 of gestation at 2–10 mg/kg/day had fetotoxic effects, and the highest dosage reduced maternal weight gain. Carbosulfan was not teratogenic in either rats or rabbits (FAO/WHO, 1985; FMC, 1986b).

17.3.7.3 Toxicity to Humans

Use Experience In experiences with technical product manufacturing, preparation of formulations, and application of products containing carbosulfan as the active ingredient, no incidences of overexposure have been reported (FMC, 1986b).

17.3.8 DIOXACARB

17.3.8.1 Identity, Properties, and Uses

Chemical Name Dioxacarb is 2-(1,3-dioxolan-2-yl)phenyl *N*-methylcarbamate. Its structure is shown in Table 17.1.

Synonyms The common name dioxacarb (ANSI, BSI, ISO, JMAF) is in general use. Trade names include Elecron®, Elocron®, Famid®, Flocron®, Gamid®, and Rovlinka®. Code designations include C 8353, I 1519, and OMS 1102. The CAS registry number is 6988-21-2.

Physical and Chemical Properties Dioxacarb has the empirical formula $C_{11}H_{13}NO_4$ and a molecular weight of 223.23. It forms white crystals with a slight odor. Dioxacarb has a melting point of 114–115°C and a vapor pressure of 3×10^{-7} mm Hg at 20°C. Its solubility at 20°C is 180 ppm in hexane, 0.6% in water, 0.9% in xylene, 8% in ethanol, 23.5% in cyclohexane, 28% in acetone, 34.5% in dichloromethane, and 55% in dimethylformamide. At 20°C, dioxacarb has a half-life of 40 min at pH 3, 3 days at pH 5, 60 days at pH 7, 20 hr at pH 9, and 2 hr at pH 10.

History, Formulations, and Uses Introduced in 1968, dioxacarb is a contact and stomach insecticide effective against a wide range of pests, including leafhoppers and planthoppers in rice, aphids, various beetles, cockroaches, and other household and industrial pests. Formulations include a wettable powder for agricultural use and wettable powders, a residual aerosol, and a bait concentrate for household hygiene applications.

17.3.8.2 Toxicity to Laboratory Animals

Except as otherwise indicated, toxicological information is proprietary data from Ciba-Geigy Limited (1986).

Basic Findings The acute toxicity of dioxacarb is summarized in Tables 17.2–17.4. Signs of acute intoxication are typical of acetylcholinesterase inhibition. Animals surviving LD 50 determinations recovered within 2–8 days. In rabbits, dioxacarb did not irritate the eyes and was slightly irritating to the skin. It did not cause a skin sensitization reaction in guinea pigs.

Dermal exposure of rabbits to dioxacarb at 1000 mg/kg/day for 21 days caused weight loss and acetylcholinesterase depression in the plasma (up to 63%) and erythrocytes (up to 29%). Blood acetylcholinesterase activity had recovered by sacrifice at 14 days after the last treatment, but slight brain acetylcholinesterase depression (up to 16%) was seen in some animals. No pathologic lesions were observed. Exposure at 100 mg/kg/day for 21 days had no observable effect.

Nose-only exposure of rats to an aerosol containing dioxacarb at 98 mg/m³ 6 hr daily for 21 days produced mild cholinergic signs, from which the animals recovered within 1 hr after the end of each exposure. The death of one female during the ninth exposure was not explained. After the last exposure period, acetylcholinesterase activity was transiently inhibited (25–38%) in females. Exposure had no effects on body weight or histopathology.

Rats given dioxacarb by gavage at 40 mg/kg/day (males) or 30 mg/kg/day (females) for 3 months initially showed acute cholinergic signs within 5 min of each administration, recovering completely within 2 hr. Cholinergic signs (which included

mydriasis, atypical for acetylcholinesterase inhibition) decreased in severity and duration over the course of the study and disappeared after 2 months. At 20 mg/kg/day, cholinergic signs were initially less severe, disappearing after week 5; no cholinergic signs were seen at 10 mg/kg/day. The highest dosages resulted in mortality in both sexes and decreased body weight in males. No hematological or urinary effects or pathologic lesions were observed at any dosage, and acetylcholinesterase activity was not depressed in blood taken 3 hr after dioxacarb administration. A no-effect level in this study was 10 mg/kg/day.

In a 3-month study, dogs were orally administered dioxacarb at 2, 5, and 20 mg/kg/day. The high dosage caused vomiting, tremors, and 67% mortality. Cholinergic signs were less severe at 5 mg/kg/day and absent at 2 mg/kg/day; no mortality occurred at these dosages. Acetylcholinesterase activity was inhibited at 1 hr postdosing; at dosages of 20, 5, and 2 mg/kg/week, the respective mean decreases were 50, 30, and 20% in the plasma and 40, 25, and 15% in the erythrocytes. At all dosages, acetylcholinesterase activity completely recovered over the course of the week between treatments. No pathologic lesions were attributable to dioxacarb at any dosage. At sacrifice, an apparent dose-related depression of brain acetylcholinesterase activity was not statistically significant. As the only effect of dioxacarb at 2 mg/kg was transient acetylcholinesterase depression with no cholinergic signs, this was considered a level causing no adverse effect.

Absorption, Distribution, Metabolism, and Excretion In rats receiving 10 daily 1 mg/kg doses of [^{14}C]dioxacarb, tissue radioactivity stabilized on the second day at the following approximate levels (ppm dioxacarb equivalents): blood, 0.3; liver, 0.7; kidney, 1.0; fat, 0.3; muscle, 0.2; and brain, 0.1. Residues in all tissues rapidly declined after dosing stopped. In rats given a single oral dose of ^{14}C-labeled dioxacarb (5 mg/kg), urinary and fecal metabolites each accounting for about 4–12% of the dose were tentatively identified as salicylic acid, salicyluric acid, 2,5-dihydroxybenzoic acid, and 2,3-dihydroxybenzoic acid. Traces of 3,4-dihydro-4-hydroxy-3-methyl-1,3-benzoxazine-2-(2H)-one also were detected in the urine. About 5% of the dioxacarb was excreted unchanged in the feces. The dose was almost completely eliminated in 24 hr, with 75% appearing in the urine and 13% in the feces. At sacrifice 9 days after dosing, residues were not detectable in the brain, fat, or muscle and were found at 2 ppm or less in the blood, liver, or kidneys.

Effects on Organs and Tissues Results of mutagenicity testing with dioxacarb are summarized in Section 17.2.3.2.

Effects on Reproduction In rats receiving dioxacarb by gavage on days 6–15 of pregnancy, a dosage of 20 mg/kg/day decreased food consumption and caused tremors in some animals during the first 3 days of treatment. Among the progeny, incidence of incompletely ossified sternebrae was slightly increased, indicating slight, nonspecific growth retardation. At a dosage of 3 mg/kg/day, maternal food consumption was increased, as were fetus weights and rates of ossification in the phalangeal nuclei and the calcanei; this finding was attributed to accelerated development due to the dams' increased food consumption and was not regarded as adverse. A no-effect level was considered to be 10 mg/kg/day. In rabbits receiving dioxacarb by gavage on days 6–18 of pregnancy, the only effects at 15 mg/kg/day were a temporary reduction in food consumption and an increase in fetal resorptions, a result considered equivocal. No effects were seen at dosages of 10 mg/kg/day or less.

17.3.8.3 Toxicity to Humans

Accidental Overexposure Apparently the only report of human injury from dioxacarb involved a female factory worker who splashed a 3% formulation into one eye and developed unilateral miosis. She was treated with atropine (1 mg), and the miosis receded in 3 hr. No illness resulted, and all systemic findings were normal (Kozler, 1975).

Use Experience Dioxacarb has never been associated with toxic reactions in applicators, even in applications resulting in skin exposure (Ciba-Geigy Limited, 1986).

17.3.9 FORMETANATE HCl

17.3.9.1 Identity, Properties, and Uses

Chemical Name Formetanate is 3-dimethylaminomethylene-aminophenyl *N*-methylcarbamate. Its structure is shown in Table 17.1.

Synonyms The common name formetanate (ANSI, BSI, ISO) is in general use. Trade names for formulations of the hydrochloride salt include Carzol® and Dicarzol®, and code designations include EP-332, FMT.HCl, SN 36056.HCl, and ZK 10970.HCl. The CAS registry numbers are 23422-53-9 HCl for the hydrochloride salt and 22259-30-9 for formetanate base.

Physical and Chemical Properties Formetanate hydrochloride has the empirical formula $C_{11}H_{16}ClN_3O_2$ and a molecular weight of 257.8. It is a colorless, odorless crystalline powder with a melting point of 200–202°C and a vapor pressure of 3.6×10^{-3} mm Hg at 25°C. Its solubility at room temperature (grams per liter) is 0.015 in ethyl acetate, 0.29 in dichloromethane, less than 1 in acetone, chloroform, or hexane, approximately 250 in methanol, and greater than 500 in water. Formetanate HCl is stable under normal storage conditions. At 22°C, it has a half-life of 1500 hr at pH 5, 23 hr at pH 7, and 2 hr at pH 9.

History, Formulations, and Uses Introduced in 1968, formetanate HCl is an acaricide and insecticide effective against spider mites, rust mites, thrips, lygus and stink bugs, and other hemipterans on a wide range of fruits and vegetables. It is available in water-soluble powder formulations.

17.3.9.2 Toxicity to Laboratory Animals

Except as otherwise indicated, toxicological information is proprietary data from Schering (1987).

Basic Findings The acute toxicity of formetanate HCl is summarized in Tables 17.2–17.4. Signs of acute intoxication are typical of acetylcholinesterase inhibition. Formetanate HCl did not irritate the skin of rabbits, but caused moderate reversible eye irritation.

Acute oral administration of formetanate HCl to rats and dogs inhibited whole-blood, plasma, erythrocyte, and brain acetylcholinesterase at doses of 1.5–2 mg/kg or higher. Inhibition was maximal from 30 min to 2 hr after administration, and recovery was complete in 6–24 hr. In a 90-day dietary study with rats, a no-effect level for acetylcholinesterase inhibition was 100 ppm.

Exposure of a cow to formetanate HCl at dietary concentrations increasing from 37.5 to 300 ppm over a 5-week period resulted in severe loss of body weight, but no other adverse effects other than weakening of rumen contractions at a dosage of 300 ppm. A no-effect level for 1-year dietary exposure of dogs to formetanate HCl was 10 ppm. Chronic dietary studies now in progress with rats and mice are currently yielding no-effect levels of 50 ppm.

Absorption, Distribution, Metabolism, and Excretion At 72 hr after acute oral administration of formetanate HCl to rats, the highest tissue residue level was 0.178 ppm in the liver (Sen Gupta and Knowles, 1970). At the end of a 10-day oral exposure period, tissue residue levels in goats did not exceed 0.1 ppm except in the liver (0.45 ppm) and kidneys (0.26 ppm). After a 30-day exposure of cows to formetanate HCl at dietary dosages of 35–80 ppm, residues were detected at less than 1 ppm in the liver and kidney but were not found in muscle or fat. No tissue residues were found after a 21-day posttreatment interval.

In rats, formetanate HCl was metabolized to *m*-formaminophenyl *N*-methylcarbamate, *m*-formaminophenol, *m*-aminophenol, *m*-acetamidophenol, and glucuronide and ethereal sulfate conjugates of *m*-acetamidophenol (Sen Gupta and Knowles, 1970). The metabolic pathway was identical in rat liver preparations *in vitro* (Ahmad and Knowles, 1970, 1971) and similar in lactating goats (Schering, 1987).

Of a single dose of formetanate HCl to rats, 75% was excreted in the urine during the first 12 hr, with peak concentrations observed at 6 hr. Within 24 hr after administration, 80% of the dose was eliminated in the urine and 6% in the feces (Sen Gupta and Knowles, 1970). When ^{14}C-labeled formetanate HCl was orally administered to lactating goats at 1.4 mg/kg/day for 10 days, 80–90% of the dose was excreted in the urine within 24 hr of the last administration, and fecal excretion ranged from 1.3 to 6.6%. Two days after exposure began, radiolabel in the milk (as formetanate HCl) plateaued at 0.46 ppm. When cows were given formetanate HCl for 30 days, residues (less than 1 ppm) were detected in the milk of animals at a dietary dosage of 80 ppm, but not at dosages of up to 35 ppm. At the highest dosage, no residues were detected in milk 7 days after exposure ended.

Biochemical Effects   Formetanate HCl inhibited rat brain monoamine oxidase *in vitro*. Inhibition ranged from 22% with β-phenylethylamine as a substrate to 54% with tryptamine (Kadir and Knowles, 1981).

Effects on Organs and Tissues   Results of mutagenicity testing with formetanate HCl are summarized in Section 17.2.3.2. In a 2-year study with rats, formetanate HCl was not carcinogenic at dietary levels of up to 200 ppm.

Effects on Reproduction   In a two-generation reproduction study with rats, formetanate HCl at a dietary dosage of 250 ppm caused signs of parental toxicity. Dosages of up to 50 ppm had no effects on growth, development, or reproductive performance. No evidence of teratogenicity was found in either rats or rabbits at maternally toxic dosages.

17.3.9.3 Toxicity to Humans

Experimental Exposures   In a repeat dermal insult patch test, only 1 of 50 volunteer subjects showed slight irritation and sensitization to a 0.1% formetanate HCl solution (Schering, 1987).

Use Experience   During many years of formetanate HCl manufacturing, no accidents have been reported during formulation, filling, or packaging. Routine medical examination of workers every 6 months has not revealed any adverse health effects from handling formetanate HCl. During 5 weeks of monitoring, all plasma and erythrocyte acetylcholinesterase values for 17 workers at a formetanate HCl production plant were within the normal range. The same results were obtained in a later 4-week surveillance program.

In the course of 3 years of field research in 280 different tests and 2 years of application of 45,000 lb of formetanate HCl in grower testing programs, no skin reactions or any other health effects were reported. Over a 12-month period, medical surveillance revealed no clinical signs of toxicity among personnel spraying formetanate HCl on trees while wearing coveralls, cap, and respirator. In a systematic 1-year survey of 136 customers using formetanate HCl by spray application, a slight headache on the part of one individual was the only report of illness (Schering, 1987).

17.3.10 ISOLAN

Cases of poisoning by isolan (see Table 17.1) have followed dermal and/or respiratory exposure but were serious only after ingestion. All reported cases involved laboratory evidence of temporary liver injury (Hayes, 1982).

17.3.11 3-ISOPROPYLPHENYL N-METHYLCARBAMATE

As reviewed by Hayes (1982), 3-isopropylphenyl N-methylcarbamate (see Table 17.1) produced typical signs of poisoning

among sprayers and villagers when it was tested for malaria control. It produced rashes, especially in males.

17.3.12 MECARBAM

17.3.12.1 Identity, Properties, and Uses

Chemical Name   Mecarbam is S-(N-ethoxycarbonyl-N-methylcarbamoylmethyl) O,O-diethyl phosphorodithioate. Its structure is shown in Fig. 17.1.

Synonyms   The common name mecarbam (BSI, ISO, JMAF) is in general use. Trade names include Afos®, Murfotox®, Murphotox®, Murotox®, and Pestan®. Code designations are MC 474 and P 474, and the CAS registry number is 2595-54-2.

Physical and Chemical Properties   Mecarbam has the empirical formula $C_{10}H_{20}O_5NPS_2$ and a molecular weight of 329.4. The pure material is a colorless, oily liquid, and the technical material is pale yellow to brown. It has a freezing point of 9°C and a vapor pressure of 3.38×10^{-3} mm Hg at 40°C. Mecarbam is slightly soluble in water; its solubility is 2% in kerosene and 4% in hexane, and it is miscible in all proportions with alcohols, ketones, aromatic hydrocarbons, and chlorinated hydrocarbons. It is stable at normal temperatures, but hydrolyzes at pH values below 3.

Formulations and Uses   Mecarbam is an insecticide and acaricide with ovicidal action. It is used to control aphids, whiteflies, red spider mites, scale insects, and mealybugs on fruit trees; olive and fruit flies; leafhoppers, planthoppers, and miners on rice; and root maggots on several vegetable crops. Mecarbam is available in emulsifiable concentrate, wettable powder, dust, granular, and oil formulations.

17.3.12.2 Toxicity to Laboratory Animals

Basic Findings   The acute toxicity of mecarbam is summarized in Tables 17.2–17.4. The symptoms of acute intoxication are typical of acetylcholinesterase inhibition.

Dermal exposure of rats to mecarbam at 1000 mg/kg/day for 21 days depressed growth and food consumption and elevated blood urea nitrogen values. At dosages of 500 mg/kg/day or higher, liver weight was increased, and decreases were observed in erythrocyte acetylcholinesterase activity and several hematological parameters. There were no abnormal histopathological findings at any dosage. A dosage of 250 mg/kg/day had no treatment-related effects (FAO/WHO, 1984).

Rats exposed by inhalation of a 50,000 mg/m³ aerosol of mecarbam 6 hr a day for 3 weeks showed tremors, respiratory irritation, and inhibition of erythrocyte acetylcholinesterase. No exposure-related effects were seen on growth, gross or microscopic characteristics of organs and tissues, urinalyses, hematology, or clinical chemistry parameters. At 10,000 mg/m³ the only effect observed was respiratory irritation (FAO/WHO, 1981).

In a 2-year study with dogs, exposure to mecarbam in the diet at up to 50 ppm (1.78 mg/kg/day did not affect mortality, growth, food consumption, urinalysis, hematology, clinical chemistry parameters, or gross or microscopic characteristics of organs or tissues. Erythrocyte, plasma, and brain acetylcholinesterase activities were depressed at a dosage of 50 ppm. At 5 ppm (0.15 mg/kg/day), slight acetylcholinesterase inhibition was seen periodically in the erythrocytes and plasma. No treatment-related effects were seen at a dosage of 1 ppm (about 0.03 mg/kg/day). A no-effect level was considered to be 0.35 mg/kg/day (FAO/WHO, 1981).

Rats given mecarbam in their diet for 2 years showed reduced growth and depressed acetylcholinesterase activity at a dosage of 4.15 ppm, but not at 0.83 ppm. They also exhibited a "hunched" appearance that was related to mecarbam dosage and duration of exposure. Treatment did not affect food consumption, urinalyses, hematology, clinical chemistry parameters, or gross or microscopic characteristics of tissues and organs. A no-effect level was 4.15 ppm in the diet (0.21 mg/kg per day) (FAO/WHO, 1981).

Absorption, Distribution, Metabolism, and Excretion Following single oral doses of [^{14}C]mecarbam to rats, tissue levels were highest in the liver and kidneys; some label was still found in the stomach up to 48 hr after administration. Rats metabolized mecarbam primarily by hydrolysis, oxidative desulfuration, and degradation of the carbamoyl moiety; O-deethylation was a minor pathway. At least 10 nonconjugated metabolites and 1 conjugate were found in the urine, but little or no unchanged mecarbam. Mecarbam orally administered to a lactating goat was metabolized mainly at the carbamoyl moiety, with minor O-deethylation; at least 6 nonconjugated metabolites appeared in the urine (FAO/WHO, 1981, 1985a, 1986b).

In rats given radiolabeled mecarbam iv, residues declined most rapidly during the first 40 min after administration; removal from the blood was nearly complete in 6 hr. Rats given single oral doses of radiolabeled mecarbam eliminated about 80–92% of the dose in the urine, 2–3% in the feces, and 0.2–5% as exhaled $^{14}CO_2$ within 48 hr. Urinary radioactivity was associated mainly with seven major polar metabolites; little or no unchanged mecarbam was found in the urine (FAO/WHO, 1981, 1985a). Mecarbam in the diet of cows for 30 days at 10 ppm was excreted at in the milk at levels not exceeding 10 ppm (FAO/WHO, 1981).

Effects on Organs and Tissues Results of mutagenicity testing with mecarbam are summarized in Section 17.2.3.2. Mecarbam was not carcinogenic in a 2-year study with rats (FAO/WHO, 1981).

Effects on Reproduction In a two-generation reproduction study with rats, mecarbam in the diet at 50 ppm depressed growth and caused slight signs of toxicity in the parents and affected the following reproductive parameters: numbers of implantations, ovarian corpora lutea, resorption sites, and liveborn pups; pup survival during lactation; and pup weight at weaning. No teratologic abnormalities were observed. Mecarbam at

2 ppm had no effect on reproductive parameters (FAO/WHO, 1981). Rats intubated with mecarbam at 3 mg/kg/day on days 6–19 of gestation showed clinical cholinergic signs and growth depression, and erythrocyte acetylcholinesterase activity was depressed at dosages of 1 mg/kg/day or higher, but no treatment-related reproductive or teratogenic effects were observed (FAO/WHO, 1984).

Factors Influencing Toxicity No potentiation of toxicity was observed when mecarbam was orally coadministered with the organophosphate compounds malathion, demeton-methyl, or dimethoate (FAO/WHO, 1981).

17.3.12.3 Toxicity to Humans

The 1986 FAO/WHO Joint Meeting on Pesticide Residues estimated a human ADI for mecarbam of 0–0.002 mg/kg body weight (FAO/WHO, 1986b).

Monitoring of Japanese citrus farmers before and after they spent 4 hr spraying fruit trees with mecarbam revealed decreases in serum pseudocholinesterase activity and in serum total cholesterol and HDL-cholesterol levels following exposure. Erythrocyte acetylcholinesterase, serum β-glucuronidase, and serum alkaline phosphatase activities were unchanged (Shiwaku *et al.*, 1982).

17.3.13 METHIOCARB

17.3.13.1 Identity, Properties, and Uses

Chemical Name Methiocarb is 3,5-dimethyl-4-(methylthio)-phenyl N-methylcarbamate. Its structure is shown in Table 17.1.

Synonyms Common names in addition to methiocarb (ISO) are mercaptodimethur (BSI, ISO), metmercapturon, and MXMC. Trade names include Draza®, Mesurol®, and Slug Guard®. Code designations are BAY 37344 and H 321, and the CAS registry number is 2032-65-7.

Physical and Chemical Properties Methiocarb has the empirical formula $C_{11}H_{15}NO_2$ and a molecular weight of 225.33. It forms a white crystalline powder with a mild odor. The melting point is 119°C, and the vapor pressure is 1.99 mm Hg at 60°C. Methiocarb is soluble in acetone and alcohol, and its solubility in water is 10 ppm at 20°C. It is unstable in highly alkaline media.

History, Formulations, and Uses Methiocarb has been in use since the 1960s as a molluscicide, acaricide, and insecticide (contact and stomach poison) for control of snails and slugs in home gardens and ornamentals; mites, thrips, aphids, leafhoppers, fruit flies, and biting insects; and some soil pests of field crops. It is also used as a bird repellent on fruit crops. Methiocarb is formulated as a wettable powder, liquid, seed dressing, bait, and hopper box treater.

17.3.13.2 Toxicity to Laboratory Animals

Basic Findings The acute toxicity of methiocarb is summarized in Tables 17.2–17.4. Acute administration produced typical signs of acetylcholinesterase inhibition.

Methiocarb given orally to rats for 4 weeks at 10 mg/kg/day caused acetylcholinesterase depression in the plasma, erythrocytes, and brain, as well as transient cholinergic symptoms; no effects were observed at 3 mg/kg/day. In rats given methiocarb orally at 4 mg/kg for 27 days, erythrocyte acetylcholinesterase activity was depressed up to 80%, but no cholinergic signs were observed. After treatment was terminated, recovery of acetylcholinesterase activity to normal levels took about 42 days (FAO/WHO, 1982). Rats given methiocarb at 50 ppm in their diet for 16 weeks showed reductions in acetylcholinesterase activity of about 30% in the plasma and 15% in the erythrocytes; no acetylcholinesterase inhibition was seen at a dosage of 10 ppm (FAO/WHO, 1985).

Dogs given methiocarb for 2 weeks at 15 ppm in their diet showed depression of plasma acetylcholinesterase activity; no effect was seen at 5 ppm (FAO/WHO, 1982). In a 29-day study with dogs, methiocarb administered orally at 0.5 mg/kg/day caused hypersalivation, vomiting, and depression of acetylcholinesterase activity by about 20% in the plasma and erythrocytes, maximal 1–2 hr after administration. Methiocarb at 0.05 mg/kg/day did not affect acetylcholinesterase activity (FAO/WHO, 1985). Methiocarb in the diet of dogs at up to 60 ppm for 2 years did not affect growth, food consumption, or gross or microscopic characteristics of organs and tissues. In another 2-year study with dogs, plasma acetylcholinesterase was inhibited at dietary levels of 15 ppm or higher, and cholinergic symptoms were seen at a dosage of 240 ppm (FAO/WHO, 1982). A dietary no-effect level for dogs was considered to be 5 ppm (0.125 mg/kg/day) (FAO/WHO, 1985).

Methiocarb in the diet of rats for 2 years at up to 600 ppm depressed body weight and inhibited plasma and erythrocyte acetylcholinesterase activity, but had no effect on mortality, food consumption, behavior, hematology, clinical chemistry, urinalyses, gross pathology, histopathology, or organ weight. At a dietary level of 200 ppm, only transient depression of erythrocyte acetylcholinesterase activity was observed. No treatment-related effects were seen on any of these parameters at a dosage of 67 ppm (FAO/WHO, 1982). A dietary no-effect level for rats was considered to be 25 ppm (1.3 mg/kg/day) (FAO/WHO, 1985).

Absorption, Distribution, Metabolism, and Excretion In dermal toxicity studies, methiocarb was not readily absorbed via the skin, even in solvents expected to enhance dermal absorption (FAO/WHO, 1982).

In a cow given five daily doses of ring-labeled methiocarb, radioactivity in the milk (due to methiocarb sulfoxide) peaked at 0.062 ppm after the third dose. Tissue residues were highest in the kidney (0.108 ppm) and liver (0.073 ppm); levels in other tissues did not exceed 0.02 ppm. Following subchronic dietary exposure of beef and dairy cattle to methiocarb, residues exceeded 0.005 ppm only in the liver (at dosages of 30 ppm or higher) and the kidney (at a dosage of 100 ppm); residues were not detected in the brain, heart, muscle, or fat. Milk collected on exposure days 28 and 29 contained methiocarb residues ranging from 0.005 ppm (at a dosage of 10 ppm) to 0.033 ppm (at a dosage of 100 ppm) (FAO/WHO, 1982).

In vitro liver, kidney, and blood preparations from rats, dogs, and humans metabolized methiocarb primarily to methiocarb sulfoxide and *N*-hydroxymethylmethiocarb. The sulfone and 4-methylthio-3,5-xylyl-*N*-hydroxymethylcarbamate also were reported (Oonnithan and Casida, 1968; Wheeler and Strother, 1971). Methiocarb was oxidized, relatively slowly, by pig liver microsomal FAD-dependent monooxygenase.

In rats, orally administered carbonyl-[^{14}C] and methylthio-[^{3}H]methiocarb were partly oxidized to the sulfoxide and sulfone; the carbamate metabolites were hydrolyzed to phenols, which were excreted in the urine as glycosidic conjugates (FAO/WHO, 1982). Rats given a single oral 5-mg dose of methiocarb eliminated up to 2.3% of the dose in the urine as unchanged methiocarb and 3.3% as its phenolic metabolites, mostly within 48 hr of administration (Van Hoof and Heyndrickx, 1975). The principal urinary metabolites in rats given ring-labeled methiocarb were conjugated methiocarb phenol and sulfoxide phenol. In dogs orally dosed with ring-labeled methiocarb, the urinary metabolites were primarily conjugates of methiocarb sulfoxide phenol and methiocarb sulfone phenol; the radioactivity in the feces was almost all unchanged methiocarb. In a dairy cow given ring-labeled methiocarb, the principal urinary metabolites were conjugated phenols of methiocarb and its sulfoxide and sulfone (FAO/WHO, 1982).

Of a single dose of carbonyl-labeled methiocarb to rats, more than 60% was eliminated as expired $^{14}CO_2$ (FAO/WHO, 1982). In another study, about 66% was eliminated as $^{14}CO_2$, about 22% in the urine, and 2.5% in the feces; elimination was about 91% complete (Krishna and Casida, 1966). Ring-labeled methiocarb was excreted almost entirely in the urine within 48 hr. Of a ring-labeled dose of methiocarb to a dairy cow, 96% appeared in the urine, 1% in the feces, and 1% in the milk within 144 hr (FAO/WHO, 1982).

Effects on Organs and Tissues Results of mutagenicity testing with methiocarb are summarized in Section 17.2.3.2. Methiocarb in the diet of rats at up to 600 ppm for 2 years was not carcinogenic (FAO/WHO, 1982).

Effects on Reproduction Carbonyl-[^{14}C]methiocarb administered ip to pregnant rats crossed the placenta; fetal radioactivity was highest in the kidneys and heart. By 8 hr after administration, pregnant rats eliminated about 10% less of the dose than did nonpregnant animals (Wheeler and Strother, 1974b). Major routes of methiocarb metabolism *in vitro* were sulfoxidation in maternal and fetal rats liver (12.3 and 23.1% of ^{14}C-labeled compound, respectively) and hydroxylation in maternal liver (7.9%). Slight sulfoxidation occurred in placental tissue, but no metabolic activity was observed for maternal or fetal brain (Wheeler and Strother, 1974a).

In a three-generation reproduction study with rats, methiocarb at up to 300 ppm in the diet had no adverse effects on fertility, litter size, pup birth weight and survival, or lactation; histopathological examination of the pups revealed no treatment-related abnormalities. Methiocarb given orally to rats at up to 10 mg/kg/day on days 6–15 of gestation was not teratogenic and did not affect reproductive parameters (FAO/WHO, 1982). In rabbits, methiocarb was not teratogenic at oral dosages of up to 10 mg/kg/day on days 6–18 of gestation, but maternal and fetal toxicity was observed at dosages of 3 mg/kg/day or higher (FAO/WHO, 1985).

Factors Influencing Toxicity In rats, toxicity was not potentiated when methiocarb was coadministered ip with trichlorfon, coumaphos, oxydemeton methyl, fenthion, propoxur, parathion, methyl parathion, malathion, azinphos methyl, or several other anticholinesterase insecticides (FAO/WHO, 1982).

Accidental Poisoning in Animals Poisoning of domestic animals by methiocarb in snail and slug baits has been reported, especially in dogs and cows, which apparently find the baits palatable (Quick, 1982; Studdert, 1985). An Australian survey found snail and slug baits to be the most common cause of poisoning in dogs and cats (Studdert, 1985), with methiocarb-containing baits accounting for 43% of such poisoning. All these cases of methiocarb poisoning involved dogs, and the incidence of poisoning and fatality rate were independent of body size. Several published case reports of methiocarb poisoning in dogs (Orton, 1973; Udall, 1973; Keck and Jaussaud, 1981; Lunder, 1981) and one of poisoning in a sheep (Giles *et al.*, 1984) indicated rapid appearance of typical cholinergic symptoms and successful treatment with atropine in cases accurately diagnosed in time.

17.3.13.3 Toxicity to Humans

The 1984 FAO/WHO Joint Meeting on Pesticide Residues estimated a human ADI for methiocarb to be 0–0.06 mg/kg body weight (FAO/WHO, 1985).

Use Experience Attempts have been made to estimate occupational exposure to methiocarb. In one study, patch monitors were placed on blueberry harvesters working 4 days after methiocarb was applied to the bushes as a bird repellent. Total dermal exposure to methiocarb was estimated at 3.8 mg/hr, with the greatest contribution (53%) from the hands (Zweig *et al.*, 1985). Another study sampled for methiocarb in the air breathed by workers in a seed-pelleting plant; depending on the pelleting process used, average methiocarb levels ranged from 0.002 to 0.23 mg/m³ (O'Keefe and Pierse, 1980).

17.3.14 METHOMYL

17.3.14.1 Identity, Properties, and Uses

Chemical Name Methomyl is *S*-methyl-*N*-[(methylcarbamoyl)oxy]thioacetimidate. Its structure is shown in Table 17.1.

Synonyms The common name methomyl (ANSI, BSI, ISO, JMAF) is in general use. Other names are metomil and mesomile. Trade names include Lannate®, Lanox®, Methavin®, and Nudrin®. Code designations have included DX 1179, OMS 1196, SD 14999, and WL 18236. The CAS registry number is 16752-77-5.

Physical and Chemical Properties Methomyl has the empirical formula $C_5H_{10}N_2O_2S$ and a molecular weight of 162.23. The pure material is a white crystalline solid with a slight sulfurous odor. The melting point is 78–79°C, and the vapor pressure is 5×10^{-5} mm Hg at 25°C. The solubility of methomyl at 25°C is 3% in toluene, 5.8% in water, 22% in isopropanol, 42% in ethanol, 73% in acetone, and 100% in methanol. Methomyl is stable in solid form and in aqueous solutions at pH 7.0 or less, it decomposes rapidly in alkaline solutions and in moist soils.

History, Formulations, and Uses Introduced in 1966, methomyl is used as a contact and stomach insecticide for broad-spectrum control of pests of vegetables, soybeans, cotton, other field crops, some fruit crops, and ornamentals. Methomyl is formulated as water-soluble powders and liquids.

17.3.14.2 Toxicity to Laboratory Animals

Some of the toxicology studies cited from du Pont (1986) were also described by Kaplan and Sherman (1976). Methomyl is also the first intermediate metabolite of thiodicarb (see Section 17.3.21).

Basic Findings The acute toxicity of methomyl is summarized in Tables 17.2–17.4. Signs of acute toxicity are typical of acetylcholinesterase inhibition. Methomyl did not cause skin irritation in rabbits or guinea pigs; mild erythema was seen in some individuals. In rabbits, methomyl produced mild eye irritation (conjunctivitis, iritic injection, and mucous membrane irritation). Ocular administration also caused miosis and other systemic cholinergic effects, less pronounced when the eye was washed. Methomyl did not cause a skin sensitization reaction in guinea pigs (du Pont, 1986).

Acute dermal administration of methomyl (in acetone) to rats decreased acetylcholinesterase activity in plasma, but not erythrocytes, at 24 and 72 hr postdosing. After 24 hr, activity was reduced 46% at 99 mg/kg and 66% at 357 mg/kg. Following acute dermal administration of analytical-grade methomyl (in acetone) to rats, the 24-hr ED 50 values for erythrocyte and plasma acetylcholinesterase activity were 0.594 and 4.085 mg/cm², respectively, and the corresponding dose–response slopes were 1.25 and 1.41 (du Pont, 1986). Methomyl was administered orally to goats at 0.95 mg/kg/day for 4 days; at 48 hr after the last dose, acetylcholinesterase activity was reduced by up to 28% in the plasma and 20% in the erythrocytes. Recovery was complete within 7 days (Osman *et al.*, 1983).

In a 3-week study with rabbits, dermal exposure to methomyl at 200 mg/kg/day produced clinical cholinergic signs, but did not affect organ weight or histopathology (du Pont, 1986). In a 29-day study, rats given methomyl at 800 ppm in the diet showed slight plasma and erythrocyte acetylcholinesterase depression on days 7–28; after 29 days, brain acetylcholinesterase activity was reduced by 12% in males and 15% in females. At dosages of 100 ppm and higher, slight brain acetylcholinesterase depression was also seen in females after 29 days. Blood acetylcholinesterase activity was unaffected by dosages of up to 400 ppm.

Methomyl in the diet of rats for 90 days decreased food consumption and body weight at mean dosages of 18.83 mg/kg/day to males and 23.95 mg/kg/day to females. At 18.83 mg/kg/day, males also showed moderate erythroid hyperplasia of the bone marrow. At mean dosages of up to 20.69 mg/kg/day to males and 23.95 mg/kg/day to females, there were no deaths or other effects on behavioral, clinical, hematological, serological, urological, or pathological observations. A no-effect level for this study, based on effects seen in males, was 50 ppm in the diet, equivalent to 3.56 mg/kg/day. In other 90-day feeding studies, methomyl had no effects on mortality, body or organ weights, food consumption, gross or microscopic pathology, or a wide variety of clinical parameters at dosages of up to 20 mg/kg/day to mice or 400 ppm to dogs (14.68 mg/kg/day for males and 12.5 mg/kg/day for females) (du Pont, 1986). In a 5-month study, transient blood acetylcholinesterase depression of 25–40% was seen in rats fed methomyl at 800 ppm; onset and return to normal were faster in males than in females. No effects on blood acetylcholinesterase were observed at dietary dosages of up to 400 ppm (du Pont, 1986).

In a 2-year study with dogs, methomyl in the diet at 1000 ppm (31.12 mg/kg/day for males and 32.67 mg/kg/day for females) resulted in clinical signs of acetylcholinesterase inhibition, increased mortality, slight to moderate anemia, evidence of compensatory hematopoiesis in the spleen and bone marrow, hemosiderin deposits, epithelial swelling of kidney tubules, and minimal to slight bile-duct proliferation. At 400 ppm (10.93 mg/kg/day for males and 13.90 mg/kg/day for females), accumulation of pigment was noted in the spleen and kidneys. No effects were seen on body weight, food consumption, blood acetylcholinesterase activity, or serological or urological parameters. A no-effect level was 100 ppm (2.94 mg/kg/day for males and 2.31 mg/kg/day for females) (du Pont, 1986).

In 22- and 24-month studies with rats, methomyl at 400 ppm (19.9 mg/kg/day for males and 26.2 mg/kg/day for females) reduced erythrocyte counts, hemoglobin values, and hematocrits in females and affected food consumption and body weights. Females receiving dosages of 200 ppm (11.18 mg/kg/day) and higher showed a dose-related decrease in hemoglobin values. Acetylcholinesterase activity was not affected. Effects on organs at 400 ppm were increased relative testis weight and tubular lesions in kidneys; at 200 ppm and higher, spleens of females showed increased extramedullary hematopoiesis; and at 100 ppm and higher, relative liver weights were increased in females. Exposure had no significant effect on mortality, nor any other effects on organs, tissues, clinical parameters, or other indices of toxicity. A no-effect level was considered to be 100 ppm (4.83 mg/kg/day for males and 5.82 mg/kg/day for females) (du Pont, 1986).

In a 2-year study with mice, dietary exposure to methomyl at 100 and 800 ppm increased mortality and decreased erythrocyte mass during the first 26 weeks. Although these dosages were reduced to 75 and 200 ppm at week 39, increased mortality in these groups persisted throughout the study. No effects were observed on clinical parameters, body weights, food consumption, gross pathology, or histopathology. A no-effect level was 50 ppm (8.7 mg/kg/day for males and 10.6 mg/kg/day for females) (du Pont, 1986).

Absorption, Distribution, Metabolism, and Excretion
Shah *et al.* (1981) assessed dermal penetration rate, distribution, retention, and excretion of [^{14}C]methomyl in mice. The penetration half-life was 13.3 min, and the label was detected in the blood, tissues, and excreta within 5–15 min after application. By 8 hr after application, more than half of the radioactivity appeared in the excreta and 6.1% in the blood; other organs and tissues contained 0.1 to 3.3%.

Methomyl can exist in two geometric configurations. The *syn* isomer is more stable and is the main one used as an insecticide. In rats, carbonyl- or oximino-labeled *syn*-methomyl was metabolized to carbon dioxide and acetonitrile at a 2:1 ratio. In contrast, the *anti* isomer was metabolized predominantly to acetonitrile. It was concluded on the basis of this and other evidence that a Beckman rearrangement of the *syn* and *anti* oximes occurs prior to formation of carbon dioxide and acetonitrile (Huhtanen and Dorough, 1976).

Methomyl was not oxidized *in vitro* by FAD-dependent monooxygenase in a pig liver microsomal preparation. In rats, methomyl was rapidly converted to methomyl methylol, oxime, sulfoxide, and sulfoxide oxime; these unstable intermediates were converted to acetonitrile and CO_2, which were eliminated primarily via respiration and in the urine. Conversion of acetonitrile to CO_2 via acetamide (for which evidence for carcinogenicity is equivocal; Jackson and Dessau, 1961) is not a significant metabolic process in mammals (Huhtanen and Dorough, 1976; Union Carbide, 1984).

When oximino-labeled [^{14}C]methomyl was administered by stomach tube to rats that had been given nonradioactive methomyl in their diet at 200 ppm, less than 10% of the label was found in the whole body 24 hr after treatment. Most of the labeled dose was exhaled as carbon dioxide, exhaled as acetonitrile, and excreted as polar compounds in the urine, in a ratio of 1:2:1. Although the urinary metabolites were not identified, the following were ruled out: methomyl, *S*-methyl-*N*-hydroxythioacetimidate, and the sulfoxide and sulfone of methomyl (Harvey *et al.*, 1973).

In lactating goats, [^{14}C]methomyl given orally at 0.95 mg/kg/day for 4 days was found in the urine 24 hr after the first dose and in the milk within 48 hr; concentrations peaked 24 hr after the last dose, at 0.35 ppm in the urine and 0.13 ppm in the milk. At the end of a 7-day recovery period, residues were 0.001 ppm in the urine, 0.01 ppm in the milk, and undetectable in the blood (Osman *et al.*, 1983). In another goat study, ^{14}C-labeled methomyl administered orally for up to 10 days was eliminated primarily as acetonitrile and carbon dioxide. About

16% of the dose was excreted in the urine, 7% in the feces, and 6% in the milk. Low total recovery (65%) was attributed to loss of acetonitrile through the skin (du Pont, 1986). In cows fed methomyl at up to 20 ppm (0.76 mg/kg/day) for 30 days, no methomyl residues were found in the organs, meat, or milk. In rumen fluid from a cow, approximately 90% of [^{14}C]methomyl was metabolized to acetonitrile; the other 10% consisted of unidentified water-soluble metabolites (du Pont, 1986).

Biochemical Effects Methomyl did not inhibit rat brain monoamine oxidase *in vitro* (Kadir and Knowles, 1981). Methomyl given ip to rats at 2 mg/kg inhibited liver carboxylesterase activity (with *o*-nitrophenyl butyrate as substrate) to about 58% of control and acetanilide amidase activity to about 20% of control (Iverson, 1977). Borady *et al.* (1983) gave rats methomyl at 40 mg/kg/day for 8 days via oral intubation, to examine the effect on fat metabolism and blood enzymes. At 24 hr postdosing, significant increases were noted in serum activities of alkaline phosphatase, glutamic-oxaloxacetic transaminase, and glutamic-pyruvic transaminase; in serum triglycerides, phospholipids, free fatty acids, and cholesterol; and in liver total lipids, cholesterol, and phospholipids (though not in liver weight or triglycerides). There was histological evidence of hepatotoxicity, and serum acetylcholinesterase activity was decreased. In mice, oral exposure to methomyl inhibited liver vitamin-B$_6$-dependent kynurenine hydrolase and kynurenine aminotransferase activities by about 27% following one dose of 1.7 mg/kg and 14% after six daily doses of 0.53 mg/kg/day (El-Sewedy *et al.*, 1982).

Effects on Organs and Tissues The results of mutagenicity testing with methomyl are summarized in Section 17.2.3.2. Methomyl was not carcinogenic in 22- and 24-month studies with rats at dietary dosages of up to 400 ppm (19.9 mg/kg/day to males and 26.2 mg/kg/day to females) or in a 2-year study with mice at mean dietary dosages of up to 93.4 mg/kg/day to males and 118.5 mg/kg/day to females (du Pont, 1986). Methomyl also did not show transforming activity in a host-mediated hamster cell culture assay (Quarles *et al.*, 1979a,b).

Effects of Reproduction In a three-generation study with rats, dietary levels of methomyl as high as 100 ppm for 90 days had no effect on reproduction or lactation. No pathological changes, gross or microscopic, were found in the young. No teratogenic or fetotoxic effects were observed after pregnant rats were given methomyl in the diet on days 6–21 of gestation at up to 400 ppm (33.9 mg/kg/day), a maternally toxic dosage. Similarly, no developmental toxicity resulted when rabbits were fed methomyl at maternally toxic dosages (50 and 100 mg/kg/day) (du Pont, 1986).

Factors Influencing Toxicity More than 20 pesticides or other anticholinesterase agents have been tested for their abilities to potentiate the toxicity of methomyl in rats, but unfortunately the statistical significance of the differences was not reported. Compounds with synergistic effects (assessed as either excess mortality or greater inhibition of blood cholinesterase activity) included carbaryl, ronnel, methyl parathion, and mevinphos. Dimethoate was antagonistic; a mixture with methomyl inhibited cholinesterase 53% less than predicted. Compounds producing only additive effects included endosulfan and diflubenzuron (du Pont, 1986). In mice, pretreatment with butylated hydroxyanisole (BHA) for 4 days reduced the LD 50 of methomyl by a factor of 2.2–3.2 (Joa and Hsu, 1981).

Ethanol administered to rats in their diet for 2 weeks (as 25% of their total calories) did not potentiate erythrocyte acetylcholinesterase inhibition by methomyl coadministered at 200 ppm (Bracy *et al.*, 1979). However, in a 12-week study with rats, 10% ethanol in the drinking water potentiated the toxicity of methomyl at 200 ppm in the diet. Potentiated effects included increased relative adrenal weights in both sexes, elevated liver triglyceride and free fatty acid contents and decreased brain acetylcholinesterase activity in males, and increased relative kidney weights and blood glucose levels in females (Antal *et al.*, 1979).

17.3.14.3 Toxicity to Humans

The 1986 FAO/WHO Joint Meeting on Pesticide Residues estimated a temporary human ADI for methomyl of 0–0.01 mg/kg weight (FAO/WHO, 1986b).

Use Experience Dr. Keith T. Maddy, in an unpublished manuscript, reported that there were more than 225 poisonings in 1972 and 1973 (some serious, but none fatal) following exposure to dry formulations of methomyl, primarily by inhalation of powder. After the compound was reformulated and marketed as a liquid concentrate, cases decreased to fewer than 10 per year. Cases reported from Australia were usually associated with dust formulations (Simpson and Penney, 1974; Simpson and Bermingham, 1977). Cases reported from a tobacco-growing area of Japan occurred primarily on the day of application and often involved rates of application higher than those recommended (Kudo, 1975). Among Japanese tea-growers reporting acute symptoms (fatigue, headache, and profuse perspiration) following pesticide use, 42% named methomyl as one of the chemicals used (Fujita, 1985).

Sallam and El-Ghawaby (1980) reported without detail 4000 cases and 30 deaths due to methomyl in Egypt in 1979.

In a plant manufacturing methomyl and propanil, 11 of 102 workers had been hospitalized for occupationally acquired illness. Workers involved in packaging methomyl reported the highest rate of hospitalization following chemical exposure (27%) and the highest frequency of cholinergic symptoms, including miosis, blurred vision, nausea or vomiting, muscle weakness, fatigue, and increased salivation. No precise dose–response relationship could be determined, and reliable cholinesterase measurements were not made (Morse *et al.*, 1979).

Accidental and Intentional Overexposure Three fishermen in Jamaica became critically ill within 5 min of eating a meal including roti, an unleavened bread made from flour, water, and salt. Symptoms were perspiration, visual disturbances, trembling, vomiting, and defecation, progressing to convulsions and coma. The men were taken to a hospital about 3 hr later and pronounced dead on arrival. Postmortem examinations revealed congestion of the stomach lining, lungs, tracheae, and bronchi. One of two other men who had shared the meal showed generalized twitching, fasciculations, and severe bronchospasms, but recovered within 2 hr after treatment; the fifth was asymptomatic. Poisoning was traced to a small, unlabeled bag of pure methomyl powder found in a tin in the fishermen's hut; the powder was probably used instead of salt in preparing the roti, which contained methomyl at about 11,000 ppm. The lethal doses were estimated at 12–15 mg/kg (Liddle *et al.*, 1979).

A 31-year-old Japanese housewife committed suicide by taking an insecticide containing methomyl in food, which was also eaten by her three children. All were found dead except a 9-year-old son, who survived. Autopsies of the woman and her 6-year old son revealed congestion of the stomach lining and lungs, with edema and hemorrhaging of tissues due to acute circulatory failures. Methomyl doses were estimated at 55 mg/kg to the mother and 13 mg/kg to the child (Araki *et al.*, 1982). Noda (1984) reported the course of therapy and symptoms for a patient who had attempted suicide by ingesting about 2.25 gm of methomyl. At 6 hr postingestion, methomyl was present in the blood at 1.61 ppm and in the urine at 10.91 ppm; at 15 hr, levels were 0.04 ppm in the blood and 0.25 ppm in the urine; and at 22 hr, methomyl was not detectable in the samples.

Volf and Hanuš (1984) reported a case in which methomyl was detected in grounds from coffee that caused cholinergic symptoms.

17.3.15 MEXACARBATE

17.3.15.1 Identity, Properties, and Uses

Chemical Name Mexacarbate is 4-dimethylamino-3,5-xylyl *N*-methylcarbamate. Its structure is shown in Table 17.1.

Synonyms The common name mexacarbate (ANSI, BSI, ISO) is in general use. The trade name is Zectran®, a code designation is D 139, and the CAS registry number is 315-18-4.

Physical and Chemical Properties Mexacarbate has the empirical formula $C_{12}H_{18}N_2O_2$ and a molecular weight of 222.29. The technical material is a tan to brown waxy powder with a slight fishy odor. The melting point is 87°C, and the vapor pressure is 2×10^{-5} mm Hg at 25°C. Mexacarbate is readily soluble in xylene, benzene, and acetone, and its solubility in water at 25°C is 1% (w/w). It hydrolyzes rapidly in alkaline solutions and degrades at temperatures above 90°C.

History, Formulations, and Uses Mexacarbate is used to control pests of ornamental plants, trees, turf, and ground cover. It is effective against a wide range of insects, as well as mites, snails, and slugs. Mexacarbate is available as an emulsifiable

concentrate for use on ornamentals and as a bait for snail and slug control, and it is registered for a number of other applications in the United States.

17.3.15.2 Toxicity to Laboratory Animals

Basic Findings The acute toxicity of mexacarbate is summarized in Tables 17.2 and 17.3. Symptoms of acute intoxication were typical of acetylcholinesterase inhibition. Mexacarbate produced mild, reversible skin and eye irritation in rabbits and did not cause a skin sensitization reaction in guinea pigs (Dodd, 1987b).

In a 21-day dermal exposure study with rabbits, dosages of up to 1000 mg/kg/day had no effects on antemortem observations, body and organ weights, food consumption, hematology, clinical chemistry, blood acetylcholinesterase activity, gross pathology, or histopathology (Dodd, 1987b).

Mexacarbate in the diet of mice at 300 ppm for 90 days caused depression of body weight, food and water consumption, and plasma and erythrocyte acetylcholinesterase activity. No treatment-related effects were seen on antemortem observations, ophthalmology, urinalyses, brain acetylcholinesterase activity, hematology, serum chemistries, organ weights, gross pathology, or histopathology. A no-effect level was 150 ppm (26 mg/kg/day for males and 40 mg/kg/day for females). A similar 90-day study with rats revealed the same treatment-related effects at dietary levels of 150 ppm or higher; no-effect levels were 4.6 mg/kg/day for males and 5.4 mg/kg/day for females. Mexacarbate in the diet of dogs at 325 ppm for 1 year resulted in increased mortality, tremors, depressed body weight and food consumption, increased liver weight and increased frequency of liver lesions, decreased heart weight, changes in several serum chemistry parameters, and inhibition of plasma, erythrocyte, and brain acetylcholinesterase. At a dosage of 90 ppm, tremors, liver histopathology, and inhibition of plasma and erythrocyte acetylcholinesterase were noted. A dietary no-effect level was 25 ppm (0.6 mg/kg/day) (Dodd, 1987b).

In a 2-year study with rats, mexacarbate at 250 ppm in the diet (11.5 mg/kg/day for males and 14.4 mg/kg/day for females) caused decreases in body weight and food consumption, inhibition of acetylcholinesterase activity in the plasma and erythrocytes, and changes in urinalyses. No treatment-related effects were seen on mortality, water consumption, organ weights, gross or histopathological lesions, ophthalmological examination, brain acetylcholinesterase activity, or other clinical chemistry parameters. A no-effect level was 80 ppm in the diet (3.5 mg/kg/day for males and 4.3 mg/kg/day for females). In a 78-week study with mice mexacarbate at 250 ppm in the diet (32.2 mg/kg/day for males and 41.2 mg/kg/day for females) depressed body weight, water consumption, and acetylcholinesterase activity in the plasma, erythrocytes, and brain. Mexacarbate had no effects on mortality, food consumption, gross or histopathological lesions, hematology, or clinical chemistry. A no-effect level was 80 ppm (10.6 mg/kg/day for males and 13.6 mg/kg/day for females (Dodd, 1987b).

Absorption, Distribution, Metabolism, and Excretion In goats given 20 mg of [^{14}C]mexacarbate per day for 10 days, tissue levels of radiolabel did not exceed 0.004 ppm except in the liver (0.2 ppm), kidney (0.06 ppm), and fetal tissues (0.3 ppm) (Chib, 1985).

In rat or human liver enzyme systems, mexacarbate was metabolized primarily to 4-methylamino-3,5-xylyl N-methylcarbamate and 4-dimethylamino-3,5-xylyl N-hydroxymethyl carbamate (which was also the major ether-extractable metabolite formed in human blood *in vitro*); 4-methylformamido-3,5-xylyl N-methylcarbamate and 4-amino-3,5-xylyl N-methylcarbamate also were reported (Oonnithan and Casida, 1968; Wheeler and Strother, 1971). Bedford (1975) observed formation of 4-dimethyl-3,5-xylyl-N-hydroxymethyl carbamate in a rat liver preparation but not in a human liver preparation, suggesting a species difference. Essac and Matsumura (1979) described an *in vitro* rat liver and intestine flavoprotein-flavin cofactor system that reduced mexacarbate to 4-N-desmethylmexacarbate; the importance of this system *in vivo* was not known.

In a dog, ring-labeled [^{14}C]mexacarbate (administered in the diet for 2 weeks) was metabolized to the sulfates and glucuronides of 4-dimethylamino-3,5-xylenol and 2,6-dimethylhydroquinone, along with a small amount of free 4-dimethylamino-3,5-xylenol (Williams *et al.*, 1964). In lactating goats given radiolabeled mexacarbate for 10 days, the major urinary metabolite was 4-dimethylamino-3,5-xylenol, which accounted for 46% of a 7-day sample. Also present was 2,6-dimethylbenzoquinone. No unchanged mexacarbate was excreted (Chib, 1985).

Rats given a single oral 10-mg dose of mexacarbate eliminated up to 2% of the dose in the urine as unchanged parent compound and 2.2% as its phenolic metabolites within 72 hr of administration (van Hoof and Heyndrickx, 1975). Rats eliminated 77% of a carbonyl-^{14}C-labeled dose of mexacarbate as ^{14}CO$_2$, 12% in the urine, and 2.5% in the feces (Krishna and Casida, 1966). By 48 hr after administration of carbonyl-labeled mexacarbate to mice, 75% of the dose was eliminated as ^{14}CO$_2$; 17% was excreted in the urine and 7% in the feces (Miskus *et al.*, 1969). Lactating goats given 20 mg of radiolabeled mexacarbate per day for 10 days eliminated 90% of the dose in the urine and 3.8% in the feces; less than 0.1 ppm ^{14}C appeared in the milk (Chib, 1985).

Biochemical Effects Mexacarbate inhibited rat brain monoamine oxidase *in vitro;* inhibition was greatest (65.3%) with dopamine as the substrate (Kadir and Knowles, 1981).

Effects on Organs and Tissues Results of mutagenicity testing with mexacarbate are summarized in Section 17.2.3.2. Mexacarbate was not carcinogenic in two independent series of chronic studies with rats and mice (NCI, 1978; Dodd, 1987b).

Effects on Reproduction In a two-generation reproduction study with rats, the only mexacarbate-related effects were decreases in adult growth and pup weight and survival during lactation at a dietary level of 250 ppm and sporadic weight decreases in adults and pups at a dosage of 80 ppm. A no-effect level was 25 ppm (1.5 mg/kg/day). In rats and rabbits, mexacarbate was not teratogenic at maternally toxic dosages (up to 6.25 mg/kg/day to rats and 10.0 mg/kg/day to rabbits); fetotoxicity was minimal in rats and absent in rabbits (Dodd, 1987b).

In vitro, maternal and fetal rat brain metabolized about 12% of [^{14}C]mexacarbate to 4-methylamino-3,5-xylyl N-methylcarbate. In maternal liver and major routes were N-demethylation (15.8%) and N-methyl hydroxylation (13.6%); fetal liver and placenta did not metabolize mexacarbate (Wheeler and Strother, 1974a). In rats injected ip with [^{14}C]mexacarbate on days 18 and 19 of gestation, distribution and placental transfer were rapid, and an equilibrium between placental and fetal concentrations was reached by 15 min after administration. Elimination of radiolabel from the fetus was initially rapid ($t_{1/2} = 22$ min), but subsequently slow; after 24 hr, 35% of the dose that had crossed the placenta remained in the fetus. The highest fetal levels were in the kidney and heart, the highest maternal level was in the liver, and brain levels were higher in the fetuses than in the dams. Pregnant rats exhaled less ^{14}CO$_2$ than did nonpregnant rats and retained up to 23% more radioactivity in the tissues at 8 hr after administration (Wheeler and Strother, 1974b).

Factors Influencing Toxicity No potentiation of toxicity was seen when mexacarbate was administered to rats jointly with malathion or O-ethyl-O(4-nitrophenyl)phenylphosphonothioate (EPN) (Dodd, 1987b).

17.3.15.3 Toxicity to Humans

Accidental and Intentional Overexposure A 17-year-old plant nursery employee was found unconscious, with miosis and irregular heartbeat, after ingesting approximately 55 gm of mexacarbate (as a 22% formulation). After hospitalization, a regular heartbeat was restored briefly, but the patient developed bradycardia and recurrent heart failure and died after about 4–4.5 hr (Reich and Welke, 1966).

In 1972, during aerial spraying of mexacarbate in Maine, a pinhole leak in a high-pressure pump line allowed a fine aerosol spray to be emitted into the fuselage, 12 feet behind the copilot's seat. After about 110 min exposure, the copilot began to experience characteristic cholinergic symptoms, including weakness, headache, stomach cramps, and a metallic taste in the mouth. Within minutes of onset, symptoms progressed to drowsiness, disturbances of vision, and respiratory difficulty. On landing, he could not stand and shook uncontrollably; en route to the hospital, he developed numbness and paralysis of the hands and arms and slurred speech. Symptoms noted on admission included miosis, flushed face, and muscular twitching. Atropine was given immediately; a blood sample taken 10 min later showed severe acetylcholinesterase depression. Symptoms subsided rapidly, and the patient was able to leave the hospital 3 hr after admission, although headache and weakness persisted for the remainder of the day. Acetylcholinesterase activity was normal 3 days after the exposure (Richardson and Batteese, 1973).

17.3.16 OXAMYL

17.3.16.1 Identity, Properties, and Uses

Chemical Name Oxamyl is *N-N*-dimethyl-2-methylcarbamoyloxyimino-2-(methylthio)acetamide. Its structure is shown in Table 17.1.

Synonyms The common name oxamyl (ANSI, BSI, ISO) is in general use. The name oxamil (JMAP) also is current. A trade name is Vydate®, and code designations include D-1410 and DPX 1410. The CAS registry number is 23135-22-0.

Physical and Chemical Properties Oxamyl has the empirical formula $C_7H_{13}N_3O_3S$ and a molecular weight of 219.3. The pure compound is a white crystalline solid with a slightly sulfurous odor. It melts at 100–102°C, changing to a different crystalline form with a melting point of 108–110°C. The vapor pressure of oxamyl (mm Hg) is 2.3×10^4 at 25°C, 3.7×10^4 at 30°C, 8.4×10^4 at 40°C, and 7.6×10^3 at 70°C. Its solubility (w/w at 25°C) is 1% in toluene, 11% in isopropanol, 28% in water, 29% in cyclohexanone, 33% in ethanol, 67% in acetone, 108% in dimethylformamide, and 144% in methanol. It is stable in solid form and in most solutions.

Formulations and Uses Oxamyl is a broad-spectrum systemic and contact insecticide, miticide, and nematicide used on many field crops, vegetables, fruits, and ornamentals. Available formulations include a water-soluble liquid and granules.

17.3.16.2 Toxicity to Laboratory Animals

Basic Findings The acute toxicity of oxamyl is summarized in Tables 17.2–17.4. Signs of acute intoxication are characteristic of acetylcholinesterase inhibition. In rabbits, oxamyl caused mild conjunctival irritation and was mildly irritating to the skin. Oxamyl did not produce a skin sensitization reaction in guinea pigs (Kennedy, 1986).

In rats given a single oral dose of oxamyl at 4.86 mg/kg, blood acetylcholinesterase activity was reduced at 5 min postdosing and maximally reduced at 4 hr, returning to normal within 24 hr (Kennedy, 1986). Rabbits dermally exposed to oxamyl at 50 mg/kg (in dimethylformamide) 6 hr daily for 15 days exhibited transitory cholinergic signs for each administration. Treatment had no effect on body or organ weights or on histopathology. In a similar study, rabbits given 10 doses of oxamyl at 50 or 100 mg/kg/day in aqueous methanol showed no treatment-related effects (Kennedy, 1986).

In female rats given oxamyl at dietary levels of 100 ppm or higher for 29 days, acetylcholinesterase activity was decreased in the plasma from day 7 on and in the brain at sacrifice; there were no clear effects on erythrocyte acetylcholinesterase levels. In males, acetylcholinesterase activity was marginally depressed in plasma and erythrocytes. Acetylcholinesterase activity was not affected by oxamyl at 50 ppm (2.5 mg/kg/day) (FAO/WHO, 1981).

Dietary exposure of rats to oxamyl at up to 150 ppm for 90 days caused no clinical cholinergic symptoms and had no effects on hematology, clinical chemistry, or histopathology. At 150 ppm, food consumption was reduced. At dietary levels of 100 ppm and higher, body and organ weights were reduced and urinalysis results were affected. In a 90-day study with dogs, oxamyl in the diet at 150 ppm slightly affected organ weights, but caused no histopathological abnormalities. In a 2-year study with dogs, oxamyl in the diet at 150 ppm reduced hemoglobin content, hematocrit, and red blood cell number; no effects were observed on acetylcholinesterase activity, organ weights, or histopathology. For both subchronic and chronic exposures, a no-effect level for oxamyl in the diet was 100 ppm, equivalent to 2.5 mg/kg/day (FAO/WHO, 1981).

In a 2-year study, rats given oxamyl in the diet at 150 ppm showed decreased food consumption and increased relative organ weights; at 100 ppm, body weight was decreased in both sexes and organ weights were affected in females. Blood acetylcholinesterase activity was decreased only at 150 ppm during the first few days of the study. No hematological, biochemical, or histopathological changes were attributed to oxamyl exposure (FAO/WHO, 1981). A dietary no-effect level for rats was determined to be 50 ppm, equivalent to 2.5 mg/kg/day (FAO/WHO, 1985).

Absorption, Distribution, Metabolism, and Excretion In rats that had received oxamyl in the diet for 18 days or more (about 2.5–7.4 mg/kg/day), a single dose of ^{14}C-labeled oxamyl (2.5–4.6 mg/kg) was degraded by two major pathways. Oxamyl was hydrolyzed to an oximino metabolite (methyl-*N*-hydroxy-*N'*,*N'*-dimethyl-l-thiooxamidate) or converted enzymatically via *N*,*N*-dimethyl-l-cyanoformamide (DMCF) to *N*,*N*-dimethyloxamic acid. Conjugates of the oximino compound, the acid, and their monomethyl derivatives constituted over 70% of the metabolites excreted in the urine and feces (Harvey and Han, 1978). In addition to these metabolites, the organosoluble compounds excreted by mice included oxamyl and methyl *N'*-methyl-*N*-[(methylcarbamoyl)oxy]-l-thiooxamidate (Chang and Knowles, 1979).

Radiolabeled oxamyl was rapidly metabolized *in vitro* in cow rumen fluid (99% within 6 hr). Metabolites were the same as found in the rat, with the addition of *N*,*N*-dimethyloxamide; after 24 hr, 80% of the radioactivity was accounted for by the oximino compound and DMCF (Belasco and Harvey, 1980). No oxamyl or DMCF residues were detected in milk or tissue samples from dairy cows fed oxamyl at up to 20 ppm for 30 days (FAO/WHO, 1981).

In 72 hr, rats eliminated 68–72% of a ^{14}C-labeled dose of oxamyl; 48–61% appeared in the urine and 6–23% in the feces. Less than 0.3% was exhaled as carbon dioxide, but incorporation of $^{14}CO_2$ accounted for more than 50% of the radioactivity remaining in the tissues (Harvey and Han, 1978). Mice injected ip with [^{14}C]oxamyl (1.16 mg/kg) excreted 75.5% of the dose within 6 hr. In 96 hr, 88.7% was excreted in the urine and 7.7% in the feces. Organosoluble radioactive material constituted 24.7% of the total radioactivity in the urine at 6 hr and 6.5% at 72 hr. Tissue activity levels ranged from 11 to 37 ng/g (Chang and Knowles, 1979). When lactating goats were given diets containing 10 ppm [^{14}C]oxamyl for 10 or 20 days, 60–70% of the radioactivity was excreted in the urine and feces, about 6% was expired, and 2–3% appeared in the milk; peak levels in milk were reached after about 10–14 days. No oximino metabolite or oxamyl was found in the milk, blood, or tissues (FAO/WHO, 1981).

Biochemical Effects   Oxamyl did not inhibit rat brain monoamine oxidase *in vitro* (Kadir and Knowles, 1981). Long-term dietary exposure of rats to oxamyl at 150 ppm did not affect aliesterase activity. In 90-day and 2-year studies with dogs, this dietary dosage increased alkaline phosphatase activity and cholesterol, but did not affect aliesterase activity (FAO/WHO, 1981).

Effects on Organs and Tissues   Results of mutagenicity tests with oxamyl are summarized in Section 17.2.3.2. Oxamyl was not carcinogenic to mice at dietary dosages of up to 75 ppm; food consumption and body weight gains were decreased at 50 and 75 ppm, but not at 25 ppm (FAO/WHO, 1985).

Effects on Reproduction   In a three-generation reproduction study with rats, oxamyl at 100 or 150 ppm increased relative testes weight and decreased litter size, viability, lactation, and weanling body weight. Weanling body weight was marginally affected at 50 ppm (the lowest dosage). None of these dosages affected fertility or gestation or produced histopathologic anomalies. Oxamyl at 100–300 ppm on days 6–15 of pregnancy decreased food consumption and body weight in the pregnant rats, but had no embryotoxic or teratogenic effects (FAO/WHO, 1981). In rabbits, oxamyl was not teratogenic at up to 4 mg/kg/day, but this dosage (the highest tested) had fetotoxic effects (FAO/WHO, 1985).

17.3.16.3 Toxicity to Humans

The 1984 FAO/WHO Joint Meeting on Pesticide Residues estimated a human ADI for oxamyl of 0–0.03 mg/kg body weight (FAO/WHO, 1985).

Accidental and Intentional Overexposure   A 53-year-old woman employed in transplanting tobacco plants apparently mistook a jug containing oxamyl for a water jar (evidently failing to notice the labeling, including skull and crossbones symbols on two sides of the square jug). She drank a "swallow" of the clear liquid and within 10 min was semiconscious. Despite reasonably prompt attention in a university medical center, she died 12 hr later (Gelbach and Williams, 1975). Hayes (1982) provided further details of this case. The woman immediately realized her mistake and took some salt water, but apparently without benefit. When she reached the hospital, she was unconscious, incontinent of feces, apneic, and without detectable blood pressure, and her pupils were constricted. Autopsy revealed thrombotic and hemolytic crisis in sickle-cell disease, undoubtedly triggered by the oxamyl; this crisis may have been

the cause of death. The same hospital had a record of a 73-year-old man who ingested oxamyl by mistake but survived.

17.3.17 PHENCYCLOCARB

When phencyclocarb (see Table 17.1) was tested for malaria control, it caused slight to moderate, brief inhibition of cholinesterase but no symptoms among sprayers (Hayes, 1982).

17.3.18 PIRIMICARB

17.3.18.1 Identity, Properties, and Uses

Chemical Name   Pirimicarb is 2-(dimethylamino)-5,6-dimethyl-4-pyrimidinyl *N,N*-dimethylcarbamate. Its structure is shown in Table 17.1.

Synonyms   The name pirimicarb (BSI,ISO) is in general use. Trade names include Abol®, Aficida®, Aphox®, Fernos®, Pirimor®, and Rapid®. A code designation is PP062, and the CAS registry number is 23103-98-2.

Physical and Chemical Properties   Pirimicarb has the empirical formula $C_{11}H_{18}N_4O_2$ and a molecular weight of 238.33. It is a colorless, crystalline solid with a melting point of 90.5°C. Its solubility (grams per liter at 25°C) is 2.75 in water, 230 in methanol, 250 in ethanol, 290 in xylene, 320 in chloroform, and 400 in acetone. Its vapor pressure (mm Hg) is 1.6×10^{-5} at 25°C, 1.7×10^{-4} at 45°C, and 1.8×10^{-3} at 65°C. Pirimicarb is stable for at least 2 years under normal storage conditions.

History, Formulations, and Uses   Pirimicarb was first synthesized in 1965 and was introduced in 1969 as a selective aphicide with contact, translaminar, vapor, and systemic activity (Baranyovits and Ghosh, 1969). It is used on a wide variety of cereal, fruit, and vegetable crops, including sugar beets and potatoes. Pirimicarb formulations include dispersible grains, dispersible powders, emulsifiable concentrates, an aerosol, an ultralow-volume spray, and a smoke generator.

17.3.18.2 Toxicity to Laboratory Animals

Basic Findings   The acute toxicity of pirimicarb is summarized in Tables 17.2–17.4. The symptoms of acute pirimicarb intoxication are typical of acetylcholinesterase inhibition. In rats given single oral doses of pirimicarb from 10 to 15% of the LD 50, blood and brain acetylcholinesterase activity was decreased by 9–25% within 15–30 min after administration (Osicka-Koprowska and Wysocka-Paruszewska, 1983). In a cat given a single iv injection of pirimicarb (20 mg/kg), plasma acetylcholinesterase activity was depressed by 72% within 5 min; this level of depression persisted for at least 4.5 hr, but cholinergic signs disappeared within 1 hr (FAO/WHO, 1977).

Pirimicarb was mildly irritating to the eyes of rabbits, but did not irritate the skin of rabbits or mice. Pirimicarb did not cause a skin sensitization reaction in guinea pigs (FAO/WHO, 1977).

Dermal exposure of rabbits to pirimicarb at 500 mg/kg for 14 days did not produce cholinergic signs. Inhalation exposure of rats for 6 hr to smoke generated from pirimicarb caused mortality at 300 mg/m^3 and clinical signs of intoxication at 75 mg/m^3 but not at 15 mg/m^3. Subchronic exposure to 0.015 mg/liter caused only slight acetylcholinesterase inhibition. Subchronic exposure to a saturated vapor of pirimicarb had to effect on rats (FAO/WHO, 1977).

In subchronic dietary studies with dogs, pirimicarb at dosages of 10 mg/kg/day or higher caused hemolytic anemia. At 50 mg/kg/day (reduced to 25 mg/kg/day) for 16 weeks, reversible changes in blood and bone marrow included reduced hemoglobin, packed cell volume, and erythrocyte count; increases in reticulocytes and normoblasts; and bone marrow hyperplasia. Plasma acetylcholinesterase activity was decreased by 80–90% at 50 mg/kg/day and 50–79% at 25 mg/kg/day. No changes were seen in gross pathology, urinalyses, or various clinical chemistry parameters. The only finding at 2 mg/kg/day was loose feces. Dogs fed pirimicarb at 4 mg/kg/day for 2 years showed a slight increase in nucleated erythrocytes in the bone marrow, but no signs of anemia and no effects on growth, food consumption, behavior, blood chemistry (including acetylcholinesterase activity), urinalyses, gross pathology, or histopathology. A no-effect level for dogs was 1.8 mg/kg/day (FAO/WHO, 1977, 1979).

Rhesus monkeys given pirimicarb orally for 13–17 weeks at 25 mg/kg/day showed a slight reduction in body weight gain. Acetylcholinesterase activity was reduced in the plasma by 63–74% at 25 mg/kg/day, 35% at 7 mg/kg/day, and 8–23% at 2 mg/kg/day, and in the erythrocytes by 31–38% at 25 mg/kg/day, 18% at 7 mg/kg/day, and 16–19% at 2 mg/kg/day. No other treatment-related effects were seen; parameters examined included mortality, behavior, hematology, bone marrow, clinical chemistry, urinalysis, organ weights, and gross examination of organs and tissues. A no-effect level for monkeys was 2 mg/kg/day (FAO/WHO, 1979).

In a 2-year study with rats, growth and plasma acetylcholinesterase activity were reduced at dietary pirimicarb levels of 250–750 ppm, and spleen weight was reduced at 750 ppm. No other treatment-related effects were seen. A no-effect level for rats was 175 ppm in the diet (9 mg/kg/day) (FAO/WHO, 1983).

Absorption, Distribution, Metabolism, and Excretion   Pirimicarb's major urinary metabolites in rats, dogs, and cows were similar, resulting from oxidative and hydrolytic mechanisms and consisting primarily of hydroxypyrimidines with modifications of the alkyl constitutents of the heterocyclic moiety. Of the administered dose, 2-dimethylamino-5,6-dimethyl-4-hydroxypyrimidine accounted for 10–16.3%, 2-methylamino-5,6-dimethyl-4-hydroxypyrimidine for 20.5–41%, 2-amino-5,6-dimethyl-4-hydroxypyrimidine for 12.9–21%, and 2-dimethylamino-6-hydroxymethyl-5-methyl-4-hydroxypyrimidine for 1.8–5.7%. The major metabolites were eliminated unconjugated (FAO/WHO, 1977).

In rats given carbonyl-labeled [^{14}C]pirimicarb by gavage or ip injection, more than 50% of the dose was expired as $^{14}CO_2$ within 5 hr, and 15% was eliminated in the urine; essentially no residues were detected at sacrifice 8 days after administration. Up to four daily administrations of pirimicarb to rats resulted in no accumulation in adipose tissue. In dogs, 86–94% of a ring-^{14}C-labeled dose of pirimicarb was recovered, 79–88% in the urine and 6-7% in the feces; recovery was 74–86% after 1 day. Of a carbonyl-labeled dose to dogs, 15–26% was recovered, primarily in the urine; the unrecovered portion was thought to be expired rapidly as $^{14}CO_2$ hr. Of pirimicarb administered to a lactating dairy cow, 96% of the dose appeared in the urine, 4% in the feces, and less than 0.3% in the milk (FAO/WHO, 1977).

Biochemical Effects   In rats given single oral doses of pirimicarb from 10 to 50% of the LD 50, serum and adrenal cortex corticosterone levels were increased, and adrenal cortex ascorbic acid content was decreased, maximally at 2 hr after administration (Osicka-Koprowska and Wysocka-Paruszewska, 1983).

Single oral doses of pirimicarb to rats (20% of the LD 50) caused significant changes in neurotransmitter levels, beginning within 5 min of administration and lasting up to 30 min. In the brain and heart, serotonin and epinephrine levels increased, while norepinephrine decreased. Dopamine in the brain also increased. Adrenal levels of epinephrine, norepinephrine, and dopamine all decreased (Biel-Zielinska et al., 1983).

Effects on Organs and Tissues   Results of mutagenicity testing with pirimicarb are summarized in Section 17.2.3.2. Pirimicarb was not carcinogenic in a 96-week study with mice at dietary dosages of up to 1600 ppm (FAO/WHO, 1983).

In a 110-week study with dogs, pirimicarb at 25–50 mg/kg/day resulted in decreased hemoglobin, increased reticulocytes, increased serum levels of unconjugated bilirubin, and possible induction of IgG antibodies (Jackson et al., 1977).

Effects on Reproduction   Pirimicarb given by gavage to fasted pregnant rats on day 18 of gestation at 2 or 20 mg/kg depressed acetylcholinesterase activity in both the fetus and the dam at 1 and 5 hr (but not 24 hr) after administration. Effects were seen in the fetal and maternal blood, liver, and brain at the high dose, but not in the maternal brain at the low dose. In preliminary studies, unfasted pregnant rats given pirimicarb at 20 mg/kg showed no acetylcholinesterase depression 5 hr after administration (Cambon et al., 1979). Pirimicarb affected acetylcholinesterase isoenzymes similarly in fetuses and dams (Cambon et al., 1980).

In a three-generation reproduction study with rats, pirimicarb at up to 750 ppm in the diet was not teratogenic and did not affect fertility, gestation, lactation, viability, or growth of pups prior to weaning. Pirimicarb in the diet of mice at 40 or 500 ppm throughout pregnancy was not teratogenic; implantations were slightly reduced at both dosages. Oral exposure of rabbits to pirimicarb at up to 5 mg/kg/day on days 1–28 of gestation had no teratogenic effects; maternal toxicity at dosages of

2.5 mg/kg/day or higher resulted in reduced fetal weights (FAO/WHO, 1977).

Factors Influencing Toxicity Coadministration of pirimicarb and azinphos-methyl to rats by gavage resulted in a slight potentiation of acute toxicity. No potentiation was observed when pirimicarb was administered with carbaryl (FAO/WHO, 1977). Benzonal at a dose of 20 mg/kg and phenobarbital at 14 mg/kg decreased the toxicity of pirimicarb, by less than twofold. In rats and cats, pretreatment with benzonal prevented the development of neuromuscular blockade and normalized spontaneous activity at the myoneural junction (Kagan *et al.*, 1983).

17.3.18.3 Toxicity to Humans

The 1982 FAO/WHO Joint Meeting on Pesticide Residues estimated a human ADI for pirimicarb to be 0–0.02 mg/kg body weight (FAO/WHO, 1983).

Use Experience Workers in the manufacture of formulated pirimicarb products showed transient cholinergic signs and depressed plasma cholinesterase activity. Investigation of plant procedures indicated that the workers had inhaled vapors generated when pirimicarb volatilized at high temperatures (65°C). This occupational exposure had no evident long-term effects (FAO/WHO, 1977).

17.3.19 PROMECARB

When tested for malaria control, promecarb (see Table 17.1) caused cholinesterase inhibition among both sprayers and villagers but no signs or symptoms in either except for contact dermatitis in two male villagers (Hayes, 1972).

17.3.20 PROPOXUR

17.3.20.1 Identity, Properties, and Uses

Chemical Name Propoxur is 2-isopropoxyphenyl-*N*-methylcarbamate. Its structure is shown in Table 17.1.

Synonyms The name propoxur (BSI, ISO) is in general use; in Japan, the common name is PHC. The previously used names aprocarb and arprocarb were withdrawn. Propoxur has also been called IMPC and IPMC. Trade names have included Baygon®, Blattanex®, Invisi-Gard®, Propogon®, Sendra®, Sendran®, Suncide®, Tendex®, Tugon Fliegenkugel®, Unden®, and Undene®. Code designations have included BAY 39007, BAY 9010, BO 58 12315, ENT 25671, and OMS 33. The CAS registry number is 114-26-1.

Physical and Chemical Properties Propoxur has the empirical formula $C_{11}H_{15}NO_3$ and a molecular weight of 209.24. The pure material is a white crystalline powder with a faint odor and a melting point of 91.5°C. Its vapor pressure (mm Hg) is 6.5 $\times$ 10^6 at 20°C and 0.01 at 120°C. The technical material is a white to cream-colored crystalline powder with a milk phenolic odor and a melting point of 86–89°C. The solubility of propoxur in water at 20°C is 0.2%. It is soluble in methanol, acetone, and many other organic solvents, but only slightly soluble in cold hydrocarbons. Propoxur is unstable in alkaline media and has a half-life at pH 10 of 40 min.

History, Formulations, and Uses Propoxur was introduced in 1959. It is a nonsystemic insecticide used primarily against household insect pests and pests of domestic animals. Its use for malaria control has tended to emphasize its high vapor toxicity to mosquitoes. It also shows nonsystemic action against some agricultural pests. Propoxur is formulated as wettable powders, dusts, granules, emulsifiable concentrates, pressurized sprays, baits, and an oil fog concentrate.

17.3.20.2 Toxicity to Laboratory Animals

Basic Findings The acute toxicity of propoxur is summarized in Tables 17.2–17.4. Signs of acute intoxication are typical of acetylcholinesterase inhibition.

In rats exposed for 6 hr to aerosols of propoxur, plasma and erythrocyte acetylcholinesterase activities were significantly depressed only at concentrations of 78 mg/m³ or higher, and cholinergic symptoms were seen only at 172 mg/m³. At 30 mg/m³, acetylcholinesterase activity was mildly depressed, and no effect was seen at concentrations of 9 mg/m³ or lower (Machemer *et al.*, 1982).

After a single 2-mg/kg ip injection of propoxur to mice, acetylcholinesterase inhibition was maximal at 15 min (47% inhibition in the brain and 54% in the blood), and recovery took approximately 4 hr (Ruppert *et al.*, 1983). In mice given a single 2-mg/kg sc injection of propoxur, acetylcholinesterase activity decreased by about 50% in the forebrain and 30% in the blood within 10 min. Activity returned to normal by 60 min after administration (Kobayashi *et al.*, 1985). A single 10-mg/kg sc injection of propoxur to mice reduced forebrain acetylcholinesterase activity by 50–26% from 10 to 180 min after administration, accompanied by increases in forebrain acetylcholine content of up to 78%. Ten daily 5-mg/kg doses did not affect these parameters 24 hr after the final injection (Kajita *et al.*, 1983).

In a study of the time course of acetylcholinesterase inhibition, rats were given propoxur as a single 5-mg/kg iv injection, a single 50-mg/kg oral dose, or 14 doses of 30 mg/kg/day followed by 28 doses of 50 mg/kg/day. Following iv administration, acetylcholinesterase activity was lowest (about 30% inhibition in the blood and 45% in the brain) after 5 min and recovered within 2 hr. A single oral administration produced maximal inhibition (by more than 60%) in the blood after 15 min and in the brain after 30 min; acetylcholinesterase activity recovered in the brain within 2 hr, but was still somewhat depressed in the blood after 12 hr. In the blood, acetylcholinesterase activity was correlated with propoxur levels following both iv and oral administration; in the brain, the correlation was seen only for iv administration. During subacute exposure, acetylcholinesterase activity gradually recovered despite continued dosing; recovery was complete within 28 days in the brain and 42 days in the blood. In a dose–response study employing single oral doses of 2.1–70.0 mg/kg, both degree and duration of acetylcholinesterase inhibition were related to dose (Krechniak and Foss, 1982).

Subchronic (12-week) inhalation exposure of rats to propoxur produced acetylcholinesterase depression in the plasma, erythrocytes, and brain at a concentration of 31.7 mg/m^3, but not at 10.7 mg/m^3 (Kimmerle and Iyatomi, 1976).

Rats given propoxur in their diet at 2000 ppm (less than 100 mg/kg/day) for 16 weeks showed reduced food consumption. At 1000 ppm, brain and blood acetylcholinesterase activity was depressed and histological changes were seen in the liver. Dietary levels of 500 ppm (about 25 mg/kg/day) did not affect these parameters or a number of other clinical laboratory measurements (Syrowatka *et al.*, 1971). Similar results were reported by others for rats and dogs (FAO/WHO, 1974; Jurek, 1978). Mice injected ip with propoxur at 20 mg/kg/day for 20 days showed hypertrophy of the intestinal epithelium, decreased size and vacuolation of liver cells, and increased size of nuclei of the neurosecretory neurocytes and the hypothalamus (Jordan *et al.*, 1975). Dogs given propoxur in their diet for 2 years showed reduced body weight at a concentration of 2000 ppm, but not at 750 ppm (Nelson *et al.*, 1984).

In a 2-year study with rats, propoxur in the diet at 750 ppm resulted in increased liver weight; a no-effect level was 250 ppm (Nelson *et al.*, 1984). In a 2-year study with mice, propoxur reduced body weight at a dietary level of 6000 ppm, but not at 2000 ppm (Nelson *et al.*, 1984).

Absorption, Distribution, Metabolism, and Excretion The half-time for *in vivo* gastric absorption of intubated propoxur by fasted mice was 8 min. Of a 1-mg/kg ring-^{14}C-labeled dose, about 25% was absorbed within 1 min, 48% in 5 min, and 74% in 60 min, by which time about half the radioactivity had been excreted in the urine and a trace amount expired as $^{14}CO_2$ (Ahdaya *et al.*, 1981).

After iv administration of 5 mg/kg radiolabeled propoxur to rats, blood and tissue concentrations were maximal at 5 min, and the half-time for elimination from the tissues was 11–16 min. Levels were consistently higher in the kidneys than in blood, liver, or brain. The metabolite 2-isopropoxyphenol was detected in the tissues within 10 min and peaked between 30 and 60 min after administration. After oral administration at 50 mg/kg, peak concentrations were seen in the blood at 15 min, the brain at 1 hr, the liver at 4 hr, and the kidneys at 6 hr. Levels were lowest in the brain and highest in the kidneys (the only tissue in which propoxur was detected 24 hr after administration) (Foss and Krechniak, 1980). Similar results were found following daily oral doses of 30–50 mg/kg/day for 6 weeks (Krechniak and Foss, 1983).

Five daily oral doses of propoxur to rats at up to 30 mg/kg/day did not induce the liver microsomal enzymes aminopyrine-*N*-demethylase, cytochrome P-450, or *p*-nitroanisole-O-de-

methylase (Nelson *et al.*, 1984). In studies with rats, propoxur was metabolized primarily to 2-hydroxyphenyl *N*-methylcarbamate and 2-isopropoxyphenol; minor metabolites included 5-hydroxy propoxur and *N*-hydroxymethyl propoxur (Krishna and Casida, 1966; Oonnithan and Casida, 1968; unpublished report cited by Machemer *et al.*, 1982). In the urine of rats subchronically exposed to propoxur, it and 2-isopropoxyphenol appeared to be eliminated as sulfate complexes (Krechniak and Foss, 1983).

Following acute inhalation exposure of rats to propoxur, the relationship of urinary excretion of 2-isopropoxyphenol to propoxur concentration was nearly linear. This metabolite was found in the urine 3 days after termination of exposure to 78 mg/m^3, 2 days after exposure to 9 mg/m^3, and 24 hr after exposure to 0.4 mg/m^3 (Machemer *et al.*, 1982). Subchronic dietary exposure to lead (at 200–600 mg/kg/day) did not affect the rate at which ring-labeled propoxur was eliminated by rats (Abd-Elraof *et al.*, 1981).

Biochemical Effects Six daily oral 1.2-mg doses of propoxur to rats reversibly stimulated oxidative miochondrial deamination of 2-phenylethylamine in the brain and liver, with a selective effect on B-type monoamine oxidase. This effect was also observed *in vitro*. Oxidation of serotonin and tyramine were not affected by propoxur (Zĕinalov, 1984, 1985). Propoxur given ip to rats at 8 mg/kg inhibited liver carboxylesterase activity (with *o*-nitrophenyl butyrate as substrate) to about 46% of control and acetanilide amidase activity to about 14% of control (Iverson, 1977). Popov and Ribarova (1979) reported that daily peroral administration of propoxur at 0.1 LD 50 resulted in increased transport and decreased resorption of glucose in the small intestines of rats. In mice, both single 10-mg/kg and repeated 5-mg/kg/day sc injections of propoxur decreased brain homogenate high-affinity choline uptake and [^{3}H]quinuclidinyl benzilate binding (Kajita *et al.*, 1983).

Effects on Organs and Tissues The results of mutagenicity testing with propoxur are summarized in Section 17.2.3.2. Propoxur did not cause transformation of hamster fetal cells in a transplacental assay (Quarles *et al.*, 1979a).

Effects on Reproduction In a three-generation reproduction study, propoxur at 6000 ppm in the diet reduced parental food consumption and growth, lactation, litter size, and growth of the pups. Effects at 2000 ppm were similar except that litter size was normal; dietary levels of 750 ppm and less did not affect fertility, litter size, or lactation. No malformations or histological abnormalities were found (FAO/WHO, 1974). In another three-generation study, propoxur at 3200 ppm also increased parental mortality and reduced pup survival, because of abandonment by the dams. Dietary levels of 100 ppm and higher were reported to increase time from mating to first delivery (Tyrkiel and Bojanowska, 1978).

Propoxur at up to 10,000 ppm in the diet of rats during gestation was not teratogenic, but reduced the number of fetuses and increased the number of resorption sites. At dosages of 3000 ppm and higher, growth of the pups was reduced and the parents were adversely affected (FAO/WHO, 1974). Studies in mice also revealed no teratological effect of propoxur at oral or ip dosages as high as 31 mg/kg/day on days 4 and 13 of gestation, which produced some embryotoxicity. Dosages of up to 10.5 mg/kg were not embryotoxic (Tyrkiel, 1978). Propoxur administered intragastrically to rats at 5–50 mg/kg/day on days 7–19 of gestation or to mice at 5–40 mg/kg on days 6–16 of gestation had no teratogenic or fetotoxic effects and did not increase fetal mortality, even at dosages toxic to the dams. In mice, a dosage of 60 mg/kg/day resulted in 70% maternal mortality and increased the mortality and decreased the weight of pups of surviving dams (Courtney *et al.*, 1985). In another study with rats, oral doses of 34 mg/kg on days 7–19 of gestation decreased maternal serum calcium and magnesium levels, decreased fetus weight, increased fetal skeletal anomalies by about 50%, and affected ossification (Roszkowski, 1982).

Among the neonatal offspring of rats fed propoxur at 1000 ppm from day 2 of gestation through weaning or from day 6 of gestation through day 15 of lactation, birth weight was reduced, development of the startle reflex was delayed, and changes were evident in electroencephalograms and visual evoked potentials, indicating some degree of CNS impairment. Litter viability and onset of the righting reflex were not affected (Rosenstein and Chernoff, 1976, 1978).

Factors Influencing Toxicity Toxicity was not potentiated when propoxur and malathion were orally coadministered to mice (Miyata and Saito, 1981). Mice given propoxur in their drinking water at concentrations increasing from 50 to 2000 ppm over 6 weeks developed tolerance to propoxur, as indicated by an increase in the LD 50 from 25.4 to 44.5 mg/kg. Tolerant animals showed induction of hepatic microsomal enzymes but not resistance to the cholinergic agonists carbachol and oxotremorine, decreased binding of [^{3}H]quinuclidinyl benzilate, or enhanced carboxylesterase activity (Costa *et al.*, 1981a,b). Rats given carbaryl in the diet at 2000 ppm for 60 days also developed tolerance to the toxic effect of propoxur; cytochrome P-450 content of their livers was increased (Neskovic, 1979). The acute ip toxicity of propoxur was reduced by prior treatment with phenobarbital and increased by prior treatment with SKF 525A (Neskovic *et al.*, 1978). Tolerance was suggested to be due to enhanced metabolic detoxification (Costa *et al.*, 1982). Mice made tolerant to propoxur showed cross-tolerance to the organophosphate disulfoton, but prior exposure to disulfoton potentiated the effects of propoxur, possibly by inhibition of carboxylesterase (Costa and Murphy, 1983). The acute toxicity of propoxur was decreased in rats given Aroclor 1242 for 30 days (Neskovic *et al.*, 1984).

The acute oral toxicity of propoxur was increased 1.3- to 4.3-fold in rats previously fed diets low in casein (4.5%, instead of 26% in diets with normal protein). The effects of subchronic dietary exposure to propoxur (at 4500 and 9000 ppm) on several biochemical parameters of the liver, serum, and brain (including acetylcholinesterase activity) were greater in the protein-deficient rats (Pużyńska, 1977, 1980).

17.3.20.3 Toxicity to Humans

The 1973 FAO/WHO Joint Meeting on Pesticide Residues estimated an ADI for propoxur of 0–0.02 mg/kg body weight (FAO/WHO, 1974).

Experimental Exposures A 42-year-old male volunteer ingested propoxur at 1.5 mg/kg body weight about 2 hr after a light breakfast. Erythrocyte acetylcholinesterase activity reached a minimum (27% of normal) 15 min after administration, at which time no cholinergic signs were observed, but discomfort described as "pressure in the head" was reported. Blurred vision and nausea developed 3 min later. After 20 min, the volunteer was pale and sweating; his pulse rate had increased from 76 to 140 per minute and his blood pressure from 135/90 to 175/95 mm Hg. Pronounced nausea, repeated vomiting, and profuse sweating developed within the next 10 min and lasted, with no change in intensity, until about 45 min after administration. During this period, erythrocyte acetylcholinesterase activity increased from 50 to 56% of its normal value. One hour after administration, the volunteer was feeling better and sweating less, but still felt nauseated and tired. Ten minutes later, his pulse and blood pressure were normal. Erythrocyte acetylcholinesterase activity reached about 95% or normal 2 hr after administration (at which time the volunteer felt well) and was normal 1 hr later. Plasma acetylcholinesterase remained entirely normal throughout the study (Vandekar *et al.*, 1971).

In the case just described, the persistence of inhibitor in the blood was determined by using plasma from the volunteer to inhibit erythrocyte acetylcholinesterase *in vitro;* the molar concentrations of propoxur were $5.0 \times 10^{-7}, 3.2 \times 10^{-7}$, and 1.5×10^{-7}, respectively, in plasma collected 0.5, 2.0, and 7.5 hr after ingestion. This rate of decrease did not correspond fully to the rate of excretion; 81% of the total amount recovered from the urine in the form of *o*-propoxyphenol was found in the first two samples, collected within 4.75 hr after ingestion. The total recovered from the urine corresponded to about 45% of the dose. It was assumed that part of the dose was vomited before it could be absorbed.

In another volunteer study, a single 0.36-mg/kg dose of propoxur produced a rapid fall in erythrocyte acetylcholinesterase to 57% of normal within 10 min and also produced abdominal discomfort, blurred vision, and moderate facial redness and sweating, lasting about 5 min. Acetylcholinesterase activity recovered to normal within 3 hr. When volunteers received dosages as high as 0.20 mg/kg every half-hour, for a total dose of 1.0 mg/kg, they were symptomless even though their maximum erythrocyte acetylcholinesterase inhibition was just as great (Vandekar *et al.*, 1971). In another study, volunteers who took doses of up to about 1.6 mg/kg before going to bed reported no untoward effects (Dawson *et al.*, 1964).

In an excretion study, three male volunteers given 50 mg

(about 0.71 mg/kg) of propoxur orally experienced no ill effects, but excreted 27.4% of the dose as 2-isopropoxyphenol in the urine the next morning (8–10 hr after administration) and 2.3% in the sample voided at noon, corresponding to concentrations of 17.9 and 2.8 ppm of 2-isopropoxyphenol. In another experiment, two men took 110 and 116 mg of the carbamate without untoward reaction. According to a nonspecific colorimetric test, they excreted more phenol in their morning urine than is likely to be excreted by persons with a normal diet. Thus, the gas chromatographic test was specific and the colorimetric test was sensitive to a dose of about 1 mg/kg of the insecticide (Dawson *et al.*, 1964).

In volunteers who received an application of radiolabeled propoxur to their ventral forearms, radioactivity was present in the urine within 4 hr, reached its greatest concentration in 8–12 hr, decreased to a low level by 48 hr, and continued at essentially this same level for more than 96 hr (Feldmann and Maibach, 1974). The average total radioactivity recovered from the urine following iv injection of propoxur was 83.8%; thus, the corrected average of 15.9% for dermal absorption must represent a good estimate of the proportion of this dose.

A 4-hr exposure to propoxur at an average concentration of 3 mg/m^3 had no overt effects on four human volunteers and did not inhibit acetylcholinesterase activity in the erythrocytes or plasma. In the 24 hr after the start of the exposure, from 2 to 4 mg of the major metabolite 2-isopropoxyphenol appeared in the urine; only trace amounts were detected after 48 hr. Detection of 2-isopropoxyphenol in the urine was proposed as a sensitive indicator of propoxur exposure (Machemer *et al.*, 1982).

Accidental and Intentional Overexposure   In one suicide case, a 36-year-old man was thought to have ingested 200 ml of a propoxur formulation of unspecified concentration. Only 10 mg of atropine was administered on the first day; the amount used on subsequent days varied from 22 to 55 mg/day. Both 2-PAM and obidoxime were administered. The patient died after 5 days without regaining consciousness. In another suicide attempt, a 32-year-old man survived ingestion of what was thought to be 150 ml of an unspecified formulation. He responded promptly to relatively small doses of atropine (Bomirska and Winiarska, 1972).

In a third case of attempted suicide, a comatose 39-year-old woman was brought to the emergency room of a hospital. Her pupils were pinpoint and unresponsive to light; white, frothy secretions were bubbling from her mouth; and rales, wheezes, and rhonchi were heard in her chest. An electrocardiogram revealed a sinus rate of 120 per minute and complete right-bundle branch block. Erythrocyte and plasma acetylcholinesterase levels (measured by the Michel method) were 0.50 and 0.81 $\triangle$pH/hr, within the normal range, and obviously did not reflect her condition. The patient did not respond to a small dose of atropine (1.2 mg iv over 10 min), although her pulse rate increased slightly. She also failed to respond to 6.5 mg of nalorphine hydrochloride, presumably given on the as-

sumption that she might have taken a narcotic. The patient was intubated, suctioned vigorously and frequently, and provided with oxygen. Eighteen hours after admission, propoxur and its main metabolite were identified in the gastric aspirate, but atropine was not administered because the patient had regained consciousness and no longer suffered from pulmonary edema. She eventually admitted having taken an unspecified amount of an "unknown insecticide" (Salisbury *et al.*, 1974).

Use Experience   Propoxur was subjected to several village trials during 1962–1966 and then to operational field trials in El Salvador (1966–1967), Iran (1967), and Nigeria (1967). The tests, conducted under medical supervision, involved 4000 person-days of spraying and employed over 30 metric tons of water-wettable powder. Recommended safety measures were limited to simple protective clothing and good personal hygiene. When work was not up to standard, the frequency of reactions rose. These reactions consisted of nausea, headache, excessive sweating, and general weakness. Brief removal from exposure led to such rapid recovery that the men could return to work in 30 min to an hour without recurrence of illness. Recovery was more rapid if the men washed contaminated skin. There were no serious cases of overexposure, but mild illness occurred in nearly all groups of sprayers and in some inhabitants of sprayed homes. In one of the tests, involving only 21 sprayers, the 4 sprayers who developed symptoms (including nausea, vertigo, vomiting, and tachycardia) did so from 1 to 7 days after contact (Montazemi, 1969). Because there is so much contrary evidence, the possibility of recent reexposure or misdiagnosis must be considered in this instance, especially because the symptoms were nonspecific. In El Salvador, some small children showed reactions when they crawled on floors that had been sprayed but not swept. In Iran, villagers who complained of transient cholinergic symptoms (headache, sweating, nausea, and vomiting) were often those who had violated instructions by entering houses during or immediately after spraying or by sweeping floors with an insufficient amount of water. Although the concentration of propoxur vapor frequently was high enough in sprayed homes or even in entire villages to kill malaria mosquitoes, no adverse effects on the inhabitants due to inhalation of vapor were observed (Vandekar and Svetličić, 1966; WHO, 1967, 1973; Vandekar *et al.*, 1968; Wright *et al.*, 1969; Motabar, 1971).

Sprayers who regularly used propoxur for malaria control showed a pronounced daily fall in whole blood acetylcholinesterase activity during work and a distinct recovery after exposure stopped. No cumulative inhibitory effect could be demonstrated. Erythrocyte acetylcholinesterase was much more sensitive than plasma enzyme. In view of the marked symptomless daily fluctuation of acetylcholinesterase activity and the absence of a cumulative inhibitory effect, routine acetylcholinesterase determinations could not be used as an early indication of excessive exposure. Instead, minor complaints, from which the men recovered in 2–3 hours, served as an early indication of overexposure (Vandekar *et al.*, 1968).

17.3.21 THIODICARB

17.3.21.1 Identity, Properties, and Uses

Chemical Name Thiodicarb is dimethyl N,N'-{thiobis-[(methylimino)carbonyloxy]}-bis(ethanimidothioate). Its structure is shown in Fig. 17.1.

Synonyms The name thiodicarb (ANSI, BSI, ISO) is in general use. Trade names are Larvin® and Nivral™, and a code designation is UC 51762. The CAS registry number is 59669-26-0.

Physical and Chemical Properties Thiodicarb has the empirical formula $C_{10}H_{18}N_4O_4S_3$ and a molecular weight of 354.5. The technical material is a white to light tan crystalline powder with a slightly sulfurous odor. The melting point is 168–174°C, and the vapor pressure is 4.3×10^5 mm Hg at 20°C. The solubility of thiodicarb (w/w at 25°C) is 35 ppm in water, 0.3% in xylene, 0.5% in methanol, 0.8% in acetone, and 15.0% in dichloromethane. It is stable under normal storage conditions, but degrades at temperatures above 60°C.

History, Formulations, and Uses Thiodicarb is a contact insecticide for control of major lepidopterous, coleopterous, and hemipterous pests on a variety of crops. Thiodicarb is available in aqueous flowable, wettable powder, dry flowable, bait, and dust formulations.

17.3.21.2 Toxicity to Laboratory Animals

Except as otherwise indicated, toxicological information is proprietary data developed by Union Carbide Agricultural Products Company, Inc. (1984) and the property of Rhône-Poulenc Ag Company.

Basic Findings The acute toxicity of thiodicarb is summarized in Tables 17.2–17.4. Signs of acute toxicity are typical of acetylcholinesterase inhibition. Thiodicarb did not irritate the skin of rabbits, producing only slight erythema in a few individuals, and did not cause a skin sensitization reaction in guinea pigs. In rabbits, thiodicarb caused temporary eye irritation, but no eye damage; in monkeys, neither irritation nor damage was observed.

A 24-hr ED 50 for erythrocyte acetylcholinesterase inhibition by thiodicarb applied to 25 mc² shaved skin of rats was 33.3 mg/kg. Inhibition was the same after dermal doses of 400 and 800 μg/cm² (Knaak and Wilson, 1985).

In rabbits dermally exposed to thiodicarb for 3 weeks at 4000 mg/kg/day, body weight was depressed and liver weight was increased; no gross or histopathologic lesions were seen, and acetylcholinesterase activity was not affected in the erythrocytes, plasma, or brain. Dosages of 1000–4000 mg/kg/day induced a dose-related macrocytic anemia; no hematological effects were seen at dosages of 500 mg/kg/day or less. Soft feces or diarrhea were seen at dosages of 1000 mg/kg/day or

higher. Thiodicarb at dosages of up to 400 mg/kg/day did not affect body weight or food consumption.

In rats exposed to thiodicarb dust by inhalation 6 hr/day for 9 days, body weight was depressed at concentrations of 20 mg/m³ or higher. Miosis and tremors were observed at concentrations of 48 mg/m³ or higher; however, acetylcholinesterase levels were not significantly depressed at concentrations of up to 200 mg/m³. The only other effect seen at 48 mg/m³ was a slight decrease in kidney weight.

In a 28-day study with rats, thiodicarb in the diet reduced plasma and erythrocyte acetylcholinesterase activity at 30 mg/kg/day, but not at 10 mg/kg/day (Union Carbide, 1984).

In dogs given thiodicarb at about 1500 ppm in the diet (38.3 mg/kg/day for males and 39.5 mg/kg/day for females) for 1 year, relative liver and spleen weights were increased, and acetylcholinesterase activity was decreased by more than 25% in the plasma, erythrocytes, and brain. Erythrocyte acetylcholinesterase activity also was transiently decreased at a dosage of 487 ppm. No other effects were observed on body or organ weights, food and water consumption, mortality, hematology, clinical chemistry, ophthalmology, gross pathology, or histopathology. A no-effect level was 487 ppm (12.8 mg/kg/day for males and 13.8 mg/kg/day for females) (Hamada, 1986).

In rats, thiodicarb in the diet for 2 years at dosages of up to 10 mg/kg/day had no effect on food consumption, organ weights, or acetylcholinesterase activity. Effects observed at 10 mg/kg/day were reduced body weight gain and increased incidence of certain nonneoplastic lesions, including pituitary cysts, thymic epithelial hyperplasia, and hemosiderosis of the mediastinal lymph nodes. At dosages of 3 mg/kg/day or higher, males also showed an increased incidence of prostatitis and hepatocellular hyperplasia. No treatment-related histopathological effects were seen in animals sacrificed after up to 19 months of thiodicarb exposure. A no-effect level, based on decreased body weight, was 3 mg/kg/day. In a similar 2-year study with mice, no effects were seen on food consumption or body weight gain at dosages of up to 10 mg/kg/day. During the last 2 months of the study, mortality was increased at 10 mg/kg/day; no effect was seen at 3 mg/kg/day.

Absorption, Distribution, Metabolism, and Excretion In a percutaneous absorption study with rats, about 22% of an applied dose of radiolabeled thiodicarb (in acetone) had penetrated the shaved skin 168 hr after administration. Thiodicarb was absorbed through the skin at rates varying from 0.27 to 0.42 μg/hr/cm² (Knaak and Wilson, 1985).

In rats, thiodicarb was rapidly degraded to methomyl, which was rapidly converted to methomyl methylol, oxime, sulfoxide, and sulfoxide oxime. These unstable intermediates were converted to acetonitrile and carbon dioxide, which were eliminated primarily by respiration and in the urine; a small fraction of the acetonitrile was further degraded to acetamide, acetic acid, and CO_2 (Huhtanen and Dorough, 1976). (Metabolism of methomyl is discussed in Section 17.3.14.2.)

In rats given a single oral dose of [¹⁴C]thiodicarb, 80% of the radioactivity was eliminated within 48 hr. After 4 days, 48% of the dose had been eliminated in the respiratory gases, 32% in the urine, and 4.5% in the feces; 11% remained in the carcass, via incorporation of $^{14}CO_2$ and acetic acid metabolites into natural products. In a dairy cow given a single oral dose of thiodicarb, 66% of the radioactivity was eliminated in the respiratory gases, 11% in the feces, 5% in the urine, and 4.6% in the milk, with 10% remaining in the carcass. The ratio of $^{14}CO_2$ to acetonitrile in the respiratory gases was 1 : 1 in the rat and 8 : 1 in the cow. When dairy cows were given radiolabeled thiodicarb at up to 100 ppm in the diet for 21 days, no carbamate residues were found in the milk or body tissue samples at any time.

Biochemical Effects   In a 6-month study with dogs, thiodicarb in the diet at 45 mg/kg/day resulted in elevated levels of SGPT, decreased levels of calcium, total protein, and globulin, and increased ratios of albumin to globulin.

Effects on Organs and Tissues   The results of mutagenicity testing with thiodicarb are summarized in Section 17.2.3.2. In 2-year studies, dietary exposure to thiodicarb at dosages of up to 10 mg/kg/day did not cause tumors in rats or mice (Union Carbide, 1984). A case study of the U.S. EPA's application of the Delaney Clause of the Federal Food, Drug and Cosmetic Act (prohibiting approval of any food additive found to be oncogenic in animals or humans) describes the rationale by which the agency calculated dietary risks from the metabolite acetamide and issued Section-409 tolerances for thiodicarb on crops used for animal feed (Wiles, 1987).

Effects on Reproduction   In a three-generation reproduction study with rats, thiodicarb in the diet at up to 10 mg/kg/day had no effect on any reproductive parameter, including fertility, gestation, viability, and lactation. Thiodicarb was not teratogenic when administered in the diet or by gavage to pregnant rats at up to 100 mg/kg/day throughout gestation, on days 6–15, or on days 6–19. Although dosages of 40 mg/kg/day or higher were maternally toxic, the only effects observed in the fetuses were dose-related reductions in body weight and ossification. thiodicarb was not teratogenic or fetotoxic when administered orally to mice on days 6–16 of gestation at up to 200 mg/kg/day or to rabbits on days 6–19 at up to 40 mg/kg/day (maternally toxic dosages in both cases) (Union Carbide, 1984; Rodwell, 1986).

17.3.21.3 Toxicity to Humans

The 1986 FAO/WHO Joint Meeting on Pesticide Residues estimated a human ADI for thiodicarb of 0–0.03 mg/kg body weight (FAO/WHO, 1986b).

Experimental Exposures   In tests with human subjects, thiodicarb did not produce allergic sensitization following repeated dermal contact (Union Carbide, 1984).

17.3.22 TRIMETHACARB

17.3.22.1 Identity, Properties, and Uses

Chemical Name   Trimethacarb is a 4 : 1 mixture of the 3,4,5- and 2,3,5- isomers of trimethylphenyl *N*-methylcarbamate. Its structure is shown in Table 17.1.

Synonyms   The common name trimethacarb is in general use. Trade names include Broot® and, formerly, Landrin®, and code designations are UC 27867 and SD 8530. The CAS registry numbers are 58784-13-7 for trimethacarb, 2686-99-9 for the 3,4,5- isomer, and 2655-15-4 for the 2,3,5- isomer.

Physical and Chemical Properties   Trimethacarb has the empirical formula $C_{11}H_{15}NO_2$ and a molecular weight of 193.25. The technical material is a buff to brown crystalline flaked powder with a mild ester odor. The melting point is 105–114°C, and the vapor pressure is 5.0×10^5 mm Hg at 23°C. Trimethacarb is not readily soluble in organic solvents, and its solubility in water at 23°C is 58 ppm. It is stable under normal storage conditions.

History, Formulations, and Uses   Trimethacarb is an insecticide and molluscicide used to control corn rootworm larvae and a wide variety of other insect pests, snails, and slugs. It is formulated as granules and a wettable powder.

17.3.22.2 Toxicity to Laboratory Animals

Except as otherwise indicated, toxicological information is proprietary data developed by Union Carbide Agricultural Products Company, Inc. (Dodd, 1987a) and the property of Rhône-Poulenc Ag Company.

Basic Findings   The acute toxicity of trimethacarb is summarized in Tables 17.2 and 17.3. Symptoms of acute toxicity are typical of acetylcholinesterase inhibition. Trimethacarb did not cause skin irritation in rabbits or an allergic skin sensitization reaction in guinea pigs. In rabbits' eyes, trimethacarb produced transient mild conjunctival irritation. One-hour exposure of rats to a saturated vapor atmosphere of trimethacarb resulted in no mortality or effects on body weights, organs, or tissues.

Dermal exposure of rabbits to trimethacarb at up to 1000 mg/kg/day for 3 weeks produced no treatment-related effects other than a slight increase in liver weight at the highest dosage.

In a 90-day study with rats, the only trimethacarb-related effects observed at dietary concentrations of up to 1200 ppm were depression of body weight, food and water consumption, and acetylcholinesterase activity in the plasma and erythrocytes. No effects were seen on ophthalmology, hematology, clinical chemistry, urinalyses, gross pathology, histopathology, organ weights, or brain acetylcholinesterase activity. A no-effect level was 300 ppm (19 mg/kg/day for males and 21 mg/kg/day for females). In a similar 90-day study with mice, trimethacarb in the diet at up to 1200 ppm had no effects other than depression of body weight and acetylcholinesterase activity in the plasma and erythrocytes. A no-effect level, based on marginal depression of acetylcholinesterase activity in females, was 600 ppm (119 mg/kg/day for males and 138 mg/kg/day for females).

In a 1-year study with dogs, trimethacarb at 2000 ppm in the diet resulted in slight body weight decreases, tremors, death of 1 of 12 dogs, and acetylcholinesterase inhibition in the plasma, erythrocytes, and brain. At 800 ppm, plasma acetylcholinesterase activity was reduced, but no effects were seen on clinical hematology, urinalyses, ophthalmology, water consumption, organ weights, or gross and microscopic tissue evaluations. A no-effect level was 200 ppm (4.9 mg/kg/day for males and 4.6 mg/kg/day for females). In a similar 2-year study, trimethacarb in the diet at 2500 ppm caused body weight loss, decreased food consumption, and inhibition of plasma acetylcholinesterase by up to 57%; 4 of 10 dogs were sacrificed in moribund condition and showed brain acetylcholinesterase depression. At 1250 ppm, plasma acetylcholinesterase was depressed by 17–31%. No effects on tissues were seen at up to 2500 ppm.

In a 2-year study with rats, trimethacarb at dietary concentrations of up to 800 ppm had no effects on mortality, body or organ weights, food consumption, hematology, acetylcholinesterase activity, or gross or microscopic characteristics of tissues at dietary concentrations of up to 800 ppm. In the first year of a large ongoing 2-year rat study, the only effects observed have been slight body weight reduction and inhibition of blood acetylcholinesterase activity at a dosage of 1000 ppm and decreased water consumption and urine volume, along with increased urine specific gravity, at dosages of 350 ppm or higher. In a similar 1-year study with mice, food consumption was decreased at a dosage of 1200 ppm, and body weights were slightly depressed at dosages of 600 ppm or higher. No effects were observed on acetylcholinesterase activity, serum chemistries, organ weights, or histopathologic findings.

Absorption, Distribution, Metabolism, and Excretion In mice given ^{14}C-labeled preparations of trimethylphenyl methylcarbamates by gavage, each isomer formed 15–20 metabolites. Hydrolytic and nonhydrolytic metabolic routes were about equally important. With carbonyl-labeled isomers, urinary metabolites included glucuronide or sulfate conjugates; 17–35% of the radioactivity was expired as CO_2 and 42–45% was excreted in the urine within 48 hr of administration (Slade and Casida, 1970). In rats given repeated doses of carbonyl-labeled 3,4,5-isomer over 3–10 days, expired CO_2 accounted for 70% of the dose. With N-methyl-labeled 3,4,5-isomer, most of the dose was excreted in the urine, primarily as conjugates (Dodd, 1987a).

Effects on Organs and Tissues Results of mutagenicity testing with trimethacarb are summarized in Section 17.2.3.2. In a transplacental host-mediated hamster cell culture system, trimethacarb induced morphologic transformation of cells (Quarles *et al.*, 1979a,b). However, trimethacarb did not cause tumors in rats at dietary concentrations of up to 800 ppm in a 2-

year study or up to 1000 ppm in the first year of another 2-year study. Trimethacarb was not carcinogenic to mice at up to 1000 ppm in the diet for 1 year (Dodd, 1987a).

Effects on Reproduction In rats, trimethacarb did not affect any indices of reproduction, including fertility, gestation, viability, or lactation, in a three-generation reproduction study at dietary concentrations of up to 800 ppm (Dodd, 1987a) and in a two-generation study at dietary concentrations of up to 1000 ppm (maternally toxic dosages) (Tyl and Dodd, 1987). No teratogenic or embryotoxic effects were observed when trimethacarb was given to rats by gavage on days 6–16 of gestation at up to 30 mg/kg/day; this dosage caused maternal toxicity and delayed ossification in the fetuses. A similar teratogenicity study in rabbits gave negative results at dosages of up to 50 mg/kg/day (a maternally toxic dosage) on days 6–18 of gestation (Dodd, 1987a).

17.3.22.3 Toxicity to Humans

Two trials for malaria control carried out in Nigeria with Landrin® lasted for 2 and 4 days, respectively. There were no complaints among the operators and residents, although in one of the trials a water shortage prevented operators from washing and bathing after work as frequently as planned. Whereas moderate to pronounced inhibition of whole-blood cholinesterase was observed in some sprayers at the end of the day's work, this was considerably less than that observed in the same sprayers when spraying propoxur at other times. A WHO committee concluded that Landrin® has proved safe enough to warrant extended field trials provided that precautionary measures similar to those for propoxur were taken (WHO, 1973).

Treatment of Poisoning Atropine is helpful and oximes may be harmful as discussed in Section 17.2.2.2.

REFERENCES

Aaronson, M. J., Tessari, J. D., Savage, E. P., and Goes, E. A. (1980). Determination of aldicarb sulfone in hydroponically grown cucumbers. *J. Food Saf.* **2,** 171–181.

Abdel-Rahman, M. S., Lechner, D. W., and Klein, K. M. (1985). Combination effect of carbaryl and malathion in rats. *Arch. Environ. Contam. Toxicol.* **14,** 459–464.

Abd-Elraof, T. K., Dauterman, W. C., and Mailman, R. B. (1981). *In vivo* metabolism and excretion of propoxur and malathion in the rat. Effect of lead treatment. *Toxicol. Appl. Pharmacol.* **59,** 324–330.

Abdel-Wahab, A. M., and Casida, J. E. (1967). Photo-oxidation of two 4-dimethylaminoaryl-methylcarbamate insecticides (Zectran and Mataicil) on bean foliage and of alkylaminophenyl methylcarbamates on silical gel chromatoplates. *J. Agric. Food Chem.* **15,** 479–487.

Abo-Khatwa, N., and Hollingworth, R. M. (1974). Pesticidal chemicals affecting some energy-linked functions of rat liver mitochondria *in vitro. Bull. Environ. Contam. Toxicol.* **12,** 446–454.

Abrahamsen, L. H., and Jerkofsky, M. (1981). Enhancement of varicella-zoster virus replication in cultured human embryonic lung cells treated with the pesticide carbaryl. *Appl. Environ. Microbiol.* **41,** 652–656.

Abrahamsen, L. H., and Jerkofsky, M. (1983). Characterization of varicella-zoster virus enhancement by the pesticide carbaryl. *Appl. Environ. Microbiol.* **45**, 1560–1565.

Ahdaya, S. M., and Guthrie, F. E. (1982). Stomach absorption of intubated insecticides in fasted mice. *Toxicology* **22**, 311–317.

Ahdaya, S. M., Shah, P. V., and Guthrie, F. E. (1976). Thermoregulation in mice treated with parathion, carbaryl, or DDT. *Toxicol. Appl. Pharmacol.* **35**, 575–580.

Ahdaya, S. M., Monroe, R. J., and Guthrie, F. E. (1981). Absorption and distribution of intubated insecticides in fasted mice. *Pestic. Biochem. Physiol.* **16**, 38–46.

Ahmad, S., and Knowles, C. O. (1970). Degradation of formetanate acaricide by rat liver preparations. *J. Econ. Entomol.* **63**, 1690–1692.

Ahmad, S., and Knowles, C. O. (1971). Formamidase involvement in the metabolism of chlorphenamidine and formetanate acaricides. *J. Econ. Entomol.* **64**, 792–795.

Ahmed, F. E., Hart, R. W., and Lewis, N. J. (1977a). Pesticide induced DNA damage and its repair in cultured human cells. *Mutat. Res.* **42**, 161–174.

Ahmed, F. E., Lewis, N. J., and Hart, R. W. (1977b). Pesticide induced ouabain resistant mutants in Chinese hamster V79 cells. *Chem.-Biol. Interact.* **19**, 369–374.

Akhundov, V. Y., Lur'e, L. M., and Ismailova, I. M. (1981). Effect of Sevin on immunologic reactivity. *Gig. Sanit.* **46**, 25–28 (in Russian).

Aldridge, W. N., and Reiner, E. (1972). "Enzyme Inhibitors as Substrates. Interaction of Esterases with Esters of Organophosphorus and Carbamic Acids." Am. Elsevier, New York.

Aleksashina, Z. A. (1969). The therapeutic properties of cholinolytics in combination with cholinesterase reactivators in Sevin poisoning of animals. *Zdravookhr. Beloruss.* **15**, 57–59 (in Russian).

Andrawes, N. R., Dorough, H. W., and Lindquist, D. A. (1967). Degradation and elimination of TEMIK in rats. *J. Econ. Entomol.* **60**, 979–987.

André, F., Gillon, J., André, C., and Jourdan, G. (1981). Prevention of reaginic antibody production and anaphylactic gastric ulcer by pesticides and by a polychlorinated biphenyl. *Environ. Res.* **25**, 381–385.

André, F., Gillon, J., André, C., Lafont, S., and Jourdan, G. (1983). Pesticide-containing diets augment anti-sheep red blood cell nonreaginic antibody responses in mice but may prolong murine infection with *Giardia muris*. *Environ. Res.* **32**, 145–150.

Anger, W. K., and Setzer, J. V. (1979). Effects of oral and intramuscular carbaryl administrations on repeated chain acquisition in monkeys. *J. Toxicol. Environ. Health* **5**, 793–808.

Anger, W. K., and Wilson, S. M. (1980). Effects of carbaryl on variable interval response rates in rats. *Neurobehav. Toxicol.* **2**, 21–24.

Antal, M., Bedö, M., Constantinovits, G., Nagy, K., and Szépvölgyi, J. (1979). Studies on the interaction of methomyl and ethanol in rats. *Food Cosmet. Toxicol.* **17**, 333–338.

Araki, M., Yonemitsu, K., Kambe, T., Idaka, D., Tsunenari, S., Kanda, M., and Kambara, T. (1982). Forensic toxicological investigations on fatal cases of carbamate pesticide methomyl (Lannate®) poisoning. *Jpn. J. Leg. Med.* **36**, 584–588 (in Japanese).

Azizova, O. M. (1976). Effect of Sevin and methyl-mercaptophos on different levels of the nervous system. *In* "Current Problems of the Hygiene of Application of Pesticides in Different Climatic and Geographical Zones" (L. I. Medved, ed.). Erevan, Abovjana (in Russian).

Baranyovits, F. L., and Ghosh, R. (1969). Pirimicarb (PP062), a new selective carbamate insecticide. *Chem. Ind. (London)*, pp. 1018-1019.

Barnett, J. B., Spyker-Cranmer, J. M., Avery, D. L., and Hoberman, A. M. (1980). Immunocompetence over the lifespan of mice exposed *in utero* to carbofuran or diazinon. I. Changes in serum immunoglobulin concentrations. *J. Environ. Pathol. Toxicol.* **4**, 53–63.

Baron, R. L. (1968). Radioactive lactose in skim milk following administration of carbonyl-^{14}C-carbaryl to a lactating cow. *J. Assoc. Off. Anal. Chem.* **51**, 1046–1049.

Baron, R. L., and Locke, R. K. (1970). Utilization of cell culture techniques in carbaryl metabolism studies. *Bull. Environ. Contam. Toxicol.* **5**, 287–291.

Baron, R. L., and Merriam, T. L. (1988). Toxicology of aldicarb. *Revs. Envir. Contam. Toxicol.* **105**, 1–70.

Baron, R. L., Casterline, J. J., Jr., and Fitzhugh, O. G. (1964). Specificity of

carbamate-induced esterase inhibition in mice. *Toxicol. Appl. Pharmacol.* **6**, 402–410.

Bedford, C. (1975). Biotransformations: Agricultural and industrial chemicals. *In* "Foreign Compound Metabolism in Mammals" (D. E. Hathaway, ed.). Chemical Society, London.

Belasco, I. J., and Harvey, J., Jr. (1980). In vitro rumen metabolism of ^{14}C-labeled oxamyl and selected metabolites of oxamyl. *J. Agric. Food Chem.* **28**, 689–692.

Belonozhko, G. A., and Kuchak, Y. A. (1969). Electrocortical reactions of rats to Sevin. *Gig. Sanit.* **34**, 298–300.

Benard, P., and Declume, C. (1979). Placental transfer and milk excretion of radioactivity in rats given orally [^{14}C]carbaryl. *Colloq.—Inst. Natl. Santé Rech. Med.* **89**, 469–475 (in French).

Bend, J. R., Holder, G. M., Protos, E., and Ryan, A. J. (1971). Water-soluble metabolites of carbaryl (1-naphthyl *N*-methylcarbamate) in mouse liver preparations and in the rat. *Aust. J. Biol. Sci.* **24**, 535–546.

Benson, W. H., and Dorough, W. (1984). Comparative ester hydrolysis of carbaryl and ethiofencarb in four mammalian species. *Pestic. Biochem. Physiol.* **21**, 199–206.

Beraud, M., Pipy, B., Derache, R., and Gaillard, D. (1979). Formation of *N*-nitrosocarbaryl, a carcinogen, through interactions between carbaryl, a carbamate insecticide, and sodium nitrite in rat gastric juice. *Food Cosmet. Toxicol.* **17**, 579–583 (in French).

Best, E. M., Jr., and Murray, B. L. (1962). Observations on workers exposed to Sevin insecticide: A preliminary report. *J. Occup. Med.* **4**, 507–517.

Biel-Zielinska, A., Zielinski, W., and Brzezinski, J. (1983). Subacute Pirimor intoxication and levels of biogenic amines in rat tissues. *Przegl. Lek.* **40**, 485–487 (in Polish).

Blase, B. W., and Loomis, T. A. (1976). The uptake and metabolism of carbaryl by isolated perfused rabbit lung. *Toxicol. Appl. Pharmacol.* **37**, 481–490.

Blevins, R. D., Lijinsky, W., and Regan, J. D. (1977a). Nitrosated methylcarbamate insecticides: Effect on the DNA of human cells. *Mutat. Res.* **44**, 1–7.

Blevins, R. D., Lee, M., and Regan, J. D. (1977b). Mutagenicity screening of five methyl carbamate insecticides and their nitroso derivatives using mutants of *Salmonella typhimurium* LT2. *Mutat. Res.* **56**, 1–6.

Bomirska, T., and Winiarska, A. (1972). Toxicology of carbamates as exemplified by intoxication with Baygon insecticide. *Pol. Tyg. Lek.* **27**, 1448–1450 (in Polish).

Borady, A. M. A., Mikhail, T. H., Awadallah, R., Ibrahim, K. A., and Kamar, G. A. R. (1983). Effect of some insecticides on fat metabolism and blood enzymes in rats. *Egypt. J. Anim. Prod.* **23**, 33–44.

Bošković, B., Vojvodić, V., Maksimović, M., Granov, A., Besarović-Lazarev, S., and Binenfeld, Z. (1976). Effect of mono- and bis-quaternary pyridinium oximes on the acute toxicity and on the serum cholinesterase inhibitory activity of dioxacarb, carbaryl and carbofuran. *Arh. Hig. Rada Toksikol.* **27**, 289–295.

Boyd, E. M., and Boulanger, M. A. (1968). Insecticide toxicology. Augmented susceptibility to carbaryl toxicity in albino rats fed purified casein diets. *J. Agric. Food Chem.* **16**, 834–838.

Boyd, E. M., and Kirjnen, C. J. (1969). The influence of protein intake on the acute oral toxicity of carbaryl. *J. Clin. Pharmacol.* **9**, 292–297.

Bracy, O. L., Doyle, R. S., Kennedy, M., McNally, S. M., Weed, J. D., and Thorne, B. M. (1979). Effects of methomyl and ethanol on behavior in the Sprague-Dawley rat. *Pharmacol., Biochem. Behav.* **10**, 21–25.

Branch, R. A., and Jacqz, E. (1986). Subacute neurotoxicity following long-term exposure to carbaryl. *Am. J. Med.* **80**, 741–745.

Bukin, A. L., and Filatov, G. V. (1965). Sevin toxicity for mammals and birds. *Veterinariia* **42**, 93–95.

Cambon, C., Declume, C., and Derache, R. (1979). Effect on the insecticidal carbamate derivatives (carbofuran, pirimicarb, aldicarb) on the activity of acetylcholinesterase in tissues from pregnant rats and fetuses. *Toxicol. Appl. Pharmacol.* **49**, 203–208.

Cambon, C., Declume, C., and Derache, R. (1980). Foetal and maternal rat brain acetylcholinesterase: Isoenzymes changes following insecticidal carbamate derivatives poisoning. *Arch. Toxicol.* **45**, 257–262.

Cambon, C., Fernandez, Y., Falzon, M., and Mitjavila, S. (1981). Variations of the digestive absorption kinetics of carbaryl with the nature of the vehicle. *Toxicology* **22,** 45–51.

Carpenter, C. P., Weil, C. S., Palm, P. E., Woodside, M. W., Nair, J. H., III, and Smyth, H. F., Jr. (1961). Mammalian toxicity of l-naphthyl-*N*-methylcarbamate (Sevin insecticide). *J. Agric. Food Chem.* **9,** 30–39.

Carricaburu, P., Lacroix, R., and Lacroix, J. (1979). Differential action of an anticholinesterase pesticide, carbaryl (*N*-methyl naphthyl carbamate), on the photopic and scotopic systems of the white mouse. *Ann. Pharm. Fr.* **37,** 445–450 (in French).

Casper, H. H., and Pekas, J. C. (1971). Absorption and excretion of radiolabeled l-naphthyl-*N*-methylcarbamate (carbaryl) by the rat. *N. D. Acad. Sci.* **24,** 160–166.

Cecil, H. C., Harris, S. J., and Bitman, J. (1974). Effects of nonpersistent pesticides on liver weight, lipids, and vitamin A of rats and quail. *Bull. Environ. Contam. Toxicol.* **11,** 496.

Challis, I. R., and Adcock, J. W. (1981). The metabolism of the carbamate insecticide bendiocarb in the rat and in man. *Pestic. Sci.* **12,** 638–644.

Chang, K.-M., and Knowles, C. O. (1979). Metabolism of oxamyl in mice and twospotted spider mites. *Arch. Environ. Contam. Toxicol.* **8,** 499–508.

Chib, J. S. (1985). "Zectran®. Metabolism of 4-dimethylamino-3,5-xylyl methyl carbamate (Mexacarbate) in lactating goats," File No. 33603. Union Carbide Agricultural Products Company, Inc., Research Triangle Park, North Carolina (unpublished).

Chin, B. H., Eldridge, J. M., and Sullivan, L. J. (1974). Metabolism of carbaryl by selected tissues using an organ-maintenance technique. *Clin. Toxicol.* **7,** 37–56.

Chin, B. H., Sullivan, L. J., Eldridge, J. M., and Tallant, M. J. (1979). Metabolism of carbaryl by kidney, liver, and lung from human postembryonic fetal autopsy tissue. *Clin. Toxicol.* **14,** 489–498.

Christensen, H. E., ed. (1977). "Registry of Toxic Effects of Chemical Substances." National Institute for Occupational Safety and Health, Rockville, Maryland.

Ciba-Geigy Limited (1986). "Dioxacarb (C 8353): Toxicological Evaluation." Ciba-Geigy Limited, Basel (unpublished).

Collins, T. F. X., Hansen, W. H., and Keeler, H. V. (1971). The effect of carbaryl (Sevin) on reproduction of the rat and the gerbil. *Toxicol. Appl. Pharmacol.* **19,** 202–216.

Comer, S. W., Staiff, D. C., Armstrong, J. F., and Wolfe, H. R. (1975). Exposure of workers to carbaryl. *Bull. Environ. Contam. Toxicol.* **13,** 385–391.

Cook, W. L., Crow, S. A., and Bourquin, A. W. (1977). Inhibitory effects of pesticides and polychlorinated compounds on representative surface slick bacteria. *Am. Soc. Microbiol., Abstr. Annu. Meet.* **77,** 243.

Corbett, J. R., Writh, K., and Baille, A. C. (1984). "The Biochemical Mode of Action of Pesticides," 2nd ed., pp. 99–140. Academic Press, London.

Costa, L. G., and Murphy, S. D. (1983). Unidirectional cross-tolerance between the carbamate insecticide propoxur and the organophosphate disulfoton in mice. *Fundam. Appl. Toxicol.* **3,** 483–488.

Costa, L. G., Hand, H., and Murphy, S. D. (1981a). Tolerance to the carbamate insecticide propoxur. *Fed. Proc., Fed. Am. Soc. Exp. Biol.* **40,** 630.

Costa, L. G., Hand, H., Schwab, B. W., and Murphy, S. D. (1981b). Tolerance to the carbamate insecticide propoxur. *Toxicology,* **21,** 267–278.

Costa, L. G., Schwab, B. W., and Murphy, S. D. (1982). Tolerance to anticholinesterase compounds in mammals. *Toxicology* **25,** 79–97.

Coulston, F. (1968). Qualitative and quantitative relationships between toxicity of drugs in man, lower mammals, and nonhuman primates. *In* "Proceedings, Conference on Nonhuman Primate Toxicology" (C. O. Miller, ed.). U.S. Govt. Printing Office, Washington, D.C.

Coulston, F., Rosenblum, I., and Dougherty, W. J. (1974). "Teratogenic Evaluation of Carbaryl in the Rhesus Monkey (*Macaca mulatta*)." International Center of Environmental Safety and Albany Medical College, Albany, New York (unpublished).

Courtney, K. D., Andrews, J. S., and Grady, M. A. (1983). "14-C-Naphthyl, 14-C-Methyl, and 14-C-Carbonyl Carbaryl Distribution in the Pregnant Mouse and Rat," U.S. Environ. Prot. Agency Rep., NTIS/PB83-193557. National Technical Information Service, Springfield, Virginia.

Courtney, K. D., Andrews, J. E., Springer, J., and Dalley, L. (1985).

Teratogenic evaluation of the pesticides Baygon, carbofuran, dimethoate and EPN. *J. Environ. Sci. Health, Part B* **B20,** 373–406.

Cranmer, M. F., Jr. (1986). Carbaryl: A toxicological review and risk analysis. *Neurotoxicology* **7,** 247–332.

Cress, R. C., and Strother, A. (1974). Effects on drug metabolism of carbaryl and l-naphthol in the mouse. *Life Sci.* **14,** 861–872.

Cummins, J. E. (1982). Nitroso-Baygon formation in nitrogen dioxide gas. *Environ. Mutagen.* **4,** 337.

Dashiell, O. L., and Kennedy, G. L. (1984). The effects of fasting on the acute oral toxicity of nine chemicals in the rat. *J. Appl. Toxicol.* **4,** 320–325.

Dawson, J. A., Heath, D. F., Rose, J. A., Thain, E. M., and Ward, J. B. (1964). Excretion by humans of phenol derived *in vivo* from arprocarb (2-isopropoxyphenyl *N*-methylcarbamate). *Bull. W.H.O.* **30,** 127–134.

Debuyst, B., and Van Larebeke, N. (1983). Induction of sister-chromatid exchanges in human lymphocytes by aldicarb, thiofanox and methomyl. *Mutat. Res.* **113,** 242–243.

Declume, C., and Benard, P. (1977). Autoradiographic study of the distribution of an anticholinesterase agent, l-naphthyl-*N*-methyl[^{14}C]carbamate, in the pregnant rat. *Toxicol. Appl. Pharmacol.* **39,** 451–460 (in French).

Declume, C., and Benard, P. (1978). Study of the pharmacokinetics of ^{14}C-carbaryl in the pregnant mouse. *Toxicol. Eur. Res.* **1,** 173–180 (in French).

Declume, C., and Derache, M. (1976). Bioavailability of ^{14}C-carbaryl after oral administration to the pregnant rat. *C. R. Hebd. Seances Acad. Sci., Ser. D* **283,** 1799–1801 (in French).

Declume, C., and Derache, M. (1977). Placental transfer on an anticholinesterase carbamate with insecticidal activity: Carbaryl. *Chemosphere* **6,** 141–146 (in French).

Declume, C., Cambon, C., and Derache, R. (1979). Acetylcholinesterase activity in fetuses and neonates after ingestion of carbamate derivatives by the pregnant rat. *Colloq.—Inst. Natl. Sante Rech. Med.* **89,** 455–460 (in French).

DeGiovanni-Donnelly, R., Kolbye, S. M., and Greeves, P. D. (1968). The effects of IPC, CIPC, Sevin and Zectran on *Bacillus subtilis. Experientia* **24,** 80–81.

Degraeve, N., Moutschen-Dahmen, M., Houbrechts, N. and Colizzi, A. (1976). The hazards of an insecticide: Carbaryl used alone and in combination with nitrites. *Bull. Soc. Sci. Liege* **45,** 46–57 (in French).

De Lorenzo, F., Staiano, N., Silengo, L., and Cortese, R. (1978). Mutagenicity of diallate, sulfallate, and triallate and relationship between structure and mutagenic effects of carbamates used widely in agriculture. *Cancer Res.* **38,** 13–15.

de Maroussem, D., Pipy, B., Beraud, M., Souqual, M.-C., and Forgue, M.-F. (1986). The effect of carbaryl on the arachidonic acid metabolism and superoxide production by mouse resident peritoneal macrophages challenged by zymosan. *Int. J. Immunopharmacol.* **8,** 155–166.

DeNorscia, R. M., and Lodge, J. R. (1973). Dietary carbaryl and reproduction in mice. *J. Anim. Sci.* **37,** 243–244.

DeProspo, J. R., Weiner, M., McCarty, J. D., Geiger, L. E., Norvell, and Fletcher, M. J. (1985). Twenty-four month dietary toxicity and oncogenicity studies with carbosulfan in mice and rats. *Toxicologist* **5,** 16.

de Saint-Georges-Gridelet, D., Léonard, A., and Lebrun, P. (1982). Cytogenetic effects of carbofuran in mammals. *Mutat. Res.* **97,** 244–245.

Dési, I. (1983). Neurotoxicological investigation of pesticides in animal experiments. *Neurobehav. Toxicol. Teratol.* **5,** 503–516.

Dési, I., Gönczi, L., Simon, G., Farkas, I., and Kneffel, Z. (1974). Neurotoxicologic studies of two carbamate pesticides in subacute animal experiments. *Toxicol. Appl. Pharmacol.* **27,** 465–476.

Deutsch-Wenzel, R. P., Brune, H., Grimmer, G., and Misfeld, J. (1985). Local application to mouse skin as a carcinogen-specific test system for nonvolatile nitroso compounds. *Cancer Lett.* **29,** 85–92.

Dieringer, C. S., and Thomas, J. A. (1974). Effects of carbaryl on the metabolism of androgens in the prostate and liver of the mouse. *Environ. Res.* **7,** 381–386.

Dikshith, T. S. S., Gupta, P. K., Gaur, J. S., Datta, K. K., and Mathur, A. K. (1976). Ninety-day toxicity of carbaryl in male rats. *Environ. Res.* **12,** 161–170.

Dodd, D. E. (1987a). "Toxicology Investigations to Support Registration of

Trimethacarb Technical." Union Carbide Agricultural Products Company, Inc., Research Triangle Park, North Carolina (unpublished).

Dodd, D. E. (1987b). "Toxicology Investigations to Support Registration of Mexacarbate Technical." Union Carbide Agricultural Products Company, Inc., Research Triangle Park, North Carolina (unpublished).

Dorough, H. W. (1967). Carbaryl-C^{14} metabolism in a lactating cow. *J. Agric. Food Chem.* **15,** 261–266.

Dorough, H. W. (1968). Metabolism of Furadan (NIA-10242) in rats and houseflies. *J. Agric. Food Chem.* **16,** 319–325.

Dorough, H. W. (1979). Metabolism of insecticides by conjugation mechanisms. *Pharmacol. Ther.* **4,** 433–471.

Dorough, H. W., and Casida, J. E. (1964). Nature of certain carbamate metabolites of the insecticide Sevin. *J. Agric. Food Chem.* **12,** 294–304.

Dorough, H. W., and Ivie, G. W. (1968). TEMIK-S^{35} metabolism in a lactating cow. *J. Agric. Food Chem.* **16,** 460–464.

Dorough, H. W., and Wiggins, O. G. (1969). Nature of the water soluble metabolites of carbaryl in bean plants and their fate in rats. *J. Econ. Entomol.* **62,** 49–53.

Dorough, H. W., Davis, R. B., and Ivie, G. W. (1970). Fate of TEMIK-carbon-14 in lactating cows during a 14-day feeding period. *J. Agric. Food Chem.* **18,** 135–142.

Dougherty, W. J., Goldberg, L., and Coulston, F. (1971). The effect of carbaryl on reproduction in the monkey (*Macaca mulatta*). *Toxicol. Appl. Pharmacol.* **19,** 365.

Douglas, G. R., Nestmann, E. R., Pooley, J. M., and Kowbel, D. J. (1982). Mutagenicity of Matacil in a battery of microbial and *in vitro* mammalian assays. *Can. J. Genet. Cytol.* **24,** 622.

Douglas, G. R., Nestmann, E. R., Bayley, J. M., Liu-Lee, V. W., Kowbel, D. J., and Blakey, D. H. (1983). Effect of *in vitro* metabolic activation on the mutagenicity of Matacil in a battery of microbial and *in vitro* mammalian assays. *Environ. Mutagen.* **5,** 384.

Drabek, J., and Bachmann, F. (1983). Proinsecticides: Structure–activity relationships in carbamoyl sulfenyl N-methylcarbamates. *In* "Pesticide Chemistry: Human Welfare and the Environment" (J. Miyamoto, P. C. Kearney, P. Doyle, and T. Fujita, eds.), Vol. 1, pp. 271–277. Pergamon, New York.

du Pont (1986). "Methomyl Toxicology Monograph," E. I. du Pont de Nemours and Company, Inc., Wilmington, Delaware (unpublished).

Earl. F. L., Miller, E., and Van Loon, E. J. (1973). Reproductive, teratogenic, and neonatal effects of some pesticides and related compounds in beagle dogs and miniature swine. *In* "Pesticides and the Environment: A Continuing Controversy" (W. B. Deichman, ed.), pp. 253–266. Intercontinental Medical Book Corp., New York.

Egert, G., and Greim, H. (1976). Formation of mutagenic nitroso-compounds from ephedrine and from the pesticides carbaryl, dodin, and prometryn in the presence of nitrite at pH 1. *Naunyn-Schmiedberg's Arch. Pharmacol.* **293,** Suppl., R66.

Eisenbrand, G., Ungerer, O., and Preussmann, R. (1975). The reaction of nitrite with pesticides. II. Formation, chemical properties and carcinogenic activity of the N-nitroso derivative of N-methyl-l-naphthyl carbamate (carbaryl). *Food Cosmet. Toxicol.* **13,** 365–368.

Elespuru, R., Lijinsky, W., and Setlow, J. K. (1974). Nitrosocarbaryl as a potent mutagen of environmental significance. *Nature (London)* **247,** 386–387.

Ellman, G. L., Courtney, K. D., Andres, V., Jr., and Featherstone, R. M. (1961). A new and rapid colorimetric determination of acetylcholinesterase activity. *Biochem. Pharmacol.* **7,** 88–95.

El-Sewedy, S. M., Zahran, M. A., Zeidan, M. A., Mostafa, M. H., and El-Bassiouni, E. A. (1982). Effect and mechanism of action of methomyl and cypermethrin insecticides on kynurenine metabolizing enzymes of mouse liver. *J. Environ. Sci. Health, Part B* **B17,** 527–539.

Epstein, S. S., Arnold, E., Andrea, J., Bass, W., and Bishop, Y. (1972). Detection of chemical mutagens by the dominant lethal assay in the mouse. *Toxicol. Appl. Pharmacol.* **23,** 288–325.

Essac, E. G., and Matsumura, F. (1979). Roles of flavoproteins in degradation of mexacarbate in rats. *Pestic. Biochem. Physiol.* **10,** 67–78.

Eto, M., Kuwano, E., Yoshikawa, M., Suiko, M., Kohno, M., Kamihata, M., and Nakatsu, S. (1982). Mutagenicity and anticholinesterase activity of possible metabolites of aryl N-methylcarbamates. *J. Fac. Agric. Kyushu Univ.* **26,** 213–219.

Eya, B. K., and Fukuto, T. R. (1986). Formamidine-S-carbamates: A new procarbamate analogue with improved ovicidal and acaricidal activities. *J. Agric. Food Chem.* **34,** 947–952.

Fahmy, M. A. H., Fukuto, T. R., Myers, R. D., and March, R. B. (1970). The selective toxicity of the new N-phosphorothioylcarbamate esters. *J. Agric. Food Chem.* **18,** 793–796.

Fait, D. W., Nachreiner, D. J., Dodd, D. E., and Frank, F. R. (1984). "Aldoxycarb Technical Acute Inhalation Toxicity Test," Rep. No. 47–114. Union Carbide Bushy Run Research Center, Export, Pennsylvania (unpublished).

Faragó, A. (1969). Suidical, fatal Sevin (l-naphthyl-N-methylcarbamate) poisoning. *Arch. Toxikol.* **24,** 309–315.

FBC (1986). "Bendiocarb." FBC Limited, England (unpublished).

Feldmann, R. J., and Maibach, H. I. (1974). Percutaneous penetration of some pesticides and herbicides in man. *Toxicol. Appl. Pharmacol.* **28,** 126–132.

Ferguson, P. W., Jewell, S. A., Krieger, R. I., and Raabe, O. G. (1982). Carbofuran disposition in the rat after aerosol inhalation. *Environ. Toxicol. Chem.* **1,** 245–258.

Ferguson, P. W., Dey, M. S., Jewell, S. A., and Krieger, R. I. (1984). Carbofuran metabolism and toxicity in the rat. *Fundam. Appl. Toxicol.* **4,** 14–21.

Fiore, M. C., Anderson, H. A., Hong, R., Golubjatnikov, R., Seiser, J. E., Nordstrom, D., Hanrahan, L., and Belluck, D. (1986). Chronic exposure to aldicarb-contaminated groundwater and human immune function. *Environ. Res.* **41,** 633–645.

FMC (1986a). "Carbofuran." FMC Corporation, Princeton, New Jersey (unpublished).

FMC (1986b). "Carbosulfan." FMC Corporation, Princeton, New Jersey (unpublished).

Food and Agriculture Organization/World Health Organization (FAO/WHO) (1968). "1967 Evaluation of Some Pesticide Residues in Food. The Monographs," WHO/Food Add./68.30. World Health Organ., Rome.

Food and Agriculture Organization/World Health Organization (FAO/WHO) (1974). "1973 Evaluation of Some Pesticide Residues in Food: The Monographs," WHO Pestic. Residue Ser. No. 3. World Health Organ., Geneva.

Food and Agriculture Organization/World Health Organization (FAO/WHO) (1977). "1976 Evaluations of Some Pesticide Residues in Food. The Monographs." Food Agric. Organ. U.N., Rome.

Food and Agriculture Organization/World Health Organization (FAO/WHO) (1978). "Pesticide Residues in Food: 1977 Evaluations: The Monographs," FAO Plant Prod. Prot. Pap. *No.* 10, Suppl. Food Agric. Organ. U.N., Rome.

Food and Agriculture Organization/World Health Organization (FAO/WHO) (1979). "Pesticide Residues in Food: 1978 Evaluations. The Monographs." FAO Plant Prod. Prot. Pap. No. 15 Suppl. Food Agric. Organ. U.N., Rome.

Food and Agriculture Organization/World Health Organization (FAO/WHO) (1980). "Pesticide Residues in Food: 1979 Evaluations: The Monographs," FAO Plant Prod. Prot. Pap. No. 20, Suppl. Food Agric. Organ. U.N., Rome.

Food and Agriculture Organization/World Health Organization (FAO/WHO) (1981). "Pesticide Residues in Food: 1980 Evaluations: The Monographs," FAO Plant Prod. Prot. Pap. No. 26, Suppl. Food Agric. Organ. U.N., Rome.

Food and Agriculture Organization/World Health Organization (FAO/WHO) (1982). "Pesticide Residues in Food: 1981 Evaluations: The Monographs," FAO Plant Prod. Prot. Pap. No. 42. Food Agric. Organ. U.N., Rome.

Food and Agriculture Organization/World Health Organization (FAO/WHO) (1983). "Pesticide Residues in Food: 1982 Evaluations: The Monographs," FAO Plant Prod. Prot. Pap. No. 49. Food Agric. Organ. U.N., Rome.

Food and Agriculture Organization/World Health Organization (FAO/WHO) (1984). "Pesticide Residues in Food: 1983 Evaluations. FAO Plant Prod. Prot. Pap. No. 56. Food Agric. Organ. U.N., Rome.

Food and Agriculture Organization/World Health Organization (FAO/WHO) (1985). "Pesticide Residues in Food: 1984 Evaluations. The Monographs," FAO Plant Production and Protection Paper, Food Agric. Organ. U.N., Rome.

Food and Agriculture Organization/World Health Organization (FAO/WHO) (1986a). "Pesticide Residues in Food: 1985 Evaluations," FAO Plant Prod. Prot. Pap. No. 72/2. Food Agric. Organ. U.N., Rome.

Food and Agriculture Organization/World Health Organization (FAO/WHO)

(1986b). "Pesticide Residues in Food: 1986 Report," FAO Plant Prod. Prot. Pap. No. 77. Food Agric. Organ. U.N., Rome.

Foss, W., and Krechniak, J. (1980). The fate of propoxur in rat. *Arch. Toxicol.*, *Suppl.* **4**, 346–349.

Fujita, Y. (1985). Studies on contact dermatitis from pesticides in tea growers. *Acta Med. Univ. Kagoshima.* **27**, 17–37.

Fukuto, T. R. (1983). Structure–activity relationships in derivatives of anticholinesterase insecticides. *In* "Pesticide Chemistry: Human Welfare and the Environment" (J. Miyamoto and P. C. Kearny, eds.), Vol. 1, pp. 203–213. Pergamon, New York.

Gaines, T. B. (1960). The acute toxicity of pesticides to rats. *Toxicol. Appl. Pharmacol.* **2**, 88–99.

Gaines, T. B. (1969). Acute toxicity of pesticides. *Toxicol. Appl. Pharmacol.* **14**, 515–534.

Gaines, T. B., and Linder, R. E. (1986). Acute toxicity of pesticides in adult and weanling rats. *Fundam. Appl. Toxicol.* **7**, 299–308.

Gelbach, S. H., and Williams, W. A. (1975). Pesticide containers. Their contribution to poisoning. *Arch. Environ. Health* **30**, 49–50.

Gentile, J. M., Gentile, G. J., Bultman, J., Sechriest, R., Wagner, E. D., and Plewa, M. J. (1982). An evaluation of the genotoxic properties of insecticides following plant and animal activation. *Mutat. Res.* **101**, 19–29.

Georgian, L., Moraru, I., Drǎghicescu, T., and Tarnavschi, R. (1985). The effect of low concentrations of carbofuran, choline salt of maleic hydrazine, propham and chlorpropham on sister-chromatid exchange (SCE) frequency in human lymphocytes in vitro. *Mutat. Res.* **147**, 296.

Giles, C. J., Pycock, J. F., Humphreys, D. J., and Stodulski, J. B. J. (1984). Methiocarb poisoning in a sheep. *Vet. Rec.* **114**, 642.

Goes, E. A., Savage, E. P., Gibbons, G., Aaronson, M., Ford, S. A., and Wheeler, H. W. (1980). Suspected foodborne carbamate pesticide intoxications associated with ingestion of hydroponic cucumbers. *Am. J. Epidemiol.* **111**, 254–260.

Gold, R. E., Leavitt, J. R. C., Holcslaw, T., and Tupy, D. (1982). Exposure of urban applicators to carbaryl. *Arch. Environ. Contam. Toxicol.* **11**, 63–67.

Goldberg, M. E., Johnson, H. E., and Knaak, J. B. (1964). Influence of SKF525-A on the behavioral and anticholinesterase effects of certain carbamates. *Biochem. Pharmacol.* **13**, 1483–1488.

Goldberg, M. E., Johnson, H. E., and Knaak, J. B. (1965). Inhibition of discrete avoidance behavior by three anticholinesterase agents. *Psychopharmacologia* **7**, 72–76.

Gonzáles Cid, M., and Matos, E. (1984). Induction of sister-chromatid exchanges in cultured human lymphocytes by Aldicarb, a carbamate pesticide. *Mutat. Res.* **138**, 175–179.

Gordon, W. A., Eckerman, D. A., Elliott, S. L., Garner, J. A., and MacPhail, R. C. (1981). Effects of decamethrin, chlordimeform, Baygon, and carbaryl in spatially controlled behavior of rats. *Toxicologist* **1**, 48.

Gray, L. E., Jr., Kavlok, R. J., Ostby, J., Ferrell, J., Rogers, J., and Gray, K. (1986). An evaluation of figure-eight maze activity and general behavioral development following prenatal exposure to forty chemicals: Effects of cytosine arabinoside, dinocap, nitrofen, and vitamin A. *Neurotoxicology* **7**, 449–462.

Guerzoni, M. E., Del Cupolo, L., and Ponti, I. (1976). Mutagenic activity of pesticides. *Riv. Sci. Tecnol. Alimenti Nutr. Um.* **6**, 161–165 (in Italian).

Gupta, M., and Bagchi, G. K. (1982). Behavioral pharmacology of Furadan and Nuvacron in mice. *Indian J. Hosp. Pharm.* **19**, 136–141.

Gupta, M., Bagchi, G. K., Gupta, S. D., Sasmal, D., Chatterjee, T., and Dey, S. N. (1984). Changes of acetylcholine, catecholamines and amino acid in mice brain following treatment with Nuvacron and Furadan. *Toxicology* **30**, 171–175.

Gupta, M., Mukherjee, S., Gupta, S. D., Dolui, A. K., Dey, S. N., and Roy, D. K. (1986). Changes of lipid spectrum in different tissues of Furadan-treated mice. *Toxicology* **38**, 69–79.

Haley, T. J., Farmer, J. H., Dooley, K. L., Harmon, J. R., and Peoples, A. (1974). Determination of the LD_{01} and extrapolation of the LD_{001} for five methylcarbamate pesticides. *J. Eur. Toxicol.* **7**, 152–158.

Hamada, N. N. (1986). "One-Year Feeding Study in Dogs with Thiodicarb Technical," Rep. No. 2100-126 from Hazleton Laboratories America, Inc., Vienna, VA, to Union Carbide Agricultural Products Company, Inc., Research Triangle Park, North Carolina (unpublished).

Hamada, N. N. (1987a). Aldicarb technical. One year feeding study in dogs. Rep. 400-706 from Hazleton Laboratories America to Union Carbide Agricultural Products Company, Inc., Research Triangle Park, North Carolina (unpublished).

Hamada, N. N. (1987b). "One-Year Oral Toxicity Study in Beagle Dogs with Carbaryl Technical," Rep. 400-715 from Hazleton Laboratories America, Inc., Vienna, VA, to Union Carbide Agricultural Products Company, Inc., Research Triangle Park, North Carolina (unpublished).

Han, J. C.-Y. (1975). Absence of nitroso formation from [^{14}C]methomyl and sodium nitrite under simulated stomach conditions. *J. Agric. Food Chem.* **23**, 892–896.

Hart, E. R. (1971). "Teratology Study. SEVIN®, Vitamin A, Aspirin, and Malathion," Report from Bionetics Research Laboratories to Union Carbide Agricultural Products Company, Inc., Research Triangle Park, North Carolina (unpublished).

Harvey, J., and Han, J. C.-Y. (1978). Metabolism of oxamyl and selected metabolites in the rat. *J. Agric. Food Chem.* **26**, 902–910.

Harvey, J., Jr., Jelinek, A. G., and Sherman, H. (1973). Metabolism of methomyl in the rat. *J. Agric. Food Chem.* **21**, 679–775.

Hassan, A. (1971). Pharmacological effects of carbaryl—I. The effect of carbaryl on the synthesis and degradation of catecholamines in the rat. *Biochem. Pharmacol.* **20**, 2299–2308.

Hassan, A., and Santolucito, J. A. (1971). Pharmacological effects of carbaryl. II. Modification of serotonin metabolism in the rat brain. *Experientia* **27**, 287–288.

Hassan, A., Zayed, S. M. A. D., and Abdel-Hamid, F. M. (1966). Metabolism of carbamate drugs. I. Metabolism of l-naphthyl-*N*-methylcarbamate (Sevin) in the rat. *Biochem. Pharmacol.* **15**, 2045–2055.

Hayes, W. J., Jr. (1971). Studies on exposure during the use of anticholinesterase pesticides. *Bull, W. H. O.* **44**, 277–278.

Hayes, W. J., Jr. (1982). Carbamate pesticides. *In* "Pesticides Studied in Man," pp. 436–462. Williams & Wilkins, Baltimore, Maryland.

Heise, G. A., and Hudson, J. D. (1985a). Effects of pesticides and drugs on working memory in rats: Continuous delayed response. *Pharmacol., Biochem. Behav.* **23**, 591–598.

Heise, G. A., and Hudson, J. D. (1985b). Effects of pesticides and drugs on working memory in rats: Continuous non-match. *Pharmacol. Biochem. Behav.* **23**, 599–606.

Hoberman, A. M. (1978). Ultrastructural study of liver tissue from mice prenatally exposed to the cholinesterase inhibitor carbofuran. *Teratology* **17**, 41A.

Hodogaya Chemical Co., Ltd. (1986). "Toxicological Information on XMC." Hodogaya Chemical Co., Ltd., Tokyo (unpublished).

Holmstedt, B. (1972). The ordeal bean of Old Calabar: The pageant of *Physostigma venenosum* in medicine. *In* "Plants in the Development of Modern Medicine" (T. Swain, ed.). Harvard Univ. Press, Cambridge, Massachusetts.

Hoque, M. Z. (1972). Carbaryl, a new chemical mutagen. *Curr. Sci.* **41**, 855–856.

Huhtanen, K., and Dorough, H. W. (1976). Isomerization and Beckman rearrangement reactions in the metabolism of methomyl in rats. *Pestic. Biochem. Physiol.* **6**, 571–583.

Hurst, H. E., and Dorough, H. W. (1978). Chemical alteration of the hydrolytic detoxication of methylcarbamates in rats. *Pharmacology* **20**, 146.

Hwang, S. W., and Schanker, L. S. (1974). Absorption of carbaryl from the lung and small intestine of the rat. *Environ. Res.* **7**, 206–211.

Imming, R. J., Shaffer, B. C., Woodard, G. (1969). "SEVIN®. Safety Evaluation by Feeding to Female Beagles from Day One of Gestation through Weaning of the Offspring," Report from Woodard Research Corporation to Union Carbide Agricultural Products Company, Inc., Research Triange Park, North Carolina (unpublished).

Innes, J. R. M., Ulland, B. M., Valerio, M. G., Petrucelli, L., Fishbein, L., Hart, E. R., Pallotta, A. J., Bates, R. R., Falk, H. L., Gart, J. J., Klein, G. M., Mitchell, I., and Peters, J. (1969). Bioassay of pesticides and industrial chemicals for tumorigenicity in mice: A preliminary note. *J. Natl. Cancer Inst. (V.S.)* **42**, 1101–1114.

Ishidate, M., Jr., and Odashima, S. (1977). Chromosome tests with 134 compounds on Chinese hamster cells in vitro: A screening for chemical carcinogens. *Mutat. Res.* **48,** 337–354.

Ishidate, M., Jr., Sofuni, T., and Yoshikawa, K. (1981). Chromosomal aberration tests *in vitro* as a primary screening tool for environmental mutagens and/or carcinogens. *Gann Monogr. Cancer Res.* **72,** 95–108.

Isshiki, K., Miyata, K., Matsui, S., Tsutsumi, M., and Watanabe, T. (1983). Effects of post-harvest fungicides and piperonyl butoxide on the acute toxicity of pesticides in mice. Safety evaluation for intake of food additives. III. *J. Food Hyg. Soc. Jpn.* **24,** 268–274 (in Japanese).

Iverson, F. (1977). Inhibition and regeneration of rat liver enzymes hydrolyzing acetanilide and *o*-nitrophenyl butyrate. *Bull. Environ. Contam. Toxicol.* **18,** 466–471.

Ivie, G. W., and Dorough, H. W. (1968). Furadan-^{14}C metabolism in a lactating cow. *J. Agric. Food Chem.* **16,** 849–855.

Iwami, T., Inokuchi, K., Sasaki, K., Kogaku, H., Taniguchi, N., Yokouchi, H., Nakajoh, T., and Terui, K. (1981). Studies on general pharmacological properties of FMC 35001 (2,3-dihydro-2,2-dimethyl-7-benzofuranyl[(dibutylamino)thiol] methyl carbamate. *Hirosaki Med. J.* **33,** 653–690 (in Japanese).

Izmirova, N., Milcheva, V., Monov, A., and Kaloyanova, F. (1981). Acute carbofuran intoxication. *Khig. Zdraveopaz.* **25,** 445–448 (in Bulgarian).

Jackson, B., and Dessau, F. I. (1961). Liver tumors in rats fed acetamide. *Lab. Invest.* **10,** 909–923.

Jackson, J. A., Chart, J. S., Sanderson, J. H., and Gaines, R. (1977). Pirimicarb induced immune haemolytic anaemia in dogs. *Scand. J. Haemotol.* **19,** 360–366.

Jao, L. T., and Hsu, S. L. (1981). Toxicological effects of butylated hydroxyanisole (BHA) and butylated hydroxytoluene (BHT) on insecticide chemicals. I. Effects of BHA and BHT on chlorpyrifos, methomyl and pentobarbital. *Proc. Natl. Sci. Counc. Repub. China* **9,** 426–432 (in Chinese).

Jaszczuk, E., and Syrowatka, T. (1980). Mutagenic action of certain pesticides on *Salmonella typhimurium*. *Rocz. Panstw. Zakl. Hig.* **31,** 305–311 (in Polish).

Jayapragasam, M., Jasmine, I., Thenammai, V., and Kasthuri, R. (1981). Biochemical changes due to carbofuran, Sevin and Rogor administration to albino rats. *Madras Agric. J.* **68,** 461–465 (in Polish).

Jeleniewicz, K., and Szczepaniak, S. (1980). Free amino acids and amino nitrogen levels in serum and blood erythrocytes of rats exposed to subacute intoxication with carbaryl. *Bromatol. Chem. Toksykol.* **13,** 237–240 (in Polish).

Jeleniewicz, K., and Szczepaniak, S. (1985). Dynamics of liver free amino acid changes in rats intoxicated with carbaryl. *Bromatol. Chem. Toksykol.* **18,** 202–208.

Jeleniewicz, K., Szczepaniak, S., and Sienkiewicz, E. (1984). Effect of acute intoxication with carbaryl on brain free amino acid levels in rats. *Bromatol. Chem. Toksykol.* **17,** 221–227.

Jerkofsky, M., and Abrahamsen, L. H. (1983). Variation in human herpesvirus susceptibility to enhancement by the pesticide carbaryl. *Appl. Environ. Microbiol.* **45,** 1555–1559.

Johnson, M. K. (1970). Organophosphorus and other inhibitors of brain "neurotoxic esterase" and development of delayed neurotoxicity in hens. *Biochem. J.* **120,** 523–531.

Jones, D. C. L., Simmon, V. F., Mortelmans, K. E., Mitchell, A. D., and Evans, E. L. (1984). "*In Vitro* and *in vivo* Mutagenicity Studies of Environmental Chemicals," Rep. No. EPA-600/1-84-003. U.S. Environ. Prot. Agency, Research Triangle Park, North Carolina.

Jordan, M., Srebro, A., Pierscinska, E., and Wozny, L. (1975). Preliminary observations on the effects on the organs of mice of administering some carbamate pesticides. *Bull. Environ. Contam. Toxicol.* **12,** 205–208.

Jurek, A. (1978). Long-term chronic toxicity of the carbamate propoxur. *Rocz. Panstw. Zakl. Hig.* **29,** 327–338.

Kadir, H. A., and Knowles, C. O. (1981). Inhibition of rat brain monoamine oxidase by insecticides, acaricides and related compounds. *Gen. Pharmacol.* **12,** 239–247.

Kajita, T., Ohkawa, T., Kobayashi, H., and Yuyama, A. (1983). Effects of a carbamate insecticide (propoxur) on brain cholinergic system in mice. *Jpn. J. Pharmacol.* **33,** Suppl., 232.

Kagan, Y. S., Rodionov, G. A., Voronina, L. Y., Velichko, L. S., Kulagin, O. M., and Peremitina, A. D. (1970). The effect of Sevin on the functional state and structure of the liver. *Farmakol. Toksikol. (Moscow)*, **33,** 219–224.

Kagan, Y. S., Kokshareva, N. V., Savateev, N. V., Linyuchev, M. N., Sergeev, V. V., Petritsyuk, V. D., and Ovsyannikova, L. M. (1983). Effect of benzonal on resistance to organophosphorus and carbamic compounds. *Farmakol. Toksikol. (Moscow)*, **46,** 101–103 (in Russian).

Kaplan, A. M., and Sherman, H. (1976). Toxicity studies with methyl *N*-[[(methylamino)carbonyl]oxy]ethanimidothioate. *Toxicol. Appl. Pharmacol.* **40,** 1–17.

Karpenko, V. N., Khokhol'kova, G. A., Pokrovskaya, T. N., Ryazanova, R. A., and Gritsevskaya, I. L. (1984). Data on hygienic characteristics of the pesticide Croneton. *Gig. Sanit.* **10,** 23–26 (in Russian).

Kazarnoskaya, M. L., and Vasilos, A. F. (1977). The effect of Sevin on the chromosomal apparatus of cells *in vitro*. *Zdravookhr. Beloruss.* **20,** 14–16 (in Russian).

Keck, G., and Jaussaud, P. (1981). Toxicological cases. Poisoning of a dog by mercaptodimethur (methiocarb). *Notes Toxicol. Vet.* **4,** 90–91 (in French).

Kennedy, G. L., Jr. (1986). Acute toxicity studies with oxamyl. *Fundam. Appl. Toxicol.* **6,** 423–429.

Khaikina, B. I., and Kuz'minskaia, U. A. (1970). The mechanism of action of Sevin on warm-blooded animals. *Vopr. Pitan.* **29,** 8–14 (in Russian).

Kikuchi, H., Suzuki, Y., and Hashimoto, Y. (1981). Increase of beta-glucuronidase activity in the serum of rats administered organophosphate and carbamate insecticides. *J. Toxicol. Sci.* **6,** 27–36.

Kimmerle, G. (1971). Comparison of the antidotal actions of tetraethylammonium chloride and atropine in acute poisoning of carbamate insecticides in rats. *Arch. Toxikol.* **27,** 311–314.

Kimmerle, G., and Iyatomi, A. (1976). Toxicity of propoxur to rats by subacute inhalation. *Jpn. J. Ind. Health.* **18,** 375–382.

Kiran, R., Sharma, M., and Bansal, R. C. (1985). In vivo effect of carbaryl on some enzymes of rat liver, kidney and brain. *Pesticides* **19,** 42–43.

Kitagawa, K., Wakakura, M., and Ishikawa, S. (1977). Light microscopic study of endocrine organs of rats treated by carbamate pesticide. *J. Toxicol. Sci.* **2,** 53–60.

Knaak, J. B., and Sullivan, L. J. (1967). Metabolism of carbaryl in the dog. *J. Agric. Food Chem.* **15,** 1125.

Knaak, J. B., and Wilson, B. W. (1985). Dermal dose–cholinesterase and percutaneous absorption studies with several cholinesterase inhibitors. *ACS Symp. Ser.* **273,** 63–79.

Knaak, J. B., Tallant, M. J., Bartley, W. J., and Sullivan, L. J. (1965). The metabolism of carbaryl in the rat, guinea pig, and man. *J. Agric. Food Chem.* **13,** 537–543.

Knaak, J. B., Tallant, M. J., and Sullivan, L. J. (1966). The metabolism of 2-methyl-2(methylthio)propionaldehyde *O*-(methylcarbamoyl)oxime in the rat. *J. Agric. Food Chem.* **14,** 573–578.

Knaak, J. B., Tallant, M. J., Kozbelt, S. J., and Sullivan, L. J. (1968). The metabolism of carbaryl in man, monkey, pig, and sheep. *J. Agric. Food Chem.* **16,** 465–470.

Knaak, J. B., Munger, D. M., McCarthy, J. F., and Satter, L. D. (1970). Metabolism of carbofuran alfalfa residues in the dairy cow. *J. Agric. Food Chem.* **18,** 832–837.

Knaak, J. B., Yee, K., Ackerman, C. R., Zweig, G., Fry, D. M., and Wilson, B. W. (1984). Percutaneous absorption and dermal dose–cholinesterase response studies with parathion and carbaryl in the rat. *Toxicol. Appl. Pharmacol.* **76,** 252–263.

Kobayashi, H., Yuyama, A., Kajita, T., Shimura, K., Ohkawa, T., and Satoh, K. (1985). Effects of insecticidal carbamates on brain acetylcholine content, acetylcholinesterase activity and behavior in mice. *Toxicol. Lett.* **29,** 153–159.

Kokshareva, N. V. (1982). Therapeutic effectiveness of diethyxime in poisoning by anticholinesterase-action carbamate pesticides. *Farmakol. Toksikol. (Moscow)* **45,** 61–64 (in Russian).

Kossakowski, S., and Lysek, C. (1982). Experimental carbaryl poisoning in rabbits. *Med. Weter.* **38,** 222–225 (in Polish).

Kossakowski, S., and Żuk, M. (1983). Distribution of Zn in an animal organism following sublethal poisonings with carbaryl. *Med. Weter.* **39,** 31–33 (in Polish).

Kossakowski, S., Žuk, M. and Dziura, A. (1982). Effect of carbaryl intoxication on thyroid function. *Bull. Vet. Inst. Pulawy* **25,** 62–65.

Kotin, P., Falk, H., Pallotta, A. J., and Hart, E. R. (1968). "Evaluation of Carcinogenic, Teratogenic and Mutagenic Activities of Selected Pesticides and Industrial Chemicals. Vol. II. Teratogenic Study in Mice and Rats," Natl. Tech. Inf. Serv. Rep. PB-223. U.S. Govt. Printing Office, Washington, D.C.

Kozler, M. (1975). The local effect of dioxacarb on the eye. *Prac. Lek.* **27,** 209–210.

Krechniak, J., and Foss, W. (1982). Cholinesterase activity in rats treated with propoxur. *Bull. Environ. Contam. Toxicol.* **29,** 599–604.

Krechniak, J., and Foss, W. (1983). Distribution, biotransformation, and elimination of propoxur following the intoxication with this agent in repeated doses. *Bromatol. Chem. Toksykol.* **16,** 205–208 (in Polish).

Krieger, R. I., Ferguson, P. W., Dey, M. S., and Jewell, S. A. (1984). Carbofuran metabolism and toxicity in the rat. *Fundam. Appl. Toxicol.* **4,** 14–21.

Krishna, J. G., and Casida, J. E. (1966). Fate in rats of the radiocarbon from ten variously labeled methyl- and dimethylcarbamate-C14 insecticide chemicals and their hydrolysis products. *J. Agric. Food Chem.* **14,** 98–105.

Krug, H. F., and Berndt, J. (1985). Inhibition by pesticides of prostaglandin formation in blood platelets. *Blut* **51,** 19–23.

Kudo, N. (1975). Pathological physiology of pesticide intoxication. Part 17. Cultivation of tobacco plants and pesticide intoxication. *J. Jpn. Assoc. Rural Med.* **24,** 436–437.

Kuhr, R. J., and Dorough, H. W. (1976). "Carbamate Insecticides: Chemistry, Biochemistry, and Toxicology." CRC Press, Boca Raton, Florida.

Kusevitskiy, I. A., Kirlich, A. Y., and Khovaeva, L. A. (1970). The action of maneb and Sevin on the thyroid gland. *Veterinariya (Moscow)* **46,** 73–74 (in Russian).

Kuz'minskaya, U. A., Ivanitskii, V. A., and Shilina, V. F. (1984). Effect of pesticides with anticholinesterase activity on the biogenic amine content in the brain. *Gig. Sanit.* **5,** 80–81.

Leavitt, J. R. C., Gold, R. E., Holcslaw, T., and Tupy, D. (1982). Exposure of professional pesticide applicators to carbaryl. *Arch. Environ. Contam. Toxicol.* **11,** 57–62.

Lechner, D. W., and Abdel-Rahman, M. S. (1985). Alterations in rat liver microsomal enzymes following exposure to carbaryl and malathion in combination. *Arch. Environ. Contam. Toxicol.* **14,** 451–457.

Lechner, D. W., and Abdel-Rahman, M. S. (1986). Kinetics of carbaryl and malathion in combination in the rat. *J. Toxicol. Environ. Health* **18,** 241–256.

Lee, M. H., and Ransdell, J. F. (1984). A farmworker death due to pesticide toxicity: A case report. *J. Toxicol. Environ. Health* **14,** 239–246.

Lee, W.-K., and Hong, S.-U. (1985). Toxicological study of carbaryl in rats. *Arch Pharmacol. Res.* **8,** 119–132.

Lee, Y. S., Cinn, Y. W., Chang, W. H., and Kim, J. S. (1981). Hypersensitivity of Korean farmers to various agrochemicals. 1. Determination of concentration for patch test of fruit-tree agrochemicals and hypersensitivity of orange orchard farmers in Che-ju Do, Korea. *Seoul J. Med.* **22,** 137–142 (in Korean).

Leeling, N. C., and Casida, J. E. (1966). Metabolites of carbaryl (l-naphthyl methylcarbamate) in mammals and enzymatic systems for their formation. *J. Agric. Food Chem.* **14,** 281–290.

Lewerenz, H. J., Plass, R., and Bleyl, D. W. R. (1980). Studies on the coergism of selected pesticides. Part I. Acute oral toxicity of combined administration. *Nahrung* **24,** 463–469 (in German).

Liddle, J. A., Kimbrough, R. D., Needham, L. L., Cline, R. E., Smrek, A. L., Yert, L. W., Bayse, D. D., Ellington, A. C., and Dennis, P. A. (1979). A fatal episode of accidental methomyl poisoning. *Clin. Toxicol.* **15,** 159–167.

Lijinsky, W., and Andrews, A. W. (1979). The mutagenicity of nitrosamides in *Salmonella typhimurium. Mutat. Res.* **68,** 1–8.

Lijinsky, W., and Schmäl, D. (1978). Carcinogenicity of N-nitroso derivatives of N-methylcarbamate insecticides in rats. *Ecotoxicol. Environ. Saf.* **2,** 413–419.

Lijinsky, W., and Taylor, H. W. (1977). Transplacental chronic toxicity test of carbaryl with nitrite in rats. *Food Cosmet. Toxicol.* **15,** 229–232.

Lijinsky, W., and Winter, C. (1981). Skin tumors induced by painting nitrosoalkylureas on mouse skin. *J. Cancer Res. Clin. Oncol.* **102,** 13–20.

Lin, T. H., North, H. H., and Menzer, R. E. (1975). Metabolism of carbaryl (l-naphthyl N-methylcarbamate) in human embryonic lung cell cultures. *J. Agric. Food Chem.* **23,** 253–256.

Lockard, J. M., Schuette, B. P., and Sabharwal, P. S. (1982). Inhibition by carbaryl of DNA, RNA and protein synthesis in cultured rat lung cells. *Experientia* **38,** 686–687.

Lox, C. D. (1984). The effects of acute carbaryl exposure on clotting factor activity in the rat. *Ecotoxicol. Environ. Saf.* **8,** 280–283.

Lucier, G. W., McDaniel, O. S., Williams, C., and Klein, R. (1972). Effects of chlordane and methylmercury on the metabolism of carbaryl and carbofuran in rats. *Pestic. Biochem. Physiol.* **2,** 244.

Lunder, H. G. (1981). Poisoning of a dog by snail poison bait, methiocarb. *Nor. Veterinaertidsskr.* **93,** 441–442 (in Norwegian).

Machemer, L., Eben, A., and Kimmerle, G. (1982). Monitoring of propoxur exposure. *In* "Education and Safe Handling in Pesticide Application" (E. A. H. van Heemstra and W. F. Tordoir, eds.), pp. 255–262. Elsevier, Amsterdam.

MacLeod, J. (1982). "Report on UCC Sperm Morphology Readings Submitted to Agricultural Products Company, Inc.; Union Carbide Corporation." Cornell University Medical College, Ithaca, New York (unpublished).

Maliwal, B. P., and Guthrie, F. E. (1981). Interaction of insecticides with human plasma lipoproteins. *Chem.-Biol. Interact.* **35,** 177–188.

Mann, J. B., and Danauskas, J. X. (1984). Human effects associated with the use of aldicarb on cotton in Sudan, Africa. *In* "The Biosphere: Problems and Solutions" (T. N. Veziroğlu, ed.), pp. 571–578. Elsevier, Amsterdam.

Marsden, P. J., Kuwano, E., and Fukuto, T. R. (1982). Metabolism of carbosulfan [2,3-dihydro-2,2-dimethylbenzofuran-7-yl (di-n-butylaminothio)methylcarbamate] in the rat and house fly. *Pestic. Biochem. Physiol.* **18,** 38–48.

Marshall, T. C., and Dorough, H. W. (1977). Bioavailability in rats of bound and conjugated plant carbamate insecticide residues. *J. Agric. Food Chem.* **25,** 1003–1009.

Marshall, T. C., and Dorough, H. W. (1979). Biliary excretion of carbamate insecticides in the rat. *Pestic. Biochem. Physiol.* **11,** 56–63.

Marshall, T. C., Dorough, H. W., and Swim, H. E. (1976). Screening of pesticides for mutagenic potential using *Salmonella typhimurium* mutants. *J. Agric. Food Chem.* **24,** 560–563.

Martin, A. R. (1982). Evaluation of pesticide effects on parameters of male reproduction in the mouse. *Diss. Abstr. Int. B* **42,** 4279.

McCarthy, J. F., Fancher, O. E., Kennedy, G. L., Keplinger, M. L., and Calandra, J. C. (1971). Reproduction and teratology studies with the insecticide carbofuran. *Toxicol. Appl. Pharmacol.* **19,** 370.

Mehendale, H. M., and Dorough, H. W. (1971). Glucuronidation mechanisms in the rat and their significance in metabolism of insecticides. *Pestic. Biochem. Physiol.* **1,** 307.

Metcalf, R. L. (1971). Structure–activity relationships for insecticidal carbamates. *Bull. W.H.O.* **44,** 43.

Metcalf, R. L., Fukuto, T. R., Collins, C., Borck, K., El-Aziz, S. A., Rumoz, R., and Cassil, C. C. (1968). Metabolism of 2,2-dimethyl-2,3-dihydrobenzofuranyl-7-N-methylcarbamate (Furadan) in plants, insects, and mammals. *J. Agric. Food Chem.* **16,** 300–311.

Michel, T., Miller, E., Olivito, V., and Van Loon, E. J. (1971). Toxic effects of carbaryl on the C.N.S. of the miniature pig. *Fed. Proc., Fed. Am. Soc. Exp. Biol.* **30,** 443.

Miller, A., III, Henderson, M. C., and Buhler, D. R. (1979). Covalent binding of carbaryl (l-naphthyl-N-methylcarbamate) to rat liver microsomes *in vitro. Chem.-Biol. Interact.* **24,** 1–17.

Miskus, P. R., Andrews, T. L., and Look, M. (1969). Metabolic pathways affecting toxicity of N-acetyl Zectran. *J. Agric. Food Chem.,* **17,** 842.

Mitsubishi Chemical Industries Limited (1986a). "Summary of Toxicological Data on BPMC (Fenobucarb)." Mitsubishi Chemical Industries Limited, Tokyo (unpublished).

Mitsubishi Chemical Industries Limited (1986b). "Summary of Toxicological Data on MIPC (Isoprocarb)." Mitsubishi Chemical Industries Limited, Tokyo (unpublished).

Miyaoka, T., Takahashi, H., Tsuda, S., and Shirasu, Y. (1984). Potentiation of acute toxicity of 2-sec-butylphenyl N-methylcarbamate (BPMC) by fenthion in mice. *Fundam. Appl. Toxicol.* **4,** 802–807.

Miyata, T., and Saito, T. (1981). Synergistic action of IBP (Kitazin p®) and malathion in mice. *J. Pestic. Sci.* **6**, 351–353.

Mogilevchik, Z. K., Rusyaev, A. P., Viatchannikov, K. A., and Buslovich, S. Y. (1970). Importance of nonspecific manifestations of pesticide poisoning in setting norms for their residual quantities. *Vopr. Gig. Toksikol. Pestits., Tr. Nauchn. Sess. Akad. Med. Nauk SSSR, 1967,* p. 49 (in Russian).

Montazemi, K. (1969). Toxicological studies of Baygon insecticides in Shabankareh area, Iran. *Trop. Geogr. Med.* **21**, 186–190.

Morbidity and Mortality Weekly Reports (MMWR) (1986). Aldicarb food poisoning from contaminated melons—California. *Morbid. Mortal. Wkly. Rep.* **35**, 264–268.

Moriya, M., Ohta, T., Watanabe, K., Miyazawa, T., Kato, K., and Shirasu, Y. (1983). Further mutagenicity studies on pesticides in bacterial reversion assay systems. *Mutat. Res.* **116**, 185–216.

Morse, D. L., Baker, E. L., Jr., Kimbrough, R. D., and Wisseman, C. L. III. (1979). Propanil-chloracne and methomyl toxicity in workers of a pesticide manufacturing plant. *Clin. Toxicol.* **15**, 13–21.

Motabar, M. (1971). Observations on the effect on operators and inhabitants following first round spraying with OMS-33 in Jareh, Iran. *Acta Med. Iran.* **14**, 81–91.

Mount, M. E., Dayton, A. D., and Oehme, F. W. (1981). Carbaryl residues in tissues and cholinesterase activities in brain and blood of rats receiving carbaryl. *Toxicol. Appl. Pharmacol.* **58**, 282–296.

Murakami, M., and Fukami, J. (1982). Carbaryl binds to proteins of human cells in culture but chlorinated organic chemicals do not. *Bull. Environ. Contam. Toxicol.* **28**, 500–503.

Murakami, M., and Fukami, J. (1983). Effects of carbaryl on nucleic acid and protein biosyntheses in cultured human cells. *J. Pestic. Sci.* **8**, 353–355.

Murray, F. J., Staples, R. E., and Schwetz, B. A. (1979). Teratogenic potential of carbaryl given to rabbits and mice by gavage or by dietary inclusion. *Toxicol. Appl. Pharmacol.* **51**, 81–89.

Myers, R. C., and Christopher, S. M. (1986). "Thiodicarb. Determination of Antidotal Effectiveness of 2-PAM and Atropine in the Rat," Rep. No. 48–180. Union Carbide Bushy Run Research Center, Export, Pennsylvania (unpublished).

Myers, W. R. (1977). "Carbaryl Insecticide. Estimation of Carbaryl Exposure to Humans," Proj. No. 111A12. Union Carbide Agricultural Products Company, Inc., Research Triangle Park, North Carolina (unpublished).

Namba, T., Nolte, C. T., Jackerel, J., and Grob, D. (1971). Organophosphate insecticides. *Am. J. Med.* **50**, 475.

National Cancer Institute (NCI) (1978). "Bioassay of Mexacarbate for Possible Carcinogenicity," Carcinogenesis Tech. Rep. Ser. No. 147, NIH Publ. No. 78–1073. U.S. Department of Health, Education, and Welfare, Washington, D.C.

National Cancer Institute (NCI) (1979). "Bioassay of Aldicarb for Possible Carcinogenicity," Carcinogenesis Tech. Rep. Ser. No. 136, NIH Publ. No. 79–1391. U.S. Department of Health, Education, and Welfare, Washington, D.C.

National Institute for Occupational Health and Safety (NIOSH) (1976). "Criteria for a Recommended Standard: Occupational Exposure to Carbaryl," Publ. No. 77–107. National Institute for Occupational Health and Safety, U.S. Department of Health, Education, and Welfare, Cincinnati, Ohio.

National Research Council (1986). "Drinking Water and Health," Vol 6, pp. 303–309. National Academy Press, Washington, D.C.

Natoff, I. L., and Reiff, B. (1973). Effect of oximes on the acute toxicity of anticholinesterase carbamates. *Toxicol. Appl. Pharmacol.* **25**, 569–573.

Nelson, D. L., and Lamb, D. W. (1977). An evaluation of methiocarb bait toxicity to dogs. *VM/SAC, Vet. Med. Small Anim. Clin.* **72**, 185–186.

Nelson, D. L., Lamb, D. W., and Mihail, F. (1984). A study of liver microsomal enzymes in rats following propoxur (Baygon) administration. *Vet. Hum. Toxicol.* **26**, 305–308.

Nelson, J., MacKinnon, E. A., Mower, H. F., and Wong, L. (1981). Mutagenicity of *N*-nitroso derivatives of carbofuran and its toxic metabolites. *J. Toxicol. Environ. Health* **7**, 519–531.

Neskovic, N. K. (1979). Effects of subacute feeding of carbaryl on mixed function oxidase and on acute toxocity of parathion and propoxur in rats. *Environ. Res.* **20**, 148.

Neskovic, N. K., Terzic, M., and Vitorovic, S. (1978). Acute toxicity of carbaryl and propoxur in mice previously treated with phenobarbital and SKF 525-A. *Arh. Hig. Rada Toksikol.* **29**, 251–256 (in Russian).

Neskovic, N. K., Vojinovic, V. D., and Vuksa, M. M. (1984). Subacute toxicity of polychlorinated biphenyl (Aroclor 1242) in rats. *Arh. Hig. Rada Toksikol.* **35**, 333–342.

New South Wales Department of Public Health, Division of Occupational Health, Sydney (1965). "Carbaryl Poisoning," WHO Inf. Circ. Toxic. Pestic. Man, No. 18. World Health Organ. Sydney, Australia.

Noda, J. (1984). Determination of methomyl by using chemical ionization mass fragmentography. A case report of methomyl poisoning and the animal experiment of its poisoning. *Jpn. J. Leg. Med.* **38**, 71–82 (in Japanese).

Nye, D. E., and Dorough, H. W. (1976). Fate of insecticides administered endotracheally to rats. *Bull. Environ. Contam. Toxicol.* **15**, 291–296.

O'Brien, R. D., and Dannelley, C. E. (1965). Penetration of insecticides through rat skin. *J. Agric. Food Chem.* **13**, 245–247.

O'Keefe, M., and Pierse, C. (1980). Exposure of seed pelleting plant workers to methiocarb. *Bull. Environ. Contam. Toxicol.* **25**, 777–781.

Olefir, A. I., and Minster, O. P. (1977). Natural immunity of the organism as a function of the intensity of pesticide exposure. *Vrach. Delo* **9**, 121–123 (in Russian).

Olson, L. J., Erickson, B. J., Hindsill, R. D., Wyman, J. A., Porter, W. P., Binning, L., Bidgood, R., and Norheim, E. (1986). Immunosuppression of mice by a pesticide ground water contaminant. Presented at the Fertilizer, Aglime, and Pest Management Conference, Madison, Wisconsin.

Önfelt, A. (1983). Spindle disturbances in mammalian cells. I. Changes in the quantity of free sulfhydryl groups in relation to survival and C-mitosis in V79 Chinese hamster cells after treatment with colcemid, diamide, carbaryl and methyl mercury. *Chem.-Biol. Interact.* **46**, 201–217.

Önfelt, A., and Klasterska, I. (1983). Spindle disturbances in mammalian cells. II. Induction of viable aneuploid/polyploid cells and multiple chromatid exchanges after treatment of V79 Chinese hamster cells with carbaryl. Modifying effects of glutathione and S9. *Mutat. Res.* **119**, 319–330.

Önfelt, A., and Klasterska, I. (1984). Sister-chromatid exchanges and thioguanine resistance in V79 Chinese hamster cells after treatment with the aneuploidy-inducing agent carbaryl ± S9 mix. *Mutat. Res.* **125**, 269–274.

Oonnithan, E. S., and Casida, J. E. (1968). Oxidation of methyl- and dimethylcarbamate insecticide chemicals by microsomal enzymes and anticholinesterase activity of the metabolites. *J. Agric. Food Chem.* **16**, 28–44.

Orlova, N. V., and Zhalbe, E. P. (1968). Experimental data concerning the problem of permissible amounts of Sevin in foodstuffs. *Vopr. Pitan.* **27**, 49–55 (in Russian).

Orton, R. G. (1973). Methiocarb poisoning in the dog. *Vet. Rec.* **93**, 478.

Orzel, R. A., and Weiss, L. R. (1966). The effect of carbaryl (l-naphthyl-*N*-methylcarbamate) on blood glucose, and liver and muscle glycogen in fasted and nonfasted rats. *Biochem. Pharmacol.* **15**, 995–998.

Oshima, H., and Bartsch, H. (1981). Quantitative estimation of endogenous nitrosation in humans by monitoring *N*-nitrosoproline excreted in the urine. *Cancer Res.* **41**, 3658–3662.

Osicka-Koprowska, A., and Wysocka-Paruszewska, B. (1983). Cholinergic effect and adrenal cortex activity in rats intoxicated with pirmor. *Przegl. Lek.* **40**, 575–577 (in Polish).

Osman, A. Z., Hazzaa, N. I., and Awad, T. M. (1983). Fate and metabolism of the insecticide ^{14}C-Lannate in farm animals. *Isot. Radiat. Res.* **15**, 111–120.

Osterloh, J., Letz, G., Pond, S., and Beeker, C. (1983). An assessment of the potential testicular toxicity of 10 pesticides using the mouse-sperm morphology assay. *Mutat. Res.* **116**, 407–415.

Otsuka Chemical Company (1987). "Toxicology of Benfuracarb." Otsuka Chem. Co., Ltd, Osaka, Japan (unpublished).

Palut, D., Grzymala, W., and Rozycki, Z. (1970). Study of the metabolism of ^{14}C-carbaryl in model animal systems. *Rocz. Panstw. Zakl. Hig.* **21**, 417–426 (in Polish).

Panciera, R. J. (1967). "Determinations of Teratogenic Properties of Orally Administered l-Naphthyl *N*-methylcarbamate (Sevin®) in Sheep," Rep. Union Carbide Agric. Prod. Co., Inc., Research Triangle Park, North Carolina (unpublished).

Parafita, M. A., and Fernandez Otero, M. P. (1983). Effect of carbaryl on microsomal cytochrome P-450 from rat liver. *IRCS Med. Sci.* **11/12,** 1046–1047.

Parafita, M. A., and Fernandez Otero, M. P. (1984a). The interaction of carbaryl with the metabolism of isolated hepatocytes. I. Effect of respiration and glycolysis. *Gen. Pharmacol.* **15,** 327–332.

Parafita, M. A., and Fernandez Otero, M. P. (1984b). The interaction of carbaryl with the metabolism of isolated hepatocytes. II. Effect on gluconeogenesis. *Gen. Pharmacol.* **15,** 333–337.

Patocka, J., and Bajgar, J. (1971). Affinity of human brain acetylcholinesterase to some organophosphates and carbamates *in vitro. J. Neurochem.* **18,** 2545–2546.

Peoples, S. A., Maddy, K. T., and Smith, C. R. (1978). Occupational exposure to Temik (aldicarb) as reported by California physicians for 1974–1976. *Calif. Dep. Food Agric. Sci. Rep.,* pp. 321–324.

Perelygin, V. M., Shpirt, M. B., Aripov, O. A., and Ershova, V, I. (1971). Effects of some pesticides on immunological reactivity. *Gig. Sanit.* **36,** 29–33 (in Russian).

Pilinskaya, M. A. (1981a). Study of the cytogenetic effect of a number of pesticides in human peripheral blood lymphocyte culture at various initial levels of chromosome aberrations. *Cytol. Genet.* **15,** 74–76.

Pilinskaya, M. A. (1981b). The significance of cytogenetic observations on occupational populations for the genetic and hygienic evaluation of pesticides. *Mutat. Res.* **97,** 211–212.

Pilinskaya, M. A. (1982). The cytogenetic effect of pesticide pirimor in a human peripheral blood lymphocyte culture in vivo and in vitro. *Cytol. Genet.* **16,** 45–49.

Pilinskaya, M. A., and Stepanova, L. S. (1984). Effect of biotransformation of the insecticide carbofuran on its cytogenetic activity *in vivo* and *in vitro. Tsitol. Genet.* **18,** 17–20 (in Russian).

Pipy, B., Beraud, M., and Gaillard, D. (1978). Relation between inhibition of phagocytosis by the rat reticuloendothelial system and the anticholinesterase effect of an insecticide, carbaryl. *J. Physiol. (Paris)* **74,** 379–385 (in French).

Pipy, B., Gaillard, D., and Derache, R. (1982). Enzymatic activities of liver serine esterases during the reticuloendothelial system phagocytosis blockade by carbaryl, an anticholinesterase insecticide. *Toxicol. Appl. Pharmacol.* **62,** 11–18.

Pipy, B., de Maroussem, D., Beraud, M., and Derache, P. (1983). Evaluation of cellular and humoral mechanisms of carbaryl-induced reticuloendothelial phagocytic depression. *RES: J. Reticuloendothel. Soc.* **34,** 395–412.

Pleština, R., and Svetličić, B. (1973). Toxic effects of two carbamate insecticides in dogs. *Arh. Hig. Rada Toksikol.* **24,** 217–225.

Podolak-Majczak, M., and Tyburczyk, W. (1984). The combined effect of sodium nitrite and carbaryl on rats. Part II. Methemoglobinemia. *Bromatol. Chem. Toksykol.* **17,** 211–214 (in Polish).

Popov, B., and Ribarova, F. (1979). Effect of the pesticide propoxur (Unden) in toxic doses on glucose transport in small intestines. *Khig. Zdraveopaz.* **22,** 584–588.

Probst, G. S., McMahon, R. E., Hill, L. E., Thompson, C. Z., Epp, J. K., and Neal, S. B. (1981). Chemically-induced unscheduled DNA synthesis in primary rat hepatocyte cultures: A comparison with bacterial mutagenicity using 218 compounds. *Environ. Mutagen.* **3,** 11–32.

Pużyńska, L. (1977). The effect of propoxur on rats fed diets differing in protein content. *Environ. Res.* **14,** 152–163.

Pużyńska, L. (1980). Brain biochemistry and learning ability of rats treated with propoxur given in diets of varying protein content. *Environ. Res.* **23,** 385–396.

Quarles, J. M., Sega, M. W., Schenley, C. K., and Lijinsky, W. (1979a). Transformation of hamster fetal cells by nitrosated pesticides in a transplacental assay. *Cancer Res.* **39,** 4525–4533.

Quarles, J. M., Sega, M. W., Schenley, C. K., and Tennant, R. W. (1979b). Rapid screening for chemical carcinogens: Transforming activity of selected nitroso compounds detected in a transplacental host-mediated culture system. *Natl. Cancer Inst. Monogr.* **51,** 257–263.

Quick, M. P. (1982). Pesticide poisoning of livestock: A review of cases investigated. *Vet. Rec.* **111,** 5–7.

Quinto, I., Martire, G., Vricella, G., Riccardi, F., Perfumo, A., Giulivo, R.,

and De Lorenzo, F. (1981). Screening of 24 pesticides by *Salmonella/* microsome assay: Mutagenicity of benazolin, metoxuron and paraoxon. *Mutat. Res.* **85,** 265.

Ramasamy, P. (1976). Carbamate insecticide poisoning. *Med. J. Malays.* **31,** 150–152.

Rappoport, M. B. (1969). Microscopic and ultrastructural changes in the thyroid gland under the action on the organism of the insecticide Sevin. *Vrach. Delo* **5,** 102–105 (in Russian).

Rappoport, M. B. (1971). Electron microscopic study of the posterior lobe of the hypophysis during multiple effects of the pesticide Sevin. *Vrach. Delo* **9,** 137–140 (in Russian).

Rashid, K. A. (1978). The relationships between mutagenic and DNA damaging activity of pesticides and their potential carcinogenesis. Ph.D. dissertation, Pennsylvania State University, University Park (unpublished).

Rashid, K. A., and Mumma, R. O. (1986). Screening pesticides for their ability to damage bacterial DNA. *J. Environ. Sci. Health, Part B* **21,** 319–334.

Ray, S. K., and Poddar, M. K. (1983a). Carbaryl-induced elevation of corticosterone level and cholinergic mechanism. *Biosci. Rep.* **3,** 973–977.

Ray, S. K., and Poddar, M. K. (1983b). Possible involvement of central cholinergic mechanisms in carbaryl-induced changes in levels of 5-hydroxyindoleacetic acid and homovanillic acid. *IRCS Med. Sci.* **11,** 168–169.

Ray, S. K., and Poddar, M. K. (1984). Effect of pentylenetetrazole on the carbaryl-induced changes of serotonin metabolism in rat-brain hypothalamus. *Biosci. Rep.* **4,** 427–432.

Ray, S. K., and Poddar, M. K. (1985a). Central cholinergic–dopaminergic interaction in carbaryl-induced tremor. *Eur. J. Pharmacol.* **119,** 251–253.

Ray, S. K., and Poddar, M. K. (1985b). Effect of pentylenetetrazole on carbaryl-induced changes in striatal catecholamines. *Biochem. Pharmacol.* **34,** 553–557.

Ray, S. K., Haque, S. J., and Poddar, M. K. (1984). Effect of carbaryl on catecholamines in brain regions. *Indian J. Exp. Biol.* **22,** 141–144.

Regan, J. D., Setlow, R. B., Francis, A. A., and Lijinsky, W. (1976). Nitrosocarbaryl: Its effect on human DNA. *Mutat. Res.* **38,** 293–302.

Reich, G. A., and Welke, J. O. (1966). Death due to a pesticide. *N. Engl. J. Med.* **274,** 1432.

Reiner, E., and Aldridge, W. N. (1967). Effect of pH on inhibition and spontaneous reactivation of acetylcholinesterase treated with a series of phosphoric acids and of carbamic acids. *Biochem. J.* **105,** 171–179.

Renzi, B. E., and Krieger, R. I. (1986). Sublethal acute toxicity of carbosulfan [2,3-dihydro-2,2-dimethyl-7-benzofuranyl-(di-*n*-butylaminosulfenyl) (methyl)carbamate] in the rat after intravenous and oral exposures. *Fundam. Appl. Toxicol.* **6,** 7–15.

Rhône-Poulenc (1987). "Toxicology of TEMIK® Aldicarb Pesticide." Rhône-Poulenc Ag Company, Research Triangle Park, North Carolina (unpublished).

Richardson, E. M., and Batteese, R. I., Jr. (1973). An incident of Zectran poisoning. *J. Maine Med. Assoc.* **64,** 158–159.

Richardson, J. A., Keil, J. E., and Sandifer, S. H. (1975). Catecholamine metabolism in humans exposed to pesticides. *Environ. Res.* **9,** 290–294.

Rickard, R. W., and Dorough, H. W. (1984). *In vivo* formation of nitrosocarbamates in the stomach of rats and guinea pigs. *J. Toxicol. Environ. Health* **14,** 279–290.

Rickard, R. W., Walter-Echols, G., Lawrence, L. J., and Dorough, H. W. (1982). Importance of pH in assessing the potential for nitrosocarbamate formation in the stomach. *Pestic. Biochem. Physiol.* **18,** 325–333.

Risher, J. F., Mink, F. L., and Stara, J. F. (1987). The toxocologic effects of the carbamate insecticide aldicarb in mammals: A review. *Environ. Health Perspect.* **72,** 267–281.

Robacker, K. M., Kulkarni, A. P., and Hodgson, E. (1981). Pesticide induced changes in the mouse hepatic microsomal cytochrome P-450-dependent monooxygenase system and other enzymes. *J. Environ. Sci. Health, Part B* **16,** 529–545.

Robens, J. F. (1969). Teratologic studies of carbaryl, diazinon, norea, disulfiram, and thiram in small laboratory animals. *Toxicol. Appl. Pharmacol.* **15,** 152–163.

Robertson, I. G. C., Sivarajah, K., Eling, T. E., and Zeiger, E. (1983). Activation of some aromatic amines to mutagenic products by prostaglandin endoperoxide synthetase. *Cancer Res.* **43**, 476–480.

Rodgers, K. E., Leung, N., Imamura, T., and Devens, B. H. (1986). Rapid *in vitro* screening assay for immunotoxic effects of organophosphorus and carbamate insecticides on the generation of cytotoxic T-lymphocyte responses. *Pestic. Biochem. Physiol.* **26**, 292–301.

Rodwell, D. E. (1986). "A Teratology Study in Rabbits with Thiodicarb," Rep. No. WIL-95002. WIL Research Laboratories, Inc., to Union Carbide Agricultural Products Company, Inc., Research Triangle Park, North Carolina (unpublished).

Rosenstein, L., and Chernoff, N. (1976). Spontaneous and evoked ECG changes observed in neonatal rats following *in utero* exposure to Baygon: A preliminary investigation. *Toxicol. Appl. Pharmacol.* **37**, 130.

Rosenstein, L., and Chenoff, N. (1978). Spontaneous and evoked EEG changes in perinatal rats following *in utero* exposure to Baygon: A preliminary investigation. *Bull. Environ. Contam. Toxicol.* **20**, 624–632.

Roszkowski, J. (1978). Immunomorphological investigations on the effect of lindane, chlorfenvinphos, and carbaryl in immune reactions. I. Experiments on rabbits. *Bull. Vet. Inst. Pulawy* **22**, 25–30.

Roszkowski, P. (1982). Effect of propoxur (2-isopropoxyphenyl *N*-methylcarbamate) on the intrauterine development and the state of the skeletal system of rat fetuses. *Ginekol. Pol.* **53**, 201–207 (in Polish).

Rotaru, G., Constantinescu, S., Filipescu, G., and Ratea, E. (1981). Experimental research on chronic poisoning by carbofuran. *Med. Lav.* **72**, 399–403.

Ruppert, P. H., Cook, L. L., Dean, K. F., and Reiter, L. W. (1983). Acute behavioral toxicity of carbaryl and propoxur in adult rats. *Pharmacol., Biochem. Behav.* **18**, 579–584.

Rybakova, M. N. (1966). Toxic effect of Sevin on animals. *Hyg. Sanit.* **31**, 402–407.

Rybakova, M. N. (1967). Comparative toxic effects of Sevin and DDT used in the treatment of food crops. *Vopr. Pitan.* **26**, 9–15 (in Russian).

Rybakova, M. N. (1968). Effect of some pesticides on the hypophysis and its gonadotropic functions. *Gig. Sanit.* **33**, 27–31 (in Russian). (*Chem. Abstr.* **70**, 19169).

Salisbury, B. G., Tate, C. F., and Davies, J. E. (1974). Baygon-induced pulmonary edema. *Chest* **65**, 455–457.

Sallam, M., and El-Ghawaby, S. H. (1980). Safety in the use of pesticides. *J. Environ. Sci. Health, Part B* **15**, 677–681.

Samaam, H. A., Nour-el-Dien, S., and Kamel, S. (1984). The potentiation of the acute toxicity of niridazole by the concurrent administration of some commonly used insecticides in rats. *J. Drug Res.* **15**, 73–78.

Sanderson, D. M. (1961). Treatment of poisoning by anticholinesterase insecticides in the rat. *J. Pharm. Pharmacol.* **13**, 435–442.

Santolucito, J. A. (1970). Comparison of chronic and acute low-level exposure effects of carbaryl in the EEG of squirrel monkeys. *Ind. Med.* **39**, 52.

Santolucito, J. A., and Morrison, G. (1971). EEG of rhesus monkeys following prolonged low-level feeding of pesticides. *Toxicol. Appl. Pharmacol.* **19**, 147–154.

Santolucito, J. A., and Whitcomb, E. (1971). Mechanical response of skeletal muscle following oral administration of pesticides. *Toxicol. Appl. Pharmacol.* **20**, 66–72.

Schein, L. G., Thomas, J. A., Donovan, M. P., and Klase, P. A. (1976). Effects of diazinon, parathion and carbofuran on the *in vitro* metabolism of ^{3}H-testosterone by rodent prostate glands and hepatic microsomal enzymes. *Pharmacologist* **18**, 243.

Schering (1987). "Formetanate Hydrochloride." Schering Aktiengesellschaft, Agrochemical Division, Berlin (unpublished).

Schmidt, N. J. (1983). Effect of the pesticide carbaryl on replication of human and simian varicella viruses. *Infect. Immun.* **39**, 1485–1487.

Schneider, W. G., Butler, G. C., Campbell, J. S., Migicousky, B. B., Morley, H. V., and Norman, M. G. (1976). "Forest Spray Program and Reye's Syndrome." Rep. of the panel convened by the government of New Brunswick.

Seiler, J. P. (1977). Nitrosation in vitro and in vivo by sodium nitrite, and mutagenicity of nitrogenous pesticides. *Mutat. Res.* **48**, 225–236.

Sen Gupta, A. K., and Knowles, C. O. (1970). Fate of formetanate-^{14}C acaricide in the rat. *J. Econ. Entomol.* **63**, 10–14.

Serrone, D. M., Stein, A. A., and Coulston, F. (1966). Biochemical and electron microscopic change observed in rats and monkeys medicated orally with carbaryl. *Toxicol. Appl. Pharmacol.* **8**, 353.

Shabanov, M., Toshkov, A., and Georgiev, D. (1983a). Influence of some new ecological factors on the course of experimental infections in laboratory animals. 2. Influence of the pesticide Sevin on experimental infection with staphylococci in rats. *Acta Microbiol. Bulg.* **12**, 65–70 (in Bulgarian).

Shabanov, M., Toshkov, A., Georgiev, D., and Ibrishimov, N. (1983b). Effect of carbaryl on an experimental *Erysipelothrix rhusiopathiae* infection in rats. *Vet.-Med. Nauki* **20**, 9–15 (in Bulgarian).

Shah, P. V., and Guthrie, F. E. (1977). Dermal absorption, distribution, and the fate of six pesticides in the rabbit. In "Pesticide Management and Insecticide Resistance" (D. L. Watson and A. W. A. Brown, eds.), pp. 547–554. Academic Press, New York.

Shah, P. V., Monroe, R. J., and Guthrie, F. E. (1981). Comparative rates of dermal penetration of insecticides in mice. *Toxicol. Appl. Pharmacol.* **59**, 414–423.

Sharaf, A. A., Temtamy, S. A., de Hondt, H. A., Belal, M. H., and Kassam, E. A. (1982). Effect of aldicarb (Temik) a carbamate insecticide, on chromosomes of the laboratory rat. *Egypt. J. Genet. Cytol.* **11**, 135–144.

Shea, T. B. (1987). Effects of carbaryl on differentiated and undifferentiated neuroblastoma cells: Inhibition of growth rates and direct cell toxicity. *Bull. Environ. Contam. Toxicol.* **38**, 143–150.

Shehata, T., Richardson, E., and Cotton, E. (1984). Assessment of human population exposure to carbaryl from the 1982 Maine Spruce Budworm Spray Project. *J. Environ. Health* **46**, 293–297.

Shimkin, M. B., Wieder, R., McDonough, M., Fishbein, L., and Swern, D. (1969). Lung tumor response in strain A mice as a quantitative bioassay of carcinogenic activity of some carbamates and aziridines. *Cancer Res.* **29**, 2184–2190.

Shiwaku, K., Hirai, K., Torii, M., and Mima, Y. (1982). Health hazards by pesticides on farmers in citrus fruit area. Fluctuations in blood enzymes and lipids by spraying work of mecarbam. *Jpn. Assoc. Rural Med.* **30**, 1028–1033.

Shtenberg, A. I., and Khovaeva, L. A. (1970). The effect of Sevin on the state of the thyroid gland of rats receiving an artificial complete diet with a varying content of iodine. *Gig. Sanit.* **35**, 119–122 (in Russian).

Shtenberg, A. I., and Ozhovan, M. V. (1971). Effect of small doses of Sevin on the reproductive function of animals in several generations. *Vopr. Pitan.* **1**, 42–49 (in Russian).

Shtenberg, A. I., and Rybakova, M. N. (1968). Effect of carbaryl on the neuroendocrine system of rats. *Food Cosmet. Toxicol.* **6**, 461–467.

Shtenberg, A. I., and Torchinskiy, A. M. (1972). Relationships between general toxic, embryotoxic, and teratogenic effects of exogenous chemicals and the possibility of predicting their influence on antenatal ontogenesis. *Vestn. Akad. Med. Nauk SSSR* **27**, 39–46 (in Russian).

Shtenberg, A. J., Ashmenskas, Y. I., and Kusevitskiy, I. A. (1972). Immunobiological reactivity changes under the effect of some pesticides belonging to the group of carbamate and dithiocarbamate compounds. *Vopr. Pitan.* **31**, 58–63 (in Russian).

Sideroff, S. I., and Santolucito, J. A. (1972). Behavioral and physiological effects of the cholinesterase inhibitor carbaryl. *Physiol. Behav.* **9**, 459.

Siebert, D., and Eisenbrand, G. (1974). Induction of mitotic gene conversion in *Saccharomyces cerevisiae* by *N*-nitrosated pesticides. *Mutat. Res.* **22**, 121–126.

Simeon, V., and Reiner, E. (1973). Comparison between inhibition of acetylcholinesterase and cholinesterase by some *N*-methyl- and *N,N*-dimethyl carbamates. *Arh. Hig. Rada Toksikol.* **24**, 199–206.

Simmon, V. F., Poole, D. C., and Newell, G. W. (1976). *In vitro* mutagenic studies of twenty pesticides. *Toxicol. Appl. Pharmacol.* **37**, 109 (abstr.).

Simmon, V. F., Mitchell, A. D., and Jorgenson, T. A. (1977). "Evaluation of Selected Pesticides as Chemical Mutagens in *in Vitro* and *in Vivo* Studies," Rep. No. EPA-600/1-77-028. U.S. Environ. Prot. Agency, Research Triangle Park, North Carolina.

Simpson, G. R., and Bermingham, S. (1977). Poisoning by carbamate pesticides. *Med. J. Aust.* **2**, 148–149.

Simpson, G. R., and Penney, D. J. (1974). Pesticide poisoning in the Namoi and Macquare valleys, 1973. *Med. J. Aust.* **1**, 258–260.

Singh, J. M. (1973). Decreased performance behavior with carbaryl—an indication of clinical toxicity. *Clin. Toxicol.* **6,** 97–108.

Slade, M., and Casida, J. E. (1970). Metabolic fate of 3,4,5- and 2,3,5-trimethylphenyl methylcarbamates, the major contitutents in Landrin insecticide. *J. Agric. Food Chem.* **18,** 467–474.

Smalley, H. E. (1970). Diagnosis and treatment of carbaryl in swine. *J. Am. Vet. Med. Assoc.* **156,** 339–344.

Smalley, H. E., Curtis, J. M., and Earl, F. L. (1968). Teratogenic action of carbaryl in beagle dogs. *Toxicol. Appl. Pharmacol.* **13,** 392–403.

Smalley, H. E., O'Hara, P. J., Bridges, C. H., and Radeleff, R. D. (1969). The effects of chronic carbaryl administration on the neuromuscular system of swine. *Toxicol. Appl. Pharmacol.* **14,** 409–419.

Sterman, A. B., and Varma, A. (1983). Evaluating human neurotoxicity of the pesticide aldicarb: When man becomes experimental animal. *Neurobehav. Toxicol. Teratol.* **5,** 493 495.

Sterri, S. H., Rognerud, B., Fiskum, S. E., and Lyngaas, S. (1979). Effect of Toxogonin and P2S on the toxicity of carbamates and organophosphorus compounds. *Acta Pharmacol. Toxicol.* **45,** 9–15.

Stevens, J. T., Stitzel, R. E., and McPhillips, J. J. (1972a). The effects of subacute administration of anticholinesterase insecticides on hepatic microsomal metabolism. *Life Sci.* (Part 2), **11** 423.

Stevens, J. T., Stitzel, R. E., and McPhillips, J. J. (1972b). Effects of anticholinesterase insecticides on hepatic microsomal metabolism. *J. Pharmacol. Exp. Ther.* **181,** 576.

Street, J. C., and Sharma, R. P. (1975). Alteration of induced cellular and humoral immune responses by pesticides and chemicals of environmental concern: Quantitative studies of immunosuppression by DDT, Aroclor 1254, carbaryl, carbofuran, and methylparathion. *Toxicol. Appl. Pharmacol.* **32,** 587–602.

Strother, A., and Wheeler, L. (1980). Excretion and disposition of [^{14}C]carbaryl in pregnant, non-pregnant and foetal tissues of the rat after acute administration. *Xenobiotica* **10,** 113–124.

Struble, C. B., Feil, V. J., Pekas, J. C., and Gerst, J. W. (1983). Biliary secretion of ^{14}C and identification of 5,6-dihydro-5,6-dihydroxycarbaryl glucuronide as a biliary metabolite of (^{14}C)carbaryl in the rat. *Pestic. Biochem. Physiol.* **19,** 85–94.

Studdert, V. P. (1985). Epidemiological features of snail and slug bait poisoning in dogs and cats. *Aust. Vet. J.* **62,** 269–271.

Sullivan, L. J., Eldridge, J. M., Knaak, J. B., and Tallant, M. J. (1972). 5,6-Dihydro-5,6-dihydroxycarbaryl glucuronide as a significant metabolite of carbaryl in the rat. *J. Agric. Food Chem.* **20,** 980–985.

Sussman, H. F., Cooke, S. B., and Block, V. (1969). Human louse infestation: Treatment with Carbacide. *Arch. Dermatol.* **100,** 82–83.

Syrowatka, T., Jurek, A., and Nazarewicz, T. (1971). Short term chronic toxicity study of o-isopropoxyphenyl-N-methylcarbamate (propoxur). *Rocz. Panstw. Zakl. Hig.* **22,** 579–589 (in Polish).

Szczepaniak, S., Sienkiewicz, E., Jeleniewicz, K., and Nowinski, H. (1980). Effect of carbaryl and chlorfenvinfos on the level of free amino acids in rat blood serum. Part II. Intoxication with a single dose corresponding to 1/5 LD 50. *Bromatol. Chem. Toksykol.* **13,** 351–353 (in Polish).

Tachibana, H., Hashimoto, K., Ishibashi, T., Ando, T., and Kitagawa, M. (1973). Studies of the learned behavior of rats as an index for toxicity. *Jpn. Ind. Hyg. Soc. Proc.* **46,** 408.

Takahashi, H., Miyaoka, T., Tsuda, S., and Shirasu, Y. (1983). Combined toxicity of malathion and carbamate insecticides in mice and rats. *J. Pestic. Sci.* **8,** 41–46.

Takahashi, H., Miyaoka, T., Tsuda, S., and Shirasu, Y. (1984). Potentiated toxicity of 2-sec-butylphenyl methylcarbamate (BPMC) by O,O-dimethyl O-(3-methyl-4-nitrophenyl)phosphorothioate (fenitrothion) in mice; relationship between acute toxicity and metabolism of BPMC. *Fundam. Appl. Toxicol.* **4,** 718–723.

Takahashi, H., Kato, A., Yamashita, E., Naito, Y., Tsuda, S., and Shirasu, Y. (1987a). Potentiations of N-methylcarbamate toxicities by organophosphorus insecticides in male mice. *Fundam. Appl. Toxicol.* **8,** 139–146.

Takahashi, H., Tanaka, J., Tsuda, S., and Shirasu, Y. (1987b). Contribution of monoaminergic nervous system in potentiation of 2-sec-butylphenyl N-methylcarbamate (BPMC) toxicity by malathion in male mice. *Fundam. Appl. Toxicol.* **8,** 415–422.

Tanaka, A. K., Umetsu, N., and Fukuto, T. R. (1985). Metabolism of benfuracarb in young cotton, bean, and corn plants. *J. Agric. Food Chem.* **33,** 1049–1055.

Tanaka, R., Fujisawa, S., Nakai, K., and Minagawa, K. (1980). Distribution and biliary excretion of carbaryl, dieldrin and paraquat in rats: Effect of diets. *J. Toxicol. Sci.* **5,** 151–162.

Tanaka, R., Fujisawa, S., and Nakai, K. (1981). Study on the absorption and protein binding of carbaryl, dieldrin and paraquat in rats fed on protein diet. *J. Toxicol. Sci.* **6,** 1–11.

Thomas, J. A., Dieringer, C. S., and Schein, L. (1974). Effects of carbaryl on mouse organs of reproduction. *Toxicol. Appl. Pharmacol.* **28,** 142–145.

Thomas, P. T., Ratajczak, H. V., Eisenberg, W. C., Furedi-Machacek, M., Ketels, K. V., and Barbera, P. W. (1987). Evaluation of host resistance and immunity in mice exposed to the carbamate pesticide aldicarb. *Fund. Appl. Toxicol.* **9,** 82–89.

Thust, R., Mendel, J., Schwarz, H., and Warzok, R. (1980). Nitrosated urea pesticide metabolites and other nitrosamides. Activity in clastogenicity and SCE assays and aberration kinetics in Chinese hamster V79-E cells. *Mutat. Res.* **79,** 239–248.

Tobin, J. S. (1970). Carbofuran: A new carbamate insecticide. *J. Occup. Med.* **12,** 16–19.

Trifonova, T. K. (1984). Effect of pesticides on reproductive function in animals. *Veterinariya* **8,** 55–56 (in Russian).

Triolo, A. J., Lang, W. R., Coon, J. M., Lindstrom, D., and Herr, D. L. (1982). Effect of the insecticides toxaphene and carbaryl on induction of lung tumors by benzo[a]pyrene in the mouse. *J. Toxicol. Environ. Health* **9,** 637–649.

Tsuda, S., Miyaoka, T., Iwasaki, M., and Shirasu, Y. (1984). Pharmacokinetic analysis of increased toxicity of 2-sec-butylphenyl methylcarbamate (BPMC) by fenitrothion pretreatment in mice. *Fundam. Appl. Toxicol.* **4,** 724–730.

Tyburczyk, W. (1981). Study on the effect of carbofuran on central nervous system. *Bromatol. Chem. Toksykol.* **14,** 289–296 (in Polish).

Tyburczyk, W., and Podolak-Majczak, M. (1984a). Effect of joint action of sodium nitrite and carbaryl in the rat. Part 1. Serotonin metabolism. *Bromatol. Chem. Toksykol.* **17,** 125–129 (in Polish).

Tyburczyk, W., and Podolak-Majczak, M. (1984b). Effect of joint action of sodium nitrite and carbaryl in the rat. Part 3. Some parameters of catecholaminergic, GABA-ergic, and cholinergic systems. *Bromatol. Chem. Toksykol.* **17,** 215–219 (in Polish).

Tyl, R. W., and Dodd, D. E. (1987). "Two-Generation Reproduction Study in CD® Albino Rats Exposed to Trimethacarb Technical by Dietary Inclusion," Rep. No. 49–172. Union Carbide Bushy Run Research Center, Export, Pennsylvania (unpublished).

Tyrkiel, E. (1978). Effect of O-isopropoxyphenyl-N-methylcarbamate (propoxur) on the embryonal development of mice. *Rocz. Panstw. Zakl. Hig.* **29,** 655–664 (in Polish).

Tyrkiel, E., and Bojanowska, A. (1978). Effect of insecticides from the carbamate group on reproduction of laboratory animals. *Rocz. Panstw. Zakl. Hig.* **29,** 181–192 (in Polish).

Tyrkiel, E., Palut, D., and Cybulski, J. (1978). Mutagenic action of N-nitroso derivatives of carbamate insecticides (carbaryl and propoxur) on mammalian cells. *Rocz. Panstw. Zakl. Hig.* **29,** 527–532 (in Polish).

Uchiyama, M., Takeda, M., Suzuki, T., and Yoskikawa, K. (1975). Mutagenicity of nitroso derivatives of N-methylcarbamate insecticides in microbiological method. *Bull. Environ. Contam. Toxicol.* **14,** 378 394.

Udall, N. D. (1973). The toxicity of the molluscicides metaldehyde methiocarb to dogs. *Vet. Rec.* **93,** 420–422.

Umetsu, N., and Fukuto, T. R. (1982). Alteration of carbosulfan [2,3-dihydro-2,2-dimethyl-7-benzofuranyl (di-n-butylaminosulfenyl) methylcarbamate] in the rat stomach. *J. Agric. Food Chem.* **30,** 555–557.

Union Carbide (1984). "Toxicology of Thiodicarb Insecticide." Union Carbide Agricultural Products Company, Inc., Research Triangle Park, North Carolina.

Union Carbide (1985). "Toxicology of Aldoxycarb Pesticides." Union Carbide Agricultural Products Company, Inc., Research Triangle Park, North Carolina.

U.S. Environmental Protection Agency (USEPA) (1978). "Summary for Reported Incidents Involving Carbofuran," Pesticide Incident Monit. Rep. No. 109. U.S. Environ. Prot. Agency, Washington, D.C.

Usha Rani, M. V., Reddi, O. S., and Reddy, P. P. (1980). Mutagenicity studies involving aldrin, endosulfan, dimethoate, phosphamidon, carbaryl and ceresan. Bull. Environ. Contam. Toxicol. 25, 277–282.

Valencia, R. (1981). "Mutagenesis Screening of Pesticides—Drosophila," Rep. No. EPA-600/1-18-017. U.S. Environ. Prot. Agency, Research Triangle Park, North Carolina.

Vandekar, M. (1965). Observations on the toxicity of carbaryl, Folithion and 3-isopropylphenyl N-methylcarbamate in a village-scale trial in southern Nigeria. Bull. W.H.O. 33, 107–115.

Vandekar, M. (1980). Minimizing occupational exposure to pesticides: Cholinesterase determination and organophosphorus poisoning. Residue Rev. 75, 67–80.

Vandekar, M., and Fajdetić, T. (1966). Studies in the toxicology of N-methylcarbamates. III. Tolerance of carbamates at different rates of intravenous infusion. Int. Congr. Occup. Health, Proc., 15th, 1966, Vol. 2, p. 529.

Vandekar, M., and Svetličić, B. (1966). Observations on the toxicity of three anticholinesterase insecticides in a village-scale trial and comparison of methods used for determining cholinesterase activity. Arh. Hig. Rada Toksikol. 17, 135–150.

Vandekar, M., and Wilford, K. (1969). The effect of cholinesterase activity of storage of undiluted whole blood sampled from men exposed to o-isopropoxyphenyl methylcarbamate (OMS-33) Bull. W.H.O. 40, 91–96.

Vandekar, M., Reiner, E., Svetličić, B., and Fajdetic, T. (1965). Value of ED 50 testing in assessing hazards of acute poisoning by carbamates and organophosphates. Br. J. Ind. Med. 22, 317–320.

Vandekar, M., Hedayat, S., Pleština, R., and Ahmady, G. (1968). A study of the safety of o-isopropoxyphenyl methylcarbamate in an operational field trial in Iran. Bull. W.H.O. 38, 609–623.

Vandekar, M., Pleština, R., and Wilhelm, K. T. (1971). Toxicity of carbamates for mammals. Bull. W.H.O. 44, 241–249.

van Hoof, F., and Heyndrickx, A. (1975). The excretion in urine of four insecticidal carbamates and their phenolic metabolites after oral administration to rats. Arch. Toxicol. 34, 81–88.

Vashakidze, V. I. (1965). Some questions of the harmful action of Sevin on the reproductive functions of experimental animals. Soobshch. Akad. Nauk Bruz. SSR 39, 471–474 (in Russian).

Vashakidze, V. I. (1967). Mechanism of action of pesticides (GranoSan, Sevin, Dinoc) on the reproductive cycle of experimental animals. Soobshch. Akad. Nauk Gruz. SSR 48, 219–224 (in Russian). (Chem. Abstr. 68, 28750).

Vashakidze, V. I. (1975). The effect of small doses of Sevin on the function of gonads under its repeated exposure to white rats. Vopr. Gig. Tr. Prof. Patol. Prom. Toksikol. pp. 253–267.

Vasilos, A. F., Dmitrienko, V. D., and Shroyt, I. G. (1972). Colchicine-like action of Sevin on the human embryo fibroblasts in vitro. Byull. Eksp. Biol. Med. 73, 91–93.

Vasilos, A. F., Dmitrienko, V. D., and Shroyt, I. G. (1975a). Disruption of the mitotic system following acute Sevin poisoning. Izv. Akad. Nauk Mold. SSR, Ser. Biol. Khim. Nauk 3, 64–67.

Vasilos, A. F., Dmitrienko, V. D., and Shroyt, I. G. (1975b). Changes in mitosis in chronic poisoning of rats with Sevin. Izv. Akad. Nauk Mold. SSR, Ser. Biol. Khim. Nauk 4, 45–47 (in Russian).

Vaughn-Dellarco, V. (1981). "Preliminary Report on the Mutagenicity of Carbaryl," Rep. No. EPA-600/6-81-001, NTIS/PB81-200768. U.S. Environ. Prot. Agency, Natl. Tech. Inf. Serv., Washington, D.C.

Verschoyle, R. D., and Barnes, J. M. (1969). Therapeutic effect of atropine and tetraethylammonium bromide against anticholinesterase insecticides in mice and rats. Bull. W.H.O. 41, 306–308.

Viter, V. F. (1978). Continuous and intermittent effect of carbaryl on certain behavior reactions of experimental animals. Gig. Sanit. 43, 33–34 (in Russian).

Volf, K., and Hanuš, V. (1984). Mass intoxication by agrochemical compound. Cesk. Patol. 20, 25–28 (in Czech).

Wakakura, M., Ishikawa, S., and Uga, S. (1978). Ultrastructural hepatic changes by carbamate pesticide (Sevin) in rats. Environ. Res. 16, 191–204.

Waters, M. D., Nesnow, S., Simmon, V. F., Mitchell, A. D., Jorgenson, T. A., and Valencia, R. (1981). Pesticides: Mutagenic and carcinogenic potential. ACS Symp. Ser. 160, 89–113.

Weil, C. S., and Carpenter, C. P. (1962). Mellon Institute Spec. Rep. 25–122 (unpublished).

Weil, C. S., Woodside, M. D., Carpenter, C. P., and Smyth, H. F., Jr. (1972). Current status of tests of carbaryl for reproductive and teratogenic effect. Toxicol. Appl. Pharmacol. 21, 390–404.

Weil, C. S., Woodside, M. D., Bernard, J. B., Condra, N. I., King, J. M., and Carpenter, C. P. (1973). Comparative effect of carbaryl on rat reproduction and guinea pig teratology when fed either in the diet or by stomach intubation. Toxicol. Appl. Pharmacol. 26, 621–638.

Weiss, L.R., and Orzel, R. A. (1967). Enhancement of toxicity of anticholinesterases by central depressant drugs in rats. Toxicol. Appl. Pharmacol. 10, 334.

Weiss, L. R., Bryand, J., and Fitzhugh, O. G. (1964). Blood sugar levels following acute poisoning with parathion and l-naphthyl-N-methylcarbamate (Sevin). Toxicol. Appl. Pharmacol. 6, 363.

Weiss, L. R., Orzel, R. A., and Fitzhugh, O. G. (1965). Hyperglycemia and drug interactions in anticholinesterase toxicity. Fed. Proc., Fed. Am. Soc. Exp. Biol. 24, 641.

Wheeler, L., and Strother, A. (1971). In vitro metabolism of the N-methylcarbamates, Zectran and Mesurol, by liver, kidney and blood of dogs and rats. J. Pharmacol. Exp. Ther. 178, 371.

Wheeler, L., and Strother, A. (1974a). In vitro metabolism of ^{14}C-pesticidal carbamates by fetal and maternal brain, liver, and placenta of the rat. Drug Metab. Dispos. 2, 533–538.

Wheeler, L., and Strother, A. (1974b). Placental transfer, excretion, and disposition of [^{14}C]Zectran and [^{14}C]Mesurol in maternal and fetal rat tissues. Toxicol. Appl. Pharmacol. 30, 163–174.

Whitehurst, W. E., Bishop, E. T., Critchfield, F. E., Gyrisco, G. G., Huddleston, E. W., Arnold, H., and Lisk, D. J. (1963). The metabolism of Sevin in dairy cows. J. Agric. Food Chem. 11, 167–169.

Whitlock, N. H., Schuman, S. H., and Loadholt, C. B. (1982). "Executive Summary and Epidemiologic Survey of Potential Acute Health Effects of Aldicarb in Drinking Water—Suffolk County, N.Y.," South Carolina Pesticide Hazard Assessment Program Center, Medical University of South Carolina, Charleston. Prepared for the Health Effects Branch, Hazard Evaluation Division, Office of Pesticide Programs, U.S. Environmental Protection Agency (unpublished).

Whorton, M. D., Milby, T. H., Stubbs, H. A., Avashia, B. H., and Hull, E. Q. (1979). Testicular function among carbaryl-exposed employees. J. Toxicol. Environ. Health 5, 929–941.

Wiles, R. (1987). Case studies of the EPA's application of the Delaney Clause in the tolerance-setting process. In "Regulating Pesticides in Food: The Delaney Paradox," Committee on Scientific and Regulatory Issues Underlying Pesticide Use Patterns and Agricultural Innovation (R. Thornton, chairman), pp. 220–225. Board of Agriculture, National Research Council, National Academy Press, Washington, D.C.

Williams, E., Meikle, R. W., and Redemann, C. T. (1964). Identification of metabolites of Zectran insecticide in dog urine. J. Agric. Food Chem. 12, 457–461.

Willigan, D. A. (1980). Letter of review and comment to R. Case on "Hepatic Changes in Mice. . . ," M. S. Thesis, A. M. Hoberman, University of Arkansas (unpublished).

Wills, J. H., Jameson, E., and Coulston, F. (1968). Effects of oral doses of carbaryl on man. Clin. Toxicol. 1, 265–271.

Wiltrout, R. W., Ercegovich, C. D., and Ceglowski, W. S. (1978). Humoral immunity in mice following oral administration of selected pesticides. Bull. Environ. Contam. Toxicol. 20, 423–431.

Wojciechowski, J. P., Kaur, P., and Sabharwal, P. S. (1982). Induction of ouabain resistance in V-79 cells by four carbamate pesticides. Environ. Res. 29, 48–53.

Wolfe, J. L., and Esher, R. J. (1980). Toxicity of carbofuran and lindane to the old-field mouse (Peromyscus polionotus) and the cotton mouse (P. gossypinus). Bull. Environ. Contam. Toxicol. 24, 894–902.

Woodruff, R. C., Phillips, J. P., and Irwin, D. (1983). Pesticide-induced complete and partial chromosome loss in screens with repair-defective females of *Drosophila melanogaster. Environ. Mutagen.* **5,** 835–846.

World Health Organization (WHO) (1967). "Safe Use of Pesticides in Public Health," Sixteenth Report of the WHO Expert Committee on Insecticides, Tech. Rep. Ser. No. 356. World Health Organ., Geneva.

World Health Organization (WHO) (1973). "Safe Use of Pesticides," 20th Report of the WHO Expert Committee on Insecticides, Tech. Rep. Ser. No. 513. World Health Organ., Geneva.

World Health Organization (WHO) (1986). "Environmental Health Criteria for Carbamate Pesticides: A General Introduction." World Health Organ., Geneva.

Wright, J. W., Fritz, R. F., Hocking, K. S., Babione, R., Gratz, N. G. Pal, R., Stiles, A. R., and Vandekar, M. (1969). *ortho*-Isopropoxyphenyl methylcarbamate (OMS-33) as a residual spray for control of anopheline mosquitos. *Bull. W.H.O.* **40,** 67–90.

Wyrobeck, A. J., Watchmaker, G., Gordon, L., Wong, K., Moore, D., II, and Whorton, D. (1981). Sperm shape abnormalities in carbaryl-exposed employees. *Environ. Health Perspect.* **40,** 67–90.

Yakim, V. S. (1967). The maximum permissible concentration of Sevin® in the air of the work zone. *Hyg. Sanit.* **32,** 32–37.

Zbinden, G., and Flury-Roversi, M. (1981). Significance of the LD_{50}-test for the toxicological evaluation of chemical substances. *Arch. Toxicol.* **47,** 77–99.

Zĕinalov, T. A. (1984). Biochemical studies of monamine oxidase activity in a hygienic assessment of effects of environmental toxic factors. *Gig. Sanit.* **6,** 49–52 (in Russian).

Zĕinalov, T. A. (1985). Stimulation of 2-phenylethylamine enzymatic deamination using 2-isopropoyl hydroxyphenyl-*N*-methylcarbamate (Baygon). *Vopr. Med. Khim.* **31,** 60–64 (in Russian).

Zweig, G., Leffingwell, J. T., and Popendorf, W. (1985). The relationship between dermal pesticide exposure by fruit harvesters and dislodgeable foliar residues. *J. Environ. Sci. Health, Part B* **20,** 27–59.

Nitro Compounds and Related Phenolic Pesticides

Thomas A. Gasiewicz
University of Rochester

18.1 INTRODUCTION

This chapter deals with a small number of compounds characterized by closely related chemical structures, a similar primary mode of toxic action in mammals, and unusually diverse applications as pesticides. Chemically, all of these compounds are substituted phenols. Biochemically, most are uncouplers of oxidative phosphorylation (see Sections 18.3.1.1 and 18.3.1.2). Practically, they find use as insecticides, acaricides, molluscicides, fungicides, bactericides, herbicides, and plant growth regulators.

The compounds can be divided into three main categories: mononitrophenols, dinitrophenols, and halophenols. There is some overlapping, for example, 2,6-diiodo-4-nitrophenol.

The toxicity of phenol and its derivatives, including the dinitrophenols and chlorophenols, has been reviewed in great detail by von Oettingen (1949).

18.2 MONONITROPHENOLS

Only a small number of pesticides are mononitrophenols. They include lampricides (3-bromo-4-nitrophenol and 3-trifluoromethyl-4-nitrophenol); one molluscicide, niclosoamide (see Section 22.3.2); some biphenyl ether herbicides such as fluorodifen and nitrofen (see Section 20.13.1); and a few fungicides including dicloran (see Section 21.8.1). They are compounds of moderate to low acute toxicity, with oral LD 50 values in adult rats ranging from 370 to >1000 mg/kg. According to Burkatskaja and Anina (1969), dichloronitrophenol is an uncoupler of oxidative phosphorylation. 2,6-Diiodo-4-nitrophenol, an anthelmintic used in veterinary medicine, certainly has this action (Kaiser, 1964). It seems possible that some mononitrophenols used as pesticides are uncouplers, and the possibility was discussed by Kawatski and McDonald (1974) in connection with 3-trifluoromethyl-4-nitrophenol but without a clear-cut result. The biology and toxicology of niclosamide (2′,5-dichloro-4′-nitrosalicyl anilide) has been reviewed by Andrews et al. (1983). All investigations on niclosamide in experimental animals and human subjects indicate low acute toxicity and no cumulative toxic effects in humans for long-term exposures. The low mammalian toxicity of all of these compounds indicates that they are not highly active, regardless of their modes of action, and their diverse uses suggest that these modes may be different. Therefore, further discussion of those that have been studied in humans may be found in specific sections of Chapters 20, 21, and 22 as indicated above.

18.3 DINITROPHENOLS

18.3.1 INTRODUCTION

18.3.1.1 Chemical Identity and Use

A number of substituted 2,4-dinitrophenols, alone or as salts of aliphatic amines (triethanolamine or isopropanolamine) or alkalies (sodium, potassium, or ammonium hydroxide), are sold under many trade names, frequently with a suffix to indicate the formulation. The details of their chemistry and use for pest control were reviewed by Kirby (1966). Some of these compounds are closely related to 2,4-dinitrophenol, which has limited use as a pesticide but has been studied extensively as a drug and in connection with its biochemical effects. The structures of 2,4-dinitrophenol and some of its analogs are listed in Table 18.1. Minor differences in chemical structure determine whether these compounds are useful as fungicides, herbicides, or insecticides. Several have more than one use. However, as far as is known, all of them have the same mode of systemic action in mammals. They do differ in the ease with which they are absorbed by the skin, and this may make an important difference in the danger they present to workers. They also differ in their ability to produce cataract.

18.3.1.2 Biochemical and Pharmacological Effects

It is interesting that of the six isomeric dinitrophenols, those with nitro groups in the 2,4- and 3,4- positions stimulate oxygen

Table 18.1
2,4-Dinitrophenols and Their Derivatives of the Form:

Name and abbreviations	R	R'
binapacryl	—C—CH=C—CH$_3$ ‖O	—CH—C$_2$H$_5$
		CH$_3$
		CH$_3$
2,4-dinitroanisole	—CH$_3$	—H$_3$
2,4-dinitrocresol (DNOC, DNC)	—H	—CH$_3$
2,4-dinitrophenol (DNP)	—H	—H
dinocap	—C—CH=CH—CH$_3$	—(CH$_2$)$_5$—CH$_3$
dinoseb (DNBP)	—H	—CH—C$_2$H$_5$
		CH$_3$

consumption, while that with nitro groups in the 2,5- position does not. On the other hand, 2,4-dinitrophenol does not produce methemoglobin, but the 2,3-, 2,5-, 2,6-, and 3,4- isomers do produce it (Magne *et al.*, 1932b). Furthermore, although 2,4- and 3,4-dinitrophenols uncouple oxidative phosphorylation in such a way that there is an increase in oxygen consumption and heat production, there is a decrease in the trapping of energy in compounds such as adenosine triphosphate necessary for muscular movement and many other vital functions.

Parker (1958) recognized three biological actions of 2,4-dinitrophenol, dinitrocresol, pentachlorophenol, and a number of other substituted phenols of what he termed "type A," namely, (*a*) inhibition of oxidative phosphorylation, (*b*) stimulation of oxidation, and (*c*) stimulation of adenosine triphosphatase activity. In isolated mitochondria, a number of effects associated with uncoupling are readily demonstrated. These include (*a*) increased respiration (loss of respiratory control); (*b*) inhibition of several exchange reactions catalyzed by mitochondria, including reactions involving adenosine diphosphate, inorganic phosphate, adenosine triphosphate, and water; (*c*) increased adenosine triphosphatase activity and release of the enzyme into the supernatant fraction; and (*d*) osmotic swelling of mitochondria. Pressman (1963) proposed that uncouplers promote the conductivity of protons within mitochondrial membranes and subsequently prevent the formation of a gradient across the membrane, while Mitchell (1961) suggested that these compounds promote the splitting of an energy-rich intermediate prior to adenosine triphosphate production. Virtually all uncouplers are poorly soluble in water, and this may be related to their mode of action. All that have been tested do in fact increase the conductivity of phospholipid bilayer membranes, acting as proton ionophores (Bakker *et al.*, 1973;

Cunarro and Weiner, 1975). Thus, an uncoupler destroys the essential proton gradient by freely exchanging protons across the mitochondrial membrane (Kessler *et. al.*, 1976). The loss of the gradient likely results in the release of mitochondrial calcium into the cytoplasm (Pettersson, 1983, 1984), which may in turn generate a variety of biochemical alterations including loss of integrity of the cellular membrane (George *et al.*, 1982; Ganote *et al.*, 1984; Deleze and Herve, 1983). It was originally thought that uncouplers penetrate the mitochondrial membrane in an un-ionized form and become ionized inside to then adsorb to catalytic proteins. Although many newer pesticides that are uncouplers are neutral molecules and do not dissociate under physiological pH, a direct interaction of the uncouplers with proteins resulting in structural and catalytic changes cannot be discounted (Weinbach and Garbus, 1969).

Eisenhardt and Rosenthal (1964) found that, if 2,4-dinitrophenol is added to a preparation of rat liver mitochondria after incubation with substrate, orthophosphate, and oxygen, and just prior to the addition of the phosphate acceptor adenosine diphosphate, steady-state phosphorylation is greatly reduced, although the initial state of rapid phosphorylation is undisturbed. The uncoupling agents do allow electron transport to continue but prevent the phosphorylation of adenosine diphosphate to adenosine triphosphate. It also should be pointed out that these agents, in most cases, do not uncouple glycolytic phosphorylation or directly affect cellular reactions other than oxidative phosphorylation.

The aminonitrophenol metabolites of 2,4-dinitrophenol do not inhibit oxidative phosphorylation (Judah and Williams-Ashman, 1951).

Most investigators consider that depletion of high-energy phosphate bonds is due mainly to prevention of their synthesis and only secondarily to acceleration of their cleavage (Cockrell and Pressman, 1979). However, Zhivkov *et al.* (1970) reached the opposite conclusion. Regardless of the relative importance of the different factors, everyone agrees that uncoupling of oxidative phosphorylation is the main cause of poisoning.

The uncoupling of oxidative phosphorylation by dinitrophenols can be detected in the tissues of poisoned animals and, at least for some compounds, it can be demonstrated *in vitro* at concentrations ≤1 μM (Ilivicky and Casida, 1969). Finally, some other pesticides (e.g., captan) do not produce uncoupling of oxidative phosphorylation *in vivo* but do have the effect at concentrations of 100 μM or more *in vitro* (Syrowatka, 1970).

Whereas the overall metabolic rate of the intact animal, and in particular the tricarboxylic acid cycle, is increased by 2,4-dinitrophenol, it inhibits the oxidation of some substrates, notably lactate, *in vitro*. Lipogenesis from pyruvate and lactate is subsequently inhibited (Rognstad and Katz, 1969). Over and above the effect of increased metabolism, it may be that the inhibition of lipogenesis makes a substantial contribution to the weight loss observed.

Although both dinitro compounds and thyroxine stimulate metabolism, the two effects can be distinguished both *in vitro* (Michel and Pairault, 1969) and in myxademateous people

(Dodds and Robertson, 1933b). An opposite conclusion, namely that the presence of endocrine secretion of the thyroid is essential for the uncoupling action of dinitrophenol, was presented by Medvedeva (1969). However, it is clear that dinitrophenols have direct effects on a variety of isolated cell types, independent of the influence of possible fluctuations of the levels of circulating thyroid hormones.

Cardus and Hoff (1963) made a careful study of oxygen consumption, ventilation, respiratory frequency, and temperature in anesthetized dogs given 2,4-dinitrophenol intravenously at doses of 0, 3, 6, and 9 mg/kg. All of the parameters tended to increase with dosage. Although ventilation correlated with oxygen consumption, an even better correlation was obtained when the temperature of the animals was taken into account. Thus, at least in the dog, ventilation is adjusted partly to provide oxygen and partly to dissipate heat.

Even at dosages that are survived, abnormal metabolism is reflected in abnormal electrocardiographic findings, namely diphasic T wave, T-wave reversal, elevation or depression of the S-T segment, and reduction in the amplitude of the R wave. At dosages of 25 mg/kg and greater, some tracings were bizarre; no characteristic waves were present (Kaiser, 1964). The oxygen consumption of the perfused rat heart was increased approximately 50% when the dinitrophenol was added to the perfusion fluid at a concentration of 10 μM (about 1.84 ppm) (Lochner and Brink, 1969).

It is interesting that, whereas 2,4-dinitrophenol causes an increase in oxygen consumption at all ambient temperatures, it leads to a more rapid than normal reduction in body temperature in mice subjected to an environmental temperature of 5°C for 1 hr (Turner, 1946). This is likely associated, in part, with the prostration caused by the compound.

Studies of infused dog kidneys indicated the possibility of a minor, direct effect of dinitrophenol on the kidney. However, studies in living dogs showed that the major effects of intravenous injection at a dose of 6 mg/kg or slightly more were extrarenal. The effects included increased diuresis and excretion of sodium, potassium, and chloride ions related to decreased resorption in the tubules. The extrarenal character of the action was demonstrated by experiments in which dinitrophenol was injected into one renal artery while urine was collected separately from both ureters (Anikin, 1969).

Following a single intraperitoneal injection of dinitrophenol, a higher concentration was reached, and the compound persisted longer in the aqueous humors, vitreous humors, and lenses of ducklings and young rabbits, which are susceptible to the cataractogenic activity of the compound, than in mature rabbits, which are not susceptible. Dinitrophenol persisted longer in these tissues of immature rabbits than in those of ducklings, a finding congruent with the fact that cataracts produced by dinitrophenol in immature rabbits persist longer than those produced in ducklings (Gehring and Buerge, 1969). A study by Rae et al. (1982) has indicated that gap junctions of lens fiber cells are particularly sensitive to the uncoupling action of dinitrophenol and that the effect is reversible upon removal of the uncoupler.

18.3.1.3 Treatment of Poisoning

Treatment of Poisoning in Animals In guinea pigs tested at 18°C, the intraperitoneal LD 50 was raised from 28 mg/kg to 31 and 35 mg/kg, respectively, when chlorpromazine was given subcutaneously at the rate of 5 mg/kg 90 and 60 min, respectively, after administration of the poison. There was a further improvement (LD 50 39 mg/kg) when the animals were cooled for 8 hr as well as being given chlorpromazine. For the most part, the rectal temperature of the animals was held at 5°C under that of poisoned control animals not subject to special cooling (Ritzmann, 1958).

Activated charcoal, tannin, magnesia, starch solution, and paraffin oil all reduced the absorption of 2,4-dinitrophenol administered orally to rats either 1 or 5 min earlier. Activated charcoal and magnesia were most effective. The maximal blood level of the poison was reached 30 min after its administration, both in controls and in those given an antidote, except after paraffin oil, where the interval was 60 min (Sen'chuk and Adamska, 1977).

Working on the thesis that the idiopathic malignant hyperpyretic syndrome sometimes seen in general anesthesia is the result of uncoupling of oxidative phosphorylation by certain anesthetics in susceptible persons, Gatz and Jones (1970) used dinitrophenol poisoning in rats as a model and found that the occurrence of hyperthermia and death could be reduced by pretreatment with haloperidol. Apparently, there has been no exploration of the possible value of haloperidol for treating animals after poisoning by a dinitrophenol has appeared.

Haloperidol was chosen on the basis of *in vitro* experiments that showed that it inhibited, whereas chlorpromazine uncoupled, oxidative phosphorylation (Gatz and Jones, 1969). However, Bacila and Medina (1962) reported that not only chlorpromazine but also promethazine, perphenazine, and neozine inhibit the effect of 2,4-dinitrophenol on the respiration of heart muscle sarcosomes. Tesic *et al.* (1972) reported that prior treatment with large doses of chlorpromazine prolonged the life of rats poisoned by subcutaneous injection of DNOC—as did prior treatment with vitamins A and E and with glucose in Tyrode's solution. It must be noted that if some neurotropic drugs really have value for treating poisoning by dinitrophenol, the basis for the action may by entirely different from that for which the drugs ordinarily are used.

Issekutz (1984) studied the effect of the β-blocker propranolol on the alterations of carbohydrate metabolism elicited by sublethal poisoning of dogs with 2,4-dinitrophenol. The infusion rate was 0.3–0.4 mg/kg/min for a total dosage of 8.5 mg/kg. Propranolol had no effect on the dinitrophenol-induced rise in body temperature, but completely blocked the rise in lactate production, the lactacidemia, and the rise in peripheral glycogenolysis. In contrast, propranolol significantly increased the participation of glucose in lactate production, prolonged the dinitrophenol-induced hyperphosphatemia, and caused a decline of plasma glucose concentration. The effects of dinitrophenol on the control animals agreed with previous findings of Hetenyi *et al.* (1955). From the effects of propranolol, Issekutz concluded that the effect of dinitrophenol poisoning on carbohydrate metabolism *in vivo* is more complex than one would expect on the basis of just *in vitro* studies. An important role of the β-adrenergic system in the control of glycogenolysis was suggested. However, it was also pointed out that propranolol may have a calcium antagonistic effect in addition to the blocking of β-receptors (Rokutanda *et al.*, 1983).

Although rats pretreated with methylthiouracil or thiouracil are less susceptible than normal rats to poisoning by dinitrocresol (Hofmann-Credner and Siedek, 1949; Barker, 1946a,b), there is no evidence that such drugs act rapidly enough to benefit an animal already poisoned by a nitro compound.

Treatment of Poisoning in Humans   Treatment is symptomatic and difficult. An effort must be made to maintain the fluid and electrolyte balance and to keep the body temperature within tolerable limits.

The poison should be removed promptly from the skin and/or gastrointestinal tract. If available, activated charcoal should be used for gastric lavage; some should be left in the stomach and a saline cathartic should be given about 1 hr later (see Section 8.2.1 and 8.2.3.1). No attempt beyond ordinary washing should be made to remove the deeply penetrated, persistent stain from the skin or hair (Hofmann-Credner and Siedek, 1949).

Forced diuresis apparently was responsible for saving an elderly man poisoned by pentachlorophenol, and its more general use was urged (Young and Haley, 1978; Haley, 1977). The administration of a large amount of fluid with careful attention to the electrolyte balance will, of course, tend to compensate for the extensive fluid and electrolyte loss even before diuresis becomes effective.

Treatment should include temperature control (see Section 8.2.2.9) and the administration of oxygen (see Section 8.2.2.2).

It has been claimed that the intravenous injection of 10 ml of a 2.5% solution of sodium methyl thiouracil rapidly reduces the metabolic rate in persons in whom the rate of metabolism has been increased by dinitrocresol (Hofmann-Credner and Siedek, 1949). Antipyretic drugs are not effective because poisoning involves peripheral metabolism, not central nervous system control of temperature. Furthermore, there is evidence from animal studies (Tainter and Cutting, 1933) that salicylates potentiate the stimulation of metabolism by nitrophenols. Therefore, control of the temperature of persons poisoned by nitrophenol should be restricted to physical measures.

The use of atropine is absolutely contraindicated. The headache, nausea, vomiting, sweating, dyspnea, pain in the chest or abdomen, and weakness or coma produced by dinitrophenol may be reminiscent of the effects of anticholinesterase compounds. However, the modes of action of the two kinds of poison are entirely different. They may be distinguished by an accurate history of exposure, by the presence of high temperature in poisoning by dinitrophenol, and by the presence of muscular fasciculations and excessive respiratory secretions in poisoning by anticholinesterase compounds.

The possibility that haloperidol or some other drug could be administered after poisoning and still compete with dinitrophenols for binding, thus blocking or mitigating their uncoupling action, should be explored in animals.

18.3.2 2,4-DINITROPHENOL

18.3.2.1 Identity, Properties, and Uses

Chemical Name   2,4-Dinitrophenol

Structure   See Table 18.1.

Synonyms   2,4-Dinitrophenol is the name in common use, although the acronym DNP is sometimes used. Trade names for the compound include Aldifen®, Fenoxyl®, Nitro Kleenup®, Solfo Black B®, and Tertrosulphus Black PB®. Code designations include NSC-1,532. The CAS registry number is 51-28-5.

Physical and Chemical Properties   2,4-Dinitrophenol has the empirical formula $C_6H_4N_2O_5$ and a molecular weight of 184.11. It forms yellow orthorhombic crystals with a melting point of 113.9°C. It sublimes upon careful heating and is volatile in steam. Its density is 1.683. At 25°C, it is practically insoluble in water (0.0587%) but soluble in benzene, alcohol, and alkaline solution. Its sodium salt is freely water-soluble.

Use   2,4-Dinitrophenol is a woodworm insecticide and wood preservative.

18.3.2.2 Toxicity to Laboratory Animals

Basic Findings   In rats and mice, 2,4-dinitrophenol produces tremor, prostration, increased respiratory rate, tonic convulsions, and rigidity of the limbs just before or immediately after death. Poisoned dogs show an increase in heart rate, respiratory rate, and body temperature, and they may vomit. Those that die show early rigor mortis (Kaiser, 1964). In a narcotized dog, the intravenous administration of 2,4-dinitrophenol at a dosage of 8.5–9 mg/kg increased the metabolic rate by 100–200%. A striking rise in plasma lactate and inorganic phosphate was observed. At the same time, the oxygen uptake of the muscle was shown to increase 5–6-fold, while its adenosine triphosphate and glycogen content decreased markedly. Death was caused by hyperthermia (Hetenyi *et al.*, 1955).

The compound is only slightly irritating to the skin or eye (Spencer *et al.*, 1948).

The acute toxicity of 2,4-dinitrophenol is shown in Table 18.2. The oral toxicity is similar to that of nicotine, the common arsenicals, and the moderately toxic organic phosphorus compounds. Rabbits absorb 2,4-dinitrophenol less readily than dinitrocresol, but the toxicity of the two compounds to guinea pigs is almost the same.

A number of investigators have found that the toxicity of 2,4-dinitrophenol is increased at increased ambient temperatures. Fuhrman *et al.* (1943) found that the subcutaneous LD 50 of the

Table 18.2
Single-Dose LD 50 for 2,4-Dinitrophenol

Species and sex	Route	LD 50 (mg/kg)	Reference
Rat	oral	50	Spencer et al. (1948)
Rat, M	oral	71	Kaiser (1964)
Rat, M	subcutaneous	44	Kaiser (1964)
Rat, M	intraperitoneal	60	Kaiser (1964)
Rat, M	intravenous	72	Kaiser (1964)
Mouse, M	oral	72	Kaiser (1964)
Mouse, M	subcutaneous	58	Kaiser (1964)
Mouse, M	intraperitoneal	52	Kaiser (1964)
Mouse, M	intravenous	56	Kaiser (1964)
Guinea pig	intraperitoneal	28	Ritzmann (1958)

compound in mice was 35.7 mg/kg at 6°C, 30.9 mg/kg at 25°C, and <8.2 at 40°C.

Dogs survived 14 oral doses by capsule at rates of 5 and 12.5 mg/kg, but another died after a single dose at this rate (Spencer et al., 1948). Only slight increases in urine albumin levels were observed in dogs administered daily oral doses of 5 or 10 mg/kg for up to 6 months (Tainter et al., 1934).

Ducklings fed 2,4-dinitrophenol at a concentration of 2500 ppm developed cataracts within 24 hr and died in 6 or more days (Spencer et al., 1948). Chickens are also susceptible. Cataract was observed in a duckling only 3.5 hr after crop intubation; with no further dosing, the lesion cleared within 3 days (Armbrecht and Saver, 1960).

Male rats fed 2,4-dinitrophenol for 6 months at a dietary level of 100 ppm (2.7–10 mg/kg/day) grew normally and appeared well; all of their laboratory findings were normal, but at autopsy the weight of their kidneys (2.36 ± 0.04 gm) was slightly greater than that of the controls (2.18 ± 0.05 gm). The kidneys and other organs were histologically normal. At a dietary level of 200 ppm (5.4–20 mg/kg/day), there was not only a slight increase in kidney weight but also a slight increase in blood urea nitrogen (228 ppm compared with 194 ppm in controls); other findings were normal. A dietary level of 500 ppm (13.5–50 mg/kg/day) caused a 5–10% deficiency in growth, which was statistically significant. Injury to the kidneys was similar to that already described, but the increase in blood urea nitrogen affected only certain individuals, the others remaining completely normal. A dietary level of 1000 ppm caused weight loss, kidney damage, and a slight decrease in the weight of the heart, all without apparent histological change. A dietary level of 2000 ppm caused marked food refusal, marked loss of weight, and death difficult to distinguish from starvation after 7 or more days. Cataracts were not observed at any dosage level (Spencer et al., 1948).

Using a mouse skin tumor model, Boutwell and Bosch (1959) suggested that 2,4-dinitrophenol may act as a promoter for carcinogenesis. It has been found to cause frameshift mutations in *Salmonella typhimurium* TA98, but only in the presence of an S-9 fraction containing drug-metabolizing enzymes

(Furukawa et al., 1985). 2,4-dinitrophenol gave a negative response in a test for unscheduled DNA synthesis in hepatocytes and the modified Ames test (Probst et al., 1981).

Absorption, Distribution, Metabolism, and Excretion In dogs given a single oral dose by capsule, the concentration in the plasma reached its highest point in 2–4 hr at a dosage of 12.5 mg/kg or more and in 2 hr at a dosage of 5 mg/kg. The concentration was markedly reduced 8 hr after dosing. At dosages of 25 mg/kg/day or less for 13 days, there was no accumulation from day to day, and the peak value came at the same interval after each daily dose (Kaiser, 1964).

2,4-Dinitrophenol is excreted unchanged and as metabolites. It is metabolized in humans, dogs, and mice to 2-amino-4-nitrophenol, 2-nitro-4-aminophenol, and 2,4-diaminophenol and their glucuronic acid conjugates (Guerbet and Mayer, 1932; Georgescu, 1932; Robert and Hagardorn, 1983, 1985). The major excretory product in human, dog, rat, and mouse is probably 2-amino-4-nitrophenol (Magne et al., 1932a; Parker, 1952; Robert and Hagardorn, 1983). The kinetics of *in vitro* nitro reduction of 2,4-dinitrophenol by rat liver homogenates have been defined by Eiseman et al. (1974).

Pathology Rats fed 1000 ppm revealed marked emaciation, slightly enlarged spleen, and small testes. Microscopic examination revealed slight congestion and cloudy swelling of the liver, very slight degeneration of the kidney tubules, and testicular atrophy. All of these changes were difficult to distinguish from those caused by starvation alone (Spencer et al., 1948). Ultrastructural lesions of the mitochondria from liver and heart have been described by Cieciura and Rydzynski (1980).

18.3.2.3 Toxicity to Humans

Therapeutic Use 2,4-Dinitrophenol was introduced in 1933 for stimulation of metabolism and promotion of weight loss (Cutting et al., 1933). It was thought that increased oxidation involved fat almost exclusively (Tainter et al., 1933, 1935). The sodium salt was given at the rate of 100 mg daily for a week, then 200 mg daily for several weeks, followed by a gradual increase in steps of 100 mg until the limit of tolerance was reached and the dose was stabilized. The objective was loss of 2 or 3 lb/week. Symptoms of excessive heat and sweating constituted warnings of excessive intake. It was estimated that the treatment was used by 100,000 people in the United States in the first 3 years after introduction of the drug (Sollmann, 1942).

In spite of success in most instances, reports of injury soon appeared. As reviewed by von Oettingen (1949), the signs of poisoning, especially those in serious cases, were similar to those seen in animals. However, a wide range of other complaints, including peripheral neuritis, neutropenia, agranulocytosis, indications of liver injury, and various rashes of the skin were reported. One sign that was observed so often that there could be no doubt of its origin was cataract (Boardman, 1935; Horner et al., 1935). Whalman (1936) collected about 100 of these cases from California alone. With one exception, the patients were women. The condition was often delayed, appearing as much as 13 months after the drug was discontinued; however, once it appeared, the lesion developed rapidly and involved marked swelling of the lens. The cataracts were further characterized by being bilateral and occurring in an age group in which the disease is uncommon. The abnormality of the lens predisposed to glaucoma, and in all instances the anterior chamber was shallow. Horner (1936) estimated that between 0.1 and 1.0% of all persons using dinitrophenol as a reducing agent developed cataract. Later, the same author (Horner, 1942), in an exhaustive review, showed that the incidence varied from 0.63 to 1.52% and averaged 0.86 in four series of 66–170 cases each.

In 1935, the Council of Pharmacy and Chemistry of the American Medical Association refused to accept the drug and warned against its uncontrolled use (Sollmann, 1942).

Until replaced by DDT, which had a longer duration of action, 2,4-dinitroanisole was used as a constituent of MYL powder for the control of lice on humans. The MYL formula consisted of 0.2% pyrethrins as a toxicant, 2.0% of IN-930 (*N*-isobutylundecylenamide) as a synergist, 0.25% Phenol-S (isopropyl cresols obtained as a by-product of thymol manufacture) as an antioxidant, 2.0% 2,4-dinitroanisole as an ovicide, and pyrophyllite as an inert diluent. The powder was applied to the entire inner surface of winter underwear at a dosage of 30 gm/suit. Thus, the dosage of 2,4-dinitroanisole was 600 mg/person. Applied in this way, MYL powder killed all lice and eggs present at the time and gave complete protection against introduced lice for at least a week (Bushland *et al.*, 1944). The medical use of 2,4-dinitroanisole is discussed here because the compound is demethylated to form 2,4-dinitrophenol, which is the active toxicant. However, both the rate of absorption and the rate of demethylation limit the concentration of toxicant, and both tests and experience showed the MYL powder was safe.

Use Experience   Most accidents caused by 2,4-dinitrophenol have been occupational in origin. The largest number occurred in France during World War I in connection with the use of this compound as an explosive. Except for the propensity of the compound for causing cataract, little or nothing now known about the clinical aspects of poisoning by 2,4-dinitrophenol was missed by Perkins (1919) in his careful review of the French experience. It is not clear why cataract was apparently more frequent following medical use of the compound. It is tempting to speculate that the difference of route of exposure was important, but sex differences cannot be excluded as a cause. With few exceptions, the reducers were women and the workers were men.

Atypical Cases of Various Origins   A single case of hemolytic anemia in a worker who impregnated wooden poles with dinitrophenol, arsenic, and sodium fluoride was reported by Saita (1949). The lowest red cell count recorded was 3,400,000. No specific hemolytic episode was noted, and other evidence for hemolysis as a basis for the anemia was incomplete. The illness, which started about 15 days after work began, was attributed to dinitrophenol because the entire syndrome was considered to resemble that usually associated with that compound and not those associated with arsenic or sodium fluoride.

Treatment of Poisoning   See Section 18.3.1.3.

18.3.3 DNOC

18.3.3.1 Identity, Properties, and Uses

Chemical Name   2,4-Dinitro-6-methylphenol.

Structure   See Table 18.1.

Synonyms   DNOC (BSI, JMAF, ISO) is the common name in use; it is an acronym for 4,6-dinitro-*o*-cresol. Other names for the compound include dinitrocresol and DNC. Trade names include Antinonin®, Dekrysil®, Detal®, Dinitrol®, Ditrosol®, Effusan®, Elgetol®, K III®, K IV®, Lipan®, Prokarbol®, Selinon®, and Sinox®. Code designations include ENT-154. The CAS registry number is 534-52-1.

Physical and Chemical Properties   DNOC has the empirical formula $C_7H_6N_2O_5$ and a molecular weight of 198.13. It forms odorless yellow prisms melting at 87.5°C with a vapor pressure of 1.05×10^{-4} torr. At 15°C, DNOC is slightly soluble in water (0.013%) but freely soluble in alkaline solution, acetic acid, alcohol, and in most other organic solvents. It is explosive when dry and strongly phytotoxic. The sodium salt appears as a red powder and is readily soluble in water.

History, Formulations, and Uses   DNOC is primarily an agricultural pesticide, but also has limited use in the dyestuffs industry. The potassium salt of DNOC was introduced as early as 1892, as the active ingredient of Antitonnin used for controlling the nun moth. Since 1925, DNOC has been used as a herbicide and occasionally as a fungicide. According to the U.S. National Institute for Occupational Safety and Health, DNOC is not currently manufactured in the United States and imports have decreased considerably since 1972 (National Institute for Occupational Safety and Health, 1978). The phenol is sold as such but usually moistened with up to 10% water to reduce the danger of explosion. Sodium or amine salts also are available. The sodium salt is formulated as a 30–40% solution in petroleum oil. Both the phenol and the salt are used as insecticides and fungicides where phytotoxicity is not a problem.

18.3.3.2 Toxicity to Laboratory Animals

Basic Findings   Signs of poisoning include hyperactivity followed by depression and fever. Fever tends to be higher in larger animals. Other signs include dyspnea and cyanoses and may include asphyxial convulsions. Death is followed almost immediately by rigor mortis. Survivors appear normal 24 hr after dosing (Heyman and Casier, 1935; Ambrose, 1947; Parker *et al.*, 1951).

Dinitrocresol is not significantly irritating to the skin or the eye (Ambrose, 1947; Spencer *et al.*, 1948). Although a 2% aqueous solution and a 5% solution in olive oil for 20 days or more were harmless (Ambrose, 1947; Spencer *et al.*, 1948), a 3% solution or a 4% solution in spray oil was fatal after only a few applications (Spencer *et al.*, 1948).

The acute oral toxicity of dinitrocresol to rats is similar to that of 2,4-dinitrophenol and is distinctly greater than that of the cyclohexyl derivatives of 2,4-dinitrophenol (see Table 18.3). Sex, age, fatness, or intake of alcohol does not influence the susceptibility of rats to dinitrocresol. A more complete listing of the exposure–effect relationships in animals can be found in reviews by the National Institute for Occupational Safety and Health (1978) and the World Health Organization (WHO) (1982).

As for 2,4-dinitrophenol, a rise in temperature was found to increase the severity of the effects of dinitrocresol. In rats, the subcutaneous LD 50 was 27.7 mg/kg at 5–10°C, 24.8 mg/kg at 18–20°C, and 19.2 mg/kg at 36–37°C (Parker *et al.*, 1951). Heat enhanced the toxic effect of any dose of dinitrocresol at a constant blood level (King and Harvey, 1953).

Male rats fed for 6 months at a dietary concentration of 100 ppm exhibited no appreciable ill effects (Spencer *et al.*, 1948), but failed to show an increase in growth noted in an earlier study (Ambrose, 1947) in rats fed 62.5 and 125 ppm. A dietary level of 200 ppm caused failure to gain weight but the difference was due largely or entirely to food refusal. Higher concentrations produced more interference with growth, and a level of 1000 ppm killed half of the rats in 10 days (Spencer *et al.*, 1948). The long-term LD 50 appeared to be about 25 mg/kg/day. However, Ambrose (1947) found repeated doses distinctly more toxic with a long-term LD 50 of about 6.6 mg/kg/day. Judging from both studies, the chronicity index does not exceed 5.0 in the rat and may be considerably less, as suggested by the work of Parker *et al.* (1951).

Burkatskaja (1965) reported repeated (and also single) respiratory exposure of cats to solid and liquid aerosols. The animals survived daily, 4-hr exposures for 2–3 months in separate experiments, but one cat died 5 days after the last exposure to 2.0

mg/m^3. Although the mortality following single and repeated exposures corresponded somewhat to dosage, death was usually delayed 4–11 days after exposure, and several laboratory results were atypical compared to findings in other animals and humans. It is not known whether the difference involves the species or something peculiar about the experimental conditions.

Cataracts were detected within 24 hr and death occurred in 48 hr in ducklings fed 2500 ppm (Spencer *et al.*, 1948). However, cataracts have not been observed in rats, even when the rats have been fed dinitrocresol for long periods or at levels that proved fatal (Spencer *et al.*, 1948).

Carcinogenic effects of dinitrocresol have not been described.

Absorption, Distribution, Metabolism, and Excretion
Dinitrocresol may be absorbed in dangerous amounts from the skin, as well as by ingestion or the inhalation of aerosols. Following a single dose by stomach tube, the concentration in the blood reaches a maximum in 2–4 hr in rats and in 4–6 hr in rabbits. Following intraperitoneal injection at the same dose, the peak appears sooner and is higher (King and Harvey, 1953). Under the conditions of their study, King and Harvey found that increasing the ambient temperatures did not increase the concentrations of dinitrocresol in the blood of animals, but it did increase the mortality.

In studying the concentration of dinitrocresol in tissues, especially the liver and kidney, it is necessary to homogenize the tissue in $5 \times 10^{-3} M$ cyanide in order to inhibit an enzyme that reduces the nitro groups (Fouts and Brodie, 1957). Even when this precaution is taken, it is found that the concentration of dinitrocresol in the serum is high in comparison with those in other tissues. There is no greater tendency for the compound to accumulate in any other tissue than in the blood, where over 90% of the compound is in the serum (Parker *et al.*, 1951).

It appears that blood levels of dinitrocresol in exposed animals do not increase to the same extent as in humans, and this may be due to a more rapid elimination in experimental animals. In rats and dogs, blood levels do not increase significantly after the second daily oral dose. Accumulation is even less in rabbits (Parker *et al.*, 1951; King and Harvey, 1953). In humans, continued dosage for 7 days, the longest period studied, caused a continuing increase in blood level. Furthermore, the dosage necessary to reach a given blood level was entirely different. In the rat, eight doses given at the rate of 5 mg/kg/day produced an average blood level of 12 ppm, whereas in humans five doses at the average rate of 1 mg/kg/day produced blood levels of 15–20 ppm (King and Harvey, 1953; Harvey *et al.*, 1951). In humans, blood levels are reduced at the rate of only about 5 ppm/week (Edson, 1957). After voluntary ingestion of 75 mg of pure dinitrocresol for 5 consecutive days, the level in blood was 1 mg/liter almost 6 weeks later. It was found that in intoxicated dinitrocresol sprayers, it took up to 8 weeks to clear the compound from the serum (Van Noort *et al.*, 1960).

The question of whether dinitrocresol is cumulative is, however, somewhat relative. The compound is cleared from the blood at different rates in different species. The time required for

Table 18.3
Single-Dose LD 50 for Dinitrocresol

Species	Route	LD 50 (mg/kg)	Reference
Rat	oral	34	Ambrose (1942)
Rat	oral	31	Spencer *et al.* (1948)
Rat	oral	26	Lehman (1951, 1952)
Rat	subcutaneous	26	Ambrose (1947)
Rat	subcutaneous	24.6	Parker *et al.* (1951)
Rat	intraperitoneal	29	Lawford *et al.* (1954)
Mouse	subcutaneous	24.2	Parker *et al.* (1951)
Mouse	intraperitoneal	24–26	Lawford *et al.* (1954)
Guinea pig	dermal	320	Spencer *et al.* (1948)
Guinea pig	intraperitoneal	23	Lawford *et al.* (1954)
Rabbit	intraperitoneal	24	Lawford *et al.* (1954)

the level of the compound in the blood to fall to half its initial value after a single injection of 10 mg/kg is about 3 hr in the rabbit, 15 hr in the rat, 20 hr in the cat, and 36 hr in the dog (Parker *et al.*, 1951). A half-life for dinitrocresol in human blood of about 150 hr has been noted in a case of acute poisoning (Jastroch *et al.*, 1978). These differences are sufficient to account for the slight accumulation seen in the rat and dog (and probably the cat) following daily doses and to account for the absence of such accumulation in the rabbit. However, these differences in half-life do not appear to be sufficiently great to influence the susceptibility of these laboratory animals; when doses are given every 24 hr, illness is a response to the peak blood level that follows each dose. In other words, the height of the baseline reached at equilibrium is negligible compared to the height of the peak superimposed on it after each daily dose. If the doses are spaced closely enough, as with hourly injections, the effects of small doses can be cumulative, even in these laboratory animals. After the administration of dinitrocresol is stopped, the rate of its disappearance from the blood of dogs is exactly the same whether they have received one or a number of daily injections. The same rule applies to the blood and tissues of rats (Parker *et al.*, 1951).

Rats do not develop a tolerance for dinitrocresol (Parker *et al.*, 1951).

The importance of the skin as a reservoir for dinitrocresol was shown by King and Harvey (1953); 48 hr after dermal dosing, rabbits still had blood levels of 2.4–7.9 ppm, whereas the compound was undetectable in the blood of rabbits dosed 24 hr earlier by other routes.

Dinitrocresol is excreted in the urine, partly (4–10%) as free dinitrocresol, partly in reduced form as unidentified conjugates, as 6-amino-4-nitro-*o*-cresol, as 6-acetamido-4-nitro-*o*-cresol,

and as hydroxyl-group conjugates. The metabolism in the rabbit may be summarized as shown in Fig. 18.1. The main metabolite in that species is 2-methyl-4-nitro-6-acetoaminophenol (Smith *et al.*, 1953).

Dinitrocresol is also metabolized in soil. At least one species, *Arthrobacter simplex,* is capable of utilizing the compound as its sole source of carbon and nitrogen in a simplified mineral salts medium (Gunderson and Jensen, 1956). Although a pseudomonad employed a different metabolic pathway, it produced the same compound in which both nitro groups were replaced by hydroxy groups prior to ring cleavage (Tewfik and Evans, 1966).

Biochemical Effects The biochemical action of dinitrocresol is the same as that of 2,4-dinitrophenol (see Section 18.3.1.2). At least the smaller laboratory animals may be fatally poisoned without ever showing an increase in body temperature. This fact and the stiffening of the skeletal muscles just before death led Parker *et al.* (1951) to conclude that the essential injury caused by the uncoupling of oxidative phosphorylation is the exhaustion of adenosine triphosphate, making contraction of the heart and the muscles of respiration impossible. In fact, respiratory and cardiac activity cease simultaneously, and at the moment of death muscular rigidity is complete. Death accompanied by rigor of the muscle is also produced by iodoacetic acid, which inhibits triosephosphate dehydrogenase and thus leads to progressive breakdown of adenosine triphosphate. This explanation involving the supply of adenosine triphosphate is consistent with the finding that the isolated rat diaphragm poisoned by dinitrocresol completely failed to contract in response to stimulus and developed rigor at a time when the level of adenosine triphosphate had reached the vanishing point (Judah, 1952). It is

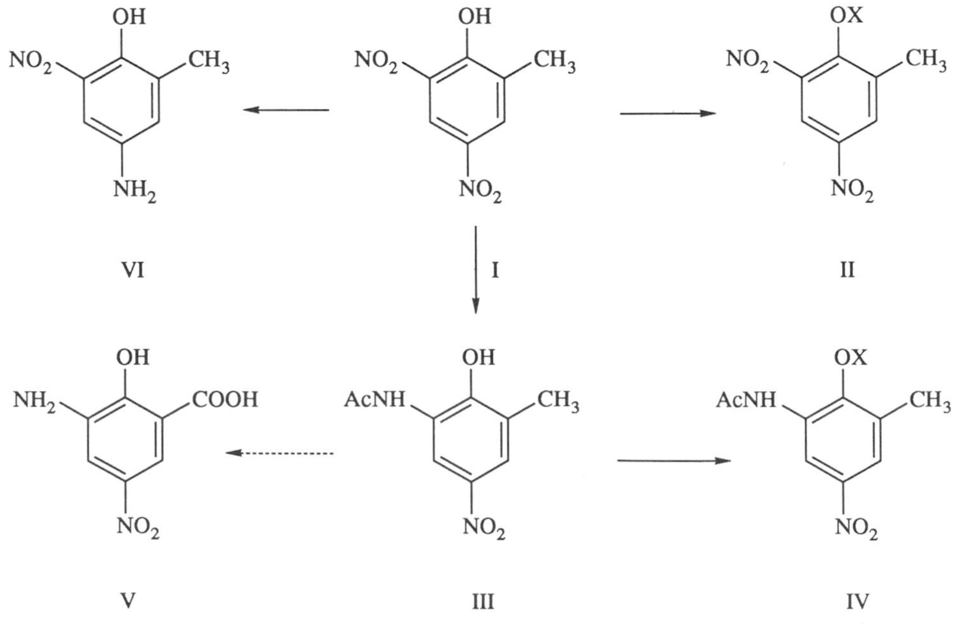

Figure 18.1 Metabolism of DNOC. Reproduced from Smith *et al.* (1953), by permission of the Editorial Board of the Biochemical Society.

also consistent with the fact that, although dinitrocresol has little effect on blood pressure until late in toxicity, death is preceded by a gradual fall in pressure (Ambrose, 1947).

The increase in body temperature that often occurs in laboratory animals and may be so striking in larger animals, including humans, contributes to a fatal outcome by hastening the consumption of adenosine triphosphate and other phosphorus compounds with high-energy bonds and (if the temperature is sufficiently high) by direct injury to the central nervous system.

The increase in metabolic rate is proportional to the dose of the toxicant absorbed, and very high levels (up to four times normal) may be reached temporarily. However, with high metabolic rates, heat production so exceeds the physiologic capabilities of heat dissipation that fatal hyperthermia may result. Dinitrocresol is much more effective in raising the body temperature if the temperature of the surroundings is 22°C (72°F) or over. If the external temperature is 16°C (61°F) or below, increased oxidation and pyrexia are not produced. On the contrary, in this situation, dinitrocresol lowers oxidation by greatly diminishing or abolishing shivering and eventually causes rapid cooling of the animals (Sollmann, 1957). Heat regulation is, therefore, disturbed in both directions, so as to exaggerate the detrimental effects of external temperature.

Effects on Organs, Tissues, and Cells Increases in chromosomal aberrations were found in human lymphycyte cultures treated with DNOC *in vitro* and in bone marrow preparations from mice treated *in vivo* (Nehez *et al.*, 1977, 1978a). The embryos fathered by treated male mice also showed an increase in chromosomal aberrations, compared to that in controls. Similar changes were found in the male germ cells. The dominant lethal percentages for different weeks after treatment indicated that damage occurred in the premeiotic phase of spermatogenesis (Nehez *et al.*, 1978a,b, 1982). 2,4-Dinitrocresol also causes an increase in mutations in *Drosophila* (Muller and Haberzettl, 1980).

18.3.3.3 Toxicity to Humans

Experimental Exposure No toxic effects were noted by any of five volunteers after the ingestion of one dose of 75 mg of dinitrocresol (0.92–1.27 mg/kg), which led to blood levels of 10 ppm or slightly less. Additional doses that raised the blood level to about 20 ppm and caused staining of the conjunctivae did not produce symptoms in all subjects. However, two volunteers who ingested doses of 75 mg of dinitrocresol per day for 5 and 7 days, respectively, experienced lassitude, headache, and malaise when their blood levels exceeded 20 ppm and briefly reached 40–48 ppm. Blood levels were almost always higher about 4 hr after ingestion than they were later in the day. Spiking of blood levels to about twice the current average was seen only in those who became sick. The average daily blood levels were still rising when dosage was discontinued; there was no indication of approaching equilibrium. This finding was consistent with the recovery of only about 1–2% of the administered daily dose in the 24-hr urine collections. Correlation between blood values and urine values was poor. Loss of stored material was slow; 40 days after the last dose, the men still had blood levels of 1.0–1.5 ppm (Harvey *et al.*, 1951).

Repeated application of 2% aqueous solution to the arms was not irritating (Ambrose, 1947).

Therapeutic Use Soon after the introduction of 2,4-dinitrophenol for stimulation of metabolism and promotion of weight loss (see Section 18.3.2.3), dinitrocresol was proposed for the same purposes on the basis that they were about equally toxic, but only about one-third as much of the latter compound was required to produce the same therapeutic effect. Contrary to the results with dinitrophenol (see Section 18.3.2.3), only four or five daily doses of DNOC at the rate of 3 mg/kg/day produced an excessive increase in metabolic rate and symptoms, including sweating, lethargy, and interference with normal sleep. The authors concluded that the safe but effective dosage of DNOC was 0.5–1.0 mg/kg/day (Dodds and Robertson, 1933a,b). It will be appreciated, however, that later studies in volunteers indicated that even a dosage of 1.0 mg/kg/day is unsafe.

Reports of illnesses and deaths produced by this kind of treatment were reviewed by von Oettingen (1949). Some cases showed the same signs seen in occupational accidents and experimental animals. However, there seemed to be a high proportion of cases with skin lesions. Cataracts and glaucoma did occur but apparently were less common then when 2,4-dinitrophenol was used for weight reduction.

Accidents and Use Experience Most cases of poisoning involving dinitrocresol have been occupational in origin. These have been most recently reviewed by the World Health Organization (1982).

The onset of illness caused by dinitrocresol often is preceded immediately by an exaggerated feeling of well-being (Bidstrup, 1952). It is easy to understand that this important warning sign is often misinterpreted by those working with the compound. The signs and symptoms of confirmed acute dinitrocresol poisoning in humans have closely paralleled those of experimental animals and include nausea, gastric distress, restlessness, sensation of heat, flushed skin, sweating, thirst, deep and rapid respiration, tachycardia, fever, cyanosis, collapse, and coma. Acute poisoning with dinitrocresol usually runs a rapid course; death or almost complete recovery within 24–48 hr is the general rule (Bidstrup and Payne, 1951).

The signs and symptoms of chronic dinitrocresol intoxication may include fatigue, restlessness, anxiety, excessive sweating, unusual thirst, and loss of weight. Yellow staining of the conjunctivae may be noted, though staining of skin is not necessarily indicative of poisoning (Bidstrup, 1952). Cataract formation is another possible sequela of chronic dinitrocresol poisoning.

Poisoning by pesticides always has been held to a low level in Great Britain. However, it is an indication of the potential danger of dinitro compounds that during the period 1946–1959 there were nine deaths from DNOC and only two from organic phosphorus compounds (Edson, 1960).

Numerous single cases or small outbreaks have been reported from other parts of the world (Valla, 1962; Prost *et al.*, 1973; Varnai and Kote, 1969; Gaultier *et al.*, 1974).

The symptoms of chronic poisoning from dinitrocresol resemble those of hyperthyroidism rather closely. Determination of metabolic rate is of no value in differentiating between these two conditions. An exposure history should provide some basis for making a distinction. In doubtful cases, this may be supplemented by urine and blood determinations for dinitrocresol content and by the use of tests for thyroid function.

Acute poisoning, whether from one dose or from repeated occupational exposure, is so rapid in onset that it will not be confused with hyperthyroidism. It may be confused with other forms of poisoning merely because of rapidity and severity. Confusion with poisoning by an organic phosphorus compound would be disastrous.

An interesting variant in poisoning by DNOC is illustrated by two accidents and two suicides that were recorded in one city of Yugoslavia during the first half of 1971. In the suicides, death was associated with acute poisoning, but autopsy showed a terminal inhalation of gastric contents. The accident victims both survived the acute phase, but each choked to death on a bolus of food. The authors of this report suggested that DNOC may, by local and/or central action, interfere with the complex reflex act of swallowing (Sovljanski *et al.*, 1971).

Atypical Cases of Various Origins   Staining of the skin, fingernails, and hair by DNOC is commonplace. However, an unusual distribution of staining of the fingernails and other nail pathology that persisted for 7 months were reported by M. R. Baran (1973) and R. L. Baran (1974). The findings were attributed to exposure to a 57% aqueous solution of DNOC for 3 hr.

Dosage Response   Through error, an ointment was prepared containing 25% DNOC; application of 50 gm of this ointment to the skin of a 4-year-old boy led to typical poisoning and death in 3.5 hr despite therapeutic intervention (Buchinskiy, 1974). Based on the average weight of 4-year-old boys, the applied dosage was about 757 mg/kg. The dangerous single oral dose of DNOC has been estimated to be 2000 mg (about 29 mg/kg). This seems consistent with the documented effect of a few repeated doses of 75 mg/person/day (about 1 mg/kg/day; see Experimental Exposure). The threshold limit value (0.2 mg/m³) indicates that occupational intake of 0.03 mg/kg/day is considered safe.

Laboratory Findings   The most striking laboratory finding is the increased basal metabolic rate. Repeated daily oral doses of 75 mg give rise, after 3 days, to a blood level of about 20 ppm (Harvey *et al.*, 1951). Symptoms appear when the concentration in the blood reaches 40 ppm or more. Cases with blood levels of 70 ppm or more terminated fatally (Corti, 1954; Steer, 1951; World Health Organization, 1982). In one of these cases, the concentration found in blood taken at autopsy next day was only

4.3 ppm, although a sample taken immediately after death contained 75 ppm (Steer, 1951). Both determinations were made in the same laboratory. The report of significant symptoms at blood levels as low as 9 ppm and of illness that apparently was not critical at levels as high as 69 ppm (Jastroch *et al.*, 1978) requires confirmation. Breakdown of the compound after death (Parker *et al.*, 1951) may explain certain low values reported for dinitrocresol in the blood and tissues of persons killed by the compound (Heyndrickx and Herman, 1957; Heyndrickx *et al.*, 1962).

Among 20 people who applied 1% DNOC to fruit trees, blood levels varied from a trace to 50 ppm (Burkatskaja, 1965). An identical range of values with an average of 27 ppm was found in 122 workers who applied a 0.75% spray. Their urinary levels of DNOC ranged from 0 to 170 ppm and averaged 48 ppm. These workers were in a good state of health and had a normal work capacity. Some of them had a fine tremor of the hands and tongue and exaggerated reflexes, but this was attributed to alcoholism. The authors of this report pointed out that such high blood levels were consistent with good health only because the work was carried out at temperatures of 1–4°C (Wassermann *et al.*, 1960).

Among 27 healthy chemical plant workers exposed to DNOC, serum concentrations of DNOC ranged from 1.0 to 8.7 ppm and averaged about 3 ppm; concentrations of DNOC in urine ranged from 0 to 4.2 ppm and averaged 1–2 ppm (Markicevic *et al.*, 1972). When workers were removed from further exposure (usually when their blood levels exceeded 15 ppm and certainly at 25 ppm), the rate of recovery was 5 ppm/week (Edson, 1957).

Applicators should observe all necessary precautions in using dinitrophenols and should have routine periodic checks of blood levels. The significance of different concentrations of dinitrocresol in whole blood is as follows:

0 to 10 ppm	trivial
11 to 20 ppm	appreciable absorption
21 to 30 ppm	unsafe
31 to 40 ppm	likely to cause some toxicity
41 to 50 ppm	dangerous
>50 ppm	critically dangerous

Corresponding values for plasma or serum are approximately twice as high (Edson, 1954).

Because dinitrocresol is excreted slowly by humans, persons who have suffered any symptoms of poisoning should be removed from risk of further absorption for a period of at least 6 weeks (Bidstrup and Payne, 1951). Workers who have blood levels greater than 20 ppm 8 hr after exposure should receive no further exposure for at least 6 weeks (Bidstrup, 1952; Bidstrup *et al.*, 1952).

Persons clearly poisoned by DNOC, including those who recover completely, may show clinical laboratory evidence of liver and kidney damage—for example, increased blood bilirubin, increased SGOT and SGPT, increased alkaline phosphatase, and azotemia (Gaultier *et al.*, 1974). However, the levels reported have been only moderately normal, and the indicated degree of specific organ injury would seem to have little influence on the outcome.

Pathology In persons who have died from the effect of DNOC, yellow staining of the organs, tissues, and fluids due to the presence of the sodium salt of DNOC may be noted. The lungs are congested and there is usually some edema and a few petechial hemorrhages. There may be similar hemorrhagic changes in the brain and gastric mucosa (Bidstrup and Payne, 1951).

Treatment of Poisoning See Section 18.3.1.3.

18.3.4 BINAPACRYL

18.3.4.1 Identity, Properties, and Uses

Chemical Name The chemical name for binapacryl is 2-*sec*-butyl-4,6-dinitrophenyl-3-methylcrotonate.

Structure See Table 18.1.

Synonyms Binapacryl (ANSI, BSI, ISO) is the common name for this chemical compound. It also is used as BINAPACRYL (JMAF). Trade names include Acricid®, Ambox®, Endosan®, Morocide®, and Niagara 9044®. Code designations include HOE-2,784. The CAS registry number is 485-31-4.

Physical and Chemical Properties The empirical formula for binapacryl is $C_{15}H_{18}N_2O_6$ and the molecular weight is 322.31. Binapacryl is a white crystalline powder with a faint aromatic odor. Its melting point is 68–69°C, and it has a density of 1.2307 and vapor pressure of 1×10^{-4} torr at 60°C. It is practically insoluble in water but is soluble in most organic solvents. Binapacryl is unstable in alkalies and concentrated acids, and it suffers slight hydrolysis on long contact with water. It is decomposed slowly by ultraviolet light.

History, Formulations, and Uses Binapacryl was introduced in 1960 by Hoechst AG. It is used primarily against red spider mites and powdery mildews of fruits. Its formulations include wettable powder (250 and 500 gm active ingredient per kilogram), emulsifiable concentrate (400 gm active ingredient per liter), suspension (500 gm active ingredient per liter), and dust (40 gm active ingredient per kilogram).

18.3.4.2 Toxicity to Laboratory Animals

Basic Findings As might be expected of an ester of dinoseb (see Section 18.3.6), binapacryl is slightly less toxic, reflecting the time necessary for its hydrolysis and its consequently slower, more gradual release. According to Bough *et al.* (1965), binapacryl is poorly absorbed by the skin. A single dermal dosage of 1000 mg/kg or 10 doses in the course of 12 days of 750 mg/kg failed to kill mice or retard their growth. However, the compound is better absorbed by the rat and is more toxic by the dermal and oral routes to rats than to mice (see Table 18.4). A slight decrease in weight gain was found in rats that received dietary levels of 100 ppm or more for 90 days. However,

Table 18.4
Single-Dose LD 50 for Binapacryl

Species and sex	Route	LD 50 (mg/kg)	Reference
Rat, M	oral	150–225	Bough *et al.* (1965)
Rat, M	oral	63	Gaines (1969)
Rat, F	oral	58	Gaines (1969)
Rat, M	dermal	810	Gaines (1969)
Rat, F	dermal	720	Gaines (1969)
Mouse, M	oral	1600–3200	Bough *et al.* (1965)
Guinea pig, F	oral	200–400	Bough *et al.* (1965)

survival, hematology, urinalysis, average organ weights, and gross and microscopic pathology, including the incidence of tumors, were unaffected by a dietary level of 200 ppm or less both at 90 days and after 2 years. The no-effect level was 50 ppm (about 2.5 mg/kg/day) [Food and Agriculture Organization/World Health Organization (FAO/ WHO), 1970].

Oral administration of binapacryl at the rate of 25 mg/kg/day to dogs caused depression and continuous paresis of the hindquarters, and the dogs died within 6 months. Those that received doses of 1.25, 2.5, and 5 mg/kg/day displayed paresis of the hindquarters lasting 5–10 hr after each dose; however, their survival, food consumption, body weight, hematology, blood biochemistry, liver function tests, urinalysis, organ weights, and gross and microscopic pathology remained normal in a 2-year study. The no-effect level was 0.25 mg/kg/day (FAO/WHO, 1970).

Absorption, Distribution, Metabolism, and Excretion Binapacryl is the dimethylacrylic ester of dinoseb (DNBP); it is metabolized to form this phenol, and its toxicity is attributed to this conversion. When binapacryl and dinoseb were given to guinea pigs by mouth at doses of 400 and 40 mg/kg, respectively, those receiving dinoseb died faster, but the concentrations of dinoseb in the blood at the time of death were in the same range (76–86 ppm) following dosages with both compounds. No unmetabolized binapacryl was detected in the blood. Rabbits administered 20 or 40 mg dinoseb/kg died with only slightly lower blood levels (36–59 ppm). Rabbits that reached a maximal blood level of 33 ppm following a dermal dosage of dinoseb at 10 mg/kg survived, and the level had fallen to 9 ppm 24 hr after the administration. Rabbits treated dermally with 750 mg binapacryl/kg also survived, and the highest average blood level observed in any group was 4 ppm (Bough *et al.*, 1965).

Following oral doses of binapacryl, the urine of both rabbits and rats contained oxidation products of the butyl side chain of dinoseb, including the acid. In addition, rat urine contained traces of free 6-aminophenol, and the urine of rabbits contained a substantial amount of this compound and its glucuronide. After a single administration of binapacryl, both rats and rabbits excreted 7–17% in the urine within 48 hr. As late as the tenth day, 0.12% of the dose was detected in the urine of rats (Ernst and Bar, 1964).

Effects on Reproduction   In a three-generation study in rats, dietary levels as high as 50 ppm (the highest fed) were without effect on reproductive performance as measured by the indices of mating, pregnancy, fertility, parturition, and lactation and by litter size, number of stillbirths, and viability, survival, and weight of weanlings. Gross and histological examinations of a sample of the F_{3b} generation revealed no change attributable to the compound (FAO/WHO, 1970).

18.3.4.3 Toxicity to Humans

Use Experience   One report (Mazzella di Bosco, 1970) states that two workers developed headache, nausea, vomiting, abdominal pain, diarrhea, and breathing difficulties after spraying tomatoes with binapacryl for 2 hr. Fever, weak pulse, and tremor were noted later. Treatment with analeptics and atropine brought considerable improvement within 24 hr, and recovery was complete within a week. The signs and symptoms were consistent with poisoning by a dinitrophenol but were not diagnostic of it. The speed of onset without any record of massive exposure and the favorable response to atropine both cast doubt on the diagnosis.

Treatment of Poisoning   See Section 18.3.1.3.

18.3.5 DINOCAP

18.3.5.1 Identity, Properties, and Uses

Chemical   Name   2,4-Dinitro-6-(1-methyl-*n*-heptyl)phenyl crotonate.

Structure   See Table 18.1.

Synonyms   The common name dinocap (BSI, CSA, ESA, ISO) is in general use. Other names include the acronyms DCPC and DNOPC. Trade names for dinocap include Arathan®, Caprane®, Crotothane®, Isocothan®, Karathane®, and Mildex®. Code designations include CR-1,639 and ENT-24,727. The CAS registry number is 39300-45-3.

Physical and Chemical Properties   Dinocap has the empirical formula $C_{18}H_{24}N_2O_6$ and a molecular weight of 364.39. It is a dark brown liquid boiling at 138–140°C. It is practically immiscible with water but is miscible with most organic solvents.

History, Formulations, and Uses   Dinocap was introduced about 1934. The technical material contains about 90% dinocap and 10% other nitrophenols, chiefly, 2,4-dinitro-6-(1-methyl-*n*-heptyl)phenol. The technical material is available as a 25% water-wettable powder, 48% liquid concentrate, and a 1% dust. It is used as an acaricide and fungicide.

18.3.5.2 Toxicity to Laboratory Animals

Basic Findings   Dinocap apparently is somewhat less toxic by the oral route than some other dinitrophenols. Oral LD 50 values of 950, 1190, 2000, and 100 mg/kg were found in male rats, female rats, male rabbits, and dogs, respectively. The intravenous LD 50 in male rats was only 2.3 mg/kg, indicating poor absorption by the oral route (Larson *et al.*, 1959). The oral LD 50 in mice has been reported to be 53 mg/kg, which indicates that this species is considerably more sensitive to dinocap than rats (Mlodecki *et al.*, 1975).

Both the growth and survival of rats were reduced by a dietary level of 2500 ppm, and growth was reduced at 1000 ppm. The spleen was enlarged in males receiving 2500 ppm, but hematological and histological examination revealed no change attributable to this or lower dietary levels. Retardation of growth by 1000 ppm occurred also in a 2-year study, but only in male rats. Other findings for this and lower dietary levels were the same. The no-effect levels were 1000 ppm in female rats and 500 ppm in male rats (Larson *et al.*, 1959).

Decreased appetite and drastic weight loss were followed by death within 6 weeks in most dogs offered dinocap at a dietary level of 1000 ppm. Dogs fared little better at 250 ppm, and moderate weight loss was evident at 100 ppm but not at 50 or 10 ppm. Hepatic necrosis occurred in dogs fed 250 and 1000 ppm. Hematological values were normal at all dietary levels (Larson *et al.*, 1959).

Results of separate studies of the cataractogenic action of dinocap in ducklings fed dietary levels ranging from 50 to 2500 ppm produced inconsistent results not explained by dosage (Larson *et al.*, 1959). Whether the erratic results were caused by impurities or other variations in the technical product or by some factor unrelated to dinocap remains unknown.

Reproductive and Prenatal Toxicity   There are reports suggesting that dinocap is teratogenic at doses well below those causing maternal toxicity. Fraczek (1979) reported that the administration of dinocap in the diet at 104–126 mg/kg/day (about 10% of the LD 50) to male and female rats for four generations decreased growth rates and reduced offspring survival in the second generation.

Dinocap was administered orally on days 7–16 of gestation to the pregnant CD-1 mouse at doses of 0, 6, 12, and 25 mg/kg/day. Treatment with the highest dose resulted in increased postnatal mortality (40 and 80% in separate experimental groups). Many of the treated pups that died were "ballooned" from extreme abdominal distention and exhibited cleft palate. Twenty-four percent of the survivors in the group treated with 25 mg/kg/day displayed torticollis (a twisting of the neck resulting in an abnormal tilting of the head). There was no treatment-related mortality in the 12 mg/kg/day treatment group, but 6% of newborn mice also showed the torticollis. No effects were observed in the control or the 6 mg/kg/day treatment group. In this same study, pregnant rats and hamsters were administered dinocap at doses up to 100 and 200 mg/kg/day, respectively. In the rat, there was reduced maternal weight gain at 100 mg/kg/day, but offspring viability and weights were unaffected. In the hamster, the only effect observed in the offspring was retarded growth. The dinocap used in this study contained 74% 2,4- and 2,6-dinitrooctylphenyl crotonates (in an approximate 2 : 1 ratio), 6% mixed nitrooctylphenols, and 0.54–0.86% mononitrooctylphenols. Nonvolatile materials accounted for 6–13% (Gray *et al.*, 1986). A study by Rogers *et al.* (1987) concluded that 2,6-dinitro-6-(1-methylheptyl)phenyl crotonate and 2,6-dinitro-4-(1-methylheptyl)phenyl crotonate, isomers of the major active ingredients of technical dinocap, are not the active teratogenic components.

Using a preparation of dinocap similar to that described in the above study, the teratogenic potential was further evaluated by Rogers *et al.* (1986). Pregnant mice were dosed with 0, 5, 10, 20, 40, 80, and 120 mg/kg/day on days 7–16 of gestation. Dams were killed on day 18 and the fetuses were examined. There were no live fetuses in the 120 mg/kg/day group. The number of live fetuses per litter was decreased and resorptions increased at 80 mg/kg/day. Gravid uterus weight and fetal weights were decreased at all doses of dinocap. Cleft palate was found in fetuses at 5 (0.4%), 20 (23.6%), 40 (75.5%), and 80 (74.1%) mg/kg/day. At the higher doses there was also an increase in supernumerary ribs and a low frequency of exencephaly and umbilical hernias.

Biochemical Effects   It would seem that part of the toxicity of dinocap observed in adult animals depends on some action other than the uncoupling of oxidative phosphorylation. Larson *et al.* (1959) reported that this compound produced an increase in oxygen consumption in female but not in male rats. By contrast, male rats were somewhat more susceptible to both single and repeated doses.

The biochemical events leading to the increased sensitivity of the fetus (especially mice) to dinocap exposure are unknown. It would be of interest to determine this relative sensitivity using pure chemical preparations rather than the technical product.

Effects on Organs and Tissues   Dinocap was not tumorigenic when fed to two strains of mice at the highest tolerated level (Innes *et al.*, 1969).

18.3.5.3 Toxicity to Humans

Experimental Exposure   Patch tests were done on the forearms of 50 persons using dinocap both as an emulsion and as a powder on each person. Exposure for 48 hr resulted in moderate irritation of 11 persons by the emulsion and of 3 by the powder. When the test was repeated on the opposite forearm 12 days later, 25 people reacted to the emulsion and 9 reacted to the powder. During the succeeding days, the reaction became worse in 3 persons where an emulsion was last applied; it became worse in 1 additional person, both where the emulsion and where the powder were last applied, and there were exacerbations at both original application sites on the opposite arm. Thus, dinocap cause both irritation and sensitization (Larson *et al.*, 1959).

Use Experience   One case of acute allergic dermatitis was ascribed to dinocap. Initial symptoms included not only generalized pruritis and erythema but also thirst and dyspnea. Symptomatic treatment provided rapid improvement, but 9 days later vesicles appeared over the patient's entire body. Cortisone treatment led to complete recovery in 1 month (Mazella di Bosco, 1970). The initial occurrence of thirst and dyspnea suggest that a moderate degree of poisoning was present, presumably as a result of heavy exposure.

Treatment of Poisoning   See Section 18.3.1.3.

18.3.6 DINOSEB

18.3.6.1 Identity, Properties, and Uses

Chemical Name   2,4-Dinitro-6-*sec*-butylphenol.

Structure   See Table 18.1.

Synonyms   The common name dinoseb (ANSI, BSI, ISO, WSSA) is in general use. Other nonproprietary names for the compound are dinitrobutylphenol (ESA) and DNBP (JMAF). Trade names include Chemox®, Dow General®, Gebutox®, Knox-Weed®, Premerge®, Sinox General®, and Supersevtox®. Code designations include ENT-1,122. The CAS registry number is 88-85-7.

Physical and Chemical Properties   Dinoseb has the empirical formula $C_{10}H_{12}N_2O_5$ and a molecular weight of 240.21. It forms dark amber, monoclinic crystals melting at 37.9–39.3°C. At 25°C, it is only slightly soluble in water (52 ppm) but readily soluble in alcohol, spray oil, and most organic solvents. It forms salts with inorganic and organic bases, some of which are water-soluble.

History, Formulations, and Uses   Dinoseb was introduced in 1945 and developed for use as a herbicide and insecticide by the Dow Chemical Company. As the ammonium or an amine salt, it is used to control annual weeds in cereals, peas, soybeans, seedling lucerne, cotton, and many other crops. As an emulsifiable concentrate, it is used in the preemergence control of weeds in peas, beans, and potatoes and as a preharvest desiccant for potatoes and legumes.

18.3.6.2 Toxicity to Laboratory Animals

Basic Findings   Both the oral and dermal toxicities of dinoseb are high (see Table 18.5). In both rabbits and guinea pigs, even a fatal dose of dinoseb caused no irritation of the skin through which it was absorbed (Spencer *et al.*, 1948; Bough *et al.*, 1965). Mice kept at 32°C were more susceptible to dinoseb (intraperitoneal LD 50, 14.1 mg/kg) than those kept at 23–24°C (LD 50, 20.2 mg/kg) (Preache and Gibson, 1975a).

A dietary level of 500 ppm caused marked food refusal and death of some rats after five or more doses. A dietary level of

Table 18.5
Single-Dose LD 50 for Dinoseb

Species and sex	Route	LD 50 (mg/kg)	Reference
Rat	oral	46	Spencer *et al.* (1948)
Rat, M	oral	25–40	Bough *et al.* (1965)
Mouse, M	oral	20–40	Bough *et al.* (1965
Guinea pig, F	oral	20–40	Bough *et al.* (1965)
Guinea pig	dermal	200–300	Spencer *et al.* (1948)
Chick, M	oral	40–80	Bough *et al.* (1965)

200 ppm (5.4–20 mg/kg/day) caused a small but statistically significant deficiency of growth; the animals appeared healthy. Their average blood urea nitrogen was 203 ppm. Except for a slight increase in liver weight, there was no gross or microscopic evidence of injury seen at necropsy. At a dietary level of 100 ppm (2.7–10 mg/kg/day) rats showed an average blood urea nitrogen value of 209 ppm, compared with 175 ppm in the controls. A dietary level of 50 ppm (1.35–5 mg/kg/day) fed to rats for 6 months had no effect on their growth, blood urea nitrogen levels, organ weights, or histologic findings (Spencer *et al.*, 1948).

A dietary level of 2500 ppm killed ducklings in 3 days with no sign of cataract formation. However, dietary levels of 1000 ppm and 300 ppm, which permitted longer survival, produced cataracts. No cataracts were seen in rats fed 6 months at rates as high as 20 mg/kg/day (Spencer *et al.*, 1948).

Absorption, Distribution, Metabolism, and Excretion At death, following a single oral dose, the plasma level of dinoseb in guinea pigs averaged 78–86 ppm. The corresponding value in rabbits after a fatal dermal dose (20–40 mg/kg) was 45–53 ppm. The plasma level of dinoseb in rabbits reached 33 ppm 8 hr after a dermal dose of 10 mg/kg, but it decreased to 9 ppm by the end of the day (Bough *et al.*, 1965).

In mice, dinoseb was absorbed faster following intraperitoneal than following oral administration, with the result that almost identical maximal plasma levels (about 100 ppm) were reached following 17.7 mg/kg intraperitoneally or 40 mg/kg orally. However, because of continuing gastrointestinal absorption, plasma levels declined less rapidly during the first 24 hr after oral than after intraperitoneal administration. Dinoseb reached the fetus but never at a concentration more than 2.5% of that in the maternal plasma. After oral administration, maximal concentrations were reached in maternal plasma and in fetuses in about 2 and 12 hr, respectively. The corresponding intervals after intraperitoneal injection were very much shorter (Gibson and Rao, 1973).

No dinoseb or metabolite was detectable in the milk of cows fed the compound at dietary levels as high as 100 ppm (McKellar, 1971).

Esters of dinoseb, including the isopropylcarbonate, dinobuton (Bandal and Casida, 1972), are rapidly hydrolyzed to form dinoseb, which is the active toxicant. Dinoseb undergoes oxidation of either of the two methyl groups on the *sec*-butyl side chain, conjugation of the phenolic products, formation of many as yet uncharacterized metabolites, and, in rats but not mice, reduction of either of the two nitro groups and acetylation of the metabolically formed *p*-amino group. Carbaryl protects rats from dinobuton, probably by inhibiting its hydrolysis to dinoseb. Microsomal enzymes of rat liver hydrolyze dinobuton and reduce the *o*-nitro group of dinoseb (Bandal and Casida, 1972). Intestinal metabolism may result in the reduction of dinoseb to diamino metabolites (Ingebrigtsen and Froslie, 1980).

Biochemical Effects The metabolism of one dinitrophenol may be modified by another. Dinoseb acts as a noncompetitive inhibitor of nitroreduction of 2,4-dinitrophenol (Eiseman *et al.*, 1974).

Dinoseb has been reported to be an inhibitor of the photosynthetic electron flow in plants (Moreland and Hilton, 1976) and to have a site of action associated with the photophosphorylating pathway in this flow (Alsop and Moreland, 1975). Additional work has indicated that dinoseb both affects the adenosine triphosphatase complex of chloroplasts and inhibits the oxidizing side of photosystem II (Younis and Mohanty, 1980; Mullet and Arntzen, 1981).

Effects on Organs, Tissues, and Cells At least some preparations of dinoseb form methemoglobin and can cause coproporphyrinuria and urobilinogenuria. Jaundice caused by this compound is thought to be hemolytic rather than hepatic in origin (Henneberg, 1973).

Dinoseb did not cause a significant increase in tumors when administered to two strains of mice at the highest tolerated rate for about 18 months (Innes *et al.*, 1969). Dinoseb has been shown to produce primary DNA damage in two prokaryotic systems but not eukaryotic systems, and no gene mutations were noted in prokaryotes or eukaryotes (Garrett *et al.*, 1986).

Reproductive and Prenatal Toxicity Dinoseb produced hyperthermia in the dams and resorptions and reduced size of the young when administered to mice intraperitoneally at the rate of 17.7 mg/kg/day or subcutaneously at the same rate. Oral doses of 20 or 32 mg/kg/day produced maternal toxicity but essentially no embryotoxicity or teratogenic effects. In this study, the only regimen that produced definite teratogenic effects (imperforate anus and acaudia) was intraperitoneal injection of 17.7 mg/kg/day on days 10–12, but not days 14–16. Intraperitoneal, subcutaneous, and oral doses of 5, 10, or 20 mg/kg/day, respectively, were without adverse effects on embryonic or fetal growth and development (Gibson, 1973).

Fetal and neonatal rats treated on days 10–12 with 8.0 and 9.0 mg/kg/day had dilated renal pelves and ureters. No effect was noted at 6.4 mg/kg/day. Pathological changes were detected in kidneys from only 3 of 28 rats (9.0 mg/kg/day) and in no ureters at 42 days postpartum (McCormack *et al.*, 1980).

These findings confirmed the original findings of Gibson (1976) noting the transient hydronephrosis following prenatal treatment with dinoseb. Thus, the hydronephrosis appears to be due to a delay in renal papillary growth and is not a permanent malformation.

Other investigations revealed an increased incidence of supernumerary ribs in rats and mice exposed *in utero* to dinoseb (Kavlock *et al.*, 1985; Giavini *et al.*, 1986). However, Kavlock *et al.* (1985) noted that there was a significant linear inverse relationship between maternal weight gain during gestation and the incidence of extra ribs in the treated groups. Thus, the possibility that the incidence of supernumerary ribs increased in response to nonspecific maternal toxicity cannot be eliminated.

Maternal mortality, fetal toxicity, and teratogenesis of a particular dosage of dinoseb were all increased by exposing pregnant mice to a temperature of 32°C for 24 hr. Ambient temperatures of 0–6°C for as much as 4 hr were without effect (Preache and Gibson, 1975a). Phenobarbital protected mice from the teratogenic effects of intraperitoneal dinoseb, and SKF 525A had the opposite effect. These actions and the different effects of different durations of starvation could be explained by their influence on the rate of metabolism and excretion of dinoseb (Preache and Gibson, 1974a, 1975b). Environmental stress did not necessarily increase teratogenicity and might decrease it. For example, forcing dams to swim for 2 hr immediately after a dose of dinoseb on day 11 caused a significant decrease in the incidence of external, soft tissue, and skeletal anomalies (Preache and Gibson, 1974b).

Hall *et al.* (1978) reported diffuse tubular atrophy of the testis and reproductive failure in rats fed levels of dinoseb up to 200 ppm in the diet. This study was extended by that of Linder *et al.* (1982). In rats fed 300 ppm, 90% of the spermatozoa demonstrated atypical morphology by 20 days of treatment. By 30 days, sperm counts were decreased as well. Histological changes in the testes included abnormal spermatozoa and spermatids and multinucleated spermatogenic cells. Reproductive failure occurred at dietary levels of 225 and 300 ppm, although mating behavior was unaffected. Reproduction was unaffected at a dietary level of 150 ppm, but there were decreased epididymal sperm counts and atypical epididymal spermatozoa. Dietary levels of dinoseb of 125, 150, and 175 ppm fed to male rats for 25 days were found to decrease sperm motility. At the highest dose level, the motility index was reduced to near zero (Linder *et al.*, 1986). In another study, the administration of dinoseb by gavage daily for 5 days at doses of 2–20 mg/kg/day produced no sperm abnormalities in mice (Osterloh *et al.*, 1983).

Studies by Spencer and Sing (1982) suggested a direct toxic effect of dinoseb on the uterus and placenta. In day 10 decidualized pseudopregnant rats fed dinoseb from days 6–9 of pseudopregnancy, uterine weights were reduced in the groups fed 100–750 ppm. Uterine protein and glycogen concentrations were reduced in a dose-dependent manner. In day 16 pregnant rats, fed dinoseb from days 6–15 of pregnancy, placental protein and glycogen concentrations were decreased at 200 ppm and greater. Fetal survival rates were reduced at 150 ppm and greater.

18.3.6.3 Toxicity to Humans

Accidental and Intentional Poisoning A workman developed convulsions while spraying an orchard with parathion and DDT. He was dead on arrival at the hospital. Autopsy revealed a yellow fluid in the stomach, and investigators showed that a portion of the contents was missing from a jug of similar material in the shed where the man had eaten lunch about an hour before being observed in convulsions. The label on the jug identified the contents as dinoseb, and this compound was identified in the stomach contents and blood at concentrations of 65% and 72.5 ppm, respectively. The case was thought to be a suicide (Hayes, 1982).

In a somewhat similar case, a man told his physician that at 0130 hr he ingested and then spat out a small quantity of fluid that he had supposed was grape juice but which proved to be dinoseb. The physician sent him home. At 0630 hr he awoke vomiting; while on his way to see his physician again 24 hr after the ingestion, the patient died (Cann and Verhulst, 1960). The report speaks of the episode as an accident but fails to explain either the long delay between the onset of vomiting and the second trip to the physician or how a fluid that stained the victim's right hand and gastric rugae yellow could have been mistaken for grape juice.

Use Experience In general, use experience with dinoseb has been good. However, a tractor driver who got some dilute spray in one eye developed pain and swelling, and 16 hr after the accident required hospitalization. His vision was seriously impaired for 3 days. Recovery was complete.

In another incident a self-employed farmer sprayed an area of new seed grass with dinoseb. During the spraying operation he noted that a jet appeared blocked. He proceeded to repair the jet without any protection for his hands. He completed the remainder of the spraying during the afternoon. He also noted that at the end of the spraying, the gauze of his face mask was heavily stained yellow. Headache, malaise, lassitude, and sweating appeared later that same afternoon. The next day he went to the nearest hospital, but the tentative diagnosis was that of an influenzal type of illness. During the next 5 days the patient showed symptoms of anorexia, excessive sweating, and intermittent shivering attacks, pains in the chest and abdomen, excessive thirst, restlessness, insomnia, loss of weight, and generalized yellow staining of the skin and sclera. It was reported that one night the patient drank 9 liters of water, and during the 5 days approximately 10 kg of weight was lost. He also demonstrated shortness of breath and hemoptysis. Six days after the incident he was admitted to a hospital. The clinical findings resulted in treatment with oxytetracycline. The urine was discolored yellow, but no dinitro compound was subsequently detected in a sample. Liver function tests were abnormal, chest X ray showed shadowing at the bases of the lungs, and there was reduction of forced expiratory volume and forced vital capacity. At the end of 1 week in the hospital his condition improved and he was discharged. Two weeks later he still complained of lethargy, night sweats, and forgetfulness. His condition slowly improved and 6 months after the initial exposure he was symptom free, although his blood urea nitrogen was reported to be elevated (Smith, 1981).

Treatment of Poisoning   See Section 18.3.1.3.

18.4 HALOPHENOLS

Phenol (C_6H_5OH) was formerly used to some extent as an oil-base roach and bedbug spray. However, chlorination increases the persistence and the insecticidal and fungicidal effectiveness of phenol. Of the simple halophenols, pentachlorophenol has been used most extensively, and it is discussed below. 2,3,4,6-Tetrachlorophenol and, to a lesser degree, 2,4,5-trichlorophenol, 2,4,6-trichlorophenol, and 2,4-dichlorophenol have been used for essentially the same purposes. Although trichlorophenol is a pesticide in its own right, much more of the compound has been manufactured as a precursor for other compounds, notably 2,4,5-trichlorophenoxyacetic acid (2,4,5-T) and hexachlorophene, than for direct use. Likewise, 2,4-dichlorophenol has mainly been used for the synthesis of 2,4-dichlorophenoxyacetic acid (2,4-D). During the manufacture of these chlorophenols, the synthesis of unavoidable by-products, the chlorinated dioxins, often results. Although purified chorophenols and their derivatives possess some toxicity in their own right, results to date indicate that it may be many orders of magnitude less than that of the trace dioxin contaminants. Thus, the effects that have been observed in humans appear to be due mainly, if not exclusively, to the presence of trace amounts of these dioxins. Detailed discussion of the halogenated dioxins and related acnegenic agents may be found in Section 18.5.

18.4.1 PENTACHLOROPHENOL

18.4.1.1 Identity, Properties, and Uses

Chemical Name   Pentachlorophenol.

Structure C_6Cl_5OH.

Synonyms   Pentachlorophenol (BSI, ISO) is the name in common use for this compound, but it is also known as PCP (JMAF, WSSA), penchlorol, and penta. Trade names for pentachlorophenol include Dowicide 7®, Dowicide EC-7®, and Santophen 20®. Trade names for the sodium salt have included Dowicide G® and Santobrite®. The CAS registry number is 87-86-5.

Physical and Chemical Properties   The empirical formula for pentachlorophenol is C_6HCl_5O and it has a molecular weight of 266.35. It forms colorless crystals with a phenolic odor and a melting point of 191°C. Its vapor pressure at 100°C is 0.12 torr. The sodium salt, sodium pentachlorophenate, has the empirical formula C_6Cl_5NaO and a molecular weight of 288.34. It forms buff-colored flakes; its solution has an alkaline reaction. Technical pentachlorophenol forms dark grayish powder or flakes

with a melting point of about 158°C. The technical product primarily is a mixture of penta- and tetrachlorophenol, but it also contains 4–6% other polychlorophenols plus traces of nonphenolic impurities such as the higher chlorinated dibenzo-p-dioxins (CDDs), polychlorinated dibenzofurans (CDFs), and polychlorobenzenes. Bromotetrachlorophenol (Timmons et al., 1984) and chlorinated diphenyl ethers (Newsome et al., 1983) may also be common contaminants of pentachlorophenol formulations. Although it is impractical to manufacture pure pentachlorophenol for use as a pesticide, the concentrations of impurities depend on details of the manufacturing process, and the concentrations have tended to decrease over a period of years (Williams, 1982). Pentachlorophenol's solubility in water is 20 ppm at 30°C. It is soluble in most organic solvents (the log octanol/water partition coefficient is 5.01), although only moderately so in carbon tetrachloride and paraffinic petroleum oils. It is volatile in steam. The sodium salt is insoluble in petroleum oils but 33% soluble in water at 25°C.

History, Formulations, and Uses   Pentachlorophenol was introduced in 1936 for timber preservation and used as a herbicide by C. Chabrolin in 1940. It is used for the control of termites and for protection against fungal rots and wood-boring insects in timber. The phenol is used as a preharvest defoliant and as an eradication herbicide. The sodium salt is used as a molluscicide. It should also be noted that pentachlorophenol is a major product resulting from the metabolism of the fungicide hexachlorobenzene in mammalian systems (van Ommen et al., 1985).

18.4.1.2 Toxicity to Laboratory Animals

Basic Findings   Signs of poisoning by the purified pentachlorophenol are exactly the same as those described for 2,4-dinitrophenol and dinitrocresol. Pentachlorophenol dissolved in fuel oil causes irritation of the skin and marked local damage followed by slow but complete recovery. Aqueous solutions of the sodium salt are less irritating (Kehoe et al., 1939; Boyd et al., 1940; Deichmann et al., 1942). The solubilities of the sodium salt are very different from those of the phenol. This fact and the ionization of the salt make its absorption different from that of the parent compound. However, once absorbed, the two materials are identical in pharmacokinetics and toxicity.

The toxicity of pentachlorophenol is similar to that of dinitrocresol (see Table 18.6). Based on inhalation exposures lasting 28–44 min and on the assumption that each rat inhaled 80 ml/min, it was calculated that the LD 50 for this route of exposure is 11.7 mg/kg, a value about one-third the intraperitoneal LD 50 determined in the same laboratory (Hoben et al., 1976a). St. Omer and Gadusek (1987) determined that young rats (10–20 days old) and adults (70 and 134 days old) were more susceptible to the toxic and lethal effects of technical pentachlorophenol that were juveniles (25–50 days old). The LD 50 values (milligrams per kilogram) ranged from 50 to 180 for preweaned rats, from 220 to 230 for juveniles, and from 80 to 120 for adults.

Table 18.6
Single-Dose LD 50 for Pentachlorophenol

Species and sex	Route	LD 50 (mg/kg)	Reference
Rat	oral	27–211[a]	Deichmann et al. (1942)
Rat	oral	78	Lehman (1951, 1952)
Rat	oral	184	Demidenko (1969)
Rat, M	oral	146	Gaines (1969)
Rat, F	oral	175	Gaines (1969)
Rat, M	oral	211	Hoben et al. (1976a)
Rat	dermal	96	Demidenko (1969)
Rat, M	dermal	320	Gaines (1969)
Rat, F	dermal	330	Gaines (1969)
Rat	subcutaneous	66	Deichmann et al. (1942)
Rat, M	intraperitoneal	34	Hoben et al. (1976a)
Mouse	oral	130	Demidenko (1969)
Mouse	oral	74	Ahlborg and Larsson (1978)
Mouse M	oral	177	Borzelleca et al. (1985)
Mouse F	oral	117	Borzelleca et al. (1985)
Mouse M	intraperitoneal	59	Renner et al. (1986)
Mouse F	intraperitoneal	61	Renner et al. (1986)
Mouse	subcutaneous	120[b]	Beechhold and Ehrlich (1906)
Rabbit	oral	70–300[a]	Deichmann et al. (1942)
Rabbit	dermal	40 >1111[a]	Deichmann et al. (1942)
Rabbit	subcutaneous	70–100	Deichmann et al. (1942)
Rabbit	intravenous	22–23	Deichmann et al. (1942)

[a]Depending in part on formulation.
[b]"Lethal dose" (mg/kg).

Many papers on the toxicity of pentachlorophenol have failed to specify the chemical composition of the sample studied. However, the results reflect improved manufacturing procedures over a period of years in the United States, and no doubt similar improvement has occurred in some other countries.

The toxicity of repeated doses of pentachlorophenol depends largely on its chlorodibenzo-p-dioxin (CDD) content. The best commercial materials available until about 1972 contained <0.05 ppm 2,3,7,8-tetrachlorodibenzo-p-dioxin (TCDD), 9–27 ppm hexachlorodibenzo-p-dioxin, and 575–2510 ppm octachlorodibenzo-p-dioxin. Such commercial material not only was positive in the rabbit ear and chick edema assays (see Section 18.5) but also in a 90-day feeding study in rats at a dosage of 30 mg/kg, depressed erythrocytes, hemoglobin, and packed cell volumes and produced degeneration and necrosis of the liver. At even lower dosages, serum alkaline phosphatase was elevated, serum albumin was depressed, and liver and kidney weights were increased. In contrast, pentachlorophenol available after about 1975 contained only 1 ppm of the hexachloro- and 26 ppm of the octachlorodibenzo-p-dioxin. Like pure pentachlorophenol, this commercial product was negative in rabbit ear and chick edema bioassays, and it produced only liver and kidney enlargement in feeding studies (Johnson et al., 1973). A number of other investigators have also reported technical pentachlorophenol to elicit a variety of other toxic effects, including hepatic damage and immune alterations that were not observed with purified pentachlorophenol preparations (Goldstein et al., 1977; Kimbrough and Linder, 1978; Kerkvliet et al., 1982a,b, 1985a,b; White and Anderson, 1985).

In a 90-day feeding study with pentachlorophenol containing 200 ppm of octachlorodibenzo-p-dioxin and 82 ppm of the other CDDs but no detectable TCDD, Knudsen et al. (1974) found that a dietary level of 200 ppm (about 10 mg/kg/day) decreased the growth of female but not male rats without decreasing food intake. Liver weight and the activity of liver microsomal enzymes were increased by dietary levels of 50 and 200 ppm. The no-toxic-effect level was considered to be 25 ppm (about 1.2 mg/kg/day). It is interesting that pentachlorophenol decreased the occurrence of calculi at the corticomedullary junction of the kidney of female rats, a condition not found in all rat colonies.

In a 2-year study of pentachlorophenol containing only 22.5 ppm CDDs, ingestion of dosages of 30 or 10 mg/kg/day by females or 30 mg/kg/day by males caused decreased growth, increased SGPT, and accumulation of pigment in the liver and kidney in one or both sexes. Ingestion of 3 mg/kg/day by females or 10 mg/kg/day by males did not result in toxic effects (Schwetz et al., 1978).

Additional information on the mammalian toxicology of pentachlorophenol and a great deal of information on its environmental and occupational implications may be found in reviews by Arsenault (1976) and Williams (1982) and in a book edited by Rao (1978).

Absorption, Distribution, Metabolism, and Excretion
Pentachlorophenol is absorbed rapidly and nearly completely by the skin and after inhalation or ingestion.

Following oral administration, rabbits show a maximal blood level in about 7 hr. Daily application of 200 mg to the skin of rabbits (followed by washing 1 hr later) led to blood levels of about 4.5 ppm, compared to about 6 ppm found in the blood of rabbits dosed orally at the rate of 3 mg/kg/day. Blood and tissue levels were only about half as high when the compound was washed from the skin within $\frac{1}{2}$ hr instead of a full hour. The blood levels at death following a large oral dose were 40–85 ppm (Deichmann et al., 1942).

Following a single oral dose, pentachlorophenol could be detected in the blood of rabbits for 3 days. Following daily oral doses, the concentration in the blood increased gradually for about 6 or 7 days and then (although there was considerable fluctuation) showed no systematic increase in spite of continued intake (Deichmann et al., 1942). In the rabbit, pentachlorophenol is more cumulative than dinitrocresol, whether judged on the basis of one or many doses. However, the degree of accumulation is small in both instances.

Oral dosing of calves with 0.05 and 0.5 mg/kg/day resulted in maximal plasma pentachlorophenol levels of 1.4 and 9.5 ppm at days 10 and 14, respectively, after the start of treatment. Following cessation of the 0.5 mg/kg/day regimen, plasma pentachlorophenol levels dropped to 0.6 ppm within 10 days (Osweiler et al., 1984).

Hoben et al. (1976b) found that, based on the half-life following a single exposure of rats to an aerosol of the sodium salt, the body burden of pentachlorophenol did not increase following as many as five daily exposures. The results suggested that prior exposure increased the ability of animals to eliminate the compound. Excretion seemed insufficient to account for all of the observed effect. Indirect evidence indicated that increased metabolism might be the explanation. These findings and conclusions are consistent with those reached earlier by Stohlman (1951) on strictly toxicological grounds.

In pentachlorophenol-treated rats, the highest residual concentrations of pentachlorophenol in tissues were in the liver and kidneys, with lower levels (less than 0.005% of the dose) being found in other tissues. This distribution likely reflects the kidneys and liver being the principal organs for the metabolism and excretion, respectively, of pentachlorophenol (Braun et al., 1979).

Renner and Mucke (1986) summarized studies investigating the metabolism of pentachlorophenol. Unchanged pentachlorophenol is excreted in the urine of the rabbit, rat, mouse, and monkey (Deichmann et al., 1942; Ahlborg et al., 1974; Braun and Sauerhoff, 1976; Braun et al., 1977, 1979; Jakobson and Yllner, 1971). In addition to free pentachlorophenol, rats excrete tetrachloro-p-hydroquinone (Ahlborg et al., 1974; Braun et al., 1977) and lesser amounts of trichloro-p-hydroquinone (Ahlborg and Thunberg, 1978). Production of tetrachloro-p-hydroquinone is promoted in rats by pretreatment with phenobarbital, 3-methylcholanthrene, and TCDD. Production of trichloro-p-hydroquinone is promoted by 3-methylcholanthrene and TCDD. Strangely enough, production of tetrachloro-p-hydroquinone also is increased during the first 24 hr after treatment with SKF 525A at a dose of 25 mg/kg (Ahlborg et al., 1978). Both metabolite and parent compound are excreted free and as glucuronides (Ahlborg and Thunberg, 1978). β-Glucuronidase of bacterial origin is strongly inhibited by tetrachloro-p-hydroquinone at concentrations less than those found in experimental animals (Ahlborg et al., 1974, 1977). β-Glucuronidase obtained from liver is not inhibited by chlorinated hydroquinones or benzoquinones (Ahlborg et al., 1977). Glucuronides of pentachlorophenol or of its metabolites can be split by boiling with hydrochloric acid (Ahlborg et al., 1974), by using enzyme obtained from liver (Ahlborg et al., 1977), or by the bacterial enzyme after extraction of unconjugated compounds (Braun et al., 1977).

One report has identified the formation of a palmitic acid conjugate of pentachlorophenol by rat liver microsomes in vitro (Leighty and Fentiman, 1982). Another study has indicated the presence of tetrachloro-p-benzoquinone (chloranil) as a metabolite in mice and rabbits (Tashiro et al., 1970).

Although tetrachloro-p-hydroquinone has been identified as a major metabolite in the rat and mouse, it has not been found in the monkey (Braun et al., 1979). Studies in humans are equivocal as to whether tetrachlorohydroquinone is a major metabolic product of pentachlorophenol (see Section 18.4.1.3).

Pentachlorophenol and its metabolites are excreted mainly in the urine and, to a much lesser extent, the feces. Something less than 0.5% of ^{14}C from radiolabeled pentachlorophenol is exhaled and can be trapped as carbon dioxide (Jakobson and Yllner, 1971; Larsen et al., 1972; Braun et al., 1977).

The oral toxicity of tetrachlorohydroquinone is much less than that of the parent compound. In mice, oral LD 50 values of 750 and 500 mg/kg were found for males and females, compared to 36 and 74 mg/kg for pentachlorophenol (Ahlborg and Larsson, 1978). Furthermore, tetrachloro-p-hydroquinone does not increase the body temperature of poisoned animals at an ambient temperature of 31°C, and it probably is not an uncoupler of oxidative phosphorylation. However, Witte et al. (1985) reported that tetrachloro-p-hydroquinone, but not purified pentachlorophenol, bound covalently to calf thymus DNA and caused single-strand breaks in bacteriophage DNA. Renner et al. (1986) reported that tetrachloro-p-hydroquinone was more toxic to mice than pentachlorophenol when given by intraperitoneal injection; for male mice the LD 50 values were 28 and 59 mg/kg, respectively.

In a study using [^{14}C]pentachlorophenol, rats that received a single dose at 10 mg/kg excreted 79.8% in the urine, 18.6% in the feces, and 0.2% in the breath as carbon dioxide, and after 9 days they retained 0.437% in their bodies and 1.4% on their cages, making a total recovery of 99.8%. Rats that received 100 mg/kg excreted 64.0% in the urine and 33.6% in the feces. At a dosage of 10 mg/kg, elimination was biphasic, with a half-life in the rapid phase of 17 hr in males and 13 hr in females. Over 99% of the pentachlorophenol in the plasma was bound to albumin, which may account for the low renal clearance (Braun et al., 1977). Other studies also have found only a small proportion of excretion via the feces. Larsen et al. (1972) found only 9.2–13.2% of the total dose in the feces of rats fed [^{14}C]pentachlorophenol.

In monkeys, there appeared to be a sex difference in the elimination of [^{14}C]pentachlorophenol. After a single oral dose at 10 mg/kg, the half-life for elimination was 40.8 and 92.4 hr in males and females, respectively. This was related to corresponding half-lives of 72.0 and 83.5 hr for clearance from plasma. The proportions of radioactivity recovered from urine and feces were similar to those in the rat, but retention in the body was distinctly greater (Braun and Sauerhoff, 1976).

Other animal studies are consistent in showing that excretion occurs largely in the urine. In certain fatal human cases, it seemed that the victim was unusually susceptible by virtue of renal deficiency (Truhaut et al., 1952a). This hypothesis was supported by experiments showing that rabbits made nephritic experimentally were very much more easily poisoned by pentachlorophenol than were normal animals (Truhaut *et al.*, 1952b).

Pentachlorophenol is also metabolized in soil. A *Flavobacterium* strain has been identified that is apparently able to utilize pentachlorophenol as its sole carbon source (Saber and Crawford, 1985; Brown *et al.*, 1986).

Biochemical Effects The biochemical action of pentachlorophenol is similar to that of the dinitro compounds, namely uncoupling of oxidative phosphorylation (Weinbach, 1957; Kanda *et al.*, 1968; Matsumura, 1972). The mechanism of uncoupling involves binding to mitochondrial protein, a matter that has been studied in detail (Weinbach *et al.*, 1965). A study of Mg^{2+}-ATPase and of Na^+,K^+-ATPase from various tissues of the rat revealed very complex reactions, suggesting that pentachlorophenol uncouples oxidative phosphorylation at low concentrations and inhibits it at high concentrations and that Na^+,K^+-ATPase is the locus of action of the poison (Desaiah, 1978). *In vivo* uncoupling of oxidative phosphorylation fully explains the clinical findings in acute exposures, namely a marked increase in metabolic rate leading to an increase in body temperature, collapse, and death with almost instantaneous onset of severe rigor mortis.

Both pentachlorophenol and 2,6-dichloro-4-dinitrophenol are potent and long-lasting inhibitors of hepatic sulfotransferase activity (Mulder and Scholtens, 1977; Meerman, 1983). High levels of pentachlorophenol or sodium pentachlorophenate in the diet (350 ppm) or pentachlorophenate in the drinking water (1.4mM) of rats for 1 week inhibited the sulfation of harmol by 30–50%. A log-linear correlation was found between the plasma concentration of pentachlorophenol and the inhibition of harmol sulfation. This property of pentachlorophenol has made it useful as a tool to study the importance of sulfotransferase reactions in the metabolism and activation of a number of carcinogenic compounds (Kedderis *et al.*, 1984; Meerman, 1985). Boberg *et al.* (1983) found that pentachlorophenol antagonized the tumorigenic effects of either 1'-hydroxysafrole or its metabolite, 1'-sulfooxysafrole, in mouse liver. Pentachlorophenol also has been shown to reduce the toxicity of *N*-hydroxy-2-acetylaminofluorene (Meerman *et al.*, 1980; Meerman and Mulder, 1981).

Pentachlorophenol is about equally bound by albumin from human, rat, and cow. However, some unidentified feature of human plasma contributes to the higher and more prolonged retention of the compound in humans (Casarett *et al.*, 1969; Hoben *et al.*, 1976c; Uhl *et al.*, 1986). The availability of free pentachlorophenol varies directly with temperature, and this may contribute to the rapid progression of poisoning once the body temperature begins to rise.

The hepatic effects of technical and pure pentachlorophenol were compared in female rats fed one or the other at dietary levels of 20, 100, and 500 ppm for 8 months. The particular sample of technical pentachlorophenol contained 8 ppm hexa-, 520 ppm hepta-, and 1380 ppm octachlorodibenzo-*p*-dioxins and 4 ppm tetra-, 42 ppm penta-, 90 ppm hexa-, 1500 hepta-,

and 200 ppm octachlorodibenzofurans; the pure sample contained less than 0.1 ppm of each of these contaminants. An increase in cytochrome P-450 and increases in related associated enzyme activities were produced by all dietary levels of technical pentachlorophenol, and porphyria was produced by dietary levels of 100 and 200 ppm; pure pentachlorophenol produced none of these changes at any feeding level. Pure and technical samples decreased weight gain to an equal degree but only at the highest dietary level (Goldstein *et al.*, 1977). Kimbrough and Linder (1978) reached essentially the same conclusion on morphological grounds. Technical pentachlorophenol produced mild alterations in the liver when fed at 20 ppm and severe lesions at 500 ppm. Pure compound produced no effect at 20 and 200 ppm and only occasional eosinophilic inclusions at 500 ppm. Ultrastructural studies of the livers of rats fed pure pentachlorophenol at 1000 ppm showed that the change involved an increase in endoplasmic reticulum and the formation of myelin figures (Kimbrough and Linder, 1975). Diffuse cloudy swelling of hepatocytes was also observed in pigs treated orally with purified pentachlorophenol at dosages of 10 and 15 mg/kg/day for 30 days. No changes were noted at a dosage of 5 mg/kg/day (Greichus *et al.*, 1979). Technical grade pentachlorophenol induces cytochrome P-450-associated monooxygenase activities in cultured at hepatocytes, whereas pure pentachlorophenol had no inducing effect (Wollesen *et al.*, 1986). Decreased serum concentrations of triiodothyronine and thyroxine were observed in calves fed 10 mg/kg/day of technical pentachlorophenol, but not analytical grade pentachlorophenol (Hughes *et al.*, 1985). Decreased serum protein concentrations, elevated serum γ-glutamyltransferase activities, and histologic changes in the thymus and Meibomian gland were also noted in calves fed the technical grade but not the analytical grade pentachlorophenol. The only toxic effect which was closely related to pentachlorophenol and not its contaminants was depressed active transport of *p*-aminohippurate measured in kidney slices *in vitro*.

Although pure pentachlorophenol itself does not apparently produce porphyria in experimental animals (Goldstein *et al.*, 1977; de Calmanovici and San Martin de Viale, 1980), it has been found to accelerate the onset of hexachlorobenzene-induced porphyria in rats (Debets *et al.*, 1980). Again, it should be recalled that pentachlorophenol is a major metabolite of hexachlorobenzene.

Effects on Organs, Tissues, and Cells Daily intake of pentachlorophenol at the highest tolerated rate for 19 months was not carcinogenic to mice (Innes *et al.*, 1969). Daily intake of pentachlorophenol containing only 22.5 ppm of CDDs for 2 years at a dosage of 30 mg/kg/day, which was sufficient to cause mild signs of toxicity, or at lesser dosages was not carcinogenic in rats (Schwetz *et al.*, 1978). Bionetics Research Laboratories administered 46.4 mg pentachlorophenol/kg/day by gavage on days 7–28 postpartum to two strains of mice. At 28 days postpartum, mice were fed diets containing 130 ppm pentachlorophenol for 78 weeks. No significant increase in the incidence of tumors was observed in the pentachlorophenol-treated mice compared to control animals (Bionetics Research Laboratories, 1968).

At a concentration of 400 ppm *in vitro,* pentachlorophenol and 2,4,6-trichlorophenol were mutagenic in some but not all bacterial systems. Some impurities [4-chloro- and 4,5,6-trichloro-2-(2,4-dichlorophenoxy)phenol] but not all had similar activity in bacterial systems. All four substances were effective in a "spot test" system in mice, but the activity of the chlorophenols was lower than that of the predioxins (Fahrig *et al.,* 1978). A statistical review of these data by an EPA panel (Cirelli, 1978) indicated that the study of Fahrig *et al.* (1978) did not provide evidence of the mutagenicity of pentachlorophenol. Pentachlorophenol was found not to cause point mutations in a sex-linked recessive lethal test in *Drosophila melanogaster* (Vogel and Chandler, 1974), point mutations in rats (Schwetz *et al.,* 1978; Fahrig *et al.,* 1978), or chromosomal aberrations (Buselmair *et al.,* 1973). Pentachlorophenol also failed to induce 6-thioguanine-resistant mutants in V79 Chinese hamster cells (Jansson and Jansson, 1986).

A number of studies have examined the effect of technical grade and purified pentachlorophenol on the immune system. Many of these have indicated that while the technical grade product elicits a variety of effects on both humoral and cell-mediated immune responses, no striking effect is seen when purified pentachlorophenol is used (White and Anderson, 1985; Kerkvliet *et al.,* 1982a,b, 1985a,b; Holsapple *et al.,* 1987). Chickens fed a purified grade of pentachlorophenol at dosages of 0, 600, 1200, or 2400 ppm showed decreased lymphoproliferative responses to concanavalin A at dosages of 600 and 1200 ppm. Chickens fed the diet containing 2400 ppm of pentachlorophenol had lower humoral responses to bovine serum albumin. Serum concentrations of IgM and IgG and the humoral responses to sheep red blood cells and Newcastle disease virus were normal (Prescott *et al.,* 1982). Total leukocyte counts and serum levels of gamma globulin and IgG were also decreased in pigs orally administered purified pentachlorophenol at dosages of 5, 10, or 15 mg/kg/day for 30 days (Hillam and Greichus, 1983). However, in the latter two studies, where significant alterations were observed, dose-related effects were not apparent.

Kerkvliet *et al.* (1982a) examined the susceptibility of adult mice fed technical or pure pentachlorophenol to Maloney sarcoma virus or primary methylcholanthrene-induced transplanted tumor growth in the spleen. Although, the response of the mice fed technical pentachlorophenol was more severe, splenic tumor development was observed in 22 and 44% of the challenged mice exposed to 50 and 500 ppm pure pentachlorophenol. Control mice did not develop splenic tumors. These investigators suggested that even pure pentachlorophenol may promote immunosuppression leading to splenic tumor development.

Effects on Reproduction   Rats fed pentachlorophenol at a dosage of 30 mg/kg/day for 62 days before mating and then continuously through lactation lost weight, and the neonatal survival and growth of their young were decreased. There were

no other apparent changes. Ingestion of 3 mg/kg/day on the same schedule had no effect on reproduction or on neonatal survival, growth, or development (Schwetz *et al.,* 1978). The feeding of lactating cattle with pentachlorophenol at dosages of 0.2 mg/kg/day for 75–84 days followed by 2 mg/kg/day for 56–60 days had no effect on milk production, feed intake, or body weight of the adult animals (Kinzell *et al.,* 1981).

A maternal dosing regimen of 50 mg/kg/day on days 6–15, 8–11, or 12–15 of gestation caused toxicity in the young in the form of resorptions, subcutaneous edema, dilated ureters, and skeletal anomalies. These effects appeared to be dose-dependent. At a maternal dosage of 5 mg/kg/day the commercial grade of pentachlorophenol produced no toxicity to the embryo or fetus (Schwetz *et al.,* 1974; Schwetz and Gehring, 1973; Chou and Cook, 1979). Larsen *et al.* (1975) showed that the concentration of radioactive pentachlorophenol or its metabolites that reached the rat fetus when administered on day 15 of gestation was very low compared to that in the maternal blood. On the basis of studies involving a dosage of 60 mg/kg on day 8, 9, 10, 11, 12, or 13 of gestation, they concluded that pentachlorophenol was slightly teratogenic but that the effect may be indirect, resulting from toxicity to the mother.

The majority of literature concerning the potential teratogenicity of pentachlorophenol has been reviewed by the EPA's Office of Pesticide Programs (Cirelli, 1978). They concluded that pentachlorophenol and possibly the hexachlorodibenzo-*p*-dioxin contaminants cause teratogenic and fetotoxic effects. The no-effect level was given as 5.8 mg/kg/day for pentachlorophenol and 0.1 μg/kg/day for hexachlorodibenzo-*p*-dioxin.

Treatment of male mice daily for 5 days by gavage with purified or technical grade pentachlorophenol at dosages of 6–50 mg/kg/day produced no sperm abnormalities when the animals were examined 35 days following the first injection (Osterloh *et al.,* 1983).

18.4.1.3 Toxicity to Humans

Experimental Exposure   In order to study its metabolism and pharmacokinetics, four men ingested sodium pentachlorophenate at a dose of 0.1 mg/kg (Braun *et al.,* 1979). In another study, pentachlorophenol was given orally to three volunteers at single doses of 3.9, 4.5, and 18.8 mg (Uhl *et al.,* 1986). In both cases the dosage was without clinical effect. The results are discussed under Laboratory Findings.

Use Experience and Accidental Poisoning in Adults   Pentachlorophenol may cause irritation of the skin, conjunctiva, and upper respiratory tract and also cause demonstrable systemic absorption, even at dosages that do not produce systemic disease. Exfoliation of the epidermal layer of the hands occurred 1–2 days after adjusting a weir dispensing 20% sodium pentachlorophenate; recovery occurred within 5 days (Nomura, 1953). Bevenue *et al.* (1967b) reported a case in which a man washed a paint brush in a solvent later shown to contain 0.4% pentachlorophenol. After his hands had been immersed for about 10 min they became painful and red, and the pain lasted 2 hr, although the hands were washed with soap and water as soon as the pain was noticed. Samples of urine collected 2 and 4 days later had pentachlorophenol concentrations of 0.236 and 0.080 ppm, respectively. Later samples showed that subsequent excretion was slow; it required about a month for the values to fall to the average for the general male population of the area.

Unlike the situation with most pesticides, nearly all poisoning of adults with pentachlorophenol has been occupational in origin, and in some instances no specific accident was identified. For example, nine men died after dipping timber by hand and without any protection in a 1.5–2% solution for periods varying from 3 to 30 days, with an average of 13 days (Menon, 1958). In another instance, one man died after working 6 days as a mixer preparing 2% cotton defoliant from a 40% concentrate. It was reported later that he had failed to wear gloves and waterproof pants that were provided and that he had not changed clothes or bathed during the period. [It should be noted that Silkowski *et al.* (1984) observed that not all types of gloves are completely impermeable to pentachlorophenol.] Even so, poisoning may have been precipitated by a single careless act. To retrieve a spigot, he reached above his wrist into a bucket of 40% solution. The material was washed off promptly with plain water and no symptoms were reported during the remainder of the afternoon. However, at about 0400 hr the next morning, his associates found him severely and typically poisoned, and he died 4 hr and 25 min later in a hospital (Hayes, 1982).

In some instances, workers have been affected as the result of what would seem to be total neglect of hygienic principles. For example, 6 workers died and 24 were hospitalized as the result of moving paper and plastic bags of pentachlorophenol powder from a freighter to a dock by means of a small boat. The men used hooks, which damaged the bags. At least part of the work was done during rain. The powder stuck to wet surfaces and contaminated the men's bare feet and hands. The powder may have contaminated an open jar of drinking water in the boat. The same work had been done twice before when there was no rain; then the men were only moderately affected, being only a little dazed and developing red areas on their skin (WHO, 1962). Cases of poisoning by ingestion have occurred, although it is claimed that one man drank a glassful of a 2% solution of the sodium salt with no effect except a hangover (Menon, 1958). In another fatal case, a 33-year-old man had been working for about 3 weeks in a chemical plant and used a jackhammer to break up large blocks of pentachlorophenol into small pieces, which were then ground into powder. The environment was described as dusty, the patient had been observed to have powder on his clothes, and precautions against cutaneous exposure to chemical dust had not been observed (Gray *et al.*, 1985).

In fatal cases the temperature is frequently extremely high (up to 42.2°C) but may be only moderately elevated (Gordon, 1956; Menon, 1958; WHO, 1962; Gray *et al.*, 1985; Wood *et al.*, 1983). Sweating, dehydration, and dyspnea are present, and there may be pain in the chest or abdomen. The pulse is rapid. Coma appears early. There is frequently a terminal spasm. Pro-

found, generalized rigor mortis is usually observed. In 20 fatal cases for which the information is available, the time from first symptoms to death ranged from 3 to 30 hr and averaged 14 hr (Gordon, 1956; Menon, 1958; Blair, 1961; Wood *et al.*, 1983; Gray *et al.*, 1985; Hayes, 1982).

Nonfatal systemic poisoning is characterized by weakness, by more or less marked loss of appetite and weight, sometimes by a feeling of constriction in the chest and dyspnea on moderate exercise, and almost always by excessive sweating. Headache, dizziness, nausea, and vomiting may be present (Truhaut *et al.*, 1952a; Nomura, 1953; Bergner *et al.*, 1965). While noting that serious poisoning by pentachlorophenol usually is fatal, Imaizumi and Atsumi (1971) reported that survivors of such poisoning show impairment of autonomic function and circulation and visual damage, including an arcuate type of scotoma. Other authors have reported complete recovery of survivors. The difference in experiences is unexplained.

Chloracne (see Section 18.5.1.3) has occurred in connection with the production (Baader and Bauer, 1951; Miura *et al.*, 1974) and use (Cole *et al.*, 1986) of pentachlorophenol and its derivatives (Sehgal and Ghorpade, 1983). Samples of technical products have been found to be contaminated with hexa-, hepta-, and octachlorodibenzo-*p*-dioxins and dibenzofurans and have been found to give a positive rabbit ear test (Goldstein *et al.*, 1977). One recent case of chloracne is of interest because of the means of exposure as well as the documentation of the concentrations of the octachlorodibenzo-*p*-dioxin. A 32-year-old male had been complaining of an acneform eruption of 6 months duration. The patient was responsible for the construction of piers for small boat marinas. These were built with lumber pretreated with pentachlorophenol. The man spent a considerable amount of time lying on the lumber in the course of construction, which was performed wearing only shorts and shoes. He noted the appearance of the acneform lesion within about 9 months of beginning work. Analysis of the pentachlorophenol preparation used, wood samples, and wood surface for octachlorodibenzo-*p*-dioxin yielded the following results: 1600 ppm, technical grade pentachlorophenol; 13 ppm, wood shavings; 11 ppm, sawdust; 160 ppm, crystals from the wood surface; and 400 ppm, yellow residue from the wood surface (Cole *et al.*, 1986).

Animal experiments have shown that the toxicity of pentachlorophenol is increased substantially by various impurities present in some formulations. However, the identity and concentrations of the impurities were unknown in connection with many earlier animal studies and almost all reported human cases. Therefore, it is impossible, in most instances, to state what contribution impurities may have to systemic poisoning in humans. On the other hand, there have been cases in which dermatitis was the main finding, and it was due almost certainly to contaminants and not to pentachlorophenol. Some reports contain nothing to indicate that the workers who made pentachlorophenol made 2,4,5-T also, but the workers did have chronic acneform dermatitis of the face, as well as a variety of other chronic symptoms not characteristic of CDDs (Vinogradova *et al.*, 1973, 1976). Another report distinguished clearly between workers who made pentachlorophenol and others who made 2,4,5-T, but both groups suffered chloracne and other skin diseases. In each instance, the urinary excretion of coproporphyrin and of alanine was increased slightly, but not statistically significantly compared to controls, and urobilinogen was not detected in the urine samples. Thus, in these cases there was no evidence of porphyria (Miura *et al.*, 1974). In neither instance was any CDD quantitated.

Baxter (1984) reported the results of a 3-year study that examined a number of biochemical parameters in 40 volunteers who had been employed in the manufacture of the sodium salt. Results were compared to those for a group who had some contact with the process but were not regularly exposed and those for another group who had no exposure. Signs of chloracne appeared in 25/40 of the exposed group and in 2/25 of the intermittently exposed group. Significantly lower levels of bilirubin were noted in the exposed group, and serum triglycerides tended to be higher and lactate dehydrogenase (LDH) values tended to be lower in this group. Only in one year was there statistical elevation of serum triglyceride values in the exposed group. There was no apparent effect on liver enzymes or a number of other biochemical tests. No determination of tissue or blood levels of pentachlorophenol, dioxins, or dibenzofurans in the workers was made.

Both hemolytic anemia (Hassan *et al.*, 1985) and aplastic anemia (Schmid *et al.*, 1963; Louwagie *et al.*, 1978; Roberts, 1963, 1981, 1983) have been reported to be associated with exposure to pentachlorophenol. In two of the cases of aplastic anemia, chronic exposure to commercial grade pentachlorophenol used for the treatment of lumber occurred over the course of approximately 1 year, and both cases culminated in death within 1 year after the development of symptoms (Roberts, 1983). An earlier case of aplastic anemia was somewhat atypical in that splenomegaly was also present (Roberts, 1963). In the case of hemolytic anemia, an insecticide containing pentachlorophenol had been used to clean wooden furniture (Hassan *et al.*, 1985). The relationship of these cases to pentachlorophenol exposure may be circumstantial only. If indeed these afflictions were due to pentachlorophenol exposure, the mechanisms are likely to be different and to reflect the diversified nature of the components of the commercial preparations. In the case of the hemolytic anemia, pentachlorophenol may act by blocking the formation of adenosine triphosphate, leading to loss of osmotic equilibrium across cell membranes and resulting in hemolysis. Hematopoietic toxicity in the form of aplastic anemia may be a result of the long-term exposure to pentachlorophenol and/or the contaminating chlorinated dibenzo-*p*-dioxins and dibenzofurans. Evidence of hematopoietic toxicity of TCDD has been noted in animals (McConnell *et al.*, 1980; Allen and van Miller, 1978).

Bauchinger *et al.* (1982) reported results of a study in which 22 male workers employed at a pentachlorophenol factory were examined for chromosome changes in peripheral lymphocytes. Compared to the results for 22 matched controls, there was a small, but significant, increase in the frequency of dicentric and acentric chromosomal changes. In contrast, in an earlier study Wyllie *et al.* (1975) noted no chromosomal aberrations in work-

ers in a plant where timber was impregnated with pentachlorophenol. This study, however, consisted of only six exposed workers and four controls. Another report by Triebig *et al.* (1981) noted decreases in the sensory nerve conduction velocities of workers in a pentachlorophenol processing factory. In this case, however, a relationship between pentachlorophenol levels in plasma and conduction velocities could not be demonstrated. On the other hand, decreased sensory nerve conduction velocities have frequently been reported for workers involved in the production of the di- and trichlorophenols and their derivatives. These workers are also exposed to the chlorinated dioxins in these processes (see Section 18.5.1.3).

Accidental Poisoning in Infants Poisoning of a 3.75-year-old girl followed daily bathing in water from an open tank on the roof of her home; this water had been contaminated by pentachlorophenol recently used to spray the roof timbers. It was unlikely that the child had ingested any water from the tank, except a small amount in brushing her teeth. The fact that the rest of the family bathed in water from the same tank but did not become ill suggests that the child might have been more susceptible for unknown reasons or that exposure on a body weight basis may have been greater than for the adults. When first seen, the girl had fever (38.9°C), intermittent delirium, and rigors during the night. She was flushed and excited but cooperative. A sample of urine taken 40 hr after hospital admission contained 60 ppm pentachlorophenol. Her temperature was normal after 24 hr, and aminoaciduria stopped after a week. Recovery was complete (Chapman and Robson, 1965).

An outbreak of poisoning in newborn infants through dermal absorption of pentachlorophenol (Smith *et al.*, 1967; Robson *et al.*, 1969; Armstrong *et al.*, 1969) is of special interest. There were nine hospitalized cases, two of which were fatal. In addition, a number of mild cases that recovered without treatment were recognized by history after the occurrence of the severe cases had focused attention on the matter.

The outstanding clinical feature of the illness was profuse sweating, which was noted even in the mild cases. Another striking feature of the disease was that the babies nursed avidly, even though fever rose as high as 39.4°C, and the respiratory rate increased as the illness progressed. Other common findings included tachycardia, hepatomegaly, progressive metabolic acidosis, proteinuria, azotemia, and irritability followed by lethargy. The lungs remained clear to auscultation, but X-ray revealed "pneumonia" or "bronchiolitis." Anorexia, vomiting, and diarrhea were notably absent.

Failure of the first serious case to respond to broad-spectrum antibiotics; consistent failure to isolate a pathogen; the dramatic response of the babies to exchange transfusion; and recurrence of cases after the nursery was reopened after it had been closed, cleaned, and disinfected gradually led to a strong suspicion that a toxic chemical was involved. There had been no change in practice regarding the management of drugs, preparation of the babies' food, use of a deodorizer in the nursery, or spraying of the hospital (but never the nursery) with an insecticide. Blame was placed on a disinfectant containing a mixture of substituted phenols that had been used for only 10 months to disinfect surfaces including the cribs in the nursery. Thin-layer chromatography of serum from sick babies revealed a phenolic substance similar to an ingredient in the disinfectant. The nursery was closed a second time. An effort was made to wash phenols from all surfaces in the nursery. Use of the disinfectant was abandoned. About 1.5 months after the nursery was reopened a second time, a second case occurred. Further search revealed that an antimildew agent containing 22.9% sodium pentachlorophenate and 4.0% trichlorocarbanilide was being used in the terminal rinse of all nursery linens and diapers at a rate of 3–4 ounces per laundry cycle. The labeling of the container recommended a rate of 1 ounce per cycle and specifically forbade use of the preparation in laundering diapers. At this point, specimens were sent to another laboratory, where gas chromatography proved that pentachlorophenol was present in the serum of sick babies, the organs of a dead infant, and the diapers and other clothing in the nursery in concentrations consistent with a diagnosis of poisoning. Gas chromatography failed to reveal any of the phenols in the disinfectant in any specimen.

The amount of pentachlorophenol in each diaper varied from 1.5 to 5.7 mg (Smith *et al.*, 1967), and the concentrations varied from 26 to 172 ppm (Barthel *et al.*, 1969). The concentration in other clothing and in crib pads was similar or even higher. A concentration of 1950 ppm was found in the front of one shirt from the clean linen storage closet (Barthel *et al.*, 1969). Exposure to fabrics contaminated to about this extent produced illness beginning after less than 5 days of continuous exposure. Other laboratory findings are given in the appropriate paragraph below.

Dosage Response The exact dosage necessary to produce illness is not known. It is clear that the largest single dosage that produces no illness whatever is little less than the fatal dosage. On the other hand, and in spite of a minimal tendency to cause cumulative effects, it is occasionally possible for continuing exposure to pentachlorophenols to cause weight loss and other symptoms without threatening life. It will be recalled that 2,4-dinitrophenol was used therapeutically to induce weight loss until its danger was recognized (see Section 18.3.2.3). A convincing episode of weight loss caused by pentachlorophenol vapor was reported in a woman whose house had been treated with pentachlorophenol as a wood preservative (Anonymous, 1970). A more complete spectrum of poisoning (fever, weakness, irritation of the throat, red faces) occurred in four families who used water from the same well for drinking and bathing. Only 4 days before onset, pentachlorophenol had been applied to rice within 2 m of the well. Analysis of the well water 5 days after onset showed a pentachlorophenol concentration of 12.5 ppm. Members of the families improved within 2–3 days after use of the well water was stopped (Ueda *et al.*, 1962). If one assumes a standard daily water intake, the measured concentration would indicate an oral dosage of 0.42 mg/kg/day for an adult, to which one would have to add an unknown dermal dosage. However, the possibility cannot be excluded that the concentration that led to illness was higher.

Although illness may be produced by the cumulative action of several doses of pentachlorophenol, the onset of critical illness tends to be sudden and the course of the disease rapid. Efficiency of excretion is an important factor in the pattern of illness caused by the compound. If excretion were much better, illness would occur only after massive doses such as those associated with suicide. If excretion were a little worse, occupational poisoning would be more common, and continuing illness of exposed persons would not be a rarity as it now is. There are few kinds of poisoning in which impending death can be averted by a single exchange transfusion, as has been done in babies poisoned by pentachlorophenol. The possibility depends on having an unusually high proportion of the toxicant in the blood and on having excretion that is almost adequate, even in life-threatening situations.

The threshold limit value for pentachlorophenol (0.5 mg/m^3) indicates that an occupational intake of 0.07 mg/kg/day is considered safe. Based on study of long-term treatment of rats with pentachlorophenol (Schwetz *et al.*, 1978), the U.S. Environmental Protection Agency (USEPA) (1984b) has recommended an acceptable daily intake level of 0.03 mg/kg/day for humans. In addition, a pharmacokinetic study in volunteers indicated that storage and excretion during exposure at the rate of 0.1 mg/kg/day would reach 99% of a steady state in 8.4 days with a maximal concentration of 0.5 ppm in the plasma. It was considered that these results confirmed the safety of the threshold limit value (Braun *et al.*, 1979). However, more recent human pharmacokinetic data do not support this value. In contrast to the study of Braun *et al.* (1979), in which elimination half-lives for pentachlorophenol of 33 and 30 hr in urine and plasma, respectively, were found in four male volunteers, Uhl *et al.* (1986) reported average half-lives in urine and blood of exposed humans to be 19 and 16 days, respectively. Results of the latter study are in general agreement with those of Bevenue *et al.* (1967a) and of Begley *et al.* (1977). (The details of these are discussed subsequently.) A half-life of 16–19 days and an estimated time lag of approximately 3 months to attain steady state indicate that in the steady state the human body burden may be a factor of 10–20 times higher than the value extrapolated from animal pharmacokinetic data (Uhl *et al.*, 1986). It also should be recalled that the metabolism of pentachlorophenol is considerably different in the experimental animals that have been used for toxicity and disposition studies. In humans, elimination appears to occur completely via pentachlorophenol and its glucuronide (see also Section 18.4.1.2), and the percentage of pentachlorophenol bound to serum proteins is higher than 96% (Uhl *et al.*, 1986). Thus, some reconsideration of the recommended threshold limit values should be made based on the newer data.

Laboratory Findings Table 18.7 presents a summary of the concentrations of pentachlorophenol found in various exposed and "nonexposed" populations.

In one case of fatal occupational poisoning with autopsy 3 days after death, pentachlorophenol was found in the following concentrations: lung, 76 ppm; blood from lung, 97 ppm; liver, 62 ppm; blood from liver, 46 ppm; and kidney, 84 ppm. A 14-year-

Table 18.7
Ranges and Mean Concentrations of Pentachlorophenol in People[a]

Population	Urine	Serum	Fat	Reference
General	ND–1.84			Bevenue et al. (1967b)
	0.004–0.007	0.07–0.46		Barthel et al. (1969)
	0.002–0.011			Cranmer and Freal (1970)
	0.001–0.007 (0.0025)		0.005–0.052 (0.025)	Shafik (1973)
	0.009–0.080 (0.020)			Dougherty and Piotrowska (1976)
		(0.016)		Pearson et al. (1976)
	tr–0.193[b]			Kutz et al. (1978)
	<0.001–0.080			Edgerton et al. (1979)
			<0.005–0.140	Ohe (1979)
	0.001–0.002 (0.0014)	0.034–0.075 (0.051)		Hernandez (1980)
	0.001–0.007 (0.0025)	0.015–0.055 (0.048)		Hernandez (1980)
	0.025–0.230 (0.016)	0.004–0.021		Atuma and Okor (1985) Kleinman et al. (1986)
Healthy occupants of PCP-treated houses				
	0.047–0.216	0.580–1.750		Centers for Disease Control (1980)
	0.002–0.087 (0.0127)	0.116–1.084 (0.330)		Centers for Disease Control (1980)
		0.025–0.66		Sangster et al. (1982)
Healthy workers or other exposed people				
	1.10–5.91			Akisada (1965)
	0.6–0.7			Bergner et al. (1965)
	0.003–35.70			Bevenue et al. (1967b)
		4.3–9.1		Bevenue et al. (1968)
	(1.6–2.6)			Casarett et al. (1969)
		2–13		Barthel et al. (1969)
	0.02–0.96			Barthel et al. (1969)
	3.5–32.5			Ueda et al. (1969)
	0.270			Cranmer and Freal (1970)
	0.041–0.335	0.406–3.550		Wyllie et al. (1975)
		(5.1)		Begley et al. (1977)
	3.6			Edgerton et al. (1979)
	0.330–0.30			Kahlman and Horstman (1983)
	0.032–3.40			Siqueira and Fernicola (1981)
	(0.24)			Kleinman et al. (1986)
	0.027–11.9			R. D. Jones et al. (1986)
Poisoned persons who recovered				
	3–10			Gordon (1956)
	2.4–17.5			Bergner et al. (1965)
		118 (two babies)		Armstrong et al. (1969)
Poisoned persons who died				
	70[c]	50[c,d]		Gordon (1956)
	55–96[c]			Gordon (1956); Truhaut et al. (1952a)
		46–97[c,d]		Blair (1961)
	28[c]	53[c,d]		Blair (1961)
			34 (infant)	Barthel et al. (1969)
	29[c]	162[c,d]		Gray et al. (1985)

[a]Values in parts per million (ppm).
[b]Phenolic residues from pesticides.
[c]Postmortem.
[d]Blood, not serum.

old child who ingested the material as a result of an occupational accident showed the following concentrations: liver, postpartem 59 ppm; blood from liver, 53 ppm; kidney, 41 ppm; and urine, 28 ppm (Blair, 1961). In a case of fatal poisoning in a 33-year-old man, tissue levels of pentachlorophenol were: blood, 162 ppm; gastric contents, 8.2 ppm; urine, 29 ppm; kidney, 639 ppm; liver, 52 ppm; lung, 116 ppm; and bile, 1130 ppm (Gray et al., 1985). In another fatal case, the concentrations were as follows: blood, 50 ppm; urine, 70 ppm; lung, 145 ppm; kidney, 95 ppm; liver 65 ppm; and brain, 20 ppm (Gordon, 1956). Concentrations were 55 and 96 ppm in urine taken at autopsy from adults (Truhaut et al., 1952a; Gordon, 1956).

An infant killed by dermal absorption had the following concentrations of pentachlorophenol in tissues: kidney, 28 ppm; adrenal, 27 ppm; heart, 21 ppm; fat, 34 ppm; and connective tissue, 27 ppm (Barthel et al., 1969). The concentration of pentachlorophenol in the serum of one acutely ill baby was 118 ppm; the concentration fell to 65 ppm during the exchange transfusion and to 31 ppm on the day after transfusion (Armstrong et al., 1969). The initial value in another infant may have been higher, for the concentration during transfusion was 118 ppm; but even in this instance the value was 31 ppm the next day. Serum values of symptomatic infants in the same nursery only a few days after the second infant had recovered varied from 7 to 26 ppm. The concentration of pentachlorophenol in the serum of nurses during the same period varied from 2 to 13 ppm. Serum values of two infants in a different nursery were 0.07–0.46 ppm. Cord blood from healthy infants contained undetectable amounts of pentachlorophenol. In the outbreak of poisoning in a nursery, a concentration of 2.44 ppm was found in urine collected from an infant on the third day of recovery after an exchange transfusion. No urine samples from acutely ill babies were available for analysis. Urine values in exposed but asymptomatic infants varied from 0.02 to 0.96 ppm. Urine values for two infants from another nursery were 0.004 and 0.007 ppm (Barthel et al., 1969).

Nonfatal cases in adults have shown 2.4–17.5 ppm pentachlorophenol in the urine and sometimes traces of albumin (Gordon, 1956; Bergner et al., 1965).

The concentrations in the urine of presumably healthy persons with varying degrees of occupational exposure ranged from 0.003 to 35.7 ppm (Akisada, 1965; Bergner et al., 1965; Bevenue et al., 1967b, 1968; Casarett et al., 1969; Barthel et al., 1969; Ueda et al., 1969; Cranmer and Freal, 1970; Wyllie et al., 1975; Begley et al., 1977; Edgerton et al., 1979; Siqueira and Fernicola, 1981; Kahlman and Horstman, 1983). Some of the urinary values reported in healthy or recently recovered workers were higher than those reported in nonfatal cases. Whether the difference is due to variation in susceptibility among workers, collection of samples at inappropriate times, or variation in the sensitivity of analytical methods is not known.

Samples of blood and urine were collected once a month for 5 consecutive months from the six employees of a plant that annually treated approximately 2,500,000 board feet of timber with pentachlorophenol. Concentrations in air samples taken in 11 different locations in the plant were reported to range from 0.000,009 to 0.015,275 mg/m³ and to average from 0.000,263 to 0.001,888 mg/m³ in different months. The individual serum values ranged from 0.406 to 3.550 ppm and were about three to four times higher in the man who operated the pressure treater than in the office manager. The average value for the former for 5 months was 2.292 ppm. The urine values ranged from 0.041 to 0.335 ppm; although they showed the same general relationship to exposure, the correlation between serum and urine samples taken from the same person on the same day was not very close. The average concentration of pentachlorophenol in the five urine samples from the operator of the pressure treater was 0.296 ppm (Wyllie et al., 1975). In a different situation where concentrations of pentachlorophenol in air ranged from 0.04 to 8.9 mg/m³, urinary values ranged from 3.5 to 32.5 ppm. Concentrations for the same person tended to be consistent from day to day (Ueda et al., 1969).

Convincing evidence was offered by Casarett et al. (1969) for a straight-line, log–log relationship between the concentrations of pentachlorophenol in plasma and those in urine. The data were drawn from the general population and from healthy workers with plasma and urine values as high as approximately 10 ppm.

Although Comstock (1974) found that urinary excretion of pentachlorophenol by persons with occupational exposure to the compound increased after accidental increase of exposure, he detected no correlation between the degree of excretion and the occurrence of symptoms compatible with poisoning. He speculated that impairment of excretion precedes the appearance of clinical illness. Although this possibility cannot be excluded by the information available in some cases, the speculation is unwarranted in fatal cases where the concentration is very high. Perhaps 40 ppm is near the threshold.

Pentachlorophenol has been detected in the blood, urine, and fat of ordinary people in tropical areas where the compound is used extensively for wood preservative, agriculture, or both. Concentrations as high as 0.052 ppm in fat (Shafik, 1973) and 0.011 ppm in urine (Cranmer and Freal, 1970) have been reported from Florida.

Based on analysis of 416 samples of urine from persons of the general population of the contiguous states of the United States, the maximal values for various pesticide-related phenolic residues ranged from a trace to 0.193 ppm (Kutz et al., 1978). Using improved analytical methods, pentachlorophenol was detected in the urine of 10 of 11 persons in the general population. The range of measurable values was 0.004 to 0.080 ppm. The presence of 2,3,4,6-tetrachlorophenol in these samples was attributed to its presence as an impurity in the technical product. The only measurable metabolites found were tetrachlorohydroquinone and tetrachloropyrocatechol. The same chemical method revealed 3.6 ppm pentachlorophenol in the urine of an exposed person. The same but no additional metabolites were found. However, the study of Uhl et al. (1986) in which human volunteers were administered [^{13}C]pentachlorophenol found no metabolites of pentachlorophenol other than the glucuronide conjugate. Palmitoylpentachlorophenol has been isolated and found to be present in human fat (Ansari et al., 1985), and pentachlorophenol has been found to be metabolized to tetrachlorohydroquinone by human liver homogenates (Juhl *et al.*, 1985).

It has been speculated that traces of pentachlorophenol in the general population may, in part, be the result of metabolism of other compounds such as hexachlorobenzene (see Section 21.9.1) (van Ommen *et al.*, 1985). However, a study by Geyer *et al.* (1987), who examined dietary levels of pentachlorophenol and hexachlorobenzene in a German population, indicated that the metabolism of 10% of the dietary hexachlorobenzene to pentachlorophenol would not significantly contribute to the total body burden of pentachlorophenols.

Judging from a limited number of samples, red blood cells contain from 0.02 to 0.12 ppm pentachlorophenol with little or no relationship to the total concentration in the whole blood. However, among workers in wood treatment plants whose plasma levels ranged from 4.3 to 9.1 ppm, the concentration in the red cells was only about 1% as great (Bevenue *et al.*, 1968).

It is worthwhile to consider in some detail the studies from which data on the half-life of pentachlorophenol can be obtained. This has important implications when extrapolations from animal data and estimates of human risk assessment are made. A study of volunteers who ingested pentachlorophenol at a rate of 0.1 mg/kg permitted a comparison with data obtained for the rat and monkey. The half-life for oral absorption in the volunteers was 1.3 hr, and that for elimination from the plasma was 30.2 hr. The half-lives for excretion of pentachlorophenol and of its glucuronide in urine were 33.1 and 12.7 hr, respectively. Approximately 74% of the dose was eliminated in the urine as the parent compound and 12% as the glucuronide. In addition, 4% of the dose was eliminated in the feces. The fact that the highest concentration of pentachlorophenol in the plasma (0.245 ppm) was reached in 4 hr, but the maximal rate of urinary excretion was delayed until 42 hr after ingestion, was considered the result of enterohepatic circulation (Braun *et al.*, 1979).

From the analysis of urine samples collected at intervals after the major portion of absorption during occupational exposure at concentrations of 0.23–0.43 mg/m³, it was concluded that the excretory half-life of pentachlorophenol is 10 hr (Casarett *et al.*, 1969).

In a recent study, pentachlorophenol was given orally to three volunteers at single doses of 3.9, 4.5, 9, and 18.8 mg. To eliminate interference by the uncontrolled absorption of pentachlorophenol from the environment, [¹³C]pentachlorophenol was taken by one of the volunteers. An average elimination half-life of 17 days was found in both urine and blood. The long elimination half-life was explained by the low urinary clearance due to the high plasma protein binding (>96%) and tubular reabsorption. The lag time necessary to attain a steady state was estimated to be about 3 months (Uhl *et al.*, 1986).

Bevenue *et al.* (1967a) described an exposure to pentachlorophenol in which a worker had dipped his hands into a 0.4% solution for 10 min, and 2 days later a urinary pentachlorophenol concentration of 0.236 ppm was detected. Within 51 days after exposure, the urinary concentration had de-

creased to 0.017 ppm. From this data, an elimination half-life of 16 days can be approximated.

Pentachlorophenol was measured in blood and urine in 18 workers before, during, and after a 20-day vacation from a wood treatment plant where they worked. Concentrations of pentachlorophenol in the blood decreased from an average of 5.1 ppm to 2.2 ppm during the vacation. Urine values showed a similar but less marked change (Begley *et al.*, 1977). An estimation of the half-lives suggests 12 days for both urine and plasma. A similar type of study was conducted by Kahlman and Horstman (1983). In this case urinary pentachlorophenol half-lives ranged from 5 to 72 days. However, 11 of 24 subjects examined also showed no detectable decrease in urinary pentachlorophenol levels, and in 6 of these individuals the urinary pentachlorophenol levels actually increased after 16 days of vacation.

The exact reasons for the above discrepencies in the estimated half-lives for pentachlorophenol in humans are not known. Although some individual variations in half-life are likely, significant differences in the time of sampling since the last significant exposure, as well as sample collection and preparation methods, are all possible variables. Clearly, this is an important issue needing to be resolved.

Pathology The pathology following acute poisoning is not characteristic, except that the high temperature of the body may be noted if autopsy is performed within a few hours after death. The organs frequently show some congestion, and there may be some cerebral edema. Degenerative changes in the liver and kidneys have been observed in a few cases (Truhaut *et al.*, 1952b; Smith *et al.*, 1967; Robson *et al.*, 1969).

Treatment of Poisoning Treatment of poisoning by pentachlorophenol is identical to that of poisoning by dinitrophenols (see Section 18.3.1.3). Oral treatment with cholestyramine, colestipol, or mineral oil has been found to be effective in decreasing the body burdens of pentachlorophenol in treated monkeys (T. Rozman *et al.*, 1982) and chickens (Polin *et al.*, 1986).

18.4.2 DICHLOROPHEN

18.4.2.1 Identity, Properties, and Uses

Chemical Name 4,4′-dichloro-2,2′-methylenediphenol.

Synonyms Dichlorophen is the common name for the use as a fungicide and bactericide. It is also known as Antiphen® when used as an antihelmintic drug. Other chemical names for the compound include di-phentane-70, bis(5-chloro-2-hydroxyphenyl)methane, 5,5′-dichloro-2,2′-dihydroxydiphenylmethane, and 2,2′-methylenebis[4-chlorophenol]. Trade names used in industry include Bio Moss Killer®, Panacide®, and Super Mosstox®. When used as a drug it is also known as Plath-Lyse®, Wespuril®, Dicestal®, Didroxane®, Hyosan®, Parabis®, Prevental G-D®, Teniathane®, Teniatol®, and Taeniatol®. It is also known under the code number G4®. The CAS registry number is 97-23-4.

Physical and Chemical Properties   Dichlorophen has the empirical formula $C_{13}H_{10}Cl_2O_2$ and a molecular weight of 269.1. It is also found as the monosodium salt ($C_{13}H_9Cl_2NaO_2$) with a molecular weight of 291.1. The pure compound forms colorless, odorless crystals melting at 177–178°C. The technical grade is a cream colored powder with a slight phenolic odor. At 25°C, dichlorophen is slightly soluble in water (30 mg/liter) but more readily soluble in acetone or ethanol.

History, Formulations, and Uses   The procedure for making dichlorophen from *p*-chlorophenol was first patented in the United States in 1944. In various industries dichlorophen is primarily used as a fungicide and bactericide for the control of mold, algae, and moss. For these purposes the monosodium salt of dichlorophen is most often used.

It is also used as Antiphen in the treatment of infection by tapeworms in humans and animals (Most, 1963), however its use for this purpose has generally been replaced by niclosamide. Since dichlorophen has antifungal and antibacterial activity, it also has been used topically in the treatment of fungal infections, such as athlete's foot, and as a germicide in soaps and cosmetics.

18.4.2.2 Toxicity in Laboratory Animals

Basic Findings   Acute oral LD 50 values for dichlorophen are 1250 mg/kg for guinea pigs, 2000 mg/kg for dogs, 1000 mg/kg for mice, and 2600 mg/kg rats (Christiansen *et al.*, 1974).

Biochemical Effects   The biochemical action of dichlorophen appears to be the same as that of 2,4-dinitrophenol (see Section 18.3.1.2). Nakaue and co-workers (1972) observed that a concentration of 2.7 μ*M* dichlorophen produced a 50% increase in the mitochondrial ATPase activity. In the same system, 0.9 μ*M* and 4.8 μ*M* pentachlorophenol and 2,4-dichlorophenol, respectively, also produced a 50% increase in ATPase activity.

18.4.2.3 Toxicity to Humans

Therapeutic Use   Most (1963) reported only mild abdominal discomfort and loose stools in several of 50 patients receiving dichlorophen at a dose of 6 g/day for 2 consecutive days. Urticarial rash has been reported in some patients, and contact allergic dermatitis and photosensitivity has been reported with topical use (Reynolds *et al.*, 1989).

18.5 TCDD AND OTHER ACNEGENIC MATERIALS

TCDD (2,3,7,8-tetrachlorodibenzo-*p*-dioxin) and a number of other closely related compounds are not pesticides or phenols, but are toxic contaminants of a few pesticides, especially her-

bicides. The chloracne and other illnesses observed in workers involved in the manufacture of 2,4,5-trichlorophenol, 2,4,5-T, and a few other compounds are believed to be due primarily, if not exclusively, to the presence of these contaminants. The contamination of 2,4,5-T with TCDD also played a predominant role in the regulation and controversy over the commercial and military use of this herbicide. Furthermore, more recent evidence indicates that prolonged, low-level exposure to these compounds may be more widespread than once believed due to the combustion of chlorinated organics and diverse types of waste materials which result in the formation of these toxic chemicals and their release into the environment. For these reasons, it is essential to include a discussion of this group of compounds.

TCDD is considered the most potent member of a group of structurally and mechanistically related halogenated aromatic hydrocarbons that may be formed as unwanted by-products in the course of synthesis and/or combustion of the chlorophenols or their derivatives, including 2,4,5-T, chloronaphthalenes, chlorobiphenyls (notably hexachlorophene), chlorodiphenyloxides, and certain chlorobenzenes. In addition to TCDD, other toxic by-products may include other halogenated (chlorinated or brominated) dibenzo-*p*-dioxins, biphenyls, and dibenzofurans, as well as the azo- and azoxy-benzenes. Although only a few of these and other polychlorinated aromatic compounds (see Fig. 18.2) have actually been demonstrated to cause chloracne in humans, most produce positive results in the rabbit ear test *in vivo* or in hyperkeratinization assays using a variety of epidermal cell culture systems. Thus, the possibility that they might produce human chloracne has not been excluded. Furthermore, although chloracne has been the most easily visualized or noted manifestation of a toxic exposure to humans, accidental poisonings of domestic livestock and results from experimental animals have shown these compounds to produce a variety of other toxic injuries, most notably tumor promotion, immune alterations, and reproductive effects, which cannot be ignored when considering human exposures.

Nearly all human exposures to this group of toxic compounds have involved highly complex mixtures of these and other chemicals. Although in some cases only a single compound may have been identified as the major toxic contaminant, it is likely that one or more other contaminating isomers and/or congeners also contributed significantly to the observed toxicity. Emphasis has been placed on TCDD partly because it is the most potent representative of this class of compounds, and because it has been most often associated with human occupational exposure to the chlorinated phenols. However, the dioxins, dibenzofurans, and other compounds in this class are structurally related and cause similar biological and toxicological effects by a similar mechanism (Poland and Knutson, 1982; Safe, 1986). Thus "dioxin" should not be considered as a single entity; the more than 500 isomers and related compounds in this group (Fig. 18.2) must be taken into account when human exposures are considered. Many health organizations are currently estimating risks to humans in terms of the "dioxin equivalent," that is, the amount of the specific chemical or mixture which would cause the same

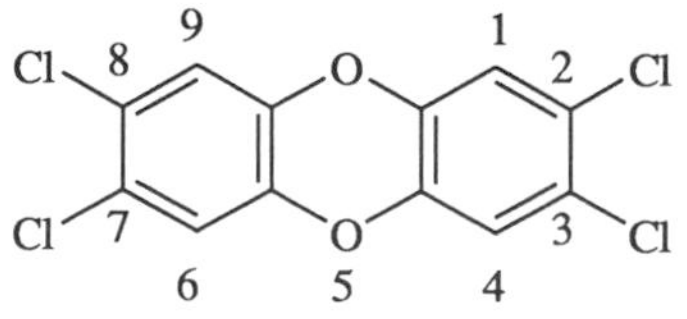

2, 3, 7, 8 -Tetrachlorodibenzo-*p*-dioxin (TCDD)

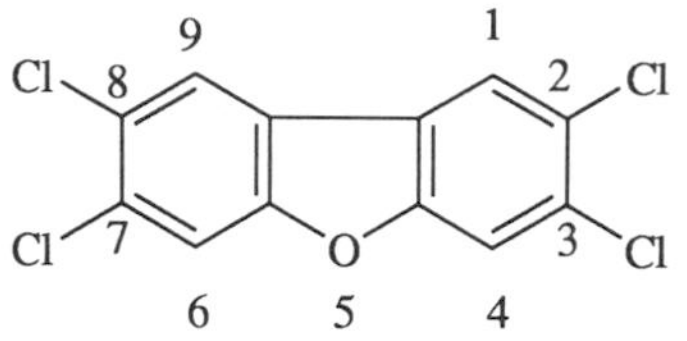

2, 3, 7, 8-Tetrachlorodibenzofuran

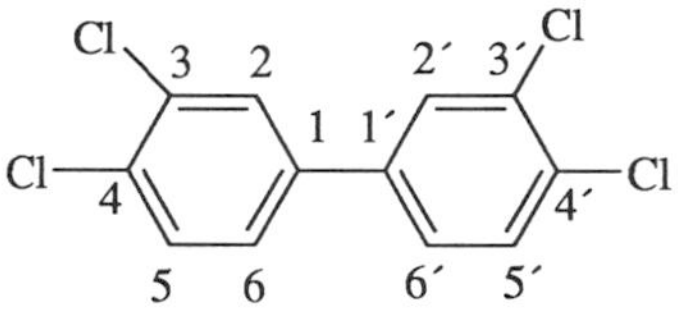

3, 3′, 4, 4′-Tetrachlorobiphenyl

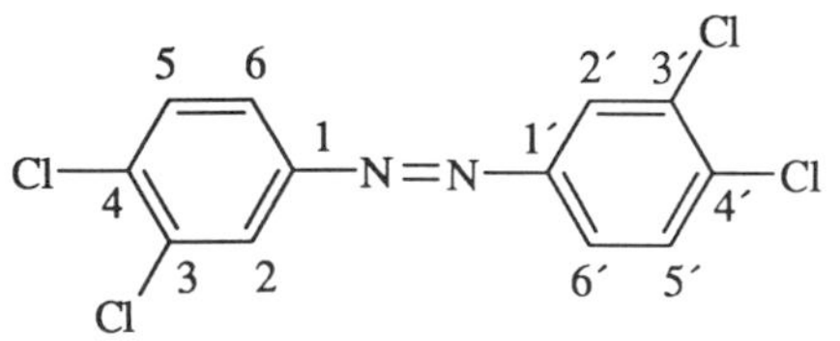

3, 3′, 4, 4′-Tetrachloroazobenzene

Figure 18.2   Chemical structure of TCDD with representative congeners.

degree of toxicity as TCDD. Depending on the source of the mixture, health risks for exposure to the total equivalents from such sources as incinerators may be many times that existing for TCDD alone from the same source (Bellin and Barnes, 1985; Eadon *et al.*, 1986; USEPA, 1987).

The most toxic isomers of this group of compounds are characterized by a planar configuration, complete halogenation of the lateral positions of the aromatic nucleus, and lack of halogenation in the peri positions. These structural requirements are important for binding to specific intracellular sites believed to be involved in toxicity and for limiting metabolism and thus detoxification of the parent compound (see Section 18.5.1.2.). When the most toxic isomer of each chemical class was administered orally to guinea pigs, the toxicity, as determined by LD 50 values, in decreasing order was found to be: dibenzo-*p*-dioxin > dibenzofuran ≥ biphenyl = naphthalene (McConnell and McKinney, 1978). Of particular importance was the fact that, at the LD 50 dose, the signs of illness, median times to death, and gross and histological lesions were essentially the same for all of the compounds, suggesting that they have the same mode of action (McConnell and Moore, 1979). To give some idea of the magnitude of the differences, naphthalenes with four chlorine atoms were about 100 times less active than 2,3,7,8-tetrachlorodibenzofuran and about 1000 times less active than TCDD. Detailed study of different isomers has

shown that TCDD is the most toxic. In general, the hexachloro isomers are less toxic than pentachloro isomers, and trichloro isomers are even less toxic (Schwetz *et al.*, 1973; McConnell and Moore, 1976; McConnell *et al.*, 1978b; Goldstein, 1980; Goldstein and Safe, 1989). If one considers all dioxins and not just the highly poisonous ones, the acute oral toxicities may differ by a factor greater than 150,000 (McConnell *et al.*, 1978b). Although the above discussion specifically refers to the oral LD 50 values, similar trends in toxicity differences have also been observed using other experimental systems and toxicological endpoints. These include thymic atrophy and weight loss (Poland and Glover, 1980; Yoshihara *et al.*, 1981; Bandiera *et al.*, 1984; Safe, 1986), cleft palate and hydronephrosis in the mouse (Weber *et al.*, 1985; Birnbaum *et al.*, 1986), suppression of humoral and cell-mediated immunity (Vecci *et al.*, 1983a; Silkworth and Grabstein, 1982), toxicity and fetal lethality in monkeys (McNulty, 1985), and epidermal hyperplasia and hyperkeratosis in the mouse (Knutson and Poland, 1982), as well as chloracne by the rabbit ear test (Schulz, 1957; Kimmig and Schulz, 1957a). However, it should be noted that quantitative differences are highly dependent on the nature of the effect as well as the specific positioning of the halogen atoms on the isomers examined. For example, the 2,3,4,7,8-pentachlorodibenzofuran is slightly more potent in producing hydronephrosis and cleft palate in fetal mice than is 2,3,7,8-tetrachlorodibenzofuran (Birnbaum *et al.*, 1986).

Many books dealing with the environmental chemistry and health effects of this large group of compounds have been published. Some of these have been edited by Kimbrough (1980), Khan and Stanton (1981), Hutzinger *et al.* (1982), Coulston and Pocchiari (1983), Tucker *et al.* (1983), Poland and Kimbrough (1984), Exner (1987), and Kimbrough and Jensen (1989).

18.5.1 TCDD

18.5.1.1 Identity, Properties, and Uses

Chemical Name   2,3,7,8-Tetrachlorodibenzo-*p*-dioxin.

Structure   See Fig. 18.2.

Synonyms   2,3,7,8-TCDD is the isomer specifically meant when the term TCDD is used alone. Although the word "dioxin" is sometimes used to indicate TCDD, this use should be discouraged because there are 75 chlorodibenzo-*p*-dioxin isomers, including 22 possible tetrachlorodibenzo-*p*-dioxins, and they differ greatly in toxicity. The CAS registry number of TCDD is 1746-01-6.

Physical and Chemical Properties   TCDD has the empirical formula $C_{12}H_4O_2Cl_4$ and a molecular weight of 321.96. It is a white, crystalline solid that melts at 300°C and begins to decompose at 700°C. Its solubility in water is 0.2 ppb. It is highly lipophilic; its octanol : water partition coefficient is 10^5. TCDD is stable in solid form under ordinary conditions of storage. Although its stability in the environment is incompletely known because of its highly lipid-soluble nature, TCDD is associated primarily if not exclusively with soil, sediments, and other organic matter. Because of this association, degradation of TCDD in the environment may be restricted. Under laboratory conditions, ultraviolet radiation degrades TCDD rapidly (Crosby and Wong, 1977). However, the reaction requires a hydrogen donor, and the limited solubility of TCDD in aqueous media may limit the occurrence of this reaction in the environment. Thus, degradation may vary considerably depending on the matrix it was originally associated with, climatic conditions, and the type of soil in the area of contamination. Although TCDD has a relatively low vapor pressure (approximately 4.5×10^{-6} Pa), it may volatilize appreciably from upper soil surfaces. The half-life of TCDD in soils under relatively dry conditions (Utah) was found to be approximately 330 days and in more moist soils and under warm conditions (Florida) was found to be approximately 190 days [Young *et al.*, 1976; International Agency for Research on Cancer (IARC), 1977]. However, recent data from soils present in contaminated areas such as Seveso, Italy, suggest an extremely long half-life, greater than 10 years (Young, 1983; Wipf and Schmid, 1983). Also, due to the lipophilic nature of TCDD, intestinal absorption into living organisms can vary significantly depending on the matrix and source of exposure (McConnell *et al.*, 1984; Umbreit *et al.*, 1986; Lucier *et al.*, 1986). A study by Shu *et al.* (1988) suggested that dermal bioavailability of TCDD from contaminated soil is very low (<1%) in the rat. In most experimental studies, TCDD has been administered in vehicles such as corn oil that enhance absorption. In some cases of environmental exposure, such as occurred in Missouri, TCDD was associated with waste oil which was sprayed on roads and horse arenas for dust control. Similarly, exposure of Japanese and Taiwanese populations to a cooking oil inadvertently contaminated with polychlorinated biphenyls and dibenzofurans resulted in significant absorption of these compounds and subsequent adverse health effects (see 18.5.1.3).

Due to the large number of isomers contained within this group of compounds, it is necessary to perform isomer-specific analysis for their quantitation. A combination of gas and liquid chromatography–mass spectrometry techniques has been used (Buser, 1975; Nestrick *et al.*, 1979; Mitchum *et al.*, 1980; Albro *et al.*, 1985). It is of interest that most recently monoclonal antibodies, directed against certain isomers, have also been developed and used for screening environmental samples (Albro *et al.*, 1979; Kennel *et al.*, 1986; Stanker *et al.*, 1987).

18.5.1.2 Toxicity to Livestock and Laboratory Animals

The way in which the toxic potency of TCDD was discovered is of interest. Because of the many cases of chloracne among workers making 2,4,5-trichlorophenol, this compound and its precursor, 1,2,4,5-tetrachlorobenzene, were studied using the highly sensitive rabbit ear test introduced by Adams *et al.* (1941) and independently by Hofmann and Neumann (1952). The pure phenol proved inactive, although the technical product

was highly active. Isolation of an active by-product was unsuccessful. Therefore, compounds were synthesized that, on the basis of theory, might be by-products of the saponification of tetrachlorobenzene. The majority of the compounds synthesized proved inactive. Only the tri- and tetrachlorodibenzofurans and 2,3,7,8-TCDD produced the characteristic changes in rabbit ear, and TCDD did so at concentrations of 10–50 ppm (Schulz, 1957; Kimmig and Schulz, 1957b; Jones and Krisek, 1962).

Outbreaks of hyperkeratosis in livestock occurred in the United States at least as early as May 1941 (Olafson, 1947) or perhaps as early as 1939 (Simpson, 1949). Olafson (1947) described a hyperkeratotic disease of cattle which he referred to as "X-disease." Symptomology, in addition to the hyperkeratosis, included severe lacrimation, diarrhea, polyuria, marked salivation, and nasal discharge. The exact cause of the syndrome was eventually established to be chlorinated naphthalenes purposely introduced into lubricants to improve their physical properties (Hansel *et al.*, 1955). In some cases these lubricants contaminated cattle feed; at other times, the animals became intoxicated by licking axle grease from farm implements (Link, 1953). Experimentally, the highly chlorinated naphthalenes and contaminated lubricants produced an identical disease not only in cattle (Bell, 1952, 1953; Sikes and Bridges, 1952; Sikes *et al.*, 1952) but also in sheep (Brock *et al.*, 1957) and swine (Huber and Link, 1962), although the skin lesions were not observed in the latter two species. A similar disease of cattle was observed in Germany between 1946 and 1948 and appeared to be related to exposure to a wood preservative (Wagener, 1951). Although the exact toxic chemical was never identified, it has been suggested that it may be related to the pentachlorophenol content of the preservatives (Conklin and Fox, 1978) and its contamination with the chlorinated dibenzo-*p*-dioxins and dibenzofurans (McConnell *et al.*, 1980) (see also 18.4.1).

Although chloracne and similar hyperkeratotic episodes have been the predominant syndromes described in exposed human and livestock populations, it has become evident that TCDD and related compounds cause other effects. In the late 1960s a chemical company in southern Missouri, which had produced 2,4,5-trichlorophenoxyacetic acid, ceased production and leased the facilities to another company which produced hexachlorophene and 2,4,5-trichlorophenol. Between February and October 1971, an estimated 21,500 gallons of contaminated waste oil were removed from this plant for disposal. Much of this material was used for spraying roads and horse arenas for dust control (Kleopfer, 1985). A number of horses (57) became ill and subsequently died. These horses exhibited extreme weight loss and alopecia. There were 26 known abortions, and many foals, exposed only *in utero*, died at birth or shortly after. Postmortem examinations showed severe emaciation, hepatic damage, gastric ulcers, atrophy of the spleen, and skin lesions (Carter *et al.*, 1975; Kimbrough *et al.*, 1977). Many cats and dogs straying in the arena areas died with the same symptoms.

Feed contaminated with halogenated dibenzo-*p*-dioxin also resulted in two major outbreaks of chick edema disease in the United States. This disease is characterized by the extracellular accumulation of body fluids (subcutaneous edema, ascites, hydrothorax, and hydropericardium) and has been observed mainly in birds, particularly chickens. The outbreaks in 1957 and 1960 were traced to the addition to chicken feed of tallow ("toxic fat") that had been scraped from hides preserved with pentachlorophenol. An outbreak in 1969 arose from an improper underground plumbing connection that permitted phenols (used in the manufacture of antimicrobial agents) to leak into a trap used to collect acidified soapstock in a vegetable oil refinery. The soapstock was later used for chicken feed. Samples of these fats have been found to be contaminated with the chlorinated dibenzo-*p*-dioxins, particularly the hexa- isomer (Cantrell *et al.*, 1969; Flick *et al.*, 1972; Firestone, 1973; Plimmer, 1973). Chick edema disease affected more than 2 million chickens in Japan during February and March 1968, and more than 400,000 chickens were reported to have died (Shoya, 1974). Oil containing about 1300 ppm polychlorinated biphenyls had been used in certain lots of feed. Contaminated food-grade rice oil from the same factory led more than 6 months later to human poisoning called "Yusho disease" (Kuratsune *et al.*, 1972) (see also Section 18.5.1.3). Polychlorinated biphenyls from a leaking transformer in a feed mill have been implicated in causing a similar syndrome in chickens in the United States (Platonow *et al.*, 1973).

Between 1973 and 1974, another livestock contamination that mimicked "X-disease" in cattle occurred in Michigan. In this case, the incident was caused by the inadvertent introduction of polybrominated biphenyls, which were used as flame retardants, into animal feed (Kay, 1977; Fries, 1984). Exposure of animals was so widespread that 18,000 cattle, 3500 pigs, 1200 sheep, and 1.5 million chickens had to be killed (Dunckel, 1975; Mercer *et al.*, 1976). To prevent further human exposure (see also Section 18.5.1.3), animal products such as milk, cheese, and eggs had to be destroyed. The main component of this mixture, 2,2′,4,4′,5,5′-hexabromobiphenyl, has subsequently been shown to produce severe hyperkeratosis of the rabbit ear (Patterson *et al.*, 1981).

Basic Findings   The extreme toxicity of TCDD, the wide differences in the susceptibility of different species, and the fact that its exact mode of action remains unknown are noteworthy characteristics of this compound. If only the LD 50 value for the guinea pig is considered, TCDD represents the most toxic synthetic compound known, being approximately 64,000 times more potent than sodium cyanide. However, other experimental animal species and strains demonstrate a considerable range of sensitivity, with the hamster being approximately 3000- to 6000-fold less sensitive than the guinea pig (Table 18.8). The signs of toxicity also differ considerably from species to species and do not point clearly in most species to any one organ or system as being responsible for death (Poland and Knutson, 1982). The same is true for necropsy findings (McConnell, 1980). Yet the compound cannot be considered a general cellular poison; compared to the intact animal, certain isolated cells are not especially susceptible. TCDD at concentrations up to 1 × 10⁻⁶ *M* (0.322 ppm) in the culture medium of several kinds

Table 18.8
Acute Toxicity of 2,3,7,8-TCDD

Species and sex	Route	LD 50 (μg/kg)	Reference
Guinea pig (Hartley)			
M	oral	0.6	Schwetz *et al.* (1973)
M	oral	2.0	McConnell *et al.* (1978b)
Yellow perch	intraperitoneal	2–4	Kleeman *et al.* (1988)
Blue gill	intraperitoneal	12–23	Kleeman *et al.* (1988)
Mink, M	oral	4.2	Hochstein *et al.* (1988)
Monkey, F	oral	<70	McConnell *et al.* (1978a)
Rat (Sprague–Dawley)			
M	oral	222	Schwetz *et al.* (1973)
F	oral	45	Schwetz *et al.* (1973)
Rat (Hans/Wistar)		>1400	Pohjanvirta *et al.* (1987)
Rabbit	oral	115	Schwetz *et al.* (1973)
Rabbit	dermal	275	Schwetz *et al.* (1973)
Mouse, M			
C57B1/6	oral	284	McConnell *et al.* (1978b)
C57B1/6	oral	182	Chapman and Schiller (1985)
DBA/2	oral	2570	Chapman and Schiller (1985)
Hamster (golden Syrian), M	intraperitoneal	>3000	Olson *et al.* (1980a)
Hamster (golden Syrian)	oral	5051	Henck *et al.* (1981)

of mammalian cells resulted in no significant effect on morphology, viability, or growth rate for, in some cells, up to 14 days (Beatty *et al.*, 1975; Knutson and Poland, 1980a). Other cell types, particularly epithelial cells, that have been examined in culture systems appear to be more sensitive to TCDD-induced alterations (Knutson and Poland, 1980b; Gierthy and Crane, 1984; Rice and Cline, 1984; Greenlee *et al.*, 1985a,b; Abernethy *et al.*, 1985; Puhvel and Sakamoto, 1987). However, within these cultured cell models, alterations in cellular differentiation, rather than cell death, are the predominant features observed. This similar finding within intact animals, along with the species-specific nature of the lesions, may partially explain the difficulty in identifying an organ system responsible for death. Thus, at least the lethal effects of TCDD likely depend on the combined effect of a number of affected organ systems, or on interference with some as yet unidentified aspect of integration of these systems.

The acute toxicity of TCDD is most unusual compared with that of most other extremely potent toxicants in that the time to death following single or multiple exposure is extended: 2–6 weeks, depending on the species (Schwetz *et al.*, 1973; McConnell and Moore, 1979). Even with doses severalfold greater than the LD 50 dose, the time to death is not shortened (Buu-Hoi *et al.*, 1972). During this period, experimental animals and livestock have been shown to exhibit a wasting-type syndrome characterized by a progressive and profound loss in body weight. When a lethal dose is administered, the body weight loss prior to death may be as much as 30–40% of the original body weight. Although initial studies suggested that hypophagia was not great enough to account for all of the weight loss (Harris *et al.*, 1973; Courtney *et al.*, 1978; Gasiewicz *et al.*, 1980; Ball and Chhabra, 1981), more recent studies indicate that a decrease in food consumption accounts for the major effect of TCDD on body weight loss (Seefeld and Peterson, 1983; Seefeld *et al.*, 1984; Huang Lu *et al.*, 1986). However, protection against TCDD-elicited toxicity or lethality was not observed in rats or guinea pigs in which body weight was maintained by the feeding of a total parenteral diet (Gasiewicz *et al.*, 1980; Huang Lu *et al.*, 1986). Thus, although decreased food consumption appears to account for the major effect of TCDD on body weight loss, additional metabolic alterations may occur which also contribute significantly to body weight loss, other signs of toxicity, and subsequent lethality.

In addition to lethality, many other signs of acute and chronic toxicity have been observed in animals. Structural, functional, and biochemical alterations to organs of the immune system, reproductive system, gastrointestinal tract, liver, kidney, bone marrow, and skin have been described. As noted above, these lesions are in general species-specific. These will be discussed in more detail in later sections.

In a 13-week study in rats, oral administration of TCDD at the rate of 1 μg/kg/day, 5 days/week, produced essentially the entire spectrum of injuries seen after a single dose, and some mortality was observed. A dosage of 0.1 μg/kg/day on the same schedule produced some of the same effects but to a lesser degree. A dosage of 0.01 μg/kg/day caused a slight increase in relative liver weight, and one-tenth of that dosage produced no detectable effect of any kind (Kociba *et al.*, 1976, 1978). Rats given 1.0 ng/kg/day for 2 years exhibited no toxicologically significant effect, while the ingestion of 10 ng/kg/day resulted in a number of lesions including hepatocellular nodules and focal alveolar hyperplasia of the lung (Kociba *et al.*, 1978). Other long-term exposure studies using 2,3,7,8-TCDD have demonstrated the production of a variety of tumors in rats as well as mice (see Mutagenesis, Genotoxicity, and Carcinogenesis).

Monkeys poisoned by TCDD at a dietary level of 0.5 ppb showed weight loss, blepharitis, loss of fingernails and eyelashes, facial alopecia with acneform eruptions, mild anemia, neutropenia, lymphopenia, and a decrease in serum cholesterol with increased serum triglycerides. At necropsy, the liver, kidneys, and adrenals showed a relative increase in weight, where-

as the thymus was reduced dramatically. There were hyperplastic and metaplastic changes of the sebaceous glands and epithelial hyperplasia of the renal pelvis, stomach, gallbladder, and bile duct. Erythroid elements of the bone marrow were reduced (Allen *et al.*, 1977; McConnell *et al.*, 1978a). Female monkeys receiving the same dietary concentration showed reproductive difficulties as they became generally incapacitated (Barsotti *et al.*, 1979). Females receiving only one-tenth as much TCDD (0.05 ppb) showed lesser but nevertheless similar signs of general toxicity. However, only two of eight were successful in producing young; the others either failed to conceive or suffered abortions or stillbirths. All of the eight controls produced normal young (Schantz *et al.*, 1979). Notably, similar results in monkeys have been reported following long-term exposure to 2,3,7,8-tetrachlorodibenzofuran and certain polychlorinated biphenyl isomers (McNulty, 1985).

Absorption, Distribution, Metabolism, and Excretion The route of exposure of humans to TCDD and related compounds may vary considerably depending on the source of the contaminated material. While dermal absorption may be the primary route for industrial workers and individuals exposed in the spraying of herbicides, oral intake and inhalation may occur for those consuming contaminated foodstuffs such as cooking oil and living or working in areas where high concentrations of these chemicals in dusts or generated aerosols may exist.

In experimental animals, the dermal absorption of TCDD has been found to be highly dependent on the nature of the formulation applied to the skin. In one study, the liver concentration of [³H]TCDD was used as the means of determining the uptake of the compound (Poiger and Schlatter, 1980). This procedure has validity, since the liver appears to be the major storage site for TCDD in the rat (Piper *et al.*, 1973; Rose *et al.*, 1976; Van Miller *et al.*, 1976). The level of TCDD was highest in the liver when it was applied in an organic solvent such as methanol or polyethylene glycol. Association of the TCDD with soil or activated charcoal greatly reduced the uptake. Similar results were observed when the induction of chloracne by TCDD in the rabbit was tested with different vehicles. Notably, the dermal LD 50 for TCDD applied to the rabbit ear was reported to be more than twice that found upon oral administration (Schwetz *et al.*, 1973).

A number of studies have examined the absorption of radiolabeled TCDD following oral administration. In these experiments, TCDD was dissolved in olive oil or in a solution of acetone and corn oil. For the rat and hamster, from 70 to 85% of orally administered TCDD was found to be absorbed (Piper *et al.*, 1973; Rose *et al.*, 1976; Allen *et al.*, 1975; Olson *et al.*, 1980b). In mice, the absorption was only 24–33% of the administered dose (Koshakji *et al.*, 1984). However, in this study the vehicle consisted of 1% ethanol, 10% Tween 80, and 89% saline. Only a few studies have examined the absorption of TCDD from environmental matrices such as fly ash, soot, and soil. Chlorinated dibenzo-*p*-dioxins and dibenzofurans appeared to be readily absorbed by guinea pigs fed contaminated soot samples from a polychlorinated biphenyl transformer fire at

Binghamton, New York (Silkworth et al., 1982). Van den Berg et al. (1985) examined the bioavailability of these compounds adsorbed on fly ash in a number of mammalian species. The uptake of the more toxic isomers resulted in concentrations in the liver corresponding to 1–10% of the total ingested material. In contrast, other investigators noted that the bioavailability of TCDD in soil samples from contaminated areas of New Jersey varied considerably but might correlate with the ease of extractability into organic solvents (McConnell et al., 1984; Umbreit et al., 1986; Lucier et al., 1986). Aging has no apparent influence on the intestinal absorption of TCDD in rats (Hebert and Birnbaum, 1987). No studies have been performed examining the absorption of these contaminants from dusts or aerosols which may be inhaled.

TCDD appears to be absorbed essentially by the lymphatic route and is transported predominantly by chylomicrons (Lakshmanan et al., 1986) and lipoproteins (Henderson and Patterson, 1988; Patterson et al., 1988). Rose et al. (1976) examined the fate of TCDD in rats following a single oral dose of 1.0 μg TCDD/kg and following repeated oral doses of 0.01, 0.1, or 1.0 μg/kg/day, 5 days/week for 7 weeks. The liver and fat contained most of the body burden of the toxin, accounting for 50 and 10 times more TCDD, respectively, than any other tissue examined. These investigators concluded that the rate of TCDD accumulation in the body was largely accounted for by the rate of accumulation in liver and fat. Other studies in rats, guinea pigs, hamsters, and mice have confirmed the major percentage distribution of TCDD into the liver and fat (Van Miller et al., 1976; Olson et al., 1980b; Gasiewicz and Neal, 1979; Gasiewicz et al., 1983a; Birnbaum, 1986; Olson, 1986). Depending on the species examined and the time of examination following treatment, the levels of TCDD in liver or adipose tissue (on the basis of total tissue) may represent 10–50% or 20–60% of the total body burden, respectively. One study showed that monkeys accumulate approximately 10% of the dose in the liver but store more than rats in the fat, skin, and muscle (Van Miller et al., 1976). High levels of radiolabeled TCDD have also been observed in the skin of treated guinea pigs (Gasiewicz and Neal, 1979; Olson, 1986) and mice (Birnbaum, 1986), although these were not as high as those observed in the monkey. Autoradiography of radiolabeled TCDD in three strains of mice showed a marked uptake and long-term retention of radioactivity in the nasal mucosa and the liver (Appelgren et al., 1983).

In a 2-year study in rats, a dosage of 0.1 μg TCDD/kg/day produced neoplasia and terminal residues of 24.0 and 8.1 ppb in liver and fat, respectively. A dosage of 0.01 μg/kg/day produced lesser toxicity and corresponding terminal residues of 5.1 and 1.7 ppb. A dosage of 0.001 μg/kg/day was without toxic effect and resulted in a residue of 0.54 ppb in the liver (Kociba et al., 1978).

The subcellular distribution of TCDD has been examined in the liver of the rat (Allen et al., 1975), guinea pig (Gasiewicz and Neal, 1979), and mouse (Vinopal and Casida, 1973). In the rat up to 90% and in the guinea pig and mouse approximately 50% of the radioactivity present following administration of radiolabeled TCDD was associated with the microsomal frac-

tion. The accumulation of lipophilic TCDD in the microsomes may be due in part to the extensive proliferation of smooth endoplasmic reticulum (SER) in the liver of TCDD-treated animals (Jones and Butler, 1974). It was suggested that the relatively lower level of TCDD in the monkey liver was the result of a lesser degree of hepatic SER proliferation following TCDD treatment (Van Miller et al., 1976). In the soluble portion of the cell, a large percentage of the TCDD is probably associated with lipoproteins (Lesca et al., 1987).

All evidence to date indicates that TCDD is only slowly metabolized in mammals and that metabolites that are formed are readily excreted. Analysis of the liver and adipose tissue of hamsters receiving radiolabeled TCDD indicated that the extractable radioactivity, which represented greater than 97% of that present in the tissues, was unmetabolized TCDD (Olson et al., 1980b). These results confirmed an earlier observation that radioactivity in the liver of treated rats was unchanged TCDD (Rose et al., 1976). More recently, 4, 8, 13, and 28% of the radioactivity in kidney, perirenal adipose tissue, liver, and skeletal muscle, respectively, from treated guinea pigs was found to be present as radiolabeled metabolites of TCDD (Olson, 1986). The in vivo covalent binding of radiolabeled TCDD to rat liver protein, ribosomal RNA, and DNA also has been reported (Poland and Glover, 1979). Twenty-four hours following the treatment of rats with radiolabeled TCDD at 7.5 μg/kg, virtually all of the radioactivity present in the liver could be extracted. The distribution of the unextractable radioactivity was as follows: protein, 60 pmol TCDD per mole of amino acid residue; RNA, 12 pmol per mole of nucleotide residue; and DNA, 6 pmol per mole of nucleotide residue. The binding of radiolabeled material to DNA is 4 to 6 orders of magnitude lower than that of most chemical carcinogens.

Whole-body half-lives for the excretion of radiolabeled TCDD and/or TCDD-derived radioactivity from rodents range from 11 to 94 days, and the corresponding values for monkeys and possibly humans are much greater (Table 18.9). In specific cases such as the guinea pig, a lower rate of metabolism of TCDD and consequently a longer whole-body half-life may contribute to the increased susceptibility of this species to the toxic effects (Table 18.8). Investigations with isolated hepatocytes have shown that control and TCDD-pretreated rats metabolized TCDD at much greater rates than control or pretreated guinea pigs (Wroblewski and Olson, 1985). The induction of hepatic mixed-function oxidase drug-metabolizing enzymes has been shown to decrease the relative sensitivity of rats to TCDD-elicited lethality (Beatty et al., 1978). Similarly, a relatively high rate of metabolism and elimination of TCDD by the hamster may contribute to the relative insensitivity of this species. However, the magnitude of some of these differences in elimination rates as compared to the LD 50 values and, for example, the finding that the half-life in the C57BL/6 mouse is similar to that in the hamster suggest that other factors in addition to metabolism and elimination play some role in the differential species sensitivity. The DBA/2 mouse possesses approximately twice as much total adipose tissue as the C57BL/6 strain, and the elimination half-life is approximately twice as long (Gasiewicz et al., 1983a).

Table 18.9
Rates and Routes of Elimination of TCDD in Various Mammals

Species	Dose (μg/kg)	Route	Half-life for elimination (days)	Relative % of TCDD-derived radioactivity at termination		Reference
				Urine	Feces	
Guinea pig	2.0	ip	30[a]	6	94	Gasiewicz and Neal (1979)
Guinea pig	1.45	oral	22–43	—	—	Nolan et al. (1979)
Guinea pig	0.56	ip	94	11	89	Olson (1986)
Rat	1.0	oral	31	<1	>99	Rose et al. (1976)
Rat	50	oral	17	20	80	Piper et al. (1973)
Rat	400	ip	—	9	91	Van Miller et al. (1976)
Mouse						
C57BL/6J	10.0	ip	11	26	74	Gasiewicz et al. (1983a)
DBA/2J	10.0	ip	24	30	70	Gasiewicz et al. (1983a)
Hamster	650	ip	11	41	59	Olson et al. (1980a)
Hamster	650	oral	15	—	—	Olson et al. (1980a)
Monkey	1	oral	365	—	—	McNulty et al. (1982)
Monkey	400	ip	—	22	78	Van Miller et al. (1976)
Monkey (infant)	400	ip	—	61	39	Van Miller et al. (1976)
Human	0.0014	oral	2120[b]	ND[c]	>99	Poiger and Schlatter (1986)

[a]Time at which 50% of the original dose was eliminated. This value is not to be confused with $t_{1/2}$ which is applicable to a component of elimination following first-order kinetics. Notably, in this study toxicity and subsequent mobilization of adipose tissue and radiolabeled TCDD contained in this tissue occurred.
[b]Results from a single individual.
[c]Not detectable. Level of detection was 9 pg TCDD ~ 1500 ml urine.

In all species examined, the major route of elimination for TCDD and/or its metabolites appears to be via the feces (Table 18.9). As noted, however, there may be considerable variation depending on the species, the dose administered, and the age of the animal. For example, approximately 78% of the material eliminated is in the feces of the adult monkey, whereas in the infant monkey the urine appears to be the major route of elimination. Following the administration of radiolabeled TCDD to rats, hamsters, mice, or guinea pigs, all of the radioactivity present in the urine and bile was found to be in metabolites of TCDD (Ramsey et al., 1982; Poiger and Schlatter, 1979; Olson et al., 1980b; Gasiewicz et al., 1983a,b; Olson, 1986). However, unchanged TCDD may account for 14–90% of the radioactivity found in the fecal material (Gasiewicz et al., 1983a,b; Olson, 1986). The presence of TCDD in feces and its absence in bile suggest that the fecal elimination of unchanged TCDD resulted from direct intestinal elimination. A number of hydroxylated metabolites of TCDD have been identified, including 2-hydroxy-3,7,8-trichlorodibenzo-p-dioxin, 2-hydroxy-1,3,7,8-tetrachlorodibenzo-p-dioxin, 1-hydroxy-2,3,7,8-tetrachlorodibenzo-p-dioxin, several other hydroxylated chlorinated dibenzo-p-dioxins and diphenyl ethers, and 4,5-dichlorocatechol (Poiger et al., 1982; Sawahata et al., 1982; Poiger and Buser, 1984; Neal et al., 1984). Many of these are excreted as glucuronide conjugates (Sawahata et al., 1982; Gasiewicz et al., 1983b). Administration of some of these purified metabolites directly into guinea pigs and rats resulted in little or no toxicity (Weber et al., 1982; Mason and Safe, 1986), indicating that the metabolism of TCDD represents a detoxification process. Indirect evidence suggests that TCDD is metabolized primarily by the cytochrome P-450-associated mixed-function oxidases and that treatment with TCDD induces these enzymes and thereby promotes TCDD metabolism (Beatty et al., 1978; Wroblewski and Olson, 1985; Poiger and Schlatter, 1985). However, the tissue uptake and rate of metabolism of TCDD do not merely correlate with genetic differences at the Ah locus in mice (Shen and Olson, 1987) (see Biochemical Effects).

It should be noted that not all of the congeners and isomers which make up this family of compounds exhibit the same half-life, metabolism, and routes of elimination as TCDD. These are highly dependent on the position and number of chlorine substitutions on the molecule as well as the species of animal examined (Birnbaum, 1985). In general, however, the most toxic isomers have long half-lives.

The few studies which have examined the transfer of TCDD to the embryo and fetus (Moore et al., 1976; Nau and Bass, 1981; Nau et al., 1986; van den Berg et al., 1987) have found limited transplacental transfer of TCDD to the fetus. Following the administration of radiolabeled TCDD to pregnant mice, exceedingly low concentrations (between 0.04 and 0.14% of the maternal dose per gram of tissue) of radioactivity were found in the fetus between days 11 and 18 of gestation. The concentrations of TCDD in fetal livers were two to four times higher than those in other fetal organs (Nau and Bass, 1981). Despite the relatively low level of transfer of TCDD to the fetus, some studies have observed significant induction of fetal hepatic microsomal enzymes (Berry *et al.*, 1976; Lucier *et al.*, 1975b). TCDD was found to be efficiently transferred to neonatal mice by lactating mothers which received TCDD during pregnancy. During the first 2 weeks, the pups received doses of TCDD via the milk which were, on a body weight basis, similar to those that had been administered to the mothers. During the third week, tissue levels in the nursing pups exceeded those of their mothers (Nau *et al.*, 1986). Other studies have obtained similar results regarding the relative efficiency of elimination of TCDD via the milk from lactating animals (Fanelli *et al.*, 1980; Arstila *et al.*, 1981; Jensen and Hummel, 1982). Thus, although the partitioning of the lipophilic TCDD into milk represents a mode of excretion for the lactating animal, it may have an impact on the nursing neonate. Significant induction of the microsomal enzymes has been observed in neonatal animals exposed to TCDD or polychlorinated biphenyls only via lactation (Lucier *et al.*, 1975a; Moore *et al.*, 1978). Moore *et al.* (1976) found that nursing of newborn rats by TCDD-treated mothers markedly increased the incidence of hydronephrosis.

Pathology and Effects on Organs, Tissues, and Cells Various lesions have been reported in TCDD-exposed animals, but the relative contribution of these lesions to lethality is as yet unknown. These lesions included hepatomegaly with hyperplasia and hypertrophy of the parenchymal cells as well as parenchymal cell necrosis, chloracne and epidermal changes, involution of the thymus and spleen, hyperplasia and hypertrophy of the epithelium of the gastrointestinal tract, urinary tract hyperplasia, edema, testicular atrophy and degeneration of the seminiferous tubules, hypocellularity of the bone marrow, hemorrhages, degenerative changes of kidney tubules and thyroid follicles, and atrophy of the zona glomerulosa of the adrenal (Buu-hoi *et al.*, 1972; Gupta *et al.*, 1973; Zinkl *et al.*, 1973; Norback and Allen, 1973; Vos *et al.*, 1974; Allen *et al.*, 1975; Croft *et al.*, 1977; McConnell *et al.*, 1978a,b; Kociba *et al.*, 1979; McConnell, 1980). The relative presence and severity of these lesions vary considerably with the dose of TCDD, length of exposure (acute versus long-term), and species of animal (McConnell, 1984).

The liver lesions observed in chickens and rabbits, and to a lesser extent in mice and rats, is relatively severe, and cellular necrosis has been observed. However, the liver of guinea pigs, cattle, and nonhuman primates shows relatively little pathologic change except for enlargement. A number of detailed studies of the hepatic lesion in rodents have been presented (Fowler *et al.*, 1973; Jones and Butler, 1974; Jones, 1975; Jones and Greig, 1975; McConnell *et al.*, 1978b; Weber *et al.*, 1983; Turner and Collins, 1983; Schecter *et al.*, 1985a). This lesion in the rat is mainly centrilobular and is characterized by parenchymal cell necrosis, the presence of large multinucleated cells, mitochondrial alterations, the accumulation of lipid droplets and eosinophilic hyaline bodies, deposition of various pigments, glycogen depletion, inflammatory cell infiltration, and the development

of fibrosis in the necrotic regions. In one study, these lesions became progressively worse up to week 16 following the administration of a single dose of 20 μg/kg and appeared thereafter to regress slowly (Weber *et al.*, 1983). Jones and Butler (1974) observed complete loss of detectable ATPase reaction of the parenchymal cells in the centrilobular region within 3 days following treatment of rats with 200 μg TCDD/kg. This remained the predominant feature throughout the 6-week study. The inhibition of hepatocyte plasma membrane ATPases was confirmed, and alterations in other membrane enzymes and proteins (see *Biochemical Effects*) were observed by Greig and Osborne (1981) and Matsumura *et al.* (1984a,b). Collectively, these studies suggest that, at least in liver, the plasma membrane is a specific subcellular site of the toxic action of TCDD. Alterations in hepatic function may be related to these membrane changes. Decreased bile flow and decreased biliary excretion of organic acids were observed to be dose-dependent and persistent following a single administration of TCDD in rats. The partial recovery of ouabain excretion 40 days after treatment coincided with the elimination of TCDD from the animal (Yang *et al.*, 1977; Peterson *et al.*, 1979a,b).

Early proliferation of smooth endoplasmic reticulum and disorganization of the rough endoplasmic reticulum are prominent features of the ultrastructural changes in hepatic parenchymal cells from most animal species following treatment with TCDD (Jones and Butler, 1974). Proliferation of the smooth endoplasmic reticulum is accompanied by an increase in the activity of a variety of enzymes found within these structures, including the microsomal mixed-function oxidases (see Biochemical Changes). Concentric membranous whorls have also been observed in rats and guinea pigs treated with TCDD (Gasiewicz *et al.*, 1980; Turner and Collins, 1983) or a mixture of chlorinated dibenzo-*p*-dioxins (Norback and Allen, 1969). The significance of the latter structures is unclear, since they may be the result of proliferative processes, degeneration of membrane components, or a combination of both.

Hyperplasia and hypertrophy of the epithelial cells of the extrahepatic bile ducts and gallbladder are more common in the species that show little liver pathology, such as monkeys, cattle, and horses, than in the species exhibiting marked hepatic alterations (McConnell *et al.*, 1978a,b, 1980; Kimbrough *et al.*, 1977).

More recent studies have implicated the heart as a major target organ of TCDD toxicity. Canga *et al.* (1988) noted decreased β-adrenergic responsiveness and increased intracellular calcium in guinea pig heart muscle following TCDD treatment. Brewster *et al.* (1987) also reported changes in atrial muscle from TCDD-treated guinea pigs but suggested that they may be secondary to overall overt toxicity. Kelling *et al.* (1987b) reported that overtly toxic doses of TCDD to rats did not alter the mechanical functioning of the heart muscle.

In intoxicated chickens, rats, and mice the livers are often darker in color and the accumulation of brown-green pigments is observed upon histological examination. Part of this discoloration is due to the accumulation of porphyrins within the liver. Examination of these livers under long-wavelength ultra-violet light has been useful in the qualitative detection of porphyrins and establishing the relative degree of intoxication (Gupta *et al.*, 1980). The more toxic isomers of these compounds are some of the most potent porphyrinogenic chemicals known (Goldstein *et al.*, 1973; Goldstein, 1979) (see *Biochemical Effects*).

It was noted earlier that a number of changes in the skin have been produced in animals following dermal or systemic exposure to TCDD. In the monkey this lesion consists of edema, alopecia, and folliculitis, which is located primarily on the face but also on the chest. Changes in the Meibomian glands of the eyelids are a characteristic indication of intoxication in monkeys. The changes observed in the skin and eyelids, as well as in the ear canal of the monkey, have a similar pathogenesis (McConnell *et al.*, 1979). Microscopically, the sebaceous glands undergo atrophy with concomitant metaplasia to a stratified squamous epithelial cell which produces keratin. The central duct of the gland enlarges due to the accumulation of keratin and may eventually rupture, resulting in a secondary inflammatory reaction. Hyperkeratosis and subsequent dilatation of the hair follicles also occurs (McConnell *et al.*, 1978a, 1979; McConnell, 1980). A similar chloracne-like lesion produced in the inner ears of rabbits has been used as a sensitive assay for the presence of acnegenic compounds (Adams *et al.*, 1941; Jones and Krizek, 1962). The hyperkeratotic lesion has been produced in hairless mice (Inagami *et al.*, 1969; Knutson and Poland, 1982; Vos *et al.*, 1982; Puhvel *et al.*, 1982) and has been shown to be very severe in intoxicated cattle (Bell, 1954). A number of investigators have shown that TCDD directly affects cultured epidermal keratinocytes and that the change involves altered differentiation (Knutson and Poland, 1982; Poland *et al.*, 1984; Hudson *et al.*, 1985, 1986; Greenlee 1984a; Greenlee and Neal, 1985; Puhvel *et al.*, 1984; Puhvel and Sakamoto, 1987).

In contrast to most other signs of TCDD toxicity, thymic atrophy and immune suppression are consistently observed in a variety of mammalian species. Morphologically, thymic atrophy is characterized by lymphocyte depletion in the cortex (Harris *et al.*, 1973; Vos *et al.*, 1973). Although TCDD exposure affects both cell-mediated and humoral immunity in the adult animal, cell-mediated immune processes appear to be more sensitive when exposure occurs during the perinatal period. In the adult animal, TCDD-elicited immune suppression has been expressed as a dosage-dependent impairment of delayed cutaneous hypersensitivity reactions (Vos *et al.*, 1973; Faith and Moore, 1977; Thomas and Hinsdill, 1979; Clark *et al.*, 1981), proliferative responses to T- and B-cell mitogens and in mixed leukocyte cultures (Vos and Moore, 1974; Sharma and Gehring, 1979; Thomas and Hinsdill, 1979; Vecci *et al.*, 1980a; Luster *et al.*, 1980), as well as graft-versus-host and allograft rejection (Vos *et al.*, 1973, 1980). The injection of certain soluble factors produced in the thymus (thymosin) does not reverse the effect of TCDD (Vos *et al.*, 1978), and natural killer-cell- or macrophage-mediated tumor cell cytolysis is not altered by TCDD exposure (Mantovani *et al.*, 1980; Dean *et al.*, 1981). In a series of investigations that demonstrated the extreme sensitivity of

cell-mediated immunity to TCDD, the generation of cytotoxic T lymphocytes was found to be suppressed at 0.4 μg/kg in C57BL/6 adult mice; this dose did not produce any thymic atrophy or any impairment of antibody or delayed hypersensitivity responses (Clark *et al.*, 1981). Thymocytes and lymph node cells from TCDD-treated mice (doses as low as 0.004 μg/kg) were also shown to suppress cytotoxic T-lymphocyte generation from peripheral lymph node cells from untreated mice, whereas direct addition of TCDD produced no suppression. When the effectiveness of TCDD in inducing the activity of microsomal enzymes and its effectiveness in suppressing cytotoxic T-lymphocyte generation were compared, the latter response was significantly reduced at a dosage as low as 0.04 ng/kg, while the enzymatic activity was increased only at dosages of 400 ng/kg or greater (Clark *et al.*, 1983). Studies utilizing fetal thymus organ cultures suggest that the TCDD-induced effects on the thymus may be due, in part, to a direct action of TCDD in this tissue (Dencker *et al.*, 1985; Hassoun, 1987). However, even more recent experiments indicate that alterations in the pre-T lymphocyte stem population present in the bone marrow may also contribute to this lesion (Fine *et al.*, 1989, 1990).

The antibody response to both T cell-dependent and -independent antigens is also diminished in TCDD-treated animals (Vecci *et al.*, 1980a,b, 1983a,b; Thomas and Hinsdill, 1979; Hinsdill *et al.*, 1980; Tucker *et al.*, 1986). Serum antibody titers to tetanus toxoid and sheep red blood cells were decreased in TCDD-treated guinea pigs and mice (Vos *et al.*, 1973; Hinsdill *et al.*, 1980). In some cases, humoral immunosuppression occurred at doses lower than those which caused thymic atrophy (Tucker *et al.*, 1986). TCDD has also been reported to alter host resistance to challenge with infectious agents or transplantable tumors. Increased susceptibility to *Streptococcus*, *Salmonella*, and *Listeria* has been reported (Thigpen *et al.*, 1975; Hinsdill *et al.*, 1980; White *et al.*, 1986), although others reported that TCDD has no effect on mortality due to these agents (Vos *et al.*, 1978; Thomas and Hinsdill, 1979). Differences in methods of dosing and dosing regimens likely account for these discrepancies. Mice also have decreased resistance to the parasite *Plasmodium yoelii* (Tucker *et al.*, 1986). Serum total hemolytic complement activity and serum C3 levels were depressed following TCDD treatment (White *et al.*, 1986). Other results utilizing thymocytes and fetal thymus suggest that the modulation of humoral immunity by TCDD may be due in part to a direct effect of TCDD on the differentiation of the B cell (Tucker *et al.*, 1986; Holsapple *et al.*, 1986a; Dooley and Holsapple, 1987; Germolec *et al.*, 1987; Kramer *et al.*, 1987; Luster *et al.*, 1988; McConkey *et al.*, 1988; McConkey and Orrenius, 1989). However, the ability of TCDD to affect stem cells formed in bone marrow may also be partly responsible for the noted alterations in T-cell immunity (Fine *et al.*, 1989, 1990).

Exposure to TCDD during immune system ontogenesis is generally thought to have a more profound effect on immune function, especially cell-mediated responses, than adult exposure (Vos and Moore, 1974). Allograft rejection times were increased and the graft-versus-host activity and lymphoproliferative responses were suppressed in both rats and mice whose mothers were administered 2 or 5 μg TCDD/kg on gestational days 14 and 17 and postnatally on days 1, 8, and 15. Animals exposed only prenatally displayed lesser alterations in these parameters, suggesting greater exposure via the milk than transplacentally (Vos and Moore, 1974). There was no decrease in these parameters after 4 months, however. In a subsequent study in which mothers were dosed with 5 μg TCDD/kg on day 18 of gestation and on postnatal days 0, 7, and 14, pups were found to have decreased lymphoproliferative responses to mitogens and delayed hypersensitivity responses, but no suppression of serum antibody titers or primary and secondary antibody responses to a T cell-dependent antigen (Faith and Moore, 1977). These alterations were seen for as long as 145 days after birth. Similar results were reported by Faith et al. (1978) and Luster et al. (1980).

In general, significant alterations in the cellular components of blood have been observed only following prolonged exposure to these halogenated compounds (McConnell, 1980). Vos et al. (1974) found little hematological change in mice exposed to an LD 50 dose. Although anemia was not observed in mice and guinea pigs following TCDD treatment (Zinkl et al., 1973), thrombocytopenia and clotting abnormalities were observed in rats exposed to lethal levels of TCDD (Weissberg and Zinkl, 1973). Female rats exposed to 0.1 μg TCDD/kg/day had no anemia after 13 weeks of treatment (Kociba et al., 1976), but mild anemia was observed following 2 years of daily treatment (Kociba et al., 1978). However, in the same studies, moderate thrombocytopenia and mild leukocytosis were observed at the end of 13 weeks and pancytopenia was noted at the end of 2 years. Additional observations have indicated that the bone marrow is a target organ for TCDD toxicity. Bone marrow hypocellularity has been noted in rats, guinea pigs, and monkeys exposed to TCDD (Kociba et al., 1976; McConnell et al., 1978a,b; Allen et al., 1977). Perinatal administration of TCDD to mice suppressed bone marrow progenitor cell proliferation (Luster et al., 1980) and inhibited hematopoiesis in vivo and in vitro by altering colony growth of stem cells (Luster et al., 1985). In the latter studies, progenitor cells were suppressed following acute exposure of mice to TCDD at dosages as low as 1.0 μg/kg.

In vivo and in vitro studies in rats indicated that TCDD has a relatively nonspecific toxic action on the kidney, depressing several major renal functions (McCormack et al., 1976; Hewitt et al., 1976; Pegg et al., 1976; Anaizi and Cohen, 1978). Proliferation of the smooth endoplasmic reticulum and peroxisomes have been observed predominantly in the S3 segment of the rat proximal tubule following treatment with TCDD or polychlorinated biphenyls (Fowler et al., 1977; Rush et al., 1986). Hyperplasia of the epithelium of the terminal portions of the collecting ducts of the renal medulla, renal pelvis, and ureter has been noted in monkeys exposed to polychlorinated biphenyls (McConnell et al., 1979).

Morphological alteration in the thyroid and decreased serum thyroxine levels (see Biochemical Effects) have been reported in animals exposed to TCDD and the polychlorinated and polybrominated biphenyls. Distention of the thyroid follicles with hypertrophy and hyperplasia of the follicular epithelium was the most striking change observed in rats (Collins et al., 1977; Rozman et al., 1986). Notably, similar changes were observed in neonatal rats exposed to polychlorinated biphenyls in utero and via the milk (Collins and Capen, 1980). In longer-term studies in rats exposed to polybrominated biphenyls and cattle exposed to technical pentachlorophenol, the morphological changes consisted of smaller thyroid follicles as well as hypertrophy of the follicular epithelium (Sleight et al., 1978; McConnell et al., 1980).

Common features of these lesions are that nearly all of the affected cells are of the epithelial type and their primary response appears to be hyperplasia and/or altered differentiation. In addition to epithelium of the urinary tract, thyroid follicles, sebaceous glands and epidermis, and extrahepatic bile ducts mentioned above, hyperplastic changes have been noted in the epithelium of the intestine and glandular stomach in a variety of species, especially the monkey (Allen et al., 1977; Kimbrough et al., 1978; Moore et al., 1979). In a variety of cell lines, the major effect of TCDD seems to be on maturation and differentiation processes rather than on cell viability. Further, and as observed in vivo, epithelial cells appear to be most affected. TCDD in the culture medium of several kinds of mammalian cells had no significant effect on morphology, viability, or growth rate (Beatty et al., 1975; Knutson and Poland, 1980a). In contrast, a mouse teratoma cell line, XB, undergoes terminal differentiation and concomitant keratinization following exposure to TCDD (Knutson and Poland, 1980b). Morphological and biochemical changes characteristic of altered differentiation patterns have been shown in epidermal cells from BALB/c mice (Puhvel et al., 1984) as well as in cell lines derived from humans (see Section 18.5.1.3). Seemingly in contrast, hypoplastic and atrophic responses occur in the thymus and bone marrow. However, evidence for a TCDD-elicited alteration of the differentiation of thymic epithelial cells has been presented (Greenlee et al., 1984b, 1985a).

Teratogenic and Reproductive Effects   Teratogenic effects resulting from TCDD exposure have been reported primarily in mice and rats, whereas the compound is highly fetotoxic in a number of experimental animals (Neubert and Dillman, 1972; Neubert et al., 1973; Allen et al., 1979; Barsotti et al., 1979). TCDD at a maternal dosage of 3 μg/kg/day injected subcutaneously on days 6–15 of gestation increased the incidence of cleft palate and kidney anomalies in three strains of mice. A dosage of 1 μg/kg/day had the same effect in the only strain in which this dose was tested (Courtney and Moore, 1971). Cleft palate with minimal fetal lethality could be produced in mice given a single maternal dose in the range of 20 to 50 μg/kg on days 8–11 of gestation (Neubert and Dillman, 1972). The no-adverse-effect level for a teratogenic response in the mouse was reported to be 0.1 μg/kg/day (Smith et al., 1976). The kidney lesions produced in pups cross-fostered to mothers treated with TCDD were similar to those of fetuses exposed in utero (Moore et al., 1973). In rats, TCDD at a subcutaneous dosage of 0.5 μg/kg/day did not produce cleft palate but did increase the incidence of kidney anomalies (Courtney and Moore, 1971). Intestinal hemorrhage has also been observed in rats exposed to TCDD *in utero* (Sparschu *et al.*, 1971; Khera and Ruddick, 1973). The no-adverse-effect level for rat embryo fetotoxicity is in the range 0.03–0.125 μg/kg/day (Sparschu *et al.*, 1971). Dosage-related cardiovascular malformations were observed in chickens, with doses of 1 pmol/egg resulting in malformations in 50% of the embryos (Cheung *et al.*, 1981).

Thyroid hormones (Lamb *et al.*, 1986), hydrocortisone (Birnbaum *et al.*, 1986), retinoic acid (Abbott and Birnbaum, 1989; Birnbaum *et al.*, 1989), and certain polychlorinated biphenyls (Birnbaum *et al.*, 1985) have been shown to increase the incidence of cleft palate in TCDD-treated mice, but one polychlorinated biphenyl mixture, Aroclor 1254, decreased the effects (Haake *et al.*, 1987a,b). The actual mechanisms of these interactions are not completely understood. There are also marked strain differences in teratogenic sensitivity to TCDD, which seem to segregate with the *Ah* locus (see Biochemical Effects) (Poland and Glover, 1980; Pratt *et al.*, 1984a; Hassoun *et al.*, 1984a,b). Like other pathologic manifestations of TCDD exposure in experimental animals, both cleft palate and hydronephrosis induced by this compound appear to be due to an effect on epithelial cells. The apical epithelial cells of the secondary palate fail to follow the normal pattern of programmed cell death following TCDD exposure (Pratt *et al.*, 1984b; Hassoun *et al.*, 1984a), and TCDD has been demonstrated to directly alter palatal epithelial cell differentiation (Abbott *et al.*, 1989). TCDD elicits hyperplasia of the ureteric luminal epithelium, resulting in hydroureter and hydronephrosis (Abbott *et al.*, 1987a,b).

Breeding of eight female monkeys which showed toxicity after 6 months of consuming a diet containing 500 ppt TCDD resulted in two pregnancies, one of which was aborted. In another study, monkeys fed 50 ppt TCDD showed slight toxicity, but four of seven pregnancies terminated in abortion (Schantz *et al.*, 1979). In a series of additional studies it was found that a short exposure to 1 μg TCDD/kg during early pregnancy results in fetal loss in rhesus monkeys (McNulty, 1978, 1984). Mares exposed to TCDD following the spraying of horse arenas with contaminated waste oil suffered abortions, and many foals exposed only *in utero* died at birth or shortly thereafter (Carter *et al.*, 1975; Kimbrough *et al.*, 1977).

In a three-generation reproduction study, no significant toxicity was seen in F_0 rats of either sex during 90 days of ingesting TCDD at a dosage of 0.1 μg/kg/day prior to mating. However, this dosage severely decreased fertility and neonatal survival. At a dosage of 0.01 μg/kg/day, fertility was significantly decreased in the F_1 and F_2 generations but not in the F_0 rats; other indications of toxicity included decreased litter size, reduced proportion of pups born alive, and reduced survival of pups to weaning. At a dosage of 0.001 μg/kg/day, no effect was seen on fertility, litter size, or postnatal body weight in any generation, and no consistent effect was seen on survival of the pups (Murray *et al.*, 1979). In another study, male rodents were exposed to mixtures of 2,4-D, 2,4,5-T, and TCDD (0.16, 1.2, and 2.4 μg/kg/day) in the diet for 8 weeks prior to mating. This ex-

posure did not reduce the ability of their unexposed mates to produce viable offspring (Lamb *et al.*, 1981a,b). Higher doses of TCDD have been associated with decreased spermatogenesis and structural damage to testis and spermatogonia (Kociba and Schwetz, 1982).

Mutagenesis, Genotoxicity, and Carcinogenesis Mutagenicity assays in microorganisms have been used to assess the genotoxic effects of TCDD. These results have been summarized by Kociba and Schwetz (1982), Hay (1982), Rogers *et al.* (1982), and Giri (1986) and indicate little, if any, potential of TCDD for mutagenic activity. In early studies, TCDD was reported to be mutagenic in *Salmonella typhimurium* strain TA1532 (Seiler, 1973) and *Escherichia coli* strain Sd-4 (Hussain *et al.*, 1972). However, a number of later studies failed to detect mutagenic activity of TCDD in *S. typhimurium* (Wassom *et al.*, 1978; Gilbert *et al.*, 1980; Geiger and Neal, 1981; Mortelmans *et al.*, 1984).

Studies of TCDD genotoxicity in eukaryotic systems have yielded equivocal results (Giri, 1986). No or only weakly positive chromosomal abnormalities were observed in bone marrow cells from male rats treated with dosages of TCDD up to 20 μg/kg (Green and Moreland, 1975; Green *et al.*, 1977; Loprieno *et al.*, 1982), and results were negative (Khera and Ruddick, 1973) or weakly positive (Murray *et al.*, 1979) in dominant lethal studies with male rats. Zimmering *et al.* (1985) found TCDD to be negative in the sex-linked recessive lethal test in the fruit fly *Drosophila melanogaster*. Although mitotic inhibition and/or chromosome aberrations have been noted in the African blood lily (Jackson, 1972), cytogenetic studies examining sister chromatid exchange and chromosome aberrations in Chinese hamster ovary cells showed negative results [National Toxicology Program (NTP), 1985]. Other investigations have found genotoxic changes in the yeast *Saccharomyces cerevisiae* (Bronzetti *et al.*, 1980, 1983), in the mouse lymphoma assay system (Rogers *et al.*, 1982), and in peripheral lymphocytes from TCDD-treated rats on exposure to α-naphthoflavone (Lundgren *et al.*, 1986). It should be noted that in the latter studies, the use of α-naphthoflavone greatly increased the sensitivity of the assay for detection of sister chromatid exchange frequencies, and a dosage-dependent increase in this frequency was observed between 0 and 3 μg TCDD/kg in female rats. The dosage–response curve for TCDD mutagenicity in the mouse lymphoma system closely resembled those generated with several DNA intercalating agents (Rogers *et al.*, 1982). Furthermore, Wahba *et al.* (1988) reported the TCDD-enhanced formation of DNA single-strand breaks in hepatic nuclei. However, as unextractable binding of TCDD-derived radioactivity to macromolecular components in rodent livers is four to six orders of magnitude less than that of most chemical carcinogens (Vinopal and Casida, 1973; Rose *et al.*, 1976; Nelson *et al.*, 1977; Guenthner *et al.*, 1979a; Poland and Glover, 1979), it seems unlikely that TCDD's effects are directly genotoxic. In addition, at concentrations found to be mutagenic in some bacteria, TCDD did not affect transfection of QB RNA, a single-stranded molecule whose transfection was found to be altered by intercalating and alkylating agents (Kondorosi et al., 1973).

TCDD has been found to produce neoplasms, especially hepatic tumors, in a number of rodent models. In a 2-year study in rats, ingestion of TCDD at a rate of 0.1 µg/kg/day increased the incidence of hepatocellular carcinoma and squamous cell carcinoma of the lung, hard palate and/or turbinates, and tongue but decreased the incidence of tumors of the pituitary, uterus, mammary gland, pancreas, and adrenal gland. A dosage of 0.01 µg/kg/day increased the incidence of hepatocellular nodules and focal alveolar hyperplasia. A dosage of 0.001 µg/kg/day was without effect (Kociba et al., 1978).

Forty-eight percent of male mice that had received TCDD by gastric tube at a rate of 0.7 µg/kg/week for 1 year developed liver tumors, compared to 33% of control mice. The average life span of the two groups was 633 and 651 days, respectively. This effect was not seen at either a lower or a higher dosage. TCDD produced chronic, ulcerous skin lesions in mice, many of which developed amyloidosis. This combination of effects was seen at a dosage of 0.007 µg/kg/week but was more frequent at higher dosages, especially 7 µg/kg/week (Toth et al., 1978, 1979).

Carcinogenicity bioassays of TCDD were sponsored by the National Cancer Institute. In one study, rats of each sex were administered TCDD by gavage 2 days/week for 104 weeks at doses of 0.01, 0.05, or 0.5 µg/kg/week. All surviving rats were killed at 105–107 weeks. In male rats, there was a dosage-related increased incidence of follicular cell adenomas or carcinomas of the thyroid. An increase in subcutaneous tissue fibromas was also noted in males of the high-dosage group. In female rats, an increased incidence of hepatocellular carcinomas and neoplastic nodules, subcutaneous tissue fibrosarcomas, and adrenal cortical adenomas was noted in the high-dosage group. In another study, mice were administered TCDD for 104 weeks at doses of 0.01, 0.05, and 0.5 µg/kg/week (males) and 0.04, 0.2, and 2.0 µg/kg/week (females). In male mice, there was an increased incidence of hepatocellular carcinomas and neoplastic nodules in the high-dosage group. In female mice, TCDD produced significant increases of hepatocellular carcinomas, hepatocellular adenomas, fibrosarcoma, histiocytic lymphoma, thyroid follicular cell adenoma, and cortical adenoma or carcinoma in the high-dosage group (NTP, 1980a,b).

The available evidence indicates that TCDD acts as a tumor promoter rather than an initiator. In early studies, TCDD was found to be a weak tumor initiator in the two-stage system of mouse skin tumorigenesis; when given concurrently with a known carcinogen in this system, it modified the response only slightly (DiGiovanni et al., 1977). In other experiments, a nontoxic dose of TCDD strongly inhibited the induction of skin tumors by 7,12-dimethylbenz[a]anthracene or benzo[a]pyrene in mice (DiGiovanni et al., 1979; Berry et al., 1979; Cohen et al., 1979). This effect is probably due to the potent ability of TCDD to induce a number of drug-metabolizing enzymes and alter the metabolism and activation of some of these compounds (see Biochemical Effects). It was shown that pretreatment with TCDD markedly reduced the formation of the presumptive ultimate carcinogenic metabolite of benzo[a]pyrene, 7,8-diol-9,10-epoxy-benzo[a]pyrene, and its covalent binding with guanosine in DNA (Cohen et al., 1979). However, TCDD was shown to be a cocarcinogen when administered to mice in conjunction with the administration of 3-methylcholanthrene (Kouri et al., 1978). Furthermore, by virtue of its ability to induce drug-metabolizing enzymes, TCDD potentiated the mutagenicity of carcinogens in bacterial systems (Felton and Nebert, 1975).

Pitot et al. (1980) showed TCDD to be a potent tumor promoter in a two-stage model of carcinogenesis in rat liver. No carcinomas were detected in four rats 32 weeks following treatment with diethylnitrosamine and partial hepatectomy. However, five of seven rats treated biweekly with 1.4 µg TCDD/kg in addition to diethylnitrosamine had hepatocellular carcinomas, and six of seven rats had an increased incidence of hepatocellular carcinomas or hepatocellular neoplastic nodules. Three of five rats treated biweekly with 0.14 µg TCDD/kg in addition to diethylnitrosamine had hepatocellular neoplastic nodules. Rats receiving only TCDD after partial hepatectomy showed no significant increase in enzyme-altered foci and no neoplasia. Similar results for the tumor-promoting capacity of TCDD were observed in studies using a mouse skin two-stage tumorigenesis model. With either 7,12-dimethylbenz[a]anthracene- or methyl-N-nitrosoguanidine-initiated mice, the effective dose of TCDD was approximately 100-fold less than that of the potent tumor promoter 12-O-tetradecanoylphorbol-13-acetate (Poland et al., 1982). A number of potent tumor promoters, including TCDD, have been shown to enhance the repair of O^6-methylguanine in rat liver DNA (Den Engelse et al., 1986).

Biochemical Effects   Studies on the multiplicity of biochemical activities modulated by TCDD have shed considerable light on the mechanism of action of this compound, which involves a hormone-like pleiotropic alteration of gene expression mediated by stereospecific binding to a soluble receptor protein (Poland and Knutson, 1982). TCDD is the most potent and persistent inducer of certain enzyme activities and is likewise effective in suppressing others. Since some of the altered activities are involved in the function and regulation of physiologically important entities, an underlying role for the TCDD-induced changes in the etiologies of various alterations has been postulated.

TCDD causes a striking change in the protein constituents of rat liver membranes (Brewster et al., 1982) and decreases bile flow and biliary excretion of indocyanine green (Hwang, 1973; Seefeld et al., 1979, 1980), ouabain (Yang et al., 1977; Hamada and Peterson, 1978; Seefeld et al., 1980), organic anions (Yang et al., 1977), and immunoglobulin A (Moran et al., 1986). Decreased ouabain excretion is paralleled by but does not appear to be caused by decreased transport ATPase activities (Peterson et al., 1979a,b). Reported alterations in renal transport are thought to be indirect results of general toxicity (Kirsch et al., 1975; Pegg et al., 1976; Anaizi and Cohen, 1978; Hook et al., 1975).

Down-regulation of epidermal growth factor receptors occurs in TCDD-treated rodent (Madhukar *et al.*, 1984) and human (Hudson *et al.*, 1985; Osborne and Greenlee, 1985) cell membranes. A good correlation was found between the degree of decline of epidermal growth factor receptors and susceptibility to toxicity in rats, mice, and guinea pigs (Madhukar *et al.*, 1984). The *in vivo* administration of TCDD also stimulated the expression of certain oncogenes (Bombick *et al.*, 1988) and protein kinase activities, especially protein kinase C (Bombick *et al.*, 1985) and protein tyrosine kinase (Bombick and Matsumura, 1987). However, TCDD did not activate protein kinase C in cultured EL4 thymoma cells (Kramer *et al.*, 1986) but apparently did activate it in murine B cells *in vitro* (Kramer *et al.*, 1987). TCDD also reduces ligand binding activities of low-density lipoprotein (Bombick *et al.*, 1984) and insulin (Matsumura *et al.*, 1984a,b) receptors, as well as concanavalin A binding (Brewster *et al.*, 1982) to rodent hepatic plasma membranes. On the basis of these data, the plasma membrane has been proposed as a primary target organelle for TCDD.

The best-characterized biochemical effect of TCDD is the selective induction and repression of a particular set of cytochrome P-450-mediated multisubstrate mixed-function oxidase activities (reviewed by Parkinson and Safe, 1981; Poland and Knutson, 1982). The specific activities stimulated or repressed are a function of species, age, sex, and tissue (Nebert and Gelboin, 1969; Hook *et al.*, 1975; Atlas *et al.*, 1977; Aitio and Parkki, 1978; Guenther and Nebert, 1978; Norman *et al.*, 1978; Liem *et al.*, 1980; Goldstein and Linko, 1984; Gasiewicz *et al.*, 1986; Kimura *et al.*, 1986). In the chick embryo, TCDD doubled the activity of aryl hydrocarbon hydroxylase at a dosage of 0.5 ng/egg and produced maximal induction at 50 ng/egg. This induction reached a plateau in 18 hr and lasted at least 5 days (Poland and Glover, 1973a). The ED 50 dose of TCDD for the induction of aryl hydrocarbon hydroxylase is approximately 0.32 μg/kg in responsive strains of mice and at least 3.2 μg/kg in nonresponsive strains. The F_1 hybrids of responsive and nonresponsive strains are intermediate in reactivity and can be distinguished quantitatively from both parents (Poland and Glover, 1975). It is of interest that the ED 50 for induction of this enzyme activity in the responsive strain is similar to that observed in both the rat (Poland and Glover, 1974) and the hamster (Gasiewicz *et al.*, 1986), the latter species being the least susceptible to TCDD toxicity. Guinea pigs, the species most susceptible to TCDD toxicity, showed little or no induction of the activities of benzo[*a*]pyrene hydroxylase or DT-diaphorase in various tissues in response to this compound (Beatty and Neal, 1978), although 4-biphenyl hydroxylase (Hook *et al.*, 1975) and the total content of cytochrome P-450 (Huang Lu *et al.*, 1986) were increased to a moderate degree.

The two major forms of cytochrome P-450 induced by TCDD and related halogenated aromatic hydrocarbons are referred to as P-450c and P-450d in rats (Thomas *et al.*, 1983), P_1-450 and P_3-450 in mice (Negishi and Nebert, 1979), and forms 4 and 6 in rabbits (Johnson and Müller-Eberhard, 1977). Analyses of the cDNAs for these cytochromes in rats and mice indicate that P-450c is equivalent to P_1-450 (Yabusaki *et al.*,

1984) and P-450-d is equivalent to P_3-450 (Kawajiri *et al.*, 1984; Kimura *et al.*, 1984). Forms 6 and 4 in rabbits are analogous to P-450c/P_1-450 and P-450d/P_3-450, respectively (Okino *et al.*, 1985). There is also notable sequence homology between these genes and the gene that encodes the human version of mouse P_1-450 (Jaiswal *et al.*, 1985a). Chromosome segregation analyses of somatic cell hybrids indicated that the genes for these inducible cytochromes are located on chromosome 9 in the mouse (Tukey *et al.*, 1984) and chromosome 15 in the human (Hildebrand *et al.*, 1985).

The induction of aryl hydrocarbon hydroxylase, as well as a variety of other cytochrome P-450-associated enzyme activities (Nebert and Jensen, 1979), occurs in many tissues, including the liver, intestine, lung, kidney, skin, testes, mammary gland, and prostate. However, the relative pattern of the cytochrome P-450-associated activities induced or repressed is very tissue and species specific (Poland and Glover, 1974; Hook *et al.*, 1975; Aitio and Parkki, 1978; Mattison and Thorgeirsson, 1978; Lee and Suzuki, 1980; Rikans *et al.*, 1979; Guenthner *et al.*, 1979b; Liem *et al.*, 1980; Tofilon and Piper, 1982; Goldstein and Linko, 1984; Cresteil *et al.*, 1987). In the kidney, this induction is localized mainly in a specific segment of the proximal tubules (Fowler *et al.*, 1975, 1977). The cells of the rat intestinal crypt region are more sensitive to the inductive effects of TCDD than are the absorptive tip cells (Schiller and Lucier, 1978). TCDD is approximately 30,000 times more potent than 3-methylchloanthrene as an inducer of hepatic aryl hydrocarbon hydroxylase (Poland and Glover, 1974). The inducing effects of TCDD can last as long as 73 days following a single dose (Poland and Glover, 1974; Kumaki *et al.*, 1977; Gasiewicz *et al.*, 1986) and may be detectable at single doses as low as 0.002 μg/kg (Kitchin and Woods, 1979).

According to Lucier *et al.* (1975b), administration of a single oral dose of 3 μg TCDD/kg to pregnant rats during middle or late pregnancy caused marked induction of maternal microsomal enzymes but had little or no effect on these enzymes in the fetus, and it was not teratogenic. However, there was marked induction of some hepatic microsomal enzymes of pups from treated mothers. Cross-fostering studies indicated that the postnatal induction resulted from exposure of the pups to TCDD via the milk. In contrast, Berry *et al.* (1976) reported substantial induction of aryl hydrocarbon hydroxylase activity in rat fetuses following a single intraperitoneal injection of 2.5 μg/kg in the mother. The distribution of [^{14}C]TCDD in the young following a single oral dose of 5 μg/kg to the mother was consistent with enzyme induction. TCDD was found in fetuses sampled on gestation days 14, 18, or 21 but at far lower concentrations than in young examined 3, 7, 10, or 14 days after birth. The induction was dosage-dependent and was especially marked in extrahepatic tissues. At 6 μg/kg, aryl hydrocarbon hydroxylase was increased 24-, 22-, and 4-fold in fetal lung, kidney, and skin, respectively. The corresponding values for the treated dam were 4-, 2-, and 2-fold (Berry *et al.*, 1977). The concentration of TCDD in the neonate, compared to that in the dam, was considered sufficient to account for the greater sensitivity of the neonate (Moore *et al.*, 1976).

TCDD also is an extremely potent enzyme inducer in many cell culture systems (Kouri *et al.*, 1978; Niwa *et al.*, 1975; Bradlaw *et al.*, 1976, 1980; Malik *et al.*, 1979). This enzyme induction is so sensitive that it has been proposed as a bioassay for detecting planar polychlorinated organic compounds (Bradlaw *et al.*, 1980; Bradlaw and Casterline, 1979; Niwa *et al.*, 1975). However, there is no correlation between cytotoxicity and enzyme induction (Beatty *et al.*, 1975; Bradlaw *et al.*, 1976; Knutson and Poland, 1980a; Yang *et al.*, 1983). These results, together with the lack of correlation between induction of certain cytochrome P-450-mediated enzyme activities and toxicity *in vivo* in different species, suggest there may be no direct connection between the induction of these particular activities and the toxicity of TCDD.

In addition to the more than 20 cytochrome P-450-associated mixed-function oxidase activities altered in response to TCDD and related compounds, a number of other enzymes are affected in a species-specific fashion. These include δ-aminolevulinic acid synthetase (Poland and Glover, 1973a,b; Goldstein *et al.*, 1973; Woods, 1973), DT-diaphorase [reduced NAD(P) : menadione oxidoreductase] (Beatty and Neal, 1976; Kumaki *et al.*, 1977), UDP-glucuronosyltransferase (Owens, 1977), glutathione-*S*-transferase B (Kirsch *et al.*, 1975), aldehyde dehydrogenase (Dietrich *et al.*, 1977), and choline kinase (Ishidate *et al.*, 1980). The analysis for functional mRNAs specific for these proteins and the use of protein synthesis inhibitors indicate that the induction of these enzymes is primarily under transcriptional control (Negishi and Nebert, 1981; Tukey *et al.*, 1981; Pickett *et al.*, 1982; Williams *et al.*, 1984; Poland and Glover, 1973a; Ishidate *et al.*, 1980; Lucier *et al.*, 1975a). In agreement, TCDD has been found to enhance liver DNA synthesis under certain conditions (Conway and Matsumura, 1975; Dickens *et al.*, 1981; Christian and Peterson, 1983) and to increase nuclear RNA polymerase activity in some tissues (Kurl *et al.*, 1982).

As noted (see Section 18.5.1.3), porphyria cutanea tarda has been observed in workers involved in the production of 2,4,5-trichlorophenol and 2,4,5-trichlorophenoxyacetic acid (Bleiberg *et al.*, 1964; Pazderova *et al.*, 1974; Pazderova-Vejlupkova *et al.*, 1981). The primary and/or synergistic role of chlorinated dioxin contaminants in the development of this porphyria in humans is not clear. However, TCDD is the most potent inducer of porphyria in mice (Goldstein *et al.*, 1973; Smith *et al.*, 1981) and rats (Goldstein *et al.*, 1976, 1982; Cantoni *et al.*, 1981; Seki *et al.*, 1987), but this effect is not observed in guinea pigs (Gupta *et al.*, 1973; McConnell *et al.*, 1978b) or rhesus monkeys (McConnell *et al.*, 1978a). As little as 1 μg TCDD/kg/week for 16 weeks (Goldstein *et al.*, 1982) or a single dose of 75 μg/kg (Smith *et al.*, 1981) has been shown to produce porphyria in rats and mice, respectively. Like porphyria cutanea tarda observed in humans, TCDD-elicited porphyria in experimental animals is characterized by the overproduction, hepatic accumulation, and increased urinary excretion of the highly carboxylated porphyrins. The primary biochemical lesion is considered to be a reduction in the activity of uroporphyrinogen decarboxylase (Elder, 1978; Jones and Sweeney, 1980; Smith *et al.*, 1981; Cantoni *et al.*, 1984a,b). However, TCDD is also the most potent of all porphyrinogens in effecting prolonged induction of δ-aminolevulinic acid synthetase, the initial and rate-limiting enzyme in the heme biosynthesis pathway. Although the induction of this enzyme occurs in the mouse and the chick embryo, in which hepatic porphyria occurs (Goldstein *et al.*, 1973; Vos *et al.*, 1974; Poland and Glover, 1973a; Sinclair and Granick, 1974), induction does not occur in the rat (Woods, 1973). Unlike many of TCDD's other effects on enzyme activities, the reduction in uroporphyrinogen decarboxylase activity does not appear to be mediated by alterations in transcription or translation; unchanged levels of immunoreactive enzyme protein were observed in one study (Elder and Sheppard, 1982), and others cited altered reaction kinetics (Kawanishi *et al.*, 1983; Cantoni *et al.*, 1984a,b). The findings that both cytochrome P-450 induction (Jones and Sweeney, 1977, 1980) and endogenous nonheme iron (Goldstein *et al.*, 1973; Sinclair and Granick, 1974; Sweeney *et al.*, 1979; Jones *et al.*, 1981; Greig *et al.*, 1984) are implicated in the pathogenesis of porphyria in mice suggest that the alterations in heme metabolism may be secondary to progressive increases in the evolution of oxygen radicals (Ferioli *et al.*, 1984; Mukerji *et al.*, 1984; Sinclair *et al.*, 1986) and/or lipid peroxidation (Jones *et al.*, 1981; Stohs *et al.*, 1983; Al-Bayati *et al.*, 1987; Shara and Stohs, 1987). Cytochrome P-450 has been shown to cause lipid peroxidation in reconstituted membrane vesicles via oxygen radical production (Ekström and Ingelman-Sundberg, 1986), and TCDD, in the presence ferric iron, stimulates the peroxidation of microsomal and lysosomal lipids (Albro *et al.*, 1986). Uncoupling of cytochrome P-450 electron transport by certain substrates has been proposed (Sousa and Marletta, 1985), and certain inducers, including TCDD, have been shown to bind to the cytochrome and inhibit catalytic activity (Voorman and Aust, 1987). Sinclair *et al.* (1986) have observed that certain TCDD-inducible P-450 isoenzymes mediate oxidation of uroporphyrinogen I to uroporphyrin. While Mohammadpour *et al.* (1988) reported that TCDD-induced lipid peroxidation segregates with the *Ah* locus in mice, Albro *et al.* (1988) indicated that although TCDD may increase hepatic lipid peroxidation in rats, the extent of increase does not account for the hepatotoxic effects of this compound.

TCDD, by virtue of its effect on the cytochrome P-450 isoenzymes, may alter arachidonic acid and prostaglandin metabolism (Kupfer *et al.*, 1979). The release of prostaglandins by the heart was found to be altered following exposure of chick embryos to TCDD *in ovo* (Quilley and Rifkind, 1986). The toxicity of 3,4,3′,4′-tetrachlorobiphenyl in chick embryo was also decreased by benoxoprofen, an inhibitor of arachidonic acid metabolism (Rifkind and Muschick, 1983). Furthermore, TCDD treatment enhances carageenan- and dextran-mediated edema in the rat paw (Katz *et al.*, 1984). Although the significance and mechanism of the latter effect is not known, arachidonic acid metabolites are known to modulate edematous and inflammatory responses.

TCDD treatment decreases the activities of hepatic Mg^{2+}- and Na^+, K^+-ATPases (Jones, 1975; Peterson *et al.*, 1979a,b) by unknown mechanisms. However, no significant differences in hepatic ATP synthesis or content, ADP/O ratio, or pyridine nucleotide content were seen in treated rats (Lucier *et al.*, 1973; Courtney *et al.*, 1978; Neal *et al.*, 1979). Also, intoxicated rats appear able to assimilate the energy content of ingested feed (Gasiewicz *et al.*, 1980; Seefeld and Peterson, 1984; Seefeld *et al.*, 1984; Potter *et al.*, 1986). The decrease in energy intake by these hypophagic animals is balanced by a reduction in energy expenditure, as evidenced by their decreased oxygen consumption and carbon dioxide production (Seefeld *et al.*, 1984a; Potter *et al.*, 1986). It should be emphasized that some earlier experiments on the metabolic effects of TCDD should be interpreted with some caution. It has only been recognized recently that the loss in body weight by TCDD-treated animals is due primarily to a decrease in food consumption (Seefeld and Peterson, 1983; Seefeld *et al.*, 1984; Huang Lu *et al.*, 1986). Depending on the parameter investigated, it may be difficult to interpret some results without the inclusion of a control group of animals that have been pair-fed to the TCDD-treated group.

TCDD causes selective alterations in rodent hepatic carbohydrate, protein, and lipid metabolism. Nitrogen balance, as assessed by urinary excretion of urea, ammonia, and creatinine and blood urea nitrogen and creatine levels, is apparently not affected by TCDD (McConnell, 1980; Christian *et al.*, 1986b). Serum protein values are generally depressed due to reduction in the albumin fraction (McConnell and Moore, 1979), although there is considerable variation among species. Increases in the plasma levels of certain amino acids handled primarily by the liver suggest that their metabolism may be reduced by TCDD exposure in rats (Christian *et al.*, 1986b). Blood glucose levels are decreased in TCDD-treated rats (Zinkl *et al.*, 1973; Schiller *et al.*, 1984; Gasiewicz *et al.*, 1980; Potter *et al.*, 1983) and mice (Chapman and Schiller, 1985), and hepatic glycogen stores are depleted (Gasiewicz *et al.*, 1980; Weber *et al.*, 1983). Hypoglycemia was observed even when treated rats were maintained on total parenteral nutrition (Gasiewicz *et al.*, 1980), suggesting that this effect is not secondary to hypophagia. It also does not appear to be a consequence of hyperinsulinemia, since the insulin level is decreased (Gorski and Rozman, 1987), probably as a result of hypophagia, in TCDD-treated rats (Potter *et al.*, 1983). Weber *et al.* (1987a,b) observed significant changes in glucose disposition in heart and brown adipose tissue in rats within 2 hr after TCDD treatment and postulated that these early events may trigger late and more overt homeostatic alterations. Serum glucose levels were unaffected in treated guinea pigs (Gasiewicz and Neal, 1979).

Qualitatively different, dosage-dependent increases in levels of serum and liver lipids, including free fatty acids, triacylglycerols, and cholesterol, are related to depletion of adipose tissue and/or fatty liver in monkeys (McConnell *et al.*, 1978b), rats (Cunningham and Williams, 1972; Zinkl *et al.*, 1973; Albro *et al.*, 1978; Gasiewicz *et al.*, 1980; Poli *et al.*, 1980; Schiller *et al.*, 1984, 1986; Christian *et al.*, 1986b), guinea pigs (Gasiewicz and Neal, 1979; Swift *et al.*, 1981; Huang Lu *et al.*, 1986), and rabbits (Lovati *et al.*, 1984). However, decreases in serum triglycerides have been reported in mice (Chapman and Schiller, 1985) and monkeys (McConnell *et al.*, 1978a). It has been suggested that hypertriacylglycerolemia and adipose tissue

depletion in guinea pigs was due to severe depression of lipoprotein lipase activity (Brewster and Matsumura, 1984, 1988) and reduction in the low-density lipoprotein receptor activities in hepatic plasma membranes (Bombick *et al.*, 1984). The observed decrease in serum ketone bodies and increases in triacylglycerols and cholesterol in TCDD-treated rats (Sweatlock and Gasiewicz, 1985; Christian *et al.*, 1986a) have been attributed to enhanced esterification of fatty acids (Christian *et al.*, 1986a), although it seems clear that other mechanisms are involved (Sweatlock and Gasiewicz, 1985). Since TCDD also decreases serum glucose concentrations in rats, the synthesis and release of liver lipid may be a compensatory response. This concept is supported by the observation of Schiller *et al.* (1986) that death occurred sooner in lethally dosed rats treated with 4-aminopyrazolo-[3,4-*d*]-pyrimidine, a chemotherapeutic agent which decreases serum lipid levels through blockage of release and/or synthesis of triacylglycerol-containing lipoproteins. The observations that (*a*) parenterally fed TCDD-treated rats exhibited more severe hepatic lesions than those fed *ad libitum* (Gasiewicz *et al.*, 1980), (*b*) TCDD-treated guinea pigs succumbed shortly after the administration of glucose (Brewster and Matsumura, 1984), and (*c*) TCDD-treated, saline-infused guinea pigs died soon after initiation of parenteral feeding (Huang Lu *et al.*, 1986) all support the concept that TCDD causes alterations, some possibly compensatory, in these species' abilities to utilize nutrients.

Several symptoms of TCDD toxicity (e.g., skin lesions, emaciation, atrophy of lymphoid tissues) resemble those of hypovitaminosis A, and TCDD and vitamin A exert opposite effects on certain enzyme activities (Thunberg *et al.*, 1980). TCDD has been found to cause dose-dependent alterations in tissue retinol and retinyl acetate storage in the Sprague–Dawley rat (Thunberg *et al.*, 1979; Hakansson and Ahlborg, 1985) and the relatively resistant Gunn rat (Thunberg and Hakansson, 1983), as well as in mice, guinea pigs, and hamsters (Hakansson, 1988). Also, TCDD toxicity in differentially sensitive strains and species appears to correlate with decreases in hepatic vitamin A storage (Thunberg, 1984). Although this depletion does not appear to be due to TCDD-induced increases in enzyme activities (Thunberg *et al.*, 1984), the exact causal relationship between the toxicity of TCDD and alterations in vitamin A metabolism has yet to be determined. It is also noteworthy that exposure of rat pups to TCDD-contaminated breast milk (dams dosed with 10 µg TCDD/kg following delivery) caused a decreased hepatic but increased renal storage of vitamin A. These effects occurred only after the pups started to eat a pelleted diet (Hakansson *et al.*, 1987).

The reproductive impairment of TCDD-treated female monkeys noted previously is associated with decreased plasma progesterone and estrogen concentrations (Barsotti *et al.*, 1979), possibly as a consequence of the induction of cytochrome P-450-dependent enzymes. Alterations in liver microsomal metabolism of a number of steroids were seen in TCDD-treated female rats (Gustafsson and Ingelman-Sundberg, 1979). However, although the hepatic metabolism of estrone and estradiol *in vitro* was altered following the treatment of pregnant rats with 1 μg/kg/day on days 7–19 of pregnancy, no alterations in circulating estradiol levels were observed (Shiverick and Muther, 1982, 1983). TCDD-induced decreases in rat hepatic and uterine estrogen receptor levels and uterine responsiveness to estradiol (Gallo *et al.*, 1986; Romkes *et al.*, 1987; Romkes and Safe, 1988) have been suggested to account for both reproductive dysfunctions and decreased incidence of spontaneous mammary and uterine tumors (Kociba *et al.*, 1978). Significantly decreased serum prolactin levels and prolactin receptor-mediated activities have also been noted in TCDD-treated rats (Jones *et al.*, 1987), but could be reversed by pimozide, a dopamine receptor antagonist (Russell *et al.*, 1988). Since dopamine is inhibitory to prolactin release by the adenohypophysis, a hypothalamic site of action of TCDD has been suggested (Russell *et al.*, 1988).

More recent data has suggested that adrenal status may be important in modulating an animal's response to TCDD. Adrenalectomy has been shown to dramatically increase mortality and greatly shorten the time to death in animals treated with TCDD (Gorski *et al.*, 1988b). Although plasma corticosterone levels are elevated following treatment (Gorski *et al.*, 1988a; Moore *et al.*, 1989), this change is apparently due to altered responsiveness of the adrenal to adrenocorticotropic hormone (ACTH) rather than any changes in ACTH concentrations (Moore *et al.*, 1989). Furthermore, TCDD alters the steroid-binding properties of the glucocorticoid receptor and adrenalectomy markedly enhances this response to TCDD (Sunahara *et al.*, 1989).

Androgen deficiency has been observed in TCDD-treated rats (Moore *et al.*, 1985) and may, in part, be causal in the male reproductive pathology described. Altered hepatic androgen metabolism has been described in TCDD-treated rats. However, the pattern of affected hydroxylation is different for each androgen examined, demonstrating the substrate-specific character of the induced enzymes (Hook *et al.*, 1975; Gustafsson and Ingelman-Sundberg, 1979; Nienstedt *et al.*, 1979). TCDD treatment also causes an overall marked depression of testosterone metabolism (Nienstedt *et al.*, 1979; Yoshihara *et al.*, 1982; Keys *et al.*, 1985), decreases the amount of cytochrome P-450 in testes of both guinea pigs (Tofilon *et al.*, 1980) and rats (Tofilon and Piper, 1982), and decreases the activities of the testicular cytochrome P-450-dependent enzymes 17-hydroxylase and 17,20-lyase in the rat (Mebus *et al.*, 1987). A role of androgen deficiency in the toxicity of TCDD is suggested by the findings that castration increased TCDD's lethality in male rats and testosterone administration to females doubled the LD 50 (Beatty *et al.*, 1978). However, these findings may be related to the maintenance of hepatic cytochrome P-450 isoenzymes that are responsible for the metabolism and detoxification of TCDD. Moore and Peterson (1988) demonstrated that although androgen catabolism rates are affected by TCDD, the *in vivo* pools of androgens are not substantially depleted. These investigators suggested that the primary cause of androgen deficiency was a TCDD-elicited decrease in testicular testosterone secretion.

TCDD-intoxicated rats exhibit adrenal hypofunction, with a prolonged depression of serum corticosterone (Balk and Piper, 1984; DiBartolomeis *et al.*, 1986a; Jones *et al.*, 1987). Adre-

nalectomy fails to protect against TCDD-elicited thymic involution (van Logten *et al.*, 1980) and in fact hastens death (Neal *et al.*, 1979). Total and mitochondrial adrenal cholesterol contents increase, due in part to both elevated plasma cholesterol and inhibition of cholesterol side-chain cleavage (DiBartolomeis *et al.*, 1986a,b, 1987). The appearance of an abnormal metabolite (11-β-hydroxyprogesterone) also suggests interference at a specific step in steroidogenesis (Balk and Piper, 1984). TCDD has been shown to decrease the number of glucocorticoid receptors in rat liver, and other congeners decrease apparent binding capacity in liver and placenta of pregnant mice (R. P. Ryan *et al.*, 1987). Decreased levels of glucocorticoid receptors in skeletal muscle from TCDD-treated rats have also been reported (Max and Silbergeld, 1987). Decreased responsiveness to dexamethasone-elicited enzyme induction in TCDD-treated rats was also interpreted as representative of a down-regulation of glucocorticoid receptors (Jones *et al.*, 1987).

The thyroid status of TCDD-treated animals is not clear, and like many toxic effects of this compound appear to be species-specific. Goiter and increased thyroid iodine uptake occur in TCDD-treated rats. Hypothyroxinemia in this species (Potter *et al.*, 1983, 1986; Henry and Gasiewicz, 1987; Byrne *et al.*, 1987) may be due in part to increased biliary excretion of thyroxine, perhaps via induction of UDP-glucuronosyltransferase (Hook *et al.*, 1975; Bastomsky, 1977; Henry and Gasiewicz, 1987). Depending on the dose and time of examination, triiodothyronine levels in plasma may be elevated (Bastomsky, 1977), decreased (Potter *et al.*, 1986; Henry and Gasiewicz, 1987), or unchanged (Potter *et al.*, 1983), while thyroid stimulating hormone levels may be greatly increased (Bastomsky, 1977; Potter *et al.*, 1986) or unchanged (Henry and Gasiewicz, 1987) in rats. Serum triiodothyronine was reduced in TCDD-treated guinea pigs fed by total parenteral nutrition (Huang Lu *et al.*, 1986), but the relatively resistant hamster exhibits an increase in both thyroxine and triiodothyronine after TCDD exposure (Henry and Gasiewicz, 1987). Despite the equivocal changes in serum triiodothyronine (the metabolically more potent thyroid hormone), TCDD intoxication may represent a functional hypothyroid state since thyroxine appears to be the more effective feedback regulator of thyroid stimulating hormone secretion (Larsen and Silva, 1983). Some of the symptoms of TCDD exposure (hypophagia, hypoglycemia, reduced basal metabolic rate, increased serum lipids) are typical of hypothyroidism. The administration of triiodothyronine or thyroxine to TCDD-treated rats and mice was observed to enhance toxicity and teratogenicity (Rozman *et al.*, 1985; Lamb *et al.*, 1986). In addition, thyroidectomy affords at least temporary protection from immunotoxicity and mortality in lethally treated rats, suggesting that the hypothyroid state may be an adaptive response to intoxication (Rozman *et al.*, 1985; Pazdernik and Rozman, 1985). McKinney *et al.* (1985) have suggested that TCDD may act as a potent and persistent thyroxine agonist, based on some common molecular properties of TCDD and thyroxine and the fact that TCDD affects tadpole growth in a thyroxine-like manner. However, the observation that the induction pattern of a group of thyroid-responsive enzymes in TCDD-treated rats is inconsistent with thyroid hormone action contradicts this hypothesis (Kelling *et al.*, 1987a). Because alteration of thyroid hormone concentrations is typical of many pathological conditions, it is not clear whether this is a direct or secondary effect of TCDD intoxication and whether it is causal or responsive to other metabolic alterations. The fact that thyroid status does not substantially alter TCDD's induction of cytochrome P-450-mediated activities in rats seems to dissociate enzyme induction from thyroid-influenced toxicity (Rozman *et al.*, 1985; Henry and Gasiewicz, 1986).

Although the mechanism of action of TCDD in producing specific pathological and biochemical lesions remains to be clarified, it is thought to be mediated by binding to a soluble intracellular protein, the *Ah* receptor (Poland *et al.*, 1976a, 1979; Whitlock, 1987). The receptor is the regulatory gene product of the *Ah* (for *aryl hydrocarbon*) locus (Nebert *et al.*, 1972; Eisen *et al.*, 1983), which was originally demonstrated to control the induction of aryl hydrocarbon hydroxylase activity by 3-methylcholanthrene in certain strains of mice (Robinson *et al.*, 1974). Mouse strains responding to 3-methylcholanthrene-elicited enzyme induction were termed "responsive," while strains that did not respond were called "nonresponsive." In crosses and backcrosses between C57BL/6 (responsive) and DBA/2 (nonresponsive) mice, inducibility segregates as a single autosomal dominant trait (Thomas *et al.*, 1972). In other strains, however, the pattern of inheritance is more complex (Thomas and Hutton, 1973). TCDD is able to induce aryl hydrocarbon hydroxylase activity in both responsive and nonresponsive mice. However, nonresponsive mice require a dose of TCDD that is approximately 10 times that required in responsive strains (Poland and Glover, 1975). It was hypothesized that the *Ah* locus is a regulatory gene whose product is a receptor that, upon binding with TCDD or polycyclic aromatic hydrocarbons, controls the induction of aryl hydrocarbon hydroxylase activity. Because of the extreme potency of TCDD, the decreased affinity of the defective receptor in nonresponsive mice could be overcome by increasing doses of TCDD. This hypothesis was confirmed by the identification in the cytosol of responsive mice of a protein with high binding affinity for TCDD (apparent K_D of approximately 0.3 nM) and for polycyclic hydrocarbon inducers. The corresponding protein from nonresponsive mice has less binding potential (Poland *et al.*, 1976a; Okey *et al.*, 1989). This protein is now referred to as the *Ah* receptor and has been found in a variety of tissues from several mammalian species (Carlstedt-Duke, 1979; Mason and Okey, 1982; Gasiewicz and Rucci, 1984; Denison *et al.*, 1985; Denison and Wilkinson, 1985; Soderkvist *et al.*, 1986; Furuhashi *et al.*, 1986; Gillner *et al.*, 1987) as well as *Drosophila* (Bigelow *et al.*, 1985). The induction of several other enzymes has been shown to be regulated by the *Ah* locus in mice. These include, in addition to cytochrome P$_1$-450, which is responsible for most of the aryl hydrocarbon hydroxylase activity, cytochrome P$_3$-450 (Negishi and Nebert, 1979), at least one form of UDP-glucuronosyltransferase (Owens, 1977; Malik and Owens, 1981), reduced NAD(P) : menadione oxidoreductase (Kumaki *et al.*, 1977), and ornithine decarboxylase (Nebert *et al.*, 1980).

The existence of the *Ah* receptor led Kumaki *et al.* (1977) to propose a mechanism of action for TCDD similar to that proposed for the regulation of gene expression by the steroid hormones (reviewed by Whitlock, 1987). Indeed, like the steroid hormone model, the TCDD–receptor complex associates with the nucleus (Greenlee and Poland, 1979; Okey *et al.*, 1979, 1980; Zacharewski *et al.*, 1989) and binds to DNA (Carlstedt-Duke *et al.*, 1981; Hannah *et al.*, 1986; Gasiewicz and Bauman, 1987; Rucci and Gasiewicz, 1988; Mason *et al.*, 1988; Henry *et al.*, 1989) and/or certain sites in the nucleus initiating the transcription of mRNAs encoding information for the synthesis of various proteins including cytochrome P-450-associated enzymes (Tukey *et al.*, 1981, 1982). TCDD-responsive domains upstream of the gene encoding cytochrome P$_1$-450 have been identified in murine hepatoma cells (P. B. C. Jones *et al.*, 1985, 1986; Neuhold *et al.*, 1986; Sogawa *et al.*, 1986; Whitlock, 1987; Durrin *et al.*, 1987; Denison *et al.*, 1988), and the TCDD-receptor complex has been demonstrated to bind specifically to these genomic regions (Fujisawa-Sehara *et al.*, 1988; Denison *et al.*, 1989; Nemoto *et al.*, 1990).

The hypothesis that the toxicity of TCDD and related compounds is mediated by their binding to the *Ah* receptor is supported by two lines of evidence. First, there are good structure–activity relationships for receptor binding and toxicity (Parkinson and Safe, 1981; Goldstein, 1980; Poland and Knutson, 1982; Holcomb *et al.*, 1988). The congeners that bind to the receptor (*in vitro*) are able to induce aryl hydrocarbon hydroxylase activity and produce the toxic syndrome. In addition, the rank-ordered ability of these compounds to bind to the *Ah* receptor correlates with their potency in inducing aryl hydrocarbon hydroxylase activity and causing toxicity. Exceptions to this relationship, such as 2,3,7-trichlorodibenzo-*p*-dioxin and polycyclic aromatic hydrocarbons such as 3-methylcholanthrene, bind to the receptor with relatively high affinity, yet have a biological potency that is lower than expected. It has been suggested that this may be due to more rapid metabolic inactivation *in vivo* (Poland *et al.*, 1976a; Knutson and Poland, 1980b). Other compounds, however, such as α-naphthoflavone, 1,6-dichlorodibenzo-*p*-dioxin and some chlorinated dibenzofurans and polychlorinated biphenyls, and 7-hydroxyellipticine, may bind to the receptor in such a manner as to be antagonistic to both the enzyme inductive and toxic effects of TCDD under certain circumstances (Blank *et al.*, 1987; Luster *et al.*, 1986; Keys *et al.*, 1986; Leece *et al.*, 1987; Bannister *et al.*, 1987; Astroff *et al.*, 1988; Fernandez *et al.*, 1988). That these relationships are far from clear is exemplified by the finding that although 2,7-dichlorodibenzo-*p*-dioxin lacks affinity for the *Ah* receptor and does not induce hepatic enzymes, it produces "TCDD-like" immunosuppression in mice (Holsapple *et al.*, 1986b).

The second line of evidence is the segregation of TCDD toxicity with the *Ah* locus in mice. After treatment with TCDD and/or related congeners, responsive mice are more susceptible to thymic atrophy (Poland and Glover, 1980), embryotoxicity and teratogenesis (cleft palate or kidney abnormalities) (Poland and Glover, 1980; Dencker and Pratt, 1981; Pratt, 1983; D'Argy *et al.*, 1984; Hassoun *et al.*, 1984a,b; Legraverend *et al.*, 1984; York and Manson, 1984; George and Manson, 1986), porphyria (Jones and Sweeney, 1980; Smith *et al.*, 1981; Greig *et al.*, 1984; Hahn *et al.*, 1988), epidermal hyperplasia and hyperkeratosis

(Knutson and Poland, 1982), suppression of cell-mediated and humoral immunity (Frank *et al.*, 1982; Silkworth and Grabstein, 1982; Clark *et al.*, 1983; Lubet *et al.*, 1984; Nagarkatti *et al.*, 1984; Vecci *et al.*, 1983a; Silkworth *et al.*, 1984, 1986), and lethality (Gasiewicz *et al.*, 1983b; Chapman and Schiller, 1985). The *Ah* locus has also been implicated in susceptibility to atherosclerosis (Paigen *et al.*, 1986) and the carcinogenesis induced by certain exogenous compounds (Kouri *et al.*, 1974, 1978; Nebert *et al.*, 1977; Duran-Reynolds *et al.*, 1978; Gurtoo *et al.*, 1978; York *et al.*, 1984; George and Manson, 1986; Paigen *et al.*, 1986).

Structure–activity and genetic relationships are also consistent with the role of the *Ah* receptor in TCDD-elicited alterations in the differentiation program of cultured epithelial cells (Knutson and Poland, 1980b; Greenlee *et al.*, 1983; Hudson *et al.*, 1983; Karenlampi *et al.*, 1983; Greenlee and Neal, 1985; Puhvel *et al.*, 1984; Rice and Cline, 1984; Willey *et al.*, 1984). However, production of epidermal hyperplasia and promotion of keratinizing skin papillomas in HRS/J hairless mice bearing a recessive mutation at the *hr* locus appear to be dependent on the interaction of the *hr* and *Ah* loci (Knutson and Poland, 1982; Poland *et al.*, 1982, 1984). TCDD-induced thymic atrophy appears in this strain independently of the *hr* locus. It has been proposed that the *Ah* receptor regulates two distinct pleiotropic responses. One consists of the induction of enzymes primarily associated with drug metabolism and occurs in most tissues that possess the *Ah* receptor. However, the receptor also regulates in a highly tissue-specific fashion an additional battery of genes, the expression of which results in toxicity. Thus, toxicity may be due to the inappropriate (for a certain tissue or stage of development) expression of this additional battery of genes (Poland and Knutson, 1982).

Although the receptor is found primarily in epithelial tissues, its presence is not directly correlated with aryl hydrocarbon hydroxylase activity or adverse effects in these tissues (Bigelow and Nebert, 1986; Gasiewicz and Rucci, 1984; Dencker, 1985). However, comparative studies of the ontogeny of the receptor (Carlstedt-Duke *et al.*, 1979; Kahl *et al.*, 1980; Gasiewicz *et al.*, 1984) have shown that these changes during development in some species are proportional to temporal changes in inducible aryl hydrocarbon hydroxylase activity (Kahl *et al.*, 1980; Lucier *et al.*, 1975b). However, Denison *et al.* (1986a) observed that the ontogeny of the *Ah* receptor in chick liver coincides with the period of tissue differentiation rather than aryl hydrocarbon hydroxylase inducibility. Dencker and Pratt (1981) have demonstrated a temporal correlation between peak *Ah* receptor concentration in mouse embryo palate and optimal inducibility of cleft palate by TCDD. The sum of available data in species other than the mouse suggests that while the presence of the *Ah* receptor is necessary for the expression of toxicity, the qualitative and quantitative characteristics of the responses generated are specific functions of the sex-, age-, tissue-, and species-related genetic constitution of each system (Dencker, 1985).

In general, the physicochemical properties of the *Ah* receptor are remarkably similar to those of steroid hormone receptors (Poland *et al.*, 1976a; Okey *et al.*, 1979, 1980; Greenlee and Poland, 1979; Carlstedt-Duke *et al.*, 1981; Gasiewicz and Neal,

1982; Poellinger *et al.*, 1983; Hankinson, 1983; Whitlock and Galeazzi, 1984; Van Gurp and Hankinson, 1984; Greenlee and Neal, 1985; Poellinger and Gullberg, 1985; Wilhelmsson *et al.*, 1986; Gasiewicz and Bauman, 1987; Cuthill *et al.*, 1987, 1988; Poland and Glover, 1987; Gudas and Hankinson, 1986; Denison *et al.*, 1986b). Nevertheless, it is clear that the *Ah* receptor is not identical to known steroid hormone receptors. It is more hydrophobic than steroid hormone receptors (Poellinger and Gullberg, 1985), and a number of studies have demonstrated that neither natural nor synthetic hormones nor several endogenous substances could compete with TCDD for specific binding (Poland *et al.*, 1976a; Guenthner and Nebert, 1977; Carlstedt-Duke *et al.*, 1978; Greenlee and Poland, 1979; Okey *et al.*, 1979, 1980; Poellinger *et al.*, 1982, 1983). In addition to the halogenated aromatic hydrocarbons such as the dioxins and dibenzofurans and the polycyclic aromatic hydrocarbons such as benzo[*a*]pyrene and 3-methylcholanthrene (Bigelow and Nebert, 1982), other ligands that bind to this protein include certain indoles (Gillner *et al.*, 1985), Sudan II dye (Lubet *et al.*, 1983), substituted diaryltriazenes (Sweatlock and Gasiewicz, 1986), certain oxidized amino acids (Rannug *et al.*, 1987), rutaecarpine alkaloids (Gillner *et al.*, 1989), ellipticines (Fernandez *et al.*, 1988), and unknown contaminants of urban airborne particulate matter (Toftgard *et al.*, 1983). The current model of the ligand binding site has the dimensions of a 6.8 × 13.7 Å envelope (Gillner *et al.*, 1985). Substituent lipophilicity was found to be the most important determinant of binding affinity, suggesting that the binding site must be highly hydrophobic (Bandiera *et al.*, 1983; Denomme *et al.*, 1985, 1986; Mason *et al.*, 1986). Polarizability of the aromatic ring system may also play an important role (McKinney *et al.*, 1983). Pretreatment with phenobarbital or polychlorinated biphenyls with phenobarbital-like, but not 3-methylcholanthrene-like, enzyme induction patterns significantly increased the concentration of TCDD receptor in hepatic cytosol from rats and C57Bl/6 mice (Okey and Vella, 1984; Denomme *et al.*, 1986). The significance of this apparent barbiturate regulation of receptor content is not known. However, some regulation of the level of the *Ah* receptor in rat liver by TCDD itself has been suggested (Sloop and Lucier, 1987). Although there have been many studies to date on the properties of the *Ah* receptor, its normal physiological function and ligand, if any, are unknown. Furthermore, although a number of genetic loci have been reported to affect the synthesis and/or functionality of the *Ah* receptor (Cobb *et al.*, 1987; Poland *et al.*, 1987; Karenlampi *et al.*, 1988), their specific role in the regulation of this receptor has yet to be determined. The receptor has been purified to approximately 20,000-fold enrichment (Perdew and Poland, 1988).

18.5.1.3 Toxicity to Humans

Human poisoning first called attention to compounds that eventually were identified as dioxins. The most commonly observed feature of this poisoning was chloracne, but other conditions frequently were reported. In some instances, it was clear that illness was a direct result of an industrial accident such as an explosion. However, due to the nature of the toxicity of this compound, chloracne and other conditions develop and resolve slowly with the result that it may be difficult to determine in an industrial situation the relative contribution of a discrete accident and of day-to-day exposure. For this reason, occupational exposures are considered separately from accidents involving the community.

Chloracne is characterized by follicular hyperkeratosis (comedones) with or without cysts and pustules. Histologically, the characteristic lesion has considerable similarity to acne commonly observed in adolescents. In chloracne, almost every follicle may be involved, with the result that there is no even partially normal skin in an involved area. It may be more disfiguring than adolescent acne. Chloracne usually occurs on the face and neck, but it may extend to the back, chest, and extremities, but not usually to the hands and feet. The genitalia may be involved in males. The lesions are reversible but only very slowly. Its duration depends to a great extent on its severity, and in the worst cases lesions may persist for up to 30 years after contact with the agent has ceased (Holmstedt, 1980). In some cases, lesions may resolve but may reappear again even after cessation of exposure to the chemical. This has been suggested to be due to delayed release of the acnegen from fat or liver stores. Healing may be complicated by scarring. Erythema and edema, and sometimes photosensitivity, may occur before the follicular hyperkeratosis is evident. Spotty pigmentation, hypertrichosis, and/or porphyria (see Biochemical Effects) may accompany chloracne, but it is not clear whether they should be regarded as part of the same syndrome. This is especially true since all reported industrial exposures were to a mixture of compounds and not pure TCDD. Certainly, chloracne often occurs alone, whereas hyperpigmentation, hypertrichosis, and porphyria without chloracne are characteristic of poisoning by hexachlorobenzene. Thus, some of the variation in the clinical picture seen in different outbreaks of poisoning may be due in part to different mixtures of chlorinated aromatic compounds and different routes of exposure. For all of these cases, and including experimental exposures, only the following substances have been shown unequivocally to have caused chloracne in humans: chloronaphthalenes (CNs), polychlorinated biphenyls (PCBs), polybrominated biphenyls (PBBs), polychlorinated dibenzofurans (PCDFs), polychlorinated dibenzodioxins (PCDDs), tetrachloroazobenzene (TCAB), and tetrachloroazoxybenzene (TCAOB).

Much more information on human exposures to TCDD than can be covered here may be found in reviews by Holmstedt (1980), Reggiani (1981), Kimbrough et al. (1984), and Fingerhut et al. (1984, 1987), as well as chapters in a book edited by Kimbrough and Jensen (1989). It is of interest that Holmstedt (1980) drew attention to the facts that the potential hazard of TCDD was set forth clearly by Schulz in 1957 (Kimmig and Schulz, 1957a) and in the same year the Boehringer Company informed its competitors about a safer procedure for the production of trichlorophenol. Reasons for the limited dissemination of the available information prior to the outbreak at Seveso were discussed.

Valuable reviews that emphasize chloracne rather than any single chemical are those of Crow (1978, 1983) and Taylor (1974, 1979).

Experimental Exposure   In a self-experiment by Schulz, two applications of a 0.01% solution of TCDD to a circumscribed area of the skin of the forearm led after 2 days to a slight dermatitis and some days later to follicular hyperkeratosis and comedones. The skin was excised and found to show typical histological lesions (Bauer et al., 1961).

In a study involving 31 volunteers, a mixture of penta- and hexachloronaphthalenes produced chloracne, whereas a mixture of mono- and dichloronaphthalene, a mixture of tri- and tetrachloronaphthalene, heptachloronaphthalene, and octachloronaphthalene were all inactive. The active mixture produced acne in each of several local areas to which it was applied, but in some instances the condition extended to distant areas. Comedones were the first stage in the experimental disease; follicular hyperkeratosis could be observed histologically within 1–3 weeks and clinical comedones within 4–6 weeks. In some instances, chloracne continued to develop after application was stopped and went on to form pustules, nodules, and abscesses. Also in some instances, the sebaceous glands became small or disappeared entirely; the glands returned months after the last application (Shelley and Kligman, 1957). Similar results were reported by Hambrick (1957) for the same mixture of penta- and hexachloronaphthalenes and for hexachloronaphthalene alone. A number of other halogenated naphthalenes were ineffective.

The development of noninflamed comedones in response to the same mixture of penta- and hexachloronaphthalenes (Halowax® 1014) was studied in eight men ranging in age from 21 to 30 years. In addition to histological studies, the metabolic state of the cells was followed by injecting [³H]thymidine, [³H]glycine, and [³H]histidine and then taking biopsies 45 min, 10 days, and 24 days later for autoradiography. Histologically, very early squamous cell proliferation in the sebaceous gland acini and acanthosis in the upper portion of the external hair root sheath were observed. Initially, the wall of the comedone was acanthotic and folded, but it finally turned into a rounded shape with loss of acanthosis. The appearance and later disappearance of acanthosis was paralleled by similar appearance of granules in the stratum granulosum. The appearance of acanthosis and granulosis was accompanied by a high uptake of [³H]thymidine (Plewig, 1970b).

Poiger and Schlatter (1986) investigated the pharmacokinetics of TCDD following the oral ingestion of 105 ng of [³H]TCDD by a 42-year-old, 92-kg volunteer. Greater than 87% of the administered dose was absorbed from the intestine. Blood levels peaked at 0.13 pg/ml within 2 hr following injection. Adipose tissue levels, measured 13 and 69 days after dosing, were 3.09 and 2.85 µg/g, respectively. The ³H-labeled material was cleared from the body with a half-life of elimination of 2120 days. ³H activity was detected only in the feces.

There have been a number of studies examining the effect of TCDD exposure on human cells in culture. Cultured human cells or cell lines derived from humans, including lymphocytes

(Atlas *et al.*, 1976), squamous cell carcinoma lines (Hudson *et al.*, 1983), a breast carcinoma cell line MCF-7 (Jaiswal *et al.*, 1985b), and lymphoblastoid cells (Nagayama *et al.*, 1985), have been shown to be inducible for aryl hydrocarbon hydroxylase activity by TCDD. As noted previously (Biochemical Effects), a major mechanism for the induction and toxicity of TCDD and related compounds appears to involve altered gene regulation that is dependent on the interaction with a receptor protein, the *Ah* receptor. The elements of this mechanistic hypothesis have been demonstrated or implicated for human cells or cell lines derived from humans. *Ah* receptors with properties similar to those observed in experimental animals have been detected in human tissues (Roberts *et al.*, 1985, 1986, 1990; Manchester *et al.*, 1987; Cook *et al.*, 1987; Cook and Greenlee, 1989; Harris *et al.*, 1989; Labruzzo *et al.*, 1989). The cytochrome P-450 regulatory elements from mouse DNA maintain responsiveness to TCDD when transfected into human cell lines (P. B. C. Jones *et al.*, 1985, 1986). This has been interpreted to indicate that the mechanisms of *Ah* receptor-dependent gene control are similar in mouse and human cells. Also, the exposure of human epidermal, thymic epithelial, and lung epithelial cells results in patterns of altered differentiation similar to those observed in rodent cells (Abernethy *et al.*, 1985; Greenlee *et al.*, 1985a,b; Hudson *et al.*, 1985, 1986; Willey *et al.*, 1984; Cook *et al.*, 1987; Milstone and LaVigne, 1984). Notably, the amounts of TCDD that caused these effects were similar in cells from both species.

Accidental Poisoning and Use Experience Chloracne is a result of exposure to industrial chemicals and is not known to be produced by any natural product or to occur spontaneously. It was first described by Herxheimer (1899) and by Thibierge (1899). The name, given by Herxheimer, reflected the initial impression that the condition was produced by free chlorine. At that time, the condition apparently was widespread, for Bettmann (1901), in discussing two cases he had seen in 1897, cited several references describing the same disease. Wauer (1918) and Teleky (1927) suggested that the condition was caused by certain chlorinated hydrocarbons. Jones and Alden (1936) described a case in a worker who distilled chlorinated biphenyls. It should be emphasized that in many cases of accidental exposure to acnegenic chemicals, chloracne was present even in the apparent absence of signs or symptoms of systemic effects. Thus, chloracne is in itself a specific marker indicating that the affected person has been exposed to the acnegen. To date, it is the most sensitive and specific indicator of overexposure to TCDD that is available for humans. Whether illness without chloracne may occur in exposed individuals is, at present, unknown.

Chloracne has been reported in workers exposed to the reaction products of chlorine and tars, mixtures of chloronaphthalenes and chlorobiphenyls, chlorodiphenoxides, chlorophenols, and "certain petroleum products" (Schwartz *et al.*, 1957; Schulz, 1968). The condition has been observed in connection with the manufacture of six pesticides: (*a*) 2,4,5-trichlorophenol (Dugois and Colomb, 1957; Jensen, 1972); (*b*) 2,4,5-T (Jirasek *et al.*, 1973, 1974); (*c*) pentachlorophenol

(Baader and Bauer, 1951; Cole *et al.*, 1986); (*d*) dichlobenil (Deeken, 1974); (*e*) methazole (Taylor *et al.*, 1977); and (*f*) propanil (Morse *et al.*, 1979). The chlorinated dibenzo-*p*-dioxins, mainly TCDD, are the acnegens associated with 2,4,5-trichlorophenol and 2,4,5-T; hexa-, hepta-, and octachlorodibenzofurans have been isolated from samples of technical grade pentachlorophenol (Goldstein *et al.*, 1978); the acnegen associated with methazole is TCAOB. It has been assumed that dichlobenil itself is an acnegen. Propanil gave a positive rabbit ear test. However, the workers who were exposed to it and developed chloracne were also exposed to TCAOB (Morse *et al.*, 1979). Because TCAOB and TCAB are formed as trace contaminants during the synthesis of 3,4-dichloroaniline or during its further conversion to certain acylphenylamide, phenylcarbamate, and phenylurea herbicides (Poland *et al.*, 1976b), it is possible that chloracne might occur in connection with the manufacture and formulation of one or more of these compounds.

It is noteworthy that among all the accidental exposures, there has been only one incident in which there was exposure to pure TCDD. Two chemists in separate laboratories synthesized large quantities of TCDD to serve as a standard in chemical analysis. Although these individuals recognized the potential hazard of this compound and precautions were taken to avoid personal contamination, these precautions apparently proved inadequate. About 8 weeks after the synthesis, chloracne began to develop. This lesion subsided 14–20 months after its appearance. Forty months after exposure the only relevant findings were a few blackheads and a blood cholesterol of 302 mg %. The second chemist actually carried out syntheses about 1 week apart. Within 5–6 weeks after the first exposure, excessive oiliness of the skin was observed. Chloracne began to appear about 8 weeks after the first exposure and appeared in two waves corresponding to the interval between syntheses. The skin lesion subsided within 16 months after onset. This patient also lost about 6.5 kg of weight and reported abdominal pains, excessive flatulence, fatigue, loss of vigor, and irritability. Excessive hair growth was also noted. Examination 42 months after exposure revealed a blood cholesterol value of 305 mg % and a type 2A hyperlipoproteinemia. A third laboratory worker, who was not directly involved with the actual synthesis but did work with dilute solutions of TCDD, did not develop chloracne but did show similar systemic symptoms as well as an elevated blood cholesterol level (310 mg %) and type 2A hyperlipoproteinemia (Oliver, 1975). It is noteworthy that for all three exposed individuals complete recovery from these symptoms has occurred. Furthermore, other chemists have successfully synthesized TCDD and related congeners without reported mishap.

The incident described just above and other accidental and experimental exposures suggest a causal relationship between TCDD and hypercholesterolemia. This abnormality occurred in all three exposed men (only 31, 41, and 33 years old, respectively) and not in their colleagues. Increased plasma cholesterol and various other changes in lipid metabolism have been observed in other workers exposed to TCDD (Walker and Martin, 1979; Jirasek *et al.*, 1976; Pazderova-Vejlupkova *et al.*, 1981), as well as in experimental animals (see Biochemical Effects).

Hyperpigmentation and hirsutism, the latter having been noted in the case of the exposure of laboratory workers, have also been reported frequently in industrial workers (Bleiberg *et al.*, 1964; Poland *et al.*, 1971; Jirasek *et al.*, 1973; Taylor *et al.*, 1977). Hirsutism involved the temples between the lateral half of the eyebrow and the temporal hair of the scalp and sometimes involved the upper and lower eyelids. These symptoms often accompany other evidences of porphyria cutanea tarda, including fragility of the skin, increased urinary excretion of the highly carboxylated porphyrins, and high porphyrin content and enlargement of the liver. In two factories, porphyria cutanea tarda developed in the workers. In a factory engaged in the manufacture of 2,4-D, 2,4,5-T, and hexachlorobenzene, among 29 workers examined before 1964 at least 19 had typical chloracne and 11 had porphyria of varying degrees of severity. When all of the 73 workers in the same plant were examined 6 years later, 48 had some degree of acne; no clinical porphyria was found, and only one worker had persistent uroporphyrinuria. Sixteen men had residual facial hirsutism, and 30 had hyperpigmentation (Bleiberg *et al.*, 1964). At one stage of the manufacturing process, the product contained 10–25 ppm TCDD. About 6 months before the second survey, a device was installed that removed most of the TCDD to a level of <1 ppm in the trichlorophenol. This reduction in TCDD explained at least partially the reduction of chloracne. It was supposed that some other by-product had been responsible for porphyria in the past, and its possible reduction as well as possible improvement in personal hygiene may have helped to reduce the incidence and severity of porphyria (Poland *et al.*, 1971). It should be noted that in cases where porphyria cutanea tarda was observed, the workers were also exposed to hexachlorobenzene (Jones and Chelsky, 1986). In other cases of occupational poisoning with TCDD, porphyria has not been observed, although chloracne was as pronounced as in the episodes where porphyria was noted.

Jirasek *et al.* (1973) described chloracne and porphyria among 80 workers making 2,4,5-T and pentachlorophenol. In this instance, four patients had severe porphyria cutanea tarda and hirsutism but did not exhibit chloracne. Notably, this was similar to the reaction of patients who had been poisoned by hexachlorobenzene (Cam, 1960; Peters *et al.*, 1982), and hexachlorobenzene is a possible contaminant of pentachlorophenol. Although compounds (hexachlorobenzene) other than TCDD are suspected to have caused the incidences of porphyria cutanea tarda in these factory workers (Jones and Chelsky, 1986), it should be pointed out that purified TCDD has been porphyrinogenic in experimental animals (see Section 18.5.1.2).

In addition to porphyria cutanea tarda, other evidence for liver dysfunction has been observed in exposed workers. Abnormal results for glucose tolerance tests, increased α_1- and γ-globulin in plasma, and decreased plasma albumin were reported (Jirasek *et al.*, 1976; Pazderova-Vejlupkova *et al.*, 1981). In addition to elevated serum lipids, altered liver function tests (serum bilirubin and transaminases) have been reported (Crow, 1978, 1981; Holmstedt, 1980; May, 1973; Hay,

1982). Goldman (1973) and Schecter *et al.* (1985b,c) described morphological alterations in a liver biopsy from an affected worker. Hepatocytes were enlarged and contained moderate-sized lipid vacuoles. A gray pigment that did not stain positive for iron was noted. However, liver function tests may remain normal even in cases of severe chloracne. Liver function tests of a total of 106 workmen exposed to TCDD in the Netherlands in 1963 did not indicate liver damage despite the prominence of chloracne. Similarly, in another episode in which cases of porphyria and moderate to severe chloracne occurred, demonstrable signs of liver dysfunction were minimal (Reggiani, 1981).

Sensory neuropathy is another clinical feature often, but not consistently, reported in affected workers. Muscular pains, fatigue, and weakness of the lower limbs with sensory changes were the common complaints. Symptoms of peripheral polyneuropathy, in some cases as verified by both electromyography and biopsy (Jirasek *et al.*, 1973, 1974, 1976; Goldmann, 1973), commenced almost concurrently with the eruption of chloracne and kept some patients immobile for as long as 2 years. Muscle tone was frequently normal or only slightly affected. Deep tendon reflexes and superficial reflexes were also reported to be normal, and there were no pyramidal signs in cases in which these parameters were examined. Subjective complaints such as sleep disturbances, headaches, decreased libido, impotence, lack of drive, and mood changes were often made. In some cases, anorexia and weight loss were reported (Jirasek *et al.*, 1973; Zack and Suskind, 1980; Goldmann, 1973; Taylor *et al.*, 1977). Singer *et al.* (1982) reported a decrease in nerve conduction velocities of sural nerves in workers exposed to phenoxy acid herbicides for an average of 7 years, compared with a similar group of nonexposed workers. Although the exact causative agent is not known, the halogenated dibenzo-*p*-dioxin contaminants were suggested. It should be noted that in some cases the skin lesions were quite disfiguring and may have contributed to depression and related personality changes in some patients. In addition, as is the case for altered liver function tests, neuromuscular effects are not a consistent feature of intoxication. May (1973) reported workers suffering from severe chloracne with no other obvious systemic illnesses.

Study of chloracne in a factory where methazole was manufactured served not only to reveal another acnegen, TCAB, but also to demonstrate how the dangers of manufacture may be distinct from those of formulation or use. Forty-one workers, all of whom had chloracne to varying degrees, were studied. Exposure to TCAB was by direct skin contact and possibly by the respiratory and oral routes following formation of aerosols during centrifugation. Family members of four workers developed chloracne due to exposure to contaminated skin, clothing, or tools. Employees of a separate plant where methazole was formulated did not develop chloracne, and animal experiments indicated that methazole is not acnegenic. On the contrary, TCAB was highly acnegenic in concentrations at least as low as 0.05% and a concentration of 0.1% caused edema and necrosis of the rabbit ear. TCAB is about half as potent as TCDD in inducing aryl hydrocarbon hydroxylase activity (Taylor *et al.*, 1977).

On February 5, 1981, an electrical malfunction in an 18-story office building in Binghamton, New York, led to overheating of a transformer. Between 180 and 200 gallons of transformer fluid leaked from the overheated transformer in a basement of the building. The fluid was originally composed of Aroclor 1254 (65%) and a mixture containing tri- and tetrachlorinated benzene (35%). Because of an unusual arrangement of the ventilation system, the entire building became contaminated by the volatilization and combustion of the fluid. Analysis showed some soot samples to contain approximately 5% PCBs. In addition, 2,168,000 ppb of PCDFs, 20,000 ppb of PCDDs, and 50,000 ppb of chlorinated biphenylenes were found in soot samples (Schecter et al., 1985c; Schechter, 1983; Buser, 1985). During the first few weeks after the accident, several hundred workers were exposed to the chemicals by virtue of their professions as office workers, cleanup workers, electricians, police, firefighters, and security workers. Serum PCB levels were initially elevated in the exposed individuals but returned to normal within 1–2 years following the accident. Elevated PCDF levels in serum were also noted, as were elevations of specific isomers of PCDFs (2,3,4,7,8-penta-, 1,2,3,4,7,8-hexa-, and 1,2,3,6,7,8-hexa-) in fat tissue which corresponded to isomers identified in soot samples. Transient serum liver enzyme elevations were found in some patients. Elevations of serum triglycerides and cholesterol concentrations were noted shortly after exposure: these returned to normal within 1 year of the incident. Three patients suffered from prolonged elevations of liver enzymes for which no apparent cause other than chemical exposure could be found. Liver biopsy samples from these patients exhibited the following ultrastructural features: increased numbers of lipid droplets and slightly increased amounts of smooth endoplasmic reticulum, abundant glycogen, pleomorphic or deformed and giant mitochondria, and the presence of crystalline structures and large, dense granules in the mitochondria. No chloracne was observed (Schecter et al., 1985a). Since the incident in Binghamton, many other electrical transformer accidents have been reported (see Rappe et al., 1986; O'Keefe and Smith, 1989). Fortunately, in these cases no apparent significant health effects have, as yet, been observed.

Several studies have been made of workers exposed to TCDD either after an interval of continuing but reduced exposure or after an interval without further exposure. As already mentioned, lessened but continuing exposure permitted a considerable degree of recovery, as evidenced by a study made 7 years after the first exposure (Poland et al., 1971). Pazderova-Vejlupkova et al. (1981) examined 55 workers 10 years after the initial outbreak. In some patients, symptoms and signs present from the very beginning of the illness gradually ameliorated during the first 3–4 years. During the first 5 years, the state of health stabilized in most patients and improved in some. Improvement occurred during the second 5 years, but no patient became entirely well. Half still had isolated cysts and comedones, and 15% still had florid chloracne. Serum lipids and α- and γ-globulin levels had normalized, but increased values of total blood protein were still noted. Results of liver function tests had improved, and increased concentrations of porphyrins

were no longer present in urine. In liver biopsies, only mild steatosis or periportal fibrosis was noted. Of even greater interest were studies of workers exposed in 1947 at a Nitro, West Virginia, plant during the manufacture of 2,4,5-trichlorophenol. These workers were reevaluated over 30 years later (Zack and Suskind, 1980; Suskind and Hertzberg, 1984). Varying degrees of chloracne still persisted in 56% of the workers, but systemic health effects were not found. No significant increase in total mortality or in mortality from malignancy or cardiovascular disease was noted. In a similar study, May (1982) evaluated workers 10 years after an explosion in which chloracne developed in 79 individuals. Only half of the affected workers still had signs of chloracne, and no other adverse health effects were observed.

Theiss et al. (1982) conducted a follow-up study of 74 individuals who had been exposed to TCDD 27 years earlier during an accident in a plant producing trichlorophenol. The overall mortality did not differ from the rate expected in three external reference populations or from that observed in two internal comparison groups. Of the 21 deceased individuals, 7 had cancer, compared with 4.1 expected. Three deaths due to stomach cancer were found, compared with 0.6 expected from regional mortality data. However, Theiss et al. were careful to point out that it was difficult to come to any firm conclusion regarding these data because of the small size of the cohort and the small number of deaths from any particular cause. Most recently, Schecter and Ryan (1987) examined the TCDD content in adipose tissue from 6 workers exposed in the same accident 32 years earlier. The average concentration was 49 ppt, 15-fold higher than the "background" human tissue TCDD levels from the same country (Germany). Assuming a half-life of 5 years for TCDD (Poiger and Schlatter, 1986), the estimated mean total body burden of TCDD for these workers at the time of the accident, and which produced chloracne, was 44 μg (range 9.7–124) or approximately 630 ng/kg body weight.

A similar study examined 2192 workers potentially exposed from 1937 through 1980 to the chlorinated dioxins during the manufacture of trichlorophenol. This group included a subgroup of 323 individuals who exhibited chloracne. No increases in total or specific cancer deaths were observed in either group (Bond et al., 1989).

Hardell and co-workers conducted four case-control studies of workers in Sweden who had been exposed to trichlorophenol or the phenoxy herbicides. These investigators suggested an increased risk of soft tissue sarcomas (Hardell and Sandström, 1979; Eriksson et al., 1981, 1990) and Hodgkin's lymphoma (Hardell et al., 1981). A cohort study of herbicide sprayers, also in Sweden, reported an excess incidence of stomach cancer (Axelson et al., 1980). Examination of the records of individuals in the United States accidentally exposed to either 2,4,5-T or trichlorophenol also suggested a relationship between exposure to these chemicals and/or associated contaminants and the development of soft tissue sarcoma (Honchar and Halperin, 1981; Cook, 1981). A more recent study of users of agricultural herbicides in the United States, including 2,4-D and 2,4,5-T, showed a 6-fold greater risk of non-Hodgkin's lymphoma in men exposed to these herbicides more than 20 days per year (Hoar *et al.*, 1986). In addition, a recent study observed that an occupational history of exposure to organic solvents, including phenoxy acids and chlorophenols, was found to be more common among 167 men diagnosed with non-Hodgkin's lymphoma than among a comparable healthy group of men (Olsson and Brandt, 1988). However, the Swedish studies were not substantiated by Milham (1982). In addition, upon review by experts, not all of the tumors diagnosed in earlier studies as being soft tissue sarcomas were found to be soft tissue sarcomas (Fingerhut *et al.*, 1984). Furthermore, preliminary results from a case-control study in New Zealand have not indicated an excess risk of soft tissue sarcoma in individuals exposed to phenoxy herbicides (Smith *et al.*, 1984). However, this study also reported a 5-fold excess of soft tissue sarcoma in persons handling animal pelts, which are sometimes preserved with trichlorophenols containing various dioxin isomers. Wiklund *et al.* (1989) also recently reported a statistically significant increased risk of Hodgkin's disease in a study of 20,245 Swedish pesticide applicators who had exposure to phenoxy acid herbicides.

Greenwald *et al.* (1984) reported a case-control study of men with soft tissue sarcomas who had had Vietnam service and military service experience and of a control group matched on the basis of dates of birth and places of residence. The study failed to show any association of soft tissue sarcoma with exposure to Agent Orange or other phenoxy herbicides contaminated with TCDD that were used in Vietnam. Two other studies conducted by the Air Force (Lathrop *et al.*, 1984) and the Veterans Administration (Kang *et al.*, 1986) reached similar conclusions regarding exposure of Vietnam veterans to herbicides and any adverse health effects. However, it should be pointed out that the latency period from the time of exposure to development of a detectable tumor may be too long for any increase in tumor incidence to be detected in this group of individuals. Furthermore, in these studies of Vietnam veterans, no actual measurement of the degree of exposure, if any, had been made. This lack of analysis may have had the effect of including a number of unexposed persons in the "exposed" population. Notably, Gross *et al.* (1984) reported detecting TCDD at levels ranging from 20 to 173 ppt in adipose tissue from three Vietnam veterans who were "heavily exposed" to Agent Orange. Tissue samples from a group of other Vietnam veterans and from controls also contained TCDD but at levels below 20 ppt. Kahn *et al.* (1988) reported on adipose tissue levels of dioxins and dibenzofurans in 10 Vietnam veterans who were heavily exposed to Agent Orange. The mean values for TCDD were 41.7 ± 16.8 ppt, whereas the values for the control subjects were 5.1 ± 1.4 ppt. A recent study from the Centers for Disease Control determined the TCDD concentrations in serum from 147 U.S. Military personnel who were involved in the application of Agent Orange. The mean value was 49 ppt (on a lipid basis) (median 26 ppt). The five highest levels ranged from 201–313 ppt. The mean concentration was 5 ppt (median 5 ppt) in a group of 49 controls (Centers for Disease Control, 1988b). A half-life for TCDD of 7.1 years (95% confidence interval 5.8–9.6 yr) was calculated in 36 members of the exposed group (Patterson *et al.*, 1989; Pirkle *et al.*, 1989). If this half-life is used to estimate the

serum concentrations at the time of exposure (approximately 20 yr earlier), then the mean for the original values was approximately 400 ppt. Although this is below those determined in some exposed residents in the contaminated Seveso area, it should be noted that some of the most heavily exposed military personnel may have had original TCDD concentrations in serum of up to approximately 2500 ppt. Although the same criticism of lack of documentation of exposure or actual tissue levels may be made of most of the epidemiologic studies performed to date, in many such studies on exposed workers, chloracne, a sentinel lesion, was used as an indicator of exposure.

Sterling and Arundel (1986) and Fingerhut *et al.* (1987) have presented reviews on the human health effects, with a focus on cancer incidence, resulting from phenoxy herbicide exposure. There are studies that show both a positive and a negative association between incidence of cancer, especially soft tissue sarcoma, and exposure to phenoxy herbicides. All of these studies have some limitations due to the small population examined or the lack of exposure assessment.

Only a few studies have examined for reproductive toxicity in dioxin-exposed workers or Vietnam veterans. In most of these studies, no significant differences in incidence in stillbirths, spontaneous abortions, or major defects were reported (IARC, 1977; Townsend *et al.*, 1982; Moses *et al.*, 1984; Lathrop *et al.*, 1984). Erickson *et al.* (1984) reported the results of studies conducted by the Centers for Disease Control in which no association was found between exposure index and birth defects overall. However, the study did show a statistically significant association with spina bifida, cleft lip, coloboma, and neoplasms in the first year of life.

A recent study examined the adipose tissue levels of TCDD in six workers exposed to this compound 32 years earlier in an industrial accident at the BASF plant in Germany. All six workers had developed persistent chloracne from the incident. The average adipose tissue concentration was 49 ppt, approximately 12 times higher than current population levels in Germany. Based on a biological half-life of TCDD in human tissue of 5 years (Poiger and Schlatter, 1986), it was estimated that the mean body burden of TCDD in these six workers at the time of the accident was 44 μg with a range of 9.7–124 (Schecter and Ryan, 1987). Another study (Ryan *et al.*, 1987a) examined the tissue levels of the PCDD and PCDF isomers in an individual who had died from acute pentachlorophenol poisoning (Gray *et al.*, 1985). Adipose tissue levels of the tetra- and penta- congeners were similar to those in the general population of North America (Ryan *et al.*, 1985; Stanley *et al.*, 1986). Concentrations of the hepta- and octa- congeners were markedly elevated, with total levels in adipose tissue of about 10–20 ng/gm lipid for hepta-PCDDs/PCDFs and octa-PCDF and about 130 ng/g lipid for octa-PCDD. These values are over 100 times greater than background levels (Stanley *et al.*, 1986). Gorski *et al.* (1984) followed the persistence of certain PCDDs and PCDFs in adipose tissue of a person with a history of long-term exposure to technical pentachlorophenol. The half-lives of 1,2,3,6,7,8-hexaCDD, 1,2,3,4,6,7,8-heptaCDD, octaCDD, and octaCDF were estimated to be about 3.5, 3, 6, and 2 years, respectively.

Poisoning Involving the Community Apparently one of the first community occurrences of chloracne and related disease was the result of contamination of rice oil by PCBs, which leaked from a heat exchange into the oil. The outbreak in Fukuoka Prefecture, Japan, was first recognized in October 1968. By the end of 1982, at least 1788 persons had been made ill from what was called "Yusho"—that is, oil disease—when its origin was traced. The epidemiological, clinical, and toxicological findings have been described in several papers and comprehensive reviews (Kuratsune, 1972, 1980, 1989; Kuratsune *et al.*, 1972; Kimbrough, 1974, 1987; Higuchi, 1976; Hirayama, 1976; Hsu *et al.*, 1985; Urabe and Asahi, 1985; Yoshimura and Hayabuchi, 1985; Murai and Kuriowa, 1971; Reggiani, 1983). Although varying degrees of chloracne, skin lesions, and hyperpigmentation were the predominant clinical features, various other signs and symptoms of illness were reported. These include liver enlargement, proliferation of smooth endoplasmic reticulum in a liver biopsy, slight increases in serum transaminases and alkaline phosphatase, serum triglycerides increased to four times the normal value, abnormal discharges of the Meibomian glands, reduced sensory nerve conduction velocity, chronic bronchitis, and excess mucus production. Some women who consumed contaminated rice oil gave birth to "coco" (heavily black-pigmented) babies (Kikuchi *et al.*, 1969). This pigmentation disappeared by the time the babies were between 2 and 5 months old. No alterations in porphyrin metabolism were observed (Strik, 1979). Fifteen years after the incident, only a few patients exhibited extensive chloracne (Urabe and Asahi, 1985).

Some oil that caused illness contained 2000–3000 ppm PCB, and patients consumed approximately 2000 mg of PCB per person. However, despite the high contamination with PCBs as well as polychlorinated quaterphenyls (PCQs), the syndrome has been attributed mainly to contaminating PCDFs (Chen *et al.*, 1981; Kashimoto *et al.*, 1981; Kuratsune, 1989). The animal data suggest that the PCB and PCQ components alone cannot cause the Yusho symptoms (Kashimoto *et al.*, 1985; Kunita *et al.*, 1985). The concentration of total PDCFs in the Yusho oil has been reported to be between 1.9 and 7.4 ppm, depending on the date of manufacture (Buser *et al.*, 1978; Kuratsune, 1980; Kunita *et al.*, 1984; Kashimoto *et al.*, 1983; Masuda *et al.*, 1982). Two major isomers, 2,3,4,7,8-penta- and 1,2,3,4,7,8-hexadibenzofuran, of the 40 isomers present in the Yusho oil are considered to be the most toxic isomers (Mason *et al.*, 1985; Safe, 1987; Nagayama *et al.*, 1985) and are those that have been shown to accumulate in humans (Kashimoto *et al.*, 1983; Lucier *et al.*, 1987; Ryan *et al.*, 1987b, 1990) and animals (Brewster and Birnbaum, 1987). These isomers have been found to constitute 8.0% and 8.5%, respectively, of the total PCDFs in the oil (Kashimoto *et al.*, 1983; Hari *et al.*, 1986). A thorough study by Hayabuchi *et al.* (1979) of 141 patients with chloracne showed that the geometric average of the total amount of oil consumed was 688 ml, corresponding to about 3.4 mg total PCDFs. However, during the period from the start of oil consumption to the appearance of skin lesions, which averaged 71 days, the average amount of oil consumed was 506 ml. The

average body burden of 2,3,4,7,8-pentachlorodibenzofuran equivalents associated with chloracne was estimated to be approximately 5.9 μg/kg (Ryan *et al.*, 1990; see also Wilson, 1987). A preliminary analysis of the oil-exposed population has suggested an increased rate of liver cancer. The authors were careful to point out that, considering the long latent period commonly needed for the development of tumors, it is still too early to draw any firm conclusion on this issue (Kuratsune *et al.*, 1987).

A second outbreak due to contamination of rice oil occurred in Taiwan in 1979. In this instance, it was never determined with certainty how the oil became contaminated. By November 1980 there were 1843 reported cases of the Yusho-like disease. The Kanechlor 400/Kanechlor 500 contamination in the oil varied from 31 to 300 ppm; the period of exposure was from 3 to 9 months, and the estimated total intake per person was 0.77–1.84 gm (Hsu *et al.*, 1985). Along with chloracne and signs and symptoms similar to those reported in the Yusho incident (Masuda, 1985; Chen *et al.*, 1985; Rogan, 1989), immunosuppression was observed. This consisted of alterations in T-cell, but not B-cell, populations (Lu and Wu, 1985; Chang *et al.*, 1981, 1982). Placental tissues from women who had been exposed 3–4 years before conception showed large increases in monooxygenase activities, particularly aryl hydrocarbon hydroxylase. Furthermore, many of the children of these poisoning victims who were exposed to the oil contaminants transplacentally and possibly through breast milk have been shown to have abnormalities similar to those of the adults, as well as developmental effects (Gladen *et al.*, 1988; Rogan *et al.*, 1988). In this poisoning incident the PCDF content of the rice oil was much lower than in the Yusho case; the values were approximately 0.14 and 5.0 ppm, respectively. However, the average consumption of oil was estimated to be much higher in the Taiwan (Yu-Cheng) incident than in the case in Japan. As in the Yusho incident, the predominant, toxic, accumulating isomers were found to be the 2,3,4,7,8-penta- and 1,2,3,4,7,8-hexachlorodibenzofurans (Kashimoto *et al.*, 1983; Lucier *et al.*, 1987). By using data from an analysis of blood samples from Yu-Cheng patients (Kashimoto *et al.*, 1983) and assuming a 1 : 1 partitioning ratio of isomers in adipose tissue and serum lipid (Patterson *et al.*, 1986), it was estimated that a body burden of 4.0 μg of 2,3,4,7,8-pentachlorodibenzofuran was necessary to produce chloracne (Ryan *et al.*, 1990).

In 1971, the spraying of contaminated waste oil to control dust on a farm road and three horse arenas in Missouri led to the fatal poisoning of 57 horses, 70 chickens, several dogs and cats, numerous rodents, and hundreds of birds and to the nonfatal poisoning of at least five people. The contamination arose from using, along with waste oil, certain oil-like wastes from a hexachlorophene manufacturing facility in southwestern Missouri. The concentration of TCDD in the surface soil was 31.8–33 ppm. In spite of removal of contaminated soil from one arena at 5 and again 11 months after application, horses continued to die of poisoning acquired there as late as 31 months after application of the spray (Carter *et al.*, 1975; Kimbrough *et al.*, 1977). Of the persons exposed, at least three children and one adult complained of skin lesions, and these were consistent with chloracne in at least two of the children. The most severely affected person was a 6-year-old girl, who suffered hematuria and painful urination, nosebleeds, headache, and diarrhea. Cystography revealed a highly contracted, edematous bladder. The patient's symptoms resolved 3–4 days after hospitalization, and hematuria and proteinuria were absent after 1 week. Cystoscopy 3 months later revealed numerous punctate hemorrhage areas in the bladder. The child was again examined 5.3 years after her exposure. Physical examination, neurological studies, urinalysis, cystography, pyelography, and clinical chemistry all gave normal results (Beale *et al.*, 1977).

The U.S. Centers for Disease Control conducted a pilot study of approximately 100 people living in another contaminated area of Missouri. The soil contamination of TCDD in this area was generally less than 1 ppm. No significant adverse effects were found in individuals who were possibly exposed to TCDD (Webb *et al.*, 1987).

More recently, another area of Missouri was identified that was also sprayed with the TCDD-contaminated waste oil for dust control. Although the original TCDD contamination was traced back to 1971, when the waste material was taken from the hexachlorophene manufacturing facility, soil concentrations of 2.2 ppm TCDD were still present more than 10 years later (Stehr *et al.*, 1985; Centers for Disease Control, 1984). Hoffman *et al.* (1986) reported on a study in which 154 exposed individuals living in the contaminated area were compared with 155 persons living in a nearby uncontaminated area; no increased clinical illness was noted in the exposed group. Trends suggesting an alteration in cell-mediated immunity were observed in this population by Knutsen (1984). The suggestion of the presence of abnormal T-cell populations is of interest, given the consistent effect of TCDD on the immune system of experimental animals (see Pathology and Effects on Organs, Tissues, and Cells). In addition, an investigation of blood samples of persons exposed to PCDFs during a transformer fire also demonstrated altered T-cell populations (Kochman *et al.*, 1986). Thirty-nine persons with a history of residential, recreational, or occupational exposure in the Missouri area had significantly higher levels of TCDD in adipose tissue biopsy samples, compared with 57 persons in the control group. Levels in the control group ranged from 1.4–20.2 ppt and in the exposed groups from 2.8 to 750 ppt (Patterson *et al.*, 1986).

The most recent nonoccupational exposure to TCDD occurred in Seveso, Italy, on July 10, 1976, where a batch reactor in a 2,4,5-trichlorophenol plant overheated and discharged its contents through a relief valve directly to the outside air. The accident was essentially the same as the one described by Jensen (1972), except that the relief valve prevented an explosion but served to distribute the contamination outdoors; in the explosion described by Jensen, contamination was confined to the factory. Other accidents involving uncontrolled overheating have occurred in the process of making 2,4,5-trichlorophenol (Hay, 1976b; Holmstedt, 1980).

The episode at Seveso has been the subject of many medical reports (Reggiani, 1978, 1980; Pocchiari *et al.*, 1979, 1983)

and of several scientific news articles (Hay, 1976a, 1977; Walsh, 1977; Revzin, 1977; Garattini, 1977). Briefly, the vapor discharged from the batch reactor drifted downwind so that the visible cloud covered an area of about 109 ha inhabited by some 2000 people. Lesser contamination affected a much larger area. The first animal deaths were reported on July 15. On the following day, some children developed skin rashes. Not until 13 days after the discharge was TCDD identified as the causal agent, and evacuation of children began 17 days after discharge. By the end of the month, 730 people of all ages had been evacuated from the most heavily contaminated area, and an additional 1300 children had been evacuated from surrounding areas.

The skin rashes (which may have been caused in part by irritation from 2,4,5-trichlorophenol) appeared on the sixth day, and at least some of them progressed to definite chloracne in about 15 people, mainly children 5–6 years old. Following screening of approximately 42,000 children, about 600 suspected cases were identified, but the total number of confirmed chloracne cases was 134. The survey revealed chloracne in children who had not been in the area until September 1976, and this was interpreted as evidence that there was still enough TCDD in the environment several months after the accident to cause chloracne. However, 1 year after the accident, only a few cases of injury persisted; these were a few with chloracne-like lesions on the armpit and a few with facial scarring from the initial chemical burn. A comparison of children who developed chloracne and children of the same area who did not develop skin lesions was reported by Caramaschi *et al.* (1981) and Mocarelli *et al.* (1986). A significant increase in the incidence of headaches, eye irritation, and gastrointestinal tract symptoms and in abnormal γ-glutamyl transpeptidase, SGPT, and aminolevulinic acid levels was noted in children with chloracne. These abnormalities were slight and disappeared with time. A significant increase in urinary D-glucaric acid levels, used to indicate increased microsomal enzyme activity, was also observed in exposed children 3 years after the accident (Ideo *et al.*, 1982). Systematic examination of pregnant women failed to reveal any embryotoxic or teratogenic effect, including chromosomal aberrations. An epidemiological study more than a year after the explosion involved 623 women who had been pregnant at the time of exposure. No unusual incidence of prenatal or postnatal mortality was observed, and the children had shown no harmful effect and had developed normally (Tuchmann-Duplessis, 1978). However, a significant increase in morphologic abnormalities, including iron-rich deposits, was found in placental tissue from exposed women whose pregnancies had been terminated (Remotti *et al.*, 1981). Results of a 4-year follow-up showed no association between TCDD exposure and the overall incidence of polydactyly and Down's syndrome in infants born to parents living in the contaminated areas. The same study, however, noted a slight correlation between exposure and occurrence of total malformations, or those affecting the heart and blood vessels or the genital system (Bruzzi, 1983). Examinations of immune capacity failed to reveal any difference between the contaminated and control groups. Examination of 156 male and 15 female plant workers revealed a transient increase in SGPT and γ-GT but no change in alkaline phosphatase or in leukocyte count. Other studies during the first 2 years after the event revealed some cases of polyneuropathy and nystagmus, but there was no evidence for a higher incidence of these conditions among those with chloracne Peripheral nerve damage was found by electromyoneurographic studies in 8 of about 200 workers in the plant, and this could not be traced to any common causes of polyneuropathy (Pocchiari *et al.*, 1979; Tognoni and Bonaccorsi, 1982; Reggiani, 1978; Filippini *et al.*, 1981). In a ten-year mortality study of the population involved in Seveso, an increased death due to a number of cancers including biliary, brain, lymphatic, and hemopoietic were observed. However, the authors were careful to point out that any interpretation of the results is hampered by the relatively short period of time between exposure and observation and the small number of deaths within each particular category (Bertazzi *et al.*, 1989).

Estimates of the amount of TCDD released varied from 0.45 to 6.80 kg. Samples that might have permitted the measurement of tissue levels were not collected. A few vegetation samples collected within the first 2 weeks after the incident contained up to 15 ppm TCDD. TCDD levels in surface soil samples taken within 3 months after the incident ranged from <0.75 to 20,000 $\mu g/m^2$. No TCDD was detected in drinking, surface, or ground water samples. The level in the unworked soil diminished sharply in the first months after the accident. However, following this period, the actual decrease in the concentration of TCDD in the soil appeared to be extremely slow, with an estimated half-life of greater than 10 years (di Domenico *et al.*, 1982; Wipf *et al.*, 1982; Wipf and Schmid, 1983; Cerquiglini Monteriolo *et al.*, 1982). Thus, although significant exposure of humans likely occurred within the first few weeks after the explosion and prior to evacuation, actual body burdens have not been determined. As in the Missouri incident, the fact that some animals died but people did not die is consistent with a species difference in susceptibility to at least the lethal effects of TCDD. Again, however, since no systematic quantitation of dose has been made, proof of differential susceptibility cannot be given at this time. Facchetti *et al.*, (1980) reported on the tissue analysis of one individual who had died from pancreatic adenocarcinoma 7 months after the Seveso accident. The following concentrations of TCDD (as ppt) were found in these tissues: fat, 1840; pancreas, 1040; liver, 150; thyroid, 85; brain, 60; lung, 60; kidney, 40; blood, 6. The subject was a resident of the most contaminated area (zone A); the mean TCDD concentration in the soil was 185.4 $\mu g/m^2$ (Facchetti *et al.*, 1980). Data from the Centers for Disease Control indicate that TCDD levels in lipid from five individuals living in zone A and exhibiting chloracne were 828, 1688, 17,274, 27,032, and 27,821 ppt. Four other individuals living in this zone with no chloracne had TCDD levels in lipid of 1772, 3054, 3729, and 10,439 ppt (Centers for Disease Control, 1988). In a recent study nine residents of the most heavily contaminated zone were examined for serum concentrations of TCDD. Values ranged from 828–27,821 ppt (on a lipid basis) with the three highest concentrations found in children with chloracne. TCDD was not detected in the serum of four out of five individuals living outside the contaminated zones (Centers for Disease Control, 1988a).

Because of the noted effect of TCDD on reproduction, hormone biochemistry, and embryo-fetal development in experimental animals (see Section 18.5.1.2), several studies have examined these parameters in populations of both sexes with potential exposure to TCDD. A positive association between possible 2,4,5-T exposures and increases in birth defects or abortions has been reported in human populations in Oregon (USEPA, 1979). New Zealand (Hanify *et al.*, 1981), and Australia (Field and Kerr, 1979). However, a lack of any such association has been reported in Arkansas (Nelson *et al.*, 1979), Hungary (Thomas, 1980), New Zealand (New Zealand Department of Health, 1980; McQueen *et al.*, 1977), and Australia (Aldred, 1978). It should be noted that 2,4,5-T or TCDD was not unequivocally identified as the causative agent in the reports in which a positive association was found. Although in 1979 there were reports of a high incidence of spontaneous abortions in a group of women living in Oregon and potentially exposed to 2,4,5-T from aerial spraying (Smith, 1979; USEPA, 1979; Newton and Norris, 1981), a panel of scientists later concluded that the basic design of the initial studies was inadequate to demonstrate any positive or negative effect of 2,4,5-T (Coulston and Olajos, 1980).

Constable and Hatch (1985) summarized studies conducted on Vietnamese populations exposed to herbicides during the military spraying of the south of Vietnam. The results of studies conducted in the north of Vietnam were consistent with an association between presumptive paternal (males who had military service in the south of Vietnam) exposure and congenital defects in offspring, particularly anencephaly and orofacial defects. For the men and women exposed in the south of Vietnam, there were reported increases in miscarriages, stillbirths, molar pregnancy, and certain types of birth defects, mainly anencephaly, anophthalmia, phocomelia, and skeletal deformities. Again, however, it should be noted that these studies were based primarily on presumptive exposure and few, if any, documentations or analyses of tissue dioxin levels of these individuals have been carried out.

A number of studies have reported the presence of a number of PCDD and PDCF isomers in samples of human tissue, mainly adipose, from "unexposed" populations in industrialized and nonindustrialized nations. In general, mean values of TCDD in industrialized nations range from nondetectable to 30 ppt, on a lipid basis (Ryan *et al.*, 1985, 1987b; Schecter *et al.*, 1985a; Graham *et al.*, 1985; Patterson *et al.*, 1986, 1987, 1988, 1989; Rappe *et al.*, 1984, 1986; Stanley *et al.*, 1986; Jensen, 1987; Thoma *et al.*, 1989; Andrews *et al.*, 1989). This body burden corresponds to an estimated average intake of approximately 0.05 ng TCDD/day (Travis and Hattemer-Frey, 1987). Notably, adipose tissue samples taken from residents of southern Vietnam, historically known to be heavily contaminated with these isomers contained in herbicide preparations, especially Agent Orange, averaged 22 ppt for the content of TCDD (Jensen,

1989). TCDD was not detected (detection limit of 2 ppt) in samples from northern Vietnam, an area with infrequent use of synthetic industrial and agricultural chemicals and not sprayed with contaminated herbicides (Schecter *et al.*, 1986, 1987). The chlorinated dioxins, in particular TCDD, have been found to be present at higher concentrations in food and wildlife samples taken from southern Vietnam (Olie *et al.*, 1989; Schecter *et al.*, 1989). Analyses of PCDDs and PCDFs in human milk samples have also been performed. All values from unexposed populations demonstrated TCDD concentrations below 2 ppt (Rappe *et al.*, 1984; Fuerst *et al.*, 1986; Heath *et al.*, 1986. Baughman (1974) reported TCDD concentrations in breast milk samples from mothers living in southern Vietnam to be as high as 40–50 ppt. Notably, these samples were taken within a few years following the discontinuation of the use of Agent Orange. Samples taken in 1984 from the same area, however, still showed elevated concentrations (2.0–6.5 ppt) (Schecter *et al.*, 1986). It should be pointed out that in most of these studies many other PCDD and PCDF isomers in addition to TCDD were detected, some at concentrations much greater than observed for TCDD.

Both the U.S. Environmental Protection Agency (EPA) and the Centers for Disease Control (CDC) have estimated the potential human health risk of TCDD exposure (USEPA, 1985; Kimbrough *et al.*, 1984). The EPA value for the "acceptable daily intake" of TCDD is 1 pg/kg/day for a 70-year lifetime. This value is based on the lowest-observed-adverse-effect-level of 1 ng/kg/day for a reproductive effect in rats (Murray *et al.*, 1979; Nisbet and Paxton, 1982). For a 1/1,000,000 cancer risk, the EPA has further estimated a 95% lower-limit criterion for a lifetime intake of 6.4 fg/kg/day (USEPA, 1984a). For the same cancer risk, the CDC estimated a "virtually safe dose" of 28 fg/kg/day. Both these estimates are based on a linear-derived multistage extrapolation model that is usually used for genotoxic agents such as ionizing radiation. Based on a nonlinear model (usually used for tumor promoters), the CDC has also estimated for this cancer risk a "virtually safe dose" of 636 fg/kg/day. It should be noted that these numbers were derived for regulatory purposes and were not intended to indicate that there will actually be an increased cancer incidence at these levels of contamination. Also note that values for acceptable daily intakes for TCDD generated by different regulatory agencies worldwide vary considerably (6.4–10,000 fg/kg/day), depending largely on the toxic effect, models chosen, and assumptions of safety factors (see Leung *et al.*, 1988).

Treatment of Poisoning   Sauna bathing followed by an acne cleansing regimen has proved useful for chloracne. At least in mild cases, vitamin A acid (retinoic acid) in the form of a solution or cream was reported to be useful (Plewig, 1970a, 1971; Taylor *et al.*, 1977). Taylor (1983) also reported successful treatment of chloracne with Accutane (13-*cis*-retinoic acid) in one patient. Accutane has been used most often in treating patients with juvenile acne (Peck *et al.*, 1979). However, it should be noted that Accutane was introduced into the medical community in 1983 despite its being a known teratogen. By 1984 reports were being published concerning spontaneous abortions and birth defects found in children exposed *in utero* to Accutane (Rosa *et al.*, 1986).

REFERENCES

Abbott, B. D., and Birnbaum, L. S. (1989). Cellular alterations and enhanced induction of cleft palate after coadministration of retinoic acid and TCDD. *Toxicol. Appl. Pharmacol.* **99**, 287–301.

Abbott, B. D., Birnbaum, L. S., and Pratt, R. M. (1987a). TCDD produces hydronephrosis in fetal mice by inducing hyperplasia of the ureteric epithelium. *Teratology* **35**, 329–333.

Abbott, B. D., Morgan, K. S., Birnbaum, L. S., and Pratt, R. M. (1987b). TCDD alters the extracellular matrix and basal lamina of the fetal mouse kidney. *Teratology* **35**, 335–344.

Abbott, B. D., Diliberto, J. J., and Birnbaum, L. S. (1989). 2,3,7,8-Tetrachlorodibenzo-p-dioxin alters embryonic palatal medial epithelial cell differentiation in vitro. *Toxicol. Appl. Pharmacol.* **100**, 119–131.

Abernethy, D. J., Greenlee, W. G., Huband, J. C., and Boreiko, C. J. (1985). 2,3,7,8-Tetrachlorodibenzo-*p*-dioxin (TCDD) promotes the transformation of C3H10T1/2 cells. *Carcinogenesis (London)* **6**, 651–653.

Adams, E. M., Irish, D. D., Spencer, H. C., and Rowe, V. K. (1941). The response of rabbit skin to compounds reported to have caused acneform dermatitis. *Ind. Med., Ind. Hyg. Sect. 2*, **10**, 1–4.

Ahlborg, U. G. (1978). Dechlorination of pentachlorophenol *in vivo* and *in vitro*. In "Pentachlorophenol. Chemistry, Pharmacology and Environmental Toxicology" (K. R. Rao, ed.), pp. 115–130. Plenum, New York.

Ahlborg, U. G., and Larsson, K. (1978). Metabolism of tetrachlorophenols in the rat. *Arch. Toxicol.* **40**, 63–74.

Ahlborg, U. G., and Thunberg, T. (1978). Effect of 2,3,7,8-tetrachlorodibenzo-*p*-dioxin on the *in vivo* and *in vitro* dechlorination of pentachlorophenol. *Arch. Toxicol.* **40**, 55–62.

Ahlborg, U. G., Lindgren, J. E., and Mercier, M. (1974). Metabolism of pentachlorophenol. *Arch. Toxicol.* **32**, 271–281.

Ahlborg, U. G., Manzoor, E., and Thunberg, T. (1977). Inhibition of β-glucuronidase by chlorinated hydroquinones and benzoquinones. *Arch. Toxicol.* **37**, 81–87.

Ahlborg, U. G., Larsson, K., and Thunberg, T. (1978). Metabolism of pentachlorophenol *in vivo* and *in vitro*. *Arch. Toxicol.* **40**, 45–53.

Aitio, A., and Parkki, M. G. (1978). Organ specific induction of drug metabolizing enzymes by 2,3,7,8-tetrachlorodibenzo-*p*-dioxin in the rat. *Toxicol. Appl. Pharmacol.* **44**, 107–114.

Akisada, T. (1965). Simultaneous determination of pentachlorophenol and tetrachlorophenol in air and urine. *Bunseki Kagaku* **14**, 101–105.

Al-Bayati, Z. A. F., Murray, W. J., and Stohs, S. J. (1987). 2,3,7,8-Tetrachlorodibenzo-*p*-dioxin-induced lipid peroxidation in hepatic and extrahepatic tissues of male and female rats. *Arch Environ. Toxicol.* **16**, 159–166.

Albro, P. W., Corbett, J. T., Harriss, M., and Lawson, L. D. (1978). Effects of 2,3,7,8-tetrachlorodibenzo-*p*-dioxin on lipid profiles in tissue of the Fisher rat. *Chem.-Biol. Interact.* **23**, 315–330.

Albro, P. W., Luster, M. I., Chae, K., Clark, G., and McKinney, J. D. (1979). A radioimmunoassay for chlorinated dibenzo-*p*-dioxins. *Toxicol. Appl. Pharmacol.* **50**, 137–143.

Albro, P. W., Crummett, W. B., Depey, A. E., Jr., Gross, M. L., Hanson, M., Harless, R. L., Hileman, F. D., Hilker, D., Jason, C., Johnson, J. J., Lamparski, L. L., Lau, B. P. Y., McDaniel, D. D., Meehan, J. L., Nestrick, T. J., Hygren, M., O'Keefe, P., Peters, T. L., Rappe, C., Ruan, J. J., Smith, L. M, Stalling, D. L., Weerasinghe, M. C. A., and Wendling, J. M. (1985). Methods for the quantitative determination of multiple, specific polychlorinated dibenzo-*p*-dioxin and dibenzofuran isomers in human adipose tissue in the parts-per-trillion range. An inter-laboratory study. *Anal. Chem.* **51**, 2717–2725.

Albro, P. W., Corbett, J. T., and Schroeder, J. L. (1986). Effects of 2,3,7,8-tetrachlorodibenzo-p-dioxin on lipid peroxidation in microsomal systems *in vitro*. *Chem.-Biol. Interact.* **57,** 301–313.

Albro, P. W., Corbett, J. T., Schroeder, J. L., and Harran, D. (1988). Comparison of the effects of carbon tetrachloride and of 2,3,7,8-tetrachlorodibenzo-p-dioxin on the disposition of linoleic acid in rat liver *in vitro*. *Chem.-Biol. Interact.* **66,** 267–285.

Aldred, J. E. (1978). "Report on the Consultative Council on Congenital Abnormalities in the Yarrom District." Minister of Health, Melbourne, Victoria, Australia (Cited in Milby *et al.*, 1980).

Allen, J. R., and van Miller, J. P. (1978). Health implications of 2,3,7,8-tetrachlorodibenzo-p-dioxin exposure in primates. *In* "Pentachlorophenol: Chemistry, Parmacology and Environmental Taxicology" (K. R. Rao, ed.), pp. 371–379. Plenum, New York.

Allen, J. R., van Miller, J. P., and Norback, D. H. (1975). Tissue distribution, excretion, and biological effects of ^{14}C tetrachlorodibenzo-p-dioxin in rats. *Food Cosmet. Toxicol.* **13,** 501–505.

Allen, J. R., Barsotti, D. A., Lalich, J. J., Van Miller, J. P., and Abrahamson, L. J. (1977). Morphological changes in monkeys consuming a diet containing low levels of 2,3,7,8-tetrachlorodibenzo-p-dioxin. *Food Cosmet. Toxicol.* **15,** 401–410.

Allen, J. R., Barsotti, D. A., Lambrecht, L. K., and van Miller, J. P. (1979). Reproductive effects of halogenated aromatic hydrocarbons on nonhuman primates. *Ann. N.Y. Acad. Sci.* **320,** 419–425..

Alsop, W. R., and Moreland, D. E. (1975). Effects of herbicides on the light-activated, magnesium-dependent APTase of isolated spinach (*Spinacia oleracea* L.) chloroplasts. *Pestic. Biochem. Physiol.* **5,** 163–169.

Ambrose, A. M. (1947). Some toxicological and pharmacological studies on 3,5-dinitro-o-cresol. *J. Pharmacol. Exp. Ther.* **76,** 245–251.

Anaizi, N. H., and Cohen, J. J. (1978). The effect of 2,3,7,8-tetrachlorodibenzo-p-dioxin on the renal tubular secretion of phenolsulfonphthalein. *J. Pharmacol. Exp. Ther.* **207,** 748–755.

Andrews, J. S., Jr., Garrett, W. A., Jr., Patterson, D. G., Jr., Needham, L. L., Roberts, D. W., Bagby, J. R., Anderson, J. E., Hoffman, R. E., and Schramm, W. (1989). 2,3,7,8-Tetrachlorodibenzo-p-dioxin levels in adipose tissue of persons with no known exposure and in exposed persons. *Chemosphere* **18,** 499–506.

Andrews, P., Thyssen, J., and Lorke, D. (1983). The biology and toxicology of molluscicides, Bayluscide. *Pharmacol. Ther.* **19,** 245–295.

Anikin, G. D. (1969). The action of 2,4-dinitrophenol on the processes of uropoiesis in dogs. *Byull. Eksp. Biol. Med.* **68,** 70–73.

Anonymous (1970). Pentachlorophenol poisoning in the home. *Calif. Health* **27,** 13.

Ansari, G. A. S., Britt, S. G., and Reynolds, E. S. (1985). Isolation and characterization of palmitoylpentachlorophenol from human fat. *Bull. Environ, Contam. Toxicol.* **34,** 661–667.

Appelgren, L.-E., Brandt, I., Brittebo, E. B., Gillner, M., and Gustafsson, J.-A. (1983). Autoradiography 2,3,7,8-tetrachloro ^{14}C-dibenzo-p-dioxin (TCDD): Accumulation in the nasal mucosa. *Chemosphere* **12,** 545–548.

Armbrecht, B. H., and Saver, S. H. (1960). Failure of 2,4-dinitro-o-cyclohexylphenol and its dicyclohexylamine salt to produce cataracts in chicks and ducklings. *Fed. Proc., Fed. Am. Soc. Exp. Biol.* **19,** 388.

Armstrong, R. W., Eichner, E. R., Klein, D. E., Barthel, W. F., Bennett, J. V., Jonsson, V., Bruce, H., and Loveless, L. E. (1969). Pentachlorophenol poisoning in a nursery for newborn infants. II. Epidemiologic and toxicologic studies. *J. Pediatr.* **75,** 317–325.

Arsenault, R. E. (1976). Pentachlorophenol and contained chlorinated dibenzodioxins in the environment. *Proc.—Annu. Meet. Am. Wood-Preserv. Assoc.* **72,** 122–148.

Arstila, A. U., Reggiani, G., Sovari, T. E., Raisaen, S., and Wipf, H. K. (1981). Elimination of 2,3,7,8-tetrachlorodibenzo-p-dioxin in goat milk. *Toxicol. Lett.* **9,** 215–219.

Astroff, B., Zacharewski, T., Safe, S., Arlotto, M. P., Parkinson, A., Thomas, P., and Levin, W. (1988). 6-Methyl-1,3,8-trichlorodibenzofuran as a 2,3,7,8-tetrachlorodibenzo-p-dioxin antagonist: Inhibition of the induction of rat cytochrome P-450 isozymes and related monooxygenase activities. *Mol. Pharmacol.* **33,** 231–236.

Atlas, S. A., Vesell, E. S., and Nebert, D. W. (1976). Genetic control of interinidividual variations in the inducibility of aryl hydrocarbon hydroxylase in cultured human lymphocytes. *Cancer Res.* **36,** 4619–4630.

Atlas, S. A., Boobis, A. R., Felton, J. S., Thorgeirsson, S. S., and Nebert, D. W. (1977). Ontogenic expression of polycyclic aromatic compound-inducible monooxygenase activities and forms of cytochrome P-450 in the rabbit. *J. Biol. Chem.* **252,** 4712–4721.

Atuma, S. S., and Okor, D. I. (1985). Gas chromatographic determination of pentachlorophenol in human blood and urine. *Bull. Environ. Contam. Toxicol.* **35,** 406–410.

Axelson, O., Sundell, L., Andersson, K., Edling, C., Hogstedt, C., and Kling, H. (1980). Herbicide exposure and tumor motality. *Scand. J. Work Environ. Health* **6,** 73–79.

Baader, H. C. E. W., and Bauer, H. J. (1951). Industrial intoxication due to pentachlorophenol. *Ind. Med. Surg.* **20,** 286–290.

Bacila, B., and Medina, H. (1962). Inhibition by phenothiazinic compounds of the effect of 2,4-dinitrophenol on respiration of heart muscle sarcosomes. *Nature (London)* **194,** 547–548.

Bakker, E. P., van den Heuvel, E. J., Wiechmann, A. H. C. A., and van Dam, K. (1973). A comparison between the effectiveness of uncouplers of exidative phosphyorylation in mitochondria and in different artificial membrane systems. *Biochem. Biophys. Acta* **292,** 78–87.

Balk, J. L., and Piper, W. N. (1984). Altered blood levels of corticosteroids in the rat after exposure of 2,3,7,8-tetrachlorodibenzo-p-dioxin. *Biochem. Pharmacol.* **33,** 2531–2534.

Ball, L. M., and Chhabra, R. S. (1981). Intestinal absorption of nutrients in rats treated with 2,3,7,8-tetrachlorodibenzo-p-dioxin (TCDD). *J. Toxicol. Environ. Health* **8,** 629–638.

Bandal, S. K., and Casida, J. E. (1972). Metabolism and photoalteration of 2-sec-butyl-4,6-dinitrophenol (DNBP herbicide) and its isopropyl carbonate derivative (dinobuton acaracide). *J. Agric. Chem.* **20,** 1235–1245.

Bandiera, S., Sawyer, T. W., Campbell, M. A., Fujita, P., and Safe, S. (1983). Comparative binding to the cytosolic 2,3,7,8-tetrachlorodibenzo-p-dioxin receptor: Effects of structure on the affinities of substituted halogenated biphenyls—a QSAR analysis. *Biochem. Pharmacol.* **32,** 3803–3813.

Bandiera, S., Sawyer, T., Romkes, M., Zmudzka, B., Safe, L., Mason, G., Keys, B., and Safe, S. (1984). Polychlorinated dibenzofurans (PCDFs): Effects of structure on binding to the 2,3,7,8-TCDD cytosolic receptor protein, AHH induction and toxicity. *Toxicology* **32,** 131–144.

Bannister, R., Davis, D., Zacharewski, Z., Tizard, I., and Safe, S. (1987). Aroclor 1254 as a 2,3,7,8-tetrachlorodibenzo-p-dioxin antagonist: Effects on enzyme induction and immunotoxicity. *Toxicology* **40,** 29–42.

Baran, M. R. (1973). Nail damage from contact with organo-synthetic pesticidal products. Concerning a case involving dinitro-o-cresol. *Bull. Soc. Fr. Dermatol. Syphiligr.* **80,** 172–173.

Baran, R. L. (1974). Nail damage caused by weed killers and insecticides. *Arch. Dermatol.* **100,** 467 (in French).

Barker, S. B. (1946a). Absence of dinitro-cresol effect in thiouracil-treated rats. *Fed. Proc., Fed. Am. Soc. Exp. Biol.* **5,** 4.

Barker, S. B. (1946b). Effect of thyroid activity on metabolic responses to dinitro-o-cresol. *Endocrinology (Baltimore)* **39,** 234–238.

Barsotti, D. A., Abrahamson, L. J., and Allen, J. R. (1979). Hormonal alterations in female rhesus monkeys fed a diet containing 2,3,7,8-tetrachlorodibenzo-p-dioxin. *Bull. Environ. Contam. Toxicol.* **21,** 463–469.

Barthel, W. F., Curley, A., Thrasher, C. L., Sedlak, V. A., and Armstrong, R. (1969). Determination of pentachlorophenol in blood, urine, tissue, and clothing. *J. Assoc. Off. Agric. Chem.* **52,** 294–298.

Bastomsky, C. H. (1977). Enhanced thyroxine metabolism and high uptake goiters in rats after a single dose of 2,3,7,8-tetrachlorodibenzo-p-dioxin. *Endocrinology (Baltimore)* **101,** 292–296.

Bauchinger, M., Dresp, J., Schmid, E., and Hauf, R. (1982). Chromosome changes in lymphocytes after occupational exposure to pentachlorophenol (PCP). *Mutat. Res.* **102,** 83–88.

Bauer, H., Schultz, K. H., and Speigelberg, U. (1961). Occupational poisoning in the production of chlorophenols. *Arch. Gewerbepathol. Gewerbehyg.* **18,** 538–555 (in German).

Baughman, R. W. (1974). Tetrachlorodibenzo-*p*-dioxins in the environment. High resolution mass spectometry at the picogram level. Ph.D. Thesis, Harvard University, Cambridge, Massachusetts.

Baxter, R. A. (1984). Biochemical study of pentachlorophenol workers. *Am. Occup. Hyg.* **28**, 429–438.

Beale, M. G., Shearer, W. T., Karl, M. M., and Robeson, A. M. (1977). Long-term effects of dioxin exposure. *Lancet* **1**, 748.

Beatty, P. W., and Neal, P. A. (1976). Induction of DT-diaphorase by 2,3,7,8-tetrachlorodibenzo-p-dioxin (TCDD). *Biochem. Biophys. Res. Commun.* **68**, 197–204.

Beatty, P. W., and Neal, R. A. (1978). Factors affecting the induction of DT—diaphorase by 2,3,7,8-tetrachlorodibenzo-p-dioxin. *Biochem. Pharmacol.* **27**, 505–510.

Beatty, P. W., Lembach, K. J., Holscher, M. A., and Neal, R. A. (1975). Effects of 2,3,7,8-tetrachlorodibenzo-p-dioxin (TCDD) on mammalian cells in tissue cultures. *Toxicol. Appl. Pharmacol.* **31**, 309–312.

Beatty, P. W., Vaughn, W. K., and Neal, R. A. (1978). Effect of alteration of rat hepatic mixed-function oxidase (MFO) activity on the toxicity of 2,3,7,8-tetrachlorodibenzo-p-dioxin (TCDD). *Toxicol. Appl. Pharmacol.* **45**, 513–519.

Beechhold, H., and Ehrlich, P. (1906). Relationships between chemical structure and anticeptic action. A contribution to "intrinsic antisepsis." *Hoppe-Seylers' Z. Physiol. Chem.* **47**, 173–179 (in German).

Begley, J., Reichert, E. L., Siemsen, A. W., Rashad, M. N., and Klemmer, H. W. (1977). Association between renal function tests and pentachlorophenol exposure. *Clin. Toxicol.* **11**, 97–106.

Bell, W. B. (1952). Further studies on the production of bovine hyperkeratosis by the administration of the lubricant. *Va. J. Sci.* **3**, 169.

Bell, W. B. (1953). The relative toxicity of chlorinated naphthalenes in experimentally produced bovine hyperkeratosis (X disease). *Vet. Med. (Kansas City, Mo.)* **48**, 135–140.

Bell, W. B. (1954). The production of hyperkeratosis (X disease) by a single administration of chlorinated naphthalenes. *J. Am. Vet. Med. Assoc.* **124**, 289–290.

Bellin, J. S., and Barnes, D. G. (1985). Health hazard assessment for chlorinated dioxins and dibenzofurans other than 2,3,7,8-TCDD. *Toxicol. Ind. Health* **1**, 235–248.

Bergner, H., Constantinidis, P., and Martin, J. H. (1965). Industrial pentachlorophenol poisoning in Winnipeg. *Can. Med. Assoc. J.* **92**, 448–451.

Berry, D. L., Zachariah, P. K., Namkung, M. J., and Juchau, M. R. (1976). Transplacental induction of carcinogen-hydroxylating systems with 2,3,7,8-tetrachlorodibenzo-p-dioxin. *Toxicol. Appl. Pharmacol.* **36**, 569–584.

Berry, D. L., Slaga, T. J., Wilson, N. M., Zachariah, P. K., Namkung, M. J., Bracken, W. M., and Juchau, M. R. (1977). Transplacental induction of mixed-function oxygenases in extra-hepatic tissues by 2,3,7,8-tetrachlorodibenzo-p-dioxin. *Biochem. Pharmacol.* **26**, 1383–1388.

Berry, D. L., Slaga, T. J., DiGiovanni, J., and Jachau, M. R. (1979). Studies with chlorinated dibenzo-p-dioxins, polybrominated biphenyls, and ploychlorinated biphenyls in a two-stage system of mouse skin tumorigenesis: Potent anticarcinogenic effects. *Ann. N. Y. Acad. Sci.* **320**, 405–414.

Bertazzi, P. A., Zocchetti, C., Pesatori, A. C., Buercilena, S., Sanarico, M., and Radice, L. (1989). Ten-year mortality study of the population involved in the Seveso incident in 1976. *Am. J. Epidemiol.* **129**, 1187–1200.

Bettmann (1901). "Chloracne," a distinct form of occupational dermatitis. *Dtsch. Med. Wochenschr.* **27**, 437–440 (in German).

Bevenue, A., Haley, T. J., and Klemmer, H. W. (1967a). A note on the effects of a temporary exposure of an individual to pentachlorophenol. *Bull. Environ. Contam. Toxicol.* **2**, 293–296.

Bevenue, A., Wilson, J., Casarett, L. J., and Klemmer, H. W. (1967b). A survey of pentachlorophenol content in human urine. *Bull. Environ. Contam. Toxicol.* **2**, 319–332.

Bevenue, A., Emerson, M. L., Casarett, L. J., and Yauger, W. L., Jr. (1968). A sensitive gas chromatographic method for the determination of pentachlorophenol in human blood. *J. Chromatogr.* **38**, 467–472.

Bidstrup, P. L. (1952). Clinical aspects of poisoning by dinitro-*ortho*-cresol. *Proc. R. Soc. Med.* **45**, 574–575.

Bidstrup, P. L., and Payne, D. J. H. (1951). Poisoning by dinitro-*ortho*-cresol. *Br. Med. J.* **2**, 16–19.

Bidstrup, P. L., Bonnell, J. A. L., and Harvey, D. G. (1952). Prevention of acute dinitro-*ortho*-cresol (DNOC) poisoning. *Lancet* **1**, 794–795.

Bigelow, S. W., and Nebert, D. W. (1982). The *Ah* regulatory gene product. Survey of nineteen polycyclic aromatic compounds' and fifteen benzo (*a*)pyrene metabolites' capacity to bind to the cytosolic receptor. *Toxicol. Lett.* **10**, 109–118.

Bigelow, S. W., and Nebert, D. W. (1986). The murine aromatic hydrocarbon responsive locus: A comparison of receptor levels and several inducible enzyme activities among recombinant inbred lines. *J. Biochem. Toxicol.* **1**, 1–14.

Bigelow, S. W., Zijlstra, J. A., Yogel, E. W., and Nebert, D. W. (1985). Measurement of the cytosolic *Ah* receptor among four strains of *Drosophila melanogaster*. *Arch. Toxicol.* **56**, 219–225.

Bionetics Research Laboratories (1968). "Evaluation of the Carcinogenic, Teratogenic, and Mutagenic Activities of Selected Pesticides and Industrial Chemicals, Vol. II. Evaluation of the Teratongenic Activity of Selected Pesticides and Industrial Chemicals in Mice and Rats," Publ. Mo. NCI-DCCP-CG 1973-1-2. Prepared by BRL, Bethesda, Maryland for National Cancer Institute.

Birnbaum, L. S. (1985). The role of structure in the disposition of halogenated aromatic xenobiotics. *Environ. Health Perspect.* **61**, 11–20.

Birnbaum, L. S. (1986). Distribution and excretion of 2,3,7,8-tetrachlorodibenzo-p-dioxin in congenic strains of mice which differ at the *Ah* locus. *Drug. Metab. Dispos.* **14**, 34–40.

Birnbaum, L. S., Weber, H., Harris, M. W., Lamb, J. C., IV, and McKinney, J. D. (1985). Toxic interaction of specific polychlorinated biphenyls and 2,3,7,8-tetrachlorodibenzo-p-dioxin: Increased incidence of cleft palate in mice. *Toxicol. Appl. Pharmacol.* **77**, 292–302.

Birnbaum, L. S. Harris, M. W., Miller, C. P., Pratt, R. M., and Lamb, J. C. (1986). Synergistic interaction of 2,3,7,8-tetrachlorodibenzo-p-dioxin and hydrocortisone in the induction of cleft palate in mice. *Teratology* **33**, 29–35.

Birnbaum, L. S. Harris, M. W., Stocking, L. M., Clark, A. M. and Morrissey, R. E. (1989). Retinoic acid and 2,3,7,8-tetrachlorodibenzo-p-dioxin selectively enhance teratogenesis in C57BL/6N mice. *Toxicol. Appl. Pharmacol.* **98**, 487–500.

Blair, D. M. (1961). Dangers of using and handling sodium pentachlorophenate as a molluscicide. *Bull.* **25**, 597–601.

Blank, J. A., Tucker, A. N., Sweatlock, J., Gasiewicz, T. A., and Luster, M. I. (1987). Alpha-naphthoflavone antagonism of 2,3,7,8-tetrachlorodibenzo-p-dioxin induced murine lymphocyte ethoxyresorufin-*O*-deethylase activity and immunosuppression. *Mol. Pharmacol.* **32**, 168–172.

Bleiberg, J., Wallen, M. Brodkin, R., and Applebaum, I. (1964). Industrially acquired porphyria. *Arch. Dermatol.* **84**, 793–601.

Boardman, W. W. (1935). Rapidly developing cataract after dinitrophenol. *J. Am. Med. Assoc.* **105**, 108.

Boberg, E. W. Miller, E. C., Miller, J. A., Poland, A., and Liom, A. (1983). Strong evidence from studies with brachymorphic mice and pentachlorophenol that 1-sulfooxysafrole is the major ultimate electrophilic and carcinogenic metabolite of 1-hydrooxysafrole in mouse liver. *Cancer Res.* **43**, 5163–5173.

Bombick, D. W., Matsumura, F. (1987). TCDD (2,3,7,8-tetrachlorodibenzo-p-dioxin) causes increases in protein tyrosine kinase activities at an early stage of poisoning *in vivo* in rat hepatocyte membranes. *Life Sci.* **41**, 429–436.

Bombick, D. W., Matsumura, F., and Madhukar, B. V. (1984). TCDD (2,3,7,8-tetrachlorodibenzo-p-dioxin) causes reduction in the low density lipoprotein (LDL) receptor activities in the hepatic plasma membrane of the guinea pig and rat. *Biochem. Biophys. Res. Commun.* **118**, 548–554.

Bombick, D. W., Madhukar, B. V., Brewster, D. W., and Matsumura, F. (1985). TCDD (2,3,7,8-tetrachlorodibenzo-p-dioxin) causes increases in protein kinases particularly protein kinase C in the hepatic plasma membrane of the rat and the guinea pig. *Biochem. Biophys. Res. Commun.* **127**, 296–302.

Bombick, D. W., Jankun, J., Tullis, K., and Matsumura, F. (1988). 2,3,7,8-Tetrachlorodibenzo-p-dioxin causes increases in expression of erb-A and levels of protein-tyrosine kinases in selected tissues of responsive mouse strains. *Proc. Natl. Acad. Sci. U.S.A.* **85**, 4128–4132.

Bond, G. G., McLaren, E. A., Lipps, T. E., and Cook, A. M., and Morrissey, R. E. (1989). Update of mortality among chemical workers with potential exposure to the higher chlorinated dioxins. *J. Occup. Med.* **31**, 121–123.

Borzellaca, J. F., Hayes, J. R., Condie, L. W., and Egle, J. L., Jr. (1985). Acute toxicity of monochlorophenols, dichlorophenols and pentachlorophenol in the mouse. *Toxicol. Lett.* **29**, 39–42.

Bough, R. G., Cliffe, E. E., and Lessel, B. (1965). Comparative toxicity and blood level studies on binapacryl and DNBP. *Toxicol. Appl. Pharmacol.* **7**, 353–360.

Boutwell, R. K., and Bosch, D. K. (1959). The tumor promoting action of phenol and related compounds for mouse skin. *Cancer Res.* **19**, 413–423.

Boyd, L. J., McGavack, T. H., Terranova, R., and Piccione, F. V. (1940). Toxic effects following the cutaneous administration of sodium pentachlorophenol. *Bull. N. Y. Med. Coll., Flower Fifth Ave. Hosp.* **3**, 323–329.

Bradlaw, D. W., and Casterline, J. L., Jr. (1979). Induction of enzyme activity in cell culture: A rapid screen for detection of planar polychlorinated organic compounds. *J. Assoc. Off. Anal. Chem.* **62**, 904–906.

Bradlaw, J. A., Garthoff, L. H., Graff, D., and Hurley, N. E. (1975). Detection of chlorinated dioxin induction of aryl hydrocarbon hydroxylase activity in rat hepatoma cell culture. *Toxicol. Appl. Pharmacol.* **33**, 166.

Bradlaw, J. A., Garthoff, L. H., Hurley, N. E., and Firestone, D. (1976). Aryl hydrocarbon hydroxylase activity of twenty-three halogenated dibenzo-p-dioxins. *Toxicol. Appl. Pharmacol.* **37**, 119.

Bradlaw, J. A., Garthoff, L. H., Hurley, N. E., and Firestone, D. (1980). Comparative induction of aryl hydrocarbon hydroxylase activity in vitro by analogues of dibenzo-p-dioxin. *Food Cosmet. Toxicol.* **18**, 627–635.

Braun, W. H., and Sauerhoff, M. W. (1976). The pharmacokinetic profile of pentachlorophenol in monkeys. *Toxicol. Appl. Pharmacol.* **38**, 525–533.

Braun, W. H., Young, J. D., Blau, G. E., and Gehring, P. J. (1977). The pharmacokinetics and metabolism of pentachlorophenol in rats. *Toxicol. Appl. Pharmacol.* **41**, 395–406.

Braun, W. H., Blau, G. E., and Chenoweth, M. B. (1979). The metabolism/pharmacokinetics of pentachlorophenol in man, and a comparison with the rat and monkey. *Dev. Toxicol. Environ. Sci.* **4**, 289–296.

Brewster, D. W., and Birnbaum, L. S. (1987). Disposition and excretion of 2,3,4,7,8-pentachlorodibenzofuran in the rat. *Toxicol. Appl. Pharmacol.* **90**, 243–252.

Brewster, D. W., and Matsumura, F. (1984). TCDD (2,3,7,8-tetrachlorodibenzo-p-dioxin) reduces lipoprotein lipase acivity in the adipose tissue of the guinea pig. *Biochem. Biophys. Res. Commun.* **122**, 810–817.

Brewster, D. W., and Matsumura, F. (1988). Reduction of adipose tissue lipoprotein lipase activity as a result of in vitro administration of 2,3,7,8-tetrachlorodibenzo-p-dioxin to the guinea pig. *Biochem. Pharmacol.* **37**, 2247–2253.

Brewster, D. W., Madhakar, B. V., and Matsumura, F. (1982). Influence of 2,3,7,8-TCDD on the protein composition of the plasma membrane of hepatic cells from the rat. *Biochem. Biophys. Res. Commun.* **107**, 68–74.

Brewster, D. W., Matsumura, F., and Akera, T. (1987). Effects of 2,3,7,8-tetrachlorodibenzo-p-dioxin on the guinea pig heart muscle. *Toxicol. Appl. Pharmacol.* **89**, 408–417.

Brock, W. E., Jones, E. W., MacVicar, R., and Pope, L. S. (1957). Chlorinated naphthalene intoxication in sheep. *Am. J. Vet. Res.* **18**, 625–630.

Bronzetti, G., Lee, I., Zeiger, E., Mailing, H., and Suzuki. (1980). Genetic effects of TCDD in vitro and in vivo using D7 strain of *S. cerevisiae*. *Mutat. Res.* **74**, 206–207.

Bronzetti, G., Bauer, C., Corsi, C., Del Carratare, R., Neeri, R., and Paoline, M. (1983). Mutagenicity study of TCDD and ashes from urban incinerator " in vitro" and "in vivo" using yeast D7 strain. *Chemosphere* **12**, 549–553.

Brown, E. J., Pignatello, J. J., Martinson, M. M., and Crawford, R. L. (1986). Pentachlorophenol degradation: A pure bacterial culture and an epilithic microbial consortium. *Appl. Environ. Microbiol.* **52**, 92–97.

Bruzzi, P. (1983). Health impact of the accidental release of TCDD at Seveso. In "Accidental Exposure to Dioxins: Human Health Aspects" (F. Coulston and F. Pocchiari, eds.), pp. 215–227. Academic Press, New York.

Buchinskiy, V. I. (1974). Fatal poisoning with dinitrocresol. *Sud.-Med. Ekspert.* **17**, 52–53 (in Russian).

Burkatskaja, E. N. (1965). The toxicity of dinitro-o-cresol for warm-blooded animals and problems of its use for industrial hygiene. *Gig. Tr. Prof. Zabol.* **9**, 56–57.

Burkatskaja, E. N., and Anina, I. O. (1969). The uncoupling action of dinitrophenol and its derivatives of oxidative phosphorylation. *Ukr. Biokhim. Zh.* **41**, 576–579.

Buselmair, W., Rohrborn, G., and Propping, P. (1973). Comparative investigations of the mutagenicity of pesticides im mammalian test systems. *Mutat. Res.* **21**, 25–26.

Buser, H.-R. (1975). Polychlorinated dibenzo-p-dioxins. Separation and identification of isomers by gas chromatography–mass spectrometry. *J. Chromatogr.* **114**, 95–108.

Buser, H.-R. (1985). Formation, occurrence and analysis of polychlorinated dibenzo furans, dioxins and related compounds. *Environ. Health Perspect.* **60**, 259–267.

Buser, H.-R., Rappe, C., and Gara, A. (1978). Polychlorinated dibenzofurans (PCDFs) found in Yusho oil and in used Japanese PCB. *Chemosphere* **7**, 439–449.

Bushland, R. C., McAlister, L. C., Jr., Jones, H. A., and Knipling, E. F. (1944). Development of a powder treatment for the control of lice attacking man. *J. Parasitol.* **30**, 377–387.

Buu-Hoi, N. P., Chanh, P.-H., Sesque, G., Agum-Gelade, M. C., and Saint-Ruf, G. (1972). Organs as targets of 'Dioxin' (2,3,7,8,-tetrachlorodibenzo-p-dioxin) intoxication. *Naturwissenschaften* **59**, 174–175.

Byrne, J. J., Carbone, J. P., and Hanson, E. A. (1987). Hypothyroidism and abnormalities in the kinetics of thyroid hormone metabolism in rats treated chronically with polychlorinated biphenyl and polybrominated biphenyl.

Cam, S. (1960). A new epidemic dermatosis of children *Ann. Dermatol. Syphiligr.* **87**, 393–397.

Canga, L., Levi, R., and Rifkind, A. B. (1988). Heart as a target organ in 2,3,7,8-tetrachlorodibenzo-p-dioxin toxicity: Decreased β-adrenergic responsiveness and evidence of increased intracellular calcium. *Proc. Natl. Acad. Sci. U.S.A.* **85**, 905–909.

Cann, H. M., and Verhulst, H. L. (1960). Fatality from acute dinitrophenol derivative poisoning. *Am. J. Dis. Child.* **100**, 947–948.

Cantoni, L., Salmona, M., and Rizzardini, M. (1981). Porphyrogenic effect of chronic treatment with 2,3,7,8-tetrachlorodibenzo-p-dioxin in female rats. *Toxicol. Appl. Pharmacol.* **57**, 156–163.

Cantoni, L., Dal Fiume, D., Rizzardini, M., and Ruggieri, R. (1984a). In vitro inhibitory effect on porphyrinogen carboxylase of liver extracts from TCDD-treated mice. *Toxicol. Lett.* **20**, 211–217.

Cantoni, L., Dal Fiume, D., and Ruggieri, R. (1984b). Decarboxylation of uropophyrinogen I and III in 2,3,7,8-tetrachlorodibenzo-p-dioxin induced porphyria in mice. *Int. J. Biochem.* **16**, 561–565.

Cantrell, J. S., Webb, N. C., and Mabis, A. J. (1969). Identification and crystal structure of a hydropericardium-producing factor: 1,2,3,7,8,9-Hexachloro-dibenzo-p-dioxin. *Acta Crystallogr., Sect. B* **150**–156.

Caramaschi, F., de Crono, G., Favarett, C., Giambelluca, S. E., Montesarchio, E., and Fara, G. M. (1981). Chloracne following environmental contamination by TCDD in Seveso, Italy. *Int. J. Epidemiol.* **10**, 135–143.

Cardus, D., and Hoff, H. E. (1963). Pulmonary ventilation response to the metabolic action of 2,4-dinitrophenol. *Arch. Int. Pharmacodyn.* **144**, 563–570.

Carlstedt-Duke, J. M. B. (1979). Tissue distribution of the receptor for 2,3,7,8-tetrachlorodibenzo-p-dioxin in the rat. *Cancer Res.* **39**, 3172–3176.

Carlstedt-Duke, J. M. B., Elfström, G., Snochowski, M., Hogberg, B., and Gustafsson, J.-A. (1978). Detection of the 2,3,7,8-tetrachlorodibenzo-p-dioxin (TCDD) receptor in rat liver by isoelectric focusing in polyacrylamide gels. *Toxicol. Lett.* **2**, 365–373.

Carlstedt-Duke, J. M. B., Elfström, G., Hogberg, B., and Gustafsson, J.-A. (1979). Ontogeny of the rat hepatic receptor for 2,3,7,8-tetrachlorodibenzo-p-dioxin and its endocrine independence. *Cancer Res.* **39**, 4653–4656.

Carlstedt-Duke, J. M. B., Harnemo, V. B., Hogberg, B., and Gustafsson, J. A. (1981). Interaction of the hepatic receptor protein for 2,3,7,8-tetrachlorodibenzo-*p*-dioxin with DNA. *Biochim. Biophys. Acta* **672**, 131–141.

Carter, C. D., Kimbrough, R. D., Liddle, J. A., Cline, R. E., Zack, M. M., and Barthel, W. F. (1975). Tetrachlorodibenzodioxin: An accidental poisoning episode in horse arenas. *Science* **188**, 738–740.

Casarett, L. J., Bevenue, A., Yauger, W. L., Jr., and Whalen, S. A. (1969). Observations on pentachlorophenol in human blood and urine. *Am. Ind. Hyg. Assoc. J.* **30**, 360–366.

Centers for Disease Control (1984). Results of a pilot study of health effects due to 2,3,7,8-tetrachlorodibenzo-*p*-dioxin contamination—Missouri. *Morbid. Mortal. Wkly. Rep.* **33**, 54–61.

Centers for Disease Control (1988a). Preliminary report. 2,3,7,8-Tetrachlorodibenzo-*p*-dioxin exposure in humans—Seveso, Italy. *Morbid. Mortal. Wkly. Rep.* **37**, 733–736.

Centers for Disease Control (1988b). Serum 2,3,7,8-TCDD levels in the Air Force health study participants-preliminary report. *Morbid. Mortal. Wkly. Rep.* **37**, 309–313.

Cerquiglini Monteriolo, S., di Domenico, A., Silano, V., Viviano, G, and Zapponi, G. (1982). 2,3,7,8-TCDD levels and distribution in the environment at Seveso after the ICMESA accident on July 10th, 1976. *In* "Chlorinated Dioxins and Related Compounds: Impact on the Environment" (O. Hutzinger, R. W. Frei, E. Merian, and F. Pocchiari, eds.), pp. 127–136. Pergamon, New York.

Chang, K. J., Hsieh, K. H., Lee, T. P., Tang, S. Y., and Tung, T. C. (1981). Immunologic evaluation of patients with polychlorinated biphenyl poisoning: Determination of lymphocyte subpopulations. *Toxicol. Appl. Pharmacol.* **61**, 58–63.

Chang, K. J., Hsieh, K. H., Tang, S. Y., and Tung, T. C. (1982). Immunologic evaluation of patients with polychlorinated biphenyl poisoning: Evaluation of delayed-type skin hypersensitive response and its relation to clinical studies. *J. Toxicol. Environ. Health* **9**, 217–223.

Chapman, D. E., and Schiller, C. M. (1985). Dose-related effects of 2,3,7,8-tetrachlorodibenzo-*p*-dioxin (TCDD) in C57BL/6J and DBA/2J mice. *Toxicol. Appl. Pharmacol.* **78**, 147–157.

Chapman, J. B., and Robson, P. (1965). Pentachlorophenol poisoning from bathwater. *Lancet* **1**, 1266–1267.

Chen, P. H., Chang, K. T., and Lu, Y. D. (1981). Polychlorinated biphenyls and polychlorinated dibenzofurans in the toxic rice–bran oil that caused PCB poisoning in Taichung. *Bull. Environ. Contam. Toxicol.* **26**, 489–495.

Chen, P. H., Wong, C.-K., Rappe, C., and Nygren, M. (1985). Polychlorinated biphenyls, dibenzofurans and quaterphenyls in toxic rice–bran oil and in the blood and tissues of patients with PCB poisoning (Yu-Cheng) in Taiwan. *Environ. Health Perspect.* **59**, 59–65.

Cheung, M. O., Gilbert, E. F., and Peterson, R. E. (1981). Cardiovascular teratogenicity of 2,3,7,8-tetrachlorodibenzo-*p*-dioxin in the chick embryo. *Toxicol. Appl. Pharmacol.* **61**, 197–204.

Chou, K., and Cook, R. M. (1979). The effects of pentachlorophenol on fetal and postpartum development in the rat. *Fed. Proc., Fed. Am. Soc. Exp. Biol.* **38**, 868.

Christian, B. J., and Peterson, R. E. (1983). Effects of 2,3,7,8-tetrachlorodibenzo-*p*-dioxin on [³H]thymidine incorporation into rat liver deoxyribonucleic acid. *Toxicology* **8**, 133–146.

Christian, B. J., Inhorn, S. L., and Peterson, R. E. (1986a). Relationship of the wasting syndrome of lethality in rats treated with 2,3,7,8-tetrachlorodibenzo-*p*-dioxin. *Toxicol. Appl. Pharmacol.* **82**, 239–255.

Christian, B. J., Menehan, L. A., and Peterson, R. E. (1986b). Intermediary metabolism of the mature rat following 2,3,7,8-tetrachlorodibenzo-*p*-dioxin treatment. *Toxicol. Appl. Pharmacol.* **83**, 360–378.

Christiansen, H. E., Luginbyhl, T. T., Hill, B. H., Jr. Georgevich, M., McGrath, D. J., Mitchell, F. L., and May, J. R. (eds.) (1974). *Toxic Substances List*, p. 581. U.S. Department of Health, Education, and Welfare, Rockville, Maryland.

Cieciura, L., and Rydzynski, K. (1980). Ultrastructure of hepatic and heart muscle mitochondria after 2,4-dinitrophenol treatment *in vivo*. *Acta Med. Pol.* **21**, 4.

Cirelli, D. (1978). Pentachlorophenol, Position Document I. *Fed. Regist.* **40**, 48446–48477.

Clark, D. A., Gauldie, M. R., Szewchuk, M. R., and Sweeney, G. (1981). Enhanced suppressor cell activity as a mechanism of immunosuppression by 2,3,7,8-tetrachlorodibenzo-*p*-dioxin (TCDD). *Proc. Soc. Exp. Biol. Med.* **168**, 290–299.

Clark, D. A., Sweeney, G., Safe, S., Hancock, E., Kilburn, D. G., and Gauldie, J. (1983). Cellular and genetic basis for suppression of cytotoxic T cell generation by haloaromatic hydrocarbons. *Immunopharmacology* **6**, 143–153.

Cobb, R. R., Stoming, T. A., and Whitney, J. B., III (1987). The aryl hydrocarbon hydroxylase (*Ah*) locus and a novel restriction-fragment length polymorphism (RFLP) are located on mouse chromosome 12. *Biochem. Genet.* **25**, 401–413.

Cockrell, R. S., and Pressman, B. C. (1979). The use of K⁺ concentration gradients for the synthesis of ATP by mitochondria. *In* "Methods in Enzymology" (S. Fleischer and L. Packer, eds.), Vol. 55, Part F, pp. 666–675. Academic Press, New York.

Cohen, G. M., Bracken, W. M., Iyer, R. P., Berry, D. L., Selkirk, J. K., and Slaga, T. J. (1979). Anticarcinogenic effects of 2,3,7,8-tetrachlorodibenzo-*p*-dioxin on benzo(*a*)pyrene and 7,12-dimethylbenz(*a*)anthracene tumor initiation and its relationship to DNA binding. *Cancer Res.* **39**, 4027–4033.

Cole, G. W., Stone, O., Gates, D., and Culver, D. (1986). Chloracne from pentachlorophenol-preserved wood. *Contact Dermatitis* **15**, 164–168.

Collins, W. T., and Capen, C. C. (1980). Fine structural lesions and hormonal alterations in thyroid glands of perinatal rats exposed *in utero* and by the milk to polychlorinated biphenyls. *Am. J. Pathol.* **99**, 125–142.

Collins, W. T., Capen, C. C., Kasza, L., Carter, C., and Dailey, R. E. (1977). Effect of polychlorinated biphenyl (PCB) on the thyroid gland of rats. *Am. J. Pathol.* **89**, 119–136.

Comstock E. G. (1974). Urinary excretion of pentachlorophenol in an occupational exposed population. *Clin. Toxicol.* **7**, 208.

Conklin, P. J., and Fox, F. R. (1978). Environmental impact of pentachlorophenol and its products—a round table discussion. *In* "Pentachlorophenol: Chemistry, Pharmacology and Environmental Toxicology" (K. R. Rao, ed.), pp. 389–394. Plenum, New York.

Constable, J. D., and Hatch, M. C. (1985). Reproductive effects of herbicide exposure in Vietnam: Recent studies by the Vietnamese and others. *Teratog., Carcinog., Mutagen.* **5**, 231–250.

Conway, C. C., and Matsumura, F. (1975). Alteration of cellular utilization of thymidine by TCDD (2,3,7,8-tetrachlorodibenzo-*p*-dioxin). *Bull. Environ. Contam. Toxicol.* **13**, 52–56.

Cook, J. C., and Greenlee, W. F. (1989). Characterization of a specific binding protein for 2,3,7,8-tetrachlorodibenzo-*p*-dioxin in human thymic epithelial cells. *Molec. Pharmacol.* **35**, 713–719.

Cook, J. C., Dold, K. M., and Greenlee, W. F. (1987). An *in vitro* model for studying the toxicity of 2,3,7,8-tetrachlorodibenzo-*p*-dioxin to human thymus. *Toxicol. Appl. Pharmacol.* **89**, 256–268.

Cook, R. R. (1981). Dioxin, chloracne and soft-tissue sarcoma. *Lancet* **1**, 618–619.

Corti, A. L. (1954). Fatal poisoning with dinitro-*o*-cresol. *Rev. Farm. (Buenos Aires)* **95**, 157–166.

Costlow, R. D., Lutz, M. F., Kane, W. W., Hurt, S. S., and O'Hara, G. P. (1986). Dinocap: Developmental toxicity studies in rabbits. *Toxicologist* **6**, 85.

Coulston, F., and Olajos, E. J. (1980). Panel Report: Panel to discuss the epidemiology of 2,4,5-T. New York City, July 10–11, 1979. *Ecotoxicol. Environ. Saf.* **4**, 96–102.

Coulston, F., and Pocchiari, F., eds. (1983). "Accidental Exposure to Dioxins: Human Health Aspects." Academic Press, New York.

Courtney, K. D., and Moore, J. A. (1971). Teratology studies with 2,4,5-T and 2,3,7,8-TCDD. *Toxicol. Appl. Pharmacol.* **20**, 396–403.

Courtney, K. D., Putnam, J. P., and Andrews, J. E. (1978). Metabolic studies with TCDD (dioxin) treated rats. *Arch. Environ. Contam. Toxicol.* **7**, 385–396.

Cranmer, M., and Freal, J. (1970). Gas chromatographic analysis of pentachlorophenol in human urine by formation of alkyl ethers. *Life Sci.* **9**, (Part 2), 121–128.

Cresteil, T., Jaiswal, A. K., and Eisen, H. J. (1987). Transcriptional control of human cytochrome P_1-450 gene expression by 2,3,7,8-tetrachlorodibenzo-*p*-dioxin in human tissue culture cell lines. *Arch. Biochem. Biophys.* **253**, 233–240.

Croft, W., Yang, K. H., and Peterson, R. E. (1977). Pathological effects of 2,3,7,8-tetrachlorodibenzo-*p*-dioxin on the common bile duct of rats. *Fed. Proc., Fed. Am. Soc. Exp. Biol.* **36**, 1060.

Crosby, D. G., and Wong, A. S. (1977). Environmental degradation of 2,3,7,8-tetrachlorodibenzo-*p*-dioxin (TCDD). *Science* **195**, 1337–1338.

Crow, K. D. (1978). Chloracne, an up to date assessment. *Ann. Occup. Hyg.* **21**, 297–298.

Crow, K. D. (1981). Chloracne and its potential clinical implications. *Clin. Exp. Dermatol.* **6**, 243–257.

Crow, K. D. (1983). Chloracne (halogen acne). *In* "Dermatoxicology" (F. N. Marzulli and H. L. Maibach, eds.), 2d ed. pp. 461–482. Hemisphere Publishing, Washington, D.C.

Cunarro, J., and Weiner, W. M. (1975). Mechanism of action of agents that uncouple oxidative phosphorylation: Direct correlation between proton-carrying and respiratory-releasing properties using rat liver mitochondria. *Biochim. Biophys. Acta* **387**, 234–240.

Cunningham, H. M., and Williams, D. T. (1972). Effect of 2,3,7,8-tetrachlorodibenzo-*p*-dioxin on growth rate and the synthesis of lipids and proteins in rats. *Bull. Environ. Contam. Toxicol.* **7**, 45–51.

Cuthill, S., Poellinger, L., and Gustafsson, J.-A. (1987). The receptor for 2,3,7,8-tetrachlordibenzo-*p*-dioxin in the mouse hepatoma cell line Hepa 1c1c7. *J. Biol. Chem.* **262**, 3477–3481.

Cuthill, S., Wilhelmssom, A., Mason, G. G. F., Gillner, M., Poellinger, L., and Gustafsson, J.-A. (1988). The dioxin receptor: A comparison with the glucocorticoid receptor. *J. Steroid Biochem.* **30**, 277–280.

Cutting, W. C., Mehrtens, H. G., and Tainter, M. L. (1933). Dinitrophenol action and uses. *JAMA, J. Am. Med. Assoc.* **101**, 193–195.

D'Argy, R., Hassoun, E., and Dencker, L. (1984). Teratogenicity of TCDD and the congener 3,3′,4,4′-tetrachloroazobenzene in sensitive and non-sensitive mouse strains after reciprocal blastocyst transfer. *Toxicol. Lett.* **21**, 197–202.

Dean, J. H., Luster, G. A., Boorman, G. A., Chae, K., Lauer, L. D., Luebke, R. W., Lawson, L. D., and Wilson, R. E. (1981). Assessment of immunotoxicity induced by the environmental chemicals 2,3,7,8-tetrachlorodibenzo-*p*-dioxin, diethylstilbestrol, and benzo(*a*)pyrene. *In* "Advances in Pharmacology" (J. Hadden, L. Chedid, P. Mullen, and F. Spreafico, eds.), pp. 35–7. Pergamon, New York.

Debets, F. M. H., Strik, J. J. T. W. A., and Olie, K. (1980). Effects of pentachlorophenol on rat liver changes induced by hexachlorobenzene, with special reference to porphyria, and alterations in mixed function oxygenases. *Toxicology* **15**, 181–195.

de Calmonovici, R. W., and San Martin de Viale, L. C. (1980). Effect of chlorophenols on porphyrin metabolism in rats and chick embryo. *Int. J. Biochem.* **12**, 1039–1044.

Deeken, J. H. (1974). Chloracne induced by 2,6-dichlorobenzonitrile. *Arch. Dermatol.* **109**, 245–246.

Deichmann, W., Machle, W., Kitzmiller, K. V., and Thomas, G. (1942). Acute and chronic effects of pentachlorophenol and sodium pentachlorophenate upon experimental animals. *J. Pharmacol. Exp. Ther.* **76**, 104–117.

Deleze, J., and Herve, J. C. (1983). Effect of several uncouplers of cell-to-cell communication on gap junction morphology in mammalian heart. *J. Membr. Biol.* **74**, 203–215.

Demidenko, N. M. (1969). Materials for establishing the maximum permissible concentration of pentachlorophenol in air. *Gig. Tr. Prof. Zabol.* **13**, 58–60.

Dencker, L. (1985). The role of receptors in 2,3,7,8-tetrachlorodibenzo-*p*-dioxin (TCDD) toxicity. *Arch. Toxicol., Suppl.* **8**, 43–60.

Dencker, L., and Pratt, R. M. (1981). Association between the presence of the *Ah*-receptor in embryonic murine tissues and sensitivity to TCDD-induced cleft palate. *Teratog., Carcinog., Mutagen.* **1**, 399–406.

Dencker, L., Hassoun, E., D'Argy, R., and Alm, G. (1985). Fetal thymus organ culture as an in vivo model for the toxicity of 2,3,7,8-tetrachlorodibenzo-*p*-dioxin and its congeners. *Mol. Pharmacol.* **27**, 133–140.

Den Engelse, L., Floot, B. G. J., Menkveld, G. J., and Tates, A. D. (1986). Enhanced repair of O^6-methylguanine in liver DNA of rats pretreated with phenobarbital, 2,3,7,8-tetrachlorodibenzo-*p*-dioxin, ethionine, or *N*-alkyl-*N*-nitrosoureas. *Carcinogenesis (London)* **7**, 1941–1947.

Denison, M. S., and Wilkinson, C. F. (1985). Identification of the *Ah* receptor in selected mammalian species and induction of aryl hydrocarbon hydroxylase. *Eur. J. Biochem.* **147**, 429–43.

Denison, M. S., Hamilton, J. W., and Wilkinson, C. F. (1985). Comparative studies of aryl hydrocarbon hydroxylase and the *Ah* receptor in nonmammalian species. *Comp. Biochem. Physiol., C* **80C**, 319–324.

Denison, M. S., Okey, A. B., Hamilton, J. W., Bloom, S. E., and Wilkinson, C. F. (1986a). *Ah* receptor for 2,3,7,8-tetrachlorodibenzo-*p*-dioxin: Ontogeny in chick embryo liver. *J. Biochem. Toxicol.* **1**, 39–49.

Denison, M. S., Vella, L. M., and Okey, A. B. (1986b). Structure and function of the *Ah* receptor for 2,3,7,8-tetrachlorodibenzo-*p*-dioxin. Species differences in molecular properties of the receptors from mouse and rat hepatic cytosols. *J. Biol. Chem.* **262**, 3987–3995.

Denison, M. S., Fisher, J. M., and Whitlock, J. P., Jr. (1988). Inducible, receptor-dependent protein–DNA interactions at a dioxin-responsive transcriptional enhancer. *Proc. Natl. Acad. Sci. U.S.A.* **85**, 2528–2532.

Denison, M. S., Fisher, J. M., and Whitlock, J. P., Jr. (1989). Protein-DNA interactions at recognition sites for the dioxin-Ah receptor complex. *J. Biol. Chem.* **264**, 16478–16482.

Denomme, M. A., Homonoko, K., Fujita, T., Sawyer, T., and Safe, S. (1985). Effects of substituents on the cytosolic binding activities and AHH induction potencies of 7-substituted 2,3-dichlorodibenzo-*p*-dioxins—a QSAR analysis. *Mol. Pharmacol.* **27**, 656–665.

Denomme, M. A., Homonko, K., Fujita, T., Sawyer, T., and Safe, S. (1986). Substituted polychlorinated dibenzofuran receptor binding affinities and aryl hydrocarbon hydroxylase induction potencies—a QSAR analysis. *Chem.-Biol. Interact.* **57**, 175–187.

Desaiah, D. (1978). Effect of pentachlorophenol on the ATPase in rat tissues. *In* "Pentachlorophenol: Chemistry, Pharmacology and Environmental Toxicology" (K. R. Rao, ed.), pp. 277–283. Plenum Press, New York.

DiBartolomeis, M. J., Moore, R. W., Peterson, R. E., and Jefcoate, C. R. (1986a). Hypercholesterolemia and the regulation of adrenal steroidogenesis in 2,3,7,8-tetrachlorodibenzo-*p*-dioxin-treated rats. *Toxicol. Appl. Pharmacol.* **85**, 313–323.

DiBartolomeis, M. J., Williams, C., and Jefcoate, C. R. (1986b). Inhibition of ACTH action on cultured bovine adrenal cortical cells by 2,3,7,8-tetrachlorodibenzo-*p*-dioxin through a redistribution of cholesterol. *J. Biol. Chem.* **261**, 4432–4437.

DiBartolomeis, M. J., Moore, R. W., Peterson, R. E., Christian, B. J., and Jefcoate, C. R. (1987). Altered regulation of adrenal steroidogenesis in 2,3,7,8-tetrachlorodibenzo-*p*-dioxin-treated rats. *Biochem. Pharmacol.* **36**, 59–67.

Dickens, M., Seefeld, M. D., and Peterson, R. E. (1981). Enhanced liver DNA synthesis in partially hepatectomized rats pretreated with 2,3,7 8-tetrachlorodibenzo-*p*-dioxin. *Toxicol. Appl. Pharmacol.* **58**, 389–398.

di Domenico, A., Viviano, G., and Zapponi, G. (1982). Environmental persistence of 2,3,7,8-TCDD at Seveso. *In* "Chlorinated Dioxins and Related Compounds: Impact on the Environment: (O. Hutzinger, R. W. Frei, E. Merian, and F. Pocchiari, eds.), pp. 105–114. Pergamon, New York.

Dietrich, R. R., Bludeau, P., Stock, T., and Roper, M. (1977). Induction of different rat liver supernatant aldehyde dehydrogenases by phenobarbital and tetrachlorodibenzo-*p*-dioxin. *J. Biol. Chem.* **252**, 6169–6176.

DiGiovanni, J., Viaje, A., Berry, D. L., Slaga, T. J., and Juchau, M. R. (1977). Tumor-initiating ability of 2,3,7,8-tetrachlorodibenzo-*p*-dioxin (TCDD) and Aroclor 1254 in the two-stage system of mouse skin carcinogenesis. *Bull. Environ. Contam. Toxicol.* **18**, 552–557.

DiGiovanni, J., Berry, D. L., Juchau, M. R., and Slaga, T. J. (1979). 2,3,7,8-Tetrachlorodibenzo-*p*-dioxin: Potent anticarcinogenic activity in CD-1 mice. *Biochem. Biophys. Res. Commun.* **86**, 577–584.

Dodds, E. C., and Robertson, J. D. (1933a). The clinical applications of dinitro-*o*-cresol. *Lancet* **2**, 1137–1139.

Dodds, E. C., and Robertson, J. D. (1933b). The clinical applications of dinitro-o-cresol. II. A study of myxoedema. *Lancet* **2**, 1197–1198.

Dooley, R. K, and Holsapple, M. P. (1987). The primary cellular target responsible for tetrachlorodibenzo-p-dioxin (TCDD) induced immunosuppression is the B-lymphocyte. *Fed. Proc., Fed. Am. Soc. Exp. Biol.* **46**, A1310.

Dougherty, R. C., and Piotrowska, K. (1976). Screening by negative chemical ionization mass spectrometry for environmental contamination with toxic residues: Application to human urines. *Proc. Natl. Acad. Sci. U.S.A.* **73**, 1777–1781.

Dugois, P., and Colomb, L. (1957). Remarks on chlorine acne. *J. Med. Lyon* **38**, 899–903 (in French).

Dunckel, A. E. (1975). An updating on the polybrominated biphenyl disaster in Michigan. *J. Am. Vet. Med. Assoc.* **167**, 838–841.

Duran-Reynolds, M., Lillie, F., Bartsch, H., and Blank, K. J. (1978). The genetic basis of susceptibility of leukemia induction in mice by 3-methylcholanthrene applied subcutaneously. *J. Exp. Med.* **147**, 459–469.

Durrin, L. K., Jones, P. B. C., Fisher, J. M., Galeazzi, D. R., and Whitlock, J. P., Jr. (1987). 2,3,7,8-Tetrachlorodibenzo-p-dioxin receptors regulate transcription of the cytochrome P_1-450 gene. *J. Cell. Biochem.* **35**, 153–160.

Eadon, G., Kaminsky, L., Silkworth, J., Aldous, K., Hilker, D., O'Keefe, P., Smith, R., Gierthy, J., Hawley, J., Kim, N., and DeCaprio, A. (1986). Calculation of 2,3,7,8-equivalent concentrations of complex environmental contaminant mixtures. *Environ. Health Perspect.* **70**, 221–227.

Edgerton, T. R., Moseman, R. F., Linder, R. E., and Wright, L. H. (1979). Multi-residue method for the determination of chlorinated phenol metabolites in urine. *J. Chromatogr.* **170**, 331–342.

Edson, E. F. (1954). Estimation of dinitro-ortho-cresol in blood. *Lancet* **1**, 981–982.

Edson, E. F. (1957). "Health Record of Dinitro—Campaigns, 1955–1956." Medical Dept., Fisons Pest Control Limited.

Edson, E. F. (1960). Applied toxicology of pesticides. *Pharm. J.* **185**, 361–367.

Eiseman, J. L., Gehring, P. J., and Gibson, J. E. (1974). Kinetics of *in vitro* nitro reduction of 2,4-dinitrophenol by rat liver homogenates. *Toxicol. Appl. Pharmacol.* **27**, 140–144.

Eisen, H. J., Hannah, R. R., Legreverend, C., Okey, A. B., and Nebert, D. W. (1983). The *Ah* receptor: Controlling factor in the induction of drug-metabolizing enzymes by certain chemical carcinogens and other environmental pollutants. *In* "Biochemical Actions of Hormones" (G. Litwack, ed.), Vol. 10, pp. 227–257. Academic Press, New York.

Eisenhardt, R. H., and Rosenthal, O. (1964). 2,4-Ditrophenol: Lack of interaction with high-energy intermediates of oxidative phosphorylation. *Science* **143**, 476–477.

Ekström, G., and Ingelman-Sundberg, M. (1986). Mechanisms of lipid peroxidation dependent upon cytochrome P-450 LM_2. *Eur. J. Biochem.* **158**, 201.

Elder, G. H. (1978). Porphyria caused by hexachlorobenzene and other polyhalogenated aromatic hydrocarbons. *Handb. Exp. Pharmakol* **44**, 157–200.

Elder, G. H., and Sheppard, D. M. (1982). Immunoreactive uroporphyrinogen decarboxylase is unchanged in porphyria caused by TCDD and hexachlorobenzene. *Biochem. Biophys. Res. Commun.* **109**, 113–120.

Erickson, J. D., Mulinare, J., McClain, P. W., Fitch, T. G., James, L. M., McClearn, A. B., and Adams, M. J. (1984). Vietnam veterans' risk for fathering babies with birth defects. *JAMA, J. Am. Med. Assoc.* **252**, 903–912.

Eriksson, M., Hardell, L., O'Berg, N., Moller, T., and Axelson, O. (1981). Soft-tissue sarcomas and exposure to chemical substances: A case-referent study. *Br. J. Ind. Med.* **38**, 27–33.

Ericksson, M., Hardell, L., and Adami, H-O. (1990). Exposure to dioxins as a risk factor for soft tissue sarcoma: A population-based case-control study. *J. Natl. Cancer Inst.* **82**, 486–490.

Ernst, W., and Bar, R. (1964). The metabolism of 2,4-dinitro-6-sec-butylphenol and its ester in animals. *Arzneim.-Forsch.* **14**, 81–84 (in German).

Exner, J. H., ed. (1987). "Solving Hazardous Waste Problems. Learning from Dioxins." Am. Chem. Soc., Washington, D.C.

Facchetti, S., Fornari, A., and Montagna, M. (1980). Distribution of 2,3,7,8-tetrachlorodibenzo-p-dioxin in the tissues of a person exposed to the toxic cloud at Seveso. *Adv. Mass. Spectrom.* **8B**, 1405–1414.

Fahring, R., Nilsson, C. A., and Rappe, C. (1978). Genetic activity of chlorophenols and chlorophenol impurities. *In* "Pentachlorophenol: Chemistry, Pharmacology and Environmental Toxicology" (K. R. Rao, ed.), pp. 325–338. Plenum, New York.

Faith, R. E., and Moore, J. A. (1977). Impairment of thymus-dependent immune functions by exposure of developing immune system to 2,3,7,8-tetrachlorodibenzo-p-dioxin (TCDD). *J. Toxicol. Environ. Health* **3**, 451–464.

Faith, R. E., Luster, M. I., and Moore, J. A. (1978). Chemical separation of helper cell function and delayed type hypersensitivity. *Cell. Immunol.* **40**, 275–284.

Fanelli, R., Bertoni, M. P., Bonfanti, M., Castelli, M. G., Chiabrando, C., Martelli, G. P., Noe, M. A., Noseda, A., Garrattini, S., Binaghi, C., Marazza, V., Pezza, F., Pozzoli, D., and Cicognetti, G. (1980). 2,3,7,8-Tetrachlorodibenzo-p-dioxin levels in cow's milk from the contaminated area of Seveso, Italy. *Bull. Environ. Contam. Toxicol.* **24**, 634–639.

Felton, J. S., Nebert, D. W. (1975). Mutagenesis of certain activated carcinogens *in vitro* associated with genetically mediated increases in monooxygenase activity and cytochrome P_1-450. *J. Biol. Chem.* **250**, 6769–6778.

Ferioli, A., Harvey, C., and DeMatteis, F. (1984). Drug-induced accumulation of uroporphyrin in chicken hepatocyte cultures. *Biochem. J.* **224**, 769–777.

Fernandez, M., Roy, M., and Lesca, P. (1988). Binding characteristics of *Ah* receptors from rats and mice before and after separation from hepatic cytosols. 7-Hydroxyellipticine as a competitive antagonist of cytochrome P-450 induction. *Eur. J. Biochem.* **172**, 585–592.

Field, B., and Kerr, C. (1979). Herbicide use and incidence of neural-tube defects. *Lancet* **1**, 1341–1342.

Filippini. G., Bordo, B., Crenna, P., Massetto, N., Musicco, M., and Boeri, R. (1981). Relationship between clinical and electrophysiological findings and indicators of heavy exposure to 2,3,7,8-tetrachlorodibenzo-p-dioxin. *Scand. J. Work Environ. Health* **7**, 257–262.

Fine, J. S., Gasiewicz, T. A., and Silverstone, A. E. (1989). Lymphocyte stem cell alterations following perinatal exposure to 2,3,7,8-tetrachlorodibenzo-p-dioxin. *Molec. Pharmacol.* **35**, 18–25.

Fine, J. S., Silverstone, A. E., and Gasiewicz, T. A. (1990). Impairment of prothymocyte activity by 2,3,7,8-tetrachlorodibenzo-p-dioxin. *J. Immunol.* **144**, 1169–1176.

Fingerhut, M. A., Halperin, W. F., Honchar, P. A., Smith, A. B., Groth, D. H., and Russell, W. O. (1984). An evaluation of reports of dioxin exposure and soft tissue sarcoma pathology among chemical workers in the United States. *Scand. J. Work Environ. Health* **10**, 299–303.

Fingerhut, M. A., Sweeney, M. H., Halperin, W. E., and Schnorr, T. M. (1987). Epidemiology of populations exposed to dioxins. *In* "Solving Hazardous Waste Problems. Learning from Dioxins" (J. H. Exner, ed.), pp. 142–161. Am. Chem. Soc., Washington, D.C.

Firestone, D. (1973). Etiology of chick edema disease. *Environ. Health Perspect.* **5**, 59–66.

Flick, D. F., Firestone, D., and Higginbotham, G. R. (1972). Studies of the chick edema disease. 9. Response of chicks fed or singly administered synthetic edema-producing compounds. *Poult. Sci.* **51**, 2026–2034.

Food and Agriculture Organization/World Health Organization (FAO/WHO) (1970). "1969 Evaluations of Some Pesticide Residues in Food." Monograph prepared by the Joint Meeting of the FAO Working Party of Experts and the WHO Expert Group on Pesticide Residues, which met in Rome, December 8–15, 1969, WHO/Food Add./70.38. World Health Organ., Geneva.

Fouts, J. R., and Brodie, B. B. (1957). The enzymatic reduction of chloramphenicol, p-nitrobenzoic acid and other aromatic nitro compounds in mammals. *J. Pharmacol. Exp. Ther.* **119**, 197–207.

Fowler, B. A., Lucier, G. W., Brown, H. W., and McDaniel, O. S. (1973). Ultrastructural changes in rat liver cells following a single oral dose of TCDD. *Environ. Health Perspect.* **5**, 141–148.

Fowler, B. A., Hook, G. E. R., and Lucier, G. W. (1975). Tetrachlorodibenzo-p-dioxin induction of renal microsomal enzyme systems. *Toxicol. Appl. Pharmacol.* **33**, 176–177.

Fowler, B. A., Hook, G. E. R., and Lucier, G. W. (1977). Tetrachlorodibenzo-*p*-dioxin induction of renal microsomal enzyme systems: Ultrastructural effects on pars recta (S3) proximal tubule cells of the rat kidney. *J. Pharmacol. Exp. Ther.* **203**, 712–721.

Fraczek, S. (1979). Toxicity studies on dinocap. Part V. Preliminary studies on effects on the reproduction. *Bromatol. Chem. Toksykol.* **12**, 351–356.

Frank, D. M., Yamashita, T. S., and Blumer, J. K. (1982). Genetic differences in methylcholanthrene mediated suppression of cutaneous delayed hypersensitivity in mice. *Toxicol. Appl. Pharmacol.* **64**, 31–41.

Fries, G. F. (1984). The PBB episode in Michigan: An overall appraisal. *CRC Crit. Rev. Toxicol.* **16**, 105–156.

Fuerst, P., Meemken, H.-A., and Groebel, W. (1986). Determination of polychlorinated dibenzodioxins and dibenzofurans in human milk. *Chemosphere* **15**, 1977–1980.

Fuhrman, G. J., Weymouth, F. W., and Fields, J. (1943). The effect of environmental temperatures on the toxicity of 2,4-dinitrophenol in mice. *J. Pharmacol. Exp. Ther.* **79**, 176–178.

Fujisawa-Sehara, A., Yamane, M., and Fujii-Kuriyama, Y. (1988). A DNA-binding factor specific for xenobiotic responsive elemtents of P-450c gene exists as a cryptic form in cytoplasm: Its possible translocation to nucleus. *Proc. Natl. Acad. Sci. U.S.A.* **85**, 5859–5863.

Furuhashi, N., Kurl, R. N., Wong, J., and Villee, C. A. (1986). A cytosolic binding protein for 2,3,7,8-tetrachlorodibenzo-*p*-dioxin (TCDD) in the uterus and deciduoma of rats. *Pharmacology* **33**, 110–120.

Furukawa, H., Kawai, N., and Kawai, K. (1985). Frameshift mutagenicity of dinitrobenzene derivatives on *Salmonella typhimurium* TA98 and Tm elevation of calf thymus DNA by dinitrobenzene derivatives. *Nucleic Acids Symp. Ser.* **16**, 5–8.

Gaines, T. B. (1969). Acute toxicity of pesticides. *Toxicol. Appl. Pharmacol.* **4**, 515–534.

Gallo, M. A., Hesse, E. J., Macdonald, G. J., and Umbreit, T. H. (1986). Interactive effects of estrodiol and 2,3,7,8-tetrachlorodibenzo-*p*-dioxin on hepatic cytochrome P-450 and mouse uterus. *Toxicol. Lett.* **32**, 123–132.

Ganote, C. E., Grinwald, P. M., and Nayler, W. G. (1984). 2,4-Dinitrophenol (DNP)-induced injury in calcium-free hearts. *J. Mol. Cell. Cardiol.* **16**, 547–557.

Garattini, S. (1977). TCDD poisoning at Seveso. *Biomedicine* **26**, 28–29.

Garrett, N. E., Stack, H. F., and Waters, M. D. (1986). Evaluation of the genetic activity profiles of 65 pesticides. *Mutat. Res.* **168**, 301–325.

Gasiewicz, T. A., and Bauman, P. A. (1987). Heterogeneity of the rat hepatic *Ah* receptor and evidence for transformation *in vitro* and *in vivo*. *J. Biol. Chem.* **262**, 2116–2120.

Gasiewicz, T. A., and Neal, R. A. (1979). 2,3,7,8-Tetrachlorodibenzo-*p*-dioxin tissue distribution, excretion, and effects on clinical chemical parameters in guinea pigs. *Toxicol. Appl. Pharmacol.* **51**, 329–339.

Gasiewicz, T. A., and Neal, R. A. (1982). The examination and quantitation of tissue cytosolic receptors for 2,3,7,8-tetrachlorodibenzo-*p*-dioxin using hydroxylapatite. *Anal. Biochem.* **124**, 1–11.

Gasiewicz, T. A., and Rucci, G. (1984). Cytosolic receptor for 2,3,7,8-tetrachlorodibenzo-*p*-dioxin. Evidence for a homologous nature among various mammalian species. *Mol. Pharmacol.* **26**, 90–98.

Gasiewicz, T. A., Holscher, M. A., and Neal, R. A. (1980). The effect of total parenteral nutrition on the toxicity of 2,3,7,8-tetrachlorodibenzo-*p*-dioxin in the rat. *Toxicol. Appl. Pharmacol.* **54**, 469–488.

Gasiewicz, T. A., Geiger, L. E., Rucci, G., and Neal, R. A. (1983a). Distribution, excretion, and metabolism of 2,3,7,8-tetrachlorodibenzo-*p*-dioxin in C57BL/6J, DBA/2J, and B6D2F1/J mice. *Drug Metab. Dispos.* **11**, 397–403.

Gasiewicz, T. A., Olson, J. R., Geiger, L. E., and Neal, R. A. (1983b). Absorption, distribution, and metabolism of 2,3,7,8-tetrachlorodibenzo-*p*-dioxin (TCDD) in experimental animals. *In* "Human and Environmental Risks of Chlorinated Dioxins and Related Compounds" (R. E. Tucker, A. L. Young, and A. P. Gray, eds.), pp. 495–525. Plenum, New York.

Gasiewicz, T. A., Ness, W. C., and Rucci, G. (1984). Ontogeny of the cytosolic

receptor for 2,3,7,8-tetrachlorodibenzo-*p*-dioxin in rat liver, lung, and thymus. *Biochem. Biophys. Res. Commun.* **118**, 183–190.

Gasiewicz, T. A., Rucci, G., Henry, E. C., and Baggs, R. (1986). Changes in hamster hepatic cytochrome P-450, ethoxycoumarin *O*-deethylase, and reduced NAD(P) : menadione oxidoreductase following treatment with 2,3,7,8-tetrachlorodibenzo-*p*-dioxin. Partial dissociation of temporal and dose–response relationships from elicited toxicity. *Biochem. Pharmacol.* **35**, 2737–2742.

Gatz, E. E., and Jones, J. R. (1969). A comparative study of the effects of chlorpromazine and haloperidol upon oxidative phosphorylation by rat brain mitochondria obtained by two different isolation procedures. *Pharmacologist* **11**, 290.

Gatz, E. E., and Jones, J. R. (1970). Haloperidol antagonism to hyperpyretic and lethal effects of 2,4-dinitrophenol in rats. *Anesth. Analg. (Cleveland)* **49**, 773–780.

Gaultier, M., Gervais, P., and Conso, F. (1974). Acute intoxication by dinitroorthocresol. *J. Eur. Toxicol.* **7**, 9–11 (in French).

Gehring, P. J., and Buerge, J. F. (1969). The distribution of 2,3-dinitrophenol relative to its cataractogenic activity in ducklings and rabbits. *Toxicol. Appl. Pharmacol.* **15**, 574–592.

Geiger, L. E., and Neal, R. A. (1981). Mutagenicity testing of 2,3,7,8-tetrachlorodibenzo-*p*-dioxin in histidine auxotrophs of *Salmonella typhimurium*. *Toxicol. Appl. Pharmacol.* **59**, 125–129.

George, J. D., and Manson, J. M. (1986). Strain-dependent differences in the metabolism of 3-methylcholanthrene by maternal, placental, and fetal tissues of C57BL/6J and DBA/2J mice. *Canc. Res.* **46**, 5671–5675.

George, M., Cherery, R. J., and Krishna, G. (1982). The effect of ionophore A23187 and 2,4-dinitrophenol on the structure and function of cultured liver cells. *Toxicol. Appl. Pharmacol.* **66**, 349–360.

Georgescu, J. (1932). Studies on the action of 1,2,4-dinitrophenol (Thermol). VI. Glucuronate content of the urine after injection of 1,2,4-dinitrophenol. *Ann. Physiol. Physicochim. Biol.* **8**, 122–126.

Germolec, D. R., Rosenthal, G. J., Silver, M. T., Wiegand, G. W., Clark, G., and Luster, M. I. (1987). Selective effects of TCDD and dexamethasone on B-cell maturation. *Fed. Proc., Fed. Am. Soc. Exp. Biol.* **46**, A5243.

Geyer, H. J., Scheunert, I., and Korte, F. (1987). Distribution and bioconcentration potential of the environmental chemical pentachlorophenol (PCP) in different tissues of humans. *Chemosphere* **16**, 887–899.

Giavini, E., Broccia, M. L., Prati, M., and Vismara, C. (1986). Effect of method of administration on the teratogenicity of dinoseb in the rat. *Arch. Environ. Contam. Toxicol.* **15**, 377–384.

Gibson, J. E. (1973). Teratology studies in mice with 2-*sec*-butyl-4,6-dinitrophenol (dinoseb). *Food Cosmet. Toxicol.* **11**, 31–43.

Gibson, J. E., (1976). Perinatal nephropathies. *Environ. Health Perspect.* **15**, 2121–2130.

Gibson, J. E., and Rao, K. S. (1973). Disposition of 2-*sec*-butyl-4,6-dinitrophenol (dinoseb). *Food Cosmet. Toxicol.* **11**, 45–52.

Gierthy, J. F., and Crane, D. (1984). Reversible inhibition of *in vitro* epithelial cell proliferation by 2,3,7,8-tetrachlorodibenzo-*p*-dioxin. *Toxicol. Appl. Pharmacol.* **74**, 91–98.

Gilbert, P., Saint-Ruf, G., Poncelet, F., and Mercier, M. (1980). Genetic effects of chlorinated anilines and azobenzenes on *Salmonella typhimurium*. *Arch. Environ. Contam. Toxicol.* **9**, 533–541.

Gillner, M., Bergman, J., Cambillau, C., Fernstrom, B., and Gustafsson, J.-A. (1985). Interactions of indoles with specific binding sites for 2,3,7,8-tetrachlorodibenzo-*p*-dioxin in rat liver. *Mol. Pharmacol.* **28**, 357–363.

Gillner, M., Brittebo, E. B., Brandt, I., Soderkrist, P., Appelgren, L.-E., and Gustafsson, J.-A. (1987). Uptake and specific binding of 2,3,7,8-tetrachlorodibenzo-*p*-dioxin in the olfactory mucosa of mice and rats. *Cancer Res.* **47**, 4150–4159.

Gillner, M., Bergman, J., Cambillau, C., and Gustafsson, J.-A. (1989). Interactions of rutaecarpine alkaloids with specific binding sites for 2,3,7,8-tetrachlorodibenzo-*p*-dioxin in rat liver. *Carcinogenesis* **10**, 651–654.

Giri, A. K. (1986). Mutagenic and genotoxic effects of 2,3,7,8-tetrachlorodibenzo-*p*-dioxin. A review. *Mutat. Res.* **168**, 241–248.

Gladen, B. C., Rogan, W. J., Ragan, H. B., and Spierto, F. W. (1988). Urinary porphyrins in children exposed transplacentally to polyhalogenated aromatics in Taiwan. *Arch. Environ. Health* **43**, 54–58.

Goldmann, P. J. (1973). Severest acute chloracne. A mass poisoning by 2,3,6,7-tetrachlorodibenzodioxin. *Hautarzt* **24**, 149–152.

Goldstein, J. A. (1979). The structure—activity relationships of the halogenated biphenyls as enzyme inducers. *Ann. N. Y. Acad. Sci.* **320**, 164–178.

Goldstein, J. A. (1980). Structure–activity relationships for the biochemical effects and the relationship to toxicity. *In* "Halogenated Biphenyls, Terphenyls, Naphthalenes, Dibenzodioxins and Related Products" (R. D. Kimbrough, ed.), Elsevier/North-Holland Biomedical Press, New York.

Goldstein, J. A., and Linko, P. (1984). Differential induction of two 2,3,7,8-tetrachlorodibenzo-p-dioxin-inducible forms of cytochrome P-450 in extrahepatic versus hepatic tissues. *Mol. Pharmacol.* **25**, 185–191.

Goldstein, J. A., and Safe, S. (1989). Mechanism of action and structure-activity relationships for the chlorinated dibenzo-p-dioxins and related compounds. *In* "Halogenated Biphenyls, Terphenyls, Naphthalenes, Dibenzodioxins and Related Products" (R. D. Kimbrough and A. A. Jensen, eds.), Elsevief/North Holland, New York.

Goldstein, J. A., Hickman, P., Bergman, H., and Vos, J. G. (1973). Hepatic porphyria induced by 2,3,7,8-tetrachlorodibenzo-p-dioxin in the mouse. *Res. Commun. Chem. Pathol. Pharmacol.* **6**, 919–928.

Goldstein, J. A., McKinney, J. D., Lucier, G. W., Hickman, P., Bergman, H., and Moore, J. A. (1976). Toxicological assessment of hexachlorobiphenyl isomers and 2,3,7,8-tetrachorodibenzofuran in chicks. II. Effects on drug metabolism and porphyrin accumulation. *Toxicol. Appl. Pharmacol.* **36**, 81–92.

Goldstein, J. A., Friessen, M., Hoss, J. R., Linder, R. E., Bergman, H., and Hickman, P. (1977). Effects of pentachlorophenol on hepatic drug-metabolizing enzymes and porphyria related to contamination with chlorinated dibenzo-p-dioxins and dibenzofurans. *Biochem. Pharmacol.* **26**, 1549–1557.

Goldstein, J. A., Friessen, M., Scotti, T. M., Hichman, P., Hass, J. R., and Bergman, H. (1978). Assessment of the contribution of chlorinated dibenzo-p-dioxins and dibenzofurans to hexachlorobenzene-induced toxicity, porphyria, changes in mixed function oxygenases, and histophathological changes. *Toxicol. Appl. Pharmacol.* **46**, 633–649.

Goldstein, J. A., Linko, P., and Bergman, H. (1982). Induction of porphyria in the rat by chronic versus acute exposure to 2,3,7,8-tetrachlorodibenzo-p-dioxin. *Biochem. Pharmacol.* **31**, 1607–1613.

Gordon, D. (1956). How dangerous is pentachlorophenol? *Med. J. Aust.* **2**, 485–488.

Gorski, J. R., and Rozman, K. (1987). Dose–response and time course of hypothyroxinemia and hypoinsulinemia and characterization of insulin hypersensitivity in 2,3,7,8-tetrachlodibenzo-p-dioxin (TCDD)-treated rats. *Toxicology* **44**, 297–307.

Gorski, J. R., Muzi, G., Weber, L. W., Pereira, D. W., Iatropoulos, M. J., and Rozman, K. (1988a). Elevated plasma corticosterone levels and histopathology of the adrenals and thymuses in 2,3,7,8-tetrachlorodibenzo-p-dioxin-treated rats. *Toxicology* **53**, 19–32.

Gorski, J. R., Rozman, T., Greim, H., and Rozman, K. (1988b). Corticosterone modulates acute toxicity of 2,3,7,8-tetrachlorodibenzo-p-dioxin (TCDD) in male Sprague–Dawley rats. *Fund. Appl. Toxicol.* **11**, 494–502.

Gorski, T., Konopka, L., and Brodzki, M. (1984). Persistence of some polychlorinated dibenzo-p-dioxins and polychlorinated dibenzofurans of pentachlorophenol in human adipose tissue. *Roczn. Panstw. Zakl. Hig.* **35**, 297–301.

Graham, M., Hileman, F., Kirk, D., Wendling, J., and Wilson, J. (1985). Background human exposure to 2,3,7,8-TCDD. *Chemosphere* **14**, 925–928.

Gray, L. E., Jr., Rogers, J. M., Kavlock, R. J., Ostby, J. S., Ferrell, J. M., and Gray, K. L. (1986). Prenatal exposure to the fungicide dinocap causes behavioral torticollis, ballooning and cleft palate in mice. *Teratog., Carcinog., Mutagen.* **6**, 33–43.

Gray, R. E., Gilliland, R. D., Smith, E. E., Lockard, V. G., and Hume, A. S. (1985). Pentachlorophenol intoxication: Report of a fatal case, with comments on the clinical course and pathologic anatomy. *Arch. Environ. Health* **40**, 161–164.

Green, S., and Moreland, F. S. (1975). Cytogenetic evaluation of several dioxins in the rat. *Toxicol. Appl. Pharmacol.* **33**, 161.

Green, S., Moreland, F., and Sheu, C. (1977). Cytogenic effect of 2,3,7,8-tetrachlorodibenzo-p-dioxin on rat bone marrow cells. U.S. FDA, Washington, D.C. *FDA By-Lines* **6**, 292.

Greenlee, W. F., and Neal, R. A. (1985). The Ah receptor: A biochemical and biologic perspective. *In* "The Receptors" (P. M. Conn, ed.), Vol. II, pp. 89–129. Academic Press, Orlando, Florida.

Greenlee, W. F., and Poland, W. (1979). Nuclear uptake of 2,3,7,8-tetrachlorodibenzo-p-dioxin in C57BL/6J and DBA/2J mice. Role of the hepatic cytosol receptor protein. *J. Biol. Chem.* **254**, 9814–9821.

Greenlee, W. G., Young, M. J., Atkins, W. M., Hudson, L. G., Dorflinger, L., and Toscano, W. A. (1983). Regulation of adenylate cyclase activity in cultured human epithelial cells by 2,3,7,8-tetrachlorodibenzo-p-dioxin (TCDD). *Toxicol. Lett.* **18**, Suppl. 1, 5.

Greenlee, W. F., Osborne, R., Hudson, L. G., and Toscano, W. A. (1984a). Studies on the mechanisms of toxicity of TCDD to human epidermis. *Banbury Rep.* **18**, 365–380.

Greenlee, W. F., Dold, K. M., and Osborne, R. (1984b). A proposed model for the actions of TCDD on epidermal and thymic epithelial target cells. *Banbury Rep.* **18**, 435–444.

Greenlee, W. G., Dold, K. M., Irons, R. D., and Osborne, R. (1985a). Evidence for direct action of 2,3,7,8-tetrachlorodibenzo-p-dioxin (TCDD) on thymic epithelium. *Toxicol. Appl. Pharmacol.* **79**, 112–120.

Greenlee, W. F., Dold, K. M., and Osborne, R. (1985b). Actions of 2,3,7,8-tetrachlorodibenzo-p-dioxin (TCDD) on human keratinocytes in culture. *In Vitro Cell. Dev. Biol.* **21**, 509–512.

Greenwald, P., Kovasznay, B., Collins, D. N., and Therriault, G. (1984). Sarcomas of soft tissue after Vietnam service. *JNCI, J. Natl. Cancer Inst.* **73**, 1107–1109.

Greichus, Y. A., Libal, G. W., and Johnson, D. D. (1979). Diagnosis and physiologic effects of pentachlorophenols on young pigs. Part 1. Effects of purified pentachlorophenol. *Bull. Environ. Contam. Toxicol.* **23**, 418–422.

Greig, J. B., and Osborne, G. (1981). Biochemical and morphological changes induced by 2,3,7,8-tetrachlorodibenzo-p-dioxin in the rat liver cell plasma membrane. *J. Appl. Toxicol.* **1**, 334–338.

Greig, J. B., Francis, J. E., Kay, S. J. E., Lovell, D. P., and Smith, A. G. (1984). Incomplete correlation of 2,3,7,8-tetrachlorodibenzo-p-dioxin hepatotoxicity with Ah phenotype in mice. *Toxicol. Appl. Pharmacol.* **74**, 17–25.

Gross, M. I., Lay, J. O., Jr., Lyon, P. A., Lippstreu, D., Kangas, N., Harless, R. L., Taylor, S. E., and Dupuy, A. E., Jr. (1984). 2,3,7,8-Tetrachlorodibenzo-p-dioxin levels in adipose tissue of Vietnam veterans. *Environ. Res.* **33**, 261–268.

Gudas, J. M., and Hankinson, O. (1986). Reversible inactivation of the Ah receptor associated with changes in intracellular ATP levels. *J. Cell Physiol.* **128**, 449–456.

Guebert, M., and Mayer, A. (1932). Studies on the action of 1,2,4-dinitrophenol (Thermol). V. Presence of 1,2,4-dinitro-phenol and its derivatives in the organs and body fluids during poisoning—urinary excretion. *Ann. Physiol. Physicochim. Biol.* **8**, 117–121.

Guenthner, T. M., and Nebert, D. W. (1977). Cytosolic receptor for aryl hydrocarbon hydroxylase induction by polycyclic aromatic compounds. *J. Biol. Chem.* **252**, 8981–8989.

Guenthner, T. M., and Nebert, D. W. (1978). Evidence in rat and mouse liver for temporal control of two forms of cytochrome P-450 inducible by 2,3,7,8-tetrachlorodibenzo-p-dioxin. *Eur. J. Biochem.* **91**, 449–456.

Guenthner, T. M., Fysh, J. M., and Nebert, D. W. (1979a). 2,3,7,8-Tetrachlorodibenzo-p-dioxin: Covalent binding of reactive metabolic intermediates principally to protein *in vitro. Pharmacology* **19**, 12–22.

Guenthner, T. M., Nebert, D. W., and Menard, R. H. (1979b). Microsomal aryl hydrocarbon hydroxylase in rat adrenal: Regulation by ACTH but not by polycyclic hydrocarbons. *Mol. Pharmacol.* **15**, 719–728.

Gunderson, K., and Jensen, H. L. (1956). Soil bacterium decomposing organic nitro compounds. *Acta Agric. Scand.* **6**, 100–114.

Gupta, B. N., Vos, J. G., Moore, J. A., Zinkl, J. G., and Bullock, B. C. (1973).

Pathologic effects of 2,3,7,8-tetrachlorodibenzo-*p*-dioxin in laboratory animals. *Environ. Health Perspect.* **5**, 125–139.

Gupta, B. N., McConnell, E. E., Harris, M. W., and Moore, J. A. (1980). Polybrominated biphenyl toxicosis in the rat and mouse. *Toxicol. Appl. Pharmacol.* **57**, 99–118.

Gurtoo, H. L., Dahms, R. P., Kanter, P., and Vaught, J. B. (1978). Association and dissociation of the *Ah* locus with the metabolism of aflatoxin B₁ by mouse liver: Cosegregation of aflatoxin B$_1$ hydroxylase with aryl hydrocarbon (benzo(*a*)pyrene) hydroxylase induction. *J. Biol. Chem.* **253**, 3952–3961.

Gustafsson, J.-A., and Ingelman-Sundberg, M. (1979). Changes in steroid hormone metabolism in rat liver microsomes following administration of 2,3,7,8-tetrachlorodibenzo-*p*-dioxin (TCDD). *Biochem. Pharmacol.* **28**, 497–499.

Haake, J. M., Mayura, F., Phillips, T., and Safe, S. (1987a). Teratogenicity of 2,3,7,8-tetrachlorodibenzo-*p*-dioxin: Antagonism by Aroclor 1254. *Toxicologist* **7**, A498.

Haake, J. M., Safe, S., Mayura, K., and Phillips, T. D. (1987b). Aroclor 1254 as an antagonist of the teratogenicity of 2,3,7,8-tetrachlorodibenzo-*p*-dioxin. *Toxicol. Lett.* **38**, 299–306.

Hahn, M. E., Goldstein, J. A., Linko, P., and Gasiewicz, T. A. (1988). The role of the *Ah* locus in hexachlorobenzene porphyria: Studies in congenic C57BL/6 mice. *Biochem. J.* **254**, 245–254.

Hakansson, H. (1988). Effects of 2,3,7,8-tetrachlorobidenzo-*p*-dioxin on the fate of vitamin A in rodents. Ph.D. Thesis, Department of Toxicology and Institute of Environmental Medicine, Karolinska Institute, Stockholm.

Hakasson, H., and Ahlborg, U. G. (1985). The effect of 2,3,7,8-tetrachlorodibenzo-*p*-dioxin (TCDD) on the uptake, distribution, and excretion of a single oral dose of [11,12-³H]retinyl acetate and on the vitamin A status in the rat. *J. Nutr.* **115**, 759–771.

Hakansson, H., Maern, F., and Ahlborg, U. G. (1987). Effects of 2,3,7,8-tetrachlorodibenzo-*p*-dioxin (TCDD) in the lactating rat on maternal and neonatal vitamin A status. *J. Nutr.* **117**, 580–586.

Haley, T. J. (1977). Human poisoning with pentachlorophenol and its treatment. *Ecotoxical. Environ. Saf.* **1**, 343–347.

Hall, L., Linder, R., Scotti, T., Bruce, R., Moseman, R., Heiderscheit, T., Hinkle, D., Edgerton, T., Chaney, S., Goldstein, J., Gage, M., Farmer, J., Bennett, L., Stevens, J., Durham, W., and Curley, A. (1978). Subchronic and reproductive toxicity of dinoseb. *Toxicol. Appl. Pharmacol.* **45**, 235–236.

Hamada, N., and Peterson, R. E (1978). Effect of microsomal enzyme inducers on 2,3,7,8-tetrachlorodibenzo-*p*-dioxin-induced depression in the biliary excretion of ouabain in rats. *Drug Metab. Dispos.* **6**, 456–464.

Hambrick, G. W., Jr. (1957). The effect of substituted naphthalenes on the pilosebaceous apparatus of rabbit and man. *J. Invest. Dermatol.* **28**, 89–103.

Hanify, J. A., Metcalf, P., Nobbs, C. L., and Worsley, R. J. (1981). Aerial spraying of 2,4,5-T and human birth malformations: An epidemiological investigation. *Science* **212**, 349–351.

Hankinson, O. (1983). Dominant and recessive aryl hydrocarbon hydroxylase-deficient mutants of mouse hepatoma line, Hepa-1, and assignment of recessive mutants to three complementation groups. *Somatic Cell. Genet.* **9**, 497–514.

Hannah, R. R., Lund, J., Poellinger, L., Gillner, M., and Gustafsson, J.-A. (1986). Characterization of the DNA-binding properties of the receptor for 2,3,7,8-tetrachlorodibenzo-*p*-dioxin. *Eur. J. Biochem.* **156**, 237–242.

Hansel, W., Olafson, P., and McEntee, K. (1955). The isolation and identification of the causative agent of bovine hyperkeratosis (X-disease) from a processed feed concentrate. *Cornell Vet.* **45**, 94–101.

Hardell, L., and Sandström, A. (1979). Case-control study: Soft-tissue sarcomas and exposure to phenoxyacetic acids or chlorophenols. *Br. J. Cancer* **39**, 711–717.

Hardell, L., Eriksson, M., Lenner, P., and Lundgren, E. (1981). Malignant lymphoma and exposure to chemicals, especially organic solvents, chlorophenols and phenoxy acids: A case-control study. *Br. J. Cancer* **43**, 169–176.

Hari, S., Obana, H., Tanaka, R., and Kashimoto, T. (1986). Comparative toxicity in rats of polychlorinated biphenyls (PCBs), polychlorinated quaterphenyls (PCQs) and polychlorinated dibenzofurans (PCDFs) present in rice oil causing "Yusho." *Eisei Kagaku* **32**, 13–21.

Harris, M. W., Moore, J. A., Vos, J. G., and Gupta, B. N. (1973). General biological effects of TCDD in laboratory animals. *Environ. Health Perspect.* **5**, 101–109.

Harris, M., Piskorska-Pliszczynska, T., Zacharewski, T., and Romkes, M., and Safe, S. (1989). Structure-dependent induction of aryl hydrocarbon hydroxylase in human breast cancer cell lines and characterization of the Ah receptor. *Cancer Research* **49**, 4531–4535.

Harvey, D. G., Bidstrup, P. L., and Bonnell, J. A. L. (1951). Poisoning by dinitro-*ortho*-cresol: Some observations on the effects of dinitro-*ortho*-cresol administration by mouth to human volunteers. *Br. Med. J.* **2**, 13–16.

Hassan, A. B., Seligmann, H., and Bassan, H. M. (1985). Intravascular haemolysis induced by pentachlorophenol. *Br. Med. J.* **291**, 21–22.

Hassoun, E. A. M. (1987). *In vivo* and *in vitro* interactions of TCDD and other ligands of the *Ah*-receptor: Effect on embryonic and fetal tissues. *Arch. Toxicol.* **61**, 145–149.

Hassoun, E., D'Argy, R., Dencker, L., Lundin, L.-G., and Borwell, P. (1984a). Teratogenicity of 2,3,7,8-tetrachlorodibenzo-*p*-dioxin in BXD recombinant inbred strains. *Toxicol. Lett.* **23**, 37–42.

Hassoun, E., D'Argy, R., Dencker, L., and Sundstrom, G. (1984b). Teratological studies on the congener 3,3′,4,4′-tetrachloroazoxybenzene in sensitive and nonsensitive mouse strains: Evidence for direct effect on embryonic tissues. *Arch. Toxicol.* **55**, 20–26.

Hay, A. (1976a). Toxic cloud over Seveso. *Nature (London)* **262**, 636–638.

Hay, A. (1976b). Seveso: The aftermath. *Nature (London)* **263**, 538–540.

Hay, A. (1977). Dioxin damage. *Nature (London)* **266**, 7–8.

Hay, A. (1982). "The Chemical Scythe: Lessons of 2,4,5-T and Dioxin." Plenum, New York and London.

Hayabuchi, H., Yoshimura, T., and Kuratsune, M. (1979). Consumption of toxic rice oil by "Yusho" patients and its relation to the clinical response and latent period. *Food Cosmet. Toxicol.* **17**, 455–461.

Hayes, W. J., Jr. (1982). "Pesticides Studied in Man." Williams and Wilkins, Baltimore.

Heath, R. G., Harless, R. L., Gross, M. L., Lyon, P. A., Dupuy, A. E., Jr., and McDaniel, D. D. (1986). Determination of 2,3,7,8-tetrachlorodibenzo-*p*-dioxin in human milk at the 0.1–10 parts-per-trillion level: Method validation and survey results. *Anal. Chem.* **58**, 463–468.

Henck, J. M., New, M. A., Kociba, R. J., and Rao, K. S. (1981). 2,3,7,8-Tetrachlorodibenzo-*p*-dioxin: Acute oral toxicity in hamsters. *Toxicol. Appl. Pharmacol.* **59**, 405–407.

Henderson, L. O., and Patterson, D. G., Jr. (1988). Distribution of 2,3,7,8-tetrachlorodibenzo-*p*-dioxin in human whole blood and its association with, and extractability from, lipoproteins. *Bull. Environ. Contam. Toxicol.* **40**, 604–611.

Henneberg, M. (1973). Studies on toxicity and toxicologic analysis of DNPP and DNBP. *Ann. Acad. Med. Lodz.* **14**, 170–171 (in Polish).

Henry, E. C., and Gasiewicz, T. A. (1986). Effect of thyroidectomy on the *Ah* receptor and enzyme induction by 2,3,7,8-tetrachlorodibenzo-*p*-dioxin in the rat liver. *Chem.-Biol. Interact.* **59**, 151–160.

Henry, E. C., and Gasiewicz, T. A. (1987). Changes in thyroid hormones and thyroxine-glucuronidation in hamsters compared with rats following treatment with 2,3,7,8-tetrachlorodibenzo-*p*-dioxin. *Toxicol. Appl. Pharmacol.* **89**, 165–174.

Henry, E. C., Rucci, G., and Gasiewicz. T. A. (1989). Characterization of multiple forms of the Ah receptor: Comparison of species and tissues. *Biochemistry* **28**, 6430–6440.

Hernandez (1980). Pentachlorophenol in log homes. *Morbid. Mortal. Wkly. Rep.* **29**, 431–437.

Herxheimer, K. (1899). On chloracne. *Muench. Med. Wochenschr.*, p. 278.

Hetenyi, G., Jr., Issekutz, B., Jr., and Winter, M. (1955). Action of 2,4-dinitrophenol on the metabolism of striated muscle with special consideration of pancreatic diabetes. *Acta Physiol. Acad. Sci. Hung.* **7**, 287–307 (in German).

Hewitt, W. R., Pegg, D. G., and Hook, J. B. (1976). Effect of 2,3,7,8-tetrachlorodibenzo-*p*-dioxin (TCDD) on renal function in rats *in vitro*. *Toxicol. Appl. Pharmacol.* **37**, 177.

Heyman, C., and Casier, H. (1935). Investigation of the action of different nitro-derivatives on metabolism and temperature. *Arch. Int. Pharmacodyn. Ther.* **59**, 20–64 (in French).

Heyndrickx, A., and Herman, M. (1957). Toxicological investigation of poisoning by dinitro-*ortho*-cresol (DNOC) with fatal outcome. *Meded. Landbouwhogesch. Opzoekingsstn. Staat Gent.* **22**, 647–653.

Heyndrickx, A., Avermaete, M., Maes, R., and Schauvliege, M. (1962). Determination of dinitro-*ortho*-cresol (DNOC) in postmortem material of a farmer. *Meded. Landbouwhogesch. Opzoekingsstn. Staat Gent.* **27**, 955–963.

Higuchi, K., ed. (1976). "PCB Poisoning and Pollution." Academic Press, New York.

Hildebrand, C. E., Gonzalez, F. J., McBride, O. W., and Nebert, D. W. (1985). Assignment of the human 2,3,7,8-tetrachlorodibenzo-*p*-dioxin-inducible cytochrome P_1-450 gene to chromosome 15. *Nucleic Acids Res.* **13**, 2009–2016.

Hillam, R. P., and Greichus, Y. A. (1983). Effects of purified pentachlorophenol on the serum proteins of young pigs. *Bull. Environ. Contam. Toxicol.* **31**, 599–604.

Hinsdill, R. S., Couch, D. L., and Speiers, R. S. (1980). Immunosuppression in mice induced by dioxin (TCDD) in feed. *J. Environ. Pathol. Health* **4**, 401–425.

Hirayama, C. (1976). Clinical aspects of PCB poisoning. *In* "PCB Poisoning and Pollution" (K. Higuchi, ed.), pp. 88–105. Academic Press, New York.

Hoar, S. K., Blair, A., Holmes, F. F., Boysen, C. D., Robel, R. J., Hoover, R., and Fraumeni, J. F., Jr. (1986). Agricultural herbicide use and risk of lymphoma and soft-tissue sarcoma. *JAMA, J. Am. Med. Assoc.* **256**, 1141–1147.

Hoben, H. J., Ching, S. A., and Casarett, L. J. (1976a). A study of inhalation of pentachlorophenol by rats. III. Inhalation toxicity study. *Bull. Environ. Contam. Toxicol.* **15**, 463–465.

Hoben, H. J., Ching, S. A., and Casarett, L. J. (1976b). A study of inhalation of pentachlorophenol by rats. IV. Distribution and excretion of inhaled pentachlorophenol. *Bull. Environ. Contam. Toxicol.* **15**, 466–474.

Hoben, H. J., Ching, S. A., Young, R. A., and Casarett, L. J. (1976c). A study of the inhalation of pentachlorophenol by rats. V. A protein binding study of pentachlorophenol. *Bull. Environ. Contam. Toxicol.* **16**, 225–232.

Hochstein, J. R., Aulrich, R. J., and Bursian, S. J. (1988). Acute toxicity of 2,3,7,8-tetrachlorodibenzo-*p*-dioxin to mink. *Arch. Environ. Contam. Toxicol.* **17**, 33–37.

Hoffman, R. E., Stehr-Green, P. A., Webb, K. B., Evans, G., Knutsen, A. P., Schramm, W. F., Staake, J. L., Gibson, B. B., and Steinberg, K. K. (1986). Health effects of long-term exposure to 2,3,7,8-tetrachlorodibenzo-*p*-dioxin. *JAMA, J. Am. Med. Assoc.* **255**, 2031–2038.

Hofmann, H. T., and Neumann, W. (1952). A method for experimental animal testing of the dermal action of chlorinated naphthalenes. *Zentralbl. Arbeitsmed. Arbeitsschutz* **2**, 169–173 (in German).

Hofmann-Credner, D. H., and Siedek, H. (1949). On the influence of vitamin A and of methylthiouracil on the action of dinitrocresol in humans. *Klin. Med. (Vienna)* **4**, 361–367 (in German).

Holcomb, M., Yao, C., and Safe, S. (1988). Biologic and toxic effects of polychlorinated dibenzo-*p*-dioxin and dibenzofuran congeners in the guinea pig. Quantitative structure–activity relationships. *Biochem. Pharmacol.* **37**, 1535–1539.

Holmstedt, B. (1980). Prolegomena to Seveso. Ecclesiastes I 18. *Arch. Toxicol.* **44**, 211–230.

Holsapple, M. P., Dooley, R. K., McNerney, P. J., and McCay, J. A. (1986a). Direct suppression of antibody responses by chlorinated dibenzodioxins in cultured spleen cells from (C57BL/6 × C3H)F1 and DBA/2 mice. *Immunopharmacology* **12**, 175–186.

Holsapple, M. P., McCay, J. A., and Barnes, D. W. (1986b). Immunosuppression without liver induction by subchronic exposure to 2,7-dichlordibenzo-*p*-dioxin in adult female B6C3F1 mice. *Toxicol. Appl. Pharmacol.* **83**, 445–455.

Holsapple, M. P., McNerney, P. J., and McCay, J. A. (1987). Effects of pentachlorophenol on the *in vitro* and *in vivo* antibody response. *J. Toxicol. Environ. Health* **20**, 229–239.

Honchar, P. A., and Halperin, W. E. (1981). 2,3,5-Trichlorophenol and soft-tissue sarcoma. *Lancet* **1**, 268–269.

Hook, G. E. R., Haseman, J. K., and Lucier, G. W. (1975). Induction and

suppression of hepatic and extrahepatic microsomal foreign-compound-metabolizing systems by 2,3,7,8-tetrachlorodibenzo-*p*-dioxin. *Chem.-Biol. Interact* **10**, 199–214.

Horner, W. D. (1936). Cataract following di-nitrophenol treatment for obesity. *Arch. Ophthalmol. (Chicago)* **16**, 447–461.

Horner, W. D. (1942). Dinitrophenol and its relation to formation of cataract. *Arch. Ophthalmol. (Chicago)* **27**, 1097–1121.

Horner, W. D., Jones, R. B., and Boardman, W. W. (1935). Cataracts following the use of dinitrophenol. Preliminary report of three cases. *JAMA, J. Am. Med. Assoc.* **105**, 108–110.

Hsu, S.-T., Ma, C.-I., Hsu, S. K.-H., Wu, S.-S., Hsu, N. H.-M, Yeh, C.-C., and Wu, S.-B. (1985). Discovery and epidemiology of PCB poisoning in Taiwan: A four-year followup. *Environ. Health Perspect.* **59**, 5–10.

Huang Lu, C.-J., Baggs, R. B., Redmond, D., Henry, E. C., Schecter, A., and Gasiewicz, T. A. (1986). Toxicity and evidence for metabolic alterations in 2,3,7,8-tetrachlorodibenzo-*p*-dioxin-treated guinea pigs fed by total parenteral nutrition. *Toxicol. Appl. Pharmacol.* **84**, 439–453.

Huber, W. G., and Link, R. P. (1962). Toxic effects of hexachloronaphthalene on swine. *Toxicol. Appl. Pharmacol.* **4**, 257–262.

Hudson, L. G., Shaikh, R., Toscano, W. A., and Greenlee, W. F. (1983). Induction of 7-ethoxycoumarin *O*-deethylase activity in cultured human epithelial cells by 2,3,7,8-tetrachlorodibenzo-*p*-dioxin (TCDD): Evidence for TCDD receptor. *Biochem. Biophys. Res. Commun.* **115**, 611–617.

Hudson, L. G., Toscano, W. A., Jr., and Greenlee, W. F. (1985). Regulation of epidermal growth factor binding in a human keratinocyte cell line by 2,3,7,8-tetrachlorodibenzo-*p*-dioxin. *Toxicol. Appl. Pharmacol.* **77**, 251–259.

Hudson, L. G., Toscano. W. A., Jr., and Greenlee, W. F. (1986). 2,3,7,8-Tetrachlorodibenzo-*p*-dioxin (TCDD) modulates epidermal growth factor (EGF) binding to basal cells from a human keratinocyte cell line. *Toxicol. Appl. Pharmacol.* **82**, 481–492.

Hughes, B. J., Forsell, J. H., Sleight, S. D., Kuo, C., and Shull, L. R. (1985). Assessment of pentachlorophenol toxicity in newborn claves: Clinicopathology and tissue residues. *J. Anim. Sci.* **61**, 1587–1603.

Hussain, S., Ehrenberg, L., Lofroth, G., and Gejvall, T. (1972). Mutagenic effects of TCDD on bacterial systems. *Ambio* **1**, 32–33.

Hutzinger, O., Frei, R. W., Merian, E., and Pocchiari, F., eds. (1982). "Chlorinated Dioxins and Related Compounds. Impact on the Environment." Pergamon, New York.

Hwang, S. W. (1973). Effect of 2,3,7,8-tetrachlorodibenzo-*p*-dioxin on the biliary excretion of indocyanine green in the rat. *Environ. Health Perspect.* **5**, 227–231.

Ideo, G., Bellati, G., Bellobuono, A., Mocarelli, P., Marocchi, A., and Brambilla, P. (1982). Increased urinary D-glucaric acid excretion by children living in an area polluted with tetrachlorodibenzoparadioxin (TCDD). *Clin. Chim. Acta* **120**, 273–283.

Ilivicky, J., and Casida, J. E. (1969). Uncoupling action of 2,3-dinitrophnols, 2-trifluoromethylbenzimidazoles and certain other pesticide chemicals upon mitochondria from different sources and its relation to toxicity. *Biochem. Pharmacol.* **18**, 1389–1401.

Imaizumi, K., and Atsumi, K. (1971). Eye lesions due to agricultural chemicals. *Ophthalmology* **13**, 717–724.

Inagami, K., Koga, T., Kikuchi, M., Hashimoto, M., Takahashi, H., and Wada, K. (1969). Experimental study of hairless mice following administration of rice oil used by a "Yusho" patient. *Fukouka Acta Med.* **60**, 548–553.

Ingebrigtsen, K., and Froslie, A. (1980). Intestinal metabolism of DNOC and DMBP in the rat. *Acta Pharmacol. Toxicol.* **46**, 326–328.

Innes, J. R. M., Ulland, B. M., Valerio, M. G., Petrucelli, L., Fishbein, L., Hart, E. R., Pallotta, A. J., Bates, R. R., Falk, H. L., Gart, J. J., Klein, M., Mitchell, I., and Peters, J. (1969). Bioassay of pesticides and industrial chemicals for tumorigenicity in mice: A preliminary note. *J. Natl. Cancer Inst. (U.S.)* **42**, 1101–1114.

International Agency for Research on Cancer (IARC) (1977). "IARC Monographs on the Evaluation of the Carcinogenic Risk of Chemicals to Man. Some Fumigants, the Herbicides 2,4-D and 2,3,5-T, Chlorinated Dibenzodioxins and Miscellaneous Chemicals," Vol. 15, pp. 41–102. IARC, Lyon, France.

Ishidate, K., Tsuruoka, M., and Nakazawa, Y. (1980). Induction of choline kinase by polycyclic aromatic hydrocarbon carcinogens in rat liver. *Biochem. Biophys. Res. Commun.* **96**, 946–952.

Issekutz, B., Jr. (1984). Effect of propranolol in dinitrophenol poisoning. *Arch. Int. Pharmacodyn. Ther.* **272**, 310–319.

Jackson, W. T. (1972). Regulation of mitosis. III. Cytological effects of 2,4,5-trichlorophenoxyacetic acid and of dioxin contaminants in 2,4,5-T formulations. *J. Cell. Sci.* **10**, 15–25.

Jaiswal, A. K., Gonzalez, F. J., and Nebert, D. W. (1985a). Human dioxin-inducible cytochrome P_1-450: Complementary DNA and amino acid sequence. *Science* **228**, 80–83.

Jaiswal, A. K., Nebert, D. W., and Eisen, H. W. (1985b). Comparison of aryl hydrocarbon hydroxylase and acetanilide 4-hydroxylase induction by polycyclic aromatic compounds in human and mouse cell lines. *Biochem. Pharmacol* **34**, 2721–2731.

Jakobson, I., and Yllner, S. (1971). Metabolism of ^{14}C-pentachlorophenol in the mouse. *Acta Pharmacol. Toxicol.* **29**, 513–524.

Jansson, K., and Jansson, V. (1986). Inability of chlorophenols to induce G-thioguanine-resistant mutants in V79 Chinese hamster cells. *Mutat. Res.* **171**, 165–168.

Jastroch, S., Knoll, W., Lange, G., Riemer, F., and Thiele, E. (1978). Results of exposure to dinitro-*o*-cresol (DNOC) among agrochemists. *Z. Gesamte Hyg. Ihre Grenzgeb.* **24**, 340–343 (in German).

Jensen, A. A. (1987). Polychlorinated biphenyls (PCBs), polychlorodibenzo-p-dioxins (PCDDs) and polychloro-dibenzofurans (PCDFs) in human milk, blood, and adipose tissue. *Sci. Tot. Environ.* **64**, 259–293.

Jensen, D. J., and Hummel, R. A. (1982). Secretion of TCDD in milk and cream following the feeding of TCDD to lactating dairy cows. *Bull. Environ. Contam. Toxicol.* **29**, 440–446.

Jensen, N. E. (1972). Chloracne: Three cases. *Proc. R. Soc. Med.* **65**, 687–688.

Jirasek, L., Kalensky, J., and Kubec, K. (1973). Chloracne and porphyria cutanea tarda during the manufacture of herbicides. *Cesk. Dermatol* **48**, 306–317 [Czech].

Jirasek, L., Kalensky, J., Kubec, K., Pazderova, J., and Lukas, E. (1974). Chloracne, porphyria cutanea tarda and other manifestations of general poisoning during the manufacture of herbicides. *Cesk. Dermatol.* **49**, 145–157.

Jirasek, L., Kalensky, J., Kubec, K., Pazderova, J., and Lukas, E. (1976). Chloracne, porphyria cutanea tarda and other intoxications by herbicides. *Hautarzt* **27**, 328–333.

Johnson, E. F., and Müller-Eberhard, U. (1977). Resolution of two forms of cytochrome P-450 from liver microsomes of rabbits treated with 2,3,7,8-tetrachlorodibenzo-p-dioxin. *J. Biol. Chem.* **252**, 2839–2845.

Johnson, R. L., Gehring, P. J., Kociba, R. J., and Schwetz, B. A. (1973). Chlorinated dibenzodioxins and pentachlorophenol. *Environ. Health Perspect.* **5**, 171–175.

Jones, E. L., and Krizek, H. A (1962). A technic for testing acnegenic potency in rabbits applied to the potent acnegen 2,3,7,8-tetrachlorodibenzo-p-dioxin. *J. Invest. Dermatol.* **39**, 511–517.

Jones, G., (1975). A histochemical study of the liver lesion induced by 2,3,7,8-tetrachlorodibenzo-p-dioxin (dioxin) in rats. *J. Pathol.* **116**, 101–105.

Jones, G., and Butler, W. H. (1974). A morphological study of the liver lesion induced by 2,3,7,8-tetrachlorodibenzo-p-dioxin in rats. *J. Pathol.* **116**, 101–105.

Jones, G., and Greig, J. B. (1975). Pathological changes in the liver of mice given 2,3,7,8-tetrachlorodibenzo-p-dioxin. *Experientia* **31**, 1315–1317.

Jones, J. W., and Alden, H. S. (1936). An acneform dermatergosis. *Arch. Dermatol. Syph.* **33**, 1022–1034.

Jones, K. G., and Sweeney, G. D. (1977). Association between induction of aryl hydrocarbon hydroxylase and depression of uroporphyrinogen decarboxylase activity. *Res. Commun. Chem. Pathol. Pharmacol.* **17**, 631–637.

Jones, K. G., and Sweeney, G. D. (1980). Dependence of the porphyrogenic effect of 2,3,7,8-tetrachlorodibenzo-p-dioxin upon inheritance of aryl hydrocarbon hydroxylase responsiveness. *Toxicol. Appl. Pharmacol.* **53**, 42–49.

Jones, K. G., Cole, F. M., and Sweeney, G. W. (1981). The role of iron in the toxicity of 2,3,7,8-tetrachlorodibenzo-p-dioxin (TCDD). *Toxicol. Appl. Pharmacol.* **61**, 74–88.

Jones, M. K., Weisenburger, W. P., Sipes, I. G., and Russell, D. H. (1987). Circadian alterations in prolactin, corticosterone, and thyroid hormone levels and down-regulation of prolactin receptor activity by 2,3,7,8-tetrachlorodibenzo-p-dioxin. *Toxicol. Appl. Pharmacol.* **87**, 337–350.

Jones, P. B. C., Galeazzi, D. R., Fisher, J. M., and Whitlock, J. P., Jr. (1985). Control of cytochrome P_1-450 gene expression by dioxin. *Science* **227**, 1499–1502.

Jones, P. B. C., Durrin, L. K., Fisher, J. M., and Whitlock, J. P., Jr. (1986). Control of gene expression by 2,3,7,8-tetrachlorodibenzo-p-dioxin: Multiple dioxin-responsive domains 5′-ward of the cytochrome P_1-450 gene. *J. Biol. Chem.* **261**, 6647–6650.

Jones, R. D., Winter, D. P., and Cooper, A. J. (1986). Absorption study of pentachlorophenol in persons working with wood preservatives. *Hum. Toxicol.* **5**, 189–194.

Jones, R. E., and Chelsky, M. (1986). Further discussion concerning porphyria cutanea tarda and TCDD exposure. *Arch. Environ. Health* **41**, 100–103.

Judah, J. D. (1952). Mode of action of the nitrophenols. *Proc. R. Soc. Med.* **45**, 574.

Judah, J. D., and Williams-Ashman, H. G. (1951). The inhibition of oxidative phosphorylation. *Biochem. J.* **48**, 33–42.

Juhl, U., Witte, I., and Butte, W. (1985). Metabolism of pentachlorophenol to tetrachlorohydroquinone by human liver homogenate. *Bull. Environ. Contam. Toxicol.* **35**, 596–601.

Kahl, G. F., Friederici, D. E., Bigelow, S. W., Okey, A. B., and Nebert, D. W. (1980). Ontogenic expression of regulatory and structural gene products associated with the *Ah* locus. Comparison of rat, mouse, rabbit, and *Sigmoden hispedis. Dev. Pharmacol. Ther.* **1**, 137–162.

Kahlman, D. A., and Horstman, S. W. (1983). Persistence of tetrachlorophenol and pentachlorophenol in exposed woodworkers. *J. Toxicol., Clin. Toxicol.* **20**, 343–352.

Kahn, P. C., Gochfeld, M., Nygren, M., Hansson, M., Rappe, C., Velez, H., Ghent-Guenther, T., and Wilson, W. P. (1988). Dioxins and dibenzofurans in blood and adipose tissue of Agent Orange-exposed Vietnam veterans and matched controls. *JAMA, J. Am. Med. Assoc.* **259**, 1161–1167.

Kaiser, J. A. (1964). Studies on the toxicity of disophenol (2,6-diiodo-4-nitrophenol) to dogs and rodents plus some comparisons with 2,4-dinitrophenol. *Toxicol. Appl. Pharmacol.* **6**, 232–244.

Kanda, M., Takahama, K., Waseda, Y., Ishii, Y., and Miyazaki, Y. (1968). Studies on the influence of organochlorine pesticides, PCP and endrin to mitochondrial respiration and oxidative phosphorylation of rat brain. *Jpn. J. Leg. Med.* **22**, 223–228.

Kang, H. K., Weatherbee, L., Breslin, P. P., Lee, Y., and Shepard, B. M. (1986). Soft tissue sarcomas and military service in Vietnam: A case comparison group analysis of hospital patients. *J. Occup. Med.* **28**, 1215–1218.

Karenlampi, S. O., Lagraverend, C., Lalley, P. A., Kozak, C. A., and Nebert, D. W. (1983). Assignment of the *Ah* locus to mouse chromosome 17. *In* "Extrahepatic Drug Metabolism and Chemical Carcinogenesis" (J. Rydstrom, J. Montelius, and M. Bengtsson, eds.), pp. 425–426. Am. Elsevier, New York.

Karenlampi, S. O., Legrarerend, C., Gudas, J. M., Carramanzana, M., and Hankinson, O. (1988). A third genetic locus affecting the *Ah* (dioxin) receptor. *J. Biol. Chem.* **263**, 10111–10117.

Kashimoto, T., Miyata, H., Kunita, N., Tung, T. C., Hsu, S. T., Chang, K. J., Tang, S. Y., Ohi, G., Nakawawa, J., and Yamamoto, S. (1981). Role of polychlorinated dibenzofuran in Yusho (PCB poisoning). *Arch. Environ. Health* **36**, 321–326.

Kashimoto, T., Miyata, H., Fukushima, S., and Kunita, N. (1983). Study on PCBs, PCQs and PCDFs in the blood of Taiwanese patients with PCB poisoning and in the causal cooking rice bran oil. *Fukuoka Acta Med.* **74**, 255–268.

Kashimoto, T., Miyata, H., Shigehiko, F., Kunita, N., Ohi, G., and Tung, T.-C. (1985). PCBs, PCQs, and PCDFs in blood of Yusho and Yu-Cheng patients. *Environ. Health Perspect.* **59**, 73–78.

Katz, L. B., Theobald, M., Bookstaff, R. C., and Peterson, R. E (1984). Characterization of the enhanced paw edema response to carrageenan and dextran in 2,3,7,8-tetrachlorodibenzo-p-dioxin-treated rats. *J. Pharmacol. Exp. Ther.* **230**, 670–677.

Kavlock, R. J., Chernoff, N., and Rogers, E. H. (1985). The effect of acute maternal toxicity on fetal development in the mouse. *Teratog., Carcinog., Mutagen.* **5,** 3–13.

Kawajiri, K., Gotoh, O., Sogawa, K., Tagashira, Y., Muramatsu, M., and Fujii-Kuriyama, Y. (1984). Coding nucleotide sequence of 3-methylcholanthrene-inducible cytochrome P-450d cDNA from rat liver. *Proc. Natl. Acad. Sci. U.S.A.* **81,** 1649–1653.

Kawanishi, S., Seki, Y., and Sano, S. (1983). Uroporphyrinogen decarboxylase: Purification, properties, and inhibition by polychlorinated biphenyl isomers. *J. Biol. Chem.* **258,** 4285–4292.

Kawatski, J. A., and McDonald, M. J. (1974). Effect of 3-trifluoromethyl-4-nitrophenol on *in vitro* tissue respiration of four species of fish with preliminary notes on its *in vitro* biotransformation. *Comp. Gen. Pharmacol.* **5,** 67–76.

Kay, K. (1977). Polybrominated biphenyls (PBB) environmental contamination in Michigan, 1973–1976. *Environ. Res.* **13,** 74–93.

Kedderis, G. L., Dyroff, M. C., and Rickert, D. E. (1984). Hepatic macromolecular covalent binding of the hepatocarcinogen 2,6-dinitrotoluene and its 2,4-isomer *in vivo*: Modulation by the sulfotransferase inhibitors pentachlorophenol and 2,6-dichloro-4-nitrophenol. *Carcinogenesis (London)* **5,** 1199–1204.

Kehoe, R. A., Deichmann-Gruebler, W., and Kitzmiller, K. V. (1939). Toxic effects upon rabbits of pentachlorophenol and sodium pentachlorophenate. *J. Ind. Hyg. Toxicol.* **21,** 160–172.

Kelling, C. K., Menahan, L. A., and Peterson, R. E. (1987a). Hepatic indices of thyroid status in rats treated with 2,3,7,8-tetrachlorodibenzo-*p*-dioxin. *Biochem. Pharmacol.* **36,** 283–291.

Kelling, C. K., Menahan, L. A., and Peterson, R. E. (1987b). Effects of 2,3,7,8-tetrachlorodibenzo-*p*-dioxin treatment on mechanical function of the rat heart. *Toxicol. Appl. Pharmacol.* **91,** 497–501.

Kennel, S. J., Jasopn, C., Albro, P. W., Mason, G., and Safe, S. A. (1986). Monoclonal antibodies to chlorinated dibenzo-*p*-dioxins. *Toxicol. Appl. Pharmacol.* **82,** 256–264.

Kerkvliet, N. I., Baecher-Steppan, L., and Schmitz, J. A. (1982a). Immunotoxicity of pentachlorophenol (PCP): Increased susceptibility to tumor growth in adult mice fed technical PCP-containing diets. *Toxicol. Appl. Pharmacol.* **62,** 55–64.

Kerkvliet, N. I., Baecher-Steppan, L., and Sheggeby, G. G. (1982b). Immunotoxicity of technical pentachlorophenol (PCP-T): Depressed humoral immune responses to T-dependent and T-independent antigen stimulation in PCP-T exposed mice. *Fundam. Appl. Toxicol.* **2,** 90–99.

Kerkvliet, N. I., Brauner, J. A., and Baecher-Steppan, L. (1985a). Effects of dietary technical pentachlorophenol exposure on T cell, macrophage, and natural killer cell activity in C57Bl/6 mice. *Int. J. Immunopharmacol.* **7,** 239–247.

Kerkvliet, N. I., Brauner, J. A., and Matlock, J. P. (1985b). Humoral immunotoxicity of polychlorinated diphenyl ethers, phenoxyphenols, dioxins, and furans present as contaminants of technical grade pentachlorophenol. *Toxicology* **36,** 307–324.

Kessler, R. J., Tyson, C. A., and Green, D. E. (1976). Mechanisms of uncoupling in mitochondria: Uncouplers as ionophores for cycling cations and protons. *Proc. Natl. Acad. Sci. U.S.A.* **73,** 3141–3145.

Keys, B., Hlavinka, M., Mason, G., and Safe, S. (1985). Modulation of rat hepatic microsomal testosterone hydroxylases by 2,3,7,8-tetrachlorodibenzo-*p*-dioxin and related toxic isostereomers. *Can. J. Physiol. Pharmacol.* **63,** 1537–1542.

Keys, B., Piskorska-Pliszczynska, J., and Safe, S. (1986). Polychlorinated dibenzofurans as 2,3,7,8-TCDD antagonists: *In vitro* inhibition of monooxygenase enzyme induction. *Toxicol. Lett.* **31,** 151–158.

Khan, M. A. Q., and Stanton, R. H. (1981). "Toxicology of Halogenated Hydrocarbons, Health and Ecological Effects." Pergamon, New York.

Khera, K. S., and Ruddick, J. A. (1973). Polychlorodibenzo-*p*-dioxins: Perinatal effects and the dominant lethal test in Wistar rats. *Adv. Chem. Ser.* **120,** 70–84.

Kukuchi, M., Hashimoto, M., Hozimi, M., Koga, K., Oyoshi, S., and Nagakawa, M. (1969). An autopsy case of stillborn of chlorobiphenyls poisoning. *Fukuoka Acta Med.* **60,** 489–495.

Kimbrough, R. D. (1974). The toxicity of polychlorinated polycyclic compounds and related chemicals. *CRC Crit. Rev. Toxicol.* **2,** 445–489.

Kimbrough, R. D., ed. (1980). "Halogenated Biphenyls, Terphenyls, Naphthalenes, Dibenzodioxins and Related Products." Elsevier/North-Holland, Amsterdam.

Kimbrough, R. D. (1987). Human health effects of polychlorinated biphenyls (PCBs) and polybrominated biphenyls (PBBs). *Annu. Rev. Toxicol.* **27,** 87–111.

Kimbrough, R. D., and Jensen, A. A. (eds.) (1989). *Halogenated Biphenyls, Terphenyls, Naphthalenes, Dibenzodioxins and Related Products.* Elsevier/North-Holland, Amsterdam.

Kimbrough, R. D., and Linder, R. E. (1975). The effect of technical and 99% pure pentachlorophenol on the rat liver. Light microscopy and ultrastructure. *Toxicol. Appl. Pharmacol.* **33,** 131–132.

Kimbrough, R. D., and Linder, R. E. (1978). The effect of technical and purified pentachlorophenol on the rat liver. *Toxicol. Appl. Pharmacol.* **46,** 151–162.

Kimbrough, R. D., Carter, C. D., Liddle, J. A., Cline, R. E., and Phillips, P. E. (1977). Epidemiology and pathology of a tetrachlorodibenzodioxin poisoning episode. *Arch. Environ. Health* **32,** 77–86.

Kimbrough, R. D., Buckley, J., Fishbein, L., Flamm, G., Kasza, L., Marcus, W., Shibko, S., and Teske, R. (1978). Animal toxicology. *Environ. Health Perspect.* **24,** 173–185.

Kimbrough, R. D., Falk, H., Stehr, P., and Fries, G. (1984). Health implications of 2,3,7,8-tetrachlorodibenzo-*p*-dioxin (TCDD) contamination of residential soil. *J. Toxicol. Environ. Health* **14,** 47–93.

Kimmig, J., and Schulz, K. H. (1957a). Occupational acne (so-called chloracne) due to chlorinated aromatic cyclic ethers. *Dermatologica* **115,** 540.

Kimmig, J., and Schulz, K. H. (1957b). Chlorinated aromatic cyclic ether as cause of the so-called chloracne. *Naturwissenschaften* **44,** 337–338 (in German).

Kimura, S., Gonzalez, F. J., and Nebert, D. W. (1984). The murine *Ah* locus. Comparison ot the complete cytochrome P_1-450 and P_3-450 cDNA nucleotide and amino acid sequences. *J. Biol. Chem.* **259,** 10705–10713.

Kimura, S., Gonzalez, F. J., and Nebert, D. W. (1986). Tissue specific expression of the mouse dioxin-inducible P_1-450 and P_3-450 genes: Differential transcriptional activation and mRNA stability in liver and extrahepatic tissues. *Mol. Cell. Biol.* **6,** 1471–1477.

King, E., and Harvey, D. G. (1953). Some observations on the absorption and excretion of 4,6-dinitro-*o*-cresol (DNOC). I. Blood dinitro-*o*-cresol levels in the rat and the rabbit following different methods of absorption. *Biochem. J.* **53,** 185–195.

Kinzell, J. H., Ames, N. K., Sleight, S. D., Krehbiel, J. D., Kuo, C., Zabik, M. H., and Shull, L. R. (1981). Subchronic administration of technical pentachlorophenol to lactating dairy cattle: Performance, general health, and pathologic changes. *J. Dairy Sci.* **64,** 42–51.

Kirby, A. H. M. (1966). Dinitroalkylphenols: Versatile agents for control of agricultural pests and diseases. *World Rev. Pest Control* **5,** 30–44.

Kirsch, R., Fleischner, G., Kamisaka, K., and Arias, I. M. (1975). Structural and functional studies of ligandin, a major renal organic anion-binding protein. *J. Clin. Invest.* **55,** 1009–1019.

Kitchin, K. T., and Woods, J. S. (1979). 2,3,7,8-Tetrachlorodibenzo-*p*-dioxin (TCDD) effects on hepatic microsomal cytochrome P-448-mediated enzyme activities. *Toxicol. Appl. Pharmacol.* **47,** 537–546.

Kleeman, J. M., Olson, J. R., and Peterson, R. E. (1988). Species differences in 2,3,7,8-tetrachlorodibenzo-*p*-dioxin toxicity and biotransformation in fish. *Fundam. Appl. Toxicol.* **10,** 206–213.

Kleinman, G. D., Horstman, S. W., Kalman, D. A., McKenzie, J., and Stansel, D. (1986). Industrial hygiene, chemical and biological assessments of exposures to a chlorinated phenolic sapstain control agent. *Am. Ind. Hyg. Assoc. J.* **47,** 731–741.

Kleopfer, R. D. (1985). 2,3,7,8-TCDD contamination in Missouri. *Chemosphere* **14,** 739–744.

Knudsen, I., Verschuuren, H. G., Den Tonkelaar, E. M., Kroes, R., and Helleman, P. F. W. (1974). Short-term toxicity of pentachlorophenol in rats. *Toxicology* **2,** 141–152.

Knutsen, A. P. (1984). Immunologic effects of TCDD exposure in humans. *Bull. Environ. Contam. Toxicol.* **33,** 673–681.

Knutson, J. C., and Poland, A. (1980a). 2,3,7,8-Tetrachlorodibenzo-*p*-dioxin: Failure to demonstrate toxicity in twenty-three cultured cell types. *Toxicol. Appl. Pharmacol.* **54,** 377–383.

Knutson, J. C., and Poland, A. (1980b). Keratinization of mouse teratoma cell line XB produced by 2,3,7,8-tetrachlorodibenzo-*p*-dioxin: An *in vitro* model of toxicity. *Cell (Cambridge, Mass.)* **22,** 27–36.

Knutson, J. C., and Poland, A. (1982). Response of murine epidermis to the 2,3,7,8-tetrachlorodibenzo-*p*-dioxin: Interaction of the *Ah* and *hr* loci. *Cell (Cambridge, Mass.)* **30,** 225–234.

Kochman, S., Bernard, J., Cazabat, A., Lavaud, F., Lorton, C., and Rappe, C. (1986). Phenotypical dissection of immunoregulatory T cell subsets in human after furan exposure. *Chemosphere* **15,** 1799–1804.

Kociba, R. J., and Schwetz, B. A. (1982). Toxicity of 2,3,7,8-tetrachlorodibenzo-*p*-dioxin (TCDD). *Drug Metab. Rev.* **13,** 387–406.

Kociba, R. J., Keeler, P. A., Park, C. N., and Gehring, P. J. (1976). 2,3,7,8-Tetrachlorodibenzo-*p*-dioxin (TCDD): Results of a 13-week oral toxicity study in rats. *Toxicol. Appl. Pharmacol.* **35,** 553–574.

Kociba, R. J., Keyes, D. G., Beyer, J. E., Carreon, R. M., Wade, C. E., Dittenber, D. A., Kalnins, R. P., Frauson, L. E., Park, C. N., Barnard, S. D., Hummel, R. A., and Humiston, C. G. (1978). Results of a two-year chronic toxicity and oncogenicity study of 2,3,7,8-tetrachlorodibenzo-*p*-dioxin in rats. *Toxicol. Appl. Pharmacol.* **46,** 279–303.

Kociba, R. J., Keyes, D. G., Beyer, J. E., Carreon, R. M., and Gehring, P. J. (1979). Long-term toxicologic studies of 2,3,7,8-tetrachlorodibenzo-*p*-dioxin (TCDD) in laboratory animals. *Ann. N. Y. Acad. Sci.* **320,** 397–404.

Kondorosi, A., Fedorcsak, I., Solymosy, F., Ehrenberg, L., and Osterman-Golkar, S. (1973). Inactivation of QB RNA by electrophiles. *Mutat. Res.* **17,** 149–161.

Koshakji, R. P., Harbison, R. D., and Bush, M. T. (1984). Studies on the metabolic fate of ¹⁴C-tetrachlorodibenzo-*p*-dioxin (TCDD) in the mouse. *Toxicol. Appl. Pharmacol.* **73,** 69–77.

Kouri, R. E., Ratrie, H., III, Atlas, S. A., Niwa, A., and Nebert, D. W. (1974). Aryl hydrocarbon hydroxylase induction in human lymphocyte cultures by 2,3,7,8-tetrachlorodibenzo-*p*-dioxin. *Life Sci.* **15,** 1585–1595.

Kouri, R. E., Rude, T. H., Joglekar, R., Dansette, P. M., Jerina, D. M., Atlas, S. A., Owens, I. S., and Nebert, D. W. (1978). 2,3,7,8-Tetrachlorodibenzo-*p*-dioxin as cocarcinogen causing 3-methylcholanthrene-initiated subcutaneous tumors in mice genetically "nonresponsive" at *Ah* locus. *Cancer Res.* **38,** 2777–2783.

Kramer, C. M., Sando, J. J., and Holsapple, M. P. (1986). Lack of direct effect of 2,3,7,8-tetrachlorodibenzo-*p*-dioxin (TCDD) on protein kinase C activity in EL4 cells. *Biochem. Biophys. Res. Commun.* **140,** 267–272.

Kramer, C. M., Johnson, K. W., Dooley, R. K., and Holsapple, M. P. (1987). 2,3,7,8-Tetrachlorodibenzo-*p*-dioxin (TCDD) enhances antibody production and protein kinase activity in murine B cells. *Biochem. Biophys. Res. Commun.* **145,** 25–33.

Kumaki, K., Jensen, N. M., Shire, J. G. M., and Nebert, D. W. (1977). Genetic differences in induction of cytosol reduced-NAD(P): menadione oxidoreductase and microsomal aryl hydrocarbon hydroxylase in the mouse. *J. Biol. Chem.* **252,** 157–165.

Kunita, N., Kashimoto, T., Miyata, H., Fukushima, S., Hori, S., and Obana, H. (1984). Causal agents of Yusho. *Am. J. Ind. Med.* **5,** 45–58.

Kunita, N., Hori, S., Obana, H., Otake, T., Nishimura, H., Kashimoto, T., and Ikegami, N. (1985). Biological effect of PCBs, PCQs and PCDFs present in oil causing Yusho and Yu-Cheng. *Environ. Health Perspect.* **59,** 79–84.

Kupfer, D., Miranda, G. K., Navarro, J., Piccolo, D. E., and Theoharides, A. D. (1979). Effects of inducers and inhibitors of monooxygenase on the hydroxylation of prostaglandins in the guinea pig. *J. Biol. Chem.* **254,** 10405–10414.

Kuratsune, M. (1972). An abstract of results of laboratory examinations of patients with Yusho and of animal experiments. *Environ. Health Perspect.* **1,** 129–136.

Kuratsune, M. (1980). Yusho. *In* "Halogenated Biphenyls, Terphenyls, Naphthalenes, Dibenzodioxins, and Related Products" (R. D. Kimbrough, ed.), pp. 287–302. Elsevier/North-Holland Press, Amsterdam.

Kuratsune, M. (1989). Yusho, with reference to Yu-Cheng. *In* "Halogenated Biphenyls, Terphenyls, Naphthalenes, Dibenzodioxins and Related Products" (R. D. Kimbrough and A. A. Jensen, eds.), Elsevier/North-Holland, New York.

Kuratsune, M., Yoshimura, T., Matsuzaka, J., and Yamaguchi, A. (1972). Epidimiologic study on Yusho, a poisoning caused by ingestion of rice oil contaminated with a commercial brand of polychlorinated biphenyls. *Environ. Health Perspect.* **1,** 119–128.

Kuratsune, M., Nakamura, T., Ikeda, M., and Hirokata, T. (1987) Analysis of deaths seen among patients with Yusho. A preliminary report. *Chemosphere* **16,** 2085–2088.

Kurl, R. N., Lund, J., Poellinger, L., and Gustafsson, J.-A. (1982). Differential effect of 2,3,7,8-tetrachlorodibenzo-*p*-dioxin on nuclear RNA polymerase activity in the rat liver and thymus. *Biochem. Pharmacol.* **31,** 2459–2462.

Kutz, F. W., Murphy, R. S., and Strassman, S. C. (1978). Survey of pesticide residues and their metabolites in urine from the general population. *In* "Pentachlorophenol: Chemistry, Pharmacology and Environmental Toxicology" (K. R. Rao, ed.), pp. 363–369. Plenum, New York.

Labruzzo, P., Yu, X. F., and Dufresne, M. J. (1989). Induction of aryl hydrocarbon hydroxylase and demonstration of a specific nuclear receptor for 2,3,7,8-tetrachlorodibenzo-*p*-dioxin in two human hepatoma cell lines. *Biochem. Pharmacol.* **38,** 2339–2348.

Lakshmanan, M. R., Campbell, B. S., Chirtel, S. J., Ekarohita, N., and Ezekiel, M. (1986). Studies on the mechanism of absorption and distribution of 2,3,7,8-tetrachlorodibenzo-*p*-dioxin in the rat. *J. Pharmacol. Exp. Ther.* **239,** 673–677.

Lamb, J. C., IV, Marks, T. A., Gladen, B. C., Allen, J. W., and Moore, J. A. (1981a). Male fertility, sister chromatid exchange, and germ cell toxicity following exposure to mixture of chlorinated phenoxy acids containing 2,3,7,8-tetrachlorodibenzo-*p*-dioxin. *J. Toxicol. Environ. Health* **8,** 825–834.

Lamb, J. C., IV, Moore, J. A., Marks, T. A., and Haseman, J. K. (1981b). Development and viability of offspring of male mice treated with chlorinated phenoxy acids and 2,3,7,8-tetrachlorodibenzo-*p*-dioxin. *J. Toxicol. Environ. Health* **8,** 835–844.

Lamb, J. C., IV, Harris, M. A., McKinney, J. D., and Birnbaum, L. S. (1986). Effects of thyroid hormones on the induction of cleft palate by 2,3,7,8-tetrachlorodibenzo-*p*-dioxin (TCDD) in C57BL/6N mice. *Toxicol. Appl. Pharmacol.* **84,** 115–124.

Larsen, P. R., and Silva, J. E. (1983). Intrapituitary mechanisms in the control of TSH secretion. *In* "Molecular Basis of Thyroid Hormone Action" (J. H. Oppenheimer and H. H. Samuels, eds.), pp. 351–385. Academic Press, New York.

Larsen, R. V., Kirsch, L. E., Shaw, S. M., Christian, J. E., and Born, G. S. (1972). Excretion and tissue distribution of uniformly labeled ¹⁴C-pentachlorophenol in rats. *J. Pharm. Sci.* **61,** 2004–2006.

Larsen, R. V., Born, G. S., Kessler, W. V., Shaw, S. M., and Van Sickle, D. C. (1975). Placental transfer and teratology of pentachlorophenol in rats. *Environ. Lett.* **10,** 121–128.

Larson, P. S., Finnegan, J. K., Smith, R. B., Jr., Haag, H. B, Hennigar, G. R., and Patterson, W. M. (1959). Acute and chronic toxicity studies on 2,4-dinitro-6-(1-methylheptyl)phenyl crotonate (Karathane). *Arch. Int. Pharmacodyn. Ther.* **119,** 31–42.

Lathrop, G. D., Wolfe, W. H., Albanese, R. A., and Moynahan, P. M. (1984). "An Epidemiologic Investigation of Health Effects in Air Force Personnel Following Exposure to Herbicides." A report prepared for the Surgeon General, United States Air Force, Washington, D. C.

Lawford, D. J., King, E., and Harvey, D. S. (1954). On the metabolism of some aromatic nitro-compounds by different species of animal. Part II. The elimination of various nitro-compounds from the blood of different species of animal. *J. Pharm. Pharmacol.* **6,** 619–624.

Lee, I. P., and Suzuki, K. (1980). Induction of aryl hydrocarbon hydroxylase activity in the rat prostate glands by 2,3,7,8-tetrachlorodibenzo-*p*-dioxins. *J. Pharmacol. Exp. Ther.* **215,** 601–605.

Leece, B., Denomme, M. A., Towner, R., Li, A., Landerg, J., and Safe, S. (1987). Nonadditive interactive effects of polychlorinated biphenyl congeners in rats: Role of the 2,3,7,8-tetrachlorodibenzo-*p*-dioxin receptor. *Can. J. Physiol. Pharmacol.* **65**, 1908–1912.

Legraverend, C., Karenlampi, S. O., Bigelow, S. W., Lalley, P. A., Kozak, C. A., Womack, J. E., and Nebert, D. W. (1984). Aryl hydrocarbon hydroxylase induction of benzo(*a*)anthracene: Regulatory gene localized to the distal portion of mouse chromosome 17. *Genetics* **107**, 447–461.

Lehman, A. J. (1951). Chemicals in foods: A report to the Association of Food and Drug Officials on current developments. Part II. Pesticides. Section I. Introduction. *Q. Bull—Assoc. Food Drug. Off. I.* **15**, (I), 122–125.

Lehman, A. J. (1952). Chemicals in foods: A report to the Association of Food and Drug Officials on current developments. Part II. Pesticides. Section II. Dermal Toxicity. Section III. Subacute and chronic toxicity. Section IV. Biochemistry. Section V. Pathology. *Q. Bull.—Assoc. Food Drug Off.* **16**, (II), 3–9; (III), 47–53; (IV), 85–91; (V), 126–132.

Leighty, E. G., and Fentiman, A. F., Jr. (1982). Conjugation of pentachlorophenol to palmitic acid by liver microsomes. *Bull. Environ. Contam. Toxicol.* **28**, 329–333.

Lesca, P., Fernandez, N., and Roy, M. (1987). The binding components for 2,3,7,8-tetrachlorodibenzo-*p*-dioxin and polycyclic aromatic hydrocarbons. Separation from the rat and mouse hepatic cytosol and characterization of a light density component. *J. Biol. Chem.* **262**, 4827–4835.

Leung, H.-W., Murray, F. J., and Paustenbach, D. J. (1988). A proposed occupational exposure limit for 2,3,7,8-tetrachlorodibenzo-*p*-dioxin. *Am. Ind. Hyg. Assoc. J.* **49**, 466–474.

Liem, H. H., Müller-Eberhard, U., and Johnson, E. F. (1980). Differential induction by 2,3,7,8-tetrachlorodibenzo-*p*-dioxin of multiple forms of rabbit microsomal cytochrome P-450: Evidence for tissue specificity. *J. Mol. Pharmacol.* **18**, 565–570.

Linder, R. E., Scotti, T. M., Svendsgaard, D. J., McElroy, W. K., and Curley, A. (1982). Testicular effects of dinoseb in rats. *Arch. Environ. Contam. Toxicol.* **11**, 475–485.

Linder, R. E., Strader, L. F., and McElroy, W. K. (1986). Measurement of epididymal sperm motility as a test variable in the rat. *Bull. Environ. Contam. Toxicol.* **36**, 317–324.

Link, R. P. (1953). Bovine hyperkeratosis (X disease). *J. Am. Vet. Med. Assoc.* **123**, 427–430.

Lochner, A., and Brink, A. J. (1969). The effects of oligomycin and 2,4-dinitrophenol on the mechanical performance and metabolism of the perfused rat heart. *Clin. Sci.* **37**, 191–204.

Loprieno, N., Sbrana, I., Rusciano, D., Lascialfari, D., and Lari, T. (1982). *In vivo* cytogenetic studies on mice and rats exposed to 2,3,7,8-tetrachlorodibenzo-*p*-dioxin. *In* "Chlorinated Dioxins and Related Compounds. Impact on the Environment" (O. Hutzinger, R. W. Frei, E. Merian, and P. Pocchiari, eds.), pp. 419–428. Pergamon, New York.

Louwagie, A. C., Cosyn, L., and Callewaert, J. (1978). Co-existence of morbus Hodgkin and aplastic anemia. *Acta Clin. Belg.* **33**, 66–68.

Lovati, M. R., Galbussera, M., Franceschini, G., Weber, G., Resi, L., Tanganelli, P., and Sirtori, C. R. (1984). Increased plasma and aortic triglycerides in rabbits after acute adminstration of 2,3,7,8-tetrachlorodibenzo-*p*-dioxin. *Toxicol. Appl. Pharmacol.* **75**, 91–97.

Lu, Y.-C., and Wu, Y.-C. (1985). Clinical findings and immunological abnormalities in Yu-Cheng patients. *Environ. Health Perspect.* **59**, 17–30.

Lubet, R. A., Connolly, G., Kouri, R. E., Nebert, D. W., and Bigelow, S. W. (1983). Biological effects on Sudan dyes. Role of the *Ah* cytosolic receptor. *Biochem. Pharmacol.* **32**, 3053–3058.

Lubet, R. A., Brunda, M. J., Taramelli, D., Dansie, D., Nebert, D. W., and Kouri, R. E. (1984). Induction of immunotoxicity by polycyclic hydrocarbons. *Arch. Toxicol.* **56**, 18–24.

Lucier, G. W., McDaniel. O. S., Hook, G. E. R., Fowler, B. A., Sonawane, B., and Faeder, R. (1973). TCDD-induced changes in rat liver microsomal enzymes. *Environ. Health Perspect.* **5**, 199–209.

Lucier, G. W., Babasaheb, R., Sonawane, B. R., McDaniel, O. S., and Hook, G. E. R. (1975a). Postnatal stimulation of hepatic microsomal enzymes following administration of TCDD to pregnant rats. *Chem.-Biol. Interact.* **11**, 15–26.

Lucier, G. W., McDaniel, O. S., and Hook, G. E. R. (1975b). Nature of the enhancement of hepatic uridine diphosphate glucuronyltransferase activity

by 2,3,7,8-tetrachlorodibenzo-*p*-dioxin in rats. *Biochem. Pharmacol.* **24**, 325–334.

Lucier, G. W., Rumbaugh, R. C., McCoy, Z., Hass, R., Harvan, D., and Albro, P. (1986). Ingestion of soil contaminated with 2,3,7,8-tetrachlorodibenzo-*p*-dioxin (TCDD) alters enzyme activities in rats. *Toxicol. Appl. Pharmacol.* **6**, 364–371.

Lucier, G. W., Nelson, K. G., Everson, R. B., Wong, T. K., Philpot, R. M., Tiernan, T., Taylor, M., and Sunahara, G. I., (1987). Placental markers of human exposure to polychlorinated biphenyls and polychlorinated dibenzofurans. *Envir. Health Perspect.* **76**, 79–87.

Lundgren, K., Andries, M., Thompson, C., and Lucier, G. W. (1986). Dioxin treatment of rats results in increased in vitro induction of sister chromatid exchanges by α-naphthoflavone: An animal model for human exposure to halogenated aromatics. *Toxicol. Appl. Pharmacol* **8**, 189–195.

Luster, M. I., Boorman, G. A., Dean, J. H., Harris, M. W., Luebke, R. W., Padarathsingh, M. L., and Moore, J. A. (1980). Examination of bone marrow, immunologic parameters and host susceptibility following pre- and postnatal exposure to 2,3,7,8-tetrachlorodibenzo-*p*-dioxin (TCDD). *Int. J. Immunopharmacol.* **2**, 301–310.

Luster, M. I., Hong, L. H., Boorman, G. A., Clark, G., Hayes, H. T., Greenlee, W. F., Dold, K., and Tucker, A. N. (1985). Acute myelotoxic responses in mice exposed to 2,3,7,8-tetrachlorodibenzo-*p*-dioxin (TCDD). *Toxicol. Appl. Pharmacol* **81**, 156–165.

Luster, M. I., Hong, L. H., Osborne, R., Blank, J. A., Clark, G., Silver, M. T., Boorman, G. A., and Greenlee, W. F. (1986). 1-Amino-3,7,8-trichlorodibenzo-*p*-dioxin: A specific antagonist for TCDD-induced myelotoxicity. *Biochem. Biophys. Res. Commun.* **139**, 747–756.

Luster, M. I., Germolec, D. R., Clark, G., Weigand, G., and Rosenthal, G. J. (1988). Selective effects of 2,3,7,8-tetrachlorodibenzo-*p*-dioxin and dibenzo-*p*-dioxin and corticosteroid on *in vitro* lymphocyte maturation. *J. Immunol.* **140**, 928–935.

Madhukar, B. V., Brewster, D. W., and Matusmura, F. (1984). Effects of *in vivo*-administered 2,3,7,8-tetrachlorodibenzo-*p*-dioxin on receptor binding of epidermal growth factor in the hepatic plasma membrane of rat, guinea pig, mouse, and hamster. *Proc. Natl. Acad. Sci. U.S.A.* **81**, 7407–7411.

Magne, H., Mayer, A., and Plantefol, L. (1932a). Pharmacodynamic action of nitro-phenols. An agent stimulating cellular oxidation; 1,2,4-dinitro-phenol (Thermol). I. General character of 1,2,4-dinitro-phenol poisoning. *Ann. Physiol. Physicochim. Biol.* **8**, 1–50.

Magne, H., Mayer, A., and Plantefol, L. (1932b). Pharmacodynamic action of nitro-phenols. An agent stimulating cellular oxidation; 1,2,4-dinitro-phenol (Thermol). VIII. Pharmacologic action of various nitro-phenols; comparison of 1,2,4-dinitro-phenol poisoning with that produced by other nitro phenols. *Ann. Physiol. Physicochim. Biol.* **8**, 157–175.

Malik, N., and Owens, I. S. (1981). Genetic regulation of bilirubin-UDP-glucuronosyltransferase induction by polycyclic aromatic compounds and phenobarbital in mice. *J. Biol. Chem.* **256**, 9599–9604.

Malik, N., Koteen, G. M., and Owens, I. S. (1979). Induction of UDP-glucuronosyltransferase in the Reuber H-4-II-E hepatoma cell culture. *Mol. Pharmacol.* **16**, 950–960.

Manchester, D. K., Gordon, S. K., Golas, C. L., Roberts, E. A., and Okey, A. B. (1987). *Ah* receptor in human placenta: Stabilization by molybdate and characterization of binding of 2,3,7,8-tetrachlorodibenzo-*p*-dioxin, 3-methylcholanthrene, and benzo(*a*)pyrene. *Cancer Res.* **47**, 4861–4868.

Mantovani, A., Vecci, A., Luini, W., Sironi, M., Candiani, G., Spreatico, F., and Garratini, S. (1980). Effect of 2,3,7,8-tetrachlorodibenzo-*p*-dioxin on macrophage and natural killer cell-mediated cytotoxicity in mice. *Biomedicine* **32**, 200–204.

Markicevic, A., Prpic-Majic, D., and Bosnar-Turk, N. (1972). Results of examinations of workers exposed to dinitro-*ortho*-cresol. *Arh. Hig. Rada Toksikol.* **23**, 1–9 (in Serbo-Croatian).

Mason, G., and Safe, S. (1986). Synthesis, biologic and toxic effects of the major 2,3,7,8-tetrachlorodibenzo-*p*-dioxin metabolites in the rat. *Toxicology* **41**, 153–159.

Mason, G., Sawyer, T., Keys, B., Bandiera, S., Romkes, M., Piskorska-Pliszczynska, J., Zmudzka, B., and Safe, S. (1985). Polychlorinated dibenzofurans (PCDFs): Correlation between *in vivo* and *in vitro* structure–activity relationships. *Toxicology* **37**, 1–12.

Mason, G., Farrell, K., Keys, B., Piskorska-Pliszczynska, J., Safe, L., and Safe, S. (1986). Polychlorinated dibenzo-*p*-dioxins: Quantitative *in vitro* and *in vivo* structure–activity relationships. *Toxicology* **41**, 21–31.

Mason, G. G. F., Wilhelmsson, A., Cuthill, G., Gillner, M., Poellinger, L., and Gustafsson, J.-A. (1988). The dioxin receptor: Characterization of its DNA-binding properties. *J. Steroid Biochem.* **30**, 307–310.

Mason, M. E., and Okey, A. B. (1982). Cytosolic and nuclear binding of 2,3,7,8-tetrachlorodibenzo-*p*-dioxin to the *Ah* receptor in extra-hepatic tissues of rats and mice. *Eur. J. Biochem.* **123**, 209–215.

Masuda, Y. (1985). Health status of Japanese and Taiwanese after exposure to contaminated rice oil. *Envir. Health Perspect.* **60**, 321–325.

Masuda, Y., Kuroki, H., Yamaryo, T., and Haraguchi, K. (1982). Comparison of causal agents in Taiwan and Fukuoka PCB poisonings. *Chemosphere* **11**, 199–206.

Matsumura, A. (1972). The relationship between chemical structures of chlorophenols and their biological activities. *Jpn. J. Ind. Health* **14**, 30–31.

Matsumura, F., Brewster, D. W., Madhukar, B. V., and Bombick, D. W. (1984a). Alteration of rat hepatic plasma membrane functions by 2,3,7,8-tetrachlorodibenzo-*p*-dioxin (TCDD). *Arch. Environ. Contam. Toxicol.* **13**, 509–515.

Matsumura, F., Madhukar, B. V., Bombick, D. W., and Brewster, D. W. (1984b). Toxicological significance of pleiotropic changes of plasma membrane functions particularly that of EGF receptor caused by 2,3,7,8-TCDD. *Banbury Rep.* **18**, 267–290.

Mattison, D. R., and Thorgeirsson, S. S. (1978). Gonadal aryl hydrocarbon hydroxylase in rats and mice. *Cancer Res.* **38**, 1368–1373.

Max, S. R., and Silbergeld, E. K. (1987). Skeletal muscle glucocorticoid receptor and glutamine synthetase activity in the wasting syndrome in rats treated with 2,3,7,8-tetrachlorodibenzo-*p*-dioxin. *Toxicol. Appl. Pharmacol.* **87**, 523–527.

May, G. (1973). Chloracne from the accidental production of tetrachlorodibenzodioxin. *Br. J. Ind. Med.* **30**, 276–283.

May, G. (1982). Tetrachlorodibenzodioxini: A survey of subjects ten years after exposure. *Br. J. Ind. Med.* **39**, 128–135.

Mazzella di Bosco, M. (1970). Some cases of occupational poisoning with dinitrophenols (binapacryl, DNOC, Karathane) in agricultural workers. *J. Eur. Toxicol.* **3**, 325–331 (in Italian).

McConkey, D. J., and Orrenius, S. (1989). 2,3,7,8-Tetrachlorodibenzo-p-dioxin (TCDD) kills glucocorticoid-sensitive thymocytes *in vivo. Biochem. Biophys. Res. Commun.* **160**, 1003–1008.

McConkey, D. J., Hartzell, P., Duddy, S. K., Hakansson, H., and Orrenius, S. (1988). 2,3,7,8-Tetrachlorodibenzo-*p*-dioxin kills immature thymocytes by Ca^{2+}-mediated endonuclease activation. *Science* **242**, 256–259.

McConnell, E. E. (1980). Acute and chronic toxicity, carcinogenesis, reproduction, teratogenesis and mutagenesis in animals. *In* "Halogenated Biphenyls, Terphenyls, Naphthalenes, Dibenzodioxins and Related Products" (R. D. Kimbrough, ed.), pp. 109–150. Elsevier/North-Holland Press, New York.

McConnell, E. E. (1984). Clinicopathologic concepts of dibenzo-*p*-dioxin intoxication. *Banbury Rep.* **18**, 27–37.

McConnell, E. E., and McKinney, J. D. (1978). Exquisite toxicity in the guinea pig to structurally similar halogenated dioxins, furans, biphenyls, and naphthalenes. *Toxicol. Appl. Pharmacol.* **45**, 298.

McConnell, E. E., and Moore, J. A. (1976). The comparative toxicity of chlorinated dibenzo-*p*-dioxin isomers in mice and guinea pigs. *Toxicol. Appl. Pharmacol.* **37**, 146.

McConnell, E. E., and Moore, J. A. (1979). Toxicopathology characteristics of the halogenated aromatics. *Ann. N.Y. Acad. Sci.* **320**, 138–150.

McConnell, E. E., Moore, J. A., and Dalgard, D. W. (1978a). Toxicity of 2,3,7,8-tetrachlorodibenzo-*p*-dioxin in rhesus monkeys (*Macaca mulatta*) following a single oral dose. *Toxicol. Appl. Pharmacol.* **43**, 175–187.

McConnell, E. E., Moore, J. A., Haseman, J. K., and Harris, M. W. (1978b). The comparative toxicity of chlorinated dibenzo-*p*-dioxins in mice and guinea pigs. *Toxicol. Appl. Pharmacol.* **44**, 335–356.

McConnell, E. E., Hass, J. R., Altman, N., and Moore, J. A. (1979). A spontaneous outbreak of polychlorinated biphenyl (PCB) toxicity in rhesus monkeys (*Macaca mulatta*): Toxicopathology. *Lab. Anim. Sci.* **29**, 666–673.

McConnell, E. E., Moore, J. A., Gupta, B. N., Rakes, A. H., Luster, M. I., Goldstein, J. A., Haseman, J. K., and Parker, C. E. (1980). The chronic toxicity of technical and analytical pentachlorophenol in cattle. 1. Clinicopathology. *Toxicol. Appl. Pharmacol.* **52**, 468–490.

McConnell, E. E., Lucier, G. W., Rumbaugh, R. C., Albro, P. W., Harvan, D. J., Hass, J. R., and Harris, M. W. (1984). Dioxin in soil: Bioavailability after ingestion by rats and guinea pigs. *Science* **223**, 1077–1079.

McCormack, K. M., Gibson, J. E., and Hook, J. B. (1976). Effect of 2,3,7,8-tetrachlorodibenzo-*p*-dioxin (TCDD) on renal function in rats *in vivo. Toxicol. Appl. Pharmacol.* **37**, 177.

McCormack, K. M., Abuelgasim, A., Sanger, V. L., and Hook, J. B. (1980). Postnatal morphology and functional capacity of the kidney following prenatal treatment with dinoseb in rats. *J. Toxicol. Environ. Health* **6**, 633–643.

McKellar, R. L. (1971). 2-*sec*-Butyl-4,6-dinitrophenol and 2-amino-6-*sec*-butyl-4-nitrophenol in milk and cream from cows fed 2-*sec*-butyl-4,6-dinitrophenol. *J. Agric. Food Chem.* **19**, 758–760.

McKinney, J. D., Gottschalk, K. E., and Pedersen, L. (1983). The polarizability of planar aromatic systems. An application to polychlorinated biphenyls (PCB's), dioxin, and polyaromatic hydrocarbons. *J. Mol. Struct.* **105**, 427–438.

McKinney, J. D., Chae, K., McConnell, E. E., and Birnbaum, L. S. (1985). Structure–induction versus structure–toxicity relationships for polychlorinated biphenyls and related aromatic hydrocarbons. *Environ. Health Perspect.* **60**, 57–68.

McNulty, W. P. (1978). "Direct Testimony before the Administrator," FIFRA Docket No. 415, EPA Exhibit No. 106. U.S. Environ. Prot. Agency, Washington, D.C.

McNulty, W. P. (1984). Fetocidal and teratogenic actions of TCDD. *In* "Public Health Risks of the Dioxins" (W. W. Lawrence and W. Kaufmann, eds.), pp. 245–253. William Kaufman, Inc., Los Altos, California.

McNulty, W. P. (1985). Toxicity and fetotoxicity of TCDD, TCDF, and PCB isomers in rhesus macaques (*Macaca mulatta*). *Environ. Health Perspect.* **60**, 77–88.

McNulty, W. P., Nielsen-Smith, J. O., Lay, J. O., Jr., Lippstreu, D. L., Kangas, N. L., Lyon, P. A., and Gross, M. L. (1982). Persistence of TCDD in monkey adipose tissue. *Food Cosmet. Toxicol.* **20**, 985–987.

McQueen, E. G., Veale, A. M. O., Alexander, W. S., and Bates, M. N. (1977). "2,4,5-T and Human Defects." Report of the Division of Public Health, New Zealand Department of Health (cited by Milby *et al.*, 1980).

Mebus, C. A., and Piper, W. N. (1986). Decreased rat adrenal 21-hydroxylase activity associated with decreased adrenal microsomal cytochrome P-450 after exposure to 2,3,7,8-tetrachlorodibenzo-*p*-dioxin. *Biochem. Pharmacol.* **35**, 4359–4362.

Mebus, C. A., Reddy, V. R., and Piper, W. N. (1987). Depression of rat testicular 17-hydroxylase and 17,20-lyase after administration of 2,3,7,8-tetrachlorodibenzo-*p*-dioxin (TCDD). *Biochem. Pharmacol.* **36**, 727–731.

Medvedeva, G. I. (1969). The participation of thyroid hormones in the realization of the action of dinitrophenols in vitro on oxidative phosphorylation in rabbit liver mitochondria. *Biokhimiya (Moscow)* **34**, 74–744.

Meerman, J. H. N. (1983). Use of pentachlorophenol as long-term inhibitor of sulfation of phenols and hydroxamic acids in the rat *in vivo. Biochem. Pharmacol.* **32**, 1587–1593.

Meerman, J. H. N. (1985). The initiation of gamma-glutamyltranspeptidase positive foci in the rat liver by *N*-hydroxy-2-acetylaminofluorene. The effect of the sulfation inhibitor pentachlorophenol. *Carcinogenesis (London)* **6**, 893–897.

Meerman, J. H. N., and Mulder, G. J. (1981). Prevention of the hepatotoxic action of *N*-hydroxy-2-acetylaminofluorene in the rat by inhibition of *N*-*O*-sulfation by pentachlorophenol. *Life Sci.* **28**, 2361–2365.

Meerman, J. H. N., Van Doorn, A. B. D., and Mulder, G. J. (1980). Inhibition of sulfate conjugation of *N*-hydroxy-2-acetylaminofluorene in isolated perfused rat liver and in the rat *in vivo* by pentachlorophenol and low sulfate. *Cancer Res.* **40**, 3772–3779.

Menon, J. A. (1958). Tropical hazards associated with the use of pentachlorophenol. *Br. J. Med.* **1**, 1156–1158.

Mercer, H. D., Teske, R. H., Condon, R. J., Furr, A., Meerdink, G., Buck, W., and Fries, G. (1976). Herd health status of animals exposed to polybrominated biphenyls (PBB). *J. Toxicol. Environ. Health* **2**, 335–349.

Michel, R., and Pairault, J. (1969). Comparative quantitative action of thyroid products and 2,4-dinitrophenol on mitochondria respiration. *C. R. Hebd. Seances Acad. Sci., Ser. D* **268**, 1549–1551.

Milby, T. H., Husting, E. L., Whorton, M. D., and Larson, S. (1980). "Potential Health Effects Associated with the Use of Phenoxy Herbicides: A Summary of Recent Scientific Literature." A report for the National Forest Products Association from Environmental Health Associated, Inc., Berkely, California.

Milham, S., Jr. (1982). Herbicides, occupation, and cancer. *Lancet* **1**, 1464–1465.

Milstone, L. M., and LaVigne, J. F. (1984). 2,3,7,8-Tetrachlorodibenzo-*p*-dioxin induces hyperplasia in confluent cultures of human keratinocytes. *J. Invest. Dermatol.* **82**, 532–534.

Mitchell, P. (1961). Coupling of phosphorylation of electron and hydrogen transfer by a chemi-osmotic type of mechanism. *Nature (London)* **191**, 144–148.

Mitchum, R. K., Moler, G. F., and Korfmacher, W. A. (1980). Combined capillary gas chromatography/atmospheric pressure negative chemical ionization/mass spectrometry for the determination of 2,3,7,8-tetrachlorodibenzo-*p*-dioxin in tissue. *Anal. Chem.* **52**, 2278–2282.

Miura, H., Omori, A., and Shibue, M. (1974). The effect of chlorophenols on the excretion of porphyrins in urine. *Jpn. J. Ind. Health* **16**, 575 (in Japanese).

Mlodecki, H., Fortak, W., Szadowska, A., Fraczek, S., Graczyk, J., and Wejmon, I. (1975). Toxicity studies on dinocap. Part I. Acute toxicity. *Bromatol. Chem. Toksykol.* **8**, 373–386.

Mocarelli, P., Marocchi, A., Brambilla, P., Gerthoux, P., Young, D. S., and Mantel, N. (1986). Clinical laboratory manifestations of exposure to dioxin in children. *JAMA, J. Am. Med. Assoc.* **256**, 2687–2695.

Mohammadpour, H., Murray, W. J., and Stohs, S. J. (1988). 2,3,7,8-Tetrachlorodibenzo-*p*-dioxin-induced lipid peroxidation in genetically responsive and non-responsive mice. *Arch. Environ. Contam. Toxicol.* **17**, 645–650.

Moore, J. A., Gupta, B. N., Zinkl, J. G., and Vos, J. G. (1973). Postnatal effects of maternal exposure to 2,3,7,8-tetrachlorodibenzo-*p*-dioxin (TCDD). *Environ. Health Perspect.* **5**, 81–85.

Moore, J. A., Harris, H. W., and Albro, P. W. (1976). Tissue distribution of ¹⁴C tetrachlorodibenzo-*p*-dioxin in pregnant and neonatal rats. *Toxicol. Appl. Pharmacol.* **37**, 146–147.

Moore, J. A., McConnell, E. E., Dalgard, D. W., and Harris, M. W. (1979). Comparative toxicity of three halogenated dibenzofurans in guinea pigs, mice, and rhesus monkeys. *Ann. N.Y. Acad. Sci.* **320**, 151–163.

Moore, R. W., and Peterson, R. E (1988). Androgen catabolism and excretion in 2,3,7,8-tetrachlorodibenzo-*p*-dioxin-treated rats. *Biochem. Pharmacol.* **37**, 560–562.

Moore, R. W., Dannan, G. A., and Aust, S. D. (1978). Induction of drug-metabolizing enzymes in polybrominated biphenyl-fed lactating rats and their pups. *Environ. Health Perspect.* **23**, 159–165.

Moore, R. W., Potter, C. L., Theobald, H. M., Robinson, J. A., and Peterson, R. E. (1985). Androgenic deficiency in male rats treated with 2,3,7,8-tetrachlorodibenzo-*p*-dioxin. *Toxicol. Appl. Pharmacol.* **79**, 99–111.

Moore, R. W., Parsons, J. A., Bookstaff, R. C., and Peterson, R. E. (1989). Plasma concentrations of pituitary hormones in 2,3,7,8-tetrachlorodibenzo *p*-dioxin-treated male rats. *J. Biochem. Toxicol.* **4**, 165–172.

Moran, R. A., Lee, C. W., Fujimoto, J. M., and Calvanico, N. H. (1986). Effects of 2,3,7,8-tetrachlorodibenzo-*p*-dioxin (TCDD) on IgA serum and bile levels in rats. *Immunopharmacology* **12**, 245–250.

Moreland, D. E., and Hilton, J. L. (1976). Actions on photosynthetic systems. *In* "Herbicides: Physiology, Biochemistry, Ecology" (L. J. Audus, ed.), 2nd ed., Vol. 1, p. 493. Academic Press, New York.

Morse, D. L., Baker, E. L., Jr., Kimbrough, R. D., and Wisseman, C. L. (1979). Propanil-chloracne and methomyl toxicity in workers of a pesticide manufacturing plant. *Clin. Toxicol.* **15**, 13–21.

Mortelmans, K., Haworth, S., Speck, W., and Zieger, E. (1984). Mutagenicity testing of Agent Orange components and related compounds. *Toxicol. Appl. Pharmacol.* **75**, 137–146.

Moses, M., Lilis, R., Crow, K. D., Thornton, J., Fischbein, A., Anderson, H. A., and Selikoff, I. H. (1984). Health status of workers with past exposure to 2,3,7,8-tetrachlorodibenzo-*p*-dioxin in the manufacture of 2,4,5-trichlorophenoxyacetic acid: Comparison of findings with and without chloracne. *Am. J. Ind. Med.* **5**, 161–182.

Most, H. (1963). Treatment of the most common worm infestations. *JAMA, J. Am. Med. Assoc.* **185**, 874–877.

Mukerji, S. K., Pimstone, N. R., and Burns, M. (1984). Dual mechanism of inhibition of rat liver uroporphyrinogen decarboxylase activity by ferrous iron: Its potential role in the genesis of porphyria cutanea tarda. *Gastroenterology* **87**, 1248–1254.

Mulder, G. J., and Scholtens, E. (1977). Phenol sulfotransferase and uridine diphosphate glucuronosyl transferase from rat liver *in vitro* and *in vivo*: 2,6-Dichloro-5-4-nitrophenol as a selective inhibitor of sulfation. *Biochem. J.* **165**, 553–559.

Muller, J., and Haberzettl, R. (1980). Mutagenicity of DNOC in *Drosophila melanogaster*. *Arch. Toxicol., Suppl.* **4**, 59–61.

Mullet, J. E., and Arntzen, C. J. (1981). Identification of a 32–34-kilodalton polypeptide as a herbicide receptor protein in photosystem II. *Biochim. Biophys. Acta* **635**, 236–248.

Murai, Y., and Kuriowa, Y. (1971). Peripheral neuropathy in chlorobiphenyl exposure. *Neurology* **21**, 1173–1176.

Murray, F. J., Smith, F. A., Nitschke, K. D., Humiston, C. G., Kociba, R. J., and Schwetz, B. A. (1979). Three-generation reproduction study of rats given 2,3,7,8-tetrachlorodibenzo-*p*-dioxin (TCDD) in the diet. *Toxicol. Appl. Pharmacol.* **50**, 241–251.

Nagarkatti, P. S., Sweeney, G. D., Gauldie, J., and Clark, D. A. (1984). Sensitivity to suppression of cytotoxic T-cell generation by 2,3,7,8-tetrachlorodibenzo-*p*-dioxin (TCDD) is dependent on the *Ah* genotype of the murine host. *Toxicol. Appl. Pharmacol.* **72**, 169–176.

Nagayama, J., Kiyohara, C., Masuda, Y., and Kuratsunc, M. (1985). Genetically mediated induction of aryl hydrocarbon hydroxylase activity in human lymphoblastoid cells by polychlorinated dibenzofuran isomers and 2,3,7,8-tetrachlorodibenzo-*p*-dioxin. *Arch. Toxicol.* **56**, 230–235.

Nakaue, H. S., Caldwell, R. S., and Buhler, D. R. (1972). Bisphenols— Uncouplers of phosphorylating respiration. *Biochem. Pharmacol.* **21**, 2273–2277.

National Institute for Occupational Safety and Health (NIOSH) (1978). "Criteria for a Recommended Standard: Occupational Exposure to Dinitro-*ortho*-cresol," DHEW Publ. No. 78-131. Natl. Inst. Occup. Saf. Health, Cincinnati, Ohio.

National Toxicology Program (NTP) (1980a). "Bioassay of 2,3,7,8-Tetrachlorodibenzo-*p*-dioxin for Possible Carcinogenicity (Gavage Study)," DHHS Publ. No. (NIH) 82-1765. Carcinogenesis Testing Program, NCI, NIH, Bethesda, Maryland, and National Toxicology Program, Research Triangle Park, North Carolina.

National Toxicology Program (NTP) (1980b). "Bioassay of 2,3,7,8-Tetrachlordibenzo-*p*-dioxin for Possible Carcinogenicity (Dermal Study)," DHHS Publ. No. (NIH) 80-1757. Carcinogenesis Testing Program, NCI, NIH, Bethesda, Maryland, and National Toxicology Program, Research Triangle Park, North Carolina.

National Toxicology Program (NTP) (1985). Unpublished results, cited in U.S. Environmental Protection Agency (1985).

Nau, H., and Bass, R. (1981). Transfer of 2,3,7,8-tetrachlorodibenzo-*p*-dioxin (TCDD) to the mouse embryo and fetus. *Toxicology* **20**, 299–308.

Nau, H., Bass, R., and Neubert, D. (1986). Transfer of 2,3,7,8-tetrachlorodibenzo-*p*-dioxin (TCDD) via placenta and milk, and postnatal toxicity in the mouse. *Arch Toxicol.* **59**, 36–40.

Neal, R. A., Beatty, P. W., and Gasiewicz, T. A. (1979). Studies of the mechanisms of toxicity of 2,3,7,8-tetrachlorodibenzo-*p*-dioxin (TCDD). *Ann. N.Y. Acad. Sci.* **320**, 204–213.

Neal, R. A., Gasiewicz, T., Geiger, L., Olson, J., and Sawahata, T. (1984). Metabolism of 2,3,7,8-tetrachlorodibenzo-*p*-dioxin in mammalian systems. *Banbury Rep.* **18,** 49–60.

Nebert, D. W. and Gelboin, H. V. (1969). The *in vivo* and *in vitro* induction of aryl hydrocarbon hydroxylase in mammalian cells of different species, tissues, strains, and developmental and hormonal states. *Arch. Biochem. Biophys.* **134,** 76–89.

Nebert, D. W., and Jensen, N. M. (1979). The *Ah* locus: Genetic regulation of the metabolism of carcinogens, drugs, and other environmental chemicals by cytochrome P-450 mediated monooxygeneases. *CRC Crit. Rev. Biochem.* **6,** 401–437.

Nebert, D. W., Goujan, F. M., and Gielen, J. E. (1972). Aryl hydrocarbon hydroxylase induction by polycyclic hydrocarbons: Simple autosomal dominant strain in the mouse. *Nature (London), New Biol.* **236,** 107–110.

Nebert, D. W., Levitt, R. C., Jensen, N. M., Lambert, G. H., and Felton, J. S. (1977). Birth defects and aplastic anemia: Differences in polycyclic hydrocarbon toxicity associated with the *Ah* locus. *Arch. Toxicol.* **39,** 109–132.

Nebert, D. W., Jensen, N. M., Perry, N. W., and Oka, T. (1980). Association between ornithine decarboxylase induction and the *Ah* locus in mice treated with polycyclic aromatic compounds. *J. Biol. Chem.* **255,** 6836–6842.

Negishi, M., and Nebert, D. W. (1979). Structural gene products of the *Ah* locus: Genetic and immunochemical evidence for two forms of mouse liver cytochrome P-450 induced by 3-methylcholanthrene. *J. Biol. Chem.* **254,** 11015–11023.

Negishi, M., and Nebert, D. W. (1981). Structural gene products of the [*Ah*] complex. Increases in large mRNAs from mouse liver associated with cytochrome P1-450 induction by 3-methylcholanthrene. *J. Biol. Chem.* **256,** 3085–3091.

Nehez, M., Selypes, A., and Paldy, A. (1977). Study of the mutagenicity of pesticides containing dinitro-*o*-cresyl. *Egeszsegtudomany* **21,** 237–243 (in Hungarian).

Nehez, M., Selypes, A., Paldy, A., and Berercsi, G. (1978a). Recent data on the examination of the mutagenic effect of a dinitro-*o*-cresol-containing pesticide by different test methods. *Ecotoxicol. Environ. Saf.* **2,** 243–248.

Nehez, M., Selypes, A., Paldy, A., and Berencsi, G. (1978b). The mutagenic effect of a dinitro-*o*-cresol-containing pesticide on mice germ cells. *Ecotoxicol. Environ. Saf.* **2,** 401–405.

Nehez, M., Salypes, A., Paldy, A., Mazzag, E., Berencsi, G., and Jarmay, K. (1982). The effects of five weeks treatment with dinitro-*o*-cresol- or triflurilin-containing pesticides on the germ cells of male mice. *J. Appl. Toxicol.* **2,** 179–180.

Nelson, C. J., Holson, J. F., Green, H. G., and Gaylor, D. W. (1979). Retrospective study of the relationship between agriculture use of 2,4,5-T and cleft palate occurrence in Arkansas. *Teratology* **19,** 377–384.

Nelson, J. O., Menzer, R. E., Kearney, P. C., and Plimmer, J. R. (1977). 2,3,7,8-Tetrachlorodibenzo-*p*-dioxin: In vitro binding to rat liver microsomes. *Bull. Environ. Contam. Toxicol.* **18,** 9–13.

Nemoto, T., Mason, G. G. F., Wilhelmsson, A., Cuthill, S., Hapgood, J., Gustafsson, J.-A., and Poellinger, L. (1990). Activation of the dioxin and glucocorticoid receptors to a DNA binding state under cell-free conditions. *J. Biol. Chem.* **265,** 2269–2277.

Nestrick, T. J., Lamparski, L. L., and Stehl, R. H. (1979). Synthesis and identification of the 22 tetrachlorodibenzo-*p*-dioxin isomers by high performance liquid chromatography and gas chromatography. *Anal. Chem.* **51,** 2273–2281.

Neubert, D., and Dillman, I. (1972). Embryotoxic effects in mice treated with 2,4,5-trichlorophenoxyacetic acid and 2,3,7,8-tetrachlorodibenzo-*p*-dioxin. *Arch. Pharmacol.* **272,** 243–264.

Neubert, D., Zens, P., Rothenwallner, A., and Merker, H. J. (1973). A survey of the embryotoxic effects of TCDD in mammalian species. *Environ. Health Perspect.* **5,** 67–79.

Neuhold, L. A., Gonzalez, F. J., Jaiswal, A. K., and Nebert, D. W. (1986). Dioxin-inducible enhancer region upstream from the mouse P1-450 gene and interaction with heterologous SV40 promoter. *DNA* **5,** 403–411.

Newsome, W. H., Iverson, F., Shields, J. B., and Hierlihy, S. L. (1983). Disposition of chlorinated diphenyl ethers isolated from technical pentachlorophenol in the rat. *Bull. Environ. Contam. Toxicol.* **31,** 613–618.

Newton, M., and Norris, L. A. (1981). Potential exposure of humans to 2,4,5-T and TCDD in the Oregon coast ranges. *Fundam. Appl. Toxicol.* **1,** 339–346.

New Zealand Department of Health (1980). Report to the Minister of Health of an investigation into allegations of an association between human congenital defects and 2,4,5-T spraying in and around Te Kuiti. *N. Z. Med. J.* **91,** 314–315.

Nienstedt, W., Parkki, M., Ootila, P., and Aitio, A. (1979). Effects of 2,3,7,8-tetrachlorodibenzo-*p*-dioxin on hepatic metabolism of testosterone in the rat. *Toxicology* **13,** 233–236.

Nisbet, I. C. T., and Paxton, M. B. (1982). Statistical aspects of three-generation studies of the reproductive toxicity of TCDD and 2,4,5-T. *Am. Stat.* **36,** 290–298.

Niwa, A., Kumaki, K., and Nebert, D. W. (1975). Induction of aryl hydrocarbon hydroxylase activity in various cell cultures by 2,3,7,8-tetrachlorodibenzo-*p*-dioxin. *Mol. Pharmacol.* **11,** 399–408.

Nolan, R. J., Smith, F. A., and Hefner, J. G. (1979). Elimination and tissue distribution of 2,3,7,8-tetrachlorodibenzo-*p*-dioxin (TCDD) in female guinea pigs following a single oral dose. *Toxicol. Appl. Pharmacol.* **48,** A162.

Nomura, S. (1953). Chlorophenol poisoning. I. Clinical examination of workers exposed to pentachlorophenol. *J. Sci. Lab., Denison Univ.* **29,** 474–483.

Norback, D. H., and Allen, J. R. (1969). Morphogenesis of the toxic fat-induced concentric membrane arrays in rat hepatocytes. *Lab. Invest.* **20,** 338–346.

Norback, D. H., and Allen, J. R. (1973). Biological responses of the nonhuman primate, chicken, and rat to chlorinated dibenzo-*p*-dioxin ingestion. *Environ. Health Perspect.* **5,** 233–240.

Norman, R. L., Johnson, E. F., and Müller-Eberhard, U. (1978). Identification of the major cytochrome P-450 form transplacentally induced in neonatal rabbits by 2,3,7,8-tetrachlorodibenzo-*p*-dioxin. *J. Biol. Chem.* **253,** 8640–8647.

Ohe, T. (1979). Pentachlorophenol residues in human adipose tissue. *Bull. Environ. Contam. Toxicol.* **22,** 287–292.

O'Keefe, P. W., and Smith, R. M. (1989). PCB capacitor/transformer accidents. *In* "Halogenated Biphenyls, Terphenyls, Naphthalenes, Dibenzodioxins and Related Products" (R. D. Kimbrough and A. A. Jensen, eds.), Elsevier/North Holland, New York.

Okey, A. B., and Vella, L. M. (1984). Elevated binding of 2,3,7,8-tetrachlorodibenzo-*p*-dioxin and 3,methylcholanthrene to the *Ah* receptor in hepatic cytosols from phenobarbital-treated rats and mice. *Biochem. Pharmacol.* **33,** 531–538.

Okey, A. B., Bondy, G. P., Mason, M. E., Kahl, G. S., Eisen, H. J., Guenthner, T. M., and Nebert, D. W. (1979). Regulatory gene product of the *Ah* locus. Characterization of the cytosolic inducer–receptor complex and evidence for its nuclear translocation. *J. Biol. Chem.* **254,** 11636–11648.

Okey, A. B., Bondy, G. P., Mason, M. E., Nebert, D. W., Forster-Gibson, C. J., Muncan, J., and Dufresne, M. J. (1980). Temperature-dependent cytosol-to-nucleus translocation of the *Ah* receptor for 2,3,7,8-tetrachlorodibenzo-*p*-dioxin in continuous cell culture lines. *J. Biol. Chem.* **255,** 11415–11422.

Okey, A. B., Vella, L. M., and Harper, P. A. (1989). Detection and characterization of a low affinity form of cytosolic Ah receptor in livers of mice nonresponsive to induction of cytochrome P1-450 by 3-methylcholanthrene. *Molec. Pharmacol.* **35,** 823–830.

Okino, S. T., Quattrochi, L. C., Barnes, H. J., Osanto, S., Griffin, K. J., Johnson, E. F., and Tukey, R. H. (1985). Cloning and characterization of cDNAs encoding 2,3,7,8-tetrachlorodibenzo-*p*-dioxin-mRNAs for cytochrome P-450 isozymes 4 and 6. *Proc. Natl. Acad. Sci. U.S.A.* **82,** 5310–5314.

Olafson, P. (1947). Hyperkeratosis (X disease) of cattle. *Cornell Vet.* **37,** 279–291.

Olie, K., Schecter, A., Constable, J., Kooka, R. M. N., Serne, P., Slot, P. C., and de Vries, P., (1989). Chlorinated dioxin and dibenzofuran levels in food and wildlife samples in the north and south of Vietnam. *Chemosphere* **19,** 493–496.

Oliver, R. M. (1975). Toxic effects of 2,3,7,8-tetrachlorodibenzo-1,4-dioxin in laboratory workers. *Br. J. Ind. Med.* **32**, 49–53.

Olson, J. R. (1986). Metabolism and disposition of 2,3,7,8-tetrachlorodibenzo-*p*-dioxin in guinea pigs. *Toxicol. Appl. Pharmacol.* **85**, 263–273.

Olson, J. R., Holscher, M. A., and Neal, R. A. (1980a). Toxicity of 2,3,7,8-tetrachlorodibenzo-*p*-dioxin in the golden Syrian hamster. *Toxicol. Appl. Pharmacol.* **55**, 67–78.

Olson, J. R., Gasiewicz, T. A., and Neal, R. A. (1980b). Tissue distribution, excretion, and metabolism of 2,3,7,8-tetrachlorodibenzo-*p*-dioxin (TCDD) in the golden Syrian hamster. *Toxicol. Appl. Pharmacol.* **56**, 78–85.

Olsson, H., and Brandt, L. (1988). Risk of non-Hodgkin's lymphoma among men occupationally exposed to organic solvents. *Scand. J. Work. Environ. Health* **14**, 246–251.

Osborne, R., and Greenlee, W. F. (1985). 2,3,7,8-Tetrachlorodibenzo-*p*-dioxin (TCDD) enhances terminal differentiation of cultured human epidermal cells. *Toxicol. Appl. Pharmacol.* **77**, 434–443.

Osterloh, J., Letz, G., Pond, S., and Becker, C. (1983). An assessment of the potential testicular toxicity of 10 pesticides using the mouse-sperm morphology assay. *Mutat. Res.* **116**, 407–415.

Osweiler, G. D., Olesen, B., and Rottinghaus, G. E. (1984). Plasma pentachlorophenol concentrations in calves exposed to treated wood in the environment. *Am. J. Vet. Res.* **45**, 244–246.

Owens, I. S. (1977). Genetic regulation of UDP-glucuronosyltransferase induction by polycyclic aromatic compounds in mice. *J. Biol. Chem.* **252**, 2827–2833.

Paigen, B., Holmes, P. A., Morrow, A., and Mitchell, D. (1986). Effect of 3-methylcholanthrene on atherosclerosis in two congenic strains of mice with different susceptibilities to methylcholanthrene-induced tumors. *Cancer Res.* **46**, 3321–3324.

Parker, V. H. (1952). Enzymic reduction of 2,4-dinitrophenol by rat-tissue homogenates. *Biochem. J.* **51**, 363–370.

Parker, V. H. (1958). Effect of nitrophenols and halogenophenols on the enzymatic activity of rat-liver mitochondria. *Biochem. J.* **69**, 306–311.

Parker, V. H., Barnes, J. M., and Denz, F. A. (1951). Some observations on the toxic properties of 3 : 5-dinitro-*ortho*-cresol. *Br. J. Ind. Med.* **8**, 226–235.

Parkinson, A., and Safe, S. (1981). Aryl hydrocarbon hydroxylase induction and its relationship to the toxicity of halogenated aryl hydrocarbons. *Toxicol. Environ. Chem.* **4**, 1–46.

Patterson, D. G., Jr., Hill, R. H., Needham, L. L., Orti, D. L., Kimbrough, R. D., and Liddle, J. A. (1981). Hyperkeratosis induced by sunlight degradation products of the major polybrominated biphenyl in Firemaster. *Science* **213**, 901–902.

Patterson, D. G., Jr., Hoffman, R. E., Needham, L. L., Roberts, D. W., Bagby, J. R., Pirkle, J. L., Falk, H., Sampson, E. J., and Houk, V. N. (1986). 2,3,7,8-tetrachlorodibenzo-*p*-dioxin levels in adipose tissue exposed and control persons in Missouri. *JAMA, J. Am. Med. Assoc.* **256**, 2683–2686.

Patterson, D. G., Jr., Hampton, L., Lapeza, C. R., Jr., Belser, W. T., Green, V., Alexander, L., and Needham, L. L. (1987). High-resolution gas chromatographic/high-resolution mass spectrometric analysis of human serum on a whole-weight and lipid basis for 2,3,7,8-tetrachlodibenzo-*p*-dioxin. *Anal. Chem.* **59**, 2000–2005.

Patterson, D. G., Jr., Needham, L. L., Dirkle, J. L., Roberts, D. W., Bagby, J., Garrett, W. A., Andrews, J. S., Falk, H., Bernert, J. T., Sampson, E. J., and Houk, V. N. (1988). Correlation between serum and adipose tissue levels of 2,3,7,8-Tetrachlorodibenzo-*p*-dioxin in 50 persons for Missouri. *Arch. Environ. Contam. Toxicol.* **17**, 139–143.

Patterson, D. G., Jr., Fingerhut, M. A., Roberts, D. W., Needham, L. L., Sweeney, M. H., Marlow, D. A., Andrews, J. S., Jr., and Halperin, W. E. (1989). Levels of polychlorinated dibenzo-*p*-dioxins (PCDDs) and dibenzofurans (PCDFs) in workers exposed to 2,3,7,8-tetrachlorodibenzo-*p*-dioxin. *Am. J. Ind. Med.* **16**, 135–146.

Pazdernik, T. L., and Rozman, K. K. (1985). Effect of thryoidectomy and thyroxine on 2,3,7,8-tetrachlorodibenzo-*p*-dioxin-induced immunotoxicity. *Life Sci.* **36**, 695–703.

Pazderova, J., Lukas, E., Nemcova, M., Spacilova, M., Jirasek, L., Kalensky, J., John, J., Jirasek, A., and Pickova, J. (1974). Chronic intoxication by chlorinated hydrocarbons produced during the manufacture of sodium 2,4,5-trichlorophenoxyacetate. *Prac. Lek.* **26**, 332–339.

Pazderova-Vejlupkova, J., Nemcova, M., Pickova, J., Jirasek, L, and Lukas, E. (1981). The development and prognosis of chronic intoxication by tetrachlorodibenzo-*p*-dioxin in men. *Arch. Environ. Health* **36**, 5–11.

Pearson, J. E., Schultz, C. D., Rivers, J. E., and Gonzalez, F. M. (1976). Pesticide levels of patients on chronic hemodialysis. *Bull. Environ. Contam. Toxicol.* **16**, 556–558.

Peack, G. L., Olsen, T. G., Yoder, F. W., Strauss, J. S., Dowing, D. T., Pandya, M., Butkus, D., and Arnaud-Battandier, J. (1979). Prolonged remissions of cystic and conglobate acne with 13-*cis*-retinoid acid. *N. Engl. J. Med.* **300**, 329–333.

Pegg, D. G., Hewett, W. R., McCormack, K., and Hook, J. R. (1976). Effect of 2,3,7,8-tetrachlorodibenzo-*p*-dioxin on renal function in the rat. *J. Toxicol. Environ. Health* **2**, 55–65.

Perdew, G. H., and Poland, A. (1988). Purification of the *Ah* receptor from C57BL/6J mouse liver. *J. Biol. Chem.* **263**, 9848–9852.

Perkins, R. D. (1919). A study of the munition intoxications in France. *Public Health Rep.* **34**, 2335–2430.

Peters, H. A., Gocman, A., Cripps, D. J., Bryan, G. T., and Dogramaci, M. D. (1982). Epidemiology of hexachlorobenzene-induced porphyria in Turkey: Clinical and laboratory follow-up after 25 years. *Arch. Neurol. (Chicago)* **39**, 744–749.

Peterson, R. E., Madhukar, B. V., Yang, K. H., and Matsumura, F. (1979a). Depression of adenosine triphosphatase activities in isolated liver surface membranes of 2,3,7,8-tetrachlorodibenzo-*p*-dioxin treated rats: Correlation with effects on ouabain biliary excretion and bile flow. *J. Pharmacol. Exp. Ther.* **210**, 275–282.

Peterson, R. E., Hamada, N., Yang, K. H., Madhukar, B. V., and Matsumura, F. (1979b). Reversal of 2,3,7,8-tetrachlorodibenzo-*p*-dioxin-induced depression of ouabain biliary excretion by pregnenolone-16*a*-carbonitrile and spironolactone in isolated perfused rat liver. *Toxicol. Appl. Pharmacol.* **50**, 407–416.

Pettersson, G. (1983). Activation of phosphorylase by anoxia and dinitrophenol in rabbit colon smooth muscle: Relation to release of calcium from mitochondria. *Acta Pharmacol. Toxicol.* **52**, 335–340.

Pettersson, G. (1984). Influence of anoxia and dinitrophenol on Ca^{2+} efflux and phosphorylase *a* activity in rabbit colon smooth muscle. *Acta Pharmacol. Toxicol.* **54**, 15–21.

Pickett, C. B., Telakowski-Hopkins, C. A., Donohue, A. M., and Lu, A. Y. H. (1982). Differential induction of rat hepatic cytochrome P-488 and glutathione *S*-transferase B messenger RNAs by 3-methycholanthrene. *Biochem. Biophys. Res. Commun.* **104**, 611–619.

Piper, W. N., Rose, J. Q., and Gehring, P. J. (1973). Excretion and tissue distribution of 2,3,7,8-tetrachlorodibenzo-*p*-dioxin in the rat. *Environ. Health Perspect.* **5**, 241–244.

Pitot, H. C., Goldsworthy, T., Campbell, H. A., and Poland, A. (1980). Quantitative evaluation of the promotion by 2,3,7,8-tetrachlorodibenzo-*p*-dioxin of hepatocarcinogenesis from diethylnitrosamine. *Cancer Res.* **40**, 3616–3620.

Platonow, N. S., Karstad, L. H., and Saschenbrecker, P. W. (1973). Tissue distribution of polychlorinated biphenyls (Aroclor 1254) in cockerels: Relation to the duration of exposure and observations on pathology. *Can. J. Comp. Med.* **37**, 90–95.

Plewig, G. (1970a). Local treatment of chlorine acne (Hallowax acne) with vitamin A acid. *Hautarzt* **21**, 465–470.

Plewig, G. (1970b). On the kinetics of conedome development in chloracne. *Arch. Klin. Exp. Dermatol.* **238**, 228–241.

Plewig, G. (1971). Vitamin A treatment of chloracne. *Hautarzt* **22**, 341–345.

Plimmer, J. R. (1973). Technical pentachlorophenol: Origin and analysis of base-insoluble contaminants. *Environ. Health Perspect.* **5**, 41–48.

Pocchiari, F., Silano, V., and Zampieri, A. (1979). Human health effects from accidental release of tetrachlorodibenzo-*p*-dioxin (TCDD) at Seveso (Italy). *Ann. N.Y. Acad. Sci.* **320**, 311–320.

Pocchiari, F., Di Domenico, A., Silano, V., and Zapponi, G. (1983). Environmental impact of the accidental release of tetrachlorodibenzo-*p*-dioxin (TCDD) at Seveso (Italy). *In* "Accidental Exposure to Dioxins: Human

Health Aspects" (F. Coulston and F. Pocchiari, eds.), pp. 5–37. Academic Press, New York.

Poellinger, L., and Gullberg, D. (1985). Characterization of the hydrophobic properties of the receptor for 2,3,7,8-tetrachlorodibenzo-*p*-dioxin. *Mol. Pharmacol.* **27**, 271–276.

Poellinger, L., Kurl, R. N., Lund, J., Gillner, M., Carlstedt-Duke, J., Hogberg, B., and Gustafsson, J.-A. (1982). High-affinity binding of 2,3,7,8-tetrachlorodibenzo-*p*-dioxin in cell nuclei from rat liver. *Biochem. Biophys. Acta* **714**, 516–523.

Poellinger, L., Lund, J., Gillner, M., Hansson, L. A., and Gustafsson, J.-A. (1983). Physicochemical characterization of specific and nonspecific polyaromatic hydrocarbon binders in rat and mouse liver cytosol. *J. Biol. Chem.* **258**, 13535–13542.

Pohjanvirta, P., Tuomisto, J., Vartjainen, T., and Rozman, K. (1987). Han/Wistar rats are exceptionally resistant to TCDD. *I. Pharmacol. Toxicol.* **60**, 145–150.

Poiger, H., and Buser, H.-R. (1984). The metabolism of TCDD in the dog and rat. *Banbury Rep.* **18**, 39–47.

Poiger, H., and Schlatter, C. (1979). Biological degradation of TCDD in rats. *Nature (London)* **281**, 706–707.

Poiger, H., and Schlatter, C. (1980). Influence of solvents and adsorbents on dermal and intestinal absorption of TCDD. *Food Cosmet. Toxicol.* **18**, 477–481.

Poiger, H., and Schlatter, C. (1985). Influence of phenobarbital and TCDD on the hepatic metabolism of TCDD in the dog. *Experientia* **41**, 376–378.

Poiger, H., and Schlatter, C. (1986). Pharmacokinetics of 2,3,7,8-TCDD in man. *Chemosphere* **15**, 1489–1494.

Poiger, H., Buser, H.-R., Weber, H., Sweifel, U., and Schlatter, C. (1982). Structure elucidation of mammalian TCDD-metabolites. *Experientia* **38**, 484–486.

Poland, A., and Glover, E. (1973a). Chlorinated dibenzo-*p*-dioxins: Potent inducers of delta-aminolevulinic acid synthetase and aryl hydrocarbon hydroxylase. II. A study of the structure activity relationship. *Mol. Pharmacol.* **9**, 736–747.

Poland, A., and Glover, E. (1973b). 2,3,7,8-Tetrachlorodibenzo-*p*-dioxin: A potent inducer of delta-aminolevulinic acid synthetase. *Science* **179**, 476–477.

Poland, A., and Glover, E. (1974). Comparison of 2,3,7,8-tetrachlorodibenzo-*p*-dioxin, a potent inducer of aryl hydrocarbon hydroxylase, with inducer 3-methylcholanthrene. *Mol. Pharmacol.* **10**, 349–359.

Poland, A., and Glover, E. (1975). Genetic expression of aryl hydrocarbon hydroxylase by 2,3,7,8-tetrachlorodibenzo-*p*-dioxin: Evidence for a receptor mutation in genetically non-responsive mice. *Mol. Pharmacol.* **11**, 389–398.

Poland, A., and Glover, E. (1979). An estimate of the maximum *in vivo* covalent binding of 2,3,7,8-tetrachlorodibenzo-*p*-dioxin to rat liver protein, ribosomal RNA, and DNA. *Cancer Res.* **39**, 3341–3344.

Poland, A., and Glover, E. (1980). 2,3,7,8-Tetrachlorodibenzo-*p*-dioxin: Segregation of toxicity with the *Ah* locus. *Mol. Pharmacol.* **17**, 86–94.

Poland, A., and Glover, E. (1987). Variation in the molecular mass of the *Ah* receptor among vertebrate species and strains of rats. *Biochem. Biophys. Res. Commun.* **146**, 1439–1449.

Poland, A., and Kimbrough, R. D., ed. (1984). "Biological Mechanisms of Dioxin Action," Banbury Rep. No. 18. Cold Spring Harbor Lab., Cold Spring Harbor, New York.

Poland, A., and Knutson, J. (1982). 2,3,7,8-Tetrachlorodibenzo-*p*-dioxin and related halogenated aromatic hydrocarbons: Examination of the mechanism of toxicity. *Annu. Rev. Pharmacol. Toxicol.* **22**, 517–554.

Poland, A., Glover, E., and Kende, A. S. (1976a). Stereospecific, high affinity binding of 2,3,7,8-tetrachlorodibenzo-*p*-dioxin by hepatic cytosol. *J. Biol. Chem.* **251**, 4936–4946.

Poland, A., Glover, E., Kende, A. S., DeCamp, M., and Giandomenico, C. M. (1976b). 3,4,3',4'-Tetrachloroazoxybenzene and azobenzene: Potent inducers of aryl hydrocarbon hydroxylase. *Science* **194**, 627–630.

Poland, A., Greenlee, W. F., and Kende, A. S. (1979). Studies on the mechanism of action of the chlorinated dibenzo-*p*-dioxins and related compounds. *Ann. N.Y. Acad. Sci.* **320**, 214–230.

Poland, A., Palen, D., and Glover, E. (1982). Tumor promotion by TCDD in skin of HRS/J hairless mice. *Nature (London)* **300**, 271–273.

Poland, A., Knutson, J. C., and Glover, E. (1984). Histologic changes produced by 2,3,7,8-tetrachlorodibenzo-*p*-dioxin in the skin of mice carrying mutations that affect the integument. *J. Invest. Dermatol.* **83**, 454–459.

Poland, A., Glover, E., and Taylor, B. A. (1987). The murine *Ah* locus: A new allele and mapping to chromosome 12. *Mol. Pharmacol.* **32**, 471–478.

Poland, A., Teitelbaum, P., and Glover, E. (1989a). [^{125}]-Iodo-3,7,8-trechlorodibenzo-*p*-dioxin-binding species in mouse liver induced by agonists for the Ah receptor: Characterization and identification. *Molec. Pharmacol.* **36**, 113–120.

Poland, A., Teitelbaum, P., Glover, E., and Kende, A. (1989b). Stimulation on *in vivo* hepatic uptake and *in vitro* hepatic binding of [^{125}]2-iodo-2,7,8-trichlorodibenzo-*p*-dioxin by the administration of agonists for the Ah receptor. *Molec. Pharmacol.* **36**, 121–127.

Poland, A. P., Smith, D., Metter, G., and Possick, P. (1971). A health survey of workers in a 2,4-D and 2,4,5-T plant, with special attention to chloracne, porphyria cutanea tarda and psychologic parameters. *Arch. Envir. Health* **22**, 316–327.

Poli, A., Grancescini, G., Puglisi, L., and Sirtori, C. R. (1980). Increased total and high density lipoprotein cholesterol with apoprotein changes resembling streptozotocin diabetes in tetrachlorodibenzodioxin (TCDD) treated rats. *Biochem. Pharmacol.* **28**, 835–838.

Polin, D., Olson, B., Bursian, S., and Lehning, E. (1986). Enhanced withdrawal from chickens of hexachlorobenzene (HCB) and pentachlorophenol (PCP) by colestipol, mineral oil, and/or restricted feeding. *J. Toxicol. Environ. Health* **19**, 359–368.

Potter, C. L., Sipes, I. G., and Russell, D. H. (1983). Hypothyroxinemia and hypothermia in rats in response to 2,3,7,8-tetrachlorodibenzo-*p*-dioxin administration. *Toxicol. Appl. Pharmacol.* **69**, 89–95.

Potter, C. L., Moore, R. W., Inhorn, S. L., Hagen, T. C., and Peterson, R. E. (1986). Thyroid status and thermogenesis in rats treated with 2,3,7,8-tetrachlorodibenzo-*p*-dioxin. *Toxicol. Appl. Pharmacol.* **84**, 45–55.

Pratt, R. M. (1983). Mechanisms of chemically-induced cleft palate. *Trends Pharmacol. Sci.* **4**, 160–162.

Pratt, R. M., Dencker, L., and Diewert, V. M. (1984a). TCDD-induced cleft palate in the mouse: Evidence for alterations in palatal shelf fusion. *Teratol., Carcinog., Mutagen.* **4**, 427–436.

Pratt, R. M., Grove, R. I., Kim, C. S., Dencker, L., and Diewert, V. M. (1984b). Mechanisms of TCDD-induced cleft palate in the mouse. *Banbury Rep.* **18**, 61–71.

Preache, M., and Gibson, J. E. (1974a). Enhancement of dinoseb-induced teratogenicity by maternal food deprivation in mice. *Toxicol. Appl. Pharmacol.* **29**, 122.

Preache, M., and Gibson, J. E. (1974b). Alteration of dinoseb-induced toxicity and teratogenicity in mice by environmental stress conditions. *Pharmacologist* **14**, 230.

Preache, M. M., and Gibson, J. E. (1975a). Effects in mice of high and low environmental temperature on the maternal and fetal toxicity of 2-*sec*-butyl-4,6-dinitrophenol (dinoseb) and on disposition of [^{14}C]dinoseb. *Teratology* **12**, 147–156.

Preache, M. M., and Gibson, J. E. (1975b). Effects of food deprivation, phenobarbital, and SKF-525A on teratogenicity induced by 2-*sec*-butyl-4,6-dinitrophenol (dinoseb) and on disposition of [^{14}C]dinoseb in mice. *J. Toxicol. Environ. Health* **1**, 107–118.

Prescott, C. A., Wilkie, B. N., Hunter, B., and Julian, R. J. (1982). Influence of a purified grade of pentachlorophenol on the immune response of chickens. *Am. J. Vet. Res.* **43**, 481–487.

Pressman, B. C (1963). Specific inhibitors of energy transfer. *In* "Energy-Linked Functions of Mitochondria" (B. Chance, ed.), pp. 181–199. Academic Press, New York.

Probst, G. S., McMahon, R. E., Hill, L. E., Thompson, Z., Epp, J. K., and Neal, S. B. (1981). Chemically-induced unscheduled DNA synthesis in primary rat hepatocyte cultures: A comparison with bacterial mutagenicity using 218 compounds. *Environ. Mutagen.* **3**, 11–32.

Prost, G., Vial, R., and Talot, F. (1973). Dinitro-orthocresol poisoning involving the liver. *Arch. Mal. Prof. Med. Trav. Secur. Soc.* **34**, 556–557.

Puhvel, S. M., and Sakamoto, M. (1987). Response of epidermal keratinocyte cultures to 2,3,7,8-tetrachlorodibenzo-*p*-dioxin (TCDD): Comparison of haired and hairless genotypes. *Toxicol. Appl. Pharmacol.* **89**, 29–36.

Puhvel, S. M., Sakamoto, M., Ertl, D. C., and Reisner, R. M. (1982). Hairless mice as models for chloracne: A study of cutaneous changes induced by topical application of established chloracnegens. *Toxicol. Appl. Pharmacol.* **64**, 492–503.

Puhvel, S. M., Ertl, D. C., and Lynberg, C. A. (1984). Increased epidermal transglutaminase activity following 2,3,7,8-tetrachlorodibenzo-*p*-dioxin: *In vivo* and *in vitro* studies with mouse skin. *Toxicol. Appl. Pharmacol.* **73**, 42–47.

Quilley, C. P., and Rifkind, A. B. (1986). Prostaglandin release by the chick embryo heart is increased by 2,3,7,8-tetrachlorodibenzo-*p*-dioxin and by other cytochrome P-448 inducers. *Biochem. Biophys. Res. Commun.* **136**, 582–589.

Rae, J. L., Thomson, R. D., and Eisenberg, R. S. (1982). The effect of 2-4 dinitrophenol on cell to cell communication in the frog lens. *Exp. Eye Res.* **35**, 597–609.

Ramsey, J. C., Hefner, J. G., Karbowski, R. J., Braun, W. H., and Gehring, P. J. (1982). The *in vivo* biotransformation of 2,3,7,8-tetrachlorodibenzo-*p*-dioxin (TCDD) in the rat. *Toxicol. Appl. Pharmacol.* **65**, 180–184.

Rannug, A., Rannug, U., Rosenkranz, H. S., Winguist, L., Westerholm, R., Agurell, E., and Grafström, A.-K. (1987). Certain photooxidized derivatives of tryptophan bind with very high affinity to the *Ah* receptor and are likely to be endogenous signal substances. *J. Biol. Chem.* **262**, 15422–15427.

Rao, K. R., ed. (1978). "Pentachlorophenol: Chemistry, Pharmacology, and Environmental Toxicology." Plenum, New York.

Rappe, C., Bergqvist, P.-A., Hansson, M., Kjeller, L.-O., Lindstrom, G., Marklund, S., and Nygren, M. (1984). Chemistry and analysis of polychlorinated dioxins and dibenzofurans in biological samples. *Banbury Rep.* **18**, 17–26.

Rappe, C., Nygren, M., Lindstrom, G., and Hansson, M. (1986). Dioxins and dibenzofurans in biological samples of European origin. *Chemosphere* **5**, 9–12.

Reggiani, G. (1978). Medical problems raised by the TCDD contamination in Seveso, Italy. *Arch. Toxicol.* **40**, 161–188.

Reggiani, G. (1980). Acute human exposure to TCDD in Seveso, Italy. *J. Toxicol. Environ. Health* **6**, 27–43.

Reggiani, G. (1981). Toxicology of 2,3,7,8-tetrachlorodibenzo-*p*-dioxin (TCDD): Short review of its formation, occurrence, toxicology, and kinetics, discussing human health effects; safety measures, and disposal. *Regul. Toxicol. Pharmacol.* **1**, 211–243.

Reggiani, G. (1983). An overview on the health effects of halogenated dioxins and related compounds—the Yusho and Taiwan episodes. *In* "Accidental Exposure to Dioxins: Human Health Aspects" (F. Coulston and F. Pocchiari, eds.), pp. 39–69. Academic Press, New York.

Remotti, G., De Virgiliis, G., Bianco, V., and Candiani, G. B. (1981). The morphology of early trophoblast after dioxin exposure poisoning in the Seveso area. *Placenta* **2**, 52–62.

Renner, G., and Mucke, W. (1986). Transformation of pentachlorophenol. Part 1. Metabolism in animals and man. *Toxicol. Environ. Chem.* **11**, 9–29.

Renner, G., Hopfer, C., and Gokel, J. M. (1986). Acute toxicities of pentachlorophenol, pentachloranisole, tetrachlorohydroquinone, tetrachlorocatechol, tetrachlororesorcinol, tetrachlorodimethoxybenzenes, and tetrachlorobenzenediol diacetates administered to mice. *Toxicol. Environ. Chem.* **11**, 37–50.

Revzin, P. (1977). Chemical fallout. *Wall Street J.* **59**, (126), Wednesday, June 29.

Reynolds, J. E. F., Parfitt, K., Parsons, A. V., and Sweetman, S. C. (1989). *Martindale. The Extra Pharmacopoeia*, pp. 50–51. Pharmaceutical Press, London.

Rice, R. H., and Cline, P. R. (1984). Opposing effects of 2,3,7,8-tetrachlorodibenzo-*p*-dioxin and hydrocortisone on growth and differentiation of cultured malignant human keratinocytes. *Carcinogenesis (London)* **5**, 367–371.

Rifkind, A. B., and Muschick, H. (1983). Benoxaprofen suppression of poly-

chlorinated biphenyl toxicity without alteration of mixed function oxidase function. *Nature (London)* **303**, 524–526.

Rikans, L. E., Gibson, D. D., and McKay, P. B. (1979). Evidence for the presence of cytochrome P-450 in rat mammary gland. *Biochem. Pharmacol.* **28**, 3039–3042.

Ritzmann, S. E. (1958). Poisoning by dinitrophenol and dinitro-*o*-cresol. *Arzneim.-Forsch.* **8**, 381–385 (in German).

Robert, T. A., and Hagardorn, A. N. (1983). Analysis and kinetics of 2,4-dinitrophenol in tissues by capillary gas chromatography–mass spectrometry. *J. Chromatogr.* **276**, 77–84.

Robert, T. A., and Hagardorn, A. N. (1985). Plasma levels and kinetic disposition of 2,4-dinitrophenol and its metabolites 2-amino-4-nitrophenol and 4-amino-2-nitrophenol in the mouse. *J. Chromatogr.* **344**, 177–186.

Roberts, E. A., Shear, N. H., Okey, A. B., and Manchester, D. K. (1985). The *Ah* receptor and dioxin toxicity: From rodent to human tissues. *Chemosphere* **14**, 661–674.

Roberts, E. A., Golas, C. L., and Okey, A. B. (1986). *Ah* receptor mediating induction of aryl hydrocarbon hydroxylase: Detection in human lung by binding of 2,3,7,8-tetrachlorodibenzo-*p*-dioxin. *Cancer Res.* **46**, 3739–3743.

Roberts, E. A., Johnson, K. C., Harper, P. A., and Okey, A. B. (1990). Characterization of the Ah receptor mediating aryl hydrocarbon hydroxylase induction in the human liver cell line Hep G2. (1990). *Arch. Biochem. Biophys.* **276**, 442–450.

Roberts, H. J. (1963). Aplastic anemia due to pentachlorophenol and tetrachlorophenol. *South. Med. J.* **56**, 632–635.

Roberts, H. J. (1981). Aplastic anemia due to pentachlorophenol. *N. Engl. J. Med.* **305**, 1650–1651.

Roberts, H. J. (1983). Aplastic anemia and red cell aplasia due to pentachlorophenol. *South. Med. J.* **76**, 45–48.

Robinson, J. R., Consodine, N., and Nebert, D. W. (1974). Genetic expression of aryl hydrocarbon hydroxylase induction. Evidence for the involvement of other genetic loci. *J. Biol. Chem.* **249**, 5851–5859.

Robson, A. M., Kissane, J. M., Elvick, N. H., and Pundavela, L. (1969). Pentachlorophenol poisoning in a nursery for newborn infants. I. Clinical features and treatment. *J. Pediatr.* **75**, 309–316.

Rogan, W. J. (1989). Yu-Cheng. *In* "Halogenated Biphenyls, Terphenyls, Naphthalenes, Dibenzodioxins and Related Products" (R. D. Kimbrough and A. A. Jensen, eds.), Elsevier/North Holland, New York.

Rogan, W. J., Gladen, B. C., Hung, K.-L., Shih, L.-Y., Taylor, J. S., Wu, Y.-C., Yang, D., Ragan, H. B., and Hsu, C.-C. (1988). Cogenital poisoning by polychlorinated biphenyls and their contamination in Taiwan. *Science* **241**, 334–336.

Rogers, A. M., Anderson, M. E., and Back, K. C. (1982). Mutagenicity of 2,3,7,8-tetrachlorodibenzo-*p*-dioxin and perfluoro-*n*-decanoic acid in L5178y mouse lymphoma cells. *Mutat. Res.* **105**, 445–449.

Rogers, J. M., Carver, B., Gray, L. E., Jr., Gray, J. A., and Kavlock, R. J. (1986). Teratogenic effects of the fungicide dinocap in the mouse. *Teratog., Carcinog., Mutagen.* **6**, 375–381.

Rogers, J. M., Gray, L. E., Jr., Carber, B. D., and Kavlock, R. J. (1987). Developmental toxicity of dinocap in the mouse is not due to two isomers of the major active ingredients. *Teratog., Carcinog., Mutagen.* **7**, 341–346.

Rognstad, R., and Katz, J. (1969). The effect of 2,4-dinitrophenol on adipose tissue metabolism. *Biochem. J.* **114**, 431–444.

Rokutanda, M., Araki, S., and Sakanasik, M. (1983). A pharmacological investigation on the possible calcium antagonistic action of propranolol. *Arch. Int. Pharmacodyn. Ther.* **262**, 99–108.

Romkes, M., and Safe, S. (1988). Comparative activities of 2,3,7,8-tetrachlorodibenzo-*p*-dioxin and progesterone as antiestrogens in the female rat uterus. *Toxicol. Appl. Pharmacol.* **92**, 368–380.

Romkes, M., Piskorska-Pliszczynska, J., and Safe, S. (1987). Effects of 2,3,7,8-tetrachlorodibenzo-*p*-dioxin on hepatic and uterine estrogen receptor levels in rats. *Toxicol. Appl. Pharmacol.* **87**, 306–314.

Rosa, F. W., Wilk, A. L., and Kelsey, F. O. (1986). Teratogen update: Vitamin A congeners. *Teratology* **33**, 355–364.

Rose, J. Q., Ramsey, J. C., Wentzler, T. H., Hummel, R. A., and Gehring, P. J. (1976). The fate of 2,3,7,8-tetrachlorodibenzo-*p*-dioxin following single and repeated oral doses to the rat. *Toxicol. Appl. Pharmacol.* **36**, 209–226.

Rozman, K., Hazelton, G. A., Klaason, C. D., Arlotto, M. P., and Parkinson, A. (1985). Effect of thyroid hormones on liver microsomal enzyme induction in rats exposed to 2,3,7,8-tetrachlorodibenzo-*p*-dioxin. *Toxicology* **37**, 51–63.

Rozman, K., Pereira, D., and Iatropoulos, M. J. (1986). Histopathology of interscapular brown adipose tissue, thyroid, and pancreas in 2,3,7,8-tetrachlorodibenzo-*p*-dioxin (TCDD)-treated rats. *Toxicol. Appl. Pharmacol* **82**, 551–559.

Rozman, T., Ballhorn, L., Rozman, K., Klaassen, C., and Greim, H. (1982). Effect of cholestyramine on the disposition of pentachlorophenol in rhesus monkeys. *J. Toxicol. Environ. Health* **10**, 277–283.

Rucci, G., and Gasiewicz, T. A. (1988). In vivo kinetics and DNA-binding properties of the *Ah* receptor in the golden Syrian hamster. *Arch. Biochem. Biophys.* **265**, 197–207.

Rush, G. F., Pratt, I. S., Lock, E. A., and Hook, J. B. (1986). Induction of renal mixed function oxidases in the rat and mouse: Correlation with ultrastructural changes in the proximal tubule. *Fundam. Appl. Toxicol.* **6**, 307–316.

Russell, D. H., Buckley, A. R., Shah, G. N., Sipes, I. G., Blask, D. E., and Benson, B. (1988). Hypothalamic site of action of 2,3,7,8-tetrachlorodibenzo-*p*-dioxin (TCDD). *Toxicol. Appl. Pharmacol.* **94**, 496–502.

Ryan, J. J., Lizotte, R., and Lau, B. P.-Y. (1985). Chlorinated dibenzo-*p*-dioxins and chlorinated dibenzofurans in Canadian human adipose tissue. *Chemosphere* **14**, 697–705.

Ryan, J. J., Lizotte, R., and Lewis, D. (1987a). Human tissue levels of PCDDs and PCDFs from a fatal pentachlorophenol poisoning. *Chemoshpere* **16**, 1989–1996.

Ryan, J. J., Schecter, A., Masuda, T., and Kikuchi, M. (1987b). Comparison of PCDDs and PCDFs in the tissues of Yusho patients with those from the general population in Japan and China. *Chemosphere* **16**, 2017–2025.

Ryan, J. J., Gasiewicz, T. A., and Brown, J. R., Jr. (1990). Human body burden of polychlorinated dibenzofurans associated with toxicity based on the Yusho and Yucheng incidents. *Fund. Appl. Toxicol.* (in press).

Ryan, R. P., Nelson, K. G., Lucier, G. W., Birnbaum, L. S., and Sunahara, G. I. (1987). 2,3,4,7,8-Pentachlorodibenzofuran and 1,2,3,4,7,8-hexachlorodibenzofuran decrease glucocorticoid receptor binding in mouse liver and placental cytosol. *Toxicologist* **7**, A501.

Saber, D. L., and Crawford, R. L. (1985). Isolation and characterization of *Flavobacterium* strains that degrade pentachlorophenol. *Appl. Environ. Microbiol.* **50**, 1512–1518.

Safe, S. (1986). Comparative toxicology and mechanism of action of polychlorinated dibenzo-*p*-dioxins and dibenzofurans. *Annu. Rev. Pharmacol. Toxicol.* **26**, 371–399.

Safe, S. (1987). Determination of 2,3,7,8-TCDD toxic equivalent factors (TEFs): Support for the use of the *in vitro* AHH induction assay. *Chemosphere* **16**, 791–802.

St. Omer, V. E. V., and Gadusek, F. (1987). The acute oral LD50 of technical pentachlorophenol in developing rats. *Environ. Toxicol. Chem.* **6**, 147–149.

Saita, G. (1949). Occupational intoxication by dinitrophenol. *Med. Lav.* **40**, 5–14 (in Italian).

Sangster, B., Wegman, R. C. C., and Hofstee, W. M. (1982). Non-occupational exposure to pentachlorophenol: Clinical findings and plasma-PCP-concentrations in three families. *Hum. Toxicol.* **1**, 123–133.

Sawahata, T., Olson, J. R., and Neal, R. A. (1982). Identification of metabolites of 2,3,7,8-tetrachlorodibenzo-*p*-dioxin (TCDD) formed on incubation of isolated rat hepatocytes. *Biochem. Biophys. Res. Commun.* **105**, 341–346.

Schantz, S. L., Barsotti, D. A., and Allen, J. R. (1979). Toxicological effects produced in nonhuman primates chronically exposed to fifty parts per trillion 2,3,7,8-tetrachlorodibenzo-*p*-dioxin (TCDD). *Toxicol. Appl. Pharmacol.* **48**, A180.

Schecter, A. (1983). Contamination of an office building in Binghamton, New York by PCBs, dioxins, furans, and biphenylenes after an electrical panel and electrical transformer incident. *Chemosphere* **12**, 669–680.

Schecter, A. (1985). Medical surveillance of exposed persons after exposure to PCBs, chlorinated dibenzo dioxins, and dibenzofurans after PCB transformer and capacitor incidents. *Environ. Health Prespect.* **60**, 333–338.

Schecter, A. J., and Ryan, J. J. (1988). Polychlorinated dibenzo-*p*-dioxin and dibenzofuran levels in human adipose tissues from workers 32 years after occupational exposure to 2,3,7,8-TCDD. *Chemosphere* **17**, 915–920.

Schecter, A. J., Ryan, J. J., Lizotte, R., Sun, W.-F., Miller, L., Gitlitz, G., and Bogdasarian, M. (1985a). Chlorinated dibenzodioxins and dibenzofurans in human adipose tissue from exposed and control New York State patients. *Chemosphere* **14**, 933–937.

Schecter, A. J., Gasiewicz, T. A., Eisen, H., and Schaffner, F. (1985b). Ultrastructural alterations in liver cells of humans, rats, and mouse hepatoma cells in response to 2,3,7,8-tetrachlorodibenzo-*p*-dioxin and related compounds. *Chemosphere* **14**, 939–944.

Schecter, A., Tierman, T., Schaffner, F., Taylor, M., Gitlitz, G., Van Ness, G. F., Garrett, J. H., and Nagel, D. J. (1985c). Patient fat biopsies for chemical analyses and liver biopsies for ultrastructural characterization after exposure to polychlorinated dioxins, furans and PCBs. *Environ. Health Perspect.* **60**, 241–254.

Schecter, A. J., Ryan, J. J., and Constable, J. D. (1986). Chlorinated dibenzo-*p*-dioxin and dibenzofuran levels in human adipose tissue and milk samples from the north and south of Vietnam. *Chemosphere* **15**, 1613–1620.

Schecter, A., Tong, H. Y., Monson, S. J., Gross, M. L., and Constable, J. (1989). Adipose tissue levels of 2,3,7,8-TCDD in Vietnamese adults living in Vietnam, 1984–87. *Chemosphere* **18**, 1057–1062.

Schecter, A. J., Kooke, R., Serne, P., Olie, K., Quang Huy, D., Hue, N., and Constable, J. (1989). Chlorinated dioxin and dibenzofuran levels in food samples collected between 1985-87 in the north and south of Vietnam. *Chemosphere* **18**, 627–634.

Schiller, C. M., and Lucier, G. W. (1978). The differential response of isolated intestinal crypt and tip cells to the inductive actions of 2,3,7,8-tetrachlorodibenzo-*p*-dioxin. *Chem.-Biol. Interact.* **22**, 199–209.

Schiller, C. M., Walden, R., Chapman, D. E., and Shoaf, C. R. (1984). Metabolic impairment associated with a low dose of TCDD in adult male Fischer rats. *Banbury Rep.* **18**, 319–331.

Schiller, C. M., Adcock, C. M., Shoaf, C. R., and Walden, R. (1986). Effects of adenine and its isomer 4-aminopyrazolo-[3,4-*d*]-pyrimidine on 2,3,7,8-tetrachlorodibenzo-*p*-dioxin-induced mortality in rats. *Toxicol. Appl. Pharmacol.* **84**, 369–378.

Schmid, J. R., Kiely, J. M., Pease, G. L., and Hargraves, M. M. (1963). Acquired pure red cell agenesis: Report of 16 cases and review of the literature. *Acta Haematol.* **30**, 255–270.

Schulz, K. H. (1957). Clinical and experimental investigation: The etiology of chloracne. *Arch. Klin. Exp. Dermatol.* **206**, 589–596 (in German).

Schulz, K. H. (1968). Clinical aspects and etiology of chloracne. *Arbeitsmed. Socialmed. Arbeitshyg.* **2**, 25–29. [English translation by Scientific Translation Service in "Effects of 2,4,5,-T on Man and the Environment" (Hearings before the Subcommittee on Energy, Natural Resources, and Environment of the Committee on Commerce, United States Senate), Serial 91-60. U.S. Govt. Printing Office, Washington, D.C., 1970.]

Schwartz, L., Tulipan, L., and Birmingham, D. J. (1957). "Occupational Diseases of the Skin." Lea & Febiger, Philadelphia, Pennsylvania.

Schwetz, B. A., and Gehring, P. J. (1973). The effect of tetrachlorophenol and pentachlorophenol on rat embryonal and fetal development. *Toxicol. Appl. Pharmacol.* **25**, 455.

Schwetz, B. A., Norris, J. M., Sparschu, G. L., Rowe, V. K., Gehring, P. J., Emerson, J. L., and Gerbig, C. G. (1973). Toxicology of chlorinated dibenzo-*p*-dioxins. *Environ. Health Perspect.* **5**, 87–99.

Schwetz, B. A., Keeler, P. A., and Gehring, P. J. (1974). The effect of purified and commercial grade pentachlorophenol on rat embryonal and fetal development. *Toxicol. Appl. Pharmacol.* **28**, 151–161.

Schwetz, B. A., Quast, J. F., Keeler, P. A., Humiston, C. G., and Kociba, R. J. (1978). Results of two-year toxicity and reproduction studies on pentachlorophenol in rats. *In* "Pentachlorophenol: Chemistry, Pharmacology and Environmental Toxicology" (K. R. Rao, ed.), pp. 301–309. Plenum, New York.

Seefeld, M. D., and Peterson, R. E. (1983). 2,3,7,8-Tetrachlorodibenzo-*p*-dioxin induced weight loss: A proposed mechanism. *In* "Human and Environmental Risks of Chlorinated Dioxins and Related Compounds" (R. E. Tucker, A. L. Young, and A. Gray, eds.), pp. 405–413. Plenum, New York.

Seefeld, M. D., and Peterson, R. E. (1984). Digestible energy and efficiency of feed utilization in rats treated with 2,3,7,8-tetrachlorodibenzo-*p*-dioxin. *Toxicol. Appl. Pharmacol.* **74**, 214–222.

Seefeld, M. D., Albrecht, R. M., and Peterson, R. E. (1979). Effects of 2,3,7,8-tetrachlorodibenzo-*p*-dioxin on indocyanine green blood clearance in rhesus monkeys. *Toxicology* **14**, 263–272.

Seefeld, M. D., Albrecht, R. M., Gilchrist, K. W., and Peterson, R. E. (1980). Blood clearance tests for detecting 2,3,7,8-tetrachlorodibenzo-*p*-dioxin hepatotoxicity in rats and rabbits. *Arch. Environ. Contam. Toxicol.* **9**, 317–327.

Seefeld, M. D., Corbett, S. W., Keesey, R. E., and Peterson, R. E. (1984). Characterization of the wasting syndrome in rats treated with 2,3,7,8-tetrachlorodibenzo-*p*-dioxin. *Toxicol. Appl. Pharmacol.* **73**, 311–322.

Sehgal, V. N., and Ghorpade, A. (1983). Fume inhalation chloracne. *Dermatologica* **167**, 33–36.

Seiler, J. P. (1973). A survey on the mutagenicity of various pesticides. *Experientia* **29**, 622–623.

Seki, Y., Kawanishi, S., and Sano, S. (1987). Role of inhibition of uroporphyrinogen decarboxylase in PCB-induced porphyria in mice. *Toxicol. Appl. Pharmacol.* **90**, 116–125.

Sen'chuk, V., and Adamska, T. (1977). The effect of some antidotes on the rate of 2,4-dinitrophenol uptake from the digestive tract into the blood. *Farmakol. Toksiko. (Moscow)* **40**, 425–427.

Shafik, T. M. (1973). The determination of pentachlorophenol and hexachlorophene in human adipose tissue. *Bull. Environ. Contam. Toxicol.* **10**, 57–63.

Shara, M. A., and Stoh, S. J. (1987). Biochemical and toxicological effects of 2,3,7,8-tetrachlorodibenzo-*p*-dioxin (TCDD) congeners in female rats. *Arch. Environ. Contam. Toxicol.* **16**, 599–605.

Sharma, R. P., and Gehring, P. J. (1979). Effects of 2,3,7,8-tetrachlorodibenzo-*p*-dioxin (TCDD) on splenic lymphocyte transformation in mice after single and repeated exposures. *Ann. N.Y. Acad. Sci.* **320**, 487–497.

Shelley, W. B., and Kligman, A. M. (1957). The experimental production of acne by penta- and hexachloronaphthalenes. *Arch. Dermatol.* **75**, 689–695.

Shen, E. S., and Olson, J. R. (1987). Relationship between the murine *Ah* phenotype and the hepatic uptake and metabolism of 2,3,7,8-tetrachlorodibenzo-*p*-dioxin. *Drug. Metab. Dispos.* **15**, 653–660.

Shiverick, K. T., and Muther, T. F. (1982). Effects of 2,3,7,8-tetrachlorodibenzo-*p*-dioxin on serum concentrations and the uterotrophic action of exogenous estrone in rats. *Toxicol. Appl. Pharmacol.* **65**, 170–176.

Shiverick, K. T., and Muther, T. F. (1983). 2,3,7,8-Tetrachlorodibenzo-*p*-dioxin (TCDD) effect on hepatic microsomal steroid metabolism and serum estradiol of pregnant rats. *Biochem. Pharmacol.* **32**, 991–995.

Shoya, S. (1974). Polychlorinated biphenyl poisoning in chickens. *Jpn. Agric. Res. Q.* **8**, 43–46.

Shu, H., Teitelbaum, P., Webb, A. S., Marple, L., Brunck, B., DeiRossi, D., Murray, F. J., and Paustenbach, D. (1988). Bioavailability of soil-bound TCDD: Dermal bioavailability in the rat. *Fundam. Appl. Toxicol.* **10**, 335–343.

Sikes, D., and Bridges, M. E. (1952). Experimental production of hyperkeratosis ("X disease") of cattle with a chlorinated naphthalene. *Science* **116**, 506–507.

Sikes, D., Wise, J. C., and Bridges, M. E. (1952). The experimental production of "X disease" (hyperkeratosis) in cattle with chlorinated naphthalenes and petroleum products. *J. Am. Vet. Med. Assoc.* **121**, 337–344.

Silkowski, J. B., Horstman, S. W., and Morgan, M. S. (1984). Permeation through five commercially available glove materials by two pentachlorophenol formulations. *Am. Ind. Hyg. Assoc. J.* **45**, 501–504.

Silkworth, J. B., and Grabstein, E. M. (1982). Polychlorinated biphenyl immunotoxicity: Dependence on isomer planarity and the *Ah* gene complex. *Toxicol. Appl. Pharmacol.* **65**, 109–115.

Silkworth, J. B., McMartin, D., DeCaprio, A., O'Keefe, P., and Kaminsky, L. (1982). Acute toxicity in guinea pigs and rabbits of soot from a polychlorinated biphenyl-containing transformer fire. *Toxicol. Appl. Pharmacol.* **65**, 425–439.

Silkworth, J. B., Antrim, L., and Kaminsky, L. S. (1984). Correlations between polychlorinated biphenyl immunotoxicity, the aromatic hydrocarbon locus, and liver microsomal enzyme induction in C57BL/6 and DBA/2 mice. *Toxicol. Appl. Pharmacol.* **75**, 156–165.

Silkworth, J. B., Antrim, L., and Sack, G., (1986). *Ah* receptor-medicated suppression of anitibody response in mice is primarily dependent on the *Ah* phenotype of lymphoid tissue. *Toxicol Appl. Pharmacol.* **86**, 380–390.

Simpson, C. F. (1949). Hyperkeratosis or X disease in Florida. *Vet. Med. (Kansas City, Mo.)* **44**, 51–52.

Sinclair, P. R., and Granick, S. (1974). Uroporphyrin formation induced by chlorinated hydrocarbons (lindane, polychlorinated biphenyls, tetrachlorodibenzo-*p*-dioxin). Requirements for endogenous iron, protein, synthesis and drug-metabolizing activity. *Biochem. Biophys. Res. Commun.* **61**, 124–133.

Sinclair, P. R., Bement, W. J., Bonkovsky, H. L., Lambrecht, R. W., Frezza, J. E., Sinclair, J. F., Urquhart, A. J., and Elder, G. H. (1986). Uroporphyrin accumulation produced by halogenated biphenyls in chick embryo hepatocytes: reversal of the accumulation of piperonyl butoxide. *Biochem. J.* **237**, 63–71.

Singer, R., Moses, M., Valciukas, J., Lilis, R., and Selikoff, I. J. (1982). Nerve conduction velocity studies of workers employed in the manufacture of phenoxy herbicides. *Environ. Res.* **29**, 297–311.

Siqueira, M. E. P. B., and Fernicola, N. A. G. G. (1981). Determination of pentachlorophenol in urine. *Bull. Environ. Contam. Toxicol.* **27**, 380–385.

Sleight, S. D., Mangkoewidjojo, S., Akoso, B. T., and Sanger, V. L. (1978). Polybrominated biphenyl toxicosis in rats fed an iodine-deficient, iodine-adequate, or iodine-excess diet. *Environ. Health Perspect.* **23**, 341–346.

Sloop, T. C., and Licier, G. W. (1987). Dose-dependent elevation of *Ah* receptor binding by TCDD in rat liver. *Toxicol. Appl. Pharmacol.* **88**, 329–337.

Smith, A. H., Francis, J. E., Kay, S. J., and Greig, J. B. (1981). Hepatic toxicity and uroporphyrinogen decarboxylase activity following a single dose of 2,3,7,8-tetrachlorodibenzo-*p*-dioxin to mice. *Biochem. Pharmacol.* **30**, 2825–2830.

Smith, A. H., Pearce, N. E., Fisher, D. O., Giles, H. J., Teague, C. A., and Howard, J. K. (1984). Soft tissue sarcoma and exposure to phenoxy herbicides and chlorophenols in New Zealand. *JNCI, J. Natl. Cancer Inst.* **73**, 1111–1117.

Smith, F. A., Schwetz, B. A., and Nitschke, K. D. (1976). Teratogenicity of 2,3,7,8-tetrachlorodibenzo-*p*-dioxin in CF-1 mice. *Toxicol. Appl. Pharmacol.* **38**, 517–523.

Smith, J. (1979). EPA halts most uses of herbicide 2,4,5-T. *Science* **203**, 1090–1091.

Smith, J. E., Loveless, L. E., and Belden, E. A. (1967). Pentachlorophenol poisoning in newborn infants. *Morbid. Mortal. Wkly. Rep.* **16**, 334–335.

Smith, J. N., Smithies, R. H., and Williams, R. T. (1953). Urinary metabolites of 4,6-dinitro-*o*-cresol in the rabbit. *Biochem. J.* **54**, 225–230.

Smith, W. D. L. (1981). An investigation of suspected dinoseb poisoning after the agriculture use of a herbicide. *Practitioner* **225**, 923–926.

Soderkvist, P., Poellinger, L., and Gustafsson, J.-A. (1986). Carcinogen-binding proteins in the rat ventral prostate: Specific and nonspecific high-affinity binding sites for benzo(*a*)pyrene, 3-methylcholanthrene, and 2,3,7,8-tetrachlorodibenzo-*p*-dioxin. *Cancer Res.* **46**, 651–657.

Sogawa, K., Fujisawa-Sehara, A., Yamane, M., and Kujii-Kuriyama, Y. (1986). Location of regulatory elements responsible for drug induction in the rat cytochrome P-450 gene. *Proc. Natl. Acad. Sci. U.S.A.* **83**, 8044–8048.

Sollman, T., ed. (1942). "A Manual of Pharmacology and Its Applications to Therapeutics and Toxicology," 6th ed. Saunders, Philadelphia, Pennsylvania.

Sollman, T., ed. (1957). "A Manual of Pharmacology and Its Applications to Therapeutics and Toxicology," 8th ed. Saunders, Philadelphia, Pennsylvania.

Sousa, R. L., and Marletta, M. A. (1985). Inhibition of cytochrome P-450 activity in rat liver microsomes by the naturally occurring flavonoid, quercetin. *Arch. Biochem. Biophys.* **240**, 345–357.

Sovljanski, M., Popovic, D., Tasic, M., and Sovljanski, R. (1971). Intoxications with dinitroorthocresol. *Arch. Hig. Rada Toksikol.* **22**, 329–332.

Sparschu, G. L., Jr., Dunn, F. L., Jr., and Rowe, V. K., Jr. (1971). Study of the teratogenicity of 2,3,7,8-tetrachlorodibenzo-*p*-dioxin in the rat. *Food Cosmet. Toxicol.* **9**, 405–412.

Spencer, F., and Sing, L. T. (1982). Reproductive toxicity in pseudopregnant and pregnant rats following postimplantational exposure: Effects of the herbicide dinoseb. *Pestic. Biochem. Physiol.* **18**, 150–157.

Spencer, H. C., Rowe, V. K., Adams, E. M., and Irish, D. D. (1948). Toxicological studies on laboratory animals of certain alkyldinitrophenols used in agriculture. *J. Ind. Hyg. Toxicol.* **30**, 10–25.

Stanker, L. H., Watkins, B., Rogers, H., and Vanderlaan, M. (1987). Monoclonal antibodies for dioxin: Antibody characterization and assay development. *Toxicology* **45**, 229–243.

Stanley, J. S., Boggess, K. E., Onstot, J., Sack, T. M., Remmers, J. C., Breen, J., Kutz, F. W., Carra, J., Robinson, P., and Mack, G. A. (1986). PCDDs and PCDFs in human adipose tissue from the EPA FY82 NHATS repository. *Chemosphere* **15**, 1605–1612.

Steer, C. (1951). Death from di-nitro-*ortho*-cresol. *Lancet* **1**, 14–19.

Stehr, P. A., Forney, D., Stein, G., Donnell, H. D., Falk, H., Hotchkiss, R., Spratlin, W. A., Sampson, E., and Smith, S. J. (1985). *Public Health Rep.* **100**, 289–293.

Sterling, T. D., and Arundel, A. V. (1986). Health effects of phenoxy herbicides. A review. *Scand. J. Work Environ. Health* **12**, 161–173.

Stohlman, E. F. (1951). The toxicity of some related halogenated derivatives of phenol. *Public Health Rep.* **66**, 1303–1312.

Stohs, S. J., Hassan, M. Q., and Murray, W. J. (1983). Lipid peroxidation as a possible cause of TCDD toxicity. *Biochem. Biophys. Res. Commun.* **111**, 854–859.

Strik, J. J. T. W. A. (1979). Porphyrins in urine as an indication of exposure to chlorinated hydrocarbons. *Ann. N.Y. Acad. Sci.* **320**, 308–310.

Sunahara, G. I., Lucier, G. W., McCoy, Z., Bresnick, E. H., Sanchez, E. R., and Nelson, K. G. (1989). Characterization of 2,3,7,8-tetrachlorodibenzo-*p*-dioxin-mediated decreases in dexamethasone binding to rat hepatic cytosolic glucocorticoid receptor. *Molec. Pharmacol.* **36**, 239–247.

Suskind, R. R., and Hertzberg, V. S., (1984). Human health effects of 2,4,5-T and its toxic contaminants. *JAMA, J. Am. Med. Assoc.* **251**, 2372–2380.

Sweatlock, J. A., and Gasiewicz, T. A. (1985). The effect of 2,3,7,8-tetrachlorodibenzo-*p*-dioxin exposure on the concentration of β-hydroxybutyrate and acetoacetate in the rat. *Chemosphere* **14**, 975–978.

Sweatlock, J. A., and Gasiewicz, T. A. (1986). The interaction of 1,3-diaryltriazenes with the *Ah* receptor. *Chemosphere* **15**, 1687–1690.

Sweeney, G. D., Jones, K. G., Cole, F. M., Basford, D., and Krestynski, F. (1979). Iron deficiency prevent liver toxicity of 2,3,7,8-tetrachloro dibenzo-*p*-dioxin. *Science* **204**, 332–334.

Swift, L. L., Gasiewicz, T. A., Dunn, G. D., Soule, P. D., and Neal, R. A. (1981). Characterization of the hyperlipidemia in guinea pigs induced by 2,3,7,8-tetrachlorodibenzo-*p*-dioxin. *Toxicol. Appl. Pharmacol.* **59**, 489–499.

Syrowatka, T. (1970). A study of the effect of fungicides on cellular energy processes. *Rocz. Panstw. Zakl. Hig.* **21**, 105–115.

Tainter, M. L., and Cutting, W. C. (1933). Miscellaneous actions of dinitrophenol—repeated administrations, antidotes, fatal doses, antiseptic tests and actions of some isomers. *J. Pharmacol. Exp. Ther.* **49**, 187–203.

Tainter, M. L., Stockton, A. B., and Cutting, W. C. (1933). Use of dinitrophenol in obesity and related conditions. *JAMA, J. Am. Med. Assoc.* **101**, 1472–1475.

Tainter, M. L., Cutting, W. C., Wood, D. A., and Proescher, F. (1934). Dinitrophenol. Studies of blood, urine and tissues of dogs on continued medication and after acute fatal poisoning. *Arch. Pathol.* **18**, 881–890.

Tainter, M. L., Cutting, W. C., and Hines, E. (1935). Effects of moderate doses of dinitrophenol on the energy exchange and nitrogen metabolism of patients under conditions of restricted dietary. *J. Pharmacol. Exp. Ther.* **55**, 326–353.

Tashiro, S., Sasamoto, T., Aikawa, T., Tokunaga, S., Taniguchi, E., and Eto, M. (1970). Metabolism of pentachlorophenol in mammals. *Nippon Nogei Kagaku Kaishi* **44**, 124–129.

Taylor, J. S. (1983). Chloracne for chlorbenzene compounds. *In* "Proceedings of the 16th International Congress of Dermatology" (A. Kukita and M. Seiji, eds.), p. 551–558. Univ. of Tokyo Press, Tokyo.

Taylor, J. S. (1974). Chloracne—a continuing problem. *Cutis* **13**, 585–591.

Taylor, J. S. (1979). Environmental chloracne: Update and overview. *Ann. N.Y. Acad. Sci.* **320**, 295–307.

Taylor, J. S., Wuthrich, R. D., Lloyd, K. M., and Poland, A. (1977). Chloracne from manufacture of a new herbicide. *Arch. Dermatol.* **113**, 616–619.

Teleky, L. (1927). Perna disease (chloracne). *Klin. Wochenschr.* **6**, 845–848 [German].

Tasic, D., Terzic, L. J., Dimitrijevic, B., Zivanov, D., and Slavic, M. (1972). Experimental investigation of the effect of environmental temperature and some medicaments on the toxic effect of dinitroorthocresol. *Acta Vet. (Belgrade)* **22**, 45–52.

Tewfik, M. S., and Evans, W. C. (1966). The metabolism of 3,5-dinitro-*o*-cresol (DNOC) by soil microorganisms. *Biochem. J.* **99**, 31P–32P.

Theiss, A. M., Frentzel-Beyme, R., and Link, R. (1982). Mortality study of persons exposed to dioxin in a trichlorophenol-process accident that occurred in the BASF AG on November 17, 1953. *Am. J. Ind. Med.* **3**, 179–189.

Thibierge, G. (1899). Generalized comedon acne. *Ann. Dermatol. Syphiligr.* **10**, 1076–1082 (in French).

Thigpen, J. E., Faith, R. E., McConnell, E. E., and Moore, J. A. (1975). Increased susceptibility to bacterial infection as a sequela of exposure to 2,3,7,8-tetrachlorodibenzo-*p*-dioxin (TCDD). *Infect. Immunol.* **12**, 1319–1324.

Thoma, H., Mucke, W., and Kretschmer, E. (1989). Concentrations of PCDD and PCDF in human fat and liver samples. *Chemosphere* **18**, 491–498.

Thomas, H. F. (1980). 2,4,5-T use and congenital malformation rates in Hungary. *Lancet* **2**, 214–215.

Thomas, P. E., and Hutton, J. J. (1973). Genetics of aryl hydrocarbon hydroxylase induction: Additive inheritance in crosses between C3H/HeJ and DBA/2J. *Biochem. Genet.* **8**, 249–257.

Thomas, P. E., Kouri, R. E., and Hutton, J. J. (1972). The genetics of aryl hydrocarbon hydroxylase induction in mice: A single gene difference between C57BL/6J and DBA/2J. *Biochem. Genet.* **6**, 157–168.

Thomas, P. E., Reik, L. M., Ryan, D. E., and Levin, E. (1983). Induction of two immunochemically related rat liver cytochrome P-450 isozymes, cytochromes P-450c and P-450d, by structurally diverse xenobiotics. *J. Biol. Chem.* **258**, 4590–4598.

Thomas, P. T., and Hinsdill, R. D. (1979). The effect of perinatal exposure to 2,3,7,8-tetrachlorodibenzo-*p*-dioxin on the immune response of young mice. *Drug Chem. Toxicol.* **2**, 77–98.

Thunberg, T. (1984). Effects of TCDD on vitamin A and its relation to TCDD toxicity. *Banbury Rep.* **18**, 333–344.

Thunberg, T., and Hakansson, H. (1983). Vitamin A (retinol) status in the Gunn rat: The effect of 2,3,7,8-tetrachlorodibenzo-*p*-dioxin. *Arch. Toxicol.* **53**, 225–233.

Thunberg, T., Ahlborg, U. G., and Johnsson, H. (1979). Vitamin A (retinol) status in the rat after a single oral dose of 2,3,7,8-tetrachlorodibenzo-*p*-dioxin. *Arch. Toxicol.* **42**, 265–274.

Thunberg, T., Ahlborg, U. G., Hakansson, H., Krantz, C., and Monier, M. (1980). Effect of 2,3,7,8-tetrachlorodibenzo-*p*-dioxin on the hepatic storage of retinol in rats with different dietary supplies of vitamin A (retinol). *Arch. Toxicol.* **45**, 273–285.

Thunberg, T., Ahlborg, U. G., and Wahlström, B. (1984). Comparison between the effects of 2,3,7,8-tetrachlorodibenzo-*p*-dioxin and six other compounds on the vitamin A storage, the UDP-glucuronosyltransferase and the aryl hydrocarbon hydroxylase activity in the rat liver. *Arch. Toxicol.* **55**, 16–19.

Timmons, L., Steele, D., Cannon, M., Grese, R., Brown, R., Merrill, E., and Jameson, C. W. (1984). Identification of bromotetrachlorophenol in commercial pentachlorophenol samples. *J. Chromatogr.* **314**, 476–481.

Tofilon, P. J., and Piper, W. N. (1982). 2,3,7,8-Tetrachlorodibenzo-*p*-dioxin-mediated depression of rat testicular heme synthesis and microsomal cytochrome P-450. *Biochem. Pharmacol.* **31**, 3663–3666.

Tofilon, P. J., Peters, P. G., Clement, R. P., Hardwicke, D. M., and Piper, W. N. (1980). Depressed guinea pig testicular microsomal cytochrome P-450 content by 2,3,7,8-tetrachlorodibenzo-*p*-dioxin. *Life Sci.* **27**, 871–876.

Toftgard, R., Lofroth, G., Carlstedt-Duke, J., Kurl, R., and Gustafsson, J.-A. (1983). Compounds in urban air compete with 2,3,7,8-tetrachlorodibenzo-*p*-

dioxin for binding to the receptor protein. *Chem.-Biol. Interact.* **46**, 335–346.

Tognoni, G., and Bonaccorsi, A. (1982). Epidemiological problems with 2,3,7,8-tetrachlorodibenzo-*p*-dioxin (TCDD). *Drug Metab. Rev.* **13**, 447–469.

Toth, K., Bence, J., and Somfai-Relle, S. (1978). Carcinogenic bioassay of the herbicide, 2,4,5-trichlorophenoxyethanol (TCPE) with different 2,3,7,8-tetrachlorodibenzo-*p*-dioxin (dioxin) content in Swiss mice. *Prog. Biochem. Pharmacol.* **14**, 82–93.

Toth, K., Somfai-Relle, S., Sugar, J., and Bence, J. (1979). Carcinogenicity testing of herbicide 2,4,5-trichlorophenoxyethanol containing dioxin and of pure dioxin in Swiss mice. *Nature (London)* **278**, 548–549.

Townsend, J. C., Bodner, K. M., Van Peenen, P. F. D., Olson, R. D., and Cook, R. R. (1982). Survey of reproductive events of wives of employees exposed to chlorinated dioxins. *Am. J. Epidemiol.* **115**, 659–713.

Travis, C. C., and Hattemer-Frey, H. A. (1987). Human exposure to 2,3,7,8-TCDD. *Chemosphere* **16**, 2331–2342.

Triebig, G., Krekeler, H., Gobler, K., and Valentin, H. (1981). Investigations on neurotoxicity of chemicals in the workplace. II. Determination of motor and sensory conduction velocity in persons occupationally exposed to pentachlorophenol. *Int. Arch. Occup. Environ. Health* **48**, 357–367 (in German).

Truhaut, R., L'Epee, P., and Boussemart, E. (1952a). Studies on the toxicology of pentachlorophenol. II. Occupational intoxications in the wood industry. Observations of two fatal cases. *Arch. Mal. Prof. Med. Trav. Secur. Soc.* **13**, 567–569 (in French).

Truhaut, R., Vitle, G., and Boussemart, E. (1952b). Studies on the toxicology of pentachlorophenol. III. Study of acute and chronic experimental intoxications in the rabbit: Influence of renal condition. *Arch. Mal. Prof. Med. Trav. Secur. Soc.* **13**, 569–574 (in French).

Tuchmann-Duplessis, H. (1978). Pollution of the environment and future generations in relation to the accident at Seveso. *Med. Hyg.* **36**, 1758–1766 (in French).

Tucker, A. N., Vore, S. J., and Luster, M. I. (1986). Suppression of B cell differentiation by 2,3,7,8-tetrachlorodibenzo-*p*-dioxin (TCDD). *Mol. Pharmacol.* **29**, 372–377.

Tucker, R. E., Young, A. L., and Gray, A. P., eds. (1983). "Human and Environmental Risks of Chlorinated Dioxins and Related Compounds." Plenum, New York.

Tukey, R. H., and Nebert, D. W. (1984). Regulation of mouse cytochrome P3-450 by the *Ah* receptor. Studies with a P3-450 cDNA clone. *Biochemistry* **23**, 6003–6008.

Tukey, R. H., Lalley, P. A., and Nebert, D. W. (1984). Localization of cytochrome P1-450 and P3-450 genes to mouse chromosome 9. *Proc. Natl. Acad. Sci. U.S.A.* **81**, 3163–3165.

Tukey, R. H., Nebert, D. W., and Negishi, M. (1981). Structural gene product of the *Ah* complex. Evidence for transcriptional control of cytochrome P1-450 induction by use of a cloned DNA sequence. *J. Biol. Chem.* **256**, 6969–6974.

Tukey, R. H., Hannah, R. R., Negishi, M., Nebert, D. W., and Eisen, H. J. (1982). The *Ah* locus: Correlation of intranuclear appearance of inducer–receptor complex with induction of cytochrome P1-450 mRNA. *Cell (Cambridge, Mass.)* **31**, 275–284.

Turner, J. N., and Collins, D. N. (1983). Liver morphology in guinea pigs administered either pyrolysis products of a polychlorinated biphenyl transformer fluid or 2,3,7,8-tetrachlorodibenzo-*p*-dioxin. *Toxicol. Appl. Pharmacol.* **67**, 417–429.

Turner, M. L. (1946). The effect of thyroxin and of dinitrophenol on the thermal response to cold. *Endocrinology (Baltimore)* **38**, 263–269.

Ueda, K., Nagai, M., and Osafune, T. (1962). Contamination of drinking water with pentachlorophenol. *Bull. Osaka Metropolitan Hyg. Sc. Ins.* **7**, 19–22 (Japanese).

Ueda, K., Nishimura, M., Aoki, H., and Mori, T. (1969). A quantitative method for urinary pentachlorophenol. *Igaku to Seibutsugaku* **79**, 89–93.

Uhl, S., Schmid, P., and Schlatter, C. (1986). Pharmacokinetics of pentachlorophenol in man. *Arch. Toxicol.* **58**, 182–186.

Umbreit, T. H., Hesse, E. J., and Gallo, M. A. (1986). Bioavailability of dioxin in soil from 2,4,5-T manufacturing site. *Science* **232**, 497–499.

Urabe, H., and Asahi, M. (1985). Past and current dermatological status of Yusho patients. *Environ. Health Perspect.* **59**, 11–16.

U.S. Environmental Protection Agency (USEPA) (1979). "Report of Assessment of a Field Investigation of Six-year Spontaneous Abortion Rates in Three Oregon Areas in Relation to Forest 2,4,5-T Spray Practice." Office of Toxic Substances, U.S. Environ. Prot. Agency, Washington, D.C.

U.S. Environmental Protection Agency (USEPA) (1984a). "Ambient Water Quality Criteria for 2,3,7,8-Tetrachlorodibenzo-*p*-dioxin," EPA/440/5-84-007. U.S. Environ. Prot. Agency, Washington, D.C.

U.S. Environmental Protection Agency (USEPA) (1984b). "Health Effects Assessment for Pentachlorophenol," EPA/540/1-86-043, U.S. Environ. Prot. Agency, Washington, D.C.

U.S. Environmental Protection Agency (USEPA) (1985). "Health Assessment Document for Polychlorinated Dibenzo-*p*-dioxins," EPA/600/8-84/014F. U. S. Environ. Prot. Agency, Washington, D.C.

U.S. Environmental Protection Agency (USEPA) (1987). "Interim Procedures for Estimating Risks Associated with Exposures to Mixtures of Chlorinated Dibenzo-*p*-dioxins and Dibenzofurans (CDDs and CDFs)," EPA/625/3-87/012. U.S. Environ. Prot. Agency, Washington, D.C.

Valla, A. (1962). Acute intoxications by 2,4-dinitrophenol and 3,5-dinitrocresol. *Arch. Mal. Prof. Med. Trav. Secur. Soc.* **24**, 478 (in French).

van den Berg, M., de Vroom, E., van Greevenbrock, M., Olie, K., and Hutzinger, O. (1985). Bioavailability of PCDDs and PCDFs adsorbed on fly ash in rat, guinea pig, and Syrian golden hamster. *Chemosphere* **14**, 865–869.

van den Berg, M., Heeremans, C., Veenhaven, E., and Olie, K. (1987). Transfer of polychlorinated dibenzo-*p*-dioxins and dibenzofurans to fetal and neonatal rats. *Fundam. Appl. Toxicol.* **9**, 635–644.

van Gurp, J. R., and Hankinson, O. (1984). Isolation and characterization of revertants from four different classes of aryl hydrocarbon hydroxylase-deficient Hepa-1 mutants. *Mol. Cell. Biol.* **4**, 1597–1604.

van Logten, M. J., Gupta, B. N., McConnell, E. E., and Moore, J. A. (1980). Role of the endocrine system in the action of 2,3,7,8-tetrachlorodibenzo-*p*-dioxin (TCDD) on the thymus. *Toxicology* **15**, 135–144.

Van Miller, J. P., Marlar, R. J., and Allen, J. R. (1976). Tissue distribution and excretion of tritiated tetrachlorodibenzo-*p*-dioxin in non-human primates and rats. *Food Cosmet. Toxicol.* **14**, 31–34.

van Ommen, B., van Bladeren, P. J., Temmink, J. H. M., and Muller, F. (1985). Formation of pentachlorophenol as the major product of microsomal oxidation of hexachlorobenzene. *Biochem. Biophys. Res. Commun.* **126**, 25–32.

Varnai, L., and Kote, Gy. (1969). Forensic medical problems of mass Krezonite poisoning. *Orv. Hetil.* **110**, 1023–1025.

Vecci, A., Mantovani, A., Sironi, M., Luini, W., Cairo, M., and Garattini, S. (1980a). Effect of acute exposure to 2,3,7,8-tetrachlorodibenzo-*p*-dioxin on humoral antibody production in mice. *Chem.-Biol. Interact.* **30**, 337–342.

Vecci, A., Mantovani, A., Sironi, M., Luini, W., Spreafico, F., and Garattini, S. (1980b). The effect of acute administration of 2,3,7,8-tetrachlorodibenzo-*p*-dioxin on humoral antibody production and cell-mediated activities in mice. *Arch. Toxicol.* **4**, 163–165.

Vecci, A., Sironi, M., Canegrati, M. A., and Garattini, S. (1983a). Comparison of the immunosuppressive effects in mice of 2,3,7,8-tetrachlorodibenzo-*p*-dioxin and 2,3,7,8-tetrachlorodibenzofuran. *In* "Chlorinated Dioxins and Dibenzofurans in the Total Environment" (G. Choudhary, L. H. Keith, and C. Rappe, eds.), pp. 397–402. Butterworth, Boston, Massachusetts.

Vecci, A., Sironi, M., Canegrati, M. A., Recchia, M., and Garattini, S. (1983b). Immunosuppressive effects of 2,3,7,8-tetrachlorodibenzo-*p*-dioxin in strains of mice with different susceptibility to induction of aryl hydrocarbon hydroxylase. *Toxicol. Appl. Pharmacol.* **68**, 434–441.

Vinogradova, V. K., Kalyaganov, P. I., Sudonina, L. T., and Yelizarov, G. P. (1973). Hygienic characteristics of working conditions and health status of workers engaged in the manufacture of sodium pentachlorophenate. *Gig. Tr. Prof. Zabol.* **17**, 11–13 (in Russian).

Vinogradova, V. K., Kalyaganov, P. I., Melnikova, L. V., Yelizarov, G. P., and Golova, I. A. (1976). The effect of health measures in industries processing "non-toxic" isomers of hexachlorocyclohexane. *Gig. Tr. Prof. Zabol.* **5**, 24–27 (in Russian).

Vinopal, J. H., and Casida, J. E. (1973). Metabolic stability of 2,3,7,8-tetrachlorodibenzo-*p*-dioxin in mammalian liver microsomal systems and in living mice. *Arch. Environ. Contam. Toxicol.* **1**, 122–132.

Vogel, E., and Chandler, J. L. R. (1974). Mutagenicity testing of cyclamate and some pesticides in *Drosophila melanogaster. Experientia* **30**, 621–623.

von Oettingen, W. F. (1949). "Phenol and Its Derivatives: The Relation between Their Chemical Constitution and Their Effect on the Organism," Natl. Inst. Health Bull. 190. U.S. Govt. Printing Office, Washington, D.C.

Voorman, R., and Aust, S. D. (1987). Specific binding of polyhalogenated aromatic hydrocarbon inducers of cytochrome P-450d to the cytochrome and inhibition of its estradiol alpha-hydroxylase activity. *Toxicol. Appl. Pharmacol.* **90**, 69–78.

Vos, J. G., and Moore, J. A. (1974). Suppression of cellular immunity in rats and mice by maternal treatment with 2,3,7,8-tetrachlorodibenzo-*p*-dioxin (TCDD). *Int. Arch. Allergy Appl. Immunol.* **47**, 777–794.

Vos, J. G., Moore, J. A., and Zinkl, J. G. (1973). Effect of 2,3,7,8-tetrachlorodibenzo-*p*-dioxin (TCDD) on the immune system of laboratory animals. *Environ. Health Perspect.* **5**, 149–162.

Vos, J. G., Moore, J. A., and Zinkl. J. G. (1974). Toxicity of 2,3,7,8-tetrachlorodibenzo-*p*-dioxin (TCDD) in C57Bl/6 mice. *Toxicol. Appl. Pharmacol.* **29**, 229–241.

Vos, J. G., Kreeftenberg, J. G., Engel, H. W. B., Minderhoud, A., and Van Noorle Jansen, L. M. (1978). Studies on 2,3,7,8-tetrachlorodibenzo-*p*-dioxin-induced immune suppression and decreased resistance to infection: Endotoxin hypersensitivity, serum zinc concentrations and effect of thymosin treatment. *Toxicology* **9**, 75–86.

Vos, J. G., Faith, R. E., and Luster, M. I. (1980). Immune alterations. *In* "Halogenated Biphenyls, Naphthalenes, Dibenzodioxins and Related Products" (R. D. Kimbrough, ed.), pp. 241–266. Elsevier/North-Holland Press, New York.

Vos, J. G., Van Leeuwen, F. X. R., and De Jong, P. (1982). Acnegenic activity of 3-methylcholanthrene and benzo(*a*)pyrene, and a comparative study with 2,3,7,8-tetrachlorodibenzo-*p*-dioxin in the rabbit and hairless mouse. *Toxicology* **23**, 187–196.

Wagener, K. (1951). Hyperkeratosis of cattle of Germany. *J. Am. Vet. Med. Assoc.* **119**, 133–137.

Wahba, Z. Z., Lawson, T. A., and Stohs, S. J. (1988). Induction of hepatic DNA single strand breaks in rats by 2,3,7,8-tetrachlorodibenzo-*p*-dioxin (TCDD). *Cancer Lett.* **29**, 281–286.

Walker, A. E., and Martin, J. V. (1979). Lipid profiles in dioxin-exposed workers. *Lancet* **1**, 446–447.

Walsh, J. (1977). Seveso: The questions persist where dioxin created a wasteland. *Science* **197**, 1064–1067.

Wassermann, M., Mihail, G., Iliescu, S., Vancea, G., Sara, V., and Iosubas, S. (1960). Conditions of work and state of health of agricultural workers using DNOC during the winter. *Concours Med.* **82**, 2537–2544 (in French).

Wassom, J. S., Huff, J. E., and Loprieno, N. (1978). A review of the genetic toxicology of chlorinated dibenzo-*p*-dioxins. *Mutat. Res.* **47**, 141–160.

Wauer, G. (1918). Occupational disease due to chlorinated hydrocarbons. *Zentralbl. Gewerbehyg. Unfallverhuet.* **6**, 100–101.

Webb, K., Evans, R. G., Stehr, P., and Ayres, S. M. (1987). Pilot study on health effects of environmental 2,3,7,8-TCDD in Missouri. *Am. J. Ind. Med.* **11**, 685–691.

Weber, G., Luzi, P., Resi, L., Tanganelli, P., Lovati, M. R., and Poli, A. (1983). Natural history of TCDD-induced liver lesions in rats as observed by transmission electron microscopy during a 32-week period after a single intraperitoneal injection. *J. Toxicol. Environ. Health* **12**, 533–540.

Weber, H., Poiger, H., and Schlatter, C. (1982). Acute oral toxicity of TCDD-metabolites in male guinea pigs. *Toxicol. Lett.* **14**, 117–122.

Weber, H., Harris, M. W., Haseman, J. K., and Birnbaum, L. S. (1985).

Tetatogenic potency of TCDD, TCDF, and TCDD–TCDF combinations in C57Bl/6N mice. *Toxicol. Lett.* **26**, 159–167.

Weber, L. W. D., Greim, H., and Rozman, K. K. (1987a). Metabolism and distribution of [^{14}C]glucose in rats treated with 2,3,7,8-tetrachlorodibenzo-*p*-dioxin (TCDD) on thermogenesis in brown adipose tissue in rats. *Toxicol. Lett.* **22**, 195–206.

Weber, L. W. D., Haart, T. W., and Rozman, K. (1987b). Effect of 2,3,7,8-tetrachlorodibenzo-*p*-dioxin(TCDD) on thermogenesis in brown adipose tissue of rats. *Toxicol. Lett.* **39**, 241–248.

Weinbach, E. C. (1957). Biochemical basis for the toxicity of pentachlorophenol. *Proc. Natl. Acad. Sci U.S.A.* **43**, 393–397.

Weinbach, E. C., and Garbus, J. (1969). Mechanism of action of reagents that uncouple oxidative phosphorylation. *Nature (London)* **221**, 1016–1018.

Weinbach, E. C., Garbus, J., and Claggett, C. E. (1965). The interaction of coupling phenols with mitochondria and with mitochondrial proteins. *J. Biol. Chem.* **240**, 1811–1819.

Weissberg, J. B., and Zinkl, J. G. (1973). Effects of 2,3,7,8-tetrachlorodibenzo-*p*-dioxin upon hemostasis and hematologic function in the rat. *Environ. Health Perspect.* **5**, 119–124.

Whalman, H. F. (1936). Dinitrophenol cataract. *Southwest. Med.* **20**, 381–385.

White, K. L., Jr., and Anderson, A. C. (1985). Suppression of mouse complement activity by contaminants of technical grade pentachlorophenol. *Agents Actions* **16**, 385–392.

White. K. L., Jr., Lysy, H. H., McCoy, J. A., and Anderson, A. C. (1986). Modulation of serum complement levels following exposures to polychlorinated dibenzo-*p*-dioxins. *Toxicol. Appl. Pharmacol.* **84**, 209–219.

Whitlock, J. P., Jr. (1987). The regulation of gene expression by 2,3,7,8-tetrachlorodibenzo-*p*-dioxin. *Pharmacol. Rev.* **39**, 147–161.

Whitlock, J. P., Jr., and Galeazzi, D. R. (1984). 2,3,7,8-Tetrachlorodibenzo-*p*-dioxin receptors in wild type and variant mouse hepatoma cells. Nuclear location and strength of nuclear binding. *J. Biol. Chem.* **259**, 980–985.

Wiklund, K., Dich, J., and Holm, L.-E., (1989). Risk of soft-tissue sarcoma, Hodgkin's disease, and non-Hodgkin's lymphoma among Swedish licensed pesticide applicators. *Chemosphere* **18**, 395–400.

Wilhelmsson, A., Wikström, A.-C. and Poellinger, L. (1986). Polyanionic-binding properties of the receptor for 2,3,7,8-tetrachlorodibenzo-*p*-dioxin. A comparison with the glucocorticoid receptor. *J. Biol. Chem.* **261**, 13456–13463.

Willey, J. C., Saladino, A. J., Ozanne, C., Lechner, J. F., and Harris, C. C. (1984). Acute effects of 12-O-tetradecanoylphorbol-13-acetate, teleicidin B, or 2,3,7,8-tetrachlorodibenzo-*p*-dioxin on cultured normal human bronchial epithelial cells. *Carcinogenesis (London)* **5**, 209–215.

Williams, J. B., Wang, R., Lu, A. Y. H., and Pickett, C. B. (1984). Rat liver DT-diaphorase: Regulation of functional mRNA levels by 3-methylcholanthrene, *trans*-stilbene oxide, and phenobarbital. *Arch. Biochem. Biophys.* **23**, 408–413.

Williams, P. L. (1982). Pentachlorophenol, an assessment of the occupational hazard. *Am. Ind. Hyg. Assoc. J.* **43**, 799–810.

Wilson, J. (1987). A dose-response curve for Yusho syndrome. *Regul. Toxicol. Pharmacol.* **7**, 364–369.

Wipf, H. K., and Schmid, J. (1983). Seveso—An environmental assessment. *In* "Human and Environmental Risks of Chlorinated Dioxins and Related Compounds" (R. E. Tucker, A. L. Young, and A. P. Gray, eds.), pp. 255–274. Plenum, New York.

Wipf, H. K., Homberger, E., Neuner, N., Ranalder, U. B., Vetter, W., and Vuilleumier, J. P. (1982). TCDD-levels in soil and plant samples from the Seveso area. *In* "Chlorinated Dioxins and Related Compounds: Impact on the Environment" (O. Hutzinger, R. W. Frei, E. Merian, and Pocchiari, F., eds.), pp. 115–126. Pergamon, New York.

Witte, I., Juhl, U., and Butte, W. (1985). DNA-damaging properties and cytotoxicity in human fibroblasts of tetrachlorohydroquinone, a pentachlorophenol metabolite. *Mutat. Res.* **145**, 71–75.

Wollesen, C., Schulzeck, S., Stork, T., Betz, U., and Wasserman, O. (1986). Effects of pure and technical grade pentachlorophenol on cultured rat hepatocytes. *Chemosphere* **15**, 2125–2128

Wood, S., Rom, W. M., White, G. L., and Logan, D. C. (1983). Pentachlorophenol poisoning. *J. Occup. Med.* **25,** 527–530.

Woods, J. S. (1973). Studies of the effects of 2,3,7,8-tetrachlorodibenzo-*p*-dioxin on mammalian hepatic delta-aminolevulinic acid synthetase. *Environ. Health Perspect.* **5,** 221–225.

World Health Organization (WHO) (1962). Pentachlorophenol poisoning in Bangkok. *WHO Inf. Circ. Toxic. Pestic. Man Nos. 8/9.*

World Health Organization (1982). Recommended health-based limits in occupational exposure to pesticides. 5. Dinitro-*o*-cresol. *World Health Org. Tech. Rep. Ser.* **677,** 85–107.

Wroblewski, V. J., and Olson, J. R. (1985). Hepatic metabolism of 2,3,7,8-tetrachlorodibenzo-*p*-dioxin (TCDD) in the rat and guinea pig. *Toxicol. Appl. Pharmacol.* **81,** 231–240.

Wyllie, J. A., Gabica, J., Benson, W. W., and Yoder, J. (1975). Exposure and contamination of the air and employees of a pentachlorophenol plant, Idaho, 1972. *Pestic. Monit. J.* **9,** 150–153.

Yabusaki, Y., Shimizu, M., Murakami, H., Nakamura, K., Oeda, K., and Ohkawa, H. (1984). Nucleotide sequence of a full-length cDNA coding for 3-methylcholanthrene-induced rat liver cytochrome P-450MC. *Nucleic Acids Res.* **12,** 2929–2938.

Yang, K. H., Croft, W. A., and Peterson, R. E. (1977). Effects of 2,3,7,8-tetrachlorodibenzo-*p*-dioxin on plasma disappearance and biliary excretion of foreign compounds in rats. *Toxicol. Appl. Pharmacol.* **40,** 485–496.

Yang, K. H., Choi, E. J., and Choe, S. Y. (1983). Cytotoxicity of 2,3,7,8-tetrachlorodibenzo-*p*-dioxin on primary cultures of adult rat hepatocytes. *Arch. Environ. Contam. Toxicol.* **12,** 183–188.

York, R. G., and Manson, J. M. (1984). Neonatal toxicity in mice associated with the *Ah*[b] allele following transplacental exposure to 3-methylcholanthrene. *Toxicol. Appl. Pharmacol.* **72,** 417–426.

York, R. G., Stemmer, K., and Manson, J. M. (1984). Lung tumorigenesis and hyperplasia in offspring associated with the *Ah*[d] allele following in utero exposure to 3-methylcholanthrene. *Toxicol. Appl. Pharmacol.* **72,** 427–439.

Yoshihara, S., Nagata, K., Yoshimura, H., Kuroki, H., and Masuda, Y. (1981). Inductive effect on hepatic enzymes and acute toxicity of individual polychlorinated dibenzofuran congeners in rats. *Toxicol. Appl. Pharmacol.* **59,** 580–588.

Yoshihara, S., Nagata, K., Wada, I., Yoshimura, H., Kuroki, H., and Masuda, Y. (1982). A unique change of steroid metabolism in rat liver microsomes induced with highly toxic polychlorinated biphenyl (pcb) and polychlorinated dibenzofuran (pcdf). *J. Pharmacol. Dyn.* **5,** 994–1004.

Yoshimura, T., and Hayabuchi, H. (1985). Relationship between the amount of rice oil ingested by patients with Yusho and their subjective symptoms. *Environ. Health Perspect.* **59,** 47–52.

Young, A. L. (1983). Long-term studies on the persistence and movement of TCDD in a natural ecosysytem. *In* "Human and Environmental Risks of Chlorinated Dioxins and Related Compounds" (R. E. Tucker, A. L. Young, and A. P. Gray, eds.), pp. 173–190. Plenum, New York.

Young, A. L., Thalken, C. E., Arnold, E. L., Cupello, J. M., and Cockerman, L. G. (1976). "Fate of 2,3,7,8-Tetrachlorodibenzo-*p*-dioxin (TCDD) in the Environment: Summary and Decontamination Recommendations, Air Force Tech. Rep. No. USAFA-TR-76-18. U.S. Air Force Academy, Colorado.

Young, J. F., and Haley, T. J. (1978). A pharmacokinetic study of pentachlorophenol poisoning and the effect of forced diuresis. *Clin. Toxicol.* **12,** 41–48.

Younis, H. M., and Mohanty, P. (1980). Inhibition of electron flow and energy transduction in isolated spinach chloroplasts by the herbicide dinoseb. *Chem.-Biol. Interact.* **32,** 179–186.

Zacharewski, T., Harris, M., and Safe, S. (1989). Induction of cytochrome P450-dependent monooxygenase activities in rat hepatoma H-4-IIE cells in culture by 2,3,7,8-tetrachlorodibenzo-*p*-dioxin and related compounds: Mechanistic studies using radiolabeled congeners. *Arch. Biochem. Biophys.* **272,** 344–355.

Zack, J. A., and Suskind, R. R. (1980). The mortality experience of workers exposed to tetrachlorodibenzodioxin in a trichlorophenol process accident. *J. Occup. Med.* **22,** 11–14.

Zhivkov, I. I., Chelibonova-Lorer, Kh., and Panaiotov, B. N. (1970). The effect of 2,4-dinitrophenol on the content and specific activity of acid-soluble nucleotides in the rat liver. *Biokhimiya (Moscow)* **35,** 484–488 (in Russian).

Zimmering, S., Manson, J. M., Valencia, R., and Woodruff, R. C. (1985). Chemical mutagenesis testing in *Drosophila*. II. Results of 20 coded compounds tested for the National Toxicology Program. *Environ. Mutagen.* **7,** 87–100.

Zinkl, J. G., Vos, J. G., Moore, J. A., and Gupta, B. N. (1973). Hematologic and chemical clinical chemistry of 2,3,7,8-tetrachlorodibenzo-*p*-dioxin in laboratory animals. *Environ. Health Perspect.* **5,** 111–118.

Synthetic Organic Rodenticides

Alain F. Pelfrene

Pennwalt, France

19.1 INTRODUCTION

Rats and mice compete with humans for food. This loss to rodents causes economic loss everywhere. In some developing countries it can cause starvation. Rodents are also hosts for human diseases, including plague, endemic rickettsiosis, leishmaniasis, spirochetosis, tularemia, leptospirosis, tick-borne encephalitis, and listeriosis. Rats occasionally bite people. Finally, rodents do a variety of other damage, mainly by gnawing.

Insofar as possible, rodent populations should be controlled by limiting their access to food and harborage. Individual animals or small groups may be removed conveniently by trapping. However, there will always be a need for poisons in rodent control.

Unfortunately, effective permanent control through poisoning is not simple. The animals must be enticed to ingest a toxicant in sufficient dosage if the effort is to succeed. But rodents rarely or ever constitute an important problem unless they have a supply of food and water. This means that, in spite of containing a foreign substance, the solid or liquid bait used should be at least as attractive to the rodents as their usual supply of food or water. The first problem may be that the intended poison makes the bait unacceptable to animals that have never encountered the poison. This is called primary bait refusal. Because of this common difficulty, many efforts to find better rodenticides have emphasized highly toxic substances of such bland taste and odor that animals always will take a lethal dose the first time. However, this is an impractical objective. At least a few animals will get only a sublethal dose on first encounter and will be conditioned thereby to avoid the poison even though it seems tasteless and odorless at first. This reaction is called secondary bait refusal or bait shyness. There is even some indication that rodents learn from the behavior of their companions in such a way that the manner of death of some of them conditions the behavior of others that have consumed no poison. Efforts to combat the problem of bait shyness involve prebaiting or changing the bait, the poison, or preferably both. A third problem with many rodenticides is that they are very nearly as dangerous to humans and useful animals as to rodents. This problem can be minimized by selecting a poison with a wide margin of safety, by coloring the bait, by combining the poison with an emetic, or by restricting the placement of baits. However, all these solutions have their limitations. There is no rat poison that cannot harm humans if sufficiently misused. The addition of a color or emetic may lead to primary bait refusal or it simply may fail in its objective. Poisons supposedly limited to unoccupied, locked premises sooner or later turn up in the hands of a child.

Considering all these difficulties, four requirements for an ideal rodenticide may be stated as follows: (a) The poison must be surely effective when incorporated into baits in such small quantity that its presence is not detected to an interfering degree. (b) Finished baits containing the poison must not excite bait shyness in any way and the necessity of prebaiting must, thereby, be avoided. (c) The manner of death must be such that surviving individuals will not become suspicious of its cause but will remain on the premises and eat freely of the bait until they themselves die. (d) The poison, in the concentration used for control, must be specific for the species to be destroyed unless its use can be made safe for humans and domestic animals by some other means.

The anticoagulant rodenticides in general and warfarin in particular fulfilled these requirements almost perfectly. Their only serious disadvantage was the appearance of resistance among some treated populations, as discussed below. Although this resistance obviously revealed a genetic potential, it would never have come to light without severe selective pressure on the populations involved. It is interesting to speculate whether resistance to any one of the acute rodenticides would become apparent if it were possible to achieve a high degree of continuing selective pressure through its use.

Part of the safety of the anticoagulant rodenticides is made possible by their cumulative properties and depends on the fact that they are offered to rodents in such a way that a single dose is harmless even to the rodents themselves. Quite aside from the important species differences in susceptibility, which favor human safety, people are protected further by the fact that, except in suicide or murder, substantial continuing exposure is far less likely than a single accidental exposure.

Although this chapter is devoted to synthetic organic rodenticides, it is necessary to recall that inorganic and botanical compounds may still be important for rodent control in some areas. Furthermore, some of them, notably arsenic, phosphorus, and strychnine, are very important as sources of human poisoning. Discussions of some inorganic and botanical rodenticides may be found in the following sections: zinc phosphide, 12.4.2; thallium sulfate, 12.7.1; arsenic trioxide, 12.12.1; phosphorus, 12.13.1; and strychnine, 13.10.1.

On the contrary, some synthetic rodenticides have other uses. The most important examples are the use of vitamin D and of certain anticoagulants as rodenticides and as drugs in human medicine. In addition, several of the organic fluorine compounds have been used experimentally or in practice as systemic insecticides and/or acaricides. MNFA is a systemic acaricide that apparently never has been promoted as a rodenticide, probably because rats are relatively resistant to the compound. However, MNFA has the same mode of action as other organic fluorides, and several species are highly susceptible to it; therefore, it is described in this chapter.

Compared to toxic substances in general, biochemical actions of the synthetic rodenticides that have been studied in humans are unusually well known. This makes it possible to assign them to groups (see the following sections) that are meaningful not only chemically but in terms of biochemical lesions. The same is not true of numerous miscellaneous compounds including crimidine (BSI, ISO) that apparently have not yet produced poisoning in humans and certainly have not been used as drugs or studied experimentally in human subjects.

19.2 FLUOROACETIC ACID AND ITS DERIVATIVES

Sodium fluoroacetate came to prominence in the United States as a result of a search for rodenticides that would not be subject to shortages imposed by World War II (Ward, 1945). This and related compounds had been considered earlier as systemic insecticides. At about the same time, it became known that fluoroacetate is the toxic material in the South African plant "gifblaar" (*Dichapetalum cymosum*). Later it was shown that the same compound is present intermittently in *Acacia georgiana*. The main toxicant in *D. toxicarium* is fluorooleic acid, but fluoropalmitic acid is present also. The ground seeds of *D. toxicarium* have been used by natives as a rat poison. It gave problems with secondary poisoning and human toxicity similar to that later associated with synthetic sodium fluoroacetate.

Under these circumstances, there were practical as well as academic reasons to study the mode of action of organic monofluoro compounds. Some of what was learned is discussed in Section 19.2.1.2. Although even an outline of what is known about the chemical class is beyond the scope of this book, it is interesting to note that some of the compounds are 10–14 times

more toxic than sodium fluoroacetate. It appears that the toxicity of all of the compounds depends on the same mechanism. These highly toxic compounds either have two carbon atoms or are metabolized to this form. It is consistent with what is known of normal metabolism that ω-monofluoro amino acids with an odd number of carbon atoms and ω-monofluoro alkanoic acids with an even number of carbon atoms are toxic. It is thought that greater fat solubility and consequent easier penetration into cells explain the fact that some long-chain ω-fluoro compounds are more toxic than fluoroacetate (Saunders, 1947; Chenoweth, 1949; Raasch, 1958; Peters, 1963a).

It seems likely that the contribution of the organic monofluoro compounds as tools for exploring intermediate metabolism has been at least as valuable as their contribution to the control of commensal rodents.

19.2.1 SODIUM FLUOROACETATE

19.2.1.1 Identity, Properties, and Uses

Chemical Name   Sodium monofluoroacetate.

Structure   See Fig. 19.1.

Synonyms   Sodium monofluoroacetate is also known as Compound-1080 or ten-eighty. The CAS registry number is 62-74-8.

Physical and Chemical Properties   The empirical formula for sodium monofluoroacetate is $C_2H_2FNaO_2$ and the molecular weight is 100.3. It forms an odorless, white, nonvolatile powder that decomposes at about 200°C. Although the compound is often said to be tasteless, dilute solutions actually tasted like weak vinegar. Sodium fluoroacetate is very water soluble and

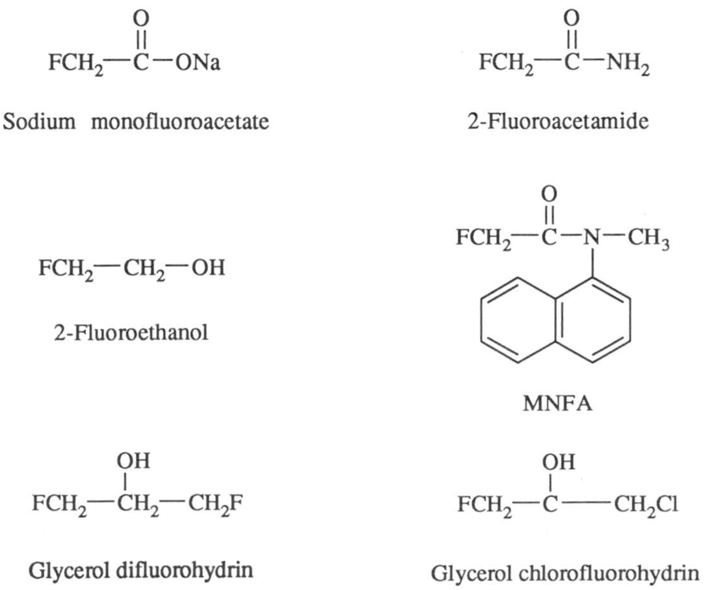

Figure 19.1   Some organic fluorine rodenticides and other organic fluorine pesticdes.

hygroscopic but is of low solubility in ethanol, acetone, and petroleum oils.

History, Formulations, and Uses Sodium monofluoroacetate was suggested for trial by the National Defense Research Committee of the U.S. Office of Scientific Research and Development in the early 1940s. It is formulated as an aqueous solution containing 0.5% nigrosine as a warning color. Sodium monofluoroacetate is used to kill rats, mice, other rodents, and predators. It is an intense mammalian poison, and it is used in many countries but only by trained personnel.

19.2.1.2 Toxicity to Laboratory Animals

Basic Findings The first paper on sodium monofluoroacetate as a rodenticide (Kalmbach, 1945) drew attention to its very high acute toxicity. LD 50 values for ordinary laboratory rats and for wild animals of the same species were reported as 2.5 and 5.0 mg/kg, respectively. The wild black rat (*Rattus rattus*), another commensal species, was much more susceptible (LD 50: 0.1 mg/kg). A LD 50 of 0.22 mg/kg has been reported for *Rattus norvegicus* (Dieke and Richter, 1946). The likelihood of danger to people, domestic animals, pets, and nontarget wildlife was pointed out. The acute toxicity of the compound to an extremely wide range of wildlife was reported by Ward and Spencer (1947). See Table 19.1.

Fluoroacetate acts mainly on the central nervous system and the heart. It seems that there are species in which fluoroacetate affects chiefly the heart, such as the rabbit, the goat, and the horse, and others in which only the central nervous system is affected, such as the dog, the guinea pig, and the frog. In the cat, the rhesus monkey, the domestic pig, and birds both systems are involved. The above results were obtained by Chenoweth and Gilman (1946) using methyl fluoroacetate instead of sodium fluoroacetate. However, since both compounds yield the fluorocitrate ion in the body, where it is converted to fluoroacetate, which is responsible for the induction of pharmacologic and toxic signs (see below), it seems that this experiment is nevertheless interesting in showing a large degree of species variability in the site of action. In all species, there was a delay of 0.5–2 hr or more between administration, either oral or intravenous, and the onset of the symptoms, and the route of administration did not significantly affect the toxicity of fluoroacetate.

Laboratory rats acquire a tolerance to sodium fluoroacetate by ingesting sublethal doses over a period of 5–14 days. However, this tolerance is lost if intake of the compound is interrupted for as little as 7 days (Kalmbach, 1945).

Tolerance of some but not all species was confirmed by several investigators, including Kandel and Chenoweth (1952). These authors found that, whereas small doses of fluoroacetate increased tolerance to challenge doses of fluoroacetate or 4-fluorobutyrate, tolerance to neither could be evoked by small doses of 4-fluorobutyrate. The citrate content of the rat brain appeared to have no relation to tolerance, and the citrate that accumulated after a small dose did not prevent the further accumulation of citrate after a larger dose.

Table 19.1
Single-Dose LD 50 for Sodium Fluoroacetate

Species	Route	LD 50 (mg/kg)	Reference
Rat	oral	0.22	Dieke and Richter (1946)
Rat	oral	2.5	Ward and Spencer (1947)
Rat	oral	1–2	Phillips and Worden (1957)
Rat	intraperitoneal	3–5	Ward and Spencer (1947)
Mouse	subcutaneous	19.3	Hutchens *et al.* (1949)
Mouse	subcutaneous	17.0	Tourtellotte and Coon (1951)
Mouse	intraperitoneal	10.0	Ward and Spencer (1947)
Mouse	intraperitoneal	16.5	Tourtellotte and Coon (1951)
Mouse	intraperitoneal	14.7	Raasch (1958)
Guinea pig	oral	0.4	Ward and Spencer (1947)
Guinea pig	intraperitoneal	0.37	Hutchens *et al.* (1949)
Rabbit	subcutaneous	0.28	Hutchens *et al.* (1949)
Dog	oral	0.06	Tourtellotte and Coon (1951)
Cow	oral	0.39	Robinson (1970)
Calf	oral	0.22	Robinson (1970)
Opossum	oral	0.79	Bell (1972)
Mallard duck	oral	4.8	Hudson *et al.* (1972)
South African clawed toad (*Xenopus laevis*)	oral	500	Chenoweth (1949)

The sensitivity of mice to sodium fluoroacetate depends on temperature. Under otherwise identical conditions, the LD 50 values were 12.1 and 5.16 mg/kg at 23 and 17°C, respectively (Misustova *et al.*, 1969). The survival of individual rats in a particular dosage group may be predicted by following their body temperature. There is a critical level that varies somewhat according to the interval after dosing. Animals that regained their initial temperature within 96 hr usually lived, but those that failed to regain normal temperature within this time usually died (Filip *et al.*, 1970). For groups of animals, the course of the temperature can be described by a computer-generated curve (Hosek *et al.*, 1970). The temperature change is correlated with citrate metabolism (Kirzon *et al.*, 1970).

Primates and birds are more resistant; rodents and carnivores are most susceptible. In general, cold-blooded vertebrates are less sensitive than warm-blooded ones (Egekeze and Oehme, 1979). Sodium monofluoroacetate in carcasses creates a secondary poisoning hazard to which carnivorous predators are extremely susceptible (Bell, 1972).

Absorption, Distribution, Metabolism, and Excretion
Using ether as a solvent, it was possible to recover 60–70% of the total dose from the body (including gastrointestinal contents) of rabbits killed by 10 times the LD 50 level. The concentration in the brain was twice that in other organs (Tomiya *et al.*, 1976). Sodium monofluoroacetate is rapidly absorbed by the gastrointestinal tract. It is not well absorbed by the intact skin, but absorption may be greater in the presence of dermatitis or other skin injury.

Biochemical Effects It was in connection with the mode of action of fluoroacetic acid that the term "lethal synthesis" was coined (Peters, 1952). Peters (1963b) later reviewed the research and extended the concept. Very briefly, no mammalian enzyme was found that was inhibited by fluoracetate *in vitro*. However *in vivo*, the ion undergoes synthesis to form fluorocitrate and this inhibits mitochondrial aconitase either *in vivo* or *in vitro*. The result is that the Krebs cycle is blocked, which leads to lowered energy production, reduced oxygen consumption, and reduced cellular concentration of ATP; furthermore, since the citrate synthetase continues to work, citrate accumulates in the tissues (Buffa and Peters, 1950). It is thought that toxicity is due not to the accumulation of citrate *per se* but to the blockage of energy metabolism. However, increased tissue and plasma concentration of citrate is probably responsible for some of the symptoms seen during acute poisoning. Citrate is a potent chelator of calcium ion, and it has been demonstrated that in cats intravenously injected with fluoroacetate at 0.03 mmol/kg the ionized calcium level in blood fell by an average of 27.2%, 40 min after the injection. There was a corresponding prolongation of the QT interval of the electrocardiogram (ECG), and treatment with $CaCl_2$ significantly prolonged the life of the treated animals as compared with unmedicated positive controls (Roy *et al.*, 1980). The characteristic delay at the onset of poisoning by sodium fluoroacetate is accounted for by the time necessary for its metabolism and biochemical mode of action.

The toxicity of fluoroacetate is entirely different from that of inorganic fluorides. It depends on the firmness of the F—C bond such that fluoroacetate is an antimetabolite.

Consistent with the theory that fluorocitrate is the active toxicant, it was found to be at least 100 times more toxic than fluoroacetate when injected directly into the brain under various experimental conditions. An intracerebral dose of 0.115 μg failed to kill rats weighing about 250 gm, and it did not cause convulsions; doses of 0.287 μg (about 0.001 mg/kg) or greater caused convulsions and killed almost all rats (Morselli *et al.*, 1968). On the other hand, a dosage of 40–60 mg/kg is necessary to kill by the intraperitoneal route, and an oral dosage of 40 mg/kg constitutes only an LD 50. The great difference was attributed to failure of fluorocitrate to reach aconitase within critical cells of the brain and heart (Peters and Shorthouse, 1971). Species differ in the degree to which the concentration of citrate increases in different organs and also in the timing of these increases (Kirzon *et al.*, 1973). These biochemical differences presumably underlie the clinical differences between species, especially the relative importance in neurological and cardiac effects.

Accumulation of citrate was evident in mice within 2 h after intraperitoneal injection of sodium fluoroacetate at a rate of 30 mg/kg, which is about 1.7 times the LD 50 in that species. The concentration of citrate increased from 48 ppm in controls to 74, 101, and 166 ppm within 2, 5, and 24 hr, respectively, after injection. The mice were dead at 24 hr (Matsumuta and O'Brien, 1963).

Whereas Williamson *et al.* (1964) agreed that the initial effect of fluoroacetate is to produce fluorocitrate, they considered that the secondary inhibition of phosphofructokinase by the accumulated citrate was actually lethal because it deprived the cell of pyruvate, which would eventually overcome the inhibition of aconitase.

Effects on Organs and Tissues Loracher and Lux (1974) concluded on the basis of studies of neuromembrane depolarization that diminished inhibitory conductance is apparently important as a causative factor in convulsions induced by sodium fluoroacetate. The decreased level of ionized calcium in blood induced by the chelating effect of citrate certainly plays a role in the depolarization of the neuromembrane, as it does on the cardiac cell membranes. The effect of sodium fluoroacetate on the heart rhythm is due, as demonstrated by Noguchi *et al.* (1966), primarily to action on the cells themselves and not on the vagus nerve. Irregularity of rhythm and a condition analogous to fibrillation were produced in cultures of heart cells that had grown until cell-to-cell contact was prevalent and beating was synchronized. The average times necessary to produce irregularity and fibrillation were 9 and 48 hr, respectively, at a concentration of 10 ppm in the medium but only 2 and 9 hr, respectively, at a concentration of 100 ppm. At a concentration of 1000 ppm, fibrillation was immediate and cytoplasmic vacuoles appeared rapidly.

Effects on Reproduction A dosage of sodium fluoroacetate just below the maternal LD 50 reduced oxygen consumption of the embryos as well as the mother but was not teratogenic (Spielmann *et al.*, 1973).

Treatment of Poisoning in Animals Hutchens *et al.* (1949) demonstrated a significant reduction of mortality in mice, guinea pigs, and rabbits (but not dogs) treated with ethanol at a rate of 800 mg/kg administered subcutaneously as a 10% solution in normal saline. The response occurred when the alcohol was given before signs of poisoning appeared and was best when given within 10 min of poisoning. In mice, sodium acetate and ethanol acted synergistically to antagonize poisoning (Tourtellotte and Coon, 1951). The beneficial effect of ethanol in rodents was confirmed by Chenoweth *et al.* (1951), but these authors found ethanol less effective in the dog and utterly useless in the monkey. In a study of a wide range of chemical substances in mice, rats, rabbits, dogs, and rhesus monkeys, they concluded that commercially available monacetin containing about 60% glycerol monoacetate was superior to any other substance tested as an antidote for poisoning by fluoroacetate. Not only did it reduce mortality, but it was able to normalize heart and brain rhythms as indicated by ECG and electroencephalogram (EEG) tracings.

Light pentobarbital anesthesia for 18–24 hr significantly reduced mortality among dogs poisoned by sodium monofluoroacetate at a rate of 0.10 mg/kg (Hutchens *et al.*, 1949; Tourtellotte and Coon, 1951).

19.2.1.3 Toxicity to Humans

Accidental and Intentional Poisoning Sodium fluoroacetate was selected by screening more than a thousand compounds for rodenticidal action during World War II (Kalmbach, 1945). It was introduced in 1946 in the United States for use by pest control operators, including persons hired for the purpose by government agencies. The poison was mixed with a dye. Solutions were supposed to be placed in shallow paper cups made in such a way that they would not tip over. These water baits were supposed to be used only in places that would be unoccupied and locked during exposure of the poison, and all cups and dead rodents were supposed to be collected and incinerated by authorized persons at the end of the exposure period. However, the regulations were not always followed. By the end of the year, at least one child who found an "empty" paper cup had died, and her 3-year-old brother had been severely poisoned. By the end of 1949 there had been at least 12 deaths and 6 cases of nonfatal poisoning. In addition, there had been 4 deaths, all in children, that probably were caused by sodium monofluoroacetate, but other sources of poisoning could not be ruled out. Of the 12 deaths clearly caused by sodium fluoroacetate, 5 involved small children who had found and often chewed on a poison cup, 3 involved juveniles who had found the poison in a soft drink bottle, and 4 were suicides of adults. Except one, each of the survivors was a child who had found a poison cup. These accidents made such an impression on the few people who had legal access to sodium fluoroacetate that they became far stricter in carrying out the recommended precautions and in selecting situations in which the compound was used at all. As a result, the safety record of the compound in the United States improved greatly.

A typical fatal case involved a 40-year-old man who was found unconscious in his bedroom. He had an 8-year history of severe depression, and his family had been warned of the possibility of suicide. When admitted to hospital, he had slight muscular spasms and nystagmus of both eyes; the heart rate was 92 per minute; rhythm was irregular. Following gastric lavage and a soft soap enema, the nystagmus became worse, and the patient had an epileptiform convulsion. The blood pressure fell to 90/40 mm Hg. Treatment consisted of plasma, oxygen, and procaine hydrochloride in the hope of desensitizing the heart. The face was flushed, and the patient vomited occasionally. The blood pressure improved to 118/75 mm Hg, but there was no decisive change until the heart and later the respiration stopped

about 17 hr after admission (Harrisson *et al.*, 1952a). Another fatal case was remarkable for its combination of prolonged survival following the ingestion of an almost certainly very large dose. Briefly, about 113,000 mg of sodium fluoroacetate was missing from a professional rat exterminator's supplies after his 17-year-old son made a solution and drank it. The boy vomited promptly and then within an hour walked into an hospital emergency room. He gradually became comatose during gastric lavage, and consciousness was never regained. Within less than 3 hr of ingestion, he had a grand mal convulsion associated with fecal incontinence. The clinical course, which lasted slightly over 5 days, was characterized by cardiac irregularity, which responded to a considerable degree to procainamide hydrochloride; dilation and failure of the heart with acute pulmonary edema, which responded surprisingly well to digitalis (lanatoside C); bouts of severe hypotension, which responded only questionably to levarterenol (norepinephrine) but somewhat better to mephentermine; cortical irritability, which responded to barbiturates and later responded more effectively to ethanol; frequent severe carpopedal spasm, controlled somewhat by calcium gluconate; and finally growing evidence of infection including a temperature reaching 42.3°C in spite of efforts to reduce it. The diagnosis based on autopsy was poisoning, bronchopneumonia with septicemia, focal infarction of the right kidney, and mediastinal emphysema (Brockmann *et al.*, 1955). The authors almost certainly were correct in believing that the patient's life was prolonged greatly by the drugs administered. It is interesting to speculate on what additional good might have been done if ethanol had been used early and especially if monoacetin had been available and put to use, and if antibiotics had been used prophylactically or even therapeutically.

Serious illness followed by full recovery occurred in a 2-year-old boy who was found licking crystals from the screw cap of a bottle of sodium fluoroacetate solution. The parents did not know whether he drank any of the solution. Almost immediately after he was found, the boy began to vomit. He was brought to hospital about 6 hr later because he began to have generalized convulsive movements and became stuporous. The parents brought along the bottle of poison they had purchased 2 years earlier from a peddler, but the handwritten label, "Rat Poison—1080" meant nothing to them or to the attending physicians. On admission, the boy was comatose and exhibiting carpopedal spasms, tetanic convulsive movements, irregular respiration, and great cardiac irregularity. While a solution of calcium gluconate was being injected, there were a few seconds of cardiac asystole. Thereafter, the irregular cardiac rhythm resumed but at a much slower rate. Tetanic convulsions stopped immediately, and the child became completely flaccid. A few hours after admission, the child became responsive and seemed to recognize his father. Vomiting continued. Very soon the boy suffered a generalized tonic clonic convulsion lasting several minutes and followed by deep coma. Briefly, the boy remained unresponsive for 4 days. Cardiac rhythm continued to change frequently during the first 3 days. Tonic convulsions lasting several minutes occurred many times every hour, sometimes about every 10 min for many successive hours. During spasm, the pupils dilated and remained inactive to light; between seizures the pupils were miotic but responsive to light. On two occasions respiration stopped and artificial respiration was required briefly.

On the evening of the fourth day, 100 hr after ingestion, the boy began to open his eyes and look about. He tried to talk but was unable to articulate. He could neither sit up nor reach for objects but appeared alert. On the fifth and sixth days, he rapidly regained all his motor ability, slowly lost his drowsiness, and became articulate. On the evening of the sixth day he was clinically well. He was discharged on the eleventh day. Reexamination 1 year later showed that the boy had had no further neurological trouble, and his mental and physical development had proceeded normally (Gajdusek and Luther, 1950).

In another case in which the initial dosage undoubtedly was smaller, there were no important clinical changes until 20 hr after ingestion, when the 8-month-old girl had a generalized seizure lasting about 1 min. In spite of treatment with phenobarbital, three additional seizures occurred during the next 12 hr. There was no further illness, and the patient was discharged 4 days later. Follow-ups revealed no change in behavior, intellect, or motor performance (Reigart *et al.*, 1975).

Any serious but reversible interference with respiration or general circulation is liable to produce some cases in which the patient survives but with severe brain damage. The cardiac arrhythmias characteristic of poisoning by sodium fluoroacetate are likely to produce such interference. An example involved an 8-year-old boy who was in status epilepticus when he entered hospital. The convulsions were controlled to some degree. There was no striking change until 14 hr after admission, when ventricular asystole occurred. Heart action was renewed but only after sufficient delay that the child suffered brain damage and was clearly mentally defective after a very long and stormy hospital course (McTaggart, 1970).

During the decade 1971–1981, 111 cases of accidental or unintentional poisoning with sodium fluoroacetate were collected by the National Poison Center of Israel. These cases included three cases of death and one case of mass accidental poisoning affecting 30 children, although the great majority of them only consumed a very small number of wheat grain baits impregnated with the compound. These latter cases did not result in clinical symptoms of poisoning (Roy *et al.*, 1982). These authors also described the clinical features of two cases of acute poisoning in which gastrointestinal disorders were rapidly followed by central nervous system manifestations (disorders of consciousness, convulsions, coma) and cardiac disorders, the most frequent cause of death. Ventricular ectopic beats preceded the ventricular arrhythmia, which was then followed by ventricular tachycardia and fibrillation. The electrocardiogram was characterized by a prolonged QT interval. A metabolic acidosis was commonly observed. Chung (1984) reported on five cases collected between 1975 and 1981 in Taiwan. The amount ingested ranged from 8 to 40 ml of a 1% formulation of sodium monofluoroacetate. All five patients survived. All cases had signs of transient cardiac dysfunction, but in addition acute renal failure was seen in three of the five patients, two of them with frank uremia. The acute renal failure was reversible.

Use Experience In spite of the great toxicity of sodium fluoroacetate, there apparently has been only one case of illness among those who used it without suicidal intent. Even in this case, the kind of illness was so atypical of poisoning and so complicated by the unrelated factor of hypertrophy of the prostate that evaluation of the case is difficult. The patient entered hospital with renal failure and other serious illness. Although he was only 59 years old, he had a 5-year history of symptoms of prostatism but no history of urinary tract infection, renal calculi, or hematuria. He had had gout for 10 years, and he had been digitalized for 12 months. For 6 months he had experienced increasing lassitude, vomiting, and pruritis. Inspection revealed rapid breathing and muscle wasting. More detailed physical examination revealed mild left ventricular failure and evidence of liver disease, hypothyroidism, extrapyramidal disease, and gout, as well as a distended bladder, caused by prostatic hypertrophy. These findings were substantiated by laboratory examinations. Following catheter drainage of the bladder, blood urea declined and renal function improved further following prostatectomy 10 days after admission. Recovery was very slow. Neurological and thyroid findings cleared within 6 months. Renal function continued to improve for about 2 years, after which the patient remained well.

Involvement of fluoroacetate was suspected because of the history of exposure, the finding of organic fluorine in the urine, and histological changes found in kidney biopsies. There was no doubt of exposure; the patient had been employed for 10 years as an exterminator of rabbits, and for about 4 weeks each year he had applied sodium fluoroacetate to pieces of carrots that served as bait for the animals. During this work, he had worn rubber gloves and he had never knowingly ingested any of the poison. The report of concentrations of 15.4 and 14.8 ppm of sodium fluoroacetate (analyzed as organic fluoride) in two samples of urine collected 2 weeks after admission and the absence of such organic fluoride in samples collected 5 weeks and 6 months later was accepted as consistent with the history of exposure. A kidney biopsy performed 4 days after admission revealed periglomerular fibrosis, some capsular adhesion and other glomerular changes plus swelling and vacuolation of tubular cells, increased interstitial fibrous tissue, a few small foci of inflammation, and mild thickening of the arterial walls. A second biopsy 4 weeks later showed little change. A third kidney biopsy 4 months after admission showed little change in the glomerular lesion, but the tubules were no longer vacuolated. However, many tubules had been lost, and many of those remaining were atrophic. Interstitial fibrosis was prominent. The kidney lesions were considered similar to those described in rats in association with acute poisoning. It was acknowledged that lower urinary tract obstruction may have been a predisposing factor (Parkin *et al.*, 1977). Even if the patient had been exposed to sodium fluoroacetate a short time before he was admitted to hospital, it is difficult to understand why excretion of organic fluoride from this source would continue 2 weeks later. Although no urinary levels of organic fluoride have been reported for other workers, one must note that 15 ppm would indicate a daily output of about 22.5 mg/person/day in a person with average urinary volume. This in turn would indicate a minimal absorption rate of about 0.32 mg/kg/day, an astonishingly high level. The renal changes previously described in rats (Cater and Peters, 1961) followed one or a few very large dosages of fluorocitrate, and the fat droplets were tiny compared to those seen in the human patient.

Dosage Response In a fatal case, 465 mg (equivalent to a dosage of over 6 mg/kg) was recovered from the stomach contents, urine, brain, liver, and kidneys (Harrisson *et al.*, 1952b). No account was taken of sodium fluoroacetate in other organs and tissues or of that removed by vomiting, lavage, and enema; therefore, the ingested dosage must have been considerably larger.

Several children varying in age from 0.66 to 8.0 years were poisoned seriously or even fatally by chewing on only one paper cup placed earlier for rat control. The cups were made to receive 15 ml of 0.33% solution, that is, 50 mg of sodium fluoroacetate. The average age of the children was 2.37 years, and the weight of such a child is abut 13 kg. Thus, the maximal dosage must have been approximately 3.8 mg/kg, but the true dosage must have been considerably smaller because part of the material originally added to the cup may have been lost and not all that dried in the cup would have been ingested. A dosage of 0.5–2.0 mg/kg must be considered highly dangerous. The estimated mean lethal dose in humans ranged from 2 to 10 mg/kg (Gajdusek and Luther, 1950; Harrison *et al.*, 1952a).

Laboratory Findings The following concentrations expressed as sodium fluoroacetate were found in samples taken at autopsy from a man who survived about 17 hr after being found unconscious; urine, 368 ppm; liver, 58 ppm; brain, 76 ppm; and kidney, 65 ppm (Harrisson *et al.*, 1952b).

A method of laboratory confirmation of poisoning by sodium fluoroacetate or fluoroacetamide poisoning in animals involved injection of an aqueous extract of the heart and kidney into guinea pigs and subsequent examination of the guinea pig kidneys for citrate. An increase in citrate constitutes a positive test (Egyed and Shlosberg, 1973). Although the method apparently has not been used in human poisoning, it should be effective.

Pathology In a fatal case, autopsy revealed petechial hemorrhages and congestion of the organs consistent with recent fits. All the findings were nonspecific, but it is interesting that they included diffuse tubular degeneration of the kidneys, which is consistent with the findings in the only case of alleged chronic human poisoning by sodium fluoroacetate.

Treatment of Poisoning Apparently, most patients who survived poisoning by sodium fluoroacetate as well as those who died of it received no medication that offered any possibility of specific antidotal action. In at least one case (unpublished), a poisoned child was treated with whiskey and survived. Unfortunately, no details are available, and there can be no assurance that the child would not have progressed equally well without treatment.

Although monacetin apparently has not been administered to a human patient, the work of Chenoweth *et al.* (1951) in various animals, especially monkeys, offered good reason to think it would be valuable for treating human poisoning. They recommended that it be injected intramuscularly at least every hour for several hours at the rate of 0.1–0.5 ml/kg per injection. There is no clinical evidence for or against the use of acetate in humans. On the contrary, acetamide has been administered to patients, and it seemed to be the reason for their survival. It is available at Accident and Emergency departments throughout New Zealand. Acetamide is administered intravenously as a 10% solution in 5% glucose. In severe cases, 500 ml is given in 30 min every 4 hr; in milder cases, 200 ml is given on the same schedule. There can be no doubt that removal of the poison and supportive care are indicated. A number of patients have shown clear-cut poisoning but survived without sequelae following such treatment. Supportive care should include continuous cardiac monitoring. There is strong clinical evidence that the danger of cardiac arrhythmia can be reduced significantly by judicious and continuing use of procainamide hydrochloride. Even so, equipment for defibrillation should be ready. There is reason to hope it would be successful if required because at least one patient was revived with only external massage of the heart. There is also clinical evidence that cortical irritability can be lessened by barbiturates. There is no basis for speculating on the value of diazepam in this connection. Contrary to the evidence in monkeys, clinical evidence in humans has indicated that ethanol is beneficial and perhaps superior to barbiturates. Whereas the effect seemed to involve needed sedation, the possibility of a more fundamental effect in the biochemical lesion was not excluded.

On the basis of laboratory studies, Chenoweth *et al.* (1951) recommended against administration of calcium, potassium, sodium chloride, bicarbonate, or acetate. They considered that any necessary replacement of fluid should be done cautiously with plasma, and they considered digitalization as definitely contraindicated. However, clinical experience argues strongly against two of these prohibitions, and there is no clinical evidence to support some of the others. Calcium gluconate has proved useful in controlling carpopedal spasm, including such spasm in a patient who survived without sequelae. Digitalis (lanatoside C) not only improved the function of a poisoned heart that had failed to the point of acute pulmonary edema but also produced no detectable side effects.

Finally, there is clinical evidence that mephentermine is more effective than levarterenol in raising blood pressure if that becomes necessary in the course of poisoning by sodium fluoroacetate.

19.2.2 FLUOROACETAMIDE

19.2.2.1 Identity, Properties, and Uses

Chemical Name 2-Fluoroacetamide.

Structure See Fig. 19.1.

Synonyms Fluoroacetamide is also known as Compound 1081. Trade names for fluoroacetamide include Fuorakil®, Fussol®, Megarox®, and Yancock®. The CAS registry number is 640.19.7.

Physical and Chemical Properties Fluoroacetamide has the empirical formula C_2H_4FNO and a molecular weight of 77.06. It is a crystalline solid that sublimes on heating but melts at 107–109°C. It is very soluble in water, moderately soluble in acetone, and sparingly soluble in aliphatic and aromatic hydrocarbons.

History, Formulations, and Uses At one time fluoroacetamide was used as a systemic insecticide for scale insects, aphids, and mites on fruits; however, it has been considered too toxic to mammals for commercial use as an insecticide. Its use as a rodenticide was suggested by Chapman and Phillips in 1955. It is used as a bait (20 gm active ingredient/kg) in areas to which the public have no access, such as sewers and locked warehouses. It is formulated as dyed cereal-based bait which is mixed with water for use.

19.2.2.2 Toxicity to Laboratory Animals

Basic Findings Fluoroacetamide is a compound of moderate to high acute toxicity depending on the species (see Table 19.2). In the WHO Recommended Classification of Pesticides by Hazards (World Health Organization, 1986), the technical material is listed in class IB, "Highly hazardous."

The compound is absorbed by the skin (Phillips and Worden, 1957). Animals acutely poisoned by this compound show listlessness, irritability, chronic convulsions, abasia, piloerection, and irregular respiration (Araki, 1972). One characteristic usually observed in animals dying from acute poisoning with fluoroacetamide as well as with sodium fluoroacetate is postmortem rigidity (Bentley and Greaves, 1960). Death generally occurs in coma after convulsions have stopped (Phillips and Worden, 1957). There is no obvious difference in susceptibility between

Table 19.2
Single-Dose LD 50 for Fluoroacetamide

Species	Route	LD 50 (mg/kg)	Reference
Rat	oral	15	Phillips and Worden (1957)
Rat	oral	13	Bentley and Greaves (1960)
Rat	dermal	20[a]	Phillips and Worden (1957)
Mouse	oral	30.62	Araki (1972)
Mouse	subcutaneous	34.20	Araki (1972)
Mouse	intraperitoneal	85	Matsumura and O'Brien (1963)
Rabbit	oral	1.5–2.0	Phillips and Worden (1957)
Rabbit	intravenous	0.25	Buckle et al. (1949)
Chicken	oral	4.25	Egyed and Schlosberg (1977)

[a] Lowest lethal dosage.

the sexes (Bentley and Greaves, 1960). The time that elapses between dosing and the onset of convulsions appears to be related to the dosage level, and fluoroacetamide seems to be much slower than sodium fluoroacetate to affect behavior (Bentley and Greaves, 1960). Subacutely poisoned animals show anorexia, emaciation, and alopecia (Araki, 1972).

Perhaps because of strain differences, investigations have reported slightly different thresholds for the largest repeated dosage tolerated by rats without clinical signs. As discussed later, the threshold for testicular injury is much lower. Phillips and Worden (1957) found that 3 mg/kg/day for 20 days was without effect on appetite or general health. Mazzanti et al. (1964) found similar results in rats on a dietary level of 50 ppm (about 2.5 mg/kg/day for 90 days). However, Steinberger and Sud (1970) reported that this same dietary level caused a reduction of food intake and of growth.

The poisoning of farm animals by effluent from a factory that manufactured fluoroacetamide caused the Ministry of Agriculture, Fisheries, and Food to recommend that the compound should not be used as an insecticide in agriculture, for home gardens, or food storage in Great Britain, and it was withdrawn from the market (Anonymous, 1964a,b; Allcroft and Jones, 1969; Allcroft et al., 1969).

Absorption, Distribution, Metabolism, and Excretion Investigators are agreed that fluoroacetamide is less toxic than fluoroacetate. This has been attributed to the fact that metabolism of the former to the latter is slow (Matsumura and O'Brien, 1963). In fact, Phillips and Worden (1957) reported that they recovered, from the urine or rats receiving fluoroacetamide at a rate of 3 mg/kg/day, 62% of the total intake unmetabolized, and they confirmed the identity of the compound by melting point and mixed melting point. This finding raises the possibility that the toxicity of fluoroacetamide (albeit lower than that of fluoroacetate) is in part inherent and does not depend entirely on metabolism to fluoroacetate. In particular, this could account for the action of fluoroacetamide on the rat testis, an effect apparently not reported for fluoroacetate.

Biochemical Effects Evidence that fluoroacetamide has essentially the same mode of action as sodium fluoroacetate is the finding that mammals poisoned by the amide contain greatly elevated levels of citrate (Matsumura and O'Brien, 1963; Egyed and Brisk, 1965; Allcroft et al., 1969; Egyed and Miller, 1971; Egyed and Shlosberg, 1973). Further evidence is offered by the fact that cockroaches convert fluoroacetamide to fluoroacetate as well as to fluorocitrate, and mouse amidase hydrolyzes fluoroacetamide (Matsumura and O'Brien, 1963).

Effects on Reproduction Selective destruction of the germinal epithelium of the testes of male rats apparently was reported first by Mazzanti et al. (1964), who studied only a single dosage level resulting from a dietary level of 50 ppm. On this diet, the body weight of 150–160-gm rats increased by 88% in 90 days but the testes were reduced to slightly less than one-third of the weight in controls. After 64 days, the tubules were almost completely lacking in seminal cells; only some spermatogonia, the Sertoli cells, and the interstitial cells were apparently undamaged. Peculiar giant cells were observed. It was noted that fluoroacetamide acts first on the more mature cells of the germinal epithelium and not on the cells where mitoses are more numerous. Dividing cells in the intestinal mucosa were undamaged.

In a later study, male rats that received a dietary level of 50 ppm (usually calculated as about 2.5 mg/kg/day but said to be about 3.4 mg/kg/day in these rats) showed a marked morphological change in the nucleus of step-13 spermatids within 24 hr, and the effects became more pronounced and the entire cell became distorted in 5 days. After 10 days of treatment, earlier-step spermatids showed degenerative changes and giant cell formation. Eventually, even spermatocytes were affected. Androgen secretion by the testis apparently was not affected. Dietary levels of 20, 10, and 5 ppm produced characteristic changes in late-stage spermatids but no effect on spermatocytes. The 5 ppm level had no effect on the weight of the testis of rats fed as long as 28 days, but higher levels led to a marked decrease in weight. Subcutaneous administration of fluoroacetamide at a rate of about 1.0 mg/kg/day produced the characteristic change in stage-13 spermatids within 4 days and a 50% reduction in the weight of the testis in 28 days. Spermatogenesis continued, and spermatocytes and young spermatids remained apparently normal, but late spermatids were distinctly abnormal. Subcutaneous doses of about 0.2, 0.04, and 0.02 mg/kg/day produced little or no change in the weight of the testis and produced progressively less histological injury so that change was barely discernible at the lowest dosages. Thus, the effect of fluoroacetamide on spermatogenesis is specific and not secondary to general toxicity, which (in the form of reduced growth) was evident only at the highest oral dosage (Steinburger and Sud, 1970). Testicular degeneration caused by fluoroacetamide has been confirmed in rats and reported in other species (Egyed, 1973).

Fluoroacetamide at an oral dosage of 15 mg/kg also interferes with reproduction in female mice, whether administered 2 days before or 10 days after fertilization; pregnancy was prolonged, prenatal mortality was increased, and the young suffered from cyanosis, respiratory distress, reduced growth, and decreased survival (Tokareva *et al.*, 1971).

Effects on Wildlife and Nontarget Species In some countries, fluoroacetamide is used to control field rodents, thus exposing nontarget species to either direct toxic effects by feeding on the baits or secondary effects by feeding on carcasses of rodents killed by the compound. These effects have been experimentally studied by Braverman (1979) on several nontarget species such as mongoose (*Herpestes ichneumon*), hyena (*Hyaena hyaena*), snakes, birds, cats, and dogs. This experiment showed a degree of susceptibility of the animals similar to that reported for sodium fluoroacetate; it also confirmed that the dog was the most sensitive species. Some species showed a relative tolerance to direct poisoning; this was the case for barn owls, buzzards, and the black kite.

A secondary poisoning study was done by offering the carnivores carcasses of jirds (*Meriones tristrami*) which had fed freely on poisoned grains. The results were quite variable; the mongoose was the most susceptible, whereas the risk of secondary poisoning to birds of prey was not high. An outbreak of poisoning by fluoroacetamide in four greylag geese (*Anser anser*) and teal (*Anas crecca*) has been reported in Israel (Shlosberg *et al.*, 1975). Clinical signs in one goose were described as severe convulsions, incoordinated twisting of the neck, total anemia, prostrating depression, and death.

Treatment of Poisoning in Animals Sodium acetate did not protect rats poisoned by fluoroacetamide. However, when administered as a mixture by mouth at a ratio of 4:1 or 9:1, acetamide raised the LD 50 of fluoroacetamide from 15 to 22 mg/kg. When acetamide was administered by mouth at a dosage of 180 mg/kg within 65 min or less after fluoroacetamide at the otherwise fatal oral dosage of 20 mg/kg, all rats survived. The same was true when the ratio (9:1) remained the same, the delay did not exceed 60 min, and the dosage of poison was as high as 35 mg/kg. However, the antidote was ineffective when the delay was 105 min or greater (Phillips and Worden, 1956). The value of acetamide was confirmed by Hashida (1971a).

When administered to rats as a mixture by mouth, L-cysteine hydrochloride was antidotal, raising the LD 50 of fluoroacetamide from 15 to 25 and 30 mg/kg, respectively, at dosage ratios of 4:1 and 9:1 (Phillips and Worden, 1957).

Acetamide at an oral dosage of 2500 mg/kg was also effective in treating chickens when given within 20 min after fluoroacetamide at a dosage of 10 mg/kg (slightly more than twice the LD 50 level). The same dosage given 30 min after the poison or 500 mg/kg given with the poison were ineffective (Egyed and Shlosberg, 1977). In limited tests, neither acetamide nor monoacetin was effective in treating poisoned sheep (Egyed, 1971).

The ineffectiveness of sodium acetate and apparently of monoacetin and the effectiveness of acetamide and L-cysteine as antidotes for poisoning by fluoroacetamide raise the possibility that the effective compounds do not prevent the biochemical lesion directly but rather competitively retard the conversion of fluoroacetamide to fluoroacetate and thus permit more time for excretion of unmetabolized fluoroacetamide.

19.2.2.3 Toxicity to Humans

Accidental and Intentional Poisoning At about 1130 hr, an 18-month-old girl removed a 120-ml bottle of 1% fluoroacetamide from a low drawer in the family kitchen and drank some of the contents. On the advice of a pharmacist, the child was given olive oil, the white of an egg, and milk at about noon and was made slightly sick. The child remained lively and played in the garden until her usual bedtime, 1830 hr. At about 2330 hr that evening the child vomited but was put back to bed when she appeared all right. Apparently the child was not checked until 1030 hr next morning, when she was found in a semiconscious state. On a physician's orders, she was taken to hospital, but convulsions occurred on the way and the patient arrived about 1130 hr in a shocked state. The child was given about 10 ml acetamide in water once, 3.7 ml of brandy in water each hour, and symptomatic treatment. She continued to have occasional convulsions and remained unconscious until she died almost 96 hr after ingesting the poison. Both the heart and kidney contained 6.3 mg of organic fluoride per gram of dry tissue; the citrate content (108 ppm in heart and 23.9 ppm in kidney) was not considered significantly high. From the evidence available, it was estimated that the baby had consumed about 300 mg of fluoroacetamide or 23 mg/kg (Great Britain Ministry of Agriculture, Fisheries and Food, 1961; WHO, 1963). Although the death occurred in 1959, it was not recorded until 1960 (Anonymous, 1962; Hearn, 1973).

Treatment of Poisoning Treatment of poisoning by fluoroacetamide should be the same as that for fluoroacetate (see Section 19.2.1.3) with due attention to removal of the poison and general care of the patient. Based on animal studies, rapid and energetic treatment with acetamide is recommended. A dosage of 315 mg/kg was effective in rats, but a much higher dosage was required in chickens. It is of special importance that the first dose be given at the earliest possible moment. Repeated administration was not used in the animal experiments but would appear wise. A combination of intravenous monoacetin (glyceryl monoacetate, 0.55 gm/kg), sodium acetate (0.12 gm/kg), and ethanol (0.12 gm/kg) has also been recommended (Dipalma, 1981). Dipalma also suggested as an alternative course the oral administration of 100 ml of monoacetin plus 500 ml of water every hour for about 2 hr.

Hemoperfusion involving fixed-bed uncoated charcoal was used in one case, but it was not helpful and the patient died (de Torrente *et al.*, 1979).

19.2.3 FLUOROETHANOL

19.2.3.1 Identity, Properties, and Uses

Chemical Name 2-Fluoroethanol.

Structure See Fig. 19.1.

Physical and Chemical Properties Fluoroethanol has the empirical formula C_2H_5OF and a molecular weight of 64.07. It is a solid melting at approximately room temperature (26.5°C). It has a density of 1.091, a boiling point of 103°C, and a flash point of 31°C.

Use Rodenticide.

19.2.3.2 Toxicity to Laboratory Animals

Fluoroethanol is a compound of high acute toxicity, as indicated by an intraperitoneal LD 50 of 5 mg/kg in the rat (Bartlett, 1952). According to Bartlett, fluoroethanol is relatively inactive and its toxicity depends on its oxidation to fluoroacetate by tissue alcohol dehydrogenase.

19.2.3.3 Toxicity to Humans

Three cases of poisoning of workers by fluoroethanol occurred in a chemical plant, in at least two instances as the result of accidental rupture of a container and rapid evaporation of the fluid. A typical patient suffered onset in about 90 min and was discharged from hospital in 4 days. All patients had tremor, severe muscular weakness, nausea, headache, and a slight swelling of the liver. (Hemorrhagic gingivitis in one patient and prediabetic hyperglycemia in another were explained by their past histories and were unrelated to poisoning.) Examination of the other 40 workers in the plant failed to reveal any complaints or clinical findings that could be related to the compound (Colamussi *et al.*, 1970).

There is no specific treatment for subacute poisoning except, of course, complete cessation of exposure. If acute poisoning should occur, it should be treated like poisoning by fluoroacetate (see Section 19.2.1.3).

19.2.4 GLIFTOR

19.2.4.1 Identity, Properties, and Uses

Chemical Name Gliftor is a mixture of 70% glycerol difluorohydrin and 30% glycerol chlorofluorohydrin.

Structure See Fig. 19.1.

Physical and Chemical Properties Glycerol difluorohydrin has a molecular weight of 112.53. Glycerol chlorofluorohydrin has a molecular weight of 96.08. The pure mixture is a colorless or slightly yellowish liquid, but the commercial mixture is colored black. Gliftor has a boiling point of 120–132°C. Is it freely miscible with water and relatively stable. The CAS registry number is 8065-71.2.

History, Formulations, and Uses Gliftor is used in the USSR to combat field rodents. It is formulated as prepared baits containing 0.5–0.7% active ingredient for use at a rate of 5–15 gm/ha.

19.2.4.2 Toxicity to Laboratory Animals

Basic Findings Gliftor has an LD 50 of only 5–7 mg/kg for rabbits. It has a low toxicity for some species; for example, the minimal lethal dosage for chickens, ducks, pigeons, thrushes, and sparrows is 1000–3000 mg/kg. However, some other useful species are susceptible. The LD 50 value for cats is the same as that for rabbits, and the compound is extremely dangerous for sheep at dosages of 14.2–28.5 mg/kg. Poisoning is characterized by agitation followed by immobility and labored breathing. Large dosages produce fibrillary twitching of the muscles (Medved, 1974). The severe hyperkinesis produced by gliftor in humans apparently has not been described in animals.

19.2.4.3 Toxicity to Humans

Accidental and Intentional Poisoning Apparently, only one case has been described in any detail. However, the patient was one of three, each of whom had consumed an estimated 30 ml of gliftor, having mistaken it for alcohol. All three suffered from choreatic hyperkinesis, but only the one most severely affected died. For 48 hr this patient's condition remained good and he did not complain. Then he suddenly developed extreme hyperemia of the face and fascicular twitching of the muscles of his arms. After 50 hr, the hyperkinesis extended to the oral region, causing difficulty in speech. As the condition became worse, the patient grimaced, stuck out his tongue, nodded his head, and waved his arms and legs. Movement of the extremities was arrhythmic and wild. The body turned left, then right around an axis. The patient seized his clothing and tore it. It took five men to keep him in bed, and it was impossible to feed him. This condition lasted 5 days. On the sixth day of severe illness, the patient developed tonic spasms, his temperature rose to 41°C, and large blisters appeared on his hands and feet. A hemorrhagic liquid flowed from the blisters where they were opened. The patient died of respiratory arrest. In spite of the severe neurological disturbances that characterized the case, no alteration of the psyche was observed (Kovalenko *et al.*, 1975).

Laboratory Findings In the fatal case, laboratory findings included a leukocytosis of 14,800 with 20% rod neutrophils, hyperglycemia up to 206 mg/100 ml, serum potassium of 2.7 mEq/liter, proteinuria, pyuria, and hematuria.

Pathology Histological examination revealed congestive and focal hemorrhage in the heart, liver, kidneys, lungs, spleen, and adrenal gland. There was centrolobular necrosis of the liver, edema of the lungs, and a moderate proliferation of neuroglia and dystrophic changes of ganglion cells in the brain (Kovalenko *et al.*, 1975).

Treatment of Poisoning Treatment of poisoning by gliftor is symptomatic. There is no evidence that specific treatment, including that suggested for fluoroacetate, is of any benefit.

19.2.5 MNFA

19.2.5.1 Identity, Properties, and Uses

Chemical Name MNFA is the acronym for *N*-methyl-*N*-(1-naphthyl)-fluoroacetamide.

Structure See Fig. 19.1.

Synonyms MNFA (JMAF) is the name in general use. The compound is also known as FAM and by the proprietary name Nissol®. Code designation include DPX-1,410 and ENT-27,403. The CAS registry number is 5903-13-9.

Physical and Chemical Properties MNFA has the empirical formula $C_{13}H_2FNO$ and a molecular weight of 217.25. It forms odorless, columnar crystals with a melting point of 88–89°C

and a boiling point of 153–154°C in 0.5 mm Hg. It is only slightly soluble in water and insoluble in *n*-hexane, petroleum ether, kerosene, and dimethylformamide.

History, Formulations, and Uses MNFA was introduced in Japan in 1965 as a systemic miticide. It is formulated as an amber-colored emulsion concentrate consisting of 25% MNFA and 75% organic solvents and as an hydrophilic powder consisting of 35% MNFA and 65% fine diamorphous powder and surfactants.

19.2.5.2 Toxicity to Laboratory Animals

Basic Findings The most striking thing to observe from Table 19.3 is the marked species difference. Guinea pigs, rabbits, cats, and dogs are highly susceptible; monkeys are highly resistant; and rats and mice are moderately resistant. Different strains of rats and mice show considerable difference even when studied in the same laboratory, and the difference may be even greater among strains studied in different laboratories—perhaps because of other variables.

The compound is readily absorbed by the skin (Hashimoto *et al.*, 1968a; Iwasaki *et al.*, 1970a,b; Namba *et al.*, 1971). Application of only 2 ml of a 25% emulsion to the skin of a rabbit (about 250 mg/kg) caused death. Daily application of only 0.25 mg/kg/day was eventually fatal (Namba *et al.*, 1971).

Onset of acute illness usually was preceded by a lag period of 2–5 hr. Monkeys showed twitching, vomiting, apprehension, auditory hallucination, slight ataxia, analgesia of the face, convulsions, and central nervous system depression; death seldom was due to respiratory failure but generally was of cardiac origin and following pulsus alternans, long sequences of ectopic beats, and ventricular tachycardia, which might progress to ventricular fibrillation. Death of other species might result from respiratory arrest following severe convulsions (dog and cat), gradual cardiac failure or ventricular fibrillation (rabbit or guinea pig), or progressive depression of the central nervous system, with either respiratory or cardiac failure as the terminal event (rat and mouse) (Hashimoto *et al.*, 1968a).

When MNFA was administered to rats by stomach tube at rates ranging from 0.625 to 10.0 mg/kg/day for 6 months, blood pressure was significantly reduced at all dosage levels in both males and females; the effect increased with increasing dosage in males, but progression was unclear in females. With the exception of blood pressure and atrophy of the testis at dosages of 5 and 10 mg/kg/day, no other effects were recorded that showed a clear dosage–response relationship, although some groups showed a *decrease* in SGOT activity. Cardiac arrhythmia was detected in only one rat and that at the lowest dosage. There was no striking effect on food intake or growth. Thus, there was no clear explanation for the death of 20 animals out of a total of 144; the highest mortality (5 out of 12) occurred among females receiving 5 mg/kg/day and not among either males or females receiving 10 mg/kg/day (Hashimoto *et al.*, 1968a).

Cardiac depression and reduced blood pressure were found

Table 19.3
Single-Dose LD 50 for MNFA

Species	Route	LD 50 (mg/kg)	Reference
Rat, M	oral	76–115[a]	Hashimoto et al. (1968a)
Rat, M	dermal	213–300[a]	Hashimoto et al. (1968a)
Rat, M	subcutaneous	41–78[a]	Hashimoto et al. (1968a)
Mouse, M	oral	200–375[a]	Hashimoto et al. (1968a)
Mouse, F	oral	198–250[a]	Hashimoto et al. (1968a)
Mouse	oral	27.42	Araki (1972)
Mouse, M	dermal	402	Hashimoto et al. (1968a)
Mouse, M	subcutaneous	250	Hashimoto et al. (1968a)
Mouse	subcutaneous	28.58	Araki (1972)
Mouse, M	intraperitoneal	164	Hashimoto et al. (1968a)
Mouse	intraperitoneal	200	Johansen and Knowles (1972)
Mouse, M	intravenous	100	Hashimoto et al. (1968a)
Guinea pig, M	oral	2.0	Hashimoto et al. (1968a)
Guinea pig, M	dermal	5.4	Hashimoto et al. (1968a)
Rabbit, M	dermal	5.0[b]	Hashimoto et al. (1968a)
Dog, M	oral	2.7[b]	Hashimoto et al. (1968a)
Dog, M	dermal	3.5[b]	Hashimoto et al. (1968a)
Cat, M	oral	2.5[b]	Hashimoto et al. (1968a)
Cat, M	dermal	4.0[b]	Hashimoto et al. (1968a)
Monkey, F	oral	300[b]	Hashimoto et al. (1968a)
Monkey, F	dermal	800	Hashimoto et al. (1968a)

[a]Values for different strains.
[b]Minimal lethal dose.

not only in rats but also in mice, guinea pigs, rabbits, dogs, and monkeys (Hashimoto et al., 1968b).

Absorption, Distribution, Metabolism, and Excretion Hydrolysis of MNFA yields fluoroacetate and N-methyl-1-naphthylamine (Noguchi et al., 1968). Differences in the toxicity of MNFA compared to that of fluoroacetate presumably are due to presence of both MNFA and N-methyl-1-naphthylamine and to the slow rate at which fluoroacetate is released by metabolism.

Biochemical Effects MNFA causes a 2- to 3-fold increase in citrate in mice 3–12 hr after injection and, therefore, presum-

ably acts through metabolism to fluoroacetate (Johannsen and Knowles, 1972). Similar increases in citrate, at least in some organs, occur in other species (Noguchi et al., 1968). The citrate content of rats fed MNFA for 6 months varied according to different patterns in different tissues and even in the same tissues of the two sexes and was more often low than high. It was, however, high in the testes of rats receiving 10 mg/kg/day (Hashimoto et al., 1968a).

Marked hypoglycemia is characteristic of acute poisoning by MNFA in most species (Hashimoto et al., 1968b); rabbit blood glucose, which normally was 112 mg/100 ml, fell to 56 mg/100 ml in 7 hr following dermal application of 2 ml of a 25% emulsion (Namba et al., 1971).

Liver homogenates from guinea pigs hydrolyze MNFA much more rapidly than do homogenates from rats and mice (Noguchi et al., 1968). The more rapid release of fluoroacetate in guinea pigs presumably accounts for this greater susceptibility.

Rabbits poisoned by single or repeated dermal doses of MNFA (2 ml of 25% emulsion) showed characteristic electrocardiographic and electroencephalographic changes. Red cell count, hemoglobin, lactate dehydrogenase, transaminases, and serum electrolytes also were altered, especially in chronic poisoning (Iwasaki et al., 1970a,b).

The ECGs of poisoned rabbits showed initial depression of the ST segment with gradual development of giant T waves. Ventricular flutter and fibrillation appeared immediately before death (Takagi, 1971).

Especially in acute poisoning, the EEG sometimes exhibited a transient convulsive pattern but always gradually lapsed into a low-voltage, relatively flat pattern (Hashimoto et al., 1968b; Namba et al., 1971). Intraperitoneal injection of 20% glucose caused temporary development of an alpha wave. It was concluded that there was a cause-and-effect relationship between hypoglycemia and the observed EEG changes. In chronic poisoning, ischemic changes in the brain were thought to contribute to the EEG changes (Namba et al., 1971).

Effects on Reproduction Significant gross and microscopic atrophy of the testes occurred in male rats receiving 5 mg/kg/day or more for 6 months but not among those receiving 2.5, 1.25, or 0.625 mg/kg/day. At worst, only Sertoli cells and a few spermatogonia survived in the testicular tubules. In many tubules, only relatively mature germinal cells were destroyed, and mitosis continued among the less mature cells. Peculiar giant cells were prominent in some tubules. In a few tubules, spermatogenesis was apparently normal (Hashimoto et al., 1968a).

Pathology In addition to the testicular changes already mentioned, histological changes were observed in duodenal mucosa, lung, and renal glomeruli of rats that had received MNFA at dosages up to 10 mg/kg/day for 6 months (Hashimoto et al., 1968a). Others have reported myocardial degeneration and changes in nerve cells in the central nervous system (Iwasaki et al., 1970a,b; Namba et al., 1971).

Treatment of Poisoning in Animals Hashimoto et al. (1970) explored several treatments of animals poisoned by MNFA and found acetamide most effective. It was administered intraperitoneally three times in 1 day at a rate of 1000 mg/kg. The LD 50 values of MNFA were increased by factors of 2.5 in mice and 3.4 in rats compared with untreated animals.

19.2.5.3 Toxicity to Humans

Use Experience Examination of 181 farmers before and 4 days after application of MNFA revealed subjective complaints among 45%, namely general malaise, headache, nausea, loss of appetite, diarrhea, insomnia, abdominal pain, and tachypnea in that order of frequency. No arrhythmia was found on ECG. Weight loss was recorded in 33.6% 3 weeks after application. Red cell count decreased in about 52%, but hemoglobin decreased in only 18.7%. Liver findings were normal (Hashida, 1971a).

Other patients poisoned by repeated exposure to dilute MNFA spray showed bradycardia, prolongation of the PQ segment, and U waves, but no detectable arrhythmia. Most of these young men complained of nausea, weakness, and fatigue, but one of five showed a profound disturbance of consciousness and was almost unable to talk (Takagi, 1971). It appears that brief exposure to MNFA spray can cause poisoning, even though some precautions are taken and no accident is recognized (Iwasaki *et al.*, 1970b).

Laboratory Findings Extreme hypoglycemia is characteristic of acute poisoning by MNFA, and this has been attributed to the same mechanism that is active in poisoning by fluoroacetate (Iwasaki *et al.*, 1970a). However, the facts that hypoglycemia is not prominent in poisoning by fluoroacetate and that simple glucose infusion is an effective treatment for poisoning by MNFA suggest that the mechanisms of poisoning by the two compounds are not identical.

In a case of poisoning in which the patient was unconscious and had a blood sugar of only 50 mg/100 ml, the EEGs recorded on the first and seventh day of hospitalization showed flat, low-voltage waves without any slow waves or spikes. Intravenous administration of 40 ml of 40% glucose solution restored the α waves, although at low voltage. The EEG returned to normal after 1 month (Hiraki *et al.*, 1972). Similar results have been reported by others (Iwasaki *et al.*, 1970a,b).

Treatment of Poisoning Every effort should be made to maintain a normal blood glucose level (Hashida, 1971a).

In addition to administration of glucose, which is of proven value, treatment should be symptomatic. Although the value of antidotes suggested for treating poisoning by fluoroacetate apparently has not been demonstrated in a human case of poisoning by MNFA, it would seem reasonable to consider them, depending on the history of exposure and the condition of the patient (see Section 19.2.1). Iwasaki *et al.* (1970a) indicated the administration of acetamide to one patient at the rate of 20,000 mg/kg; they thought that repeated doses of 40% glucose aided in the patient's recovery but failed to comment on the value of the acetamide.

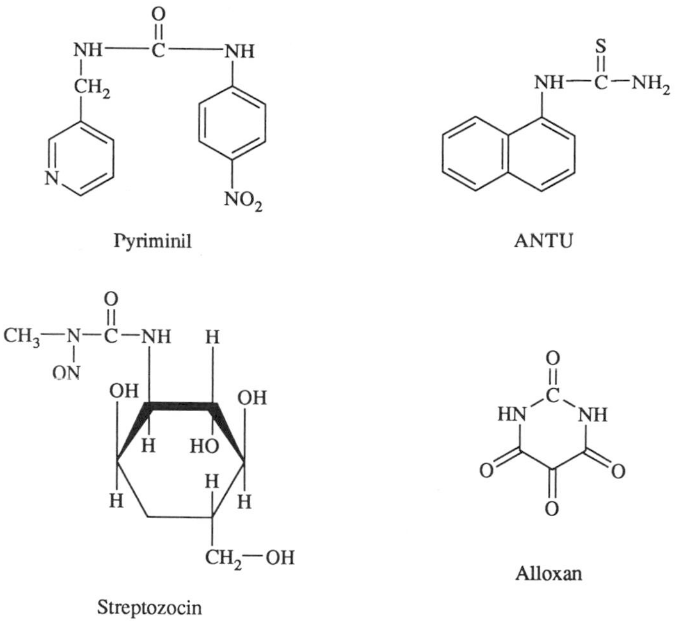

Figure 19.2 ANTU, a thiourea rodenticide, and three substituted ureas known to cause diabetes in one or more species.

19.3 SUBSTITUTED UREAS

One of the compounds that has been promoted as a rodenticide relatively safe for other mammals is pyriminil, a substituted urea (see Fig. 19.2). It is not clear whether this group of compounds has been explored extensively with a view to selecting the one with the best combination of effectiveness for killing rodents and safety for humans and useful animals. However, it has become apparent that pyriminil and some other substituted ureas are specific poisons for the β cells of the pancreas and, therefore, cause diabetes mellitus. This effect may not be related to the mode of action of pyriminil as a rodenticide, but it has great bearing on the overall safety of the material.

19.3.1 PYRIMINIL

19.3.1.1 Identity, Properties, and Uses

Chemical Name N-(3-Pyridylmethyl)-N'-(4-nitrophenyl)-urea.

Structure See Fig. 19.2.

Synonyms Pyriminil is also known as PNU, pyrinuron, and RH-787. It was sold under the trade name Vacor®, Rat killer®, DLP-787 20% bait, and DLP-787 10% House Mouse Tracking Powder. The CAS registry number is 53558-25-1.

Physical and Chemical Properties Pyriminil has the empiric formula $C_{13}H_{12}N_4O_3$ and a molecular weight of 272.27. It decomposes at 223°C.

History, Formulations, and Uses Pyriminil was introduced in 1975 and developed as an acute rodenticide. It was used to control Norway rats, roof rats, and house mice; it was especially effective against rodents resistant to anticoagulant poisons. Pyriminil was sold for indoor use only as a prepared bait containing 2% active ingredient and a 10% tracking powder. The product was withdrawn from the market by the U.S. manufacturer in 1979 (Chappelka, 1980), but it is still manufactured on a small scale for local use—in the People's Republic of China, for example.

19.3.1.2 Toxicity in Laboratory Animals

There are great differences in the susceptibility of different species to pyriminil (technical material) as shown in Table 19.4 (Peardon, 1974).

The marked susceptibility of Norway rats was of course the basis for its use as a rodenticide. Cats also are very susceptible.

Apparently, a good description of the signs of acute poisoning in laboratory animals has not been published. A simple list of signs and symptoms in dogs has been given in the distributing company's technical bulletin. The onset of the symptoms may be delayed 4–48 hr. They include nausea and emesis, depression, initial constriction of pupils followed later by dilated pupils and visual impairment with slow pupillary response to light, ataxia, fine to coarse tremors, hind-limb weakness, decreased reflexes, deep breathing, and dehydration. Similar symptoms have been reported in a horse that had eaten at least 250,000 mg (about 250 mg/kg). The animal showed severe muscular fasciculations, dilated pupils, and profuse sweating within 24 hr after ingestion. Laboratory tests revealed severe hyperglycemia (418 mg/100 ml) and indications of liver injury (elevated liver enzymes). The animal was treated with intravenous nicotinic acid (2.2 mg/kg) followed by four subsequent injections of 1 gm and recovered; it was considered clinically

Table 19.4
Single-Dose LD 50 for Pyriminil in Various Species

Species	Sex	Oral LD 50 (mg/kg)
Albino rat	M	12.3
Norway rat	M	4.75
Roof rat	M	18.0
Cotton rat	M, F	20–60
Albino mouse	M	84
House mouse	M	98
Deer mouse	M	10–20
Guinea pig	M	30–100
Rabbit	M	300
Dog	M	500
Cat	M, F	62
Rhesus monkey	M, F	2000–4000
Pig	M	500
Vole	M, F	205
Chicken	M	710
Pigeon	M, F	1780

normal 3 months later. Three other poisoned horses showed the same signs as well as intense abdominal pain, hind-limb weakness, ataxia, and persistent inappetence (Russell *et al.*, 1978). Peoples and Maddy (1979) have reported without details poisoning in domestic animals (two horses, three cats, and 17 dogs) in California. The case of a 22-kg dog seen eating a full 30-gm packet of Vacor (780 mg active ingredient) is mentioned. Immediately following ingestion, the dog vomited but became blind 2 days later.

Absorption, Distribution, Metabolism, and Excretion
Pyriminil is rapidly absorbed by rats, mice, and dogs after oral administration. Blood levels peaked in 1–6 hr, depending on species and site of the radiolabel ^{14}C. Gastrointestinal transit of ^{14}C is more rapid in dogs than in rats. Urinary and fecal excretions are of similar importance in all three species. Tissue distribution of two ^{14}C labels (nitrophenyl and pyridyl) varied, especially in dogs. The liver contained more of the dose than any other single organ (Deckert *et al.*, 1978a). Rats tolerated, metabolized, and eliminated single or multiple sublethal dosages (5 mg/kg) but were less efficient than dogs in detoxifying dosages in excess of 20 mg/kg. It was concluded that the tolerance of dogs for the compound depended on their efficient hepatic extraction, metabolism, and excretion of it (Deckert *et al.*, 1978b).

Several metabolites of pyriminil have been identified (Deckert *et al.*, 1978a, 1979). These include aminopyriminil, *p*-aminophenyl urea, *p*-acetamidophenyl urea, *p*-nitroaniline, *p*-phenylenediamine, *p*-acetamidoaniline, nicotinic acid, nicotinuric acid, and nicotinamide. The concentrations of these metabolites varied from one species to another. The presence of the parent compound in rat and human urine suggests that they may be more sensitive to the compound than the dog because of less efficient metabolism (Deckert *et al.*, 1979).

Biochemical Effects Repeated, sublethal doses of pyriminil increased the urinary and fecal excretion of a later dose of the compound tagged with ^{14}C; however, the same animals showed increased hexobarbital sleeping time and other evidence of inhibition of certain liver microsomal enzymes, especially *p*-nitroanisole *O*-demethylase. Whatever microsomal enzymes are responsible for metabolism of pyriminil are induced by pretreatment with 3-methylcholanthrene, which increases the biliary excretion of the metabolites and decreases pyriminil toxicity 50-fold (Deckert *et al.*, 1977, 1978a).

Mild pyriminil-induced hyperglycemia was observed in rats; it was also shown to be reversible by insulin (Deckert *et al.*, 1977). The diabetogenic effects of pyriminil were also confirmed in patients poisoned by the product. This effect is the result of a direct toxic action on the β cells of the pancreas. Wilson and Gaines (1983) have demonstrated that pyriminil at concentrations ranging from 10^{-2} to 10^{-5} *M* preferentially intoxicates rat pancreatic β cells in culture, within 1 hr of contact. It was also shown in this study that nicotinamide can reduce pyriminil-induced β cell injury, thus confirming previous findings by Karam *et al.* (1980) that nicotinamide could partially reverse pyriminil inhibition of glucose-stimulated insulin secretion by freshly isolated islets of Langerhans from the rat.

In addition to its diabetogenic effect, pyriminil has a direct effect on glucose metabolism. The erythrocytes of patients poisoned by the compound showed a marked depression of glucose consumption as well as decreased uptake of methylene blue in the presence of glucose. In addition, a 0.1 mM concentration *in vitro* caused decreased utilization of glucose and decreased uptake of methylene blue by erythrocytes from normal people and rabbits (Lee and Lee, 1977).

Treatment of Poisoning in Animals The mechanism of action of pyriminil remains uncertain, but it is of interest that alloxan, streptozotocin, and dithizone (see Sections 4.2.8.1 and 19.3), all of which can induce diabetes mellitus in experimental animals, are substituted ureas. However, it would appear that some species such as dogs, cats, and laboratory primates are refractory to both the diabetogenic and neurotoxic effects of pyriminil (Karam *et al.*, 1980).

Whereas 6-aminonicotinamide is not a substituted urea, it is toxic to β cells and it is a recognized antagonist of nicotinamide (Herken, 1971). Because nicotinamide can prevent the toxic effect of streptozotocin (Ganda *et al.*, 1976), alloxan (Rossini *et al.*, 1975), and N-3-pyridylmethyl-N'-4-nitrophenyl urea (Deckert *et al.*, 1977), it seems possible that all of these compounds act as nicotinamide antagonists.

19.3.1.3 Toxicity to Humans

Accidental and Intentional Poisoning There are many reports of human poisonings in the literature describing the main clinical and laboratory features of those poisonings.

A 25-year-old man with a history of psychiatric disturbances attempted suicide by injecting an unknown amount of pulverized methaqualone tablets and ingesting two packets of rat poison each containing 737 mg of pyriminil. Seven days later he was admitted to a local hospital for treatment of a staphylococcal abscess of the left antecubital fossa. He received antibiotics and had rapid clinical improvement. It was recorded that since attempting suicide the patient had noticed lassitude, anorexia, abdominal bloating, constipation, and the onset of painful paresthesia with numbness of his legs and difficulty in walking. A random plasma glucose level on admission was 309 mg/100 ml, and check samples taken on subsequent days were slightly higher. Ketones and glucose were present in the urine. On the fourth hospital day insulin therapy was started. The diabetes gradually was controlled, although tolerance for carbohydrate and need for insulin were erratic. An upper gastrointestinal tract series done on the tenth hospital day showed gastric and proximal small bowel hypomobility bordering on atony. The patient was discharged on hospital day 19 on a regimen of insulin and temporary thoridiazine.

The patient remained well for 16 days and then returned because of nausea and vomiting. He was found to have severe autonomic and peripheral polyneuropathy characterized by orthostatic hypotension, greatly diminished response to pinprick and vibratory sensation in the lower extremities, and other changes. Although the diabetes was now better controlled, the serum sodium was low (116 mEq/liter), and the syndrome of inappropriate antidiuretic hormone (SIADH) was demonstrated. The hyponatremia responded to fluid restriction, and the orthostatic hypotension was improved by support stockings.

Ten months after the suicide attempt, the patient experienced two episodes of weakness and lethargy that were relieved by eating. He had lost about 18 kg and appeared cachetic (45 kg, 174 cm) but alert and well oriented. His gait was ataxic and there was substantial muscle wasting. A very thorough examination showed reduced disappearance rate of intravenous glucose and depressed C-peptide response to intravenous glucose when compared with a normal control but no impairment of glucagon release after stimulation by intravenous arginine. Nerve conduction studies demonstrated severe sensory and mild motor neuropathy. Quadriceps capillary basement membrane thickness was in the diabetic range. Insulin was discontinued and tolbutamide prescribed. Following discharge, the patient regained 5 kg and experienced subjective improvement of his neuropathy (Prosser and Karam, 1978).

Whereas most clinical studies have placed greatest emphasis on the diabetogenic action of pyriminil, its injury to the nervous system was no less remarkable, as emphasized in a paper by LeWitt (1980a). This injury often involved autonomic impairment (postural hypotension often severe enough to cause fainting when the patient sat up, impaired pupillary responses, impotence, decreased sweating, urinary retention, dysphagia, and gastrointestinal hypomobility), peripheral neuropathy (loss of muscle-stretch reflexes, sensory loss, neurogenic myopathy), and encephalopathic and dyskinetic features (loss of cortical function ranging from confusion to coma, cerebellar ataxia, tremor, motor hyperactivity, nystagmus, and diffuse electroencephalographic changes). In addition, some cases involved chest or epigastric pain and some showed ischemic electrocardiographic changes. Cardiac arrhythmias were occasionally the cause of death. Neurological disorders often appeared within hours after ingestion. Occasionally, onset was delayed or insidious. Symptoms related to different parts of the nervous system began and later improved at different times in the same patient, and the order of progression varied from case to case. Neurological improvement took many months, and full recovery was uncommon; orthostatic hypotension in particular tending to persist. Causes of delayed death included inanition, sepsis, aspiration pneumonia, and insulin-induced hypoglycemia.

Accidental ingestion of pyriminil by a 25-month-old boy resulted in acute vomiting, lethargy, seizures, hypoglycemia (followed by hyperglycemia and glucose intolerance), and autonomic and peripheral neuropathy (Johnson *et al.*, 1980).

A review of reports unpublished in 1978 indicated seven deaths and two nonfatal cases in Korea and four fatal and 11 nonfatal cases in the United States. At least in the United States, all the cases were in adults; all but one were attempted suicide; all the survivors developed diabetes mellitus and autonomic nervous system dysfunction, chiefly dysphasia, dystonia, and bowel and bladder dysfunction. Hypothermia and paresthesias were seen. A later review revealed nearly 90 cases in the United States and over 250 in Korea (Fretthold *et al.*, 1980).

A case of acute poisoning (approximately 67 mg/kg) in a 42-year-old man with all the signs already described but characterized by a severe orthostatic hypotension with full spontaneous recovery 11 months after hospitalization was reported by Osterman *et al.* (1981). Gallanosa *et al.* (1981) have compared the main features of four cases reported with enough details in the literature with those of one case of their own.

Dosage Response   A dose as low as 780 mg was fatal within 150 days. A dose of 2340 mg was fatal within 1 day, but a patient survived 40 days after ingesting 7020 mg. One patient survived 2340 mg, and at least two survived 1560 mg but not without characteristic, persistent illness. The smallest dose known to have produced characteristic illness was 390 mg (about 5.6 mg/kg) (LeWitt, 1980b).

Laboratory Findings   The most important findings for guiding treatment and often for diagnosis include early transient hypoglycemia followed by persistent hyperglycemia, glycosuria, ketosis, and elevation of serum amylase and lipase activities. *p*-Nitroaniline at a concentration of 5.1 ppm has been reported in the liver of a person who died after accidentally ingesting pyriminil (Osteryoung *et al.*, 1977). In the case of a 7-year-old boy who was found dead in bed a day after another child saw him ingest a packet of pyriminil, unchanged compound at a concentration of 1.5 ppm was found in the urine hydrolysate and two metabolites were found in the liver and some other samples. Aminopyriminil (nitro group metabolized to an amine) was found at concentrations of 5.6, 1.4, 0.3, and 0.6 ppm in liver, kidney, spleen, and urine, respectively. Acetamidopyriminil (amino group conjugated with acetic acid) was found in traces in the blood and liver (Fretthold *et al.*, 1980).

Karam *et al.* (1980) reported (in addition to the clinical features) autopsy findings from several cases of acute poisoning, including that of a 7-year-old boy. All three cases showed extensive islet degeneration of the pancreatic tissue with generalized destruction of β cells and sparing of α and Δ cells as well as of the exocrine glandular tissue.

Islet-cell surface antibodies were detected in four of the six reported cases. It may be that these antibodies are the result rather than the cause of β-cell destruction.

Pathology   Loss of β cells of the pancreas has been observed generally in persons killed by pyriminil (Prosser and Karam, 1978; Karam *et al.*, 1980; LeWitt, 1980a; Fretthold *et al.*, 1980). Lesions of the nervous system have not been found so regularly. In one case reported by LeWitt (1980a) no lesions of the central or peripheral nervous system were found; in another case, cerebral edema and neuropathic changes restricted to the sensory spinal roots were found. Autopsy of a 39-year-old man who survived 19 days revealed (*a*) severe loss of ganglion cells and rare degenerating neurons in the paravertebral sympathetic ganglia, (*b*) marked loss of neurons in the sensory spinal ganglia

with multiple residual nodules of Nageotte, (*c*) marked degeneration of the sensory roots and posterior columns, (*d*) slight perivascular lymphatic infiltrates in both the sympathetic and sensory ganglia, (*e*) swelling of nerve fibers and thinning of the myelin sheaths of the sural nerve, and (*f*) isolated degenerated and regenerating fibers in the skeletal muscles (Papasozomenos, 1980).

Treatment of Poisoning   Patients who develop diabetes mellitus clearly must be treated for that condition in the usual way. There is good reason from animal experiments to believe that diabetes could be prevented if the patient were given large, repeated doses of nicotinamide beginning promptly after ingestion of the poison. However, cases have ended in diabetes and neuropathy when nicotinamide was started 9 and 14 hr, respectively, after ingestion. Nicotinamide was considered possibly beneficial in the case of an infant, even through administration was started something over 12 hr after ingestion of pyriminil (Johnson *et al.*, 1980). However, the fact that the child received the poison "on a piece of gum" offered by another child suggests that the initial dose was small, and complete recovery may have been due to that fact alone (Pont *et al.*, 1979).

The dose and duration of the treatment with nicotinamide are still uncertain (Anonymous, 1979). Nicotinic acid has also been tried as an antidote (Pont *et al.*, 1979), but its use is contraindicated because (*a*) it is toxic in humans, (*b*) it protects animals only against alloxan and not streptozotocin (Ganda *et al.*, 1976), and (*c*) its vasodilatory effects may complicate the control of blood pressure.

Cases that require insulin may progress so that insulin is no longer required but the patient can be maintained on sulfonylureas.

Orthostatic hypotension secondary to pyriminil may respond to dihydroergotamine (0.5 mg intramusculary) in cases where sympathomimetic drugs are ineffective (Benowitz *et al.*, 1979).

In one case of lasting anorexia, treatment with cyproheptadine was beneficial (LeWitt, 1980b).

19.4 THIOUREAS

The development of ANTU as a poison for adult Norway rats was described by Richter (1945). The entire development was a result of a chance observation associated with studying the taste of phenylthiourea, which is bitter to most people but tasteless to a few who inherit this specific lack of sensation as a Mendelian recessive trait. When an attempt was made to explore this taste difference in animals, it was found that if a few crystals were placed on the tongues of rats, all of them died overnight. The wide and prolonged use of phenylthiourea for taste and inheritance tests without any untoward effect indicated its safety for humans, whereas the result in rats suggested that it might serve as a rat poison. Further study revealed that rats detect and reject phenylthiourea too effectively for it to be practical as poison. This led to a systematic search for other thiourea derivatives with high toxicity but little or no taste. All monosubstituted thiourea derivatives tested produced pulmonary edema and pleural effusion in the laboratory rat (Dieke *et al.*, 1947). The toxicity of thiourea to wild Norway rats was enhanced by a single aromatic substitution on one of the nitrogen atoms. Two or more substitutions on one or both nitrogen atoms lowered the toxicity, as was also true of substitution on the sulfur atom. ANTU was chosen as the most suitable compound.

Although the dog is susceptible to ANTU, most animals, including monkeys, are resistant. This offered the hope that humans would be resistant also, and extensive field trials in areas of Baltimore led to no toxic symptoms either in workers or in the over 500,000 persons living in treated areas (Richter, 1945).

A disadvantage of ANTU as a rodenticide is that young Norway rats and roof rats of all ages are too resistant to the compound for it to be practical for their control. Another disadvantage is the prompt appearance of both tolerance and bait refusal in adult Norway rats that have received a nonfatal dose. Tolerance is completely lost within 30 days, but refusal may last longer (Richter, 1945, 1946). Gaines and Hayes (1952) found that bait shyness lasted at least 4 months under field conditions.

Several interesting observations were made during the survey of thioureas. All of these compounds produce hyperplasia of the thyroid gland. Whereas nonlethal doses of unsubstituted thiourea have little effect on pigmentation or hair growth, phenylthiourea destroys pigment both in the skin and in the hair but without affecting growth of the hair, and ANTU completely stops pigment production and growth of hair. Withdrawal of the substituted thioureas is followed in less than 10 days by recovery of pigment and hair growth. Finally, different strains of Norway rats on different diets showed thiourea LD 50 values as different as 4 and 1830 mg/kg. The difference was modified but not eliminated by placing the rats on the same diet as that of the most susceptible ones. Age differences in the susceptibility of Norway rats to thiourea are similar to those with ANTU (Richter, 1945; Dieke and Richter, 1945).

19.4.1 ANTU

19.4.1.1 Identity, Properties, and Uses

Chemical Name   1-(1-Naphthyl)-2-thiourea.

Structure   See Fig. 19.2.

Synonyms   ANTU, an acronym for α-naphthylthiourea, is the approved common name (BSI, ISO) for this compound. Trade names include Anturat®, Bantu®, Kill Kantz®, Krysid®, Rattrak®, and Rat-tu®. Code designations for ANTU include Chemical-109 and U-5227. The CAS registry number is 86-88-4.

Physical and Chemical Properties   ANTU has the empirical formula $C_{11}H_{10}N_2S$ and a molecular weight of 202.27. Pure ANTU forms colorless crystals and the technical grade is a gray crystalline powder with a bitter taste. Its melting point is 198°C

(pure). Its solubility in water is 25°C is 0.06 gm/100 ml; in acetone, 2.43 gm/100 ml; and in triethylene glycol, 8.6 gm/100 ml (technical).

History, Formulations, and Uses   ANTU was discovered as a rodenticide in 1945. The formulations include baits (10–30 gm/kg) and tracking powders (200 gm/kg). It is used specifically against the Norway rat. In some countries it has been withdrawn from use because of the carcinogenicity of β-naphthylamines present as impurities (Worthing and Walker, 1983).

19.4.1.2 Toxicity to Laboratory Animals

Basic Findings   Different investigators have been in good agreement about the acute oral toxicity of ANTU to Norway rats. Dieke and Richter (1945) and Lehman (1951, 1952) found oral LD 50 values of 6.9 and 6 mg/kg, respectively. There is a wide variation in susceptibility among different species, especially to intraperitoneal administration (see Table 19.5). The Norway rat is particularly susceptible, the young being slightly more resistant than the adults.

Absorption, Distribution, Metabolism, and Excretion   Early studies on the metabolism of phenylthiourea and of diphenylthiourea suggest the basis of the toxicity of mono-

Table 19.5
Single-Dose LD 50 for ANTU[a]

Species	Route	LD 50 (mg/kg)	Reference
Rat	intraperitoneal	10	Boyd and Neal (1976)
Rat	intraperitoneal	7	Lisella *et al.* (1971)
Rat	intraperitoneal	5	DuBois *et al.* (1947)
Norway, domestic I	intraperitoneal	2.5	
Norway, domestic II	intraperitoneal	6.25	
Norway, wild, adult	intraperitoneal	6.20–8.10	
Norway, wild, young	intraperitoneal	16–58	
Alexandrine	intraperitoneal	250	
Norway, wild	oral	6.9	
Mouse	intraperitoneal	56	
Rabbit	intraperitoneal	400	
Guinea pig	intraperitoneal	140	DuBois *et al.* (1947)
Guinea pig	intraperitoneal	350	
Dog	intraperitoneal	16	
Dog	dermal	38	
Cat	oral	500	
Monkey	intraperitoneal	175	
Monkey	oral	4250	
Chicken	intraperitoneal	2500	
Chicken	oral	4250	

[a]From IARC (1983).

substituted thioureas. It was shown by Dieke *et al.* (1947) that the oral LD 50 of the phenyl compound is 8.6 mg/kg, whereas a dosage of 2000 mg/kg of the diphenyl compound did not produce illness. Both rats and rabbits excrete little phenylthiourea as compounds with the —C≡S group intact (Carrol and Noble, 1949; Williams, 1959). In rabbits, the proportion of such compounds was only about 12%, but the corresponding proportion was about 70–80% for diphenylthiourea. These observations suggest that toxicity was associated with desulfuration *in vivo* (Williams, 1959). It has been speculated that ANTU acts on the lung by the release of hydrogen sulfide (Petit *et al.*, 1970), but this seems highly unlikely because rats rendered tolerant to ANTU are not tolerant to hydrogen sulfide (or carboxyl sulfide or phosgene) (Caroll and Noble, 1949).

Biochemical Effects By using a mixture of ^{35}S- and ^{14}C-labeled ANTU, it was possible to show that some of the sulfur and a smaller proportion of the carbon were covalently bound to macromolecules of the lung and liver following *in vivo* administration. By contrast, practically no radioactive carbon was bound when an equal amount of the almost nontoxic, ^{14}C-labeled oxygen analog of ANTU (α-[^{14}C]naphthylurea) was administered. In the presence of NADPH, ANTU was metabolized by either lung or liver microsomes *in vitro* in such a way that the rates of binding of ^{35}S or of ^{14}C to macromolecules of the microsomes were greater than those associated with boiled microsomes or with normal microsomes without NADPH. Binding in the presence of active enzyme and NADPH was covalent and accompanied by a decrease in the level of cytochrome P-450 detectable as its carbon monoxide complex. Pretreatment of rats at the rate of 2 mg/kg/day for 5 days produced a decrease of their microsomal enzyme activity as measured by metabolism of parathion. All such pretreated rats survived a dosage of ANTU (10 mg/kg) which killed 6 of 10 controls, and binding of ^{35}S by proteins of the liver and especially the lungs of the pretreated animals was less than that of the controls. Pretreatment with 4-ipomeanol protected all rats from an otherwise uniformly fatal dose of [^{35}S]ANTU and caused a slight reduction of covalent binding of ^{35}S to lung (but not liver) proteins. Finally, rats pretreated with dimethylmaleate, which depletes tissue stores of glutathione, were killed by ANTU at 5 mg/kg, a dosage which was harmless to controls. In every instance, rats killed by ANTU showed a hydrothorax of at least 4 ml, whereas those protected by pretreatment with ANTU or ipomeanol developed no hydrothorax. These findings were interpreted as evidence that (*a*) the toxicity of ANTU depends on metabolic activation and on covalent binding of the reactant(s) to lung macromolecules and (*b*) tolerance to ANTU is the result of inhibition of microsomal enzymes and consequent reduction in the metabolic activation of a challenge dose (Boyd and Neal, 1976). An extension of this reasoning would attribute the normal tolerance of young Norway rats to ANTU to their relative lack of microsomal enzyme activity.

Further study showed that about half of the atomic sulfur released from ANTU reacted with cysteine side chains of microsomal protein to form a hydrodisulfide. The other moiety released by microsomal enzymes is α-naphthylurea (Lee *et al.*, 1980).

Effects on Organs and Tissues ANTU induced reverse mutations in *Salmonella typhimurium* strain TA1538 in the presence but not in the absence of Aroclor- or phenobarbital-induced rat liver microsomal preparations. A preparation purified by thin-layer chromatography was as active as a technical grade material, thus excluding the attribution of activity to impurities. ANTU also transformed Syrian hamster embryo cells *in vitro* without the addition of an activating system (Kawalek *et al.*, 1979).

ANTU was tested for carcinogenicity (Fitzburgh and Nelson, 1947) and mice (Innes *et al.*, 1969) by administration in the diet. No tumor was reported in either study, but the International Agency for Research on Cancer (IARC) (1983) found that both studies were inadequate to evaluate the carcinogenicity of ANTU to experimental animals.

Pathology As far as the rat lung is concerned, ANTU causes marked edema of the subepithelial spaces of the alveolar walls without erosion or other damage to type I and type II epithelial cells. Thus, edema caused by ANTU differs morphologically and presumably in mechanism from that produced by injection of epinephrine or by an injection of a mixture of fibrinogen and thrombin into the cerebrospinal cistern (Hatakeyama and Shigei, 1971). The edema caused by intraperitoneal ANTU in rats is dosage-related in the range of 3–50 mg/kg. Although interstitial edema was the first observable change, bleeding and scalloping of endothelial cells were observed within 2 hr, and epithelial damage was apparent electron microscopically within 6 hr following 50 mg/kg. The injury was apparently similar to but more rapid than that caused by 99% oxygen at 1 atmosphere pressure (Meyrick *et al.*, 1972). Not only pulmonary edema but also pleural effusion shows a dosage–response relationship (Sobonya and Kleinerman, 1973).

Using a different approach, Böhm (1973) demonstrated changes which he interpreted as indicating increased permeability to colloidal carbon in the pulmonary arterioles as well as capillaries and venules of rats within 3.25 hr after an intraperitoneal injection of ANTU at a rate of 10 mg/kg.

In anesthetized sheep given 20, 50, 75, or 100 mg/kg ANTU intravenously, the first phase of the response consisted of transient increases in pulmonary artery pressure and plasma and lymph thromboxane B$_2$ concentrations. These changes were not dependent on the dose of ANTU administered. At 2–4 hr after administration, pulmonary artery pressure and thromboxane concentrations were normal or near normal. ANTU produces a two-phase response with the steady state characterized by a dose-dependent increase in lung microvascular permeability (Havill *et al.*, 1982). These authors, on the basis of experimental results in sheep, suggest that the severe pulmonary hypertension that follows ANTU administration may be mediated by vasoconstrictor products of arachidonic acid metabolism and that the complement or coagulation systems may be involved as well, resulting in pulmonary microemboli.

O'Brien *et al.* (1985) have reported that isolated lungs from rats treated 4 hr earlier with ANTU had decreased conversion of angiotension I to angiotension II and that the extent of decrease was related to the dose of ANTU administered and to the perfusate flow rate.

It may be that permeability of membranes of the kidney as well as those of the lung and pleura is increased inasmuch as urinary excretion of albumin occurs (Patil and Radhakrishnamurty, 1977).

Treatment of Poisoning in Animals Mortality of rats caused by 5 mg/kg of ANTU was reduced when allythiourea, isopropylthiourea, ethylenethiourea, or ethylidenethiourea was administered simultaneously with or a very short time after the ANTU. The first two compounds reduced the survival time of rats that died, but the last two compounds slightly prolonged it (Meyer and Saunders, 1949). Although the reduction in mortality was statistically significant, the degree of protection was small. Furthermore, these results in the rat may be more closely related to the phenomenon of tolerance than to antidotal action in the usual sense. In any event, Carroll and Noble (1949) found that tolerance to phenylthiourea and ANTU could be produced not only by small dosages of the compounds themselves but also by a number of related and some apparently unrelated compounds. The ability of the effective thiourea-like substances to confer protection was unrelated to their acute toxicities or antithyroid activities. Protected rats failed to develop pulmonary edema or pleural effusion following dosages of toxic thioureas lethal to untreated rats. Thyroidectomized rats could be made tolerant as readily as intact rats. Following a large dose, phenylthiourea was excreted in the urine of a tolerant rat in sufficient quantity to kill a normal animal.

19.4.1.3 Toxicity to Humans

Accidental and Intentional Poisoning The absence of a report of uncomplicated poisoning is noteworthy in view of the extensive use of ANTU in Baltimore and some other places and the fact that an occasional bait must have been eaten by children.

Several series of cases were reported from France, where chloralose was used either alone for killing crows or rats or in combination with ANTU for killing rats. In one series of 22 cases, all showed some degree of coma and motor agitation, both characteristic of chloralose poisoning; however, more intense pulmonary symptoms were present where ANTU was involved. The low toxicity of ANTU for humans is indicated by the fact that all the patients recovered, although all had ingested the poison with suicidal intent and, therefore, in relative high dosages (Tempé and Kurtz, 1972). In another series of cases involving chloralose, 14 involved ANTU also, 1 involved chloralose only, and the presence or absence of ANTU was not established in the remainder. In addition to the respiratory difficulty that may be present with any coma, 11 of the 14 persons poisoned by a combination of chloralose and ANTU required intubation mainly because of tracheobronchial hypersecretion, and 9 of them required artificial respiration. All survived

(Favarel-Garrigues and Boget, 1968). The authors characterized the beginning of tracheobronchial hypersecretion as a secretory storm that started early and sometimes suddenly. The secretion was a white froth that, unlike edema fluid, was not sticky or high in protein. The mildness of X-ray changes contrasted with the clinical gravity of the situation. Oxygenation of the blood was always more nearly complete than in acute pulmonary edema. The hypersecretion disappeared rapidly, often in less than an hour. Apparently, if patients poisoned by a combination of chloralose and ANTU are treated properly, their illness is no more protracted than in poisoning by chloralose alone (see Section 19.7.1).

Use Experience Laubstein (1962) reported a case of eczema that he attributed to occupational exposure to ANTU.

On the basis that β-naphthylamine is an impurity in ANTU, Case (1966a), in a lecture delivered on December 30, 1965, raised the possibility that persons who distribute ANTU may be in danger of bladder cancer. No epidemiological evidence was offered. Later, Case (1966b), in the course of a discussion at a meeting of the Section of Occupational Medicine of the Royal Society of Medicine, mentioned that an investigation of the occupational history of two rodent operators who were suffering from bladder tumors had revealed that different batches of ANTU differed in the degree of contamination with naphthylamine, and some of the contaminant was β-naphthylamine. As a result, the Ministry of Agriculture, Fisheries and Food recommended in May 1966 that the use of ANTU be restricted to professional operators, and in November 1966 an advisory committee recommended that use of the compound stop until their investigation was complete (Anonymous, 1966).

In 1982, Davies *et al.* reported 14 cases of urothelial tumors observed among 51 rodent operatives exposed to ANTU in the United Kingdom between 1961 and 1980.

In the United States as a whole, the age-adjusted death rate for cancer of the bladder increased from 3.1 to 4.1 per 100,000 from 1931 to 1945, when ANTU was discovered, and it continued to increase more slowly until 1953, when it reached 4.4. Since 1953 the values have varied around slightly over 4.3 as a mean. The *declining* increase in rate from 1945 to 1953 occupied a period less than the average latent period for cancer of the bladder among men with heavy exposure to naphthylamine used in the manufacture of dyes. Thus there is no evidence for any carcinogenic action of ANTU in the general population. Because ANTU had been used so extensively in Baltimore, as described by Richter and his colleagues, the matter was investigated there. Because of the wide fluctuations in rates based on small frequencies, it was not practical to compare death rates for single years; therefore the data were combined for 3-year periods. For 1949–1965, the rate per 100,000 population varied from the earliest value of 4.4 to 2.9 with no definite trend but certainly with no increase.

Dosage Response The threshold limit value is 0.3 mg/m³ of air over an 8-hr work shift (OSHA standard).

Treatment of Poisoning   If treatments were required, it would have to be symptomatic.

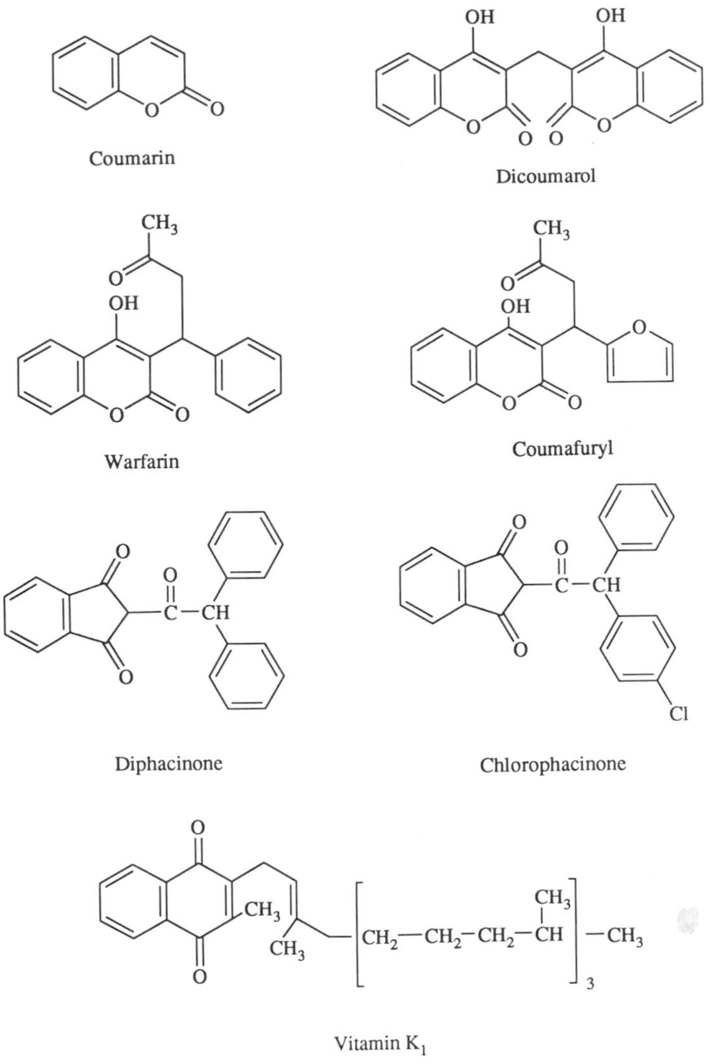

19.5 ANTI-VITAMIN K COMPOUNDS

As reviewed by Link (1944, 1959), knowledge of the anti-vitamin K compounds began not with vitamin K but with hemorrhagic disease of cattle, which was first recognized in the 1920s on the prairies of North Dakota and neighboring Alberta. It was found that the condition was not caused by a microorganism or a nutritional deficiency but was associated with sweet clover that had gone bad. Hence the condition was known as "sweet clover poisoning." When cattle or sheep had improperly cured hay made from the common varieties of sweet clover (*Melilotus* spp.) as their only food, the clotting power of their blood decreased in about 15 days and they often died of internal hemorrhage in 30–50 days. If the disease had not progressed too far, it could be reversed by substituting good hay or by transfusion of blood freshly drawn from normal cattle. Link first learned of the problem in December 1932. During the following February, a Wisconsin farmer came to his laboratory with a dead heifer, a milk can containing blood with no power to clot, 100 pounds of spoiled sweet clover, and the all too common, tragic story of cattle dying on an isolated farm.

In Link's laboratory, a practical bioassay for hemorrhagic effect was developed. It was not until June 1939 that the active poison was isolated and crystallized. Using improved methods of isolation developed after the identity of the compound was known, it was shown that the compound was present in spoiled hay at a concentration of about 60 ppm. The structure was shown to be 3,3′-methylene-bis(4-hydroxycoumarin), later known as dicoumarol or by the trade name Dicumarol®, and it was synthetized in April 1940. The biological synthesis during spoilage of the hay can be rationalized as an oxidation of coumarin (the compound responsible for the characteristic sweet smell and bitter taste of sweet clover) and the subsequent condensation of two molecules of 4-hydroxycoumarin with formaldehyde (see Fig. 19.3).

When synthetic dicoumarol became available in quantity, the essentials of its pharmacological action were established quickly. Between 1940 and 1942, it was rapidly adopted for treatment of thromboembolic disease in humans. About 50 clinical reports were published between 1941 and 1944.

In 1942, Link himself set up field trials to test the suitability of dicoumarol as a rat poison. Tests by O'Connor (1948) using a concentration of 0.44 mg/g were reported as highly successful. However, tests carried out by the U.S. Public Health Service (Hayes and Gaines, 1950) led to the same conclusion as those of Link: that dicoumarol was impractical as a rat poison.

While the medical and possible rodenticidal uses of dicoumarol were being explored, over 100 analogs of the compound were synthesized in Link's laboratory; they were arranged according to chemical classification and assigned numbers by Overman *et al.* (1944). In the hope of finding a therapeutic agent other than dicoumarol, the anticoagulant activity of

Figure 19.3   Coumarin, dicoumarol, some synthetic rodenticides, and a natural form of vitamin K.

some of those analogs was reappraised using not only rabbits (the species used to detect the hemorrhagic agent of sweet clover poisoning) but also rats, mice, and dogs. Work between 1946 and 1948 identified compounds No. 42 and No. 63 as much more potent than dicoumarol in the rat and dog and as capable of producing a more uniform anticoagulant response and of maintaining a more severe hypoprothrombinemia without visible bleeding than was possible with dicoumarol. Partly on the basis of these observations and partly on the basis of lack of taste and odor, ease of manufacturing the pure compound, and convertibility to a stable water-soluble salt, compound No. 42 was selected.

Early in 1948 it was proposed as a rodenticide and promoted by the Wisconsin Alumni Research Foundation (WARF). It soon became evident that compound 42 was an important rodenticide.

Link (1959) recalled that, although late in 1950 he proposed warfarin for clinical trial, fear of using a highly successful rat poison as a drug prevented significant progress until April 1951,

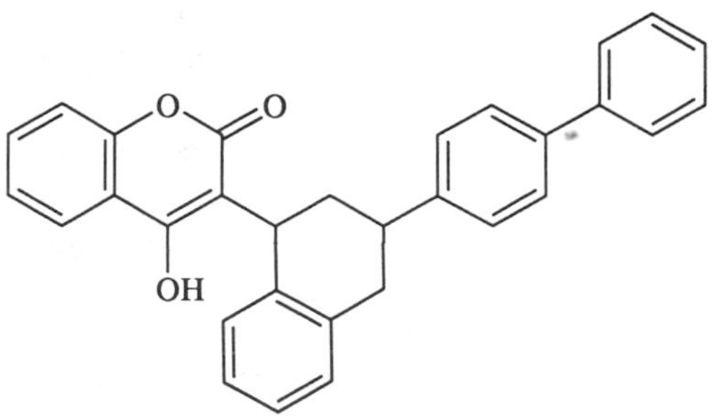

Difenacoum

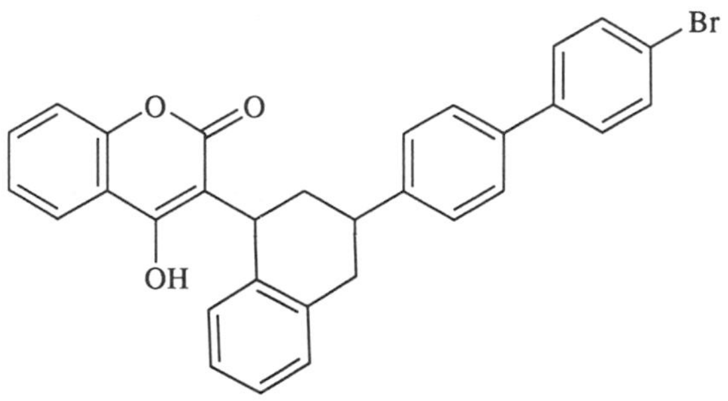

Brodifacoum

Figure 19.4 Two second-generation anticoagulant rodenticides.

when knowledge of an unsuccessful suicide effectively treated by vitamin K and transfusion of fresh whole blood (Holmes and Love, 1952) brought reassurance. Progress was so rapid that warfarin was used in 1955 for treating then-President Eisenhower.

The use of Dicumarol as a drug and the use of warfarin as a drug and as a rodenticide did not go unnoticed by those who sought a compound even more effective than warfarin—and free of patent restrictions. The result was a number of alternative compounds available either as drugs or rodenticides, or, in the case of diphacinone, used like warfarin for both purposes.

The appearance of rats resistant to warfarin and to other early anticoagulant rodenticides has stimulated the search for more potent, fast-acting compounds. These are usually called "single-dose rodenticides" or "second-generation" anticoagulants, among which difenacoum and brodifacoum are coumarin derivatives (Fig. 19.4).

Coumarin compounds are relatively free of untoward effects when used therapeutically and have been given for long periods without signs of toxicity. Occasional adverse reactions include gastrointestinal disturbances (especially diarrhea), necrosis of the small intestine, elevated transaminase, urticaria, dermatitis, leukopenia, and alopecia, but not all of these with every compound.

19.5.1 WARFARIN

19.5.1.1 Identity, Properties, and Uses

Chemical Name 3(α-acetonylbenzyl)-4-hydroxycoumarin.

Structure See Fig. 19.3.

Synonyms The name warfarin (BSI, ICPC, ISO) is in common use except in France, where the compound is called cumafène; in the USSR, where it is called zoocoumarin; and in Japan, where it and coumatetralyl both are spoken of as coumarins (JMAF). During development, warfarin was known as Compound-42 or WARF-42. As a drug, the sodium salt is called Coumadin®. Trade names for the rodenticide have included Arthrombine-K®, Dethmore®, and Panwartin®. The CAS registry number is 81-81-2.

Physical and Chemical Properties Warfarin has the empirical formula $C_{19}H_{16}O_4$ and a molecular weight of 308.32. It forms tasteless, odorless, and colorless crystals with a melting point of 159–161°C. It is practically insoluble in water and benzene, moderately soluble in alcohols, and readily soluble in acetone and dioxane. The sodium salt is fully soluble in water.

History, Formulations, and Uses The history of warfarin is outlined in Section 19.5. It is formulated as a dust (10 gm of active ingredient per kilogram) for use in holes and runs and as a powder (1 gm and 5 gm of active ingredient per kilogram) for mixing with bait to a final concentration of 50 ppm for control of the common rat or 250 ppm for control of the ship rat and mice. Warfarin also is available in many forms of prepared bait.

19.5.1.2 Toxicity to Laboratory Animals

Animals intoxicated by warfarin exhibit increasing pallor and weakness reflecting blood loss. Appetite and body weight are not specifically affected. The blood loss may be evident in the form of bloody sputum, bloody or tarry stools, petechiae, or externally visible hematomata. Hematoma formation is more common than free hemorrhage. If a hematoma is superficial, it will be marked by swelling and discoloration. However, in laboratory animals, hematomata in muscle septa are frequently so large that the entire upper or lower leg is grossly swollen, even though the lesion is so deep that no color is evident beneath the skin. There is no typical location for hematoma formation, the location of bleeding being apparently a matter of chance in the absence of obvious trauma. Bleeding associated with the central nervous system may be of such location and extent as to cause paralysis of the hindquarters several days before death occurs. Pregnant rats appear slightly more susceptible than nonpregnant ones (Hayes and Gaines, 1950). This may be related to obvious morphological factors, but the decreased metabolism of warfarin in pregnant rats suggests the presence of an inhibitory factor (MacDonald and Kaminsky, 1979).

Warfarin may be the only compound for which a log time–log dosage curve with all three segments has been demonstrated experimentally; the 90-day dose LD 50 in rats is only 0.077 mg/kg/day, and the chronicity index is 20.8. Rats tolerated for 300 days a daily dosage slightly greater than the extrapolated 90-day LD 0.01 dosage, specifically 0.02 mg/kg/day. Thus, in spite of its considerable cumulative effect, there is a level of intake that is safe for the rat. The same phenomenon permits the use of warfarin as an anticoagulant drug.

Other investigators have reported completely different results in the same species. Pyorala (1968), who made elaborate studies of the different susceptibility of male and female rats to warfarin, reported LD 50 values of 62–102 mg/kg for males and 21–33 mg/kg for females. Hagan and Radomski (1953) reported values of 323 and 58 mg/kg in males and females, respectively. Why these values differ by one or two orders of magnitude from those reported by others is not clear.

Warfarin is a racemic mixture whether it is used as a rodenticide or as a drug. Almost all published toxicity figures are for the mixture. However, West et al. (1961) were able to separate the isomers and to determine their absolute configuration. Based on prothrombin time measured 24 hr after a single oral dose, the $(-)($S$)$ isomer was 5.5 times as active as the $(+)(R)$ isomer. Based on mortality within 10 days after starting daily dietary intake, the $(-)(S)$-warfarin was 8.5 times as active as the $(+)(R)$ isomer (Elbe et al., 1966).

According to data collected by the French Veterinary Toxicological Information Centre, approximately 70% of the calls received in 1981 concerned dogs poisoned by anticoagulant rodenticides, especially warfarin (Lorgue et al., 1985).

Absorption, Distribution, Metabolism, and Excretion   Absorption of warfarin from the skin of rats is slow but measurable. Three dermal doses at the rate of 50 mg/kg had about the same pharmacological effect as three oral doses at 0.6 mg/kg (Sanger and Becker, 1975). Because of either species or formulation differences, the results were very different with guinea pigs and rabbits that received a 0.5% solution of the sodium salt in water (with 8% alcohol and 0.1% of a surface-active agent); single applications at rates of 0.7 and 0.25 mg/kg caused a marked change in prothrombin times in guinea pigs and rabbits, respectively. In fact, one dermal dose at the rate of 0.25 mg/kg was about as effective in rabbits as an oral dose of 2.0 mg/kg (Fristedt and Sterner, 1965).

There is great individual variation in the binding of warfarin by the serum proteins of laboratory rats. The rate of excretion showed a strong positive correlation with the concentration of free drug in the plasma (Yacobi and Levy, 1975).

Ninety-six hours after intraperitoneal injection of warfarin, the concentrations of activity in the kidney, liver, and pancreas were 3, 12, and 15 times, respectively, greater than that in the blood (Link et al., 1965). The significance of the pancreatic accumulation remains obscure.

Warfarin is readily hydroxylated in vitro and in vivo by rat liver microsomal enzymes to form 6-, 8-, and especially 7-hydroxywarfarin. Formation of another metabolite is catalyzed by the soluble fraction of liver in either the presence or absence of oxygen (Ullrich and Staudinger, 1968; Ikeda et al., 1986a,b). Formation of all these metabolites is stimulated by phenobarbital, chlordane, or DDT. The metabolism is a true detoxication. The inducers can increase the LD 50 of warfarin by more than 10-fold (Ikeda et al., 1968a).

A later study of rats that had received [^{14}C]warfarin revealed the following compounds in the urine: unchanged warfarin (6.6%); 4'-hydroxywarfarin (21%); 6-hydroxywarfarin (15.4%); 7-hydroxywarfarin (8.9%); a glucuronide of 7-hydroxywarfarin (3.0%); and an intramolecular condensation product, 2,3-dihydro-2-methyl-4-phenyl-5-oxo-gamma-pyranol (3.2-c)(1)benzopyran (DHG) (6.6%). These metabolites were found in the feces also but in different relative concentrations (Barker et al., 1970). No radioactive carbon dioxide derived from warfarin has been found in exhaled air (Link et al., 1965). Many of the same metabolites were excreted by guinea pigs, but the proportions were different. Salicylic acid, not found in the rat, was found in guinea pig urine. Of all metabolites recovered, only 4'-hydroxywarfarin and DHG showed anticoagulant activity. That of 4'-hydroxycoumarin was slight. That of DHG showed two peaks, of which the second was stronger. This suggests metabolism of the compound, perhaps back to warfarin (Deckert, 1973).

Rats injected intraperitoneally with [^{14}C]warfarin excreted approximately 90% of the activity in 14 days, about half in the urine and half in the feces (Link et al., 1965).

Approximately 10% of the activity from [^{14}C]warfarin was excreted in the bile of rats within 5 hr after intraperitoneal injection, but little radioactivity appeared in the feces. Nearly all of the metabolites in the bile were conjugated; they could be released with about equal ease by incubation with β-glucuronidase or with gut flora (Powell et al., 1977; Elmer et al., 1977). The metabolites identified were the same as those found slightly later in the urine.

When guinea pigs were injected with 1 or 2 mg of [^{14}C]warfarin, about 50% of the activity was recovered from urine excreted during the first 12 hr and 87% was found in urine within 7 days. A smaller percentage of large doses was excreted promptly (Deckert, 1973).

The action of warfarin (and of fumarin and coumatetralyl as well) on the smooth muscle of the isolated intestine of the rabbit, of the rat (Rattus rattus and Rattus norvegicus), and of Bandicota bengalensis was studied in vitro. There was a fairly identical reduction in peristaltic activity by all three compounds in all four species. The effect was reversible, thus indicating no permanent damage to the tissue (Renapurkar and Deoras, 1982). Warfarin is bound to albumin, but can be displaced from albumin by several compounds, including metals (Brodie, 1964; Chakrabarti, 1978).

Resistance to Warfarin   Genetic resistance to warfarin among rodents, lagomorphs, and humans is discussed in Section 3.1.3.2.

Two cases of intriguing warfarin resistance in humans were reported by Kempin (1983). Both patients under anticoagulant therapy could not be kept within therapeutic range. The common factor that was found was heavy daily intake of broccoli (250–450 mg/day). Broccoli is an important dietary source of vitamin K (200 μg/100 gm). When the vegetable was removed from the diet, the anticoagulant therapy became effective.

Biochemical Effects Warfarin has two actions: inhibition of synthesis of vitamin K-dependent factors (VII, proconvertin; IX, Christmas factor; and X, Stuart factor) and decrease of the production of prothrombin (factor II) in the liver (Coon and Willis, 1972). In addition, warfarin induces capillary damage. There is unconfirmed evidence that these two actions are produced by the two moieties of the molecule. Thus 4-hydroxycoumarin inhibits the formation of prothrombin and reduces the clotting power of the blood, whereas there is some evidence that at sufficient dosage benzalacetone produces capillary damage and leads to bleeding upon the very slightest trauma. Significantly enough, vitamin K has an antidotal action against both actions of warfarin up to a certain point (Varon and Cole, 1966).

The basis for the change in vitamin K_1 metabolism associated with poisoning and the alteration of this metabolism in resistant animals probably involves a warfarin-binding protein in the microsomal membranes of the liver. Thierry et al. (1970) found that ribosomes isolated from the livers of resistant rats bind only one-third to one-fifth as much warfarin as ribosomes from normal rats, regardless of whether warfarin is injected before the rats are killed for study or is added to the in vitro preparation. Lorusso and Suttie (1972) found that, when [^{14}C]warfarin at a concentration of 0.786 ppm was incubated with microsomal preparations, the concentrations reached were 42.0 and 17.7 pmol/mg of protein, depending on whether the preparations were prepared from normal or from warfarin-resistant rats, respectively. Furthermore, the warfarin was bound firmly to membranes of normal rats but loosely to those of warfarin-resistant rats. Vitamin K deficiency caused a 24% increase in the amount of warfarin bound, but this was overcome in animals given vitamin K_1 1 hr before being killed for in vitro study. Warfarin binding in vitro was reduced 90% in animals injected with warfarin 22 hr before being killed. Although the binding protein was a part of microsomal membranes, it seemed unrelated to cytochrome P-450.

A protein which may be the same as the one just discussed has been isolated and shown to have a molecular weight of about 30,000. It may become adherent to ribosomes in the course of their preparation for biochemical study (Searcey and Graves, 1976).

Binding of warfarin to cytochromes P-450 and P-448 occurs also and may help to explain changes in the rate of metabolism of warfarin following induction of microsomal enzymes by phenobarbital and other compounds. The stereochemical aspects of the metabolism of warfarin have been studied in great detail (Kaminsky et al., 1976; Pohl et al., 1976a,b, 1977).

Formation of 7- and 8-hydroxywarfarin is promoted by other cytochromes. The same type of cytochrome is mainly responsible for the formation of each corresponding metabolite, regardless of how the activity of liver microsomal enzymes has been induced (Fasco et al., 1979).

Warfarin has been reported to inhibit (Biezunski, 1970) or to promote (Bernacki and Bosmann, 1970) the synthesis of liver microsomal protein and other liver protein. The contradictory results may be explained by differences in procedure, but exactly how is unclear. It is also unclear what bearing the results have on the pharmacological action of warfarin.

Warfarin causes a relative increase in vitamin K_1 oxide in the plasma or liver of people (Shearer et al., 1973) and rats (Matschiner et al., 1970). The oxide is a naturally occurring compound. In vitamin K-deficient but otherwise normal rats, the oxide and vitamin K_1 are equally effective, but the oxide is not therapeutic in warfarin-treated rats. It has been proposed that coumarin and related anticoagulants act by inhibiting the conversion of the oxide back to the active vitamin and that the oxide per se is inhibitory. Involvement of the vitamin K_1–vitamin K_1 oxide cycle in the action of warfarin seems very likely, since the effect of warfarin on this cycle is greatly reduced in resistant rats. The hypothesis that warfarin inhibits prothrombin synthesis by causing accumulation of the oxide does not appear tenable (Caldwell et al., 1974). However, it seems likely that the brevity of the action of vitamin K in the treatment of poisoning is the result of its irreversible conversion to the epoxide (Shearer and Barkhan, 1979).

The superiority of vitamin K_1 over vitamin K_3 in treating warfarin poisoning has been established experimentally (Penumarthy and Oehme, 1978).

Far more detail than can be discussed here regarding vitamin K and vitamin K-dependent proteins is available in a book edited by Suttie (1979).

Although L-histidine at a dietary level of 40 ppm was without effect on rats, it potentiated the lethal action of warfarin (50 ppm) in both laboratory and field tests (Rao, 1979). The biochemical basis for this action of histidine should be explored.

Effects on Organs and Tissues A possible oncogenic effect of prolonged warfarin therapy was speculated by Krauss (1982) based on a report by Gore and associates (1982) of an increased incidence of cancer in patients occurring 3 or more years after a pulmonary embolism. This highly speculative deduction made from a very limited number of cases has been criticized by Zacharski (1982) who cited results from two cohort studies (Michaels, 1974; Annegers and Zacharski, 1980). In those studies no increased incidence of malignancies was observed in patients who had received long-term anticoagulant treatments and had been followed for several thousand patient-years.

Pathology Animals killed by warfarin show most extreme pallor of the skin, muscles, and all the viscera. In addition, evidence of hemorrhage may be found in any part of the body but usually only in one location in a single autopsy. Such blood as remains in the heart and vessels is grossly thin and forms a poor clot or no clot. In a report of a boxer dog poisoned with a mixture of warfarin and calciferol, delayed necrosis of the tip of the tongue and large areas of necrosed skin were seen. It is difficult, however, to attribute the damaging effect on the walls of the vessels to warfarin alone, since calciferol also can induce such lesions (Edlin, 1982).

Treatment of Poisoning in Animals A diet containing selenium at a concentration of 2.5 mg/kg of feed was protective against the toxic effects of aflatoxin B$_1$ (a bifuranocoumarin) and warfarin in pigs given four daily oral doses of 0.2 mg/kg of body weight. Selenium is a component of glutathione peroxidase, an enzyme that prevents the production of free radicals (Davila *et al.*, 1983).

19.5.1.3 Toxicity to Humans

Experimental Exposure When nine normal men and five normal women were given a single oral dose of warfarin at the rate of 1.5 mg/kg, maximal concentration in plasma was reached in 2–12 hr. Maximal depression of prothrombin activity was between 36 and 72 hr. Their individual increases in prothrombin time were proportional to their half-times for disappearance of warfarin from the plasma. In other words, the pharmacological effect was greatest in those with slower excretion. The half-times for disappearance from the plasma varied from15 to 58 hr with a mean of 42 hr. Absorption of warfarin from the gastrointestinal tract was apparently complete; no warfarin was found in the stool even after massive doses, and plasma levels and prothrombin activity responses were virtually identical following oral and intravenous administration at the same rates (O'Reilly *et al.*, 1963).

Having established the absolute configuration of the four warfarin alcohols, Chan *et al.* (1972) administered them to volunteers. Reduction of the alcohols was stereoselective. The rate of elimination of one of the isomers (*R,S*) was much slower than that of the others, and its effect was more sustained. The resulting metabolites were biologically active but not as active as warfarin itself.

Six normal subjects were given a single dose of warfarin at the rate of 1.5 mg/kg. Three weeks later, the same people were given 200 mg of phenylbutazone three times a day for at least 8 days; on the fourth day, warfarin was repeated at 1.5 mg/kg. Compared to warfarin alone, administration of warfarin with phenylbutazone increased the prothrombin time even though the plasma concentration and biological half-life decreased. The result (in the face of an obvious inactivation of warfarin) was attributed to displacement of warfarin by phenylbutazone from binding to plasma albumin, making more free drug momentarily available to receptor sites in the liver (O'Reilly and Aggeler, 1968). The mutual displacement of phenylbutazone and warfarin from human plasma albumin has been studied *in vitro* (Solomon *et al.*, 1968).

As shown by study in seven volunteers, the action of triclofos (trichloroethyl sodium phosphate) is similar to that of phenylbutazone. A dosage of triclofos at the rate of 22 mg/kg/day prolonged the prothrombin time even though the dosage of warfarin was reduced. Trichloroacetic acid, a metabolite of triclofos, accumulated in the plasma to an average concentration of 80 ppm. The displacement of warfarin from albumin by trichloroacetic acid was sufficient to account for the observed potentiation of warfarin (Sellers *et al.*, 1972). At least in the rat, sodiumsalicylate has a similar effect (Coldwell *et al.*, 1974) but

phenobarbital does not significantly influence the binding capacity of the plasma for warfarin (Ikeda *et al.*, 1968a).

In a similar study with 10 male volunteers, both phenobarbital and glutethimide lowered the plasma warfarin concentration and reduced the half-life of warfarin by nearly 50%; chloral betaine had a slight effect also. Phenobarbital and glutethimide significantly reduced the hypoprothrombinemia response of warfarin, but results with chloral betaine were indistinguishable in this regard from results for placebo-treated and untreated controls (MacDonald *et al.*, 1969).

The effects of cimetidine (a drug used to treat peptic ulcer) on the kinetics and dynamics of warfarin were studied in seven volunteers. It was shown clearly that cimetidine acted by inhibition of drug metabolism without significant effect on the binding of warfarin to plasma protein (Breckenridge *et al.*, 1979).

Therapeutic Use Use of warfarin as a drug offers greater dosage and, therefore, greater opportunity for side effects than pest control operators encounter. Of course, bleeding is the most common complication of treatment. Most of it is clinically insignificant. Probably many cases remain unpublished. According to one study, the incidence among hospitalized patients was 10%, and it was 40% among ambulatory patients. The incidence of serious hemorrhage was estimated at 2–10% in hospitalized and ambulatory patients, respectively. A series of case reports illustrated some of the circumstances leading to serious hemorrhage. It was concluded that the complication can be kept at a minimum by careful selection of patients, informed and adequate supervision by the physician, and reliable laboratory control (Pastor *et al.*, 1962).

Although the diagnosis in most cases of hemorrhage is obvious, there are exceptions. For example, two cases of intestinal hemorrhage leading to an initial diagnosis of acute abdomen have been reported (Cocks, 1960).

Macular, papular, pruritic, or vesicular rashes due to warfarin are unusual, but those that do occur often are in patients who had taken the drug without untoward effect for 3 or more months. The skin returned to normal slowly after medication was stopped, but the dermatitis recurred within 2 or 3 days when medication was renewed (Schiff and Kern, 1968).

Necrosis of the skin and subcutaneous tissues of localized areas has been attributed to warfarin only rarely and not always convincingly. For example, in a case reported by Vaughan *et al.* (1969) a totally unexplained illness suggestive of but not proved to be thrombophlebitis and pulmonary embolism preceded warfarin therapy by 6 weeks and may have been the underlying cause of the complication attributed circumstantially to warfarin. In two other cases, a more persuasive interpretation was made, namely that anticoagulants (heparin and warfarin) acted as neither the preparatory nor the provoking substance for the localized necrosis attributed to their use, but that underlying disease processes, including intravascular coagulation, sepsis, or localized inflammation, triggered a localized purpuric reaction that was then intensified by the warfarin therapy (Martin *et al.*, 1970).

An entirely different kind of complication has involved potentiation of warfarin by disulfiram (Rothstein, 1968) or interference with its action by other drugs including griseofulvin (Cullen and Catalano, 1967) and phenobarbital (Robinson and MacDonald, 1966) or by insecticides. In one case, medical use of warfarin was nullified by use of 5% toxaphene and 1% lindane to dust sheep. Response to warfarin returned to normal within about 3 months after exposure to the insecticides (Jeffery *et al.*, 1976). Of course, discontinuing a drug that promotes the metabolism of warfarin has the same effect as introducing a drug such as disulfiram that interferes with metabolism of the anticoagulant.

The success of cardiac value prostheses requires anticoagulation to prevent immobilization of the valve by thrombi and to minimize the chance of emboli. Installation of such prostheses in young women to correct rheumatic mitral or aortic stenosis increases their chance of surviving and reproducing, but it necessarily complicates any pregnancies they may have.

Anticoagulants also may be used in women of childbearing age to treat thrombophlebitis, embolic disease, and a few other conditions. It has long been recognized that administration of any anticoagulant during pregnancy increases the danger of hemorrhage either during the course of gestation or during delivery. It gradually has become evident that warfarin also is teratogenic in humans (DiSaia, 1966; Keber *et al.*, 1968; Tejani, 1973; Becker *et al.*, 1975; Shaul *et al.*, 1975; Pettifor and Benson, 1975; Sherrod and Harrod, 1978). At least 29 cases of congenital anomaly have been attributed to warfarin (Hall *et al.*, 1980). Most if not all of the recognized cases have involved nasal hypoplasia ranging from barely recognizable to very severe. Many of the babies had chondrodysplasia punctata, and this defect of cartilage development may be the basis not only of the nasal deformity but also of defects of the bones such as meningocele, deformities of the limbs, and a high arched palate seen much more rarely in babies of women treated with warfarin during the first trimester. Other teratogenic effects reported in one or more cases include microphthalmia, blindness, hydrocephalus, persistent truncus arteriosus, and mental retardation. Of 423 reported pregnancies in which coumarin derivatives were used, not over two-thirds resulted in apparently normal infants, one-sixth resulted in abortion or stillbirth, and one-sixth resulted in abnormal liveborn infants of which 29 showed fetal embryopathy. The critical period of exposure seemed to be between 6 and 9 weeks of gestation. Five cases of typical embryopathy and eight other cases showed central nervous system abnormalities following exposure to coumarin derivatives during gestation, but no critical period of exposure was evident (Hall *et al.*, 1980; Stevenson *et al.*, 1980).

Twenty-nine of 423 pregnancies is a high incidence of teratogenic effect even if one takes into account that only medically reported cases were available for consideration. A different kind of evidence for the teratogenic action of warfarin involved a family with no history of consanguinity, birth defects, or mental retardation that produced one normal child in a pregnancy without warfarin and two deformed children in separate pregnancies in which warfarin was used (Sherrod and Harrod, 1978). On the other hand, inasmuch as defects occur in only

about one-third of instances, none may be found in some small series of cases (Chong *et al.*, 1984).

The use of heparin during gestation does not result in a significantly better outcome of pregnancy than that obtained with warfarin. In 135 published cases, about two-thirds were apparently normal, one-eighth were stillborn, and one-fifth (of whom one-third died) were premature (Hall *et al.*, 1980).

Kaplan (1985) and Zakzouk (1986) reviewed the subject of warfarin-associated malformations and established that, based on the timing of warfarin exposure, second- and third-trimester exposure predisposes to central nervous system abnormalities whereas first-trimester exposure is associated with the warfarin embryopathy: midface and nasal hypoplasia, optic atrophy, hypoplasia of the digits, and mental impairment. In addition, Kaplan reports a case of Dandy-Walker malformation associated with warfarin exposure confined to weeks 8–12 of gestation. Four previous cases of such association were known but the gestational exposure period was much longer.

Not only has hereditary resistance of people to warfarin been observed (O'Reilly, 1970) but also exceptional susceptibility, also presumably on a hereditary basis, has been reported (Solomon, 1968).

Accidental and Intentional Poisoning A 32-year-old man was murdered by feeding him warfarin for 13 days. On the fourth day after intake started, the victim began having severe nosebleeds. Later, he bled from the mouth. Two days before death, he complain of pain in his limbs. His symptoms became worse and he died of circulatory failure on day 15 (Pribilla, 1966).

The initial symptoms in an attempted suicide using warfarin were back pain and abdominal pain. The onset occurred 1 day after the sixth daily dose. A day after onset, vomiting and attacks of nose bleeding occurred. On the second day of illness, when admitted to hospital, the patient was observed to have a generalized petechial rash (Holmes and Love, 1952).

In Korea, a family of 14 persons lived for a period of 15 days on a diet consisting almost entirely of corn (maize) meal containing warfarin. The first symptoms appeared 7–10 days after the eating of warfarin was begun. Massive bruises or hematomata developed at the knee and elbow joints and on the buttocks in all cases. Extensive gum and nasal hemorrhage usually appeared about a day later, and by day 15 blood loss was extensive (Lange and Terveer, 1954).

A suicidal gesture that was reported and treated after only a single ingestion of a heaping tablespoonful of 0.5% warfarin produced no illness and not even an increase in prothrombin time (Kellum, 1952).

There have been at least two attempted murders with warfarin (Nilsson, 1957; Ikkala *et al.*, 1964). In each instance there were recurrent bouts of hemorrhagic difficulty, including hematuria, epistaxis, severe bruises without any history of trauma, and intestinal hemorrhage. Abdominal or back pain was present. Each patient recovered promptly in hospital, but one had relapses for nearly a year and the other had bouts of poisoning for 2.5 years following repeated doses. An anticoagulant drug was suspected from the first in both cases, but finding the source proved difficult. Solution of each case was essentially epidemiological, but measurement of warfarin in the plasma was decisive in one case. Faced with the evidence, the daughter-in-law of a 73-year-old woman and the wife of a 69-year-old man both confessed to the police.

Although numerous accidental ingestions by children and adults have been reported to the New York Poison Control Center, no known injury from these ingestions has been observed (Jacobziner and Raybin, 1960).

An outbreak of hemorrhagic disease due to the use of warfarin-contaminated talcum was described in Vietnam (Martin-Bouyer et al., 1983). Of the 741 cases located in Ho-Chi-Minh City, all in infants (55% under 2 months of age), 177 died. Eleven samples of baby powder were analyzed and concentrations of warfarin ranged from 1.7 to 6.5%. The percutaneous penetration of warfarin contained in the contaminated talc was studied in a young healthy female baboon, treated twice daily with a topical application of 3 gm of talc containing 3% warfarin (188 mg/kg/day of warfarin). One control animal was treated with uncontaminated talc. On the fifth day the treated animal began to show signs of intoxication with profuse bleeding and died. At necropsy there were two large subcutaneous hematomata on the skull and the peritoneal cavity with filled with unclotted blood. On day 3 of treatment a blood sample showed severe disturbances of the hepatic coagulation factors. Electron microscopy showed an increased number of swollen and misshapen mitochondria in the hepatocytes (Dreyfus et al., 1983).

Warfarin was administered to an 11-month-old baby girl by her psychologically disturbed mother. Upon hospitalization the parameters of coagulation were elevated (prothrombin time 53 sec, control 12 sec); the child had multiple hematomata and had a bloody discharge from her left ear. Treatment with vitamin K_1 and infusion of fresh frozen plasma stopped the bleeding (White, 1985).

Use Experience   The safety record of warfarin used as a rodenticide has been excellent. One case of poisoning has been attributed to extensive, prolonged skin contact in the process of preparing and distributing baits. Unlike most solid bait, which is prepared by mixing ground grain with starch containing warfarin powder, this bait was prepared by pouring a 0.5% solution of the sodium salt over dried bread. The hands of the 23-year-old farmer who used this method were wet with the solution each of the 10 times he made bait during a 24-day period, and he did not wash his hands until several hours after each application. Two days after the last contact with rodenticide, gross hematuria appeared. Next day hemotomata were noticed on the arms and legs; there was dull pain in both groins. The hematuria subsided after 3 days of rest but recurred along with nose bleeding when the man returned to work. When he was admitted to hospital, prothrombin, clotting, and bleeding times were abnormally long and anemia was severe (hemoglobin, 8.1%; red cell count. 2.9 million/mm³). The patient responded promptly to treatment with vitamin K_1 (Fristedt and Sterner, 1965).

Atypical Cases of Various Origins   Mogilner et al. (1974) described three fatal cases of what they considered to represent Reye's syndrome. One of the young children was said to have ingested warfarin that she found by the road on her way to kindergarten 4 days before hospital admission; warfarin was found in the urine and traces were present in the blood. In another case "significant amounts of warfarin were found in the urine and also in autopsy samples of liver and kidney tissue"; no source of the rodenticide was reported, and no information was given that would permit evaluation of the validity of the chemical analysis. There was no indication of warfarin in the third case. The authors considered that it was justified "to add warfarin to the long and varied list of etiological or precipitating factors in Reye's syndrome."

The death of a 2-year-old boy was attributed to warfarin poisoning on his death certificate but probably was the result of beating, with pneumonia as a terminal event (Hayes and Vaughn, 1977).

Dosage Response   A total dose of about 1000 mg of warfarin consumed in 13 days (about 1.1 mg/kg/day) was fatal (Pribilla, 1966).

Serious illness followed the ingestion of 1.7 mg warfarin/kg/day for 6 consecutive days with suicidal intent. This would correspond to eating almost 1 pound of bait (0.025% warfarin) each day for 6 days. All signs and symptoms were caused by hemorrhage and, following multiple small transfusions and massive doses of vitamin K, recovery was complete (Holmes and Love, 1952).

In the Korean cases, the dosage of the different individuals was determined to vary from about 1 to 2 mg warfarin/kg/day. As a result of this exposure and without benefit of treatment, 2 of the 14 persons died. A 19-year-old girl, who was in a state of shock and severe hemorrhage 2 days after the warfarin diet was discontinued, recovered following a blood transfusion and small daily doses of vitamin K. The remaining 11 members of the family recovered within a week after exposure, although only small daily doses of vitamin K were given and they all had shown marked signs of poisoning when they first accepted treatment. There was reason to think that those who died had received slightly higher dosages than those who survived (see Table 2.9 in Hayes, 1975). Recovery of the 12 survivors was complete. The entire episode was made possible only by a series of unusual events and by the extraordinary apathy of the family, resulting in their totally ignoring unmistakable signs of illness (Lange and Terveer, 1954).

A single intravenous therapeutic dose of the sodium derivative (40–60 mg or about 0.7 mg/kg) in humans may produce some increase in prothrombin time within 2 hr and usually produces a substantial increase within 14 hr. The average maximal response is on the fourth day. Spontaneous recovery to normal occurs about 8 days after a single therapeutic dose. Thus significant depression of prothrombin level is maintained for 3–6 days. In the treatment of thromboembolic disease, a maintenance dose of about 2–10 mg/day is required to keep the prothrombin level between 10 and 30% of normal. Patients have been thus maintained for years. If human susceptibility to warfarin were different (as it is in a few genetically determined cases), the therapeutic dosage could be adjusted accordingly. It is interesting, however, that the upper limit of the usual maintenance dosage for humans (about 0.14 mg/kg/day) is an LD 95 for the rat. The inherently lesser susceptibility of humans to the compound undoubtedly contributes to its safety as a rodenticide. The threshold limit value of 0.1 mg/m³ indicates that occupational intake of warfarin at the rate of 0.014 mg/kg/day is considered safe.

Laboratory Findings   Metabolites of warfarin including 5-, 6-, 7-, and 8-hydroxywarfarin and two aliphatic side-chain alcohols have been identified in the urine of normal volunteers who had received a single oral dose at the rate of 1.5 mg/kg (Lewis and Traeger, 1970; Chan *et al.,* 1972). This is, however, not a common way to confirm poisoning.

Adequacy of treatment with warfarin usually is followed by measuring prothrombin time. In case of poisoning, the prothrombin time is greatly prolonged. The coagulation time is definitely increased by the Lee-White method and slightly increased by the capillary tube method. Bleeding time often is normal. Urine may be normal in appearance but may contain many red cells on microscopic examination, or it may be grossly hemorrhagic. The red cell count and hemoglobin gradually fall if bleeding continues. In terminal cases a state of shock develops.

Sixty-nine euthyroid patients being treated with warfarin for thromboembolic disease showed no evidence of hyperthyroid condition, and 14 of them showed a hypothyroid tendency associated with an elevation of the thyroxine-binding capacity of plasma globulin. However, no clinical evidence of thyroid dysfunction was reported, and it was uncertain whether the small changes in laboratory tests of thyroid function were caused by warfarin (Braverman and Foster, 1969).

Plasma levels of warfarin were 6.8 and 11.2 ppm 4 and 7 hr, respectively, after the ingestion of 500 mg of warfarin sodium in a suicide attempt. Plasma levels declined thereafter, and the half-time for disappearance was calculated as 46 hr. Part of the dose was removed by gastric lavage soon after ingestion. This and other appropriate treatment prevented any increase in bleeding tendency (Cole and Bachman, 1976).

Pathology   Apparently there is only one complete description of human pathology associated with uncomplicated warfarin poisoning, that of Pribilla (1966). The findings in that case were strikingly different from typical findings in the rat: exsanguination was less complete, as indicated by the fact that the liver was not tan in color and bleeding was far more generalized and not restricted to one or a few large hematomata. The two factors may be related in that bleeding into the organs may have interfered with their function and hastened death. In addition to generalized bleeding (due mainly to deficiency of coagulation), evidence of capillary damage and of parenchymal injury of the liver was found in the human case. In spite of the obvious differences between the findings in human and rat, the similarity was also striking because subserosal and intraseptal bleeding was prominent in the human case.

Treatment of Poisoning   After blood has been taken for prothrombin and other differential diagnostic tests, vitamin K_1 in a dose of 5–10 mg should be given three times on the first day of treatment irrespective of symptoms. The vitamin should be given intravenously slowly, usually by infusion. Smaller doses should be continued until the prothrombin time has reached normal. In a seriously ill patient, a small transfusion of carefully matched whole blood should be given initially and repeated daily until the patient has returned to normal. Such a patient should be given vitamin K_1 also. If it were ever necessary to treat a patient in shock from blood loss resulting from warfarin poisoning, frequent small transfusions and a complete consideration of the blood chemistry would be in order. Any large hematomata should be the subject of a surgical consultation, but any surgical action should be taken only after the clotting power of the blood is restored to normal.

The progress of the patient should be followed by the prothrombin test. Tests should be made at least twice daily until a return to normal is clearly established.

19.5.2 COUMAFURYL

19.5.2.1 Identity, Properties, and Uses

Chemical Name   3-[-1(2-furanyl)-3-oxobutyl]-4-hydroxy-2*H* -1-benzopyran-2-one.

Structure   See Fig. 19.3.

Synonyms   Coumafuryl is the common name approved by ISO. Other names for the compound include fumarin (BSI) and tomarin (Turkey). Trade names include Fumarin®, Fumasol®, Krumkil®, Lurat®, Ratafin®, Rat-a-way®, and Tomarin®. The CAS registry number is 117-52-2.

Physical and Chemical Properties   The empirical formula for coumafuryl is $C_{17}H_{14}O_5$, and the molecular weight is 298.28. It is a crystalline solid melting at 124°C.

Use   Coumafuryl is an anticoagulant rat poison.

19.5.2.2 Toxicity in Laboratory Animals

Coumafuryl is very similar to warfarin (see Fig. 19.3). The oral LD 50 for rats is quoted as 0.4 mg/kg (Wiswesser, 1976).

19.5.2.3 Toxicity to Humans

It is inevitable that a number of children and perhaps others have ingested coumafuryl. In fact, McLeod (1970) reported that coumafuryl and warfarin were among the pesticides most often ingested by persons (mainly children) admitted to a large hospital in New Orleans. However, these two compounds were the least hazardous pesticides in terms of morbidity.

Treatment of Poisoning   Treatment is the same as that for warfarin (see Section 19.5.1.3).

19.5.3 DIPHACINONE

19.5.3.1 Identity, Properties, and Uses

Chemical Name   2(Diphenylacetyl)indan-1,3-dione.

Structure   See Fig. 19.3.

Synonyms   Diphacinone (ANSI, BSI, ISO) is the common name in use except in Turkey and Italy, where diphacin is used, and in the USSR, where ratindan is used. Other nonproprietary names include dipazin and diphenacin. As a drug, the compound is known as diphenadione. Trade names for formulated baits containing diphacinone include Diphacine®, Ramik®, Promar®, and Gold Crest®. The CAS registry number is 82-66-6.

Physical and Chemical Properties   Diphacinone has the empirical formula $C_{23}H_{16}O_3$ and a molecular weight of 340.40. Its technical grade is a yellow crystalline powder melting at 145°C; it is slightly soluble in water (0.3 mg/liter) and soluble in acetone (29 gm/liter) and toluene (73 gm/liter). Diphacinone is rapidly decomposed in water by sunlight.

History, Formulations, and Uses   The rodenticidal activity of diphacinone was described in 1952. It is formulated as prepared weather-resistant baits (pellets or meal) in concentrations of 50 mg/kg. A dry concentrate (1 gm/kg) for mixing with cereal bait is also available. All formulations are for professional application only. Diphacinone is used to control mice, rats, prairie dogs (*Cynomys* spp.), ground squirrels, voles, and other rodents.

19.5.3.2 Toxicity to Laboratory Animals

In a study of bishydroxycoumarin, ethyl biscoumacetate, and 17 analogs of indandione in rabbits, diphacinone was found to be the most hypoprothrombinemic. A marked response lasting about 7 days was produced by a dosage of only 0.05 mg/kg. The acute oral LD 50 ranges from 0.3 to 2.3 mg/kg in the rat and from 3.0 to 7.5 mg/kg in the dog. It was found to be 14.7 mg/kg for cats and 150 mg/kg for pigs. In mice and rabbits the oral LD 50 is 340 mg/kg and 35 mg/kg, respectively. For the mallard duck, it is 3158 mg/kg. The LD 50 associated with 14 daily oral doses in rats was 0.1 mg/kg (Correll *et al.*, 1952). Acute percutaneous LD 50 for rats is less than 200 mg/kg. In a 21-day subchronic percutaneous study in rabbits the no-effect level was 0.1 mg/kg daily. Diphacinone is neither a skin and eye irritant nor a skin sensitizer. An acute inhalation of diphacinone dust in

the rat has shown an LC 50 of less than 2000 mg/m³ of air. Diphacinone is not mutagenic in the Ames test.

Sprague–Dawley rats were fed for 21 days on a diet containing 1, 2, or 4 ppm diphacinone. All animals in the 2 and 4 ppm groups died and postmortem examination revealed massive internal hemorrhages. On day 21, the prothrombin clotting time of the animals in the 1 ppm group was not affected. A second study was performed in which the rats were fed for 90 days on a diet containing 0.0313, 0.625, 0.125, 0.25, or 0.5 ppm of diphacinone, or approximately 0.002, 0.003, 0.006, 0.013, and 0.025 mg/kg/day. One male in the 0.25 ppm group died on day 17 of treatment and another male in the 0.0625 ppm group on day 20 from a subdural hemorrhage. However, the mean prothrombin clotting times of the animals surviving the treatment period were not affected. The only parameter that showed some variation was the fibrinogen level, which was lower in the 0.5 ppm group (Elias and Johns, 1981).

The most interesting aspect of the toxicity of diphacinone involves species difference. The oral LD 50 of the compound for vampire bats (*Desmodus rotundus*) was 0.91 mg/kg, whereas a dosage of 5 mg/kg produced no sign of illness in cattle (Elias *et al.*, 1978). The blood of beef cattle given a single intraruminal injection of the compound at a rate of 1 mg/kg became toxic to these bats and remained toxic for 3 days without harming the cattle. As indicated by examination before and 2 weeks after treatment, cattle dosed in this way on three ranches in Mexico experienced a 93% reduction in vampire bat bites. Bioassays of milk and liver indicated that there was no residue problem (Thompson *et al.*, 1972). Residue studies indicated that people may safely eat meat, including liver and kidney, from treated cattle (Bullard *et al.*, 1976).

Absorption, Distribution, Metabolism, and Excretion
When ¹⁴C-labeled diphacinone was administered orally to mice, radioactivity reached its highest levels in the liver and lungs. The concentration in the liver reached its maximum in 7.5 and 3.0 hr in males and females, respectively (Cahill and Crowder, 1979). In another study, rats and mice were orally administered ¹⁴C-labeled diphacinone at dosages of 0.2 and 1.5 mg/kg. Male and female animals had similar rates of elimination. In rats, about 70% of the dose was excreted in the feces and 10% in urine in 8 days. The same elimination pattern was observed in mice. Eight days after the administration of the compound in rats and 4 days in mice, the liver had the highest level of residues, but kidneys and lung also contained significant levels of residues; brain, fat, and muscles had the lowest levels. Diphacinone is not extensively metabolized in rats, less than 1% of the dose being expired as CO_2 hr. The metabolism pattern in rats involved mainly hydroxylation and conjugation reactions (Yu *et al.*, 1982).

Mode of Action   Diphacinone inhibits the K-enzyme complex (liver-synthesized coagulation proteins: factors II, VII, and X), and this inhibition phase lasts approximately 30 days in dogs, as opposed to the relatively short effect of warfarin (Mount and Feldman, 1983). The prolonged action of diphacinone may be due to protein binding in the liver or low excretion rate or a combination of both factors.

Treatment of Poisoning in Animals   In dogs the results of the usual vitamin K oral therapy after diphacinone poisoning were poor. Dogs treated with a sufficient quantity of vitamin K relapsed fatally several days after the corrective treatment stopped. The response to treatment seems to vary according to the amount of exposure to the rodenticide. The recommended therapeutic dose of vitamin K_1 is 5 mg/kg of body weight in subcutaneous injections for at least 5 consecutive days (Mount and Feldman, 1983).

19.5.3.3 Toxicity to Humans

Therapeutic Use   Diphacinone has been used as a therapeutic agent because it has a relatively long duration of action. Its half-life in humans is 15–20 days. A single oral dose of diphacinone of 4 mg/person produced a clearly detectable reduction of pro-thrombin about 14 hr after ingestion and slightly more reduction a day later, with recovery to normal by the third day. A smaller, uncertain reduction was produced by 2 mg/person. A single 20-mg dose caused hypoprothrombinemia that was definite in 14 hr, marked in 48 hr, and persisted from 6 to 10 days. The recommended initial dose for therapy was 20 mg followed by daily doses of 2–4 mg (Field *et al.*, 1952). The drug was in use until a few years ago. Although there were no adverse effects except occasional nausea and not unexpected hemorrhagic complications at high dosage levels, caution was advised because of its close relation to phenindione, which has caused agronulocytosis, hepatitis with jaundice, nephropathy with acute renal tubular necrosis, severe exfoliative dermatitis, and massive generalized edema [American Medical Association (AMA), 1977]. The drug ceased to be listed in the AMA Drug Evaluations of 1980.

Treatment of Poisoning   Treatment is the same as that for warfarin, but based on experimental data from animals it would seem advisable to increase the dose of vitamin K as well as the duration of the corrective treatment.

19.5.4 BRODIFACOUM

19.5.4.1 Identity, Properties, and Uses

Chemical Name   3-[3-(4'-bromo-[1,1'-biphenyl]-4-yl)-1,2, 3,4-tetrahydro-1-naphthylenyl]-4-hydroxy-2H-1-benzopyran-2-one.

Structure   See Fig. 19.4.

Synonyms   Brodifacoum is the approved common name (ISO-BSI). Trade names for the formulated material include Ratak®, Volak®, and Talon®. The code names are WBA 8119 and PP 581. The CAS registry number is 56073-10-0.

Physical and Chemical Properties   The empirical formula for brodifacoum is $C_{31}H_{23}BrO_3$ and the molecular weight is 523.4. It is an off-white to fawn-colored odorless powder with a melting point of 228–232°C. It is of very low solubility in water (less than 10 mg/liter at 20°C and pH 7). Brodifacoum is slightly soluble in alcohols and benzene and soluble in acetone. It is stable at room temperature. It has a very low vapor pressure of less than 1.33×10^{-7} kPa (1×10^{-6} mm Hg) at 25°C.

History, Formulations, and Uses   The rodenticidal properties of brodifacoum were described in 1976. It is an indirect anticoagulant active against rats and mice including strains resistant to warfarin and other anticoagulants (Rennison and Hadler, 1975). It is also used to control other wild rodents. Brodifacoum is formulated as ready-to-use baits of low concentration (20 and 50 mg/kg of bait). A single ingestion is usually sufficient to kill.

19.5.4.2 Toxicity to Laboratory Animals

Brodifacoum is extremely toxic to a number of mammalian species. The oral and dermal LD 50 values of the technical material are given in Table 19.6.

In chicken the oral LD 50 is reported to be 4.5 mg/kg and in the mallard duck it is 2.0 mg/kg.

In a 42-day feeding study in rats a concentration of 0.1 ppm did not induce any adverse effect (Worthing and Walker, 1983).

Several cases of poisoning in domestic animals have been reported. One day after being seen to ingest brodifacoum-containing bait, a 17-kg cocker spaniel developed depression and icterus accompanied by accelerated pulse and rapid and labored respiration. Despite supportive therapy, the dog died the same day. The autopsy confirmed the icter and showed approximately 1 liter of unclotted blood in the thoracic cavity and 100 ml in the pericardial sac. Numerous hemorrhagic areas were seen in the serous membranes (Stowe *et al.*, 1983). A 4-year-old cross-bred bitch was noticed to be depressed and weak the day following the laying of Talon® baits (0.005% brodifacoum); she was found dead in her kennel the next morning. The actual dose of brodifacoum ingested was unknown but it was estimated that the maximum quantity of bait eaten could have been 900 gm, resulting in an intake of 45 mg of active ingredient. At autopsy the thoracic cavity contained approximately 1.8 liter of unclotted

Table 19.6
Single-Dose LD 50 for Brodifacoum

Species	Route	LD 50 (mg/kg)
Rat, M	oral	0.27
Rat	dermal	50.00
Mouse, M	oral	0.40
Guinea pig, F	oral	0.28
Rabbit, M	oral	0.30
Dog	oral	0.25–1.0
Cat	oral	~0.25

blood and a single clot was adherent to the base of the heart and to the aorta. Subcutaneous bruising was present on the rib cage. Brodifacoum was found in the liver at a concentration of 0.8 mg/kg (McSporran and Phillips, 1983).

The acute oral toxicity of brodifacoum was examined in sheep. An LD 50 of 11 mg/kg was considered a good estimate (Godfrey *et al.*, 1985).

Absorption, Distribution, Metabolism, and Excretion
Brodifacoum is absorbed through the gastrointestinal tract. When orally administered to male Sprague–Dawley rats at doses ranging from 0.1 to 0.33 mg/kg, brodifacoum exhibited a remarkably steep dose–response curve; 0.1 mg/kg failed to show an effect on the plasma prothrombin level within 24 hr, whereas 0.2 mg/kg reduced the prothrombin complex activity to 7% of normal values and 0.33 mg/kg reduced it to 4% of normal. Concentrations in the liver were rapidly established and remained relatively constant for at least 96 hr. The mean liver/serum concentration ratio is approximately 20. Disappearance from serum is slow with a half-life of 156 hr or even more. The slow disappearance from the plasma and liver and the large liver/serum ratio probably contribute to the higher toxicity of brodifacoum than of warfarin. These particular features may also explain the efficacy of brodifacoum against warfarin-resistant rats (Bachmann and Sullivan, 1983).

Six weeks after intravenous administration of a single 1 mg/kg dose of brodifacoum to male New Zealand White rabbits, the prothrombin complex activity was still lower than 30% of normal (in the early part of the study, subcutaneous injections of vitamin K were given to prevent lethal hemorrhage). In the same study (Park and Leck, 1982), it was shown that in the rabbit, the maximal antagonism of vitamin K_1 by warfarin was produced by a dose of 63 mg/kg, whereas a similar result was obtained with only 1 mg/kg brodifacoum. It was shown that, in warfarin-resistant and warfarin-sensitive rats, brodifacoum produced the same rate of degradation of prothrombin complex activity as warfarin and significantly reduced the activity of clotting factors II, VII, IX, and X without affecting factor V. It was also demonstrated that brodifacoum has the same mechanism of action as warfarin: reduction of vitamin K-dependent clotting factor synthesis by interruption of the vitamin K-epoxide cycle (Leck and Park, 1981). In mongrel dogs, the elimination of brodifacoum follows a classical experimental decay with a distributive half-life of 1.4 days and an elimination half-life phase of 8.7 days (Murphy *et al.*, 1985).

Factors Influencing Toxicity Pretreatment of rats daily by intraperitoneal injection of phenobarbital at 80 mg/kg for 2 consecutive days followed by a single administration of brodifacoum at 0.2 mg/kg by stomach tube reduced the anticoagulant effects, although the reduction was less marked than in the case of warfarin (Bachmann and Sullivan, 1983). It is also known that a very large number of drugs of different chemical structures can interact with coumarin anticoagulant therapy in humans (Koch-Weser and Sellers, 1971).

Pathology Necropsies of poisoned dogs have shown that, in addition to large collections of unclotted blood, a number of lesions were also present, including bile stasis with large amounts of brown pigment accumulated in the portal triads and in the macrophages of the periportal regions and congestion of the spleen with accumulation of golden brown pigment, believed to be hemosiderin, in the red pulp (Stowe *et al.*, 1983).

Treatment of Poisoning in Animals Treatment should be as for other anticoagulant rodenticides: vitamin K_1 at dosage of 2.5–5.0 mg/kg and transfusion of fresh whole blood. Because of the long-lasting effect of brodifacoum, vitamin K therapy must be continued for at least 2–3 weeks.

19.5.4.3 Toxicity to Humans

Brodifacoum has not been used therapeutically in humans. Cases of attempted suicide have been reported. A 31-year-old mentally disturbed woman ingested over a 2-day period approximately thirty 50-gm packages of Talon® (approximately 75 mg of brodifacoum). Two days later she was brought to the hospital's psychiatric unit, without any physical signs or symptoms. The routine laboratory tests showed a prothrombin time of 72 sec (control, 12 sec) and an activated partial thromboplastin time greater than 100 sec (normal, 25–35 sec). In spite of prolonged administration of large amounts of vitamin K_1 and repeated infusion of fresh frozen plasma, the depression of the prothrombin complex activity persisted for more than 45 days after the ingestion (Lipton and Klass, 1984). Jones *et al.* (1984) have reported a similar case in a 17-year-old boy who attempted suicide by ingesting approximately 7.5 mg (0.12 mg/kg) brodifacoum. He was first seen for a gross hematuria, rapidly followed by epistaxis and gum bleeding. The prothrombin time and the activated partial thromboplastin time were considerably prolonged. The levels of plasma clotting factors II, VII, IX, and X were decreased. Factor V was normal. Vitamin K_1 and plasma therapy were instituted and had to be continued for 55 days until the patient's coagulation remained normal and stable.

Dosage Response From the two cases of poisoning reported above, it can be seen that the total doses ingested were in one case 75 mg and in the second one 7.5 mg and that the effects on the clotting factors were maximum in both cases, the clinical signs being almost absent in the woman who absorbed 75 mg of brodifacoum (although it was ingested over a 48-hr period). Therefore it would seem that, above a certain threshold, the response is maximum. This was also shown in rabbits given 1 and 10 mg/kg brodifacoum (Park and Leck, 1982). Murphy *et al.* (1985) have shown that in dogs serum concentrations below 12 mg/ml caused no measurable coagulopathic effects after cessation of vitamin K therapy.

Treatment of Poisoning Continued administration of vitamin K_1 for periods of several weeks with regular monitoring of the coagulation parameters is necessary. In the early phase of the poisoning, infusion of fresh-frozen plasma is advisable.

19.5.5 CHLOROPHACINONE

19.5.5.1 Identity, Properties, and Uses

Chemical Name 2-[4-Chlorophenyl)phenylacetyl]-1*H*-indene-1,3(2*H*)-dione.

Structure See Fig. 19.3.

Synonyms Chlorophacinone is the approved common name (BSI, ISO). Trade names for the formulated products include Caid®, Liphadione®, Raviac®, Drat®, Quick®, Lepit®, Rozol®, and Saviac®. The CAS registry number is 3691-35-8.

Physical and Chemical Properties Chlorophacinone has the empirical formula $C_{23}H_{15}ClO_3$ and a molecular weight of 364.8. It forms a yellow crystalline solid with a melting point of 140°C. It is slightly soluble in water (100 mg/liter at 20°C) and soluble in acetone, ethanol, and methanol. It is stable under normal storage conditions and noncorrosive.

History, Formulations, and Uses Chlorophacinone is an anticoagulant rodenticide used to control rats, mice, voles, and other wild rodents. It is formulated as ready-to-use baits based on whole, cracked, or milled grain at concentrations of active ingredient ranging from 0.005 to 0.25%. It can also be used as a tracking powder. An oil concentrate is also available.

19.5.5.2 Toxicity to Laboratory Animals

The acute oral LD 50 is reported to be 2 mg/kg in the rat, 1 mg/kg in the mouse, and 50 mg/kg in the rabbit. In the duck, the oral LD 50 is 100 mg/kg. Chlorophacinone is of low acute toxicity to wild birds (LD 50 of 430 mg/kg). The acute dermal LD 50 in the rabbit is 200 mg/kg (Sax, 1984). It is absorbed through the skin of the rabbit; a solution of 5 mg in 2 ml of liquid paraffin applied to 100 Cm² of shaved skin of a rabbit caused a slight reduction of prothrombin (Worthing and Walker, 1983). Administration of 15 daily doses of 2.25 mg to gray partridges produced no detectable ill-effects. Chlorophacinone is not an eye or skin irritant.

Absorption, Distribution, Metabolism, and Excretion Chlorophacinone is absorbed through the gastrointestinal tract. After oral administration, 90% is eliminated in the feces within 48 hr in the form of metabolites (Hartley and Kidd, 1983).

Mode of Action Chlorophacinone is an anticoagulant agent depressing hepatic synthesis of prothrombin and clotting factors VII, IX, and X. Direct damage to capillary permeability occurs concurrently. The ultimate effect of these actions is to induce widespread internal hemorrhage. In addition, chlorophacinone is an uncoupler of oxidative phosphorylation. Unlike the coumarin derivatives, chlorophacinone may causes symptoms and signs of neurologic and cardiopulmonary injury in laboratory rats, which often lead to death before hemorrhage occurs. Chlo-rophacinone is characterized by its long-lasting depressive action on coagulation.

19.5.5.3 Toxicity to Humans

Chlorophacinone has not been used therapeutically. Only two reports of human intoxication are known. They both involve suicidal attempts. One of them concerns a 37-year-old woman who ingested about 250 ml of a 0.25% concentrate formulation (about 625 mg of chlorphacinone). Despite intensive therapy with vitamin K_1 (phytomenadione, natural form of vitamin K), the anticoagulant effect of chlorophacinone persisted for at least 45 days. An interesting fact is that it was discovered during this episode that the synthetic analog of vitamin K was ineffective (Murdoch, 1983). The second report concerns a 28-year-old man who ingested an unknown amount of a chlorophacinone-based rodenticide. Again, the most striking feature in this case was the unusually prolonged and severe anticoagulant effect, even under adequate therapy; it required 4 weeks for prothrombin level to come back to normal (Dusein *et al.*, 1984).

Treatment of Poisoning Intoxication by chlorophacinone is treated by massive and prolonged administration of natural vitamin K.

19.5.6 DIFENACOUM

19.5.6.1 Identity, Properties, and Uses

Chemical Name 3-[3-(1,1′-biphenyl)4-yl-1,2,3,4-tetrahydro-1-naphthalenyl]-4-hydroxy-2*H*-1-benzopyran-2-one.

Structure See Fig. 19.4.

Synonyms Difenacoum is the approved common name. Trade names include Neosorexa® and Ratak®. The CAS registry number is 56073-07-5.

Physical and Chemical Properties Difenacoum has the empirical formula $C_{31}H_{24}O_3$ had a molecular weight of 444.5. It is an off-white powder with a melting point of 215–219°C. It is slightly soluble in water (less than 10 mg/liter at pH 7) and soluble in organic solvents (50 g/liter in acetone and chloroform and 600 mg/liter in benzene).

History, Formulations, and Uses The rodenticidal properties of difenacoum were first described in 1975. It is formulated as a 1 gm/kg concentrate and as a ready-to-use bait containing 50 mg of active ingredient per kilogram of bait. It is an indirect anticoagulant, more potent than the early compounds. It is used to control rats and mice resistant to other anticoagulants with varying degrees of activity.

19.5.6.2 Toxicity to Laboratory Animals

The oral LD 50 is 1.8 mg/kg in male rats, 0.8 mg/kg in male mice, and 50 mg/kg in female guinea pigs. The LD 50 value for

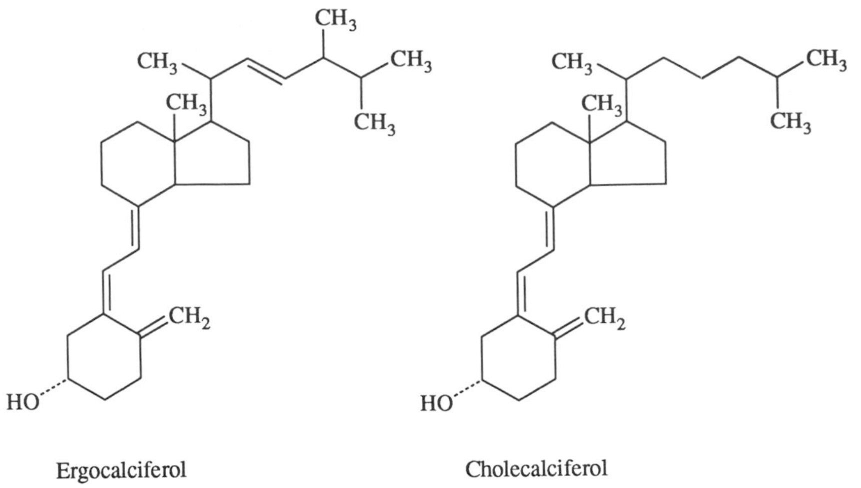

Figure 19.5 Two forms of vitamin D used as rodenticides.

oral administration in pigs is reported to be above 80 mg/kg and it is 100 mg/kg in cats. The acute dermal LD 50 is 50 mg/kg in rats and 1000 mg/kg in rabbits. The cumulative oral LD 50 in male rats over a 5-day period is 0.16 mg/kg/day.

Difenacoum and brodifacoum have been suspected of being responsible for secondary toxicity in barn owls feeding on rodents poisoned by these "second-generation" anticoagulants, a phenomenon which was not seen with warfarin baits (Wenz, 1984).

Biochemical Effects Like brodifacoum and warfarin, difenacoum was shown to inhibit vitamin K-dependent steps in the synthesis of clotting factors II, VII, IX, and X, and it is suspected that coumarin anticoagulants block the vitamin K_1 epoxide cycle by inhibiting the vitamin K_1 epoxide reductase. The latter is confirmed by the observation that difenacoum and brodifacoum produce an accumulation of tritiated vitamin K_1 epoxide in rats and rabbits administered tritiated vitamin K_1 (Park and Leck, 1982). Like brodifacoum, difenacoum has a much longer duration of action than warfarin.

Treatment of Poisoning in Animals Prolonged administration of vitamin K_1 over several weeks is the treatment of choice. Since the effect of vitamin K_1 is usually delayed as it only permits the formation of new prothrombin, initial treatment with transfusion of fresh-frozen plasma or a small quantity of matched fresh blood is recommended in order to provide enough prothrombin to prevent further hemorrhage (Park and Leck, 1982; Barlow *et al.*, 1982).

19.5.6.3 Toxicity to Humans

A case of an attempted suicide in a 17-year-old girl is reported in the literature. She was admitted to hospital having ingested 500 gm of the rat bait Neosorexa or about 25 mg of difenacoum. Upon admission she had a prolonged prothrombin time. She was treated with vitamin K_1 for 45 days. The clotting activity returned to normal 30 days after the beginning of treatment (Barlow *et al.*, 1982).

Treatment of Poisoning In case of threatening hemorrhage, transfusion of fresh blood or fresh-frozen plasma is the initial step. Intravenous and oral administration of vitamin K_1 for a prolonged period of time (several weeks) with regular monitoring of coagulation is necessary.

19.6 VITAMIN D-RELATED COMPOUNDS

19.6.1 ERGOCALCIFEROL

19.6.1.1 Identity, Properties, and Uses

Chemical Name 9,10-Secoergosta-5,7,10(19),22-tetraen-3-ol.

Structure See Fig. 19.5.

Synonyms The common name calciferol is approved by BPC (British Pharmacopeia Commission), ergocalciferol by USP (U.S. Pharmacopeia). It is also known as vitamin D_2, but for safety reasons it is prohibited in some countries to mention the identity of these compounds as vitamin D on rodenticide labels [Food and Agriculture Organization (FAO), 1979]. Other names include activated ergosterol, De-rat Concentrate®, Deratol®, and Hi-Deratol®. The trade name is Sorexa C.R.® for a combination of calciferol and warfarin.

Physical and Chemical Properties The empirical formula is $C_{28}H_{44}O$ and the molecular weight is 396.63. It forms colorless prismatic crystals. The melting point is 115–118°C. It is insoluble in water and soluble in most organic solvents; solubility at 7°C is 69.5 g/liter in acetone. It is slightly soluble in vegetable oils. Deterioration of pure, crystalline vitamin D_2 is negligible after storage for 9 months in evacuated amber ampules at refrigerator temperature. However, calciferol tends to decompose in the presence of air and moisture. The stability of corn oil solutions is, however, satisfactory (Greaves *et al.*. 1974).

History, Formulations, and Uses   The rodenticidal properties of calciferol were described by Greaves *et al.* (1974). The commercial rodenticide was introduced in the United Kingdom in 1974 as a combination of calciferol and warfarin formulated as a ready-to-use bait on canary seed (1 gm of calciferol and 250 mg of warfarin per kilogram). It is also available as an oil concentrate (20 gm/liter). Calciferol is used as a rodenticide for control of commensal rats and mice. Toxicity tests with calciferol combined with warfarin suggest that an additive effect between the compounds could exist. One interesting advantage of calciferol is that it is toxic to warfarin-resistant rodents. A second advantage is that it kills more rapidly—within 1 week instead of the 1–3 weeks that are often required with anticoagulants (Greaves *et al.*, 1974).

19.6.1.2 Toxicity to Laboratory Animals

Basic Findings   The acute oral LD 50 of calciferol is 56 mg/kg for rats and 23.7 mg/kg for mice. When administered daily for 5 consecutive days to laboratory rats, the LD 50 falls to 7 mg/kg/day. Lethal doses have also been reported by Gill and Redfern (1979) for the multimammate rat *Mastomys natalensis;* they range from 78 to 107 mg/kg (mean 96 mg/kg) in males and from 108 to 137 mg/kg (mean 119) in females when administered for 1 day at a concentration of 0.1% in bait. Similar values were reported by Greaves *et al.* (1974) for wild rodents. When calciferol was given at doses of 100 mg/kg by stomach tube on one or more days, laboratory rats and mice became visibly ill within 3 days. The clinical signs are characterized by loss of appetite, listlessness, piloerection, hunched position, absence of reaction to external stimuli, weight loss, priapism, and frequent micturition (Gillman *et al.*, 1960).

Absorption, Distribution, Metabolism, and Excretion   The action of calciferol is to raise blood calcium levels by stimulating the absorption of calcium from the intestine and mobilizing skeletal reserves. This mechanism is slow and takes many hours to build up an effective level; the period of latency between the ingestion of calciferol and the development of hypercalcemia and occurrence of lethal lesions is of the order of several days, usually 4 or 5 (Greaves *et al.*, 1974).

Calciferol has a long biological half-life in mammals and hypercalcemia induced by overdosage may continue for 6–9 months (Buckle *et al.*, 1972). The various tissues of the body store vitamin D for varying periods. The depletion of stores in the body is caused partly by its fecal excretion and partly by its destruction in the body.

Biochemical Effects   Caciferol is the most important factor for the optimal absorption of calcium. It is responsible for the synthesis of a protein that binds calcium in the intestinal mucosa, especially in the duodenum. In the absence of calciferol, calcium cannot be absorbed.

Effects on Organs and Tissues   All forms of vitamin D are toxic when given in sufficiently large amounts. Excessive doses of calcifeol mobilize the phosphorus and calcium from the tissues, thus broadly having an opposite effect to normal doses. The soft tissues tend to become calcified while the bone tends to be rarefied.

The soft tissues most affected are the renal tubules and the media of the small renal arteries and of the large vessels, especially the aorta. The bronchi, lungs, heart and coronaries, and stomach also are affected. In dogs, there is atrophy of the testes and the prostate while the parathyroids are smaller than normal. The histochemical effects of vascular injuries induced by calciferol orally administered to male and female Wistar rats for 5 consecutive days at doses ranging from 25,000 to 150,000 IU (1 mg of calciferol is equivalent to 40,000 IU) were studied by Gillman *et al.* (1960). By day 15 of the experiment—that is, day 10 after the last day of calciferol administration—necrosis of the spleen was observed in many rats that died or were sacrificed. Among the survivors, there were indications that the damaged spleen had regenerated completely by day 25. The heart was severely injured very early in the experiments. Similarly, the coronary arteries were observed showing early dilation, injury to the internal elastic membranes, and associated early calcification. These changes were associated with sclerotic repair. In the aorta, there was an apparent relationship between the intensity of the reaction and the doses of calciferol received by the rats. By day 20, a very large concentration of calcium accumulated in the aorta (13–14% calcium compared to 22% in the femur). Similar observations were made by Grant *et al.* (1963), who also showed that this phenomenon was a three-step process involving early widespread alterations in many organs and tissues, followed by spontaneous recurrent resolution and reappearance of calcification for many months, even after a single episode of acute intoxication. These authors also showed distinct differences in the time of onset and rate and extent of calcification of various tissues.

Nikodemusz *et al.* (1981) have shown that in six male and six female common vole (*Microtus arvalis*), single acute oral dosing with calciferol (80–620 mg/kg) induced morphological changes representing varying degrees of parenchymal degeneration and calcification in the kidneys, lungs, and heart. Calcium deposits were observed in the esophageal and gastric mucosae, as well as in the aortic media. These lesions were not observed in the group receiving 80 mg/kg of calciferol. The approximate lethal dose by the oral route was estimated as 120 mg/kg in males and 280 mg/kg in females. The survival time ranged from 53 to 94 hr. Tarrant and Westlake (1984) have also shown that feeding laboratory-reared male rats (*Rattus norvegicus*) and male and female quail (*Coturnix coturnix japonica*) a diet containing 0.1% calciferol (the recommended field concentration) for 2 days induced in both species a similar pattern of calcium deposits in the kidneys, beginning on the second day after the animals were returned to a standard, calciferol-free diet.

Effects on Reproduction   Adult female New Zealand White rabbits had been intramuscularly treated with ergosterol in cottonseed oil in divided doses every other day for a total of 1.5 million IU. Three other groups of five rabbits each received intramuscular injections of ergosterol daily for the duration of the gestational period for a total of 2.5–3.5 million and 4.5 million IU. At autopsy all the females given 2.5 million IU and above died spontaneously within 65 days after their first injection of calciferol and all that were pregnant aborted during the first 12 days of pregnancy or delivered macerated fetuses. All aortas had various degrees of pathological changes, including those from females treated with 1.5 million IU. A total of 14 abnormalities of the aorta were observed in the 34 offspring whose mothers had been treated with excessive levels of ergocalciferol. Aortic lesions that appeared similar to the supravalvular aortic stenosis seen in humans were noted in six rabbits. The blood levels of ergocalciferol in the mothers and their offspring were seven and nine times greater than those in the control classes and their offspring, respectively, indicating that transplacental passage occurred (Friedman and Roberts, 1966). A similar experiment was carried out by Friedman and Mills (1969) on 15 pregnant New Zealand White rabbits given divided doses of intramuscular ergocalciferol every other day, starting on the second day of insemination and throughout the pregnancy for a total of 750,000 IU. Characteristic malformations were observed in the offspring. These were represented by premature closure of cranial structures, small skulls compared with the controls, and narrowing of the body of the mandible. The maxillary and mandibular central incisors showed severe enamel hypoplasia. Some cases of anodontia and abnormal palatal shape were noted. Similar craniofacial malformations are frequently associated with supravalvular aortic stenosis in children.

Several additional studies of the effects of vitamin D on reproduction and fetal development in rats and rabbits have been reported. Latore (1961) found that excess ergocalciferol reduces fertility in rats when administered on days 0–7 of gestation but not when administered on days 8–21. Nebel and Ornstein (1966) have demonstrated that ergocalciferol administered to rats (*Rattus rattus*) in daily doses of 20,000 IU for 1–3 weeks significantly affected the genital cycle, fertility, and early pregnancy from both the morphological and functional points of view in direct relation to the beginning and duration of ergocalciferol administration. Ornoy *et al.* (1968) showned that vitamin D_2 (ergocalciferol) given to pregnant albino rats at daily doses of 4000, 20,000, or 40,000 IU, from day 9 to day 21 of pregnancy crosses the placental barrier and induces alterations of the mineral composition of the fetal bones at the 40,000 IU level only. In the same treated group, placentas, fetuses, and fetal bones were found to be smaller than those in the untreated groups. However, it seems from the experimental data that pregnant rats are more tolerant to rather high levels of ergocalciferol than nonpregnant females (Potvliege, 1962; Ornoy *et al.*, 1968).

Factors Influencing Toxicity   In commercially available preparations, calciferol is often associated with warfarin in a 4 : 1 ratio because it has been shown that this mixture produced a marked increase in mortality in Norway rats (Greaves *et al.*,

1974), thus suggesting an additive effect of the two compounds. At the LD 50 level, toxicity of the mixture is intermediate between the toxicities of calciferol and warfarin.

Treatment of Poisoning in Animals   It seems that the only case of poisoning of a domestic animal reported is that of a 4-year-old boxer dog seen several days following ingestion of a warfarin–calciferol mixture. Despite treatment with vitamin K, antibiotics, and vitamins, the end of the tongue became necrotic and had to be removed and large areas of the skin were also necrosed, indicating generalized vascular damage. The dog made a slow recovery (Edlin, 1982). It is likely that treatment with vitamin K had prevented the hemorragic manifestations of warfarin toxicity from showing but that the vascular injuries due to calciferol were responsible for the necrotic effects.

19.6.1.3 Toxicity to Humans

Therapeutic Use   As a vitamin, calciferol is used to prevent and to cure rickets, tetany, spasmophilia, and osteoporomalacia. Several decades ago, vitamin D was recommended for the treatment of lupus vulgaris (skin tuberculosis limited to the face); massive doses were used, sufficient to provoke a mild degree of hypervitaminosis. The purpose was to induce calcification of the subcutaneous lesions in order to stop their progression. In the case of rickets, the recommended preventive dose was 500–1500 IU/day, and the curative dose was 1000–3000 IU/day; it was estimated that 10,000 IU represents a toxic dose. The minimal toxic overdose does not appear to be many times greater than the optimum curative dose (Harris, 1955).

Many cases of vitamin D_2 as well as D_3 poisoning in humans have been reported. The oldest ones were analyzed by Bicknell and Prescott (1953). More recent cases have been reported, all related to accidental or inadvertent overdosing. A 69-year-old woman with hypoparathyroidism was treated with a twice-weekly dose of 50,000 IU of calciferol. However, for 4 weeks before admission to hospital she had mistakenly taken 300,000 IU (7.5 mg) a day. On examination she was lethargic and mentally confused, with muscular hypotonia. In this report two other similar cases concerning elderly women are reported; one had received 100,000 IU (2.5 mg) calciferol orally on alternate days for 3 months and the other had received 400,000 IU (10 mg) a day by mouth and 600,000 IU of calciferol once a week by injection during the 2 months before admission to the hospital. All three patients had elevated serum calcium. All three of them were treated with intravenous injections of porcine calcitonin, which caused serum calcium to fall back to a normal level within 2–3 days (Buckle *et al.*, 1972). Davies and Adams (1978) have also reported eight cases of severe vitamin D poisoning. In six patients the therapy was unnecessary, and in two others inadequate supervision of treatment resulted in overdosage. Paterson (1980) reported 21 cases of hypercalcemia due to vitamin D poisoning; among them two patients died while intoxicated. Overall, the clinical symptoms induced by chronic poisoning include, in various associations and intensity, loss of appetite, loss of weight greater than would be expected from the loss of appetite, nausea, vomiting, and constipation or diarrhea. Abdominal pain may be so severe as to lead to unnecessary laparotomies. Headaches are usual and one special form has been noticed. This is a tightness across the back of the head which goes on to acute sensitiveness of the scalp. Mental confusion and loss of memory may also be seen. Epileptiform fits are a rare complication. Metastatic calcification has been described along with vascular and renal calcification. An unusual, albeit typical case has been reported by Cohen *et al.* (1979): a case of deafness due to a long-term overdosage for the treatment of pseudohypoparathyroidy (2.5 mg of calciferol daily for 4 years). The patient had a 3-month history of deafness, weight loss, anorexia, and weakness. She had extensive calcification of the tympanic membranes, corneas, kidneys, and blood vessels. She had also, of course, high serum calcium, which was successfully treated with calcitonin and prednisolone and a low-calcium diet. She was discharged from hospital symptom-free except for the deafness. Hypercalcemia is the earliest sign of vitamin D overdosage. It was suggested at one point that increased intake of vitamin D through consumption of fish liver in Norway might be correlated with an increased probability of myocardial infarction (Linden, 1974). However, this hypothesis, based on a retrospective study of a number of patients with myocardial infarction, angina pectoris, and degenerative joint diseases, was later criticized because of serious bias and shortcomings in the methodology (Lindahl and Lindwall, 1975). A prospective study, performed in the same area of northern Norway, has not confirmed the existence of a higher risk of myocardial infraction related to vitamin D intake or status of the population (Vik *et al.*, 1979).

Use Experience and Dosage Response   There is no known report of accidents occurring with calciferol used as a rodenticide. It is difficult to estimate the minimum toxic dose in humans; however, from the reported cases of overdosage, it would seem that 0.15 mg/kg/day for 3 weeks may lead to clinical signs of poisoning.

Treatment of Poisoning   Treatment of acute and chronic overdosages with calciferol requires that hypercalcemia be brought down to a normal level quickly; intravenous injection of calcitonin is the specific treatment to be applied under close monitoring of the serum calcium level. Steroid therapy is also often effective but slower, normocalcemia being achieved after 5–7 days. Other methods are available but they are not devoid of problems: Chelation with sodium edetate is only temporary in its effect and is nephrotoxic. Sodium phosphate is also effective but may be responsible for metastatic calcifications (Buckle *et al.*, 1972). One case of vitamin D_2 poisoning in an elderly woman was successfully treated by inducing the hepatic microsomal enzymes with 500 mg/day of glutethimide. The mechanism of action is still unknown (Iqbal and Taylor, 1982), but this approach is rather slow since the serum calcium level did not fall back to normal values until day 12 of treatment.

19.6.2 CHOLECALCIFEROL

19.6.2.1 Identity, Properties, and Uses

Chemical   Name   9,10-Secocholesta-5,7,10(19)-trien-3-betaol.

Structure   See Fig. 19.5.

Synonyms   Activated 7-dehydrocholesterol, oleovitamin D_3, cholecalciferol natural vitamin D_3. The trade name for the rodenticide is Quintox®.

Physical and Chemical Properties   The empirical formula is $C_{27}H_{44}O$ and the molecular weight is 384.62. It forms fine needles. The melting point is 84–85°C. It is practically insoluble in water, soluble in the usual organic solvents, and only slightly soluble in vegetable oils. It is oxidized and inactivated by moist air within a few days. However, the formulated product is stable over 1 year at ambient temperatures in sealed packages.

History, Formulations, and Uses   Cholecalciferol is formulated for use as a rodenticide as a grain bait containing 750 ppm (0.075%) of active ingredient and commercialized under the trade name Quintox®. It is a single-feeding and multifeeding rodenticide used for controlling anticoagulant-resistant rats and mice. There is a period of time between feeding and death similar to but perhaps shorter than that observed with anticoagulant rodenticides. The rodenticidal activity of cholecalciferol is comparable to that of ergocalciferol.

19.6.2.2 Toxicity to Laboratory Animals

The two forms of calciferol are equally toxic to most mammals. The acute oral LD 50 of cholecalciferol is 43.6 mg/kg for *Rattus norvegicus* and 42.5 mg/kg for mice (*Mus musculus*). In the dog the oral LD 50 is 88 mg/kg.

Absorption, Distribution, and Excretion   Cholecalciferol after absorption from the intestine is transported to the liver, where it is metabolized to 25-hydroxycholecalciferol by an NADPH-dependent reaction. This metabolite is then transferred to the kidney and converted to 24-, 25-, or 1,25-dihydrocholecaliferol by mitochondrial mixed-function oxidases (McClain *et al.*, 1980). After their intestinal absorption, ergocalciferol (vitamin D_2) and cholecalciferol (vitamin D_3) undergo an identical metabolic C pathway (Fournier *et al.*, 1985). The metabolism and pharmacokinetics of one metabolite of cholecalciferol, 24,25-dihydrocholecalciferol, have been reviewed by Jarnargin *et al.* (1985); the excretion curve shows an initial fast phase with a plasma half-life of 0.55 hr and a second slow phase with a plasma half-life of 73.8 hr in the rat. The clearance from plasma, liver, and kidney but not intestine follows a two-compartment model. The most potent form of vitamin D_3, 1,25-dihydrocholecalciferol, has been shown to be responsible for the stimulation of intestinal absorption of calcium and the metabolism of calcium in bone. However, Frolick and Deluca (1973) have shown that, when given orally to rats, 1,25-dihydrocholecalciferol is rapidly modified during its passage through the intestine, thus reducing its physiological activity to a large extent.

Effects on Organs and Tissues Moderately excessive doses of cholecalciferol, 100, 300, 2000, and 4000 IU/kg of feed, given for 4 months to experimental Yorkshire pigs rapidly produced gross arterial lesions (fibromuscular interstitial thickening of the coronaries, especially at the branching sites). Macrophages, plasma cells, and mast cells were observed to accumulate in the subendothelial space. The extent of these lesions, resembling those commonly seen in atherosclerosis in humans, was more or less dose-related (Toda *et al.*, 1985). Since both forms of vitamin D (ergocalciferol and cholecalciferol) follow the same metabolic pathway, it is expected that they are responsible for inducing the same lesions.

Effects on Reproduction Calcitriol (1,25-dihydrocholecalciferol), which is the most biologically active metabolite of cholecalciferol, has been administered to pregnant rats and rabbits at daily doses of 0.02–0.08 and 0.30 μg/kg from days 7–15 of gestation in the rat and from days 7–18 in the rabbit. In rats no adverse effect on fertility, litter parameters, and offspring was observed. Hypercalcemia and hypophosphatemia were observed in pregnant rats of the middle and high-dose groups, as well as hypercalcemia in pups. Calcitriol induced maternal mortality and fetotoxicity in rabbits treated with 0.3 μg/kg/day. Two litters at the highest dose and one litter at the middle dose levels contained fetuses with multiple abnormalities (McClain *et al.*, 1980).

19.6.2.3 Toxicity to Humans

Experimental Oral Exposure The active metabolite 1,25-dihydrocholecalciferol was administered either orally or intravenously to four healthy volunteers and three patients with hypoparathyroidism. After an oral dose, the highest serum concentration of radioactivity was reached after 4 hr. The route of administration had little apparent effect on the serum concentration or on the rapid phase of elimination, but the slow phase of excretion was longer after oral administration. The highest urinary excretion rate was observed during the first 24 hr and was little affected by the route of administration. The half-life of 1,25-dihydrocholecalciferol was 3–5 days. On average, 40% of the dose of 1,25-dihydrocholecalciferol was excreted within 10 days (Mawer *et al.*, 1976).

Therapeutic Use Cholecalciferol being the natural form of vitamin D, the therapeutic uses are those outlined for ergocalciferol.

Accidents and Use Experience These are the same as those mentioned for ergocalciferol. There is no known report of an

Figure 19.6 Miscellaneous synthetic organic rodenticides.

accident specifically attributable to cholecalciferol used as a rodenticide. However, intoxication from overdosage during therapeutic use of vitamin D₃ is well known and signs and symptoms have been well studied (Navarro *et al.*, 1985).

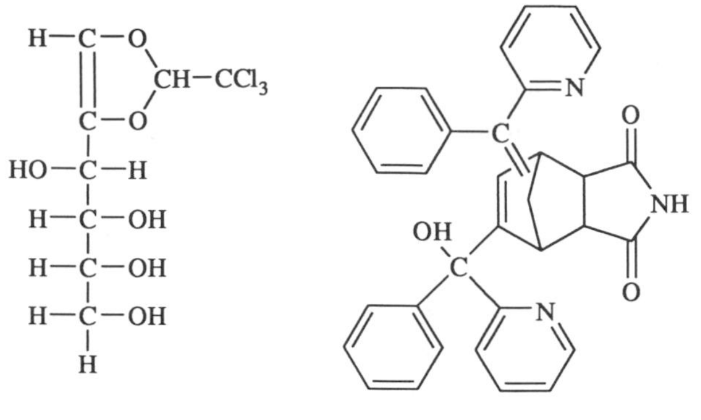

19.7 MISCELLANEOUS SYNTHETIC ORGANIC RODENTICIDES

As far as is known, the miscellaneous synthetic organic rodenticides (see Fig. 19.6) are unrelated to one another or to other groups of pesticides either pharmacologically or chemically. The two that have been studied in humans are remarkable. Chloralose is an anesthetic, albeit one with the property of inducing myoclinic seizures. With the possible exception of this compound, anesthetics have nothing to offer for killing vertebrate pests. Far too many animals become anesthetized before consuming a fatal dose, and they later recover. In fact, the possibility of recovery seems to be taken into account in the British practice of recovering birds affected by the compound.

Norbormide is of interest as one of the most selective poisons known. Its limitation is not any lack of toxicity to species of the genus *Rattus* but the problem of secondary bait refusal (Greaves, 1966).

19.7.1 CHLORALOSE

19.7.1.1 Identity, Properties, and Uses

Chemical Name 1,2-*O*-(2,2,2-Trichloroethylidene)-α-D-glucofuranose.

Structure See Fig. 19.6.

Synonyms Chloralose (BSI) is the common name in use. Other nonproprietary names include α-chloralose. α-D-glucochloralose, anhydroglucochloral, chloroalosane, and glucochloral. Trade names include Alphakil® and Somio®. The CAS registry number is 15879-93-3.

Physical and Chemical Properties Chloralose has the empirical formula $C_8H_{11}Cl_3O_6$ and a molecular weight of 309.54. It forms a crystalline powder that melts at 187°C. It is soluble in ether and glacial acetic acid, slightly soluble in chloroform, and almost insoluble in petroleum ether. Its solubility in water at 15°C is 0.44%. Chloralose reduces Fehling's solution only after prolonged heating. It is hydrolyzed into its two components by acids.

History, Formulations, and Uses Chloralose has been in use in Europe for many years. Its narcotic properties are employed to immobilize depredating birds and render them easier to kill by other means. Baits contain about 1.5% of the compound.

It has been reported that chloralose is also used on seed grain as a bird repellent. It is used against mice in baits of up to 40 gm/kg. All baits should contain a warning dye.

Chloralose is used in medicine as a soporific and formerly was used as an anesthetic.

19.7.1.2 Toxicity to Laboratory Animals

The oral LD 50 values of chloralose in rats and mice are in the range of 300–400 mg/kg. Cats are more susceptible (100 mg/kg) and dogs more resistant (600–1000 mg/kg) (Cornwell, 1969). The compound is more toxic to many birds than to mammals. Oral LD 50 values have been determined for the starling (75 mg/kg), redwing blackbird (32 mg/kg), yellow-headed blackbird (133 mg/kg), crow (42 mg/kg), pigeon (178 mg/kg), house finch (56 mg/kg), house sparrow (42 mg/kg), mallard duck (42 mg/kg), mourning dove (42 mg/kg), and white-crowned sparrow (56 mg/kg) (Schafer, 1972).

Hanriot and Richet, who advocated chloralose as a soporific, found that dogs survived oral dosages as high as 610 mg/kg but were killed by dosages of 660 mg/kg and greater. Cats survived oral dosages of 65 mg/kg or lower but one was killed by a dosage of 71 mg/kg and all were killed by 140 mg/kg or more. Dogs survived intravenous injection of 120 mg/kg or less but were killed by 150 mg/kg. A dosage of 12.5 mg/kg produced severe symptoms in a cat (Hanriot and Richet, 1897).

After some delay, animals poisoned by chloralose show incoordination, vertigo, tremor, and failure to recognize objects. The sense of pain is lost but there is increased reactivity to touch, sound, or electric shock. If stimulated, the animals respond reflexively and with full force. If artificial respiration is withheld, animals that have received a sufficient dosage die of repiratory failure (Hanriot and Richet, 1897). Thus it was recognized very early that although response to chloralose is somewhat similar to that to chloral, it is also similar to the response to strychnine in the sensitization to external stimuli.

Chloralose is metabolized to chloral, $CH(OH)_2$—CCl_3 (Cornwell, 1969), oxidized to trichloroacetic acid, and reduced to trichloroethanol (Marshall and Owens, 1954; Owens and Marshall, 1955). The latter metabolite is responsible for much of the hypnotic effect of chloral hydrate; all tissues studied so far are capable of forming it from chloral hydrate (Butler, 1949). Trichloroethanol combines with glucuronic acid in the liver to form the pharmacologically inactive urochloralic acid, which is readily excreted in the urine (Lees, 1972).

Chloralose was not tumorigenic in two strains of mice that received it at the highest tolerated level for 18 months (Innes *et al.*, 1969).

Treatment of Poisoning in Animals Administration of analeptic drugs or stimulants of the central nervous system such as methylamphetamine (0.5–4 mg/kg of body weight, orally or intramuscularly) or ephedrine (2.5 mg/kg of body weight subcutaneously) has been recommended and successfully applied in poisoned dogs (Bennett, 1972, Smith and Boyd, 1972), although this had already been criticized (Shepherd, 1971) on pharmacological and biochemical grounds. In addition, supportive therapy to correct any hypothermia and respiratory problems may be indicated in severely poisoned animals.

19.7.1.3 Toxicity to Humans

Therapeutic Use Chloralose was introduced in 1888 and 1893 as an anesthetic and soporific. Its anesthetic use was soon dropped, presumably because an effective dosage tended to cause excessive muscular activity. However, this same feature was regarded as an advantage in connection with a soporific. Thus Sollman (1901) considered chloralose preferable to chloral except for insomnia due to exaggerated reflex irritability. He pointed out that chloralose is a stronger hypnotic. heightens the reflexes, has less action on the heart, and produces practically no local irritation.

Chloralose has gone out of fashion in the United States because its action is somewhat delayed compared to that of chloral (Sollman, 1942) and perhaps because activation of reflexes was not considered an appropriate property of a soporific.

Accidental and Intentional Poisoning Most reported cases of poisoning by chloralose have occurred in France, where the compound is used medically as a soporific and sedative and also used as a poison to kill crows and rats. Tempé and Kurtz (1972) listed 60 brands of poison based on chloralose, of which 31 also contained ANTU (see Section 19.4.1.3). In their series of 22 acute intoxications by chloralose, only one was caused by the compound intended for use as a drug; the others were caused by rat poisons.

Most cases of poisoning have involved attempted—generally unsuccessful—suicide. A few cases of mild accidental poisoning of children have been recorded (Gaultier *et al.*, 1962).

The characteristic effect of chloralose is coma, which may be preceded by vomiting, vertigo, trembling, and a sensation of inebriation. In massive intoxication, the coma may appear in some minutes but usually appears in one to several hours after ingestion of chloralose (Favarel-Garrigues and Boget, 1968; Tempé and Kurtz, 1972). The patient may be calm and limp or may be agitated. Cornette and Franck (1970) saw only cases in agitated coma with varying degrees of myoclonia. The myoclonia was always reinforced by stimulation, and it occurred predominantly in the arm or leg that was stimulated. There was a bilateral, symmetrical seizure, occasionally with hypersalivation and incontinence of urine. However, tonic spasm or tonic clonic convulsions were not seen. These authors never encountered a case of hypotonic or "calm" coma seen by some others. They attributed the difference to better treatment, but it would seem difficult to exclude differences in dosage as a cause. Favarel-Garrigues and Boget (1968) specifically noted that this form of coma usually but not always occurred in massive intoxications, and one almost always saw hyperreactivity, clonic jerks, and a state of agitation in such cases during recovery. Tempé and Kurtz (1972) reported similar experience. The reflexes are active in agitated coma. In 9 of the 22 cases reported by Tempé and Kurtz (1972), 6 showed a positive Babinski test bilaterally. Reflexes are diminished or absent in massive intoxication.

Authors have not agreed on whether the most severe seizures caused by chloralose are truly epileptic (Moene *et al.*, 1969) or are bilateral, synchronous myoclonic disturbances (Cornette and Franck, 1970). That the latter view is correct seems to depend not on any difference in clinical severity but on a lack of correlation of the EEG with the physical disturbance.

Hypersecretion of the respiratory tract apparently is the most life-threatening aspect of intoxication. It may occur in the absence of ANTU but is more common and more severe when ANTU is involved. This hypersecretion may appear early, suddenly, and severely, but it also disappears in less than an hour. Unlike pulmonary edema, the secretion is not sanguineous, and it is poor in albumin. The mild appearance on X ray contrasts with the clinical severity (Favarel-Garrigues and Boget, 1968).

Even in the apparent absence of infection, the temperature may be elevated as high as 41°C (Moene *et al.*, 1969).

Reawakening requires several hours in mild poisoning, 12–14 hr in severe poisoning, and as much as 96 hr in massive poisoning. The return of consciousness may be gradual but usually is sudden and may be accompanied by headache, stiffness, and weakness. Recovery without sequelae is the rule (Favarel-Garriques and Boget, 1968; Tempé and Kurtz, 1972). Moene *et al.* (1969) reported a death caused by uncomplicated poisoning, but it is indicative of the toxicity of chloralose that the victim succeeded in his suicide with this compound only on his third attempt within a period of about 4 months. Death due to circulatory collapse occurred on the evening of the fifth hospital day.

Dosage Response Eleven patients, who were thought to have taken doses ranging from 640 to 2880 mg, all survived with appropriate treatment (Cornette and Franck, 1970). In another case involving chloralose intended as a rat poison, a dose thought to be 3000–4000 mg was survived (Boudouresque *et al.*, 1966). Other reports of nonfatal dosages have fallen within the range of 2000–9000 mg, but one kind of rat poison came in 20-gm packets and at least one person may have survived that dose. The dose in a fatal case was unknown (Moene *et al.*, 1969; Gras *et al.*, 1975). Tempé and Kurtz (1972) considered that toxic

signs could result from 400 mg but that most cases resulted from ingestion of about 1000 mg.

Laboratory Findings In two cases in which the dosage was known with considerable certainty, about 45% of the amount ingested was recovered from urines passed within the first 24 hr, about 90% in the form of the glucose conjugate (Gras *et al.*, 1975).

The EEG picture in acute poisoning by chloralose is characteristic, involving slow waves and numerous spikes that usually are bilaterally symmetrical and synchronous. The pattern is changed dramatically by diazepam, which converts it to delta activity without the rapid rhythms commonly seen with that medication. The tracing always becomes normal, often within 24 hr. The acute EEG record does not correspond to the myoclonic movements that, as observed visually or by EMG, are usually isolated, brief asymmetrical, and asynchronous (Boudouresque *et al.*, 1966; Cornette and Franck, 1970; Tempé and Kurtz, 1972).

Treatment of Poisoning The myoclonic seizures respond to intravenous injection of 10 mg of diazepam, but this may have to be repeated once or twice. Recovery without sequelae is the rule (Boudouresque *et al.*, 1966; Cornette and Franck, 1970; Tempé and Kurtz, 1972).

19.7.2 NORBORMIDE

19.7.2.1 Identity, Properties, and Uses

Chemical Name 6-(α-hydroxy-α-2-pyridylbenzyl)-7-(α-2-pyridylbenzylidene)-norbor-5-ene-2,3-dicarboximide.

Structure See Fig. 19.6.

Synonyms Norbormide (ANSI, BSI, ISO) is the common name for this compound. Trade names include Shoxin® and Raticate®. Code designations include McN-1,025 and S-6,999. The CAS registry number is 991-42-4.

Physical and Chemical Properties Norbormide has the empirical formula $C_{33}H_{25}N_3O_3$ and a molecular weight of 511.55. It is a white crystalline powder melting at 190–198°C. Its solubility at 30°C in ethanol is 14 mg/liter; in chloroform, more than 150 mg/liter; in diethyl ether, 1 mg/liter; and in 0.1 N HCl, 29 mg/liter. Norbormide is stable at room temperature and to boiling. It is hydrolyzed by alkali and is noncorrosive.

History, Formulations, and Uses Norbormide was introduced in 1964 by the McNeil Laboratories, Inc. It is a selective rodenticide, lethal to rats but not to other rodent species. It usually is concentrated in prepared baits of cereal at 5–10 gm/kg. Baits containing the compound should contain a warning dye.

19.7.2.2 Toxicity to Laboratory Animals

Basic Findings Norbormide shows a remarkable selectivity both in toxicity and in pharmacological effect. Oral LD 50 values for both wild and domestic Norway rats ranged from 5.3 to 15.0 mg/kg (Roszkowski et al., 1964; Roszkowski, 1965; Greaves, 1966; Niu, 1970). Corresponding values for roof rats and Hawaiian rats were 52 and about 10 mg/kg, respectively. Oral LD 50 values were much higher in other rodents and lagomorphs—for example, hamster, 140 mg/kg; guinea pig, 620 mg/kg; mouse, 2,250 mg/kg; and rabbit, about 1000 mg/kg. The oral toxicity was low in all other species tested; in the dog, cat, monkey, sheep, pig, and chicken no effect was detectable at 1000 mg/kg (Roszkowski et al., 1964; Roszkowski, 1965; Niu, 1970).

Rats given an overdose of norbormide died within 15 min to 4 hr. At first, the animals assumed a hunched position. Later there was locomotor impairment due to weakness but not paralysis of the hind legs. Struggling, labored breathing, and, in some instances, a mild convulsion preceded death (Roszkowski et al., 1964).

Many analogs have been studied and none found as toxic to rats as norbormide (Poos et al., 1966).

Dogs survived daily doses of norbormide corresponding to a dietary level of 10,000 ppm for 15–60 days, but they lost appetite and looked ill. Dogs tolerated a dosage corresponding to a dietary level of 1000 ppm for 60 days without ill effect (Roszkowski et al., 1964).

Even in laboratory rats, susceptibility to the compounds was greatly reduced when it was mixed into the diet rather than being given by stomach tube. This may be explained in part by tolerance. The oral LD 50 determined after a 1-day rest period was less than doubled in rats pretreated for 1–7 days at the rate of 2 mg/kg/day. The degree of tolerance was small, but it was statistically significant. When the rest period was 5 days, no tolerance remained (Roszkowski, 1965). In any event, primary bait refusal can be a very serious problem in the use of norbormide (Maddock and Schoff, 1967).

Mode of Action and Cause of Death Some sex and species differences in susceptibility could be explained by differences in metabolism or absorption. For example, the oral LD 50 values for male and female laboratory rats were 5.3 and 15.0 mg/kg, respectively, although the intravenous values (0.65 and 0.63 mg/kg, respectively) did not differ significantly. The very low susceptibility of mice to oral doses (LD 50, 2250 mg/kg) was due in part to poor absorption, as indicated by the intraperitoneal LD 50 of only 390 mg/kg. However, differences in absorption could not account for many observed species differences. For example, anesthetized dogs showed no detectable response to intravenous injection at the rate of 40 mg/kg.

Species differences in response of the peripheral blood vessels to norbormide seemed to account for most of the observed species differences in its toxicity. The compound caused an extreme, irreversible vasoconstriction in laboratory rats, and this was considered the cause of death. The effect was demonstrated by direct observation or flow experiments, or both, in the ear, eye, skin, mesentary, and heart and undoubtedly occurred in other organs. It resulted from either systemic or appropriate local administration. Only vessels of relatively small caliber were visibly constricted. Spiral rat aortic segments and duodenal strips did not respond to norbormide.

The mechanism of action was best demonstrated in the heart. Isolated myocardial strips showed no loss of contraction or responsiveness when norbormide was added to the bath. However, when norbormide was injected into the aorta of isolated rat hearts, the coronary flow rate decreased greatly and the heart slowed and developed arrhythmia. The effects were not inhibited or reversed by sodium nitrite or other vasodilators.

Following vasoconstriction and presumably as a result of vascular injury, an erythematous but not typically inflammatory lesion began to develop in the rat skin 6 hr after intradermal injection of 0.1 ml of 0.1% solution. The lesion became maximal in 24–48 hr. Sometimes an area of central necrosis was observed. A concentration of 0.01% produced the effect only inconsistently.

Except in rats, vasoconstriction was not seen even at high dosage levels. Why rats respond differently remains obscure (Roszkowski, 1965). A number of the observations just discussed were confirmed by Niu (1970), who reached the same general conclusion regarding the importance of vasoconstriction in the rat.

An oral or intraperitoneal dosage of 1020 mg/kg caused a doubling of blood glucose levels and a decrease of liver and muscle glycogen when coma began 0.5–2 hr after treatment. The same dosage had no effect on the glucose levels of two strains of mice, nor did it produce illness. Insulin counteracted the hyperglycemic effect of norbormide in rats but did not protect against toxic manifestations and death, suggesting that the hyperglycemia is secondary (Patil and Radhakrishnamurty, 1973).

19.7.2.3 Toxicity to Humans

Because the toxicity of norbormide to different species corresponds to its ability to cause peripheral vasoconstriction in them, it was a meaningful test to inject three volunteers intradermally with 0.1 ml of 0.1% solution. Skin treated in this way showed no response not seen in controls (Roszkowski, 1965).

In a study that has been cited for many years but apparently was first published by Hayes (1982), Dr. Kazwya Kamoya of the Showa Medical School in Tokyo administered norbormide to volunteers orally at doses ranging from 20 to 300 mg. No sign or symptom was produced. It was concluded that body temperature and blood pressure decreased slightly and temporarily following the larger doses. Actually, the largest fall in temperature observed at any dose was 0.7°C, and this occurred after doses of 20 and 80 mg, whereas the largest fall after a dose of 120 mg or more was only 0.3°C. Systolic (but not diastolic) blood pressure possibly fell after 120 mg of norbormide and certainly fell after larger doses. The largest decreases recorded were from 132/76 to 100/74 after 200 mg and from 120/80 to 96/80 after 300 mg. The lowest values were measured 1 hr after ingestion, and the values were essentially normal at 2 hr in each instance.

It seems unlikely that poisoning by norbormide will occur. If it does, treatment must be symptomatic.

REFERENCES

Allcroft, R., and Jones, J. S. L. (1969). Fluoroacetamide poisoning. I. Toxicity in dairy cattle: Clinical history and preliminary investigations. *Vet. Rec.* **84**, 399–402.

Allcroft, R., Salt, F. J., Peters, R. A., and Shorthouse, M. (1969). Fluoroacetamide poisoning. II. Toxicity in dairy cattle: Confirmation of diagnosis. *Vet. Rec.* **84**, 403–409.

American Medical Association (AMA) (1977). "AMA Drug Evaluations," 3rd ed. Publishing Sciences Group, Littleton, Massachusetts.

American Medical Association (AMA) (1980). "AMA Drug Evaluations," 4th ed. Am. Med. Assoc., Chicago, Illinois.

Annegers, J. F., and Zacharski, L. R. (1980). Cancer morbidity and mortality in previously anticoagulated patients. *Thromb. Res.* **18**, 399–403.

Anonymous (1962). Poisoning cases in 1960. *Pharm. J.* **189**, 453–455.

Anonymous (1964a). Fluoroacetamide. *Lancet* **1**, 442–443.

Anonymous (1964b). Fluoroacetamide. *Lancet* **1**, 759.

Anonymous (1966). A dangerous rodenticide. *Lancet* **2**, 1183.

Anonymous (1979). Pesticidal diabetes (editorial). *Br. Med. J.* **2**, 292–293.

Araki, S. (1972). Studies on organofluorine pesticides from the medico-legal viewpoint. *Jpn. J. Leg. Med.* **26**, 203–219 (in Japanese).

Bachmann, K. A., and Sullivan, T. J. (1983). Dispositional and pharmacodynamic characteristics of brodifacoum in warfarin-sensitive rats. *Pharmacology* **27**, 281–288.

Barker, W. M., Hermodson, M. A., and Link, K. P. (1970). The metabolism of 4-C^{14}-warfarin sodium by the rat. *J. Pharmacol. Exp. Ther.* **171**, 307–313.

Barlow, A. M., Gay, A. L., and Park, B. K. (1982). Difenacoum (Neosorexa) poisoning. *Br. Med. J.* **285**, 541.

Bartlett, G. R. (1952). The mechanism of action of monofluoroethanol. *J. Pharmacol. Exp. Ther.* **106**, 464–467.

Becker, M. H., Genieser, N. B., Finegold, M., Miranda, D., and Spacman, T. (1975). Chondrodysplasia punctata. Is maternal warfarin a factor? *Am. J. Dis. Child.* **129**, 356–359.

Bell, J. (1972). The acute toxicity of four common poisons to the opossum, *Trichosurus vulpecula. N. Z. Vet. J.* **20**, 212–214.

Bennett, D. (1972). Accidental poisoning in a retriever puppy by a new rodenticide. *Vet. Rec.* **91**, 609–610.

Benowitz, N. L., Byrd, R., Schambelan, M., Rosenberg, J., and Roizen, M. (1979). Rodenticide induced orthostatic hypotension and its successful management with dihydroergotamine. *Clin. Res.* **27**, 73a.

Bentley, E. W., and Greaves, J. H. (1960). Some properties of fluoroacetamide as a rodenticide. *J. Hyg.* **58**, 125–132.

Bernacki, R. J., and Bosmann, H. B. (1970). Warfarin and vitamin K accelerate protein and glycoprotein synthesis in isolated rat liver mitochondria *in vitro. Biochem. Biophys. Res. Commun.* **41**, 498–505.

Bicknell, F., and Prescott, F. (1953). "The Vitamins in Medicine," 3rd ed. Heinemann, London.

Biezunski, N. (1970). Action of warfarin injected into rats on protein synthesis *in vitro* by liver microsomes as related to its anticoagulating action. *Biochem. Pharmacol.* **19**, 2645–2652.

Blus, L. J., Henny, C. J., and Grove, R. A. (1985). Effects of pelletized anticoagulant rodenticides in California quail. *J. Wildl. Dis.* **21**, 391–395.

Böhm, G. M. (1973). Changes in lung arterioles in pulmonary oedema induced in rats by alpha-naphthyl-thiourea. *J. Pathol.* **110**, 343–345.

Boudouresque, J., Roger, J., Naquet, R., Billé, J., Guin, P., Vigouroux, R.,

and Gosset, A. (1966). Acute chloralose poisoning. Myoclonic seizures. EEG follow-up. *Rev. Neurol.* **114**, 312–317 (in French).

Boyd, M. R., and Neal, R. A. (1976). Studies on the mechanism of toxicity and of development of tolerance to the pulmonary toxin, α-naphthylthiourea (ANTU). *Drug. Metab. Dispos.* **4**, 314–322.

Boyle, C. M. (1960). Case of apparent resistance of *Rattus norvegicus* Berkenhout to anticoagulant poisons. *Nature (London)* **188**, 517.

Braithwaite, G. B. (1982). Vitamin K and brodifacoum. *J. Am. Vet. Med. Assoc.* **181**, 531–534.

Braverman, L. E., and Foster, A. E. (1969). Effect of chronic coumadin administration on thyroid hormone in serum. *J. Nucl. Med.* **10**, 511–513.

Braverman, Y. (1979). Experiments on direct and secondary poisoning by fluoroacetamide (1081) in wildlife and domestic carnivores. *J. Wildl. Dis.* **15**, 319–325.

Breckenridge, A. M., Challiner, M., Mossman, S., Park, B. K., Serlin, M. J., Siberon, R. G., Williams, J. R. B., and Willoughby, J. M. T. (1979). Cimetidine increases the action of warfarin in man. *Br. J. Clin. Pharmacol.* **8**, 392P–393P.

Brockmann, J. L., McDowell, A. V., and Leeds, W. G. (1955). Fatal poisoning with sodium fluoroacetate. Report of a case. *JAMA, J. Am. Med. Assoc.* **159**, 1529–1532.

Brodie, B. B. (1964). Displacement of one drug by another from carrier or receptor sites. *Proc. R. Soc. Med.* **58**, 946–955.

Buckle, F. J., Heap, R., and Saunders, B. C. (1949). Toxic fluorine compounds containing the C—F link. Part III. Fluoroacetamide and related compounds. *J. Chem. Soc., London,* pp. 912–916.

Buckle, R. M., Gamber, T. R., and Pullen, I. M. (1972). Vitamin D intoxication treated with porcine calcitonin. *Br. Med. J.* **3**, 205–207.

Buffa, P., and Peters, R. A. (1950). The *in vivo* formation of citrate induced by fluoroacetate poisoning and its significance. *J. Physiol. (London)* **110**, 488–500.

Bullard, R. W., Thompson, R. D., and Holguin, G. (1976). Diphenadione residues in tissues of cattle. *J. Agric. Food Chem.* **24**, 261–263.

Butler, T. C. (1949). Reduction and oxidation of chloral hydrate by isolated tissues *in vitro. J. Pharmacol. Exp. Ther.* **95**, 360–362.

Cahill, W. P., and Crowder, L. A. (1979). Tissue distribution and excretion of diphacinone in the mouse. *Pestic. Biochem. Physiol.* **10**, 259–267.

Caldwell, P. T., Ren, P., and Bell, R. G. (1974). Warfarin and metabolism of vitamin K. *Biochem. Pharmacol.* **23**, 3353–3362.

Carroll, K. K., and Noble, R. L. (1949). Resistance to toxic thioureas in rats treated with anti-thyroid compounds. *J. Pharmacol. Exp. Ther.* **97**, 478–483.

Case, R. A. M. (1966a). Tumours of the urinary tract as an occupational disease in several industries. *Ann. R. Coll. Surg. Engl.* **39**, 213–235.

Case, R. A. M. (1966b). Occupational bladder cancers (Discussion). *Proc. R. Soc. Med.* **59**, 1252.

Cater, D. B., and Peters, R. A. (1961). The occurrence of renal changes resembling nephrosis in rats poisoned by fluocitrate. *Br. J. Exp. Pathol.* **42**, 278–279.

Chakrabarti, S. K. (1978). Influence of heavy metals on the *in vitro* interaction between human serum albumin and warfarin. *Biochem. Pharmacol.* **27**, 2957–2959.

Chan, K. K., Lewis, R. J., and Trager, W. F. (1972). Absolute configuration of the four warfarin alcohols. *J. Med. Chem.* **15**, 1265–1270.

Chapman, C., and Phillips, M. A. (1955). Fluoroacetamide as a rodenticide. *J. Sci. Food Agric.* **6**, 231–232.

Chappelka, R. (1980). The rat poison Vacor. Letter to the editor. *N. Engl. J. Med.* **302**, 1147.

Chenoweth, M. B. (1949). Monofluoroacetic acid and related compounds. *Pharmacol. Rev.* **1**, 383–424.

Chenoweth, M. B., and Gilman, A. (1946). Studies on the pharmacology of fluoroacetate. *J. Pharmacol. Exp. Ther.* **87**, 90–103.

Chenoweth, M. B., Kandel, A., Johnson, L. B., and Bennett, D. R. (1951). Factors influencing fluoroacetate poisoning. Practical treatment with glycerol monoacetate. *J. Pharmacol. Exp. Ther.* **102**, 31–49.

Chong, M. K. B., Harvey, D., and DeSwiet, M. (1984). Follow-up study of children whose mothers were treated with warfarin during pregnancy. *Br. J. Obstet. Gynaecol.* **91**, 1070–1073.

Chung, H. M. (1984). Acute renal failure caused by acute monofluoroacetate poisoning. *Vet. Hum. Toxicol.* **26**, Suppl. 2, 29–32.

Cocks, J. R. (1960). Anticoagulants and the acute abdomen. *Med. J. Aust.* **1**, 1138–1141.

Cohen, H. N., Fogelman, I., Boyle, I. T., and Doig, J. A. (1979). Deafness due to hypervitaminosis D. *Lancet* **1**, 985.

Colamussi, V., Bonari, R., and Benini, F. (1970). Minor poisoning from fluoro-ethanol (description of three cases). *Arcisp. S. Anna Ferrara* **23**, 447–458.

Coldwell, B. B., Buttar, H. S., Paul, C. J., and Thomas, B. H. (1974). Effect of sodium salicylate on the fate of warfarin in the rat. *Toxicol. Appl. Pharmacol.* **28**, 374–384.

Cole, E. R., and Bachmann, F. (1976). Spectrophotometric assays for warfarin sodium and dicumarol. *Arch. Intern. Med.* **136**, 474–479.

Coon, W. W., and Willis, P. W. (1972). Some aspect of the pharmacology of oral anticoagulants. *Clin. Pharmacol. Ther.* **11**, 312–336.

Cornette, M., and Franck, G. (1970). Clinical and electroencephalographical aspects of acute chloralose poisoning. Review of 11 recent cases. *Rev. Neurol.* **123**, 268–272 (in French).

Cornwell, P. B. (1969). Alphakil—a new rodenticide for mouse control. *Pharm. J.* **202**, 74–75.

Correll, J. T., Coleman, L. L., Long, S., and Willy, R. F. (1952). Di-phenylacetyl-1,3-indandione as a potent hypoprothrombinemic agent. *Proc. Soc. Exp. Biol. Med.* **80**, 139–143.

Cullen, S. I., and Catalano, P. M. (1967). Griseofulvin–warfarin antagonism. *JAMA, J. Am. Med. Assoc.* **199**, 582–583.

Davies, J. M., Thomas, H. F., and Manson, D. (1982). Bladder tumours among rodent operatives handling ANTU. *Br. Med. J.* **285**, 927–931.

Davies, M., and Adams, P. H. (1978). The continuing risk of vitamin D intox-ication. *Lancet* **2**, 621–623.

Davila, J. C., Edds, G. T., Osuna, O., and Simpson, C. F. (1983). Modification of the effects of aflatoxin B1 and warfarin in young pigs given selenium. *Am. J. Vet. Res.* **44**, 1877–1883.

Deckert, F. W. (1973). Warfarin metabolism in the guinea-pig. I. Pharmacolog-ical studies. *Drug. Metab. Dispos.* **1**, 704–710.

Deckert, F. W., Moss, J. N., Sambuca, A. S., Seigel, M. C., and Steigerwalt, R. B. (1977). Nutritional and drug interactions with Vacor rodenticide in rats. *Fed. Proc., Fed. Am. Soc. Exp. Biol.* **36**, 990 (Abstr. 77-1300).

Deckert, F. W., Godfrey, W. J., Lisk, D. C., Steigerwalt, R. B., and Udinsky, J. R. (1978a). Metabolic interactions with RH-787 (Vacor rodenticide). *Fed. Proc., Fed. Soc. Exp. Biol.* **37**, 424.

Deckert, F. W., Hagerman, L. M., Lisk, D. C., Steigerwalt, R. D., and Udinsky, J. R. (1978b). The disposition of (14C)-RH-787 (Vacor roden-ticide) in rodents and dogs. *Toxicol. Appl. Pharmacol.* **45**, 313.

Deckert, F. W., Geyer, W., Godfrey, W. J., Lisk, D. C., Steigerwalt, R. B., and Udinski, J. R. (1979). Partial metabolic fate of 14C-RH-787 (Vacor roden-ticide) in dogs, rats, and humans. *Toxicol. Appl. Pharmacol.* **48**, A163.

de Torrente, A., Rumack, B. H., Blair, D. T., and Anderson, R. J. (1979). Fixed-bed uncoated charcoal hemoperfusion in the treatment of intoxica-tions. Animal and patient studies. *Nephron* **24**, 71–77.

Dieke, S. H., and Richter, C. P. (1945). Acute toxicity of thioureas to rats in relation to age, diet, strain, and species variation. *J. Pharmacol. Exp. Ther.* **83**, 195–202.

Dieke, S. H., and Richter, C. P. (1946). Comparative assays of rodenticides on wild Norway rats. *Public Health Rep.* **61**, 672–679.

Dieke, S. H., Allen, G. S., and Richter, C. P. (1947). The acute toxicity of thioureas and related compounds to wild and domestic Norway rats. *J. Pharmacol. Exp. Ther.* **90**, 260–270.

Dipalma, J. R. (1981). Human toxicity from rat poisons. *Am. Fam. Physician* **24**, 186–189.

DiSaia, P. J. (1966). Pregnancy and delivery of a patient with a Starr-Edwards mitral valve prothesis. *Obstet. Gynecol. (N.Y.)* **28**, 469–471.

Dreyfus, M., Dubouch, P., Pierson, K., Neveu, Y., Martin, E., and Tchernia, G. (1983). Warfarin-contaiminated talc. *Lancet* **1**, 1110.

Dusein, P., Manigaud, G., and Taillandier, J. (1984). Severe and prolonged hypoprothrombinemia following chlorophacinone poisoning. *Presse Med.* **13**, 1845 (in French).

Edlin, J. (1982). Rat bait poisoning in a boxer. *Vet. Rec.* **110**, 136.

Egekeze, J. O., and Oehme, F. W. (1979). Sodium monofluoroacetate (SMFA, compound 1080): A literature review. *Vet. Hum. Toxicol.* **21**, 411–416.

Egyed, M. N. (1971). Experimental acute fluoroacetamide poisoning in sheep. III. Therapy. *Refuah Vet.* **28**, 70–73.

Egyed, M. N. (1973). Clinical, pathological, diagnostic and therapeutic aspects of fluoroacetate research in animals. *Fluoride* **6**, 215–224.

Egyed, M. N., and Brisk, Y. (1965). Experimental fluoroacetamide poisoning in mice, rats and sheep. *Refuah Vet.* **22**, 273–274.

Egyed, M. N., and Miller, G. W. (1971). Experimental acute fluoroacetamide poisoning in guinea pig and sheep. *Fluoride* **4**, 137–142.

Egyed, M. N., and Shlosberg, A. (1973). Diagnosis of field cases of sodium fluoroacetate and fluoroacetamide poisoning in animals. *Refuah Vet.* **30**, 112–115.

Egyed, M. N., and Shlosberg, A. (1977). The efficiency of acetamide in the prevention and treatment of fluoroacetamide poisoning in chickens. *Fluor-ide* **10**, 34–37.

Elbe, J. N., West, B. D., and Link, K. P. (1966). A comparison of the isomers of warfarin. *Biochem. Pharmacol.* **15**, 1003–1006.

Elias, D. J., and Johns, B. E. (1981). Response of rats to chronic ingestion of diphacinone. *Bull. Environ. Contam. Toxicol.* **27**, 559–567.

Elias, D. J., Thompson, R. D., and Savarie, P. J. (1978). Effects of the anti-coagulant diphacinone on suckling calves. *Bull. Environ. Contam. Toxicol.* **20**, 71–78.

Elmer, G. W., Powell, M. L., and Trafer, W. F. (1977). Warfarin metabolism by rat intestinal microflora. *Lloydia* **40**, 610–611.

Fasco, M. J., Piper, L. J., and Kaminsky, L. S. (1979). Cumene hydroperoxide-supported microsomal hydroxylations of warfarin. A probe of cytochrome P-450 multiplicity and specificity. *Biochem. Pharmacol.* **28**, 97–103.

Favarel-Garrigues, J. C., and Boget, J. C. (1968). Acute poisonings by chlo-ralose and ANTU-based rodenticides. *Concours Med.* **90**, 2289–2298 (in French).

Field, J. B., Goldfarb, M. S., Ware, A. G., and Griffith, G. C. (1952). Effect in man of a new indandione anticoagulant. *Proc. Soc. Exp. Biol. Med.* **81**, 678–681.

Filip, J., Novak, L., Sikulova, J., and Kolacny, I. (1970). Body temperature during fluoroacetate poisoning in rats. *Physiol. Bohemoslov.* **19**, 123–127.

Fitzburgh, O. G., and Nelson, A. A. (1947). Chronic oral toxicity of alpha-naphthylurea. *Proc. Soc. Exp. Biol. Med.* **64**, 305–310.

Food and Agriculture Organization (FAO) (1979). "Rodenticides: Analyses, Specifications, Formulations," FAO Plant Prod. Prot. Pap. No. 16. Food Agric. Organ. U. N., Rome.

Fournier, A., Garabedian, M., Grégoire, I., Sebert, J. L., and Pruna, A. (1985). Vitamin D: Its metabolism and its biological properties. *Ann. Med. Interne* **136**, 154–163 (in French).

Fretthold, D., Undinsky, J. R., Deckert, F. W., and Sunshine, I. (1980). Post-mortem findings for a Vacor poisoning case. *Clin. Toxicol.* **16**, 175–180.

Friedman, W. F., and Mills, L. F. (1969). The relationship between vitamin D and the craniofacial and dental anomalies of the supravalvular aortic stenosis syndrome. *Pediatrics* **43**, 12–18.

Friedman, W. F., and Roberts, W. C. (1966). Vitamin D and the supravalvular aortic stenosis syndrome. The transplacental effects of vitamin D on the aorta of the rabbit. *Circulation* **34**, 77–85.

Fristedt, B., and Sterner, N. (1965). Warfarin intoxication from precutaneous absorption. *Arch. Environ. Health* **11**, 205–208.

Frolick, C. A., and Deluca, H. F. (1973). The stimulation of 1,25-di-hydrocholecalciferol metabolism in vitamin D-deficient rat by 1,25-di-hydrocholecalciferol treatment. *J. Clin. Invest.* **52**, 543–548.

Gaines, T. B. (1969). Acute toxicity of pesticides. *Toxicol. Appl. Pharmacol.* **4**, 515–534.

Gaines, T. B., and Hayes, W. J., Jr. (1952). Bait shyness to ANTU in wild Norway rats. *Public Health Rep.* **67**, 306–311.

Gajdusek, D. C., and Luther, G. (1950). Fluoroacetate poisoning. A review and report of a case. *Am. J. Dis. Child.* **79**, 310–320.

Gallanosa, A. G., Spyker, D. A., and Curnow, R. T. (1981). Diabetes mellitus associated with autonomic and peripheral neuropathy after Vacor rodenticide poisoning. A review. *Clin. Toxicol.* **18**, 441–449.

Ganda, O. P., Rossini, A. A., and Like, A. A. (1976). Studies on streptozotocin. *Diabetes* **25**, 596–603.

Gaultier, M., Fournier, E., and Gervais, P. (1962). Pesticides poisonings: Activities of an antipoison center over an eighteen-month period. *Concours Med.* **84**, 6505–6512 (in French).

Gill, J. E., and Redfern, R. (1979). Laboratory test of seven rodenticides for the control of *Mastomys natalensis. J. Hyg.* **83**, 345–352.

Gillman, T., Grant, R. A., and Hathorn, M. (1960). Histochemical and chemical studies of calciferol induced vascular injuries. *Br. J. Exp. Pathol.* **41**, 1–18.

Godfrey, M. E. R., Laas, F. J., and Rammel, C. G. (1985). Acute toxicity of brodifacoum to sheep. *N. Z. J. Exp. Agric.* **13**, 23–25.

Gore, J. M., Appelbaum, J. S., Greene, H. L., Dexter, L., and Dalen, J. E. (1982). Occult cancer in patients with acute pulmonary embolism. *Ann. Intern. Med.* **96**, 556–560.

Grant, R. A., Gillman, T., and Hathorn, M. (1963). Prolonged chemical and histochemical changes associated with widespread calcifications of soft tissues following brief acute calciferol intoxication. *Br. J. Exp. Pathol.* **44**, 220–232.

Gras, G., Pellissier, C., and Fauran, F. (1975). Analytical toxicology of chloralose. Application to 3 cases of acute poisoning. *Eur. J. Toxicol.* **8**, 371–377 (in French).

Great Britain Ministry of Agriculture, Fisheries and Food (1961). Memorandum on the working of the agriculture (poisonous substances) regulations during 1960. Reissued in *WHO Inf. Circ. Toxic. Pestic. Man* No. 9, pp. 51–55.

Greaves, J. H. (1966). Some laboratory observations on the toxicity and acceptability of norbormide to wild *Rattus norvegicus* and on feeding behavior associated with sublethal dosing. *J. Hyg.* **64**, 275–285.

Greaves, J. H., Redfern, R., and King, R. E. (1974). Some properties of calciferol as a rodenticide. *J. Hyg.* **73**, 341–351.

Hagan, E. C., and Radomski, J. L. (1953). The toxicity of 3-(acetonyl-benzyl)-4-hydroxycoumarin (warfarin) to laboratory animals. *J. Am. Pharm. Assoc.* **42**, 379–382.

Hall, J. G., Pauli, R. M., and Wilson, K. M. (1980). Maternal and fetal sequelae of anticoagulation during pregnancy. *Am. J. Med.* **68**, 122–140.

Hanriot and Richet, C. (1897). Chloraloses. *Arch. Int. Pharmacodyn.* **3**, 191–211 (in French).

Harris, L. J. (1955). "Vitamins in Theory and Practice," 4th ed. Cambridge Univ. Press, London and New York.

Harrisson, J. W. E., Ambrus, J. L., Ambrus, C. M., Rees, E. W., Peters, R. H., Reese, L. C., and Baker, T. (1952a). Acute poisoning with sodium fluoroacetate (compound 1080). *JAMA, J. Am. Med. Assoc.* **149**, 1520–1522.

Harrisson, J. W. E., Ambrus, J. L., and Ambrus, C. M. (1952b). Fluoroacetate (1090) poisoning. *Ind. Med. Surg.* **21**, 440.

Hartley, D., and Kidd, H. (1983). "The Agrochemicals Handbook." The Royal Society of Chemistry, Nottingham, England.

Hashida, K. (1971a). Studies on organofluorine pesticide intoxication. I. Experimental and clinical studies on the therapy of organofluorine pesticide intoxication. *J. Okayama Med. Soc.* **83**, 273–293 (in Japanese).

Hashida, K. (1971b). Studies of organofluorine pesticide intoxication. II. Results of health examinations of farmers using an organofluorine pesticide. *J. Okayama Med. Soc.* **83**, 295–310 (in Japanese).

Hashimoto, Y., Makita, T., Miyata, H., Noguchi, T., and Ohta, G. (1968a). Acute and subchronic toxicity of a new fluorine pesticide, *N*-methyl-*N*-(1-naphthyl)fluoroacetamide. *Toxicol. Appl. Pharmacol.* **12**, 536–547.

Hashimoto, Y., Noguchi, T., Mori, T., and Kitagawa, H. (1968b). Some pharmacologic properties of a new fluorine pesticide, *N*-methyl-*N*-(1-naphthyl)-monofluoroacetamide. *Toxicol. Appl. Pharmacol.* **13**, 174–188.

Hashimoto, Y., Makita, T., Mori, T., Nishibe, T., Noguchi, T., and Watanabe, S. (1970). Preclinical experiments on the antidote against monofluoroacetic acid derivatives poisoning in mammals. *In* "Proceedings of the Fourth International Congress of Rural Medicine—Whither Rural Medicine" (H. Kuroiwa *et al.*, eds.), pp. 59–62. Japanese Association of Rural Medicine, Tokyo.

Hatakeyama, H., and Shigei, T. (1971). Fine-structured changes of alveolar walls in fibrin-induced, so-called neurogenic pulmonary edema of the rat: Comparative representation with adrenaline and ANTU-induced edema. *Jpn. J. Pharmacol.* **21**, 673–675.

Havill, A. M., Gee, M. H., Washburne, J. D., Premkumar, A., Ottaviano, R., Flynn, J. J., and Spath, J. A. (1982). Alpha-naphthylthiourea produces dose-dependent lung vascular injury in sheep. *Am. J. Physiol.* **243**, 505–511.

Hayes, W. J., Jr. (1975). "Toxicology of Pesticides." Williams & Wilkins, Baltimore, Maryland.

Hayes, W. J., Jr., and Gaines, T. B. (1950). Control of Norway rats with residual rodenticide warfarin. *Public Health Rep.* **65**, 1537–1555.

Hayes, W. J., Jr., and Vaughn, W. K. (1977). Mortality from pesticides in the United States in 1973 and 1974. *Toxicol. Appl. Pharmacol.* **42**, 235–252.

Hearn, C. E. D. (1973). A review of agricultural pesticide incidents in man in England and Wales, 1952–1971. *Br. J. Ind. Med.* **30**, 253–258.

Herken, H. (1971). Antimetabolic action of 6-aminonicotinamide on the pentose phosphate pathway in the brain. *In* "Mechanisms of Toxicity" (W. N. Aldridge, ed.). Macmillan, London.

Hiraki, K., Iwasaki, I., and Namba, M. (1972). Electroencephalograms in pesticide poisoning cases. *Jpn. J. Leg. Med.* **14**, 333–340 (in Japanese).

Holmes, R. W., and Love, J. (1952). Suicide attempt with warfarin, a bishydroxycoumarin-like rodenticide. *JAMA, J. Am. Med. Assoc.* **148**, 935–937.

Hosek, B., Novak, L., and Misustova, J. (1970). Mathematical evaluation of the course of body temperature in mice after the administration of sodium fluoroacetate. *Physiol. Bohemoslov.* **19**, 129–133.

Hudson, R. H., Turcker, R. K., and Haegele, M. A. (1972). Effect of age on sensitivity: Acute oral toxicity of 14 pesticides to mallard ducks of several ages. *Toxicol. Appl. Pharmacol.* **22**, 556–561.

Hutchens, J. O., Wagner, H., Podolsky, B., and McMahon, T. M. (1949). The effect of ethanol and various metabolites in fluoroacetate poisoning. *J. Pharmacol. Exp. Ther.* **95**, 62–70.

Ikeda, M., Conney, A. H., and Burns, J. J. (1968a). Stimulatory effect of phenobarbital and insecticides on warfarin metabolism in the rat. *J. Pharmacol. Exp. Ther.* **162**, 338–343.

Ikeda, M., Ullrich, V., and Staudinger, H. (1968b). Metabolism *in vitro* of warfarin by enzymic and nonenzymic systems. *Biochem. Pharmacol.* **17**, 1663–1669.

Ikkala, E., Myllyla, G., Nevanlinna, H. R., Pelkonen, R., and Pyorala, K. (1964). Hemorrhagic diathesis due to criminal poisoning with warfarin. *Acta Med. Scand.* **176**, 201–203.

Innes, J. R. M., Ulland, B. M, Valerio, M. G., Petrucelli, L., Fishbein, L., Hart, E. R., Pallotta, A. J., Bates, R. R., Falk, H. L., Gart, J. J., Klein, M., Mitchell, I., and Peters, J. (1969). Bioassay of pesticides and industrial chemicals for tumorigenicity in mice: A preliminary note. *J. Natl. Cancer Inst. (U.S.)* **4**, 1101–1114.

International Agency for Research in Cancer (IARC) (1983). "Monograph on the Evaluation of the Carcinogenic Risk of Chemicals to Humans. Miscellaneous Pesticides," Vol. 30. Int. Agency Res. Cancer, Lyon, France.

Iqbal, S. J., and Taylor, W. H. (1982). Treatment of vitamin D2 poisoning by induction of hepatic enzymes. *Br. Med. J.* **285**, 541–542.

Iwasaki, I., Nawa, H., Hara, H., Takagi, S., and Hyodo, K. (1970a). Agricultural organofluoride poisoning. I. Carbohydrate metabolism. *Fluoride* **3**, 121–127.

Iwasaki, I., Namba, M., Nawa, H., Hara, A., Takagi, S., and Hyodo, K. (1970b). Studies on organofluoride poisoning. IV. Electroencephalographic (EEG) observations. *Fluoride* **3**, 133–136.

Jacobziner, H., and Raybin, H. W. (1960). Oil of wintergreen, warfarin sodium, and potassium permanganate intoxications. *N. Y. State J. Med.* **60**, 3873–3875.

Jarnargin, K., Zeng, S. Y., Phelps, M., and Deluca, H. F. (1985). Metabolism and pharmacokinetics of 24,25-dihydroxyvitamin D3 in the vitamin D3-replete rat. *J. Biol. Chem.* **260**, 13625–13630.

Jeffery, W. H., Ahlin, T. A., Goran, C., and Hardy, W. R. (1976). Loss of warfarin effect after occupational insecticide exposure. *JAMA, J. Am. Med. Assoc.* **236**, 2881–2882.

Johannsen, F. R., and Knowles, C. O. (1972). Citrate accumulation in twospotted spider mites, house flies, and mice following treatment with the acaricide 2-fluoro-*N*-methyl-*N*-(1-naphthyl)acetamide. *J. Econ. Entomol.* **65,** 1754–1756.

Johnson, D., Kubic, P., and Levitt, C. (1980). Accidental ingestion of Vacor rodenticide. The symptoms and sequelae in a 25-month-old child. *Am. J. Dis. Child.* **134,** 161–164.

Jones, E. C., Growe, G. H., and Naiman, S. C. (1984). Prolonged anticoagulation in rat poisoning. *JAMA, J. Am. Med. Assoc.* **252,** 3005–3007.

Kalmbach, E. R. (1945). "Ten-eighty," a war-produced rodenticide. *Science* **102,** 232–233.

Kaminsky, S. S., Piper, L. J., and Fasco, M. J. (1976). The binding of R and S warfarin to hepatic cytochromes P-450. *Fed. Proc., Fed. Am. Soc. Exp. Biol.* **35,** 1709.

Kandel, A., and Chenoweth, M. B. (1952). Tolerance to fluoroacetate and fluorobutyrate in rats. *J. Pharmacol. Exp. Ther.* **104,** 248–252.

Kaplan, L. C. (1985). Congenital Dandy-Walker malformation associated with first trimester warfarin: A case report and literature review. *Teratology* **32,** 333–337.

Karam, J. H., Prosser, P. R., and LeWitt, P. A. (1978). Islet cell surface antibodies in a patient with diabetes mellitus after rodenticide ingestion. *N. Engl. J. Med.* **299,** 1191.

Karam, J. H., LeWitt, P. A., Young, C. W., Nowlain, R. E., Frankel, B. J., Fujiya, N., Freedman, Z. R., and Grodsky, G. M. (1980). Insulinopenic diabetes after rodenticide (Vacor) ingestion. A unique model of acquired diabetes in man. *Diabetes* **29,** 971–978.

Kawalec, J. C., Andrews, A. W., and Pienta, R. J. (1979). 1-Naphthylthiourea: A mutagenic rodenticide that transforms hamster embryo cells. *Mol. Pharmacol.* **15,** 678–684.

Keber, I. J., Warr, O. S., III, and Richardson, C. (1968). Pregnancy in a patient with a prosthetic mitral valve associated with a fetal anomaly attributed to warfarin sodium. *JAMA, J. Am. Med. Assoc.* **203,** 223–225.

Kellum, J. M. (1952). Warfarin for suicide. *JAMA, J. Am. Med. Assoc.* **148,** 1443.

Kempin, S. J. (1983). Warfarin resistance caused by broccoli. *N. Engl. J. Med.* **308,** 1229–1230.

Kirzon, M. V., Timeiko, V. N., and Artiushkova, V. A. (1970). The content of citric acid in various organs of rats in fluoroacetate poisoning. *Vopr. Med. Khim.* **16,** 543–549 (in Russian).

Kirzon, M. V., Timeiko, V. N., and Artiushkova, V. A. (1973). Accumulation of citric acid in different organs of rabbits and cats in sodium fluoroacetate poisoning. *Vopr. Med. Khim.* **19,** 471–474 (in Russian).

Koch-Weser, J., and Sellers, E. M. (1971). Drug interactions with coumarin anticoagulants. Parts I and II. *N. Engl. J. Med.* **285,** 487–498, 547–558.

Kovalenko, L. I., Bulkina, V. A., and Panteleev, R. I. (1975). Three cases of giftor poisoning. *Gig. Tr. Prof. Zabol.* **12,** 53–54 (in Russian).

Krauss, J. S. (1982). Warfarin, pulmonary embolism and cancer. *Ann. Intern. Med.* **97,** 282.

Lange, P. F., and Terveer, J. (1954). Warfarin poisoning. *U.S. Armed Forces Med. J.* **5,** 872–877.

Latore, G. (1961). Effect of overdose of vitamin D2 on pregnancy in the rat. *Fertil. Steril.* **12,** 343–345.

Laubstein, H. (1962). Contact dermatitis from a rodenticide. *Berufs-Dermatosen* **10,** 154–160 (in German).

Leck, J. B., and Park, B. K. (1981). A comparative study of the effects of warfarin and brodifacoum on the relationship between vitamin K1 metabolism and clotting factor activity in warfarin-resistant rats. *Biochem. Pharmacol.* **30,** 123–128.

Lee, P. W., Arnau, T., and Neal, R. A. (1960). Metabolism of α-naphthylthiourea by rat liver and rat lung microsomes. *Toxicol. Appl. Pharmacol.* **53,** 164–178.

Lee, T. H., and Lee, M. W. (1977). Inhibitory effect of a rodenticide RH-787 on the glucose metabolism of erythrocytes. *Korean J. Intern. Med.* **20,** 597–601 (in Japanese).

Lees, P. (1972). Pharmacology and toxicology of alphachloralose: A review. *Vet. Rec.* **91,** 330–333.

Lehman, A. J. (1951). Chemicals in foods. A report to the Association of Food

and Drug Officials on current developments. Part II. Pesticides. Section I. Introduction. *Q. Bull.—Assoc. Food Drug Off.* **15**(I), 122–123.

Lehman, A. J. (1952). Chemicals in foods. A report to the Association of Food and Drug Officials on current developments. Part II. Pesticides. Section II. Dermal Toxicity. Section III. Subacute and chronic toxicity. Section IV. Biochemistry. Section V. Pathology. *Q. Bull.—Assoc. Food Drug Off.* **16** (II), 3–9; (III), 47–53; (IV), 85–91; (V), 126–132.

Lewis, R. J., and Traeger, W. F. (1970). Warfarin metabolism in man: Identification of metabolites in urine. *J. Clin. Invest.* **49,** 907–913.

LeWitt, P. A. (1980a). The neurotoxicity of the rat poison Vacor: A clinical study of 12 cases. *N. Engl. J. Med.* **302,** 73–77.

LeWitt, P. A. (1980b). The rat poison Vacor. *N. Engl. J. Med.* **302,** 1147.

Lindahl, O., and Lindwall, L. (1975). Vitamin D and myocardial infarction. *Br. Med. J.* **2,** 560.

Linden, V. (1974). Vitamin D and myocardial infarction. *Br. Med. J.* **3,** 647–650.

Link, K. P. (1944). The anticoagulant from spoiled sweet clover hay. *Harvey Lect.* **39,** 162–216.

Link, K. P. (1959). The discovery of dicumarol and its sequels. *Circulation* **19,** 97–107.

Link, K. P., Berg, D., and Barker, W. M. (1965). Partial fate of warfarin in the rat. *Science* **150,** 378.

Lipton, R. A., and Klass, E. M. (1984). Human ingestion of a "superwarfarin" rodenticide resulting in a prolonged anticoagulant effect. *JAMA, J. Am. Med. Assoc.* **252,** 3004–3005.

Loracher, C., and Lux, H. D. (1974). Impaired hyperpolarising inhibition during insulin hypoglycaemia and fluoroacetate poisoning. *Brain Res.* **69,** 164–169.

Lorgue, G., Rampaud, M., Keck, G., and Jaussaud, P. (1985). Toxicological data on wild and domestic animals poisoned with rodenticides. *Acta Zool. Fenn.* **173,** 213.

Lorusso, D. J., and Suttie, J. W. (1972). Warfarin binding to microsomes isolated from normal and warfarin-resistant rat liver. *Mol. Pharmacol.* **8,** 197–203.

Lund, M. (1964). Resistance to warfarin in the common rat. *Nature (London)* **203,** 778.

Lund, M. (1967). Resistance of rodents to rodenticides. *World Rev. Pest Control* **6,** 131–138.

MacDonald, M. G., and Kaminsky, L. S. (1979). Development of the hepatic monoxygenase system and metabolism of warfarin in the perinatal rat. *Pediatr. Res.* **13,** 370.

MacDonald, M. G., Robinson, D. S., Sylvester, D., and Jaffe, J. J. (1969). The effects of phenobarbital, chloral betaine and glutethimide administration on warfarin plasma level and hypoprothrombinemic responses in man. *Clin. Pharmacol. Ther.* **10,** 80–84.

Maddock, D. R., and Schoof, H. F. (1967). Laboratory and field evaluation of norbormide against wild rats. *Pest Control* **35**(8), 22, 24, 26, 28.

Marshall, E. K., and Owens, A. H. (1954). Absorption, excretion and metabolic fate of chloral hydrate. *Bull. Johns Hopkins Hosp.* **95,** 1–18.

Martin, C. M., Engström, P. F., and Chandor, S. B. (1970). Skin necrosis associated with warfarin sodium. *Calif. Med.* **113,** 78–80.

Martin-Bouyer, G., Linh, P. D., Tuan, L. C., Barin, C., Khahn, N. B., Hoa, D. Q., Tourneau, J., and Guerbois, H. (1983). Epidemic of haemorrhagic disease in Vietnamese infants caused by warfarin-contaminated talc. *Lancet* **1,** 230–232.

Matschiner, J. T., Bell, R. G., Amoletti, J. M., and Knauer, T. E. (1970). Isolation and characterization of a new metabolite of phylloquinone in the rat. *Biochim. Biophys. Acta* **201,** 309–315.

Matsumura, F., and O'Brien, R. D. (1963). A comparative study of the modes of action of fluoroacetamide and fluoroacetate in the mouse and American cockroach. *Biochem. Pharmacol.* **12,** 1201–1205.

Mawer, E. B., Backhouse, J., Davies, M., Hill, L. F., and Taylor, C. M. (1976). Metabolic fate of administered 1,25-dihydrocholecalciferol in controls and in patients with hypoparathyroidism. *Lancet* **1,** 1203–1205.

Mazzanti, L., Lopez, M., and Berti, M. G. (1964). Selective destruction in testes induced by fluoroacetamide. *Experientia* **20,** 492–493.

McClain, R. M., Langhoff, L., and Hoar, R. M. (1980). Reproduction studies with 1α,25-dihydroxyvitamin D_3 (calcitriol) in rats and rabbits. *Toxicol. Appl. Pharmacol.* **52,** 89–98.

McLeod, A. R. (1970). An epidemiological study of pesticide poisonings admitted to Charity Hospital, New Orleans. *J. La. State Med. Soc.* **122,** 337–343.

McSporran, K. D., and Phillips, C. A. (1983). Brodifacoum poisoning in a dog. *N. Z. Vet. J.* **31,** 185–186.

McTaggart, D. R. (1970). Poisoning due to sodium fluoroacetate ("1080") *Med. J. Aust.* **2,** 641–642.

Medved, L. I., ed. (1974). "Handbook of Pesticides (Hygiene of Use and Toxicology)." Urogai Publishing House, Kiev, U.S.S.R.

Meyer, B. J., and Saunders, J. P. (1949). The effects of thioureas and related compounds on alphanaphthylthiourea (ANTU) toxicity to rats. *J. Pharmacol. Exp. Ther.* **97,** 432–440.

Meyrick, B., Miller, J., and Reid, L. (1972). Pulmonary oedema induced by ANTU, or by high or low oxygen concentrations in rat—an electron microscopic study. *Br. J. Exp. Pathol.* **45,** 347–358.

Michaels, L. (1974). The incidence and course of cancer in patients receiving anticoagulant therapy: Retrospective and prospective study. *J. Med.* **5,** 98–106.

Misustova, J., Novak, L., and Hosek, B. (1969). Influence of lowered environmental temperature on metabolic and lethal effects of sodium fluoroacetate in mice. *Physiol. Bohemoslov.* **18,** 319–324.

Moene, Y., Cuche, M., Trillet, M., Motin, J., and Michel, D. (1969). Diagnostic problems from acute poisoning by chloralose (review of 6 cases). *J. Med. Lyon* **50,** 1483–1484, 1487–1488, 1491–1493.

Mogilner, B. M., Freeman, J. S., Blashar, Y., and Pincus, F. E. (1974). Reye's syndrome in three Isareli children. Possible relationship to warfarin toxicity. *Isr. J. Med. Sci.* **10,** 1117–1125.

Morselli, P. L., Garattini, S., Marucci, F., Mussini, E., Rewersky, W., Valzelli, L., and Peters, R. A. (1968). The effect of injections of fluorocitrate into the brains of rats. *Biochem. Pharmacol.* **17,** 195–202.

Mount, M. E., and Feldman, B. F. (1983). Mechanism of diphacinone rodenticide toxicosis in the dog and its therapeutic implications. *Am. J. Vet. Res.* **44,** 2009–2017.

Murdoch, D. A. (1983). Prolonged anticoagulation in chlorophacinone poisoning. *Lancet* **1,** 355–356.

Murphy, M. J., Ray, A. C., Woody, B., and Reagor, J. C. (1985). Serum brodifacoum concentrations and coagulopathic effects in anticoagulant poisoned dogs treated with vitamin K1. *Toxicologist* **5,** 88 (Abstr. 351).

Namba, M., Fujii, Y., Hara, A., Nawa, H., Iwasaki, I., and Hiraki, K. (1971). Organic fluorine poisoning. *Jpn. J. Clin. Med.* **29,** 864–870 (in Japanese).

Navarro, M., Acevedo, C., Espinosa, L., Pena, A., Picazo, M. L., and Larraudi, M. (1985). Vitamin D_3 intoxication with irreversible sequelae. *An. Esp. Pediatr.* **22**(2), 99–106.

Nebel, L., and Ornstein, A. (1966). Effect of hypervitaminosis D2 on fertility and pregnancy in rats. *Isr. J. Med. Sci.* **2,** 14–21.

Nikodemusz, E., Nechay, G., and Imre, R. (1981). Histopathological changes resulting from intoxication by some pesticides in the common vole (*Microtus arvalis* Pallas). *Acta Vet. Acad. Sci. Hung.* **29,** 317–326.

Nilsson, I. M. (1957). Recurrent hypoprothrombinaemia due to poisoning with a dicumarol-containing rat killer. *Acta Haematol.* **17,** 176–182.

Niu, M. (1970). Pharmacological action of norbormide. *Jpn. J. Pharmacol.* **66,** 224–236 (in Japanese).

Noguchi, T., Ohnyki, Y., and Okigaki, T. (1966). Effect of sodium fluoroacetate on myocardial cells *in vitro. Nature (London)* **209,** 1197–1198.

Noguchi, T., Hashimoto, Y., and Miyata, H. (1968). Studies of the biochemical lesions caused by a new fluorine pesticide, N-methyl-N-(1-naphthyl)monofluoroacetamide. *Toxicol. Appl. Pharmacol.* **13,** 189–198.

O'Brien, R. F., Makarski, J. S., and Rounds, S. (1985). Studies of the mechanism of decreased angiotensin I conversion in rat lungs injured with alphanaphthylthiourea. *Exp. Lung Res.* **8,** 243–259.

O'Connor, J. A. (1948). The use of blood anti-coagulants for rodent control. *Research (London)* **1,** 334–336.

O'Reilly, R. A. (1970). The second reported kindred with hereditary resistance to oral anticoagulant drugs. *N. Engl. J. Med.* **282,** 1448–1451.

O'Reilly, R. A., and Aggeler, P. M. (1968). Phenylbutazone potentiation of anticoagulant effect: Fluorometric assay of warfarin. *Proc. Soc. Exp. Biol. Med.* **128,** 1080–1081.

O'Reilly, R. A., Aggeler, P. M., and Leong, L. S. (1963). Studies on the coumarin anticoagulant drugs: The pharmacodynamics of warfarin in man. *J. Clin. Invest.* **42,** 1542–1551.

Ornoy (Ornstein), A., Menczel, J., and Nebel, L. (1968). Alterations in the mineral composition and metabolism of rat fetuses and their placentas induced by maternal hypervitaminosis D2. *Isr. J. Med. Sci.* **4,** 827–832.

Osterman, J., Zmyslinski, R. W., Hopkins, C. B., Cartee, W., Lin, T., and Nankin, H. R. (1981). Full recovery from severe orthostatic hypotension after Vacor rodenticide ingestion. *Arch. Intern. Med.* **141,** 1505–1507.

Osteryoung, J. G., Whittaker, J. W., Tessari, J., and Boyes, V. (1977). The identification of p-nitroaniline as a metabolite of the rodenticide Vacor in human liver. *In* "Fate of Pesticides in Large Animals" (G. W. Ivie and H. W. Dorough, eds.), pp. 253–256. Academic Press, New York.

Overman, R. S., Stahmann, M. A., Huebner, C. F., Sullivan, W. R., Spero, L., Doherty, D. G., Miyoshi, I., Grae, L., Roseman, S., and Link, K. P. (1944). Studies on the hemorrhagic sweet clover disease. XIII. Anticoagulant activity and structure in the 4-hyroxycoumarin group. *J. Biol. Chem.* **153,** 5–24.

Owens, A. H., and Marshall, E. K. (1955). Further studies on the metabolic fate of chloral hydrate and trichlorethanol. *Bull. Johns Hopkins Hosp.* **97,** 320–326.

Papasozomenos, S. (1980). The rat poison Vacor. *N. Engl. J. Med.* **302,** 1146–1147.

Park, B. K., and Leck, J. B. (1982). A comparison of vitamin K antagonism by warfarin, difenacoum and brodifacoum in the rabbit. *Biochem. Pharmacol.* **31,** 3635–3639.

Parkin, P. J., McGiven, A. R., and Bailey, R. R. (1977). Chronic sodium monofluoroacetate (compound 1080) intoxication in a rabbiter. *N. Z. Med. J.* **85,** 93–96.

Pastor, B. H., Resnick, M. E., and Rodman, T. (1962). Serious hemorrhagic complications of anticoagulant therapy. *JAMA, J. Am. Med. Assoc.* **180,** 747–751.

Paterson, C. R. (1980). Vitamin D poisoning: Survey of causes in 21 patients with hypercalcemia. *Lancet* **1,** 1164–1165.

Patil, T. N., and Radhakrishnamurty, R. (1973). Effect of norbormide on blood glucose levels in albino rats. *Indian J. Biochem. Biophys.* **10,** 206–208.

Patil, T. N., and Radhakrishnamurty, R. (1977). Biochemical changes induced by α-naphthylthiourea in albino rats. *Indian J. Biochem. Biophys.* **14,** 24.

Peardon, D. L. (1974). RH-787, a new selective rodenticide. *Pest Control* **42** (9), 14, 16, 18, 27.

Penumarthy, L., and Oehme, F. W. (1978). Treatment and prothrombin responses during warfarin toxicosis in rats and mice. *Toxicology* **10,** 377–401.

Peoples, S. A., and Maddy, K. T. (1979). Poisoning of man and animals due to ingestion of the rodent poison Vacor. *Vet. Hum. Toxicol.* **21**(4), 266–268.

Peters, R. A. (1952). Significance of biochemical lesions in the pyruvate oxidase system. *Br. Med. Bull.* **9,** 116–122.

Peters, R. A. (1963a). Organo-fluorine compounds present in certain plants and their effect on animals. *Biochem. J.* **88,** 55P.

Peters, R. A. (1963b). "Biochemical Lesions and Lethal Synthesis." Macmillan, New York.

Peters, R. A., and Shorthouse, M. (1971). Oral toxicity of fluoroacetate and fluorocitrate in rats. *J. Physiol. (London)* **216,** 40P–41P.

Petit, L., Leperchey, F., and Fournier, E. (1970). Experimental toxicology of isothioureas. *Poumon Coeur* **26,** 893–894 (in French).

Pettifor, J. M., and Benson, R. (1975). Congenital malformation associated with the administration of oral anticoagulants during pregnancy. *J. Pediatr.* **86,** 459–462.

Phillips, M. A., and Worden, A. N. (1956). Toxicity of fluoroacetamide. *Lancet* **2,** 731.

Phillips, M. A., and Worden, A. N. (1957). The mammalian oral toxicity of fluoroacetamide. *J. Soc. Food Agric.* **8,** 653–657.

Pohl, L. R., Nelson, S. D., Porter, W. R., Trager, W. F., Fasco, M. J., Baker, F. D., and Fenton, J. W., II (1976a). Warfarin—stereochemical aspects of its metabolism by rat liver microsomes. *Biochem. Pharmacol.* **25,** 2153–2162.

Pohl, L. R., Bales, R., and Trager, W. F. (1976b). Warfarin: Stereochemical aspects of its metabolism *in vivo* in the rat. *Res. Commun. Chem. Pathol. Pharmacol.* **15**, 233–256.

Pohl, L. R., Porter, W. R., Trager, W. F., Fasco, M. J., and Fenton, J. W., III (1977). Stereochemical biotransformation of warfarin as a probe of the homogeneity and mechanism of microsomal hydroxylases. *Biochem. Pharmacol.* **26**, 109–114.

Pont, A., Rubino, J. M., Bishop, D., and Peal, K. (1979). Diabetes mellitus and neuropathy following Vacor ingestion in man. *Arch. Intern. Med.* **139**, 185–187.

Poos, G. I., Mohrbacher, R. J., Carson, E. L., Paragamian, V., Puma, B. M., Rasmussen, C. R., and Roszkowski, A. P. (1966). Structure–activity studies with the selective rat toxicant norbormide. *J. Med. Chem.* **9**, 537–540.

Potvliege, P. R. (1962). Hypervitaminosis D2 in gravid rats. *Arch. Pathol.* **73**, 371–382.

Powell, M. L., Pope, B., Elmer, G. W., and Trager, W. F. (1977). Biliary excretion of warfarin metabolites and their metabolism by rat gut flora. *Life Sci.* **20**, 171–178.

Pribilla, O. (1966). Murder caused by warfarin. *Arch. Toxicol.* **21**, 235–249.

Prosser, P. R., and Karam, J. H. (1978). Diabetes mellitus following rodenticide ingestion in man. *JAMA, J. Am. Med. Assoc.* **239**, 1148–1150.

Pyorala, K. (1968). Sex differences in the clotting factor response to warfarin and in the rate of warfarin metabolism in the rat. *Ann. Med. Exp. Biol. Fenn.* **46**, 23–34.

Pyorala, K., and Nevanlinna, H. R. (1968). The effect of selective and non-selective inbreeding on the rate of warfarin metabolism in the rat. *Ann. Med. Exp. Biol. Fenn.* **46**, 35–44.

Raasch, M. S. (1958). 5-Fluoronorvaline and 6-fluoronorleucine. *J. Org. Chem.* **23**, 1567–1568.

Rao, M. B. K. (1979). Potentiation of warfarin toxicity of roof rats (*Rattus rattus*) by L-histidine and by vitamin K adsorbers. *Pestic. Sci.* **10**, 221–226.

Reigart, J. R., Brueggeman, J. L., and Keil, J. E. (1975). Sodium fluoroacetate poisoning. *Am. J. Dis. Child* **129**, 1224–1226.

Renapurkar, D. M., and Deoras, P. J. (1982). Effects of anticoagulant rodenticides on rat intestine *in vitro*. *Pestology* **6**, 11–13.

Rennison, B. D., and Hadler, M. R. (1975). Field trials of difenacoum against warfarin-resistant infestations of *Rattus norvegicus*. *J. Hyg.* **74**, 449–455.

Richter, C. P. (1945). The development and use of alpha-naphthyl thiourea (ANTU) as a rat poison. *JAMA, J. Am. Med. Assoc.* **129**, 927–931.

Richter, C. P. (1946). Biological factors involved in poisoning rats with alpha-naphthyl thiourea (ANTU). *Proc. Soc. Exp. Biol. Med.* **63**, 364–372.

Robinson, D. S., and MacDonald, M. G. (1966). The effect of phenobarbital administration on the control of coagulation achieved during warfarin therapy in man. *J. Pharmacol. Exp. Ther.* **153**, 250–253.

Robinson, W. H. (1970). Acute toxicity of sodium monofluoroacetate to cattle. *J. Wildl. Manage.* **34**, 647–648.

Rossini, A. A., Arcangeli, M. A., and Cahill, G. F. (1975). Studies on alloxan toxicity on the beta cell. *Diabetes* **24**, 516–522.

Roszkowski, A. P. (1965). The pharmacological properties of norbormide, a selective rat toxicant. *J. Pharmacol. Exp. Ther.* **149**, 288–299.

Roszkowski, A. P., Poos, G. I., and Mohrbacher, R. J. (1964). Selective rat toxicant. *Science* **144**, 412–413.

Rothstein, E. (1968). Warfarin effect enhanced by disulfiram. *JAMA, J. Am. Med. Assoc.* **206**, 1574–1575.

Roy, A., Teitelman, U., and Bursztein, S. (1980). Evaluation of the role of ionized calcium in sodium fluoroacetate ("1080") poisoning. *Toxicol. Appl. Pharmacol.* **56**, 216–220.

Roy, A., Raikhlin-Eisenkraft, B., Teitelman, U., and Hazani, A. (1982). Poisoning by fluoroacetate and fluoroacetamide. A description of two cases. *Harefuah* **48**, 523–524.

Russell, S. H., Monin, T., and Edwards, W. C. (1978). Rodenticide toxicosis in a horse. *J. Am. Vet. Med. Assoc.* **172**, 270–271.

Sanger, G., and Becker, K. (1975). Dermal absorption of warfarin in man and rat. *Umwelthygiene* **1**, 156–158 (in German).

Saunders, B. C. (1947). Toxic properties of ω-fluorocarboxylic acids and derivatives. *Nature (London)* **160**, 179–181.

Sax, I. N. (1984). "Dangerous Properties of Industrial Material," 6th ed. Van Nostrand-Reinhold, New York.

Schafer, E. W. (1972). The acute oral toxicity of 369 pesticidal, pharmaceutical and other chemicals to wild birds. *Toxicol. Appl. Pharmacol.* **21**, 315–330.

Schiff, B. L., and Kern, A. B. (1968). Cutaneous reactions to anticoagulants. *Arch. Dermatol.* **98**, 136–137.

Searcey, M. T., and Graves, C. B. (1976). Subcellular distribution and warfarin-binding protein from Sprague-Dawley and Warfarin-resistant rats. *Fed. Proc., Fed. Am. Soc. Exp. Biol.* **35**, 1763.

Sellers, E. M., Lang, M., Koch-Weser, J., and Coleman, R. W. (1972). Enhancement of warfarin-induced hypoprothrombinemia by triclofos. *Clin. Pharmacol. Ther.* **13**, 911–915.

Shaul, W. L., Emery, H., and Hall, J. G. (1975). Chondrodysplasia punctata and maternal warfarin use during pregnancy. *Am. J. Dis. Child.* **129**, 360–362.

Shearer, M. J., and Barkhan, P. (1979). Vitamin K, and therapy of massive warfarin overdose. *Lancet* **1**, 266–267.

Shearer, M. J., McBurney, A., and Barkhan, P. (1973). Effect of warfarin anticoagulation on vitamin-K metabolism in man. *Br. J. Haematol.* **24**, 471–479.

Shepherd, D. (1971). Bemegride sodium and alphachloralose poisoning. *Vet. Rec.* **88**, 375.

Sherrod, P. S., and Harrod, M. J. E. (1978). Warfarin embryopathy in siblings. *Am. J. Hum. Genet.* **30**, 104A.

Shlosberg, A., Egyed, M. N., Mendelsohn, H., and Langer, B. (1975). Fluoroacetamide (1081) poisoning in wild birds. *J. Wildl. Dis.* **11**, 534–536.

Smith, I. A., and Boyd, J. H. (1972). Another case of poisoning by alpha-cloralose. *Vet. Rec.* **91**, 662.

Sobonya, R. E., and Kleinerman, J. (1973). Recurrent pulmonary edema induced by α-naphthyl thiourea. *Am. Rev. Respir. Dis.* **108**, 926–932.

Sollman, T. (1901). "A Text-Book of Pharmacology and Some Allied Sciences." Saunders, Philadelphia, Pennsylvania.

Sollman, T. (1942). "A Manual of Pharmacology and Its Applications to Therapeutics and Toxicology." Saunders, Philadelphia, Pennsylvania.

Solomon, H. M. (1968). Variations in metabolism of coumarin anticoagulant drugs. *An. N.Y. Acad. Sci.* **15**, 932–935.

Solomon, H. M., Schrogie, J. J., and Williams, D. (1968). The displacement of phenylbutazone-^{14}C and warfarin-^{14}C from human albumin by various drugs and fatty acids. *Biochem. Pharmacol.* **17**, 143–151.

Spielmann, H., Meyer-Wendecker, R., and Spielmann, F. (1973). Influence of 2-deoxy-D-glucose and sodium fluoroacetate on respiratory metabolism of rat embryos during organogenesis. *Teratology* **7**, 127–134.

Steinberger, E., and Sud, B. N. (1970). Specific effects of fluoroacetamide on spermiogenesis. *Biol. Reprod.* **2**, 369–375.

Sterner, R. T. (1979). Effects of sodium cyanide and diphacinone in coyotes (*Canis latrans*): Applications as predaticides in livestock toxic collars. *Bull. Environ. Contam. Toxicol.* **23**, 211–217.

Stevenson, R. E., Burton, M., Ferlanto, G. J., and Taylor, H. A. (1980). Hazards of oral anticoagulants during pregnancy. *JAMA, J. Am. Med. Assoc.* **243**, 1549–1551.

Stowe, C. M., Metz, A. L., Arendt, T. D., and Schultman, J. (1983). Apparent brodifacoum poisoning in a dog. *J. Am. Vet. Med. Assoc.* **182**, 817–818.

Suttie, J. W., ed. (1979). "Vitamin K Metabolism and Vitamin K-Dependent Proteins." University Park Press, Baltimore, Maryland.

Takagi, S. (1971). Studies on agricultural organofluoride poisoning. Part III. Influence of an organofluoride on the electrocardiogram. *J. Okayama Med. Soc.* **81**, 641–650 (in Japanese).

Tarrant, K. A., and Westlake, G. E. (1984). Histological technique for the identification of poisoning in wildlife by the rodenticide calciferol. *Bull. Environ. Contam. Toxicol.* **32**, 175–178.

Tejani, N. (1973). Anticoagulant therapy with cardiac valve prothesis during pregnancy. *Obstet. Gynecol.* **42**, 785–793.

Tempé, J. D., and Kurtz, D. (1972). Acute chloralose poisoning. *Concours Med.* **94**, 801–813 (in French).

Thierry, M. J., Hermodson, M. A., and Suttie, J. W. (1970). Vitamin K and warfarin distribution and metabolism in the warfarin-resistant rat. *Am. J. Physiol.* **219**, 854–859.

Thompson, R. D., Mitchell, G. C., and Burns, R. J. (1972). Vampire bat control by systemic treatment of livestock with an anticoagulant. *Science* **177**, 806–807.

Toda, T., Ito, M., Toda, Y., Smith, T., and Kummerov, F. (1985). Angiotoxicity in swine of a moderate excess of dietary vitamin D3. *Food Chem. Toxicol.* **23**, 585–592.

Tokareva, T. G., Turov, I. S., and Alekseyev, A. N. (1971). The action of fluoroacetamide on albino mouse fecundity (preliminary report). *Zh. Mikrobiol., Epidemiol. Immunobiol.* **48**, 24–26 (in Russian).

Tomiya, K., Shimoda, R., Kakihara, Y., and Kanda, M. (1976). Studies on extraction of toxic materials from organs of victims of fatal intoxication by organofluorine pesticides. *Jpn. J. Leg. Med.* **29**, 237–238 (in Japanese).

Tourtellotte, W. W., and Coon, J. M. (1951). Treatment of fluoroacetate poisoning in mice and dogs. *J. Pharmacol. Exp. Ther.* **101**, 82–91.

Ullrich, V., and Staudinger, H. (1968). Metabolism *in vitro* of warfarin by enzymic and nonenzymic systems. *Biochem. Pharmacol.* **17**, 1663–1669.

Varon, M. L., and Cole, L. J. (1966). Hemopoietic colony-forming units in regenerating mouse liver suppression by anticoagulants. *Science* **153**, 643–644.

Vaughan, E. D., Jr., Moore, R. A., Warren, H., Moler, D. N., and Gillenwater, J. Y. (1969). Skin necrosis of genitalia and warfarin therapy. *JAMA, J. Am. Med. Assoc.* **210**, 2282–2283.

Vik, T., Try, K., Thelle, D. S., and Forde, O. H. (1979). Tromso heart study: Vitamin D metabolism and myocardial infarction. *Br. Med. J.* **2**, 176.

Ward, J. C. (1945). Rodenticides—present and future. *Soap Sanit. Chem.* **21**(9), 117, 119, 127.

Ward, J. C., and Spencer, D. A. (1947). Notes on the pharmacology of sodium fluoroacetate–compound 1080. *J. Am. Pharm. Assoc., Sci. Ed.* **36**, 59–62.

Wenz, C. (1984). New chemicals under fire. *Nature (London)* **1**, 741.

West, B. D., Preist, S., Schroeder, C. H., and Link, K. P. (1961). Studies on the 4-hydroxycoumarin. XVII. The resolution and absolute configuration of warfarin. *J. Am. Chem. Soc.* **83**, 2676–2679.

White, S. T. (1985). Surreptitious warfarin ingestion. *Child Abuse Neglect* **9**, 349–352.

Williams, R. T. (1959). "Detoxication Mechanisms," 2nd ed. Wiley, New York.

Williamson, J. R., Jones, E. A., and Azzone, G. F. (1964). Metabolite control in perfused rat heart during fluoroacetate poisoning. *Biochem. Biophys. Res. Commun.* **17**, 696–702.

Wilson, G. L., and Gaines, K. L. (1983). Effects of the rodenticide Vacor on cultured rat pancreatic beta cells. *Toxicol. Appl. Pharmacol.* **68**, 375–379.

Wiswesser, W. J. (1976). "Pesticide Index," 5th ed. Entomol. Soc. Am. College Park, Maryland.

World Health Organization (WHO) (1986). "The WHO Recommended Classification of Pesticides by Hazards," VBC/86.1. World Health Organ., Geneva.

World Health Organization (WHO) (1963). Fluoroacetamide poisoning case. *WHO Inf. Circu. Toxic. Pestic. Man* No. 11, p. 9.

Worthing, C. R., and Walker, S. B. (1983). "The Pesticide Manual," 7th ed. Br. Crop Prot. Counc., Lavenham, U.K.

Yacobi, A., and Levy, G. (1975). Comparative pharmacokinetics of coumarin anticoagulants. XIV. Relationship between binding, distribution, and elimination kinetics of warfarin in rats. *J. Pharm. Sci.* **64**, 1660–1664.

Yu, C. C., Atallah, Y. H., and Whitacre, D. M. (1982). Metabolism and disposition of diphacinone in rats and mice. *Drug Metab. Dispos.* **10**, 645–648.

Zacharski, L. R. (1982). Warfarin and cancer. *Ann. Intern. Med.* **97**, 784.

Zakzouk, M. S. (1986). The congenital warfarin syndrome. *J. Laryngol. Otol.* **100**, 215–219.

Zimmerman, A., and Matschiner, J. T. (1972). The biochemical basis of hereditary resistance to warfarin in the rat. *Fed. Proc., Fed. Am. Soc. Exp. Biol.* **31**, 714.

Herbicides

James T. Stevens and Darrell D. Sumner
CIBA-GEIGY Corporation

20.1 INTRODUCTION

The use of herbicides for control of noxious weeds and unwanted vegetation increased in the United States and internationally for the past 30 years. In fact, in 1985 over 755 million pounds of herbicides were produced in the United States, as opposed to 378 million pounds of insecticides and 109 million pounds of fungicides (Cappuccilli, 1985). The estimated U.S. production for 1987 will be 748 million, 304 million, and 100 million pounds for herbicides, insecticides, and fungicides, respectively (Delvo, 1987). The data illustrate that production of herbicides seems to have reached a plateau which is tied to a decreasing acreage planted. Still, with so great an annual consumption of herbicides, despite their designated target, the potential for adverse effects on humans or the environment is worthy of concern.

The spectrum of control of unwanted plants for a given herbicide is inherent in the chemical and biological properties of an agent. Because of the marked differences between plants and animals, it is not surprising to find materials which have high plant toxicity and low mammalian toxicity. The triazine herbicides inhibit the Hill reaction of photosynthesis (Ashton and Crafts, 1973) and usually exhibit minimal mammalian toxicity. However, it does not follow that every herbicide has low mammalian toxicity. Some herbicides, such as arsenic compounds, are protoplasmic poisons toxic to all forms of life. Finally, other herbicides are toxic to both plants and animals, even though they interfere with different biochemical systems in the two classes. This may be true in some instances where toxicity to both plants and animals depends on the same property of the toxicant. For example, it seems likely that the ability of paraquat to undergo rapid metabolism with the production of superoxide is responsible for the toxicity to both plants and animals; however, the point of attack is different, involving photosynthesis in the plant and membranes of epithelial cells in the alveolar wall in animals (Hayes, 1982).

A continual effort exists to develop more efficacious herbicides without significant mammalian toxicity. Progress has been rapid, with rather profound changes in the agents available since the publication of this chapter in 1982 (Hayes, 1982). The approximate distribution of herbicides by class is shown in Fig. 20.1. It can be seen that, on the basis of pounds sold, the amides, primarily of the subclass acetamides, hold an impressive 30% of the market share. This is followed by the triazines with 22%, thiocarbamates with 13%, and dinitroanilines with 11%. The chlorophenoxy herbicides as well as several other classes of materials that were once more popular possess less notable portions of the market. It is important to state that toxicological problems with certain chemicals have played a major role in altering the status quo of herbicides and will continue to have significant impact in the future.

The trend is toward the use of more selective agents with significantly less mammalian toxicity and significantly increased selective phytotoxicity. Indeed, some new chemicals that recently have completed the development process have herbicidal efficacy in the tablespoon per acre range as opposed to the pound per acre level that has been traditional. New agents will continue to evolve for herbicide use with the objective of finding more efficacious and less hazardous materials and eliminating chemicals for which the risks exceed the benefits.

20.2 INORGANIC AND ORGANOMETALLIC COMPOUNDS

The use of nonspecific chemicals such as common salt and smelter waste on roadsides and paths to rid them of vegetation has occurred for some hundreds of years (Hayes, 1982). Likewise, a systematic effort to develop selective herbicides has some history dating from 1896, when a French vintner noticed that Bordeaux mixture used to combat fungus on grape plants blackened a weed that grew among the vines. From this early beginning with modest successes, more selective and effective herbicides evolved.

Inorganic chemicals were prominent in this early development. They include such compounds as ammonium sulfamate, ammonium sulfate, ammonium thiocyanate, calcium cyanamide, cupric sulfate, cupric nitrate, ferrous sulfate, a mixture of magnesium sulfate and potassium chloride called kainit, potassium cyanate, sodium arsenite, sodium tetraborate, sodium chlorate, sodium chloride, sodium dichromate, sodium nitrate, borax, and sulfuric acid (Audus, 1964; Ashton and Crafts, 1973). Arsenic trioxide, a smelter waste; and iron sulfate, a

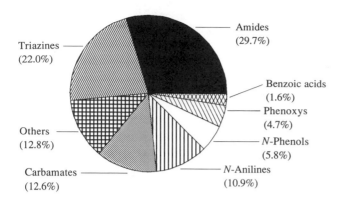

Figure 20.1   Herbicide use by class in the United States. The estimated pounds used derived from Delvo (1987).

by-product of the steel industry; and waste oils were of low commercial value (Crafts, 1961). This typified most of the agents used. In general, however, these inorganics were used as nonselective herbicides; they are especially effective against perennial weeds (Anderson, 1983).

Many inorganic herbicides are irritants, and a few, notably sulfuric acid and chlorates, are caustic. These caustic compounds rarely are ingested. However, arsenicals continue to be prominent in accidental and intentional poisoning.

Not only have some closely related inorganic salts been used, but also some organic compounds of the same elements, notably arsenic, are now used (Kearney and Kaufman, 1976).

Notably, cacodylic acid (dimethylarsinic acid), DSMA (disodium methanearsonate), and MSMA (monosodium methanearsonate) are sold today. Cacodylic acid is a nonselective postemergence agent used in general weed control, whereas both DSMA and MSMA are used as selective postemergence herbicides in cotton (Anderson, 1983). Toxicologically, these agents resemble inorganic arsenicals but they are generally less toxic (Murphy, 1986). Interestingly, however, in rats cacodylic acid is metabolized and excreted in its organic form (Stevens *et al.*, 1977).

In fact, there is no evidence that these organic arsenicals are carcinogenic in animals or humans, unlike the inorganic arsenicals. The use of these herbicides in California during the 3-year period between 1975 and 1977 resulted in 34 reports of exposure (Peoples *et al.*, 1979). Nine of these cases resulted in systemic symptoms, whereas the remainder were eye and skin irritations. Recovery was prompt in all cases. Despite this generally good toxicology profile for these agents, MSMA has been noted to cause severe peripheral neuropathy after exposure in at least one individual (Hessl and Berman, 1982). The clinical manifestations of symmetrical peripheral neuropathy, altered sensory and deep tendon reflexes, and muscle wasting are consistent with arsenic intoxication.

20.3 HERBICIDAL OILS AND SIMPLE ALIPHATICS

Because all plants are protected by a cuticle which is difficult for aqueous sprays to penetrate, oils proved to be efficacious general contact sprays (Crafts, 1961). Although discarded motor oil has been used for weed and dust control on or along highways, thinner oils such as Stoddard solvent, diesel oil, and various oils of high aromatic content (50% or more) have been found to provide excellent herbicidal control for mixed populations. In addition, it was noted that the fortification of oils without sufficient aromatics with dinitrocresol, dinitrobutylphenol, pentachlorophenol, or similar entities facilitated the spraying operation and coverage (Crafts, 1961).

The toxicity of motor oil is less than that of kerosene but otherwise similar. The toxicity of other herbicidal oils is essentially identical to that of kerosenes of different aromatic content. However, the fortification of the oils with unique aromatics may further complicate an already compounded toxicology profile.

A simple aliphatic used as a contact aquatic herbicide is acrolein (2-propenal) or $CH_2{=}CH{-}CHO$. This product is severely irritating to the skin, causes distress and irritation upon inhalation, and is highly lacrimatory (Craft, 1961). The oral LD 50 is 46 mg/kg in the rats (Sine and Meister, 1987).

20.4 CHLOROPHENOXY HERBICIDES

The chlorophenoxy moiety of these herbicides contains from one to three chlorine substitutions and occasionally a methyl substitution also. The remainder of the molecule generally is a simple acid such as acetic, propionic, or butyric; a few of the compounds involve more complex acids or esters. The herbicides that are named as acids frequently are manufactured and used in the form of metal salts, alkylamine salts, or esters. 2,4-D, 2,4,5-T, MCPA, and silvex will be discussed in detail. Other representatives of this class which will not be considered include

dichlorprop (BSI, ISO, WSSA) or
2-(2,4-dichlorophenoxy) propionic acid
2,4-DB (BSI, WSSA) or
4-(2,4-dichlorophenoxy) butyric acid
mecoprop (BSI, CSA, ISO, WSSA) or
2-(2-methyl-4-chlorophenoxy) propionic acid
MCPB (BSI, ISO, WSSA) or
4-(2-methyl-4-chlorophenoxy) butyric acid

The acid forms of the compounds known to have affected people are shown in Fig. 20.2.

Chlorophenoxy compounds (along with certain benzoic and picolinic acid derivatives) are plant growth regulators (Ashton and Crafts, 1973). Specifically, they act as synthetic auxins or plant hormones, altering the plant's metabolism and hence growth characteristics. They cause growth reactions very much like those of the approximately 12 naturally occurring indole auxins. The chlorophenoxy herbicides are more active and persistent than the indoles, and thus they elicit abnormal growth that interferes with the transport of nutrients and destroys the plant (Van Overbeek, 1964). Selectivity is based on inherent differences between the responses of enzyme systems of crops and weeds to these synthetic auxins (Crafts, 1961). The chlo-

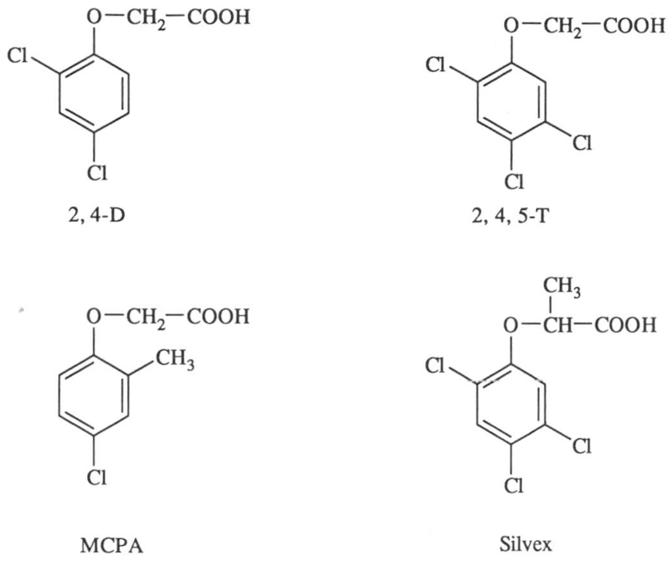

Figure 20.2   Acid forms of some chlorophenoxy herbicides.

rophenoxy compounds are much used for control of broadleaf weeds in cereal crops and pastures. 2,4,5-T has been used for control of woody plants along highways and utilities' rights-of-way (Sine and Meister, 1987).

In the body, the salts or esters of chlorophenoxy compounds are hydrolyzed fairly rapidly, so the mammalian toxicity of each compound depends mainly on the acid involved. However, different derivatives of the same compound may have very different properties as herbicides. Simple alkyl esters (e.g., isopropyl or butyl) are highly volatile and may be dangerous to neighboring crops. Other esters (e.g., butoxyethanol or tetrahydrofurfuryl) have low volatility, so their ultimate distribution is easier to control.

Although the chlorophenoxy herbicides act as growth hormones in plants, they have no hormonal action in animals. The mechanism of toxic action in animals is poorly understood, although in several instances mammalian toxicity has proved significant. The contamination of several of the chlorophenoxy herbicides with 2,3,7,8-tetrachlorodibenzo-*p*-dioxin (TCDD) has brought significant attention to this class of herbicides (see Section 18.5).

20.4.1 2,4-D

20.4.1.1 Identity, Properties, and Uses

Chemical Name   2,4-D is 2,4-dichlorophenoxyacetic acid.

Structure   See Fig. 20.2.

Synonyms   The common name 2,4-D (BSI, ISO) is in general use. Trade names include Chloroxone®, Esteron®, Salvo®, Weedar®, and Weedone®. The CAS registry number for the acid is 94-75-7.

Physical and Chemical Properties   2,4-D has the empirical formula $C_8H_6Cl_2O_3$ and a molecular weight of 221.04. It is a

white powder with a slight phenolic odor. It melts at 140.5°C. The isopropyl ester is an almost colorless liquid with a boiling point of 130°C at 1 mm Hg and a vapor pressure of 10.5×10^{-3} mm Hg at 25°C. The solubility of 2,4-D in water is 620 ppm at 25°C. It is soluble in aqueous alkali and alcohols but insoluble in petroleum oils. The isopropyl ester is practically insoluble in water but is soluble in alcohols and most oils. The solubility of the sodium salt in water is 4.5%; the amine salts range in solubility from 1.2 gm/100 ml for allylamine to 440 gm/100 ml for triethanolamine.

History, Formulations, and Uses   Some controversy surrounds the discovery of 2,4-D for herbicidal use. It is often stated that the effects of 2,4-D were discovered in England in 1942; however, the use of growth-regulating substances as selective herbicides was suggested by Ezra Jacob Kraus of the University of Chicago in 1941 (Hamner and Tukey, 1944). Although 2,4-D is effective alone against broad-leaved weeds such as lamb's-quarters, pigweed, smartweed, and ragweed, it is often used in combination with other herbicides, particularly linuron. It is available as the dimethylamine salt at 1.75 and 2 pounds acid equivalent/gallon and the isooctyl butoxyethanol esters at 2 pounds acid equivalent/gallon (Sine and Meister, 1987).

20.4.1.2 Toxicity to Laboratory Animals

Basic Findings   2,4-D is a compound of only moderate oral toxicity to rats, mice, guinea pigs, and rabbits; however, the dog appears to be more sensitive. Monkeys tolerated 214 mg/kg without serious effect (Hill and Carlisle, 1947). The oral LD 50 values for a variety of species as well as the dermal LD 50 and inhalation LC 50 values in the rat are presented in Table 20.1.

Large doses of 2,4-D quickly kill animals, apparently through ventricular fibrillation. At lower doses, when death is slow, various signs of muscular involvement, including myotonia, stiffness of the extremities, ataxia, paralysis, and coma, are seen; this is accompanied by a reduction in body temperature and metabolic rate. Repeated administration at levels that may or may not lead to death results in anorexia, loss of weight, vomiting, depression, roughness of coat, and general tenseness and muscular weakness (Hill and Carlisle, 1947; Drill and Hiratzka, 1953; Rowe and Hymas, 1954).

2,4-D was not found to elicit systemic toxicity in a 21-day dermal toxicity study in rabbits; some irritation at the application site was noted. When water was used as a solvent, only mild irritation was observed, but oil was found to be irritating (Kay *et al.*, 1965). Further, 2,4-D was found not to be a sensitizer in the standard guinea pig sensitization test.

Repeat administration at dietary levels of 3000 ppm or more was found lethal to rats, whereas 1000 ppm was tolerated longer. A level of 1000 ppm for 113 days caused depressed growth, increased mortality, and slight increase in liver weight. A dietary level of 300 ppm (about 15 mg/kg/day) for 113 days caused no clinical, laboratory, or histological changes (Rowe and Hymas, 1954). In an additional 90-day study in the Fischer 344 rat, an increase in kidney and thyroid weights was noted at

Table 20.1
Acute Toxicity of 2,4-D

Species	Route	LD 50 (mg/kg)	Reference
Rat	oral	666	Hill and Carlisle (1947)
Rat, M	oral	375	Rowe and Hymas (1954)
Rat, M	oral	395	T. B. Gaines (personal communication, 1978)
Rat, F	oral	390	T. B. Gaines (personal communication, 1978)
Rat, M	oral	855	Gorshkov (1971)
Rat, F	oral	625	Gorshkov (1971)
Rat	oral	1200	Loktionov *et al.* (1973)
Rat	oral	730	Loktionov *et al.* (1973)
Rat	oral	1000	Markosyan (1973)
Rat, M	dermal	>2000	T. B. Gaines (personal communication, 1978)
Rat, F	dermal	>2000	T. B. Gaines (personal communication, 1978)
Rat	inhalation	1790 mg/m^3	Mullison (1986)
Mouse	oral	375	Hill and Carlisle (1947)
Mouse	oral	300	Loktionov *et al.* (1973)
Mouse	oral	360	Loktionov *et al.* (1973)
Rabbit	oral	800	Hill and Carlisle (1947)
Guinea pig	oral	1000	Hill and Carlisle (1947)
Guinea pig	oral	469	Rowe and Hymas (1954)
Dog	oral	100	Drill and Hiratzka (1953)

doses of 5, 15, and 45 mg/kg/day. A no-observable-effect level (NOEL) was established at 1 mg/kg/day (Mullison, 1986).

The compound proved slightly less toxic in one 2-year study; dietary levels of 1250, 625, 125, 25, and 5 ppm had no significant effect on the growth, survival, organ weights, hematological values, or tumor incidence of rats compared to the results for those receiving no 2,4-D (Hansen *et al.*, 1971). In a second 2-year study, a feeding level of 30 mg/kg/day (approximately 600 ppm) reduced growth without reducing feed intake or survival. However, this feeding level did elicit an increase in kidney weight and volume of urine accompanied by the excretion of coproporphyrin and uroporphyrin. Mineralized deposits in the renal pelvis were also noted. A dietary level of 10 mg/kg/day (approximately 200 ppm) produced minimal mineralization in the renal pelvis as well as increased excretion of coproporphyrin during the early part of the study. The no-observable-effect level was 3 mg/kg/day (approximately 60 ppm) (Kociba *et al.*, 1979). These kidney effects may result from overload of renal tubular secretion at higher doses (Bjoerklund and Erne, 1971; Berndt and Koschier, 1973).

Repeated administration of 20 mg/kg/day produced mortality in dogs after 18 or more days; 25 mg/kg resulted in deaths within 6 days. Clinical signs consisted of bleeding gums and necrotic changes in the buccal mucosa. These signs were accompanied by a reduction in the lymphocyte count in the blood (Hill and Carlisle, 1947; Drill and Hiratzka, 1953).

Despite these findings in earlier studies in dogs, no effect related to the herbicide was found in a 2-year study in dogs maintained at dietary levels of 500, 100, 50, 10, and 0 ppm 2,4-D (Hansen *et al.*, 1971). The dose of 500 ppm is approximately equal to 12 mg/kg/day.

Absorption, Distribution, Metabolism, and Excretion

Studies with ^{14}C-labeled, 2,4-D showed that the compound reached its highest concentration in the tissues of rats within 6–8 hr after ingestion. The concentration began to fall immediately (sharp peak) when the dosage was 1 mg/rat (about 4 mg/kg); the concentration was maintained until about 17 hr after administration, when the dosage was 100 mg/rat. Within cells, the compound is found mainly in the soluble fraction, and it is excreted mainly unchanged (Khanna and Fang, 1966).

Erne (1966) found that the half-times for urinary excretion were 3 hr in rats, 8 hr in calves and hens, and about 12 hr in pigs. The excretion of small doses of 2,4-D is rapid in sheep also, 96% being excreted unchanged in the urine and <1.4% appearing in the feces within 72 hr (Clark *et al.*, 1964).

Buslovich *et al.* (1973) reported that the retention half-life in the rat was 53.1 hr for the sodium salt and 72 hr for the diethylamine salt following doses at the LD 50 level. Administration of the isooctyl ester of 2,4-D to rats resulted in rapid conversion to 2,4-D acid and rapid excretion in the urine, supporting the metabolic equivalence of the ester to 2,4-D (Mullison, 1986).

The proportion of 2,4-D excreted within 3 days was inversely proportional to dosage within the range from $\frac{1}{10}$ to $\frac{1}{100}$ of LD 50, increasing from 28% at the highest dosage to 75% at the lowest. The compound is excreted unchanged in the urine (Shafik *et al.*, 1971). The decreasing efficiency of excretion at higher dosage levels has been confirmed (Senczuk and Pogorzelska, 1975).

Biochemical Effects

Blood cholesterol levels of rats and rabbits are reduced by repeated, tolerated administration of 2,4-D (Gorshkov, 1971). Clofibrate, an analog of 2,4-D, has been used in human medicine to reduce cholesterol levels. *In vitro* cholesterol synthesis can be inhibited by 2,4-D (Gamble *et al.*, 1974; Olson *et al.*, 1974). Vainio *et al.* (1983) found that 2,4-D and MCPA (as well as the clofibrate as a positive control) induced the proliferation of hepatic peroxisomes, decreased serum lipid levels, and increased hepatic carnitine acetyltransferase and catalase activities. 2,4-D and MCPA both decreased lipoprotein activity in the adipose tissue. The authors surmised that the chlorophenoxy herbicides caused hypolipidemia not by enhancing the storage of peripheral lipids in adipose tissue but by enhancing lipid utilization in the liver.

Myotonia is one of the most characteristic effects of 2,4-D overdose. It has been produced in rats, mice, rabbits, and dogs. Clinically, this response is manifest within 30–45 min of administration. The signs include spasm, opisthotonus, and hind-limb effects with gradual recovery (Bucher, 1946).

It appears that the biochemical mechanism of myotonia produced by 2,4-D may involve enhanced enzyme activity. A K^+-independent p-nitrophenylphosphatase (basic p-NPPase) activity of microsomes isolated from normal rat skeletal muscle was increased by 2,4-D, but the activities of certain related enzymes were unchanged. Similar observations were made in muscle microsomes from rats made myotonic by intraperitoneal injection of 2,4-D at a rate of 200 mg/kg. It is thought that increased basic p-NPPase activity is related to increased passive flux of K^+ and that this might lead to myotonia through a compensatory decrease in Cl^- conductance (Brody, 1973).

Mutagenicity   No gene mutations were induced by tolerable oral doses of 2,4-D in host-mediated tests in mice using yeast and *Salmonella* as indicator cells (Zetterberg *et al.*, 1977). Further, Rashid *et al.* (1984) showed that the amino acid conjugates of 2,4-D (alanine, aspartic acid, leucine, methionine, and tryptophan) were not promutagens in the Ames *Salmonella typhimurium* test. 2,4-D did not increase the frequency of recessive lethals in *Drosophila* (Vogel and Chandler, 1974) or increased it only slightly (Magnusson *et al.*, 1977). As discussed at greater length in connection with 2,4,5-T, 2,4-D failed to induce an increase of micronuclei in mouse bone marrow erythrocytes, a test for chromosome breaking (Jenssen and Renberg, 1976).

By contrast, Pilinskaya (1974) reported a significant increase in aberrant metaphases in bone marrow cells from mice treated with 100–300 mg/kg doses but no increase in chromosomal aberrations in such cells from mice receiving 10–50 mg/kg. An increase in chromosomal aberrations was seen at all but the lowest concentrations when human lymphocyte cultures were exposed to 2,4-D at concentrations ranging from 50 to 0.002 ppm; however, the degree of change did not correspond to dose. Turkula and Jalal (1985) further showed that 50 μg/ml of 2,4-D incubated with cultured human lymphocytes significantly increased the rate of sister chromatid exchange; however, concentrations of 100 and 250 μg/ml did not elicit a response.

Oncogenicity   2,4-D did not cause a significant increase in tumors following oral administration to two strains of mice at maximal tolerated levels for 18 months (Innes *et al.*, 1969). In a lifetime study in Fisher 344 rats completed in 1986, rats were fed levels of 1, 5, 15, and 45 mg/kg/day. A slight but statistically significant increase in brain tumors (astrocytomas) was noted in male rats at 45 mg/kg/day (Mullison, 1986). The significance of this finding is uncertain.

The compound did cause some inhibition of Ehrlich ascites tumor in mice, and the animals survived slightly longer than controls (Walker *et al.*, 1972). However, the growth of two transplantable sarcomas was not inhibited (Bucher, 1946).

Effects on Reproduction   In a standard three-generation reproduction test in rats, a dietary level of 1500 ppm did not affect fertility of either sex or litter size but did reduce sharply the survival of pups to weaning and the weight of those that did survive. Dietary levels of 500 ppm (about 25 mg/kg/day) and 100 ppm were without deleterious effect (Hansen *et al.*, 1971).

Schwetz *et al.* (1971) found no teratogenic effect in rats given doses up to 87.5 mg/kg/day of 2,4-D acid or equimolar doses of three esters. At the highest dose, fetotoxic effects were noted; however, there was little or no effect on fertility, gestation, viability, and lactation indices, and there was no observable effect on neonatal growth and development. Unger *et al.* (1981) found that doses as high as 87.5 mg/kg/day of either the propylene glycol butyl ester or the isoctyl esters of 2,4-D did not affect the dam, embryo, or fetus. No remarkable anomalies were noted other than an increase in the occurrence of fourteenth rib buds with the 87.5 mg/kg/day of both esters; the no-effect level in these studies was 25 mg/kg/day.

At a high dose of 110 mg/kg/day, 2,4-D was found to be teratogenic and embryotoxic in mice (Baage *et al.*, 1973). Collins and Williams (1971) also noted terata in a non-dose-related manner in hamsters. However, investigators have not reported the same or consistent results in rats. Khera and McKinley (1972) found an increased frequency of skeletal defects. However, the changes were compatible with normal weight gain and viability in young after weaning (Khera and McKinley, 1972). On the contrary, Aleksashina *et al.* (1973) reported that 2,4-D was not teratogenic, but a large single dose did reduce growth and survival and caused other toxic effects in the fetus. Daily administration of 0.5 mg/kg reduced growth but not survival, and 0.1 mg/kg was without effect. Konstantinova *et al.* (1975) found that an oral dosage of 2,4-D as high a 50 mg/kg did not increase embryonal mortality or malformations, but it did increase the proportion of fetuses with hemorrhage of the internal organs. Konstantinova (1976) further explained these hemorrhages as a response to depression of oxidation and phosphorylation resulting in tissue hypoxia.

No congenital malformations occurred in lambs whose mothers received 2000 mg of 2,4-D per day during the first 30, 60, or 90 days of gestation (Binns and Johnson, 1970).

The fetal toxicity of 2,4-D depends largely on the derivative. When each compound was administered to rats as a single dose at half the LD 50 rate or daily throughout pregnancy at the highest level tolerated by the dam, the amine and sodium salts did not affect the development of the embryos, but the ammonium salt and especially the butyl ester of 2,4-D caused a significant increase in postimplantation mortality (Aleksashina *et al.*, 1979).

Behavioral Effects   The electroencephalogram (EEG) of rats given 2,4-D intraperitoneally at the rate of 200 mg/kg showed a reversible shortening and even elimination of the desynchronization reaction of the cortex and reticular formation. The inhibition of desynchronization began within 10 min after injection and was over in 60 min (Desi and Sos, 1962).

Pathology Animals killed by 2,4-D show irritation of the stomach or abomasum, minor liver and kidney injury, and sometimes congestion of the lungs (Drill and Hiratzka, 1953; Rowe and Hymas, 1954).

Electron microscopy of muscle demonstrated that mitochondrial proliferation and accumulation of glycogen occurred within 2 hr in rats following intraperitoneal injection of 2,4-D at a rate of 300 mg/kg. This proliferation may either return to normal or lead to irreversible mitochondrial degeneration and consequent loss of myofibrils. Muscle contractions enhanced the development of these lesions (Heene, 1968). Detailed descriptions have been given of the histological and histochemical changes caused by a single large dose and the slightly different changes produced gradually by repeated administration of moderate doses (Heene, 1975; Dux et al., 1977). It was considered that the myopathy produced by 2,4-D is a suitable model for studying primary myopathies in animals and humans (Heene, 1975). Further, Danon et al. (1976) have shown that myopathic changes correlate directly with the cumulative duration of the myotonia in rats and guinea pigs administered large doses.

20.4.1.3 Toxicity to Humans

Experimental Exposure When ^{14}C-labeled 2,4-D was injected intravenously into volunteers, 100% was recovered in the urine. The rate of excretion ranged from about 3 to 5% of the dose per hour during the first 12 hr; it then declined gradually, but a trace was still detectable in urine collected 96–120 hr after injection. Following dermal application, only 5.8% appeared in the urine within 5 days (Feldmann and Maibach, 1974), supporting limited dermal absorption.

Of six volunteers, none experienced any ill effect either subjectively or as measured by clinical and laboratory tests after ingesting one dose of 2,4-D at the rate of 5 mg/kg. Absorption was rapid; the compound appeared in the blood within 1 hr and reached its maximal level of 25–50 ppm in 7–12 hr in different men. 2,4-D appeared in the urine within 2 hr. Ninety-six hours after ingestion, 76% of the dose had been excreted unchanged in the urine. The average half-life was 33.0 hr (Kohli et al., 1974b). The results of a separate study with five volunteers were similar, except that disposal of the compound was more rapid. It disappeared from the plasma with an average half-life of 17.7 hr. Most of the excreted material was free acid, but some was conjugated (Sauerhoff et al., 1977c).

Frank et al. (1985) evaluated the exposure and urinary excretion of 2,4-D esters in six human volunteers. These studies involved exposure evaluation after aerial application to conifers during 1981 and 1982. During this program the highest daily exposure observed, based on urinalysis, was approximately 22 μg/kg (body weight). The no-effect level of 10 mg/kg, based on animal work, afforded an ample margin of safety for these workers.

Draper and Street (1982) examined the potential respiratory and dermal exposure of applicators of 2,4-D, dicamba, and a dicamba isomer from a ground boom sprayer application. It was found that airborne residues did not exceed 2.2 μg/m^3 in application vehicle cabs; however, dermal exposure to 2,4-D, as indicated by the amount rinsed from each applicator's hands after work, ranged from 1.2 to 18 mg. The elimination of 2,4-D occurred maximally between 16 and 40 hr after terminating exposure.

Occupational exposure to 2,4-D was evaluated in 45 commercial lawn care specialists who applied the herbicide 6 days/week for at least 3 weeks (Yeary, 1986). The urinary excretion over a 24-hr period was considered a reasonable estimate of absorption. The urinary levels ranged from the limit of detection, 0.01 ppm, to 2.29 ppm with a median of 0.18 ppm. This value translates to 0.00138 mg/kg with an ample margin of safety below the WHO/FAO acceptable daily dietary intake of 0.3 mg/kg.

Therapeutic Use 2,4-D has been used to treat the fungal infection producing coccidioidomycosis. In one patient with this fatal disease, moderate doses (up to 2000 mg/day intravenously) may have had some beneficial effect but clearly were not curative, and higher doses proved toxic (Seabury, 1963).

Accidental and Intentional Poisoning In a suicide involving ingestion of 50 gm of 2,4-D, the patient was conscious but dazed when first seen by a physician 1 hr after ingestion. Nine hours after ingesting the herbicide, the patient was in deep coma with generalized muscle hypotonia, relaxation of sphincters, loss of reflexes, and hypotension. He also exhibited pendular eye movements. Despite symptomatic care and diuresis, respiration became rapid and superficial, mydriasis appeared, and the patient died 12 hr after ingestion (de Larrard and Barbaste, 1969). Semicoma was noted in another suicide case; the patient died in about 2.25 days (Curry, 1962). Although the dose ingested was not known, it is believed that a dose of at least 6 gm would be necessary to produce death (Murphy, 1986).

A 46-year-old farmer accidentally ingested 2,4-D. His symptoms included a badly burned tongue and throat, nausea, vomiting, profuse sweating, and a burning sensation in his mouth, chest, and the lower part of his abdomen. Gastric lavage was performed in hospital about 1 hr after ingestion. Twelve hours after admission his face was still flushed and he vomited frequently despite antiemetic therapy. He began to complain of aching and tender muscles. Twenty-four hours after admission difficult respiration and cyanosis were evident. He had lost the use of his intercostal muscles and was breathing with his diaphragm; his arm muscles showed fibrillary twitching. He was treated with oxygen under intermittent positive pressure. To allay cardiac arrhythmia the patient was given quinidine sulfate every 4–6 hr, and this was accompanied promptly by decreased muscular tenderness. Thirty hours after admission, respiration became noticeably less labored, although X-rays revealed patchy, basilar pneumonitis, for which he received penicillin. Laboratory findings (see subsequent text) reflected muscle injury. Eleven days after admission the patient was still complaining of muscle soreness, fatigue, and insomnia, and he was moderately depressed. Two weeks after admission, the patient was discharged. Loss of sexual potency was discovered and lasted about 4 months. During 36 months of follow-up, there was no sign or symptom of polyneuropathy (Berwick, 1970).

One nonfatal case involving a mixture of 2,4-D and dichlorprop apparently was clinically typical, except that impairment of memory and change in color vision were reported (Brandt, 1971).

It is noteworthy that although myotonia is perhaps the most characteristic sign of poisoning by 2,4-D in animals, it is unusual in poisoned people, even though they often suffer marked muscle dysfunction and injury. However, marked myotonia as well as muscle weakness persisted for 2 months in a 39-year-old man who had ingested a mixture of 2,4-D and mecoprop (Park et al., 1977; Prescott et al., 1979).

Fraser et al. (1984) reported a suicide by a 61-year-old woman who ingested an unknown quantity of Killex®. This material is a liquid containing 100 gm/liter of dicamba, mecoprop, and 2,4-D as amine salts. Details of the clinical course were not presented, although tissue concentrations were monitored (see Table 20.2). Osterloh et al. (1983), in a study of a fatal overdose of 2,4-D, MCPP, and chlorpyrifos, described the clinical course as well as plasma levels consistent with the previously reported fatalities due to chlorophenoxy herbicides.

Use Experience   2,4-D can cause irritation of mucous membranes or even of the skin, but this is rarely manifest in humans. However, five female forestry workers who applied a mixture of 2,4-D and 2,4,5-T with paint brushes developed severe toxic contact eczema on the exposed parts of the skin (Jung and Wolf, 1977).

One case of acute poisoning from accidental inhalation has been reported. It involved transient loss of consciousness, urinary incontinence, and vomiting followed by myalgia, muscular hypertonia, fever, headache, and constipation. The most interesting feature was intermittent nodal tachycardia, which, along with the muscular hypertonia, gradually subsided during the administration of quinidine (Paggiaro et al., 1974).

According to Tsapko (1966), workers who entered a grain field 1 hr after it had been sprayed from the air with a mixture of

2,4-D amine salt and ammonium nitrate experienced general weakness, headache, dizziness, stomach pains, nausea, brief loss of consciousness, and moderate leukopenia. Even 14 days after application of the sodium salt, some agricultural workers complained of headache and a burning sensation in the mouth. A far wider but apparently less severe range of complaints was reported by Fetisov (1966) among various groups exposed to 2,4-D. Of particular interest was partial or complete loss of the senses of taste and smell.

Two men who used a mixture of 2,4-D and dicamba "without appropriate precautions" experienced weakness, dizziness, headache, abdominal pains, nausea, transient changes in the electrocardiogram (ECG), brief reduction of blood pressure, and transient albuminuria (Kolny and Kita, 1978).

Histories of individuals exposed to phenoxy acids and/or chlorophenols showed 19 of 52 patients with soft tissue sarcomas as opposed to 19 of 206 in matched controls. The relative risk was 5.3 for phenoxy acids and 6.6 for chlorophenols (Hardell and Sandström, 1978, 1979). As a follow-up to a study on Swedish railway workers, a cohort of 348 was evaluated (Axelson et al., 1980). An increase in tumor mortality among people exposed to phenoxy acids was more pronounced; however, no particular type of tumor predominated. These studies in Sweden were further built upon by Coggon and Acheson (1982) in the United States, who suggested a biological association between phenoxy herbicides (or their contaminants) and soft tissue sarcomas. Smith et al (1984) reported a relative risk of 1.3 with 90% confidence limits of 0.6–2.5 in regard to soft tissue sarcoma in a population occupationally exposed to phenoxy herbicides. However, this result leaves open the issue of a cause–effect relationship. Additional work by Pearce et al. (1986) in New Zealand suggested further than the phenoxy herbicides might be the cause of an increase in the occurrence of non-Hodgkin's lymphoma in occupationally exposed persons. Independently in the United States, Hoar et al. (1986) found an excess of non-Hodgkin's lymphoma in a Kansas farm population apparently associated with the use of 2,4-D. The possible association of non-Hodgkin's lymphoma with chlorophenoxy herbicides is a subject of much debate.

Table 20.2
Concentration of 2,4-D in Human Organs and Fluids Taken at Autopsy

Blood (ppm)	Brain (ppm)	Liver (ppm)	Muscle (ppm)	Kidney (ppm)	Urine (ppm)	Reference
400[a]	45	150			390	Curry (1962)
669	12.5	183	70	63	270	Nielsen et al. (1965)[b]
23	100	116				Geldmacher-von Mallinckrodt and Lautenbach (1966)[c]
58	93	408	118	193		Dudley and Thapar (1972)
520		540			670	Fraser et al. (1984)[d]

[a]Heart blood, 400 ppm; peripheral blood, 260 ppm.
[b]This paper also reported: spleen, 134 ppm; small intestine fat, 129 ppm; and large intestine fat, 36 ppm.
[c]This paper also reported: stomach, 56 ppm; small intestine, 20 ppm; lung, 88 ppm; and heart, 63 ppm.
[d]This paper also reported 340 mg/liter in the bile.

Atypical Cases of Various Origins   Three cases of peripheral neuropathy among men very recently exposed to 2,4-D were seen at one clinic in a single month (Goldstein *et al.*, 1959). In view of the extensive use of this compound, this distribution of cases would lead one to predict hundreds of similar cases per year in the United States alone. Actually, it seems that only two other cases have been reported (Todd, 1962; Berkley and Magee, 1963). No valid toxicological or epidemiological evidence was given to support a causal relationship in the five cases. In no instance has systematic poisoning, involving as it does a massive dosage, been associated with peripheral neuropathy.

The illness of a 57-year-old farmer was attributed to 2,4-D. It had been applied with a hand sprayer as a 40% aqueous solution; although part of the spraying was against the wind, no accident had been recognized. At home after work, the farmer vomited, was weak, sweated profusely, and had oliguria. In hospital, he was found to have a temperature above 38°C; white cells and albumin were found in his urine. A low fever persisted, and on day 18 diarrhea with fresh blood but no colic occurred. The diarrhea persisted for 30 days but the patient finally recovered completely (Monarca and Di Vitto, 1961). The history of minimal exposure, atypical symptomatology, and prolonged course suggest that the relation to 2,4-D was circumstantial only.

In a review of 22 cases of aplastic anemia in childhood, Hughes (1962) recorded this condition in a 5-year-old child who "was heavily contaminated with weed killer (containing '2,4-D' and possibly arsenicals) 6 weeks before onset of pallor and facile bruising."

Workers who had been exposed for 2 years to the sodium salt of 2,4-D began to experience an unpleasant sensation in the throat and nasopharynx and later showed atrophic changes in the mucosa. A 4- to 5-year contact caused dry cough and dyspnea. X ray revealed basal emphysema and other changes. Later, toxic hepatitis with enlargement and dysfunction of the liver appeared. Most patients showed dysproteinemia and elevated cholinesterase levels. Autonomic polyneuritis occurred (Belomyttseva, 1969). Somewhat similar findings were reported by Amirov *et al.* (1968), Bashirov (1969), and Bashirov and Ter-Bagadasarova (1970), but such effects have not been encountered in Western Europe or the United States. Similar acute illness with sequelae lasting at least 2 years was reported by Kaskevich and Soboleva (1978) and by Bezuglyi *et al.* (1979).

A report by Ceppi (1974) mentioned allergic dermatitis, squamous lesions of the limbs, allergic hypersensitivity, rhinitis, dermatitis, and urticaria but leaves in doubt the nature of exposure and even the identity of the compounds involved.

Dosage Response   One man survived 6 days after consuming an estimated "one pint of pure 2,4-D in a kerosene-like solvent" (Dudley and Thapar, 1972). The fatal dose in one case was estimated at 355 mg/kg (Hayes 1982). In another case, an estimate of the retained dose (the victim had vomited) as more than 80 mg/kg was based on chemical analysis of gastrointestinal contents, tissues, and urine (Nielsen *et al.*, 1965). Berwick

(1970) reported survival following an ingested dose estimated at 110 mg/kg. Even more remarkable, a man survived an absorbed dosage of about 100 mg/kg of 2,4-D plus 200 mg/kg of mecoprop, as estimated by material recovered from the urine (Park *et al.*, 1977; Prescott *et al.*, 1979).

A patient given 3600 mg of 2,4-D (66.6 mg/kg) intravenously suffered coma, fibrillary twitching of some muscles, hyporeflexia, and urinary incontinence. Seven hours after infusion, the patient could be roused but lapsed back into deep sleep. Twenty-four hours after administration he was eating well but still complained of profound muscular weakness; within an additional 24 hr, all effects of the herbicide had dissipated. The same patient had experienced no side effects from 18 previous intravenous doses during 33 days; each of the last 12 doses in this series was 800 mg or more, the last being 2000 mg (about 37 mg/kg) (Seabury, 1963). Another man, Ezra Jacob Kraus of the University of Chicago, reported at a scientific meeting that he had had no ill effect from oral doses of 500 mg/day (about 7 mg/kg/day) for 21 days, and this statement was summarized by others (Mitchell *et al.*, 1946; Assouly, 1951).

The threshold limit value (10 mg/m³) indicates that occupational intake at a rate of about 1.4 mg/kg/day is considered safe.

Laboratory Findings   Soon after ingestion, one would expect the concentration of 2,4-D in the organs and urine to increase while the concentration in the blood declines. The values in Table 20.2 are consistent with this expectation and suggest that death occurred in different cases when excretion had reached different—but always early—stages of completion.

Concentrations of 2,4-D found at autopsy of persons who ingested a mixture of 2,4-D and 2,4,5-T and probably died mainly from the effects of 2,4,5-T are discussed in Section 20.4.2.3.

Some details of the serum and urine levels of 2,4-D and dicamba are presented under Laboratory Findings in Section 20.5.1.3 in connection with a case of ingestion of a mixture of these compounds. The highest concentrations of 2,4-D in serum and urine were 1031 and 1900 ppm, respectively, and the patient survived what in all likelihood was mainly 2,4-D poisoning. Three hours after the ingestion of a mixture of 2,4-D and mecoprop, their plasma concentrations were 400 and 751 ppm, respectively. The patient recovered following forced alkaline diuresis, which reduced the plasma half-life of 2,4-D from 220 to 4.7 hr and that for mecoprop from 39 to 14 hr (Park *et al.*, 1977; Prescott *et al.*, 1979). It is interesting that the highest concentration of 2,4-D in the serum in those nonfatal cases was substantially higher than the concentrations in autopsy blood shown in Table 20.2.

Positive analyses for 2,4-D were reported in 5 of 33 men and in 3 of 37 women who had died of other causes. The highest value (0.02 ppm) was for the kidney. The occurrence of the compound in people was attributed to its persistence on fodder fed to cattle (Fedorova *et al.*, 1977). If the analytical results were dependable, the agricultural practices must have been remarkable.

Urinary levels of 2,4-D in exposed workers ranged from 0.10 to 0.19 ppm (Shafik *et al.*, 1971) or 8 ppm (Kolmodin and Erne, 1979).

A farmer who accidentally swallowed a mouthful of concentrated weed killer received a dose of 2,4-D estimated at 110 mg/kg. He suffered fibrillary twitching and paralysis of intercostal muscles requiring oxygen under positive pressure. In this case, there was marked elevation of serum glutamic-oxaloacetic transaminase, serum glutamic-pyruvic transaminase, lactate dehydrogenase, aldolase, and creatinine phosphokinase levels, all interpreted as evidence of generalized skeletal muscle damage. Hemoglobinuria and myoglobinuria also were observed. Laboratory findings returned to normal in 1 month or earlier (Berwick, 1970).

Pathology   Autopsy findings are few and not diagnostic. Congestion of all organs and severe degenerative changes of brain ganglion cells, perhaps due to anoxia, but no other abnormality, were found in one case (Nielsen *et al.*, 1965). Degeneration of the convoluted tubules, protein in the glomerular spaces, and a little fatty degeneration of the kidneys were the only lesions found in the body of a man who survived more than 2 days after intentionally drinking 2,4-D (Curry, 1962). Degenerative changes of kidney tubules and liver and severe congestion of the upper gastrointestinal tract (perhaps caused by kerosene) were reported by Dudley and Thapar (1972), who remarked especially on perivascular areas of acute demyelination, occasionally with central petechiae confined almost entirely to the white matter. The lesions were considered identical to those sometimes seen in carbon monoxide poisoning. Interpretation is complicated by the fact that hypoxia and/or the atrophic state of the brain cannot be excluded as causes. It must be added that the patient had shown progressive senile dementia for some years prior to ingestion, and the brain weighed only 1210 gm. It is of interest that muscle changes were looked for in this case but not found.

Treatment of Poisoning   With one exception, treatment is entirely symptomatic. The exception involves quinidine sulfate, which may be of value not only for preventing cardiac arrhythmia but also for treating the dysfunction of skeletal muscle. Sodium sulfate may be useful as a cathartic if bowel movement has not occurred 4 hr after exposure, if the victim is conscious (Morgan, 1982). In severe poisonings, forced *alkaline* diuresis may save the victim's life; such treatment reduced the plasma half-life of 2,4-D for up to 4.7 hr and produced gradual clinical improvement over a 48-hr period; the patient survived without permanent sequelae (Park *et al.*, 1977; Prescott *et al.*, 1979; Morgan, 1982).

20.4.2 2,4,5-T

20.4.2.1 Identity, Properties, and Uses

Chemical Name   2,4,5-T is 2,4,5-trichlorophenoxyacetic acid.

Structure   See Fig. 20.2.

Synonyms   The common name 2,4,5-T (BSI, ISO, WSSA) is in general use. Trade names include Estron® 245, Estron® Brush Killer, Marks Brushwood Killer®, Shellstar® Brush Killer, Weedar® 2,4,5-T, and Weedone® 2,4,5-T. The CAS registry number for the acid is 93-76-5.

Physical and Chemical Properties   2,4,5-T has the empirical formula $C_8H_5Cl_3O_3$ and a molecular weight of 255.49. The pure acid forms white crystals that melt at 156.6°C; the technical acid is 98% pure with a melting point of 150–151°C. The acid has a water solubility of 278 ppm at 25°C. The salts with alkali metals and amines are water-soluble but insoluble in petroleum oils. The esters are soluble in oils but not in water. The technical acid is stable and noncorrosive.

History, Formulations, and Uses   Hamner and Tukey (1944) apparently were first to demonstrate the effectiveness of 2,4,5-T as a selective herbicide. Its action is similar to that of 2,4-D, but it is more effective on woody species. In combination with 2,4-D, it was used exclusively as a defoliant during the Vietnam War. 2,4,5-T now is used mainly in the form of esters. Available formulations include emulsifiable concentrates and water-soluble concentrates usually containing about 20–800 gm of acid equivalent per liter.

20.4.2.2 Toxicity to Laboratory Animals

Basic Findings   Signs of poisoning in dogs include a mild spasticity rather than myotonia; otherwise, the signs of poisoning by 2,4,5-T and 2,4-D are similar (Drill and Hiratzka, 1953). The compound has only moderate acute toxicity, as indicated by LD 50 values of 500, 389, and 381 mg/kg in rats, mice, and guinea pigs, respectively (Rowe and Hymas, 1954), and slightly greater than 100 mg/kg in dogs (Drill and Hiratzka, 1953).

All dogs were killed by 20 mg/kg/day after 4.9 or more days. Terminally, they showed a reduction of circulating lymphocytes. Dogs survived 10 mg/kg/day or less for 90 days without illness or change in body weight, organ weights, or blood count (Drill and Hiratzka, 1953).

When rats were fed a dietary level of 2000 ppm of 2,4,5-T containing <0.05 ppm of a contaminant, TCDD, some of them became sick and a few died. The minimal cumulative fatal dosage was about 900 mg/kg (Chang *et al.*, 1974).

Dietary concentrations of 5000 ppm or higher were fatal to chicks in less than 3 weeks, but they tolerated 5000 ppm for 1 week and resumed a normal growth rate when returned to uncontaminated feed. The birds were able to discriminate between contaminated and uncontaminated feed; when given a choice, they rejected the contaminated material and grew normally. Chicks offered feed containing 2000 ppm had only a reduced feed consumption and growth rate, but survived. A level of 100 ppm was without adverse effect (Whitehead and Pettigrew, 1972).

Absorption, Distribution, Metabolism, and Excretion
Less than 0.1 ppm of 2,4,5-T was present in a sheep given the compound 3 days earlier at the rate of 25 mg/kg. Similar results were obtained for sheep and cattle that received repeated doses of 0.75 mg/kg/day. However, when the compound was administered to sheep at a rate of 250 mg/kg/day until they were acutely poisoned, tissue levels as high as 368 ppm were found in the kidney and lower levels were found in liver, muscle, and fat (Clark and Palmer, 1971). In a similar way, Leng (1972) also found very low tissue levels in animals that had received nontoxic dosages (dietary levels of 180–1800 ppm) for 28 days.

[^{14}C]2,4,5-T injected intravenously into mice at a rate of about 3 mg/kg in early pregnancy did not reach the fetus to a significant degree; a higher concentration than that in the maternal blood was noted in the maternal kidneys and the visceral yolk sac epithelium. In late pregnancy, [^{14}C]2,4,5-T also concentrated in the kidneys and yolk sac, but slowly passed the placenta and achieved a concentration in the fetal organs similar to that in the maternal ones (Lindquist and Ullberg, 1971). Similar results were found in a later study, which revealed no passage of 2,4,5-T to embryonic mouse and hamster tissues up to day 10 or 11 of gestation. During this early period, the visceral yolk sac placenta is the only route to the embryo. On days 11–18, when the chorioallantoic placenta develops and matures, there was a steady increase in the transport of the herbicide. Cleft palate was detected in fetuses from dams treated on day 13 or 14 of gestation; this was concomitant with a significant concentration of herbicide in the fetus (Dencker, 1976).

At relatively high dosage levels, about 0.5–9.0% of the 2,4,5-T excreted by rats is in the form of 2,4,5-trichlorophenol (Shafik et al., 1971). When both rats and dogs were given a lower dosage (5 mg/kg) of [^{14}C]2,4,5-T, a small amount of one metabolite was found in the urine of rats, but three unidentified metabolites were found in the urine of dogs (Piper et al., 1973). No radioactive carbon dioxide was detected in air exhaled by rats that had received an oral dose of [^{14}C]2,4,5-T (Fang et al., 1973). When 2,4,5,-T was administered orally to rats and mice at a rate of 50 mg/kg, they excreted it mainly in the urine and mainly as the free acid; however, conjugates with glycine and taurine were found also, as well as the hydrolysis product 2,4,5-trichlorophenol (Grunow and Boehme, 1974).

Only a slow disappearance of 2,4,5-T from mice could be detected by gas chromatographic analysis of whole bodies at intervals following subcutaneous injection at the rate of 100 mg/kg. Disappearance of 2,4-D was considerably faster (Zielinski and Fishbein, 1967).

2,4,5-T was excreted only slowly by rats following an oral dose at the rate of 50 mg/kg. The highest rate of excretion was reached by some animals during the first day but by most on the second day, when it averaged 18.7% of the dose for all rats. In subsequent days, excretion decreased gradually to 0.4–2.0% on the seventh day. An average of 57.6% was accounted for within 7 days, mainly in the free form but partly as a conjugate (Grunow et al., 1971). However, the proportion of intake that can be accounted for in the urine decreases as the dosage increases. Thus, 100% of the dose of 2,4,5-T was recovered in the urine of rats following a dose of 10^{-5} times the LD 50 per day for 3 days, but only 49% was recovered within the 7-day sampling period following 10^{-1} LD 50 per day for 3 days (Shafik et al., 1971).

When rats were given a single oral dose of [^{14}C]2,4,5,-T, it was found that the half-life for radioactivity in the plasma was progressively shorter and the volume of distribution was progressively less at the lower dosages. The half-lives for disappearance of radioactivity from the entire body also were proportional to dosage, the values being 28.9, 19.3, 13.1, and 13.6 hr at dosages of 200, 100, 50, and 5 mg/kg, respectively (Piper et al., 1972, 1973). Results were essentially similar following intravenous injection at rates of 100 and 5 mg/kg. For 30 hr after injection, the half-life of 2,4,5-T in the plasma was 23 hr for the higher dosage and 4 hr for the lower dosage. It is of great interest that, when the actual concentration in the plasma resulting from the higher dosage decreased to the initial level resulting from the lower dosage, the half-life for the higher dosage decreased so that it was statistically indistinguishable from that associated with the lower dosage (Sauerhoff et al., 1976a).

Studies with isolated, perfused rat kidneys showed that a small dose of 2,4,5-T was excreted effectively by the kidney tubules without markedly affecting renal function, but a large dose was nephrotoxic and interfered with its own excretion (Koschier and Acara, 1978). Retention of 2,4,5-T in the body and in the kidney in particular was explained at least in part by its binding to plasma proteins and to microsomal and cytosolic fractions of the renal cortex. One specific microsomal and two specific cytosolic binding sites have been characterized chemically (Koschier et al., 1979).

At dosages of 10, 1, and 0.04 mg/kg there was no significant difference in rate of excretion, which was rapid, averages of 75 and 8.2% of the radioactivity being recovered in the urine and feces, respectively, during the first 24 hr. Averages of 85 and 11% were recovered in urine and feces during 7 days. There was no detectable difference in the rate of elimination in pregnant and nonpregnant rats. However, radioactivity was detected in fetuses of different ages and in milk as well as in all organs of adults or of milk-fed newborns. The maximal concentrations in different tissues generally were reached in 6–12 hr after dosing and then declined rapidly so that very little activity remained in the organs after 3 days (Fang et al., 1972, 1973).

In dogs given [^{14}C]2,4,5-T at the rate of 5 mg/kg, the half-life for elimination from the body was 86.6 hr, compared to 13.6 hr in rats given the same dosage. This offers a plausible explanation of why the compound is more toxic in dogs than in rats (Piper et al., 1973). Some further light on the different ability of rats and dogs to excrete the compound comes from in vitro studies of kidney slices (Hook et al., 1974). Low clearance in the dog may be related to very tight binding of the herbicide to plasma protein (Hook et al., 1976).

When 2,4,5-T was fed to cows for 2–3 weeks at each of a series of increasing dietary levels ranging from 10 to 1000 ppm, the concentration of residues in milk corresponded to intake. The average residues found in milk at the highest level were 0.42 ppm 2,4,5-T and 0.23 ppm 2,4,5-trichlorophenol. The concentrations did not increase with duration or exposure but decreased rapidly after removal of the chemical from the feed (Bjerke *et al.*, 1972).

2,4,5-T undergoes enterohepatic circulation, and this has a marked effect on its pharmacokinetics. A mathematical model that accurately predicts excretion with or without the diversion of bile through a cannula is available (Colburn, 1978).

Mehlman *et al.* (1976) have further characterized this process in rats, dogs, and humans. It was found that lower doses of [^{14}C]2,4,5-T (up to 50 mg/kg) were eliminated as a first-order process; however, higher doses of 100 and 200 mg/kg appeared to saturate metabolic or elimination processes, resulting in a marked alteration in the elimination half-life ($t_{\frac{1}{2}}$). Remarkable differences in elimination were also noted among species at comparable doses. The $t_{\frac{1}{2}}$ for elimination in the dog was found to be 77 hr, as opposed to 23 hr in humans and 5 hr in rats. These differences in the kinetics of elimination appear to have some association with the acute toxicity as manifest in these three species, since the dog, then the human, is generally more sensitive to the chlorophenoxy herbicides than the rat (see Section 20.4.1).

At least part of the species difference in the teratogenicity of 2,4,5-T depends on difference in ability of the dams to excrete the compound and resulting differences in the interval during which it can reach the fetus. In mice, which are especially susceptible to teratogenesis by this compound, only about 10% of a dose at the rate of 100 mg/kg was excreted in an hour. After four daily doses at this rate, the 2,4,5-T accumulated in both maternal tissues and fetuses. In contrast to its slow excretion in the mouse, 2,4,5-T was rapidly excreted in the guinea pig, about 50% in 15 hr after a single oral dose. This high rate prevented the compound from reaching the fetus. When fetal guinea pigs were injected *in utero*, they excreted 2,4,5-T about as fast as the mothers (Ebron and Courtney, 1976). In the mouse, [^{14}C]2,4,5-T was obvious in fetal as well as maternal tissues 30 min after the dam received 100 mg/kg on day 13 of pregnancy. The concentrations were maximal at 8 hr and virtually absent at 24 hr. Autoradiographs demonstrated activity in the fetal liver, skin, eyes, and the ventricles of the brain. After 48 hr, activity was still detectable in fetal muscle but not the palate (Courtney *et al.*, 1977). Under similar conditions, no metabolite of 2,4,5-T was found in the tissues. Within 7 days, 35–44% of the radioactivity was excreted in the urine as the parent compound and 22–33% as highly polar metabolites; 3–6% was excreted unchanged in the feces and 1–2% as polar metabolites (Koshakji *et al.*, 1978).

Biochemical Effects   2,4,5-T is taken up *in vitro* by slices of rat or rabbit renal cortex. Details of the process indicate that it is energy dependent and involves the organic anion mechanism (Berndt and Koschier, 1973). This effect can be demonstrated after administration of a single oral dose to the intact rat at 45–90 mg/kg but not after single or repeated doses at 20 mg/kg (Koschier and Berndt, 1977). Binding of 2,4,5-T to plasma protein and to certain kidney proteins is extensive and could

limit its rate of excretion and contribute to its nephrotoxicity (Koschier *et al.*, 1979).

2,4,5-T and 2,4-D altered the synthesis of cholesterol and fatty acids in rat liver homogenates (Olson *et al.*, 1974). This result is not astonishing, because clofibrate, one of the more widely used hypocholesteremic agents in human medicine, is an analog of these herbicides; the drug usually is administered at the rate of 2000 mg/person/day. A possible mechanism for the action of such compounds has been proposed (Gamble, 1975; Vainio *et al.*, 1983).

2,4,5-T caused an increase in liver size and in the amount of RNA and protein in the liver. These actions were detectable following a single oral dose at the rate of 167 mg/kg and increased at higher dosage levels. The effect was reversible when dosing was stopped. So far, unlike the situation with clofibrate, induction of microsomal enzymes by 2,4,5-T has not been detected (Rip and Cherry, 1976). Similar results were reported by Chang *et al.* (1974).

Dosage as high as 1000 mg/kg/day failed to produce any indication of porphyria in rats (Miura *et al.*, 1978). The level of ^{131}I in the serum and also the absolute thyroid count in male rats were depressed 24 hr after a single oral dose of 2,4,5-T at the rate of 100 mg/kg. There were marked disturbances of electrolytes. These changes suggested widespread changes in membrane function (Sjöden *et al.*, 1977).

Mutagenicity   In gene mutation tests, 2,4,5-T was not mutagenic in a host-mediated assay in mice or in spot tests with indicator bacteria (Buselmaier *et al.*, 1973). Furthermore, 2,4,5-T was found to be negative in a dominant lethal assay in mice (Buselmaier *et al.*, 1973). It was not clastogenic in a sex-linked lethal test in *Drosophilia*, although it caused a decline in fertility in male flies (Vogel and Chandler, 1974). 2,4,5-T has been evaluated in several assays to examine clastogenic or chromosomal aberration potential. In micronucleus tests with red cells from bone marrow of mice 24 hr and 7 days following intraperitoneal injection of 2,4,5-T at the rate of 100 mg/kg, there was no increase in micronuclei compared to controls. However, a weak toxic effect on mitotic activity was indicated by a decrease in the percentage of young (polychromatic) cells in the samples. Gas chromatographic analysis showed that <5% of the test substance present in the plasma appeared in the cells. It was considered that the results did not exclude the possibility that 2,4,5-T is inherently mutagenic but did indicate that it does not constitute any cytogenic hazard to humans (Jenssen and Renberg, 1976).

A different result was reported by Majumdar and Golia (1974), namely a significant increase in sex-linked recessive lethals from 0.05% in flies on control diet to 0.66% in flies reared in a concentration of 1000 ppm 2,4,5-T. Similar results were reported by Magnusson *et al.* (1977). Yefimenko (1974) reported that in rats single oral doses at rates as high as 1 mg/kg did not cause general toxic effects, changes in the function of spermatozoa, or changes in the mitotic activity of bone marrow cells, but a dose of 0.01 mg/kg did produce chromatid aberrations and adhesion of chromosomes. With repeated doses given by stomach tube, the threshold for general toxic and gonadotropic action was 0.1 mg/kg/day. However, the chromosomal lesions disappeared at the end of the experiment, due, it was said, to adaptive mechanisms. In view of the negative results of other investigators for mice, except occasionally at very high dose levels, the possibility of a contaminant or some other unrecognized variable in this instance cannot be excluded. Certainly, a formulation factor was involved in a study by Dävring and Hultgren (1977). A commercial formulation of a 2,4,5-T ester caused about five times as much chromosome damage in bone marrow cells of mice dosed intraperitoneally as was found after 2,4,5-T acid; however, the solvent and the emulgators in the formulation had the same effect. Because similar solvents and emulsifiers are likely to be used in formulating a wide range of pesticides and other chemicals, it is obscure what bearing the result has regarding 2,4,5-T.

Mongolian gerbils were injected intraperitoneally with 2,4,5-T at rates of 100, 70, 50, 30, 10, or 0 mg/kg/day for 5 days and killed for examination 24 hours after the last dose of herbicide and 2 hours after an intraperitoneal injection of Colcemid (demecolcine). For each dosage group, 500 bone marrow cells in metaphase were examined for chromosome aberrations. At the higher dosage levels, increases in chromatid gaps, chromatid breaks, and fragments were found. At the highest level the percentage of abnormal metaphases was 21.5%, compared to 1.4% in each of two sets of controls. There was a good dosage–response relationship down to a total dosage of 250 mg/kg, which resulted in 4.4% abnormal metaphases. There was no significant difference at total dosages of 50 and 250 mg/kg (Majumdar and Hall, 1973).

In the cell transformation test, concentrations of 1.75 and 2.25 mM almost stopped growth of mouse L 929 cells *in vitro*, and particles appeared in the cytoplasm, mainly around the nucleus. The effects were dose dependent, with little or no effect at 0.25 mM (64 ppm). On prolonged incubation in 2.25 mM medium, the cells became rounded and detached from the substrate. When the test medium was replaced by control medium, the particles disappeared, the cells resumed their fibroblast-like structure, and cell multiplication was resumed after a lag period (Dragsnes *et al.*, 1975).

Injection of Ehrlich ascites tumor-bearing mice with 2,4,5-T for 5 or 6 days at rates of 62, 78, 80, or 85 mg/kg/day caused a slight inhibition of tumor development, and this was dosage related. At a dosage of 70 mg/kg/day for 5 days, survival time was increased by 41% but mortality was unchanged (Walker *et al.*, 1972).

Oncogenicity   2,4,5-T did not cause a significant increase in tumors following oral administration to two strains of mice at the maximal tolerated level for 18 months (Innes *et al.*, 1969). In two 2-year studies in rats, the incidence of tumors was not increased at any dosage level tested, including one (30 mg/kg/day) that produced toxic effects without increasing mortality (Hansen *et al.*, 1971; Kociba *et al.*, 1979).

Effects on Reproduction   A study carried out under contract

by a commercial laboratory was the cause, or at least the signal, for a tremendous amount of concern about the safety of 2,4,5-T. Results of the Bionetics Study were generally known by July 1969, although a summary was not published until the following year (Courtney *et al.*, 1970). Briefly, 2,4,5-T was found to be teratogenic (cleft palate) and fetocidal in two strains of mice when administered either subcutaneously or orally and in one strain of rats (cystic kidney) when administered orally. Even in 1969, it became known that the sample of 2,4,5-T used in the study contained 30 ppm TCDD, and it was alleged that this was the cause of the observed toxicity.

As a result, new tests were carried out with a much improved technical grade of 2,4,5-T containing only 0.5 ppm TCDD obtained from a different commercial source and also with an analytical grade sample containing <0.05% TCDD. Doses were given subcutaneously in mice and orally in rats on days 6–15 of gestation in both species. At the lowest dosage tested (100 mg/kg/day), even the analytical grade 2,4,5-T caused an increase in cleft palates in the one strain of mice in which it was tested. The same dosage of technical 2,4,5-T had the same effect in all three strains of mice studied. The results were also positive but less clear-cut for a relative enlargement of the pelvis of the kidney referred to as "hydronephrosis." TCDD alone at a dosage as low as 0.001 mg/kg/day produced the same changes. When analytical grade 2,4,5-T and TCDD were combined at dosage of 100 and 0.001 mg/kg/day, respectively, there was no potentiation. In the rat, 2,4,5-T was not teratogenic or fetotoxic. TCDD produced the same change in the kidney as that seen in the mouse. Prenatal administration of 2,4,5-T did not affect postnatal growth and development of the rat (Courtney and Moore, 1971). The teratogenicity in mice of 2,4,5-T containing ≤0.1 ppm TCDD was confirmed in connection with levels as low as 35 mg/kg/day (Roll, 1971) and even 15 mg/kg/day (Gaines *et al.*, 1975).

Several papers have reported no-effect levels for the teratogenic action of 2,4,5-T containing ≤0.1 ppm TCDD: 20 mg/kg/day (Roll, 1971; Beck, 1977) and 40 mg/kg/day (Frohberg, 1974). However, these negative findings may have been the statistical result of using a limited number of animals (see Section 2.2.7.1). In what was certainly the most thorough study of the subject in any one species, tests were replicated 6–10 times in four inbred and 35 times in one outbred strain of mice. The number of litters studied per strain ranged from 236 to 1485. Treatment was by gavage on days 6–14 of pregnancy, and dosages ranged from 15 to 120 mg/kg/day. Cleft palate was demonstrated at 15 mg/kg/day in one strain at 30 mg/kg/day in the other four, the lowest dosage tested in each instance. There were significant differences between strains; the ED 50 for litters containing at least one pup with cleft palate was 105 and 25 mg/kg/day for BALB/c and A/Jax mice, respectively (Gaines *et al.*, 1975).

Frohberg (1974) reported both teratogenicity and fetal toxicity in mice from 80 mg/kg/day orally and from a calculated dose of 37 mg/kg/day associated with exposure for 5 hr/day to an aerosol at a concentration of 216 mg/m^3; these levels were toxic to the dams also. As might be expected, 2,4,5-T is teratogenic in mice when administered subcutaneously (Baage *et al.*, 1973).

Although relative expansion of the renal pelvis in mice was first considered a teratogenic effect, it later became recognized as evidence of delayed maturity that was partially reversible (Moore, 1973). The delay in maturity is not only morphological but also enzymatic. Renal alkaline phosphatase tended to be subnormal in 17-day-old fetuses from dams treated with 2,4,5-T, but was significantly more nearly normal in 18-day-old fetuses (Highman *et al.*, 1977, 1979).

Neubert and Dillman (1972) reported that doses as low as 10–15 mg/kg/day reduced fetal weight in mice. In contrast, rats that had an increased incidence of skeletal defects following maternal doses of 100–150 mg/kg/day showed normal weight gain and viability (Khera and McKinley, 1972).

2,4,5-T containing no detectable TCDD was still found to be fetocidal and teratogenic to hamsters when administered orally on days 6–10 of gestation at a dose of 100 mg/kg/day. At 80 mg/kg/day the same sample reduced the number of pups per litter and fetal weight and survival, but did not cause terata. At 40 mg/kg/day, the number of young per litter was slightly decreased. Commercial 2,4,5-T containing 0.1 ppm TCDD was no more toxic or teratogenic than samples containing no detectable contaminant. However, a sample containing 0.5 ppm TCDD was teratogenic at a dose of 40 mg/kg/day, and a sample containing 45 ppm TCDD was teratogenic at a dose of only 20 mg/kg/day (Collins and Williams, 1971). At the much lower dose of 2 mg/kg, 2,4,5-T was not teratogenic (Gale and Ferm, 1973).

Most authors have reported a lack of teratogenic effect of 2,4,5-T in the rat. A lack of fetotoxic effect at doses as high as 24 mg/kg/day on days 6–16 of pregnancy was established by Emerson *et al.* (1971), using a regular commercial product containing 0.5 ppm TCDD. Even a dose of 50 mg/kg/day was not teratogenic but did lead to a slight increase of delayed ossification of skull bones. A level of 100 mg/kg/day killed a high proportion of dams; the few young that survived showed toxic effects but no terata (Sparschu *et al.*, 1971). Konstantinova (1974, 1976) reported that a dose of 0.1 mg/kg/day during the entire pregnancy of rats was the threshold dose for reduced growth and increased pathomorphological changes and mortality in the fetus. A dose of 0.01 mg/kg/day was without effect. Sokolik (1973) reported cleft palate, hydronephrosis, brachydactylia, and gastrointestinal hemorrhage in newborn rats following administration of the butyl ester of 2,4,5-T to the dams at rates as low as 50 mg/kg/day, but he considered that traces of dioxin probably were responsible.

In a three-generation reproduction study carried out at dietary levels of 30, 10, 3, and 0 ppm, the parent rats were fed for 90 days before first breeding. Neonatal survival was significantly decreased in some but not all matings at dietary levels of 30 and 10 ppm. Some groups of weanlings at the 30 ppm level showed increased liver weight and decreased thymus weight. Hydronephrosis was seen in diminishing incidence through the generations. A dietary level of 3 ppm produced no significant effect (Smith *et al.*, 1978).

Rabbits that received 2,4,5-T (0.5 ppm TCDD) by capsule on days 6–18 of pregnancy at rates of 0, 10, 20, and 40 mg/kg/day showed no teratogenic or embryotoxic effects (Emerson *et al.*, 1971).

Whereas the teratogenicity of 2,4,5-T to mice is well established, 2,4,5-T was not found to be teratogenic to the rhesus monkey at oral doses of 0.05, 1.0, and 10.0 mg/kg/day from day 22 to day 38 of gestation. The formulation used contained 0.05 ppm TCDD. The mothers showed no toxicity. Not all the infant monkeys were killed near term. Those permitted to live for a year grew and behaved normally, and they showed no deformities at autopsy (Dougherty *et al.*, 1973, 1975). The two higher doses are greater than those likely to be absorbed by workers who manufacture and formulate the compound.

Behavioral Effects   It has been reported that male, but not female, offspring of rats treated with 2,4,5-T at 100 mg/kg on day 7, 8, or 9 of pregnancy walked around and groomed more in an open-field behavior test than did the offspring of controls (Sjöden and Söderberg, 1972).

The administration of 2,4,5-T into incubating chicken eggs resulted in behavioral manifestation in the hatchlings (Sanderson and Rogers, 1981). Single doses produced no morphological effects; however, 7 mg/kg elicited a retardation of learning, and 13 and 27 mg/kg increase motor activity.

Factors Influencing Toxicity   Food intake, growth, and feed efficiency ratio were decreased in rats receiving 6% instead of 20% casein diets during gestation. This injury was additive with that produced by dietary levels of 250 and 1000 ppm 2,4,5-T. The young were poorly nourished, but no teratogenic effect was found (Hall, 1972).

Pathology   Dogs killed by 2,4,5-T may show diffuse redness of the intestine on gross examination and some necrosis and inflammation histologically. There also may be diffuse hepatic necrosis and mild renal tubular degeneration. When death is delayed, pneumonia may be found at autopsy (Drill and Hiratzka, 1953). The findings are not diagnostic.

When mice received 2,4,5-T by stomach tube on days 6–14 of pregnancy at rates of 60 or 120 mg/kg/day, some of them became sick or even moribund. In these mice, including some sacrificed as little as 2 days after beginning treatment, two distinct heart lesions, atrophy of the thymus, reduction in the size of splenic follicles, hypertrophy of the thyroid, and other changes were observed (Highman *et al.*, 1976).

The administration to broiler chickens of 2,4,5-T at a concentration of 1000 ppm in drinking water led to renal changes detectable as early as 14 days after exposure started. Progressive changes in the proximal convoluted tubules have been described in detail. However, they are fully reversible, even after as much as 8 weeks of administration (Bjoerklund and Erne, 1971).

20.4.2.3 Toxicity to Humans

Experimental Exposure   Eleven men in two separate experiments experienced no clinical effect after each voluntarily ingested 2,4,5-T at a dosage of 5 mg/kg. Most did report a metallic taste lasting 1–2 hr after ingestion (Gehring *et al.*, 1973; Kohli *et al.*, 1974a). What was learned is discussed under Laboratory Findings.

Accidental and Intentional Poisoning A 48-year-old man who had attempted suicide previously tried again by drinking a "large amount" of a mixture of one-third 2,4-D, one-third 2,4,5-T butyl ester, and one-third inert ingredients. The man was found in a drowsy, incoherent state vomiting repeatedly. When admitted to hospital 3 hr later, the patient was semiconscious but still vomiting. He was perspiring heavily. Blood pressure was 90/60 mm Hg, pulse was regular and forceful at 134/min, and respirations were 28/min. Moist rales were heard in the base of the right lung. Response to painful stimuli was very sluggish. The clinical course, which lasted 43 hr in hospital, was characterized by increasing temperature (40.36°C rectally just prior to death), increasing rates of pulse and respiration, falling blood pressure, respiratory alkylosis (pH 7.53), hemoconcentration, profuse sweating, oliguria, a rising blood urea nitrogen, restlessness, and deepening coma. Progressive shock was unresponsive to pressor amines. Autopsy revealed numerous small foci of submucosal hemorrhage and moderate congestion and edema of the mucosa of the small intestine, congestion of the lungs and consolidation of an area of the right middle lobe, and some congestion of other organs. Microscopic examination showed acute necrosis of the mucosa of the large and especially the small intestine; the muscle coat of the intestine appeared focally coagulated. The alveoli in the area of pneumonitis contained polymorphonuclear and red blood cells, and some of the contiguous terminal bronchioles were inflamed. Individual myocardial fibers were moderately separated by what appeared to be coagulated fluid; there was no inflammation, and no appreciable pathology of the myocardial fibers was noted. Central midzonal areas of acute necrosis and slight fatty infiltration of the liver were observed (Hayes, 1982).

Use Experience Apparently, most if not all occupational illness associated with 2,4,5-T was actually the result of TCDD present as a contaminant in the factory environment (see Section 18.5.1.3).

No change in cholinesterase or in tributyrinase levels was found among men who formulated 2,4,5-T and 2,4-D (Bonderman *et al.*, 1971).

Eczema attributed to a mixture of 2,4,5-T and 2,4-D is mentioned in Section 20.4.1.3. A statistical correlation between the occurrence of soft tissue sarcomas and exposure to phenoxy acids and/or chlorophenols in Sweden, New Zealand, and the United States also is discussed under Use Experience in Section 20.4.1.3. The implications for non-Hodgkin's lymphoma in the agricultural population are also considered.

Military Use of 2,4,5-T and Its Impact on Civilian Uses It seems likely that 2,4,5-T would have received far less toxicological attention and its civilian use would have been less restricted if it had never been used in the Vietnam War. Military research during World War II provided much of the information on herbicides that was turned to civilian use after that war and that led to important changes in agriculture and in the maintenance of highway, railroad, and power line rights-of-way (House *et al.*, 1967). However, times had changed when 2,4,5-T and some other herbicides were put to the military use of minimizing ambush at least as early as 1962 and more extensively in 1966.

In 1969, as the result of public pressure and potential adverse effects including reports of birth defects in South Vietnam, the white House science advisor, Dr. Lee A. DuBridge, took the highly unusual action of announcing partial curtailment in both the civilian and military use of 2,4,5-T (Nelson, 1969). Accordingly, on the following day the Secretaries of Agriculture; Health, Education, and Welfare; and Interior jointly announced the suspension of the registration of 2,4,5-T for "I. All uses in lakes, ponds, or on ditch banks. II. Liquid formulations for use around the house, recreation areas, and similar sites." A notice for cancellation of registration was issued on the following May 1 for "I. All granular 2,4,5-T formulations for use around the home, recreation areas and similar sites. II. All 2,4,5-T uses on crops intended for human consumption."

There followed a series of hearings (U.S. Senate, 1970) and reports by the Department of Defense (Cutting *et al.*, 1970), the Herbicide Assessment Commission (HAC) for the American Association for the Advancement of Science (Meselson *et al.*, 1972; Boffey, 1971), the Advisory Committee on 2,4,5-T (Wilson *et al.*, 1971), and the National Research Council Committee on the Effects of Herbicides in Vietnam (1974). The Advisory Committee report summarized what really was known about birth defects in Vietnam.

Summarizing the Vietnam data on human embryotoxicity, it can be said that (1) the sample of births surveyed was from year to year a variable but usually very small fraction of the total number, (2) it was quite unrepresentative of the geographic and ethnic distributions, (3) the heavily sprayed and otherwise exposed areas were greatly underrepresented, and (4) the birth records were not trustworthy and, therefore, the rates of stillbirth, and especially of congenital malformation, derived from them were equally unreliable. For example, the overall congenital malformation rate found in South Vietnam, 4.91/1000 livebirths, is about half of what was reported in other studies in various parts of Asia . . . , and possibly a quarter of what might actually exist at term. A further indication that the newborn children were not carefully examined is the absence of Down's syndrome in the list of specific malformations compiled by the Army survey, despite the fact that some Oriental populations have been reported to have an incidence of this condition not unlike that in Western populations . . . .

Finally, there is, and can be, no precise knowledge or reasonable approximation of the exposure to 2,4,5-T experienced by pregnant Vietnamese women, including what amounts they ingested or absorbed and when this may have occurred during pregnancy. Thus, any attempt to relate birth defects or stillbirths to herbicide exposure is predestined to failure. It can only be concluded that the birth records that have been surveyed, and probably any that will be surveyed in the future, for South

Vietnam for the period 1960 to 1970 cannot answer positively the questions about possible adverse prenatal effects following human exposure to 2,4,5-T. It must be emphasized, however, that the searches that have been made almost certainly would have revealed any marked increase in the incidence of birth defects or the introduction of a striking defect such as that produced by thalidomide. In spite of considerable effort, no such occurrences were found.

Recommendations by the Advisory Committee on 2,4,5-T included

1. That registration for use of 2,4,5-trichlorophenoxyacetic acid and its esters be restored to the status existing prior to April 1970, with the following exceptions.

2. That certain specific limitations and qualifications be added to the previously existing registration, as follows:

a. A permissible residue of not more than 0.1 ppm of 2,4,5-T on the edible parts of food products and in potable water for human consumption be accepted. It is recognized that very few foods tested to date have contained this level of residue, but it is probable that some of the reports of no residue in the past were due to limited sensitivity of the analytical method. In view of recent and future advances in methodology, which tend to make zero residues of anything increasingly unlikely, a more realistic policy would be the setting of safe tolerance limits at this time.

b. A limit of 0.5 ppm of contamination with 2,3,7,8-tetrachlorodibenzo-p-dioxin be set for existing inventories of 2,4,5-T, except as specified in item c below, and a limit of 0.1 ppm of contamination with this dioxin be established in all future production of 2,4,5-T. Surveillance should be maintained by requiring that a manufacturer submit a reference sample and a certified analysis of each future production lot to the Environmental Protection Agency.

c. All formulations to be used around the home and in recreational areas as of present date should be limited to 0.1 ppm of the dioxin, TCDD, and also should bear a conspicuous warning, e.g., " This compound may be dangerous to pregnant women and animals and its use must be such as to reduce the possibility of exposure to an absolute minimum."

The Department of Defense, the Advisory Committee on 2,4,5-T, the Herbicide Assessment Commission of the American Association for the Advancement of Science, and the National Research Council Committee on the Effects of Herbicides in Vietnam could find no evidence that 2,4,5-T had contributed to human teratogenesis. Some investigators of the teratogenic effects of 2,4,5-T in animals specifically pointed out that the required dose was so high that people were unlikely to encounter so much and, therefore, unlikely to be affected (Roll, 1973; Baage *et al.,* 1973). There are, to be sure, a few published reports that express no doubt that military use of 2,4,5-T caused abortions, deformed babies, increased postnatal mortality, poisoned about 1,293,000 people of whom about 300 died, increased the incidence of chromosomal aberrations, caused cancer in infants of exposed mothers, and increased the proportion of persons in hospitals in Hanoi with primary liver cancer (compared to the total with cancer of any kind) from 2.9% for the period of 1955–1961 to 10% for the period of 1962–1968 (Rose and Rose, 1972; Ton That *et al.,* 1973; Dmitriyev, 1974).

In a limited study by Kaye *et al.* (1985) in 10 males with a history of exposure to 2,4,5-T as Agent Orange, eight individuals were studied because they had fathered children with congenital defects. Although all individuals had normal karyotypes, a statistically significant increase in chromosome breaks was observed in exposed males compared to their unexposed wives and children. However, a lot of questions remain unanswered in regard to this cause–effect relationship.

Of course, not all reports of human teratogenesis associated with 2,4,5-T concerned military use of the compound or an effort to discourage that use. However, once the alleged relationship had been publicized, it was inevitable that it would be considered in connection with civilian situations. The Advisory Committee on 2,4,5-T considered such a report from Globe, Arizona, and one from Swedish Lapland, but could find no evidence that 2,4,5-T had contributed. Some of the cases about which questions were raised involved coincidence that seems to cry out for explanation. Thus, Sare and Forbes (1972) reported two babies with fatal myelomeningocele, who were born within a month of one another in the same hospital and whose parents lived on adjoining farms where cistern water was used for drinking and where 2,4,5-T had been sprayed during the first trimester of the mothers' pregnancies. Later, Sare (1972) reported a case of headache and diplopia in a sprayman and attributed the difficulty to 2,4-D. An editorial in the same journal (Anonymous, 1972) attempted to encourage reporting at the same time that it pointed out the basic facts of the epidemiology of teratogenesis. Other clusters of cases of birth defects or abortion, conditions that long have been endemic, were reported (Field and Kerr, 1979). In at least one instance, superficial investigation and heavy political pressure led to restrictions on the use of the compound (Smith, 1979). However, when the investigations were thorough, the allegations could not be substantiated (New Zealand Department of Health [summary available as an Editorial, 1977]; National Health and Medical Research Council, 1978; Robinson, 1979; Smith, 1979). Robinson (1979) summarized the situation as follows: "It should be pointed out that the UK, New Zealand, Canada, West Germany, and many other countries have formed special committees that have reviewed the use of 2,4,5-T and found no reason to ban its use."

A retrospective study of the relationship between agricultural use of 2,4,5-T and the occurrence of cleft lip and/or cleft palate in Arkansas for the period of 1943–1974 was made, even though no local complaint of such a relationship was reported. The overall prevalence of facial clefts was similar to that reported by others, including reports prior to the introduction of 2,4,5-T. No significant relationship was found between exposure and deformity. There was a trend of increasing frequency in progressive years in high-, medium-, and low-exposure groups. This was attributed to better case findings as a result of continuing efforts of the Crippled Children's Services of the Arkansas Social and Rehabilitative Services (Nelson *et al.,* 1979).

Hanify *et al.* (1981) investigated the rate of birth malformations in the Northland region of New Zealand and found no evidence of correlation between malformation of the central nervous system and the spraying of 2,4,5-T.

Not all reverberations from the Vietnam War involved birth defects. A listing of the complaints of a few veterans of that war is that of Bogen (1979). These complaints, which were almost entirely subjective in character and which were accepted without epidemiological support, were attributed without evidence to TCDD. Further attempts of Sare and Forbes (1977) to implicate 2,4,5-T or TCDD were met by reasoned criticism (Becroft, 1977; Bates, 1977) but without success (Sare, 1979).

An excellent summary of the safety of 2,4-D and 2,4,5-T is that of Turner (1977). Additionally, Pearn (1985) has provided a review of teratogenic potential as ascertained from epidemiology studies. Such studies reported in Hungary, Italy, New Zealand, the United States, Europe, and Australia have not revealed any positive evidence to indicate that a human/herbicide teratogenic syndrome exists.

Atypical Cases of Various Origins   It is remarkable and commendable, in view of the extensive propaganda circulated by the media regarding alleged human teratogenesis associated with 2,4,5-T, how few reports of such cases found their way into the scientific literature. One report that was published was that of Funazaki (1971) from the Department of Surgery, Saku General Hospital, Nagano Prefecture, Japan. Funazaki wrote that, while in the People's Republic of Vietnam, he personally observed several cases of abnormalities in infants whose mothers had been exposed to the defoliating agents in the northern part of South Vietnam during pregnancy and who had later moved to North Vietnam. The children suffered from Down's syndrome and were said to have characteristic chromosome changes. It does not seem to have occurred to Dr. Funazaki that seeing "several" such cases was epidemiologically meaningless because the syndrome occurs spontaneously in all races that have been studied. Nearly all cases are environmental in origin, inasmuch as older mothers are much more likely than young mothers to bear such infants. The syndrome, which has been recognized for over a hundred years, has not, in fact, been associated with any environmental chemical in people, and it has not been reproduced in experimental animals, either by a chemical or in any other way. A different version was published the next year (Funazaki, 1972), and later the same author with colleagues reported an increase in chromatid aberrations in human white cells cultured with 2,4,5-T at concentrations of 1 × 10^{-8} and 1 × 10^{-5} M (Fujita et al., 1975).

Dosage Response   A dose of 5 mg/kg was harmless to volunteers. A threshold limit value (10 mg/m^3) indicates that occupational intake of 1.4 mg/kg/day is considered safe.

Laboratory Findings   In one case of suicide with 2,4-D and 2,4,5-T, the concentrations of these compounds in the first sample of vomitus collected in hospital over 3 hr after ingestion were 480 and 1148 ppm, respectively. The ratio of the compounds in the formulation was 1 : 1; that in the first basin of vomitus was 1 : 2.4; and that in the second basin was 1 : >13.2 (actually <15 and 199 ppm). No 2,4-D was detectable in the

tissues, whereas the following concentrations of 2,4,5-T were found: blood, 506 ppm; liver, 109 ppm; kidney, 51 ppm; brain, 8 ppm; heart, 43 ppm; skeletal muscle, 21 ppm; diaphragm, 29 ppm; and fat, 11 ppm. These values attest to the excretion of 2,4-D and the retention of an appreciable amount of 2,4,5-T in the course of 2 days. The undetectability of 2,4-D in the tissues in this case was in marked contrast to the presence of substantial concentrations of the compound in the tissues of persons killed by 2,4-D alone (see Table 20.2), and death in this case must therefore be ascribed largely to 2,4,5-T.

In another case in which death took place within 16 hr after ingestion of a "large dose" of a 3 : 2 mixture of 2,4-D and 2,4,5-T, the concentrations of 2,4-D were 826, 21, 12, and 82 ppm in blood, liver, spleen, and kidneys, respectively, and the corresponding values for 2,4,5-T were 182, 4.8, 4.6, and 22 (Coutselinas et al., 1977). The greater rapidity of death in this case presumably was the reason for the persistence of 2,4-D in the samples.

Following ingestion of 2,4,5-T at a rate of 5 mg/kg by five volunteers, maximal concentration in the plasma averaging approximately 57 ppm was reached in approximately 15 hr. Thereafter, the concentration in the plasma decreased by an apparent first-order process. Excretion followed a similar pattern, the half-life being 23.06 hr. Essentially all of the compound was absorbed and excreted unchanged in the urine. No metabolite was detected. While in the body, about 65% was in the plasma, where 98.7% was reversibly bound to protein. An average of 26.8% of the dose was recovered in the urine during the first 12 hr and 88.5% during the first 96 hr. This would indicate an average urinary concentration of about 125 ppm during the first 12 hr. Utilizing the kinetic constraints found in the single-dose study, it was calculated that, following daily intake, the concentration in plasma would reach essentially a plateau in 3 days and, if expressed as parts per million, would range from 12.7 to 22.5 times the dosage expressed as milligrams per kilogram per day times the daily dosage if that dosage were evenly distributed throughout the day (Gehring et al., 1973).

Many of these results were confirmed in a separate study in which one man took 2 mg/kg, one took 3 mg/kg, and six took 5 mg/kg. In this instance, about half of the dose was recovered in 48 hr, and only 63% was recovered in 96 hr. Using the same computer program, the average half-life was calculated as 18.8 hr (Kohli et al., 1974a).

The concentration of 2,4,5-T in the urine of exposed workers ranged from 0.05 to 3.6 ppm (Shafik et al., 1971). In another country, the average concentration was 4.5 ppm (Kolmodin and Erne, 1979).

Treatment of Poisoning   Treatment is similar to that of poisoning by 2,4-D (see Section 20.4.1.3).

20.4.3 MCPA

20.4.3.1 Identity, Properties, and Uses

Chemical Name   MCPA is 4-chloro-2-methylphenoxyacetic acid.

Structure See Fig. 20.2.

Synonyms The common name MCPA (BSI, ISO) is in general use, except in the USSR, where dicotex and metaxon are used. It is sometimes called MCP. Trade names have included Agritox®, Agroxone®, Chiptox®, Cornox®, DedWeed®, Empal®, Hedonal® M, Hommotuho®, Kilsen, Mephanac®, Phenoxylene® Plus Rohomene®, Ruonox®, Shamrox®, Weedar®, Weedone®, and Weed-Rhap®. The CAS registry number is 94-74-6.

Physical and Chemical Properties MCPA has the empirical formula $C_9H_9ClO_3$ and a molecular weight of 200.63. The pure material is a white crystalline solid with a melting point of 118–119°C. Crude MCPA is 85–95% pure and melts between 100 and 115°C. The solubility of MCPA in water at room temperature is 825 ppm, but it forms soluble salts with alkali metals and organic bases.

History, Formulations, Uses, and Production MCPA was introduced in 1945 by Imperial Chemical Industries, Ltd. It is a hormone-type herbicide used to control annual and perennial weeds in cereals, grassland, and turf. Available formulations include aqueous concentrates of the salts, emulsifiable concentrates of the ester (all at 24–60%), and water-soluble powders of the sodium salt at 75–80% MCPA.

20.4.3.2 Toxicity to Laboratory Animals

Basic Findings MCPA is a compound of low acute toxicity as shown in Table 20.3.

In a 7-month feeding study, a dietary level of 2500 ppm reduced feed intake and retarded growth rate of rats, especially during the first week of feeding. Some animals died, usually with infection, suggesting that this dose reduced resistance. A smaller effect of the same kind was caused by 1000 ppm. Levels of 400 ppm or more increased the relative weight of the liver of both males and females, and 100 ppm or more increased kidney weights. These changes were reflected in histological change. In another study, 60 mg/kg/day did not affect liver or kidney weight. A dose of 150 mg/kg caused an increase in the weights of both liver and kidney within 3 weeks, but the liver returned to normal during a 2-week recovery period, and the kidney recovered more slowly. Leukocyte counts and differentials were unaffected by MCPA, but erythrocyte count, hemoglobin, and packed cell volume were reduced by dietary levels of 400 ppm or more. It was thought that these changes were due to an increased rate of breakdown of red cells, as no histological abnormality of the bone marrow was manifest.

When the esters were fed to male and female rats and mice at dietary levels up to 2560 ppm or more for 3 months, the higher levels reduced weight gain, increased the urinary excretion of coproporphyrin, increased the weight of the liver and disturbed its function, and produced anemia. Acidophilic changes in liver cells were seen in animals killed for examination. The maximal no-effect level was 120 ppm (5.9 and 15.4 mg/kg/day in rats and mice, respectively) for the n-butyl ester and 160 ppm (7.8

Table 20.3
Single-Dose LD 50 for MCPA

Species	Route	LD 50 (mg/kg)	Reference
Rat, M	oral	700[a]	Rowe and Hymas (1954)
Rat, M	oral	1200[b]	Rowe and Hymas (1954)
Rat	oral	800	Gurd et al. (1965)
Rat, M	oral	914[c]	Oshima et al. (1974)
Rat, M	oral	612[d]	Oshima et al. (1974)
Rat, F	oral	962[d]	Oshima et al. (1974)
Rat, M	subcutaneous	500	Hattula et al. (1977)
Rat	intraperitoneal	300	Gurd et al. (1965)
Mouse	oral	550	Gurd et al. (1965)
Mouse, M	oral	1182[c]	Oshima et al. (1974)
Mouse, M	oral	1050[d]	Oshima et al. (1974)
Mouse	intraperitoneal	350	Gurd et al. (1965)

[a] Acid.
[b] Amine salt.
[c] n-Butyl ester in olive oil.
[d] Allyl ester in olive oil.

and 20.5 mg/kg/day in rats and mice, respectively) for the allyl ester (Oshima et al., 1974). This estimate of a no-effect level later was changed to 40 ppm (2.81–3.35 mg/kg/day in rats and 5.99–6.7 mg/kg/day in mice) (Oshima and Imai, 1976).

Verschuuren et al. (1975) agreed with other investigators that a dietary level of 400 ppm retarded growth and increased the relative weight of the kidneys. The next smallest dose they tested (50 ppm) was a 90-day, no-effect level in both rats and rabbits.

Dermal application of MCPA to rabbits caused moderate erythema and loss of elasticity of the skin at a wide range of doses. The skin returned to normal in the course of 2 weeks after application was stopped. High mortality, weight loss, and histological changes in the liver, kidneys, spleen, and thymus were caused by daily dermal applications at rates of 1000 and 2000 mg/kg/day. Weight loss occurred at 500 mg/kg/day (Verschuuren et al., 1975).

Absorption, Distribution, Metabolism, and Excretion [^{14}C]MCPA was injected intravenously into pregnant mice, which were then studied by autoradiography at intervals of 5 min to 72 hr. The distribution pattern was characterized by a high concentration in the blood up to 4 hr and an accumulation in the visceral yolk sac epithelium up to 24 hr after injection. The radioactive substance passed the placenta, but the fetal tissues never reached the concentration of the maternal tissues. There was no site of concentration in the fetal tissues.

Radioactivity was eliminated from fetuses and mothers by 24 hr after injection (Lindquist, 1974).

When administered to rats by stomach tube, the highest concentrations of [^{14}C]MCPA in the tissues were reached in 2–8 hr and then declined rapidly. During the first 24 hr 92.3% of the dose was recovered in the urine and 6.8% in the feces (Elo, 1976). Elo *et al.* (1982) using [^{14}C]MCPA found significant penetration into the rat brain. These workers studied the penetration of MCPA in both control and MCPA-intoxicated rats (sodium salt administered subcutaneously at a toxic level of 200–500 mg/kg). The results indicated that MCPA intoxication caused selective damage to the blood–brain barrier.

When cows were fed MCPA at a dietary level of 1000 ppm, <0.05 ppm of the parent compound and 0.06 ppm of 2-methyl-4-chlorophenol were found in the milk. The concentration of phenols dropped rapidly to undetectable levels when feeding was stopped (Bjerke *et al.*, 1972).

Biochemical Effects   A single subcutaneous dose of MCPA changed the distribution of a standard dose of [^{14}C]MCPA administered intravenously somewhat later. The subcutaneous dose occupied binding sites on plasma protein in such a way that, relative to values for controls, the [^{14}C]MCPA reached lower concentrations in the plasma and kidney and greater concentrations in the liver, brain, spinal fluid, testis, lung, heart, and muscle. The effect was hardly detectable at a subcutaneous dosage of 25 mg/kg and progressively—in fact disproportionately—greater at dosages up to 500 mg/kg. The change in distribution tended to be maximal at 3.5–4.5 hr after the subcutaneous dose, and it remained at about this level for 12 hr and then declined gradually (Elo and Ylitalo, 1977, 1979).

Mutagenicity   MCPA was negative in a gene mutation bacterial test system, even in the presence of microsomal enzymes (Rasanen *et al.*, 1977). MCPA was negative for mutagenesis in spot tests and in host-mediated tests (Buselmaier *et al.*, 1973). The compound produced no detectable increase in the frequency of recessive lethals (chromosomal aberrations) in *Drosophila* (Vogel and Chandler, 1974; Magnusson *et al.*, 1977). MCPA induced mitotic recombination and gene conversion in *Saccharomyces* but only at low pH and a high dosage that killed 95% or more of the cells (Zetterberg, 1978, 1979).

Effects on Reproduction   A single oral dose of MCPA at half the LD 50 rate increased the intrauterine mortality of the young of rats to which it was administered on day 9 or 10 of pregnancy, except in dams that had received phenobarbital for 3 days prior to MCPA (Buslovich *et al.*, 1979).

Pathology   In rats, oral doses of MCPA in the LD 50 range produced hyperemia and parenchymal cell degeneration in the liver and disappearance of the white pulp of the spleen with marked depletion of lymphocytes. Changes were similar but less marked in rats receiving the compound in their drinking water at concentrations as high as 1000 ppm (Hattula *et al.*, 1977). Depletion of lymphocytes may be related to susceptibility to infection, which has been noted in some other experiments.

20.4.3.3 Toxicity to Humans

Accidental and Intentional Poisoning   A man with a long history of tuberculosis and depressive psychosis was found in bed frothing at the mouth and jerking his limbs. On admission to hospital, he was in deep coma, unresponsive to painful stimuli. The pupils were small and unreactive. There was no gross hypertonia, but at times there would be twitching of the face followed by clonic-tonic convulsions. Pulse and respiration were rapid; blood pressure was normal. Paraldehyde was given intramuscularly. Grand mal fits did not recur, but myoclonic twitching of both arms and legs continued. In spite of gastric lavage and symptomatic care, no urine was passed, the blood pressure declined gradually, and the patient died some 20 hr after admission. MCPA was found in the tissues after autopsy had failed to show the cause of death (Popham and Davies, 1964)

A 65-year-old blacksmith with a 40-year history of dyspnea and cough with purulent sputum and a 7-year history of congestive cardiac failure treated with digoxin was found unconscious near an empty 57-ml bottle of 25% MCPA. The man had been depressed by his chronic illness and had attempted suicide unsuccessfully 9 years earlier. When admitted to hospital 2 hr after being found, he was unresponsive to all stimuli, and all limbs were flaccid. Blood pressure was 80/60 mm Hg. The heart was normal, except for extrasystoles. The lung findings reflected his chronic disease. The stomach was washed out. The blood pressure responded to therapy at first but later fell gradually. The patient remained deeply unconscious and died 20.5 hr from the time he was found unconscious (Johnson and Koumides, 1965).

In a state of depression, a 61-year-old man drank MCPA but reported it before he became ill. Shortly afterward, he vomited, his speech became slurred, his face began to twitch, and his limbs began to jerk. On arrival at hospital, he was deeply unconscious, although it was only 1.5 hr since he had been asymptomatic. Probably because of phenolic impurities in the formulation, his breath smelled phenolic, copious secretions poured from his mouth, and the tongue and fauces were edematous and covered with mucus but not burned. Blood pressure was only 90/60 mm Hg. The pupils were constricted and did not react to light. Reflexes were diminished. There was generalized fibrillary twitching of skeletal muscle and clonic spasms of the limbs, but no major convulsions occurred. Treatment included gastric lavage, measures to maintain blood pressure, and the induction of diuresis. Urine output averaged 4 liters/day for the next 3 days. Involuntary movement persisted for 12 hr and unconsciousness for 72 hr. In addition to the central nervous system abnormality and irritation of the upper gastrointestinal tract, evidence of kidney and liver injury was observed, as well as anemia and pneumonia. Proteinuria was present during the first 2 weeks. After 1 week, glycosuria (up to 2 gm/100 ml) appeared and gradually subsided over the next 3 weeks. SGPT and SGOT were elevated on the seventh day but returned to normal in another week. Recovery was apparently complete but certainly slow (Jones *et al.*, 1967).

Ingestion of a mixture of 2,4-D and MCPA produced neither the muscle involvement sometimes seen in poisoning by 2,4-D nor the convulsions sometimes seen in poisoning by MCPA. The illness began with nausea, vomiting, and loss of consciousness and ended just over 4 days later with sudden circulatory collapse (Geldmacher-von Mallinckrodt and Lautenbach, 1966).

Use Experience In general, MCPA has not been a source of difficulty. In one factory in the USSR, it was considered the cause of contact dermatitis in 11% of 158 workers. Sensitization was not involved (Telegina and Bikbulatove, 1970). In addition, Timonen and Palva (1980) reported acute leukemia in an individual who had been chronically exposed to MCPA.

Although there was much discussion of epidemiology studies with 2,4-D in Sections 7.4.1.2 and 20.4.1.3, MCPA is a more frequently used herbicide outside the United States and has been the focal point for several studies. As MCPA is the most commonly used phenoxy acid in Sweden, it was the focus of a study of 354,620 men who were employed in agriculture and forestry according to a national census in 1960 (Wiklund and Holm, 1986). This cohort was divided into six subcohorts exposed to phenoxy acid herbicides. The reference cohort was 1,725,845 men employed in other industries. All persons were followed up during the period 1961–1979. A total of 331 cases of soft tissue sarcoma was observed in the study population versus 1508 cases in the reference group. The relative risk ratio was determined to be 0.9 ± 0.1. Therefore, the agricultural and forestry group does not thus far exhibit any greater risk of soft tissue sarcomas than the general male work population. In Denmark, Lynge (1985) reported on an epidemiology study conducted in two production facilities where MCPA was the predominant phenoxy herbicide produced. The worker population consisted of 3390 males and 1069 females. The analysis, which focused on soft tissue sarcomas and malignant lymphomas, revealed an excess in soft tissue sarcomas but not malignant lymphomas. Further, the total cancer risk among persons employed in the manufacture and packaging of phenoxy herbicides was equivalent to that of the Danish population.

Atypical Cases of Various Origins A condition diagnosed as acute benign pericarditis occurred in a 43-year-old farmer 12 hr after he had applied MCPA. Onset was characterized by intense dyspnea, retrosternal pain intensified by deep inspiration, and severe asthenia. The man did not consult a physician until 4 days later, at which time a pericardial rub and ECG findings suggested pericarditis. The heart was enlarged on X ray. No treatment was given. Ten days after onset, the pain stopped. Five days later the pericardial rub was gone, and the heart had returned to normal size. No infection was identified by serological tests. No recurrence or complications occurred during the next 3 years. The condition was attributed to an allergic reaction. In the same paper, another case similar in having pain, pericardial rub, and cardiac enlargement but differing in having fever (40°C), cough, and expectoration was attributed to allergy to a lindane and copper seed dressing employed several days prior to

onset. Again, prolonged follow-up revealed no sequelae (Alix *et al.*, 1974). The possibility that such different compounds would cause pericarditis, especially in the absence of any symptoms characteristic of poisoning, is remote.

A less serious illness in a 34-year-old woman was attributed to 3 days of occupational exposure to MCPA without any recognized accident. She did not feel well the first day. She experienced pain, nausea, vomiting, and itching and burning of the skin. On the third day of exposure, she developed hyperemia of the face and trunk and a micropunctate rash on the extremities. The rash later became vesicular in the underarm region. When the patient was seen again 2.5 months later, her liver was thought to be enlarged, a condition apparently not present during the acute illness (Khibin *et al.*, 1968). Somewhat similar cases were reported by Zakharov *et al.* (1968), and in some of them allergy tests were positive for MCPA.

A 64-year-old man who regularly took digoxin and nitroglycerine tablets developed hematomata and felt lethargic 2 weeks after a hand sprayer containing MCPA leaked on his back and wet his clothes. He waited 2 months before consulting a physician. Muscular weakness, hemorrhagic gastritis, and slight signs of liver damage were found on examination. The bone marrow morphology was normal. He was transfused with packed red cells and treated with prednisolone and later methenolone. Five months later he was free of symptoms (Palva *et al.*, 1975). The case apparently involved abnormal blood loss with resulting anemia. No evidence to justify a diagnosis of aplastic anemia was supplied. The white cell count on admission was 16,300 cells/mm³. The relation of the case to MCPA is obscure.

A somewhat similar case involved a 48-year-old farmer who sprayed only about 400 ml of a mixture of MCPA (34%) and the sodium and potassium salts of 2-methoxy-3,6-dichlorobenzoic acid (3%) in 40 liters of water. The work required only about ½ hr. No accident was recognized, although a light wind blew mist on the man's face and arms. Intermittent nausea, a feeling of fullness, and loss of appetite appeared a day or two after exposure, and the patient complained of feeling his heart beat in his neck. On the sixth day after exposure, vomiting of coffee ground material sometimes was followed by cramping epigastric pain. Gastroscopy 2 days later revealed a gastroesophageal prolapse and an erosive-hemorrhagic gastroduodenitis. A second gastroscopy 10 days later showed that the lesions had healed. At last report, 1½ years after exposure, the patient was healthy (Huep and Hesselman, 1979).

Dosage Response Death of two men followed ingestion of an estimated 85 ml of 25% solution by one and 57 ml by the other (Popham and Davies, 1964; Johnson and Koumides, 1965). The dose in the first case is estimated to be about 300 mg/kg and in the second case was stated to be 250 mg/kg. In contrast, another man survived after he ingested about 1900 mg/kg, of which he vomited an unknown portion (Jones *et al.*, 1967). How much the very poor health of the first two patients and the initial good health of the third patient contributed to the death of the first two and the survival of the third is unknown.

Laboratory Findings In a suicide, specimens taken at autopsy contained the following concentrations of MCPA: blood, 230 ppm; liver, 146 ppm; heart, 154 ppm; and brain, 32.8 ppm (Popham and Davies, 1964). In another case, the concentrations in autopsy specimens of blood and urine were 180 and 800 ppm, respectively (Johnson and Koumides, 1965).

About 50% of the total dose was detected in the urine of four volunteers within 48 hr after each ingested 5 mg of MCPA. Five days after ingestion, the concentration in the urine was below the detectable level of 0.02 ppm. Minor changes in serum enzymes were explained by other causes and could not be attributed to MCPA (Fjeldstad and Wannag, 1977).

Pathology Autopsy showed that there had been no irritation of the gastrointestinal tract. Nothing was found morphologically that would be helpful in diagnosing poisoning (Popham and Davies, 1964; Johnson and Koumides, 1965).

Treatment of Poisoning Treatment is similar to that of poisoning by 2,4-D (see Section 20.4.1.3).

20.4.4 SILVEX

20.4.4.1 Identity, Properties, and Uses

Chemical Name 2-(2,4,5-Trichlorophenoxy)propionic acid.

Structure See Fig. 20.2.

Synonyms Silvex (ANSI and WSSA) also is known as fenoprop (BSI, ISO) and 2,4,5-TCPPA (JMAF, USSR). Trade names, some of which are restricted to specific salts or esters, include Aqua-Vex®, Fruitone T®, Kurosal®, Miller Nu Set®, O-X-D®, and Weed-B-Gon®. The CAS registry number is 93-71-2.

Physical and Chemical Properties Silvex has the empirical formula $C_9H_7Cl_3O_3$ and a molecular weight of 269.53. It occurs as crystals or white powder melting at 181.6°C. It solubility in water at 25°C is 140 ppm, and its solubility in acetone, methanol, and ether is 15.2, 10.5, and 7.13%, respectively. It is less soluble in benzene (0.16%), carbon tetrachloride (0.024%), and heptane (0.017%). The lower alkyl esters are slightly volatile, but the acid and its propylene and butyl esters are practically nonvolatile. The formulations are noncorrosive.

History, Formulations, and Uses The plant growth-regulating action of salts of silvex was first reported in 1945 (Hayes, 1982). In 1953 the Dow Chemical Company introduced a low volatile ester. It is now available as salts as well as esters. Different formulations and application rates are used for control of brush, aquatic weeds, and weeds in certain crops, including a wide range of annual weeds in cereals. The triethanolamine salt has been used to reduce preharvest drop of apples.

20.4.4.2 Toxicity to Laboratory Animals

Basic Findings The oral LD 50 of silvex in the rat was 650 mg/kg. The values for the active ingredient in various ester formulations ranged from 600 to 621 mg/kg in rats and were 1410 mg/kg in mice, 1250 in guinea pigs, and 752–819 in rabbits. Signs of illness were essentially the same as those observed in animals poisoned by 2,4-D and 2,4,5-T, namely loss of appetite and weight, depression, roughness of coat, general tenseness, and muscular weakness particularly of the hindquarters (Rowe and Hymas, 1954).

Male rats fed a potassium salt of silvex at an acid-equivalent rate of 7.9 mg/kg/day for 2 years grew slower than controls and the weights of their kidneys were increased compared to those of controls. Some increase in relative kidney weight could not be excluded in male rats fed levels of 0.26, 0.8, and 2.6 mg/kg/day. However, in the absence of any untoward effect on general appearance, mortality, tumor incidence, blood and clinical laboratory findings, or gross or microscopic morphology, it was considered that any change in kidney weight was adaptive (Sauerhoff et al., 1977b).

A mild degeneration and necrosis of hepatocytes was found in male and female dogs receiving 8.2 and 9.9 mg/kg/day, respectively, and in males receiving 2.6 mg/kg/day. Increased SGPT and SGOT levels were found in female dogs at the high level. No change at any dosage level was found in food consumption, growth, hematological evaluation, blood urea nitrogen, alkaline phosphatase, bromsulfophthalein retention, and organ weights. The no-adverse-effect level for silvex acid equivalent was 0.9 mg/kg/day in dogs (Sauerhoff et al., 1977b).

Absorption, Distribution, Metabolism, and Excretion Orally administered silvex was extensively if not completely absorbed. Clearance of silvex from the plasma was linear with a half-life of 16.2 hr in rats following intravenous injection at a rate of 5 mg/kg but was nonlinear after a dosage of 50 mg/kg. Urinary excretion of radioactivity accounted for 80.5 and 68.7% of the [^{14}C]silvex administered at dosages of 5 and 50 mg/kg, respectively, and the corresponding values for fecal excretion were 13.7 and 26.4%. Total recoveries at the two dosage levels were 94.1 and 95.1%. Significant amounts of silvex were excreted in the bile and underwent enterophepatic circulation. Rats killed 8 or 216 hr after injection contained greater radioactivity in liver and kidney than in brain, fat, or muscle. The fact that urinary excretion was saturated at a dosage of 50 mg/kg indicates that the effects of large dosages of silvex cannot be used validly to predict the effects of small dosages (Sauerhoff et al., 1976b, 1977a).

The highest concentration of silvex in the milk of cows fed the compound at a dietary level of 1000 ppm for 2 weeks or more was 0.12 ppm. The residue decreased rapidly after the cows returned to uncontaminated feed (Bjerke et al., 1972).

Effects on Organs and Tissues When administered to mice during days 12–15 of gestation at a dosage of 400 mg/kg/day, silvex reduced fetal weight and caused an average of 3–7% cleft palate, depending on the vehicle and route of administration. It was considerably less active than 2,4,5-T in causing cleft palate (Courtney, 1977). In fact, an earlier study (Moore and Courtney, 1971) concluded that silvex is nonteratogenic in the mouse as well as in the rat.

When administered orally to mice at the highest tolerated dosage, silvex did not cause a significant increase in tumors (Innes *et al.*, 1969).

20.4.4.3 Toxicity to Humans

Experimental Exposure Seven men and one woman ingested the free acid of silvex at a dosage of 1 mg/kg. There were no untoward effects; clinical, chemical, and hematological findings remained normal (Sauerhoff *et al.*, 1977b). The fate of the compound in these volunteers is discussed under Laboratory Findings.

Laboratory Findings Among eight volunteers who ingested silvex at a rate of 1 mg/kg, the peak plasma level of silvex (about 4–6 ppm) was reached in 2–4 hr. The clearance of silvex from the plasma was biphasic; the average half-life of the first phase, which lasted about 40 hr, was 4.0 hr, and that of the second phase was 16.5 hr. Excretion of silvex and its conjugate(s) in the urine was also biphasic; the average half-lives for silvex *per se* being 5.0 and 25.9 hr for the first and second phases, respectively. Small amounts (3.2% or less) of silvex and/or silvex conjugate(s) were eliminated in the feces. Within 24 hr, an average of 65% of the administered dose had been excreted in the urine. In the different volunteers 66.6–95.1% (mean 80.3%) of the dose was recovered from the urine plus feces within 168 hr (Sauerhoff *et al.*, 1977b). No 2,4,5-trichlorophenol or any conjugate of it was detected in the urine.

Based on the pharmacodynamics following a single dose, it was concluded that daily intake at the same rate would lead to a steady state after five doses at an average plasma level of 5.06 ppm (Sauerhoff *et al.*, 1977b). It should be noted that, although a dosage of 1 mg/kg is small compared to those often used in animal experiments, it is somewhat larger than workers are likely to receive and is massive compared with anything ordinary people might receive.

Treatment of Poisoning Treatment is similar to that of poisoning by 2,4,-D (see Section 20.4.1.3).

20.5 OTHER ORGANIC ACIDS AND DERIVATIVES

Besides chlorophenoxy acid herbicides and their derivatives, other herbicides based on acetic, proprionic, benzoic, and some other acids include benazolin (BSI, ISO), chloramben (ANSI, BSI, ISO, WSSA), chlorfenac (BSI, ISO) [fenac (WSSA)], chlorfenprop-methyl (BSI, ISO), chlorflurenol (ISO) [chlorfen-

ecol (BSI)], chlorthal (BSI, ISO) [DCPA (WSSA)], dalapon (ANSI, BSI, ISO, WSSA), dicamba (ANSI, BSI, ISO, WSSA), dodicin (BSI, ISO), endothal (BSI, ISO) [endothall (ANSI)], flurenol (BSI, ISO), naptalam (BSI, ISO, WSSA), 2,3,6-TBA (BSI, ISO, WSSA), TCA (BSI, ISO, WSSA), and tricamba (ANSI, BSI, ISO). Excluding endothal, the oral LD 50 values for the other 13 compounds in the rat range from 970 to 12,800 and average 4638 mg/kg. The toxicity of endothal is of a different order of magnitude, that is, 52 mg/kg.

20.5.1 DICAMBA

20.5.1.1 Identity, Properties, and Uses

Chemical Name Dicamba is 3,6-dichloro-2-methoxybenzoic acid.

Structure See Fig. 20.3.

Synonyms The common name dicamba (ANSI, BSI, ISO, WSSA) is in general use, except in the USSR, where the name is dianat. Trade names include Banfel®, Banvel®, Banvel CST®, Banvel D®, Banvel XG®, and Mediben®. Code designations include Compound B and Velsicol 58-CS-11. The CAS registry number is 1918-00-9.

Physical and Chemical Properties Dicamba has the empirical formula $C_8H_6Cl_2O_3$ and a molecular weight of 221.04. The pure material is a white crystalline solid with a melting point of 114–116°C. The technical acid is a pale buff crystalline solid. The vapor pressure of dicamba is 3.75×10^{-3} mm Hg at 100°C. The sodium salt has a solubility of 38 gm acid equivalent/100 ml; the solubility of the dimethylamine salt is more than 72 gm acid equivalent/100 ml. The acid is stable and resistant to hydrolysis and oxidation under normal conditions.

History, Formulations, and Uses Dicamba was introduced about 1965 by the Velsicol Chemical Corporation. It is a translocatable, postemergence herbicide used to control weeds in cereals; it is also used to control docks in established grassland and to control bracken and brush. Dicamba is available in formulations containing 20 gm dicamba plus 250 gm MCPA or 2,4-D per liter, and 27.5 gm dicamba plus 425 gm mecoprop per liter, all as potassium salts; it is a component of many other formulations.

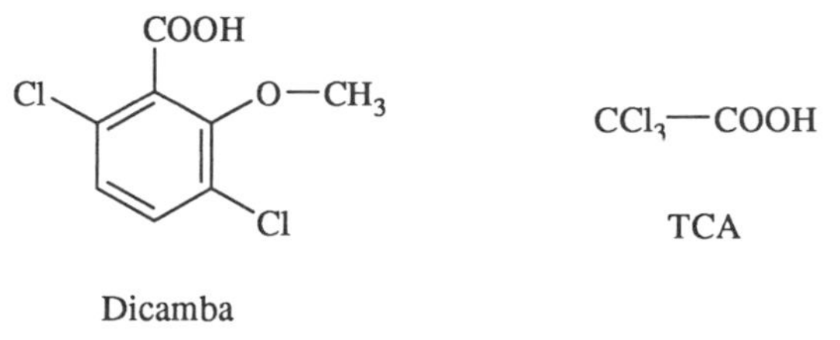

Figure 20.3 Some other organic acid herbicides.

20.5.1.2 Toxicity to Laboratory Animals

Basic Findings   Dicamba is a compound of low acute toxicity. See Table 20.4. Signs of acute poisoning include myotonic muscular spasms, urinary incontinence, and dyspnea, cyanosis, and exhaustion following repeated spasms. Most survivors recovered in 2–3 days and thereafter showed normal weight gain. Survivors of oral or dermal doses showed no macroscopic pathology, but most of those that survived an intraperitoneal dose showed visceral adhesions, and most that survived subcutaneous doses had centrally necrotic or fluid-filled abscesses.

Dicamba produced conjunctival swelling and corneal clouding if it entered the eye; the effect cleared in 5–7 days.

The dimethylamine salt of dicamba administered undiluted to the skin of rabbits and rats is mildly irritating when continued daily for 2 weeks; there is no evidence of percutaneous absorption (Beste, 1983). The dimethylamine salt of dicamba can be extremely irritating to the eye.

A dietary level as high as 3162 ppm did not produce illness or retard growth. However, there was a slight increase in the absolute and relative weight of the liver at dietary levels as low as 1000 ppm. The no-effect level was 316 ppm (corresponding to dosage of 43 to 19 mg/kg/day as the rats grew older and ate less) (Edson and Sanderson, 1965).

Dicamba (acid) at a concentration of 800 ppm in the diet was well tolerated over a 3-month period. Further 500 ppm (approximately 25 mg/kg) in the diet administered to rats and dogs for a 2-year interval produced no observable effects on survival, body weight, food consumption, organ weight, hematology, or histology compared to concurrent controls (Beste, 1983).

Absorption, Distribution, Metabolism, and Excretion
[^{14}C]Dicamba was excreted rapidly by rats, mainly in the urine, whether administered orally or subcutaneously. However, 1–2% appeared in the feces following subcutaneous injection, indicating some true fecal excretion. About twice that proportion appeared in the feces when dicamba was fed, indicating that about 2% was unabsorbed. After subcutaneous injection, 70% or more of the dose was excreted in 5 hr and over 92% in 3 days. The compound in the urine was not degraded, but at a dietary

Table 20.4
Single-Dose LD 50 for Dicamba

Species	Route	LD 50 (mg/kg)	Reference
Rat, M	oral	757	Edson and Sanderson (1965)
Rat, F	oral	1414	Edson and Sanderson (1965)
Rat, M	intraperitoneal	80	Edson and Sanderson (1965)
Mouse, F	oral	1189	Edson and Sanderson (1965)
Mouse	oral	1190	Golovan' (1970)
Guinea pig	oral	566	Edson and Sanderson (1965)
Guinea pig	oral	3000	Golovan' (1970)
Rabbit	oral	566	Edson and Sanderson (1965)
Rabbit	oral	2000	Golovan' (1970)

level of about 1000 ppm about one-fifth was conjugated with glucuronic acid. The proportion was slightly less at higher dietary levels. When the compound was ingested daily in the feed, the concentrations in different organs reached a steady state within 2 weeks. Storage was proportional to dosage at dietary levels up to 1000 ppm. When daily intake stopped, storage declined rapidly (Tye and Engel, 1967).

Following oral administration of dicamba to a cow, it was possible in 7 days to account for 73% of the dose by excretion of the unchanged compound in the urine; none was detected in the feces or milk. The concentrations in the urine were essentially uniform for 6 days and then fell to a very low level on the seventh day (St. John and Lisk, 1969); this is an unusual pattern suggesting that there may be a maximal rate of excretion.

Effects on Reproduction   Dicamba in the three-generation reproduction study in rats did not affect the reproductive capacity (Beste, 1983).

20.5.1.3 Toxicity to Humans

Experimental Exposure   The thresholds for smell and taste are 250.8 and 218.8 ppm, respectively; the threshold for specific taste is about 515.9 ppm (Golovan', 1970).

Accidental and Intentional Poisoning   What apparently was the only serious case of poisoning involving dicamba was the result of an attempted suicide with a mixture of that compound and 2,4-D. The only details available concern the result of analysis of samples of serum and urine that were collected in an unusually systematic way. During the first 14 days, urinary output exceeded 1.5 liters/day, except perhaps on the first day, when the sample (1.238 liters) probably was incomplete. The initial concentration of dicamba in the serum (46.4 ppm) was small compared to the initial concentration of 2,4-D (1006 ppm). A semilogarithmic plot (not shown) of the data revealed that the curve for dicamba in serum fell much faster than the curve for 2,4-D during the first 3 days. However, beginning early on the fourth day the rate of loss of 2,4-D increased markedly and that for dicamba increased only slightly, so that during days 4 and 5 the curves were much more similar in slope; they also had similar but much more gradual slopes on day 6 and later. Likewise, the rates of change in the concentrations of the two compounds in the urine were different during the first 3 days and similar thereafter. The highest concentration of dicamba in the urine (second sample, day 1) was 280 ppm, whereas the highest concentration of 2,4-D (overnight sample, days 3 and 4) was 1900 ppm, having risen from an initial value of 145 ppm. Dicamba reached undetectable levels in both serum and urine in 2 weeks but, because the 2,4-D values started much higher, these were still measurable for more than 3.5 weeks (Rivers et al., 1970). The initially slow fall of 2,4-D in the serum and the 3-day increase of its concentration in the urine suggest that it was essentially all absorbed when sampling began. On days 4 and 5, when excretion was maximal, the half-life for disappearance of dicamba from the serum was 12.00 hr, and that for 2,4-D was

4.46 hr. The fastest excretion of both compounds was associated with a good flow of urine but certainly with no striking diuresis (<2.5 liters/day). On the contrary, a greater diuresis (>3.1 liters/day) on days 8–11 had little or no effect on the rate of excretion that started on day 6. A computer-assisted pharmacokinetic study of this case produced curves in reasonably good agreement with the observed results (Young and Haley, 1977).

Two cases associated with use of a mixture of dicamba (2.8%) and 2,4-D (36%) are discussed in Section 20.4.1.3.

Treatment of Poisoning   Treatment is entirely symptomatic.

20.5.2 TCA

20.5.2.1 Identity, Properties, and Uses

Chemical Name   TCA is trichloroacetic acid or its sodium salt.

Structure   See Fig. 20.3.

Synonyms   TCA is the name approved by BSI and ISO for sodium trichloroacetate. In Australia, New Zealand, and Canada TCA stands for the free acid; this is also the usage approved by WSSA. (TCA has also been used as a synonym for calcitonin, but the molecules and their uses are so entirely different that confusion seems unlikely.) Trade names include Konesta®, NaTA®, Natal®, Tecane®, and Varitox®. The CAS registry number for the acid is 76-03-9; for sodium trichloroacetate, it is 650-51-1.

Physical and Chemical Properties   Trichloroacetic acid has the empirical formula $C_2HCl_3O_2$ and a molecular weight of 163.4. Sodium trichloroacetate is $C_2Cl_3NaO_2$ with a molecular weight of 185.36. The acid forms colorless crystals that melt at 57–58°C; the boiling point is 197.5°C. Technical TCA is a yellowish, slightly deliquescent powder. Sodium trichloroacetate is soluble in ethanol and many organic solvents. Its solubility in water at room temperature is 120 gm/100 ml. The acid has a solubility in water at 25°C of 1306 gm/100 ml; it is soluble in ethanol and diethyl ether.

History, Formulations, and Uses   Sodium trichloroacetate was introduced as an herbicide in 1947 by E. I. du Pont de Nemours and Company and Dow Chemical Company. It is a preemergence herbicide used on couch grass and on wild oats in sugar beets, peas, and kale and as a postemergence herbicide for control of grass seedlings and certain established perennial grasses and cattails.

20.5.2.2 Toxicity to Laboratory Animals

The oral LD 50 values of the sodium salt are 3320 mg/kg in rats and 4970 in mice (Woodard *et al.*, 1941). The oral LD 50 in the rabbit is reported as 4000 mg/kg (Beste, 1983). In addition, prolonged contact with the skin can result in chemical burns, and dust is very irritating to the nose and throat. Fassett (1963)

quoted an Atomic Energy Commission report indicating that 0.0035 mg applied to the rabbit cornea caused immediate, severe coagulation necrosis. A single application of TCA to the rat tail produced no change, but repeated application produced such severe necrosis that part of the tail dropped off (Gzhegotskiy and Doloshitskiy, 1971).

Animals poisoned by an oral dose of TCA quickly pass into a state of narcosis or seminarcosis and within 36 hr either recover completely or die without coming out of narcosis (Woodard *et al.*, 1941).

Rats tolerated a feeding level of 0.1% (1000 ppm) for 126 days without adverse effects, whereas 0.3% resulted in reduction in body weight gain (Beste, 1983).

20.5.2.3 Toxicity to Humans

The sodium salt of TCA caused an occupational problem when it was used for 5.5 months each year to control grass and weeds in pavement in the tropics. The workers had been provided with good dermal protection but with no face shields, goggles, or masks. The eight members and one foreman of a spray team complained of coughing and/or pains in the chest, and some complained of sore throat and burning eyes. Many symptoms were worse at night. The foreman, who had been employed 2.5 years, had irritation of the trachea, and he was fatigued and short of breath at night. His eyes itched by day and even more so by night, when they also burned. On windy days his eyes became markedly swollen (Faerber, 1962).

Trichloroacetic acid is a metabolite of trichloroethylene (see Section 14.7.8).

Treatment of poisoning is symptomatic.

20.6 ORGANIC PHOSPHORUS HERBICIDES

Only a few organic phosphate pesticides, especially DEF and merphos, are useful as herbicides. These are trithiobutyl phosphates, and as such they are different from insecticides. Although they are weak inhibitors of acetylcholinesterase, there is no reason to think that their primary mode of action in mammals is different from that of the organic phosphorus insecticides, which are discussed in Chapter 16. On the average, they are compounds of low oral toxicity (LD 50, 325–1475 mg/kg). However, one of them, merphos, produces polyneuropathy in humans as well as in experimental animals (see Section 16.10.1).

Glyphosate, glycerol phosphonic acid, is the only current member of a second type of phosphorus-containing herbicides. This contact agent for nonselective weed control is discussed below. Like the thiobutyl phosphates, it is not a significant inhibitor of cholinesterase; unlike merphos (see Section 16.10.1), it is not known to cause polyneuropathy.

20.6.1 GLYPHOSATE

20.6.1.1 Identity, Properties, and Uses

Chemical Name   Glyphosate is *N*-(phosphonomethyl) glycine.

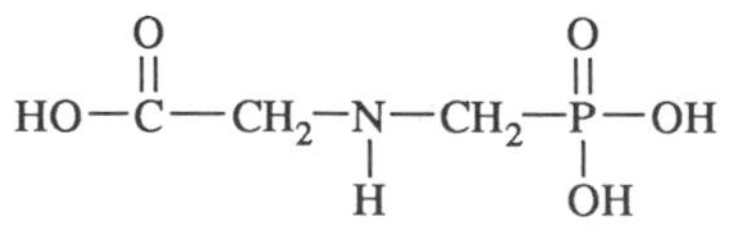

$$HO-\overset{\overset{\displaystyle O}{\|}}{C}-CH_2-\underset{\underset{\displaystyle H}{|}}{N}-CH_2-\overset{\overset{\displaystyle O}{\|}}{\underset{\underset{\displaystyle OH}{|}}{P}}-OH$$

Figure 20.4   The organic phosphorus herbicide glyphosate.

Structure   See Fig. 20.4.

Synonyms   The common name glyphosate (ANSI, BSI, ISO, WSSA) is in general use. Trade names include Glifonox®, Glycel®, Rodeo®, Rondo®, and Roundup®. Its code designation is MON-0573. The CAS registry number is 1071-83-6.

Physical and Chemical Properties   Glyphosate has the empirical formula $C_3H_8NO_5P$ and a molecular weight of 169.1. It is a white and odorless solid that melts at 200°C and has a negligible vapor pressure. The solubility of glyphosate in water is 1.2% at 25°C. It is not generally soluble in organic solvents. It is not liable to significant photodecomposition or volatilization; it is stable up to temperatures of 60°C.

History, Formulations, and Uses   Glyphosate was first introduced as a herbicide in 1971 by Monsanto Agricultural Company. It is a very broad spectrum herbicide, is relatively nonselective, and is very effective on deep-rooted perennial species and on annual and biennial species of grasses, sedges, and broadleaf weeds. It is available as an aqueous solution of the isopropylaniline salt.

20.6.1.2 Toxicity to Laboratory Animals

Response to Single Dose   The acute oral LD 50 of glyphosate in the rat is 5600 mg/kg; the dermal LD 50 in the rabbit is greater than 5000 mg/kg. In addition, the inhalation LC 50 in the rat for the formulated product is greater than 12.2 mg/liter for 4 hr of exposure (Beste, 1983).

Irritation and Sensitization   Glyphosate is slightly irritating to the rabbit eye and nonirritating to the rabbit skin. Formulations might be slightly more irritating (Beste, 1983).

Response to Repeated Doses   Glyphosate was fed to dogs and rats at levels of 200, 600, and 2000 ppm for 90 days. Body weight, food consumption, behavioral reactions, mortality, clinical pathology, and pathology were essentially unaffected (Beste, 1983). Further 2-year feeding studies in rats and dogs at levels of 30, 100, and 300 ppm did not elicit adverse effects.

Metabolism   Glyphosate is metabolized to aminomethyl phosphonic acid (Wagner, 1983).

Biochemical Effects   Olorunsogo and Bababunmi (1980), using intact mitochondria isolated from rat liver, found that glyphosate, like thyroxine, acts as a uncoupler of oxidative phosphorylation. This occurs as a result of both interactions with oxidative phosphorylation and energy-dependent transhydrogenase reaction.

Mutagenicity   Vigfusson and Vyse (1980) examined the effect of glyphosate on the rate of sister chromatid exchanges in human lymphocytes *in vitro*. The frequency of sister chromatid exchange was enhanced by glyphosate only at very high concentrations.

Carcinogenicity   The Environmental Protection Agency has classified glyphosate as a Category C (possible human) carcinogen (National Research Council, 1987). This category is reserved for chemicals for which there is no evidence of carcinogenicity in humans and only limited evidence in animals (a tumorigenic response in one species).

Effects on Reproduction   The teratogenic potential of glyphosate has been evaluated in the rabbit (Wagner, 1983); no teratogenic effects were noted at the highest level tested (30/mg/kg/day).

20.6.1.3 Toxicity to Humans

Experimental Exposure   The irritation, sensitization, photoirritation, and photosensitization potential of glyphosate was studied in 346 volunteers. A formulation that contained 41% glyphosate was applied to intact or Draize-type abraded skin. Single and 21-day cumulative irritancy and modified Draize-type skin irritation assays were performed. A phototoxicity study and a modified photo Draize skin sensitization study were also performed. On unabraded skin, glyphosate showed no greater irritation potential than either an all-purpose cleaner, a dishwashing detergent, or a baby shampoo. When tested on abraded skin, glyphosate resulted in a slightly greater incidence of erythema at 24 hr; however, the 48-hr reading indicated that the irritancy potential was similar to that of the cleaner and dishwashing liquid. In the 21-day cumulative irritancy assay, glyphosate and the baby shampoo were less irritating than either the cleaner or the dishwashing liquid. No evidence of skin sensitization was seen. Glyphosate demonstrated no potential for photoirritation or photosensitization (Maibach, 1986).

Use Experience   No known cases of poisoning have been reported or observed (Beste, 1983).

Treatment of Poisoning   Treatment, if required, is entirely symptomatic.

20.7 AMIDES

Amides have the general structure R_1—C(O)—N(R_2,R_3). Of the R_2 and R_3 substitutions, one usually is a large, often aromatic moiety while the other usually is a hydrogen, methyl, chloromethyl, ethyl, or other small group. The R_1— substitution ranges from chloromethyl to a five-carbon aliphatic chain or a ring. There is at least one thioamid (chlorthiamid) characterized by —C(S)— rather than by —C(O)—; it also differs by being a simple amine (—NH$_2$). Amide herbicides are now sold in greater tonnage than any other herbicides; examples include alachlor (ANSI, BSI, ISO, WSSA), which is currently the largest-selling herbicide in the United States; allidochlor (BSI, ISO), which has been discontinued; benzoylpropethyl (BSI, ISO); butachlor (ANSI, BSI, JMAF, WSSA); carbetamide (BSI, ISO), which has been discontinued; chloranocryl (ISO), also discontinued; chlorthiamid (BSI, ISO); diphenamid (ANSI, BSI, CSA, ISO, MAPJ, WSSA), flamprop-methyl (BSI, ISO); metolachlor (ANSI, ISO, WSSA), which is second in the class of herbicides in the United States; monalide (BSI, ISO); naptalam (ISO, WSSA): pentanochlor (BSI, ISO) [solan (ANSI)]; propachlor (BSI, ISO, WSSA); and propanil (BSI, ISO, WSSA) (see Fig. 20.5). The oral LD 50 values of these 14 compounds in the rat range from 700 to >10,000 and average >2771 mg/kg. Kearney and Kaufman (1976) recognized chloracetamides as a separate group characterized by ClH$_2$C— as the R$_1$— group. Examples include alachlor and metolachlor.

20.7.1 ALACHLOR

20.7.1.1 Identity, Properties, and Uses

Chemical Name Alachlor is *N*-methoxymethyl-2′,6′-diethyl-2-chloroacetanilide.

Structure See Fig. 20.5.

Synonyms The common name alachlor (ANSI, BSI, ISO, WSSA) is in general use. Trade names include Alanex®, Alanox®, Lasso®, and Lazo®. A code designation is CP-50,144. The CAS registry number is 15972-60-8.

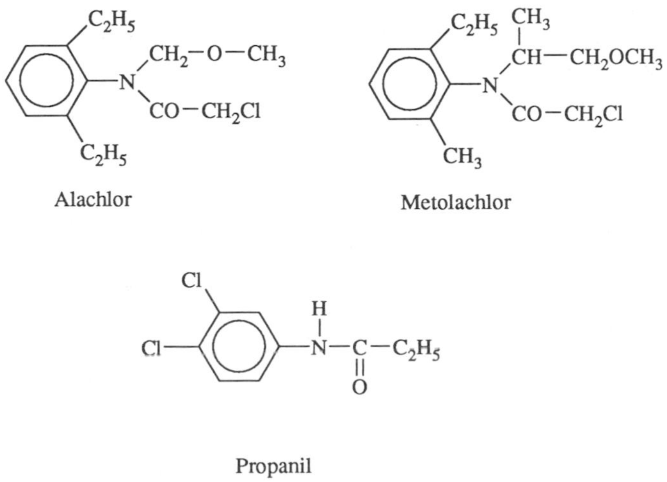

Figure 20.5 Selected amide herbicides.

Physical and Chemical Properties Alachlor has the empirical formula C$_{14}$H$_{20}$NO$_2$Cl and a molecular weight of 269.77. It is a crystalline solid with a melting point of 40–41°C and has a vapor pressure of 2.2 × 10^{-5} mm Hg at 25°C. The solubility of alachlor in water is 242 ppm at 25°C. Alachlor is soluble in ether, acetone, benzene, chloroform, ethanol, and ethyl acetate and is slightly soluble in heptane. Alachlor is relatively stable, with its first detectable heat evolution at 105°C.

History, Formulations, and Uses Alachlor was introduced in 1969 by Monsanto. It is a selective pre- and early postemergence herbicide for annual broadleaf control in crops such as beans, beets, cabbage, corn, cotton, ornamentals, peanuts, peas, potatoes, sorghum, soybeans, sugarcane, sunflowers, and tobacco.

Alachlor is available as 15% granular, 4 lb/gal emulsifiable concentrate and 4 lb/gal flowable formulations; it is also sold as a prepack formulation containing 2.5 lb (active ingredient) of alachlor and 1.5 lb (active ingredient) of atrazine per gallon. A microencapsulated formulation is also available.

20.7.1.2 Toxicity to Laboratory Animals

Irritation and Sensitization Standard rabbit eye and skin irritation tests with technical grade alachlor found the product nonirritating to the eyes and slightly irritating to the skin (Beste, 1983). Alachlor has been identified as a skin sensitizer (Monsanto, 1985).

Response to Single Dose The oral LD 50 value for alachlor in the rat is reported to be 1800 mg/kg (Morgan, 1982; Hodogaya Chemical Co., Ltd., 1986); Beste (1983) records a value of 903 mg/kg. The dermal LD 50 in the rat is reported to be greater than 2000 mg/kg (Hodogaya Chemical Co., Ltd., 1986). A more definitive dermal LD 50 value in rabbit is 13,300 mg/kg (Beste, 1983).

Response to Repeated Doses Ninety-day administrations to rats and dogs were well tolerated at levels of approximately 10 and 5 mg/kg/day, respectively, without any detectable treatment-related effects (Beste, 1983). In Special Review of Alachlor, the U.S. Environmental Protection Agency issued Position Document 1 (Office of Pesticide Programs, 1984a), which included several unpublished findings developed by Monsanto, the sole manufacturer of alachlor. The EPA issued the Registration Standard for the product in the same year (Office of Pesticide Programs, 1984b). Notably, these studies revealed alachlor to be hepatotoxic to dogs fed the product at levels of 5, 25, 50, and 75 mg/kg for 6 months. A no-observable-effect level was established at 1 mg/kg/day in a 1-year dog study. In a 2-year rat feeding study in the Long-Evans strain conducted for Monsanto, which was completed in 1982, oncogenicity (discussed below), hepatotoxicity, and an ocular lesion, referred to as the uveal degeneration syndrome (UDS), were noted. UDS was seen at all doses tested (14, 42, and 126 mg/kg/day). In a second study the no-observable-effect level for UDS was established at 2.5 mg/kg/day. UDS was found to be irreversible.

Absorption, Distribution, Metabolism, and Excretion   In the rat, alachlor is metabolized and eliminated as conjugates of mercapturic acid, glucuronic acid, and sulfate in the urine and feces. The elimination of the product in both male and female rats is approximately equally distributed between the urine and feces. Nearly 90% of the administered dose is eliminated in 10 days; however, a significant portion is eliminated in 48 hr. Elimination is characterized in two phases: a rapid phase with a half-life of 0.2–10.6 hr and a slow phase with a half-life of 5–16 days (Office of Pesticide Programs, 1984a).

Radioactivity in rat tissues was concentrated in the highly perfused organs such as the spleen, liver, kidney, and heart. Additional relatively high levels of radioactivity were found in the eyes, brain, stomach, and ovaries. Further quantities of labeled material were found at the primary sites for tumor formation in this species, giving more credence to a cause-and-effect relationship.

In addition, dermal penetration studies in the rhesus monkey with an emulsifiable concentrate formulation of alachlor revealed that 50% of the applied dose was absorbed in 24 hr, whereas in an *in vitro* study using human skin over 12% of a microencapsulated formulation was absorbed over the same period (Office of Pesticide Programs, 1984a).

Biochemical Effects   Nicolau (1983) showed that 90 days of exposure to alachlor at a feeding level of 50 ppm resulted in minor alterations of the circadian rhythms of RNA, DNA, and protein in the rat testis. An isolated decrease in the thyroid RNA as well as the disappearance of the circadian rhythm in adrenal protein content was also noted. The significance of these findings is not clearly understood.

Mutagenesis   Position Document 1 of the EPA's Special Review process (Office of Pesticide Programs, 1984a) indicated that tests were available to cover the three primary areas of mutagenicity assessment (gene mutation, chromosomal aberration, and others including primary DNA damage tests). In the area of gene mutation, the *S. typhimurium* test with the TA1538, TA1537, TA1535, TA98, and TA100 strains with and without S9 metabolic activation was negative. In addition, tests with *E. coli* strain WP2 *hcr* and the rec-assay in *B. subtilis* strains M45 and H17 did not reveal any evidence of a mutagenic response. In the area of chromosomal aberrations, an *in vivo* bone marrow cytogenic test was found negative. Alachlor was evaluated in human lymphocytes *in vitro* and in rat bone marrow cells *in vivo* for chromosomal endpoints (Georgian *et al.,* 1983). A dose-dependent increase was noted in the lymphocyte cultures (40 ppm was the highest dose). In the cytogenetic evaluation in Wistar rats, a dose-dependent response in clastogenic effects was also noted at levels of 1.25 and 2.50 mg/kg (body weight). An *in vitro/in vivo* hepatocyte DNA repair study in rats suggested that alachlor was weakly genotoxic (Office of Pesticide Programs, 1984a).

Carcinogenesis   Position Document 1 of the Office of Pesticide Programs (1984a) concluded that alachlor produced oncogenic effects in laboratory animals. The tumorigenic effects included lung tumors in mice and stomach, thyroid, and nasal turbinate tumors in rats. The study in mice utilized the CD-1 strain of mouse; alachlor was administered in the diet at levels comparable to 26, 78, 260 mg/kg/day. At the highest feeding level, female mice exhibited a significant increase in bronchoalveolar tumors; no tumors were noted in the males or at the two lower feeding levels in females.

Two chronic feeding studies were conducted with alachlor in the Long–Evans strain of rat. The feeding levels used in the first study were equivalent to 14, 42, and 126 mg/kg/day for 2 years. In this study, a dose-related increase (42 and 126 mg/ kg/day) was observed for nasal turbinate adenomas in both sexes. There was also a significant increase in malignant stomach tumors (mostly mixed carcinoma–sarcoma) in both sexes at the highest feeding level. Further, follicular cell neoplasias were increased in the males administered the highest feeding level.

The second study appeared to be divided into two phases. In the first phase, Long-Evans rats were fed levels of 126 mg/kg/day in the diet. Part of this group was terminated after only 5–6 months, whereas the remainder continued on diet for 2 years. In this study, as in the first, the incidence of nasal turbinate adenomas after 2 years of feeding was significantly elevated at 126 mg/kg/day. In the first study, the incidence of these adenomas for the 126 mg/kg/day group was approximately 55 and 21% in males and females, respectively, and in the second study the incidence was approximately 69 and 44%, respectively; no tumors were noted in the control animals. Interestingly, the administration of alachlor for 5–6 months at 126 mg/kg/day was sufficient to elicit a 60% incidence of these adenomas in male rats as well as a 41% incidence in females. Likewise, malignant stomach tumors were noted in females at 126 mg/kg/day—46% in the first study and 61% in the second study. No malignant stomach tumors were seen in the control rats of either sex in either study. The reproducibility was somewhat different in the case of males; in the first study the incidence was 34% and in the second study only 4%. The administration of alachlor for 5–6 months at 126 mg/kg/day was inadequate to elicit malignant stomach tumors. Finally, the response noted in thyroid follicular tumors in the first study was even more pronounced in the second study. In fact, there was an apparent increase in follicular cell carcinomas in the second study not noted in the first. In the second phase of this second study, Long–Evans rats were administered levels of 0.5, 2.5, and 15 mg/kg/day (equivalents) in their diets for 2 years. Feeding the level of 15 mg/kg/day for 2 years resulted in an increase in the incidence of adenomas of the nasal turbinates (33% in the males and 29% in the females, versus 0% in the controls of both sexes). In this phase of the second study, no malignant stomach tumors were noted at the 15 mg/kg/day feeding level and the incidence of follicular cell adenomas and/or carcinomas was unremarkable.

The EPA (Office of Pesticide Programs, 1984b) concluded, based on these study results, that alachlor should be classified as

Category B2, a probable human carcinogen. In fact, based on the tumor incidence in the rat study, the EPA (Office of Pesticide Programs, 1986) has derived a quantitative oncogenicity potency factor estimate (Q_1^*) of 1×10^{-1} (1/mg/kg/day), which would place alachlor near the top of the list for pesticides (National Research Council, 1987). The National Research Council (1987) reported a slightly higher value of 5.95×10^{-2} (1/mg/kg/day).

Effects on Reproduction   The Office of Pesticide Programs (1984a) in their Position Document 1 reviewed the data base for alachlor in regard to reproductive effects and teratogenicity.

Alachlor administration to rats over three generations at feeding levels equivalent to 3, 10, and 30 mg/kg/day resulted in a NOEL for reproductive effects of 10 mg/kg/day. Renal effects were noted in the second-generation parental males as well as the third-generation offspring at 30 mg/kg/day; these effects consisted of kidney discoloration, chronic nephritis, and increased relative and absolute kidney weight.

In a rat teratology study, doses of 50, 150, and 400 mg/kg/day were administered without any evidence of a teratogenic effect. Maternal and fetal toxicities were noted at 400 mg/kg/day; therefore, the no-observable-effect level was set at 150 mg/kg/day. The rabbit teratology study conducted was deemed not adequate to make an assessment.

20.7.1.3 Toxicity to Humans

Use Experience   The Office of Pesticide Programs (1984a) reported on an epidemiological study conducted in a Monsanto production area to investigate the ocular status of workers exposed to alachlor; no attempt was made to evaluate the potential oncogenic effects in this population. There was no evidence of an increase in ocular lesions similar to the irreversible uveal degeneration syndrome noted in rats. Full details of the study were not available.

Treatment of Poisoning   There is no antidote for alachlor. Treatment would be symptomatic (Morgan, 1982). However, it is possible that an individual could become allergic to alachlor (Monsanto, 1985), as exhibited by a skin reaction. In such cases the sensitized person should avoid further contact.

20.7.2 ALLIDOCHLOR

20.7.2.1 Identity, Properties, and Uses

Chemical Name   Allidochlor is 2-chloro-*N,N*-dialkyl acetamide.

Structure $Cl-CH_2-C(O)-N(CH_2-CH=CH_2)_2$.

Synonyms   The common name CDAA has been approved by WSSA. The common name allidochlor is approved by BSI and ISO. Allidochlor was sold under the trade name Randox® as a 4 lb/gal emulsifiable concentrate or a 20% granule. The CAS registry number is 93-71-0.

Physical and Chemical Properties   Allidochlor (CDAA) has the empirical formula $C_8H_{12}ClNO$ and a molecular weight of 173.6. It is an oily amber liquid with a slightly irritating odor. It is soluble in organic solvents and has a vapor pressure of 9.4×10^{-3} mm Hg at 20°C. Its solubility in water at 25°C is 2 mg/100 ml.

History, Formulations, and Uses   Allidochlor was introduced by Monsanto in 1956 for weed control in corn, sorghum, and a variety of other crops. It was sold as a 4 lb/gal emulsifiable concentrate (EC) and a 20% granule. Its use was discontinued by the manufacturer in 1984.

20.7.2.2 Toxicity to Laboratory Animals

Symptomatology   Poisoning in rats is characterized by apparent discomfort, salivation, coma, and convulsions. Hepatic degeneration was observed at necropsy.

Response to Single Dose   Monsanto found the acute rat LD 50 of technical material to be 290 mg/kg; the LD 50 values for the EC and granular formulations are 210 mg/kg and 1900 mg/kg, respectively. The rabbit dermal LD 50 values for the technical, EC, and granular formulations were reported to be 830, 590, and 4750 mg/kg, respectively.

Irritation and Sensitization   CDAA technical and Randox EC are considered corrosive or severely irritating to eyes and skin. The Randox granular is considered severely irritating to skin and moderating irritating to eyes.

20.7.2.3 Toxicity to Humans

Use Experience   Allidochlor has been associated with severe contact dermatitis from occupational exposure. In three separate cases, contamination of work shoes from spills resulted in persistent swelling and violaceous edema of the exposed feet. Hemorrhagic bullae, crusting, and an exudative intertrigo were also observed. In two of the three cases, similar but milder lesions were observed on the hands and in covered areas where repeated exposure could be expected—that is, under the watch band or pocket areas on thighs and buttocks. In two of the three cases, Randox produced violent blistering in patch tests (Spencer, 1966).

20.7.3 METOLACHLOR

20.7.3.1 Identity, Properties, and Uses

Chemical Name   Metolachlor is 2-chloro-2'-ethyl-6'-methyl-*N*-(2-methoxy-1-methylethyl)acetanilide.

Structure   See Fig. 20.5.

Synonyms   The common name metolachlor (ANSI, BSI, ISO, WSSA) is in general use. Its trade name is Dual®. A code designation is CGA-24,705. The CAS registry number is 51218-45-2.

Physical and Chemical Properties Metolachlor has the empirical formula $C_{15}H_{22}NO_2Cl$ and a molecular weight of 283.8. It is a liquid, white to tan in color, and odorless. Metolachlor has a boiling point of 100°C at 0.001 mm Hg and a vapor pressure of 1.3×10^{-6} mm Hg at 20°C. Its solubility in water is 530 ppm at 20°C and it is miscible with most organic solvents.

History, Formulations, and Uses Metolachlor was first registered with the Environmental Protection Agency in 1976. It is a selective herbicide for control of annual grass weeds, yellow nutsedge, and certain broadleaf species in corn, peanuts, and soybeans. Metolachlor is sold as Dual in formulations containing 5, 15, and 25% (active ingredient) as granulars as well as an 86.4% emulsifiable concentrate. It is sold in a prepack with atrazine as Bicep®, Primagran®, and Primextra. Milocep® is a prepack of metolachlor and propazine, Codal® is a mixture of metolachlor and prometryn, and Cotoran Multi® is a combination of metolachlor and fluometuron.

20.7.3.2 Toxicity to Laboratory Animals

Symptomatology Lethal or near-lethal single oral doses of metolachlor administered as an emulsifiable concentrate to rats elicited the following toxic signs: piloerection, epistaxis, salivation, lacrimation, chromodacryorrhea, diarrhea, polyuria, constricted or dilated pupils, ptosis, rigid muscle tone, convulsions, tremors, hypoactivity, ataxia, exophthalmus, hypersensitivity to touch, respiratory gurgle, and straub tail.

The results of some acute toxicity tests with technical metolachlor are presented in Table 20.5.

Irritation and Sensitization Metolachlor technical has been found to be nonirritating to rabbit eye and minimally irritating to rabbit skin in standard tests (CIBA-GEIGY, 1982a). Metolachlor technical has been shown to have sensitization properties in a standard guinea pig test (CIBA-GEIGY, 1982a).

Response to Repeated Doses The administration of metolachlor in the diet to dogs for 6 months was well tolerated with a no-observable-effect level established at 100 ppm or 2.5 mg/kg/day (Environmental Protection Agency, 1986). In a 21-day subchronic dermal toxicity study with rabbits using the 8

Table 20.5
Acute Toxicity of Metolachlor Technical

Species	Route	LD 50	Reference
Rat	oral	2,780 mg/kg	CIBA-GEIGY (1982a)
Rat	inhalation	1.75 mg/liter for 4 hr	Sine and Meister (1987)
Rabbit	dermal	>10,000 mg/kg	Sine and Meister (1987)
Dog	oral	19 (emetic ED 50)	(Office of Pesticide Programs, 1987)

lb/gal emulsifiable concentrate, no systemic effects were observed at treatment levels as high as 540 mg/kg. Slight redness at the site of application and a reduction in body weight gain were signs noted at the 1080 mg/kg application level (Beste, 1983).

Metabolism in Animals Metolachlor is metabolized in rats by thio conjugation at the acetylchloro group or ether hydrolysis followed by oxo conjugation (CIBA-GEIGY, 1984).

Mutagenicity The available data for metolachlor would clearly indicate that the product is not mutagenic. The gene mutation potential was evaluated in an Ames *Salmonella* assay with and without metabolic activation; no mutagenic properties were seen (CIBA-GEIGY, 1984). Chromosomal aberration potential was examined in two test systems: the dominant lethal in mice (CIBA-GEIGY, 1984) and an *in vivo* cytogenetic study (Environmental Protection Agency, 1986). Neither test gave any indication of a clastogenic potential for metolachlor. Finally, DNA repair tests were evaluated; metolachlor did not exhibit potential to cause damage to DNA in these tests (Environmental Protection Agency, 1986).

Oncogenicity The oncogenic potential for metolachlor has been evaluated in two bioassays in the rat and two bioassays in the mouse. Since metolachlor has been considered as a possible substitute for alachlor, the Office of Pesticide Programs (1984a) summarized the results of these studies in the Alachlor Position Document 1. Both 2-year studies were conducted in the CD-1 mouse at feeding levels as high as 3000 ppm (approximately 420 mg/kg/day); neither study gave any indication of a tumorigenic response. In the first rat study conducted in the Sprague-Dawley-derived rat, a weak oncogenic response was noted in female rats at the highest feeding level tested, 3000 ppm or approximately 300 mg/kg/day (Environmental Protection Agency, 1986). The incidence of benign liver tumors went from 2% in the control to 15% in the 300 mg/kg/day group. In the second study in Sprague–Dawley-derived rats, the results of the first study were reproduced. No tumors of any type were seen in male rats; however, a weak, benign liver tumor response was noted in the female. The incidence went from 0% in the control females to 10% at 30 mg/kg/day. The EPA classification of this compound as a Category C oncogen is pending (National Research Council, 1987). A quantitative potency factor Q_1^* based on these liver lesions was calculated to be 2.1×10^{-3} (Office of Pesticide Programs, 1984a).

Effects on Reproduction A two-generation reproduction study conducted in Sprague–Dawley rats revealed a reproductive no-observable-effect level (NOEL) at 300 ppm (15 mg/kg) and a lowest-effect level (LEL) at 1000 ppm or 50 mg/kg (Environmental Protection Agency, 1986). In addition, in a rat teratology study there was no evidence of teratogenicity or fetotoxicity at the highest dose evaluated, 360 mg/kg; in a rabbit teratology study the maternal NOEL was established at 120 mg/kg and no evidence of teratogenicity or fetotoxicity was noted at the highest dose tested, 360 mg/kg.

20.7.3.3 Toxicity to Humans

Accidental Poisonings Irritation of skin, eyes, or mucous membranes may result from overexposure. Ingestion can cause nausea, vomiting, abdominal distress, or diarrhea. Significant exposure by other routes has been reported to result in headache and nausea; these symptoms usually disappear within 24 hr. A skin sensitization reaction may occur in susceptible individuals (CIBA-GEIGY, 1984).

There has been a limited number of cases of accidental exposure to metolachlor. Most of these have involved eye and skin exposures to adult males during the course of product use. Three previously unpublished cases are as follows.

An adult male developed symptoms of nausea, headache, and burning sensation in his chest following approximately a 15-hr exposure over 2 consecutive days when he served as a flagman, marking rows in a field where the 8 lb/gallon emulsifiable concentrations of metolachlor (Dual® 8E) was being used. The individual was not wearing any protective clothing or equipment. During observation in the hospital emergency room, his symptoms subsided and he was released within 3 hr with prescriptions for prochlorperazine suppositories and an analgesic.

In a second case, while pouring water into a beaker previously used for measuring Dual® 8E, a farmer accidentally took water from the beaker into his mouth; none of the material was swallowed and he immediately rinsed his mouth. The next morning, the farmer had severe nausea and headache; both subsided during the day without treatment.

In a third situation, Dual® 8E in a small amount splashed out of a vent hole and into a worker's eye while he was lifting a barrel that had been accidentally tipped over. The eye was immediately washed; the result was some temporary redness of the eye and surrounding area.

Treatment of Poisoning There is no specific antidote to counteract the toxic effects of metolachlor or related products of similar chemistry. Laboratory studies have shown that metolachlor has a high affinity for activated charcoal (CIBA-GEIGY, 1982a). Therefore, if ingestion is less than 10 mg/kg of body weight, it is probably best treated by administering 30–50 gm of activated charcoal in 3–4 ounces of water. If diarrhea has not already developed, follow the charcoal administration in 4 hr with a suitable saline laxative.

For ingestion of more than 10 mg/kg of body weight, especially when ingestion occurred less than an hour before treatment, induce emesis or lavage stomach. Following emesis or lavage, a suspension of 30–50 gm of activated charcoal in 3–4 ounces of water can be left in the stomach.

Skin reactions have been successfully treated with antihistamines and ointments containing an anti-inflammatory agent. Severe contamination of eyes may require specialized ophthalmologic attention.

20.7.4 PROPANIL

20.7.4.1 Identity, Properties, and Uses

Chemical Name Propanil is N-(3,4-dichlorophenyl) propanamide.

Structure See Fig. 20.5.

Synonyms Propanil is the common name approved by BSI, ISO, JMAF, and WSSA, except in Austria, Germany, and the Republic of South Africa. Trade names include Bay 30130, Chem Rice®, Drexel Prop-Job®, DPA®, Erban, FW-734, Herbax®, Propanex®, Propanilo®, Riselect®, Stam Supernox, Stampede® 3E, Stam F-34®, Stam M-4®, Strel®, Surcopur®, Surpur®, S10165, and Vertac®. A code designation is FW-734. The CAS registry number is 709-98-8.

Physical and Chemical Properties The empirical formula for propanil is $C_9H_9Cl_2NO$, and the molecular weight is 218.09. Propanil is a white crystalline solid with a melting point of 92–93°C. The vapor pressure is 9×10^{-5} mm Hg at 60°C. The technical product is a brownish crystalline solid with a melting point of 88–91°C. Propanil is soluble in ethanol, 54% at 25°C, and in isophorone, 60% at 25°C. Solubility in water at room temperature is 225 ppm. The compound is stable in emulsion concentrates but is hydrolyzed in acid and alkaline media to 3,4-dichloroaniline and propionic acid.

History, Formulations, and Uses Propanil first was described in 1960 and also was introduced that year by Rohm and Haas Company. It is used as a herbicide in rice or potato fields.

20.7.4.2 Toxicity to Laboratory Animals

Basic Findings The acute oral LD 50 values for propanil in rats and dogs are 1384 and 1217 mg/kg, respectively. In both species, deaths occurred over a 3-day period and were characterized by central nervous system depression. In a 13-week study, some rats were killed by a dietary level of 50,000 ppm, and feed consumption, growth, and hemoglobin concentrations were reduced at levels of 3300 ppm and higher. In a 2-year study, a dietary level of 1600 ppm caused a significant decrease in growth and a relative increase in the weight of the spleen and liver in female rats and of the testes in the males. A dietary level of 400 ppm (about 19 mg/kg/day) was a no-effect level (Ambrose et al., 1972).

In a 2-year study in dogs, a dietary level of 4000 ppm depressed growth in spite of increased food intake. There was a slight increase in the relative weight of the heart but no histological abnormality in that or other organs and no change in hematology or in liver and kidney function tests. A dietary level of 600 ppm (about 12.6 mg/kg/day) was a no-effect level (Ambrose et al., 1972).

Absorption, Distribution, Metabolism, and Excretion When propanil was fed to a cow for 4 days, 1.4% of the total dose was recovered in the feces, but none was detected in the urine or milk. *In vitro,* propanil was metabolized rapidly by liver microsomes, but it was stable in rumen fluid (Gutenmann and Lisk, 1975).

Biochemical Effects   Mice killed by an oral dose of propanil showed cyanosis as well as central nervous system depression. The cyanosis was the result of methemoglobinemia caused by the metabolite 3,4-dichloroaniline (DCA). TOCP, an esterase inhibitor, prevented cyanosis but did not protect against CNS depression or death (Singleton and Murphy, 1973). Sex and species differences in the formation of methemoglobin have been explained to a considerable degree by *in vitro* studies of (*a*) the ability to form DCA from propanil and (*b*) the ability to activate DCA to metabolites that form methemoglobin (Chow and Murphy, 1974, 1975).

Effects on Reproduction   In a three-generation study, male and female rats were fed propanil for 11 weeks before the parent generation was mated. Dietary levels as high as 1000 ppm were without effect on fertility, gestation, viability, or lactation (Ambrose *et al.,* 1972).

20.7.4.3 Toxicity to Humans

Use Experience   Of 28 production workers exposed to dichloroaniline and propanil, 17 had chloracne caused by tetrachloroazobenzene (see Fig. 18.2). The chloracnegenic activity of both propanil and its precursor was demonstrated by rabbit ear test (Morse and Baker, 1979). Kimbrough (1980) reported that 3,4,3',4'-tetrachloroazobenzene and 3,4,3',4'-tetrachloroazoxybenzene are responsible for the chloracnegenic activity characteristics of propanil.

Because of the danger of chloracne, the manufacturer recommends that personnel involved in the use of propanil must wear full protective equipment at all times, including neoprene-coated gloves, rubber work shoes and overshoes, latex rubber apron, goggles to protect eyes, respirator or mask approved for toxic dust or organic vapors, and overalls or rubber suit.

20.8   CARBAMATE HERBICIDES

The herbicidal carbamates differ from the insecticidal ones by having a bulky substitution on the nitrogen rather than on the oxygen atom. Examples include asulam (ANSI, BSI, ISO, WSSA), barban (ANSI, BSI, ISO, WSSA), carbetamide (ANSI, BSI, ISO, WSSA), chlorpropham (BSI, ISO, WSSA), desmedipham (ANSI, BSI, ISO, WSSA), phenisopham (BSI, ISO), phenmedipham (ANSI, BSI, ISO, WSSA), propham (BSI, CSA, ISO, WSSA), and swep (ANSI, WSSA). The herbicidal carbamates are not inhibitors of cholinesterase, and their mammalian toxicity usually is much lower than that of the insecticidal carbamates. For these nine compounds the oral LD 50 values in the rat range from 550 to 11,000 mg/kg; however, the majority of these compounds have oral LD 50 values in excess of 4000 mg/kg.

No characteristic or distinctive toxic effect and, of course, no mode of action of the carbamate herbicides have been noted in mammals.

20.8.1 PHENMEDIPHAM

20.8.1.1 Identity, Properties, and Uses

Chemical Name   Phenmedipham is methyl-3-*m*-tolycarbamoloxyphenyl carbamate.

Structure   See Fig. 20.6.

Synonyms   Phenmedipham is the common name approved by BSI, ANSI, BSI, ISO, JMAF, and WSSA. Its trade names are Betanal®, EP-452, Kemifam®, and Spin-aid®. Its code designation is SN38584 (Schering AG). The CAS registry number is 13684-63-4.

Physical and Chemical Properties   The empirical formula for phenmedipham is $C_{16}H_{16}N_2O_4$ and the molecular weight is

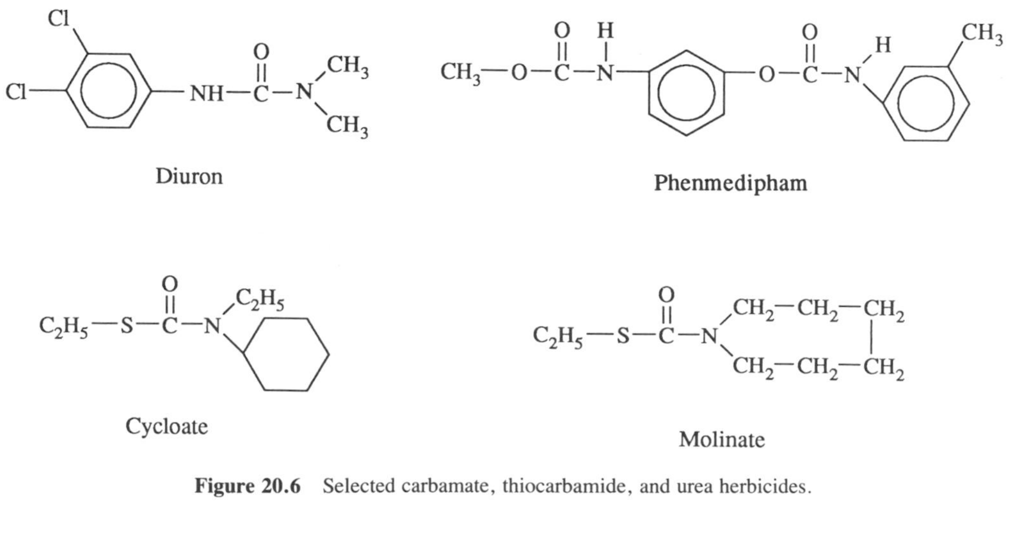

Diuron

Phenmedipham

Cycloate

Molinate

Figure 20.6   Selected carbamate, thiocarbamide, and urea herbicides.

300.3. The compound forms colorless crystals which have a melting point of 143–144°C. The technical product is 95% pure and has a melting point of 140–144°C and a vapor pressure of 10^{-11} mm Hg at 25°C. At room temperature the solubility of phenmedipham is 3 mg/liter in water, about 200 gm/kg in acetone, and about 50 gm/kg in methanol, 20 gm/kg in chloroform, 2.5 gm/kg in benzene, and about 500 mg/kg in hexane. No changes were observed in the compound when held for 6 days at 50°C.

History, Formulations, and Uses Phenmedipham first was described by F. Arndt and C. Kötter in 1967 and was introduced by Schering AG in 1968. It is used to control weeds of beet crops, particularly sugar beets.

20.8.1.2 Toxicity to Laboratory Animals

Acute oral LD 50 values are >8000 mg/kg in rats and mice and >4000 mg/kg in guinea pigs and dogs. The acute dermal LD 50 is >4000 mg/kg in rats. Rats fed at rates of 125, 250, and 500 mg/kg/day for 120 days survived, but food intake was decreased in a dosage-dependent way (Worthing, 1987).

20.8.1.3 Toxicity to Humans

Use Experience Two farmers came separately to the same department of dermatology for diagnosis. One had used phenmedipham for 8 or 9 years without recognized difficulty in spite of a long history of photodermatitis. However, what was considered an exacerbation of photodermatitis began only a few days after he used phenmedipham in 1978, and a patch test required 14 days to subside. The second farmer presented with a severe, spreading, bullous dermatitis of both hands a few days after he used the compound. He too had used it for 8 or 9 years without difficulty, but a patch test was positive (Nater and Grosfeld, 1979).

Treatment of Poisoning Treatment is symptomatic.

20.9 THIOCARBAMATES

The thiocarbamates include the following herbicides: butylate (WSSA), cycloate (WSSA), diallate (BSI, ISO, WSSA), EPTC (BSI, ISO, MAFJ, WSSA), molinate (BSI, ISO, WSSA), orbencarb (ISO), pebulate (BSI, ISO, WSSA), Thiocarbazil (proposed), thiobencarb (ANSI, BSI) or benthiocarb (JMAFF, WSSA), triallate (BSI, ISO, WSSA), and vernolate (WSSA). The oral LD 50 values of these 9 compounds in the rat range from 395 to >10,000; the majority of these compounds have an oral LD 50 >1000 mg/kg.

20.9.1 CYCLOATE

20.9.1.1 Identity, Properties, and Uses

Chemical Name Cycloate is *S*-ethyl cyclohexylethylthiocarbamate.

Structure See Fig. 20.6.

Synonyms The common name cycloate approved by BSI, ISO, and WSSA is in general use, except in the USSR, where ronit is used. Trade names include Eurex® and Ro-Neet®. A code designation is R-2063. The CAS registry number is 1134-23-2.

Physical and Chemical Properties Cycloate has the empirical formula $C_{11}H_{21}NOS$ and a molecular weight of 215.36. It is a clear liquid with a boiling point of 145°C at 10 mm Hg and a vapor pressure of 6.2×10^{-3} mm Hg at 25°C. The solubility of cycloate in water at 22°C is 100 ppm, but it is miscible with acetone, benzene, 2-propanol, kerosene, methanol, xylene, and most other organic solvents. It is stable and noncorrosive.

History, Formulations, and Uses Cycloate was introduced in the early 1960s by the Stauffer Chemical Company. It is used to control annual broad-leaved weeds and grasses and to control nut grass in sugar beets and spinach by preplant soil incorporation. Available formulations include an 80% emulsifiable concentrate and 10% granules.

20.9.1.2 Toxicity to Laboratory Animals

Oral LD 50 values were 2323 and 2285 mg/kg in rats and mice, respectively. Mortality reached 20% in 4 months in rats receiving 232 mg/kg/day, but a dosage of 116 mg/kg/day was without effect. However, repeated dermal application at the rate of 115 mg/kg/day caused hyperemia and edema of the skin of rabbits (Rebrin and Aleksandrova, 1971).

Cycloate is converted to the sulfoxide by microsomal enzymes and then cleared so rapidly by the liver soluble-glutathione system that the sulfoxide is not detectable in the liver (Casida *et al.*, 1975). According to Aleksandrova and Klisenko (1978), the urinary metabolites include cyclohexylamine and dicyclohexylamine, which are toxic, but the parent compound is entirely cleared from the body in 24 hr.

20.9.1.3 Toxicity to Humans

Use Experience Physiological and hematological investigations of workers exposed to cycloate aerosols and vapors at concentrations as high as 6.2 mg/m³ for 5 consecutive days revealed no effects (Rebrin and Aleksandrova, 1971).

Treatment of Poisoning Treatment is symptomatic.

20.9.2 MOLINATE

20.9.2.1 Identity, Properties, and Uses

Chemical Name Molinate is *S*-ethyl *N*,*N*-hexamethylene thiocarbamate.

Structure See Fig. 20.6.

Synonyms   The common name molinate is approved by BSI, ISO (except in Germany), JMAF, and WSSA. Yalan is the name used in the USSR. A trade name for molinate is Ordram® and a code designation is R-4572. The CAS registry number is 2212-67-1.

Physical and Chemical Properties   Molinate has the empirical formula $C_9H_{15}NOS$ and a molecular weight of 187.3. It is a clear liquid with an aromatic odor and a boiling point of 202°C. The vapor pressure is 5.6×10^{-3} mm Hg at 25°C. Molinate is soluble in acetone, benzene, 2-propanol, methanol, and xylene. Its solubility in water at 21°C is 800 mg/liter. It is noncorrosive and stable to hydrolysis.

History, Formulations, and Uses   Molinate was introduced in 1954 by the Stauffer Chemical Company. It is used to control weeds in rice paddies. Formulations for the product include an emulsifiable liquid (8 lb active ingredient per gallon) and granules (10% active ingredient).

20.9.2.2 Toxicity to Laboratory Animals

Basic Findings   The acute oral LD 50 in rats is 720 mg/kg, and the acute dermal LD 50 in rabbits is >10,000 mg/kg (Worthing, 1987). Sine and Meister (1987) report an acute oral LD 50 in rats of 549–955 mg/kg and an acute dermal LD 50 in rabbits of 3536 mg/kg.

Absorption, Distribution, Metabolism, and Excretion
Molinate is metabolized to the corresponding sulfoxide by mouse liver microsomal enzymes and is then cleaved by the soluble-glutathione system. The sulfoxide can be detected as a transient metabolite in the livers of mice injected with the compound (Casida *et al.*, 1975).

Excretion of ring-labeled [^{14}C]molinate by rats is 95–96% complete in 48 hr. Approximately 88% was in the urine plus cage wash and 11% in the feces. Less than 1% of the dose was found in the expired air. Molinate mercapturate constituted 35% and 3- and 4-hydroxymolinate, almost entirely as *O*-glucuronides, constituted 26.9% of the urinary ^{14}C. Tissue levels were approximately 13.8% of the administered dose after 1 day and 3.7% after 7 days (DeBaun *et al.*, 1978a,b).

Effects on Reproduction   Administration of molinate to young male rats at a rate of 3.6 mg/kg/day for 2 months caused changes in the spermatozoa but did not decrease fertility. When these rats were mated to normal females, many of the embryos were resorbed and postnatal mortality was increased (Voytenko and Medved', 1973; Anina *et al.*, 1975). Resorption of embryos suggests a dominant lethal effect, but the postnatal mortality probably occurred through some other mechanism.

20.9.2.3 Toxicity to Humans

Accidental and Intentional Poisoning   After 60 kg of molinate was applied to 2 ha of paddy fields, four families, including a total of 17 people, began to notice an odor in a nearby well, which was their source of water. Then eight people, including five children, developed nausea, diarrhea, abdominal pain, fever, weakness, and conjunctivitis, and four others had abdominal pain only. Recovery occurred when the families stopped using water from the well. Chemical analysis was not done until 15 days later, by which time the average molinate concentration in five samples was 0.006 ppm. The material disappeared only slowly; an odor was still present after 1 month (Minakawa *et al.*, 1978).

Treatment of Poisoning   Treatment is entirely symptomatic.

20.10 DITHIOCARBAMATES

The dithiocarbamate herbicides include metam (BSI, ISO, WSSA) [carbam (MAF)] and sulfallate (BSI, ISO) [CDEC (WSSA)]. The oral LD 50 values of these compounds in the rat are 1700 and 850 mg/kg, respectively.

Sulfallate has been discontinued (Sine and Meister, 1987); this product when administered in the feed was carcinogenic to Osborne–Mendel rats and to B6C3F1 mice, inducing mammary gland tumors in females of both species, tumors of the forestomach in male rats, and lung tumors in male mice [National Cancer Institute (NCI), 1978a].

Metam in the form of sodium salt has been shown to elicit allergic contact dermatitis. Karlsmark *et al.* (1982) describe a case of a 21-year-old male who wore no protective equipment during his work but repeatedly accidentally soaked his clothing and footwear with the herbicide solution. This individual developed a bullous, allergic, contact dermatitis; the probable sensitizing group in metam was considered to be methyldithiocarbamate.

20.11 UREAS AND GUANIDINES

Herbicidal ureas have the general structure R_1—NH—C(O)—N—R_2,R_3 or, in the case of thioureas, R_1—NH—C(S)—N—R_2,R_3. Guanidines have the form R_1—NH—C(NH)—R_2,R_3. The R_1 substitution is a bulky moiety, often a substituted or unsubstituted benzene ring; the R_2 and R_3 substitutions often are methyl or methoxy groups but may be larger, e.g., a butyl or a substituted benzene group. Examples of ureas include benzthiazuron (BSI, ISO) (discontinued), buturon (BSI, ISO), chlorbromuron (ANSI, BSI, ISO, WSSA) (discontinued in the United States), chlorotoluron (ISO) [chlortoluron (BSI)], chloroxuron (ANSI, BSI, ISO, WSSA) [chloroxifenidim (USSR)], cycluron (BSI, ISO, WSSA) (discontinued), difenoxuron (BSI, ISO), diuron (ANSI, BSI, CSA, ISO, WSSA), fenuron (ANSI, BSI, ISO, WSSA), fluometuron (ANSI, BSI, ISO, WSSA), isonoruron (BSI, ISO), linuron (ASA, BSI, ISO, WSSA), methabenzthiazuron (BSI, ISO), metobromuron (ANSI, BSI, ISO, WSSA), metoxuron (BSI, ISO), monolinuron (BSI, ISO, WSSA), monuron (ANSI, BSI,

ISO, WSSA), neburon (ANSI, BSI, ISO, WSSA), noruron (WSSA) [norea (ANSI, BSI, WSSA)], and siduron (ANSI, BSI, ISO, WSSA). The oral LD 50 values of these compounds range from >500 to 11,000 mg/kg.

Linuron has been reported (National Research Council, 1987) to cause an oncogenic response in one sex of one species (EPA Class C oncogen).

20.11.1 DIURON

20.11.1.1 Identity, Properties, and Uses

Chemical Name Diuron is 3-(3,4-dichlorophenyl)-1,1-dimethylurea.

Structure See Fig. 20.6.

Synonyms The common name diuron (ANSI, BSI, CSA, ISO, WSSA) is in general use, except in the USSR, where dichlorfenidion is used. The compound also has been referred to as DCMU and DMU. Trade names have included Cekiuron® (Cequisa), Crisuron®, Dailon®, Diater®, Di-on®, Direx® 4L, Diurex®, Duirol®, Karmex®, Rout®, Unidron®, and Vonduron® Diuron Weed Killer. The CAS registry number is 330-54-1.

Physical and Chemical Properties Diuron has the empirical formula $C_9H_{10}Cl_2N_2O$ and a molecular weight of 233.10. It is a white, odorless solid with a melting point of 158–159°C and a vapor pressure of 3.1×10^{-6} mm Hg at 50°C. The solubility of diuron in water is 42 ppm at 25°C. It has a low solubility in hydrocarbons; its solubility in acetone is 5.3% at 27°C. Diuron is stable to oxidation and moisture. Its rate of hydrolysis is negligible at ordinary temperatures and under neutral conditions. It decomposes at 189–190°C and is noncorrosive.

History, Formulations and Uses Diuron was introduced in 1954 by E. I. du Pont de Nemours and Company. It is a photosynthesis inhibitor that is used mainly for general weed control on noncrop areas. It is also used selectively in the control of germinating broadleaf and grass weeds in sugarcane, citrus, pineapples, cotton, asparagus, and temperate climate tree and bush fruits. It is also used as a soil sterilant. Available formulations include an 80% wettable powder and a 40% flowable water suspension, as well as a 4 lb/gal formulation. It is also available in formulations containing 50% diuron and 30% amitrole as well as mixed with MSMA, sodium metaborate, bromacil, and/or chloropropham.

20.11.1.2 Toxicity to Laboratory Animals

Basic Findings Diuron is a compound of low acute toxicity. Hodge et al. (1967) found an oral LD 50 of 3400 mg/kg in the rat. In normal juvenile rats fed ordinary laboratory chow or a purified diet containing 26% protein, respectively, Boyd and Krupa (1970) found values of 1017 and 2390 mg/kg.

Within 2 hr of an oral dose of diuron in the LD 50 range, rats were drowsy and ataxic. At 24 hr, animals that eventually died were prostrate and breathed slowly. Animals that subsequently survived were irritable and hyperreflexic. At 24 hr, diarrhea and diuresis appeared, along with reduced intake of food and water, leading to weight loss. Measurement revealed hypothermia, glycosuria, proteinuria, and aciduria. The intensity of all signs was dosage dependent. The immediate cause of death was respiratory failure. Recovery was quite evident in survivors at 48 hr, and most signs of toxicity had disappeared by 72 hr (Boyd and Krupa, 1970).

Ten daily doses at a rate of 1000 mg/kg/day depressed growth and increased erythropoiesis, but were not fatal.

Skin irritation and sensitization tests in guinea pigs proved negative.

In feeding studies, some increase in mortality may have been attributable to a dietary level of 8000 ppm. There was no dosage-related mortality at 5000 ppm or less. At 2500 ppm for 2 years, both rats and dogs showed growth retardation, slight anemia, presence of abnormal pigment, increased erythropoiesis, and splenic hemosiderosis. Some rats showed splenic enlargement, and dogs showed liver enlargement. No histological changes were seen, and there was no evidence of carcinogenicity. In 2-year studies, no effect was seen on dietary levels of 25, 125, and 250 ppm, with the exception of a trace of abnormal blood pigment in some rats and dogs at 125 and 250 ppm and a trend toward reduced erythrocyte counts in dogs at 250 ppm (Hodge et al., 1967). Although the abnormal blood pigment was virtually identical to sulfhemoglobin formed in vitro by simple sulfide, the identity of the sulfur-containing compound that leads to formation of sulfhemoglobin in diuron-fed animals is unknown. It also is unknown whether the formation of abnormal hemoglobin is related to the hemolysis of red cells that occurs and that is compensated at least in part by hyperplasia of the bone marrow.

Absorption, Distribution, Metabolism, and Excretion Diuron is absorbed from the gastrointestinal and respiratory systems. Whether it is absorbed from the skin is unknown.

The majority of metabolites excreted in the urine retain the urea configuration and result from hydroxylation and dealkylation of the parent compound. Six of these compounds were isolated and identified, and four others were identified chromatographically by comparison with standards (Boehme and Ernst, 1965).

Biochemical Effects Diuron and all other herbicidal substituted ureas caused induction of one or more microsomal enzymes. With diuron, dosage-related induction was seen in rats fed dietary levels ranging from 100 to 2000 ppm. Induction was maximal during the first 3 weeks and then decreased during the remainder of the 13-week feed period, except that O-demethylase activity remained high (Kinoshita and DuBois, 1970). Bankowska and Bojanowska (1972, 1973a,b) confirmed the fact of induction and showed that it was associated with morphological changes detectable by electron microscopy and that it promoted the detoxication of parathion *in vivo*.

Effects of Reproduction   There were no untoward findings in a three-generation study in rats maintained at a dietary level of 125 ppm (about 6 mg/kg/day in adult, nonlactating rats but higher in young or lactating animals) (Hodge *et al.*, 1967). This is consistent with the finding of Khera *et al.* (1979) that rats that received diuron by gastric tube on days 6–15 of pregnancy at a rate of 250 mg/kg/day produced young with wavy ribs and other minor variants in the rate of bone development. The effect was not increased at 500 mg/kg/day and was absent at 125 mg/kg/day.

Factors Influencing Toxicity   Rats maintained on a protein-deficient diet were more susceptible than normal rats to poisoning by diuron. The oral LD 50 values were 437, 2390, and 1017 mg/kg for rats on 3.5% casein, 26% casein, and laboratory chow, respectively. The kind of illness caused by diuron was the same in protein-deficient and in normal animals (Boyd and Krupa, 1970).

20.11.1.3 Toxicity to Humans

Accidental and Intentional Poisoning   In a suicide attempt, a 39-year-old woman ingested a herbicidal preparation that contained 56% diuron and 30% amitrole. In view of the volume ingested, the dosages were 38 and 20 mg/kg for diuron and amitrole, respectively. In hospital, the patient showed no signs of intoxication. In a urine specimen taken some hours after ingestion, no unmetabolized diuron could be demonstrated, but 1-(3,4-dichlorophenyl)-3-methylurea and 1-(3,4-dichlorophenyl)urea were isolated and identified. Some 3,4-dichloroaniline probably was present also (Geldmacher-von Mallinckrodt and Schüssler, 1971).

Use Experience   In use, diuron has given no significant difficulty but may irritate the skin, eye, or nose.

The threshold limit value of 10 mg/m³ indicates that occupational intake at a rate of about 1.4 mg/kg/day is considered safe.

Treatment of Poisoning   Treatment is symptomatic.

20.12 SUBSTITUTED PHENOLS

Substituted phenols are used not only as herbicides but also as insecticides and fungicides; they are discussed as a group in Chapter 18. The substituted phenols used as herbicides include most of the dinitrophenols and pentachlorophenol (see Section 18.4.1). Bromofenoxim (BSI,, ISO) (oral LD 50 in rat, 1217 mg/kg) is one example of a substituted phenol without remarkable acute toxicity. Bromoxynil (ANSI, BSI, ISO, WSSA), dichlorbenil (ANSI, BSI, CSA, ISO, WSSA), and oxynil (ANSI, BSI, ISO, WSSA), halogenated cyano-substituted phenols (see Section 20.15), have LD 50 values in the rat of 260,

3160, and 110 mg/kg, respectively, whereas the dinitrophenol dinoseb (BSI, ISO, WSSA) (see Section 18.3.6) has an oral LD 50 value in the rat of 40–60 mg/kg. Dinoseb is an uncoupler of oxidative phosphorylation. Dinoseb administration at the levels of 225 and 300 ppm for 50 days to male rats produced severe effects on the testes, spermatocytes, and reproductive performance in male rats (Linder *et al.*, 1982). Embryo- and fetotoxicity of the conceptus of rats administered dinoseb during gestation at levels of 200 ppm or greater were noted by Spencer and Sing (1982).

Jung *et al.* (1983) describe 14 cases of human poisoning. Eleven adults and three infants were admitted to the hospital after ingesting dinoseb. Severe cases of poisoning appeared clinically similar to cases of thyroid crisis; however, the course sometimes was oligosymptomatic. A yellow discoloration of the skin, hair, and scleras was frequently noted. High temperatures enhanced the toxicity. Early gastric lavage appeared to be effective in treatment of dinoseb poisoning; hemoperfusion might further improve prognosis.

20.13 DIPHENYL ETHERS

Diphenyl ethers have the form R_n—C_6H_n—O—C_6H_n—R'_n. Substitutions on the benzene rings can include —Cl, —Br, —F, —NO$_2$, —CH$_3$, —O—CH$_3$, and others. Such herbicides include acifluorfen (ANSI, BSI, ISO, WSSA) (oral LD 50 in rat, 1300 mg/kg); bifenox (ANSI, WSSA) (oral LD 50 in rat, >6400 mg/kg); diclofop-methyl (ANSI, BSI, ISO) (oral LD 50 in rat, 557–580 mg/kg); fluazifop-butyl (BSI, ISO) (oral LD 50 in rat, 3328 mg/kg); fluorodifen (ANSI, BSI, ISO, WSSA) (oral LD 50 in rat, 9000 mg/kg), discontinued; nitrofen (BSI, ISO, WSSA) (oral LD 50 in rat, 2630 mg/kg); and oxyfluorfen (ANSI, WSSA) (oral LD 50 in rat, >5000 mg/kg). Of these compounds, only nitrofen appears to have been studied in humans.

20.13.1 NITROFEN

20.13.1.1 Identity, Properties, and Uses

Chemical Name   2,4-Dichloro-1-(4-nitrophenoxy)benzene.

Structure   See Fig. 20.7.

Synonyms   Nitrofen (BSI, ISO, WSSA) and 2,4-dichlorophenyl-*p*-nitrophenyl ether are the names most commonly used. Other chemical designations include 2,4-dichloro-4'-nitrodiphenyl ether; 2,4-dichloro-4'-nitrophenyl ether; 4-(2,4-dichlorophenoxy)nitrobenzene; 4'-nitro-2,4-dichlorodiphenyl ether; 4-nitro-2',4'-dichlorophenyl ether; nitrofene; and nitrofen. Trade names for the compound include FW 925, Mezotox®, Niclofen®, Nip®, Nitraphen®, Nitrochlor®, Nitrophene®, Tok®, Tok® 2, E, E25, WP50, Tokkorn®, and Trizilin®. The CAS registry number is 1836-75-5.

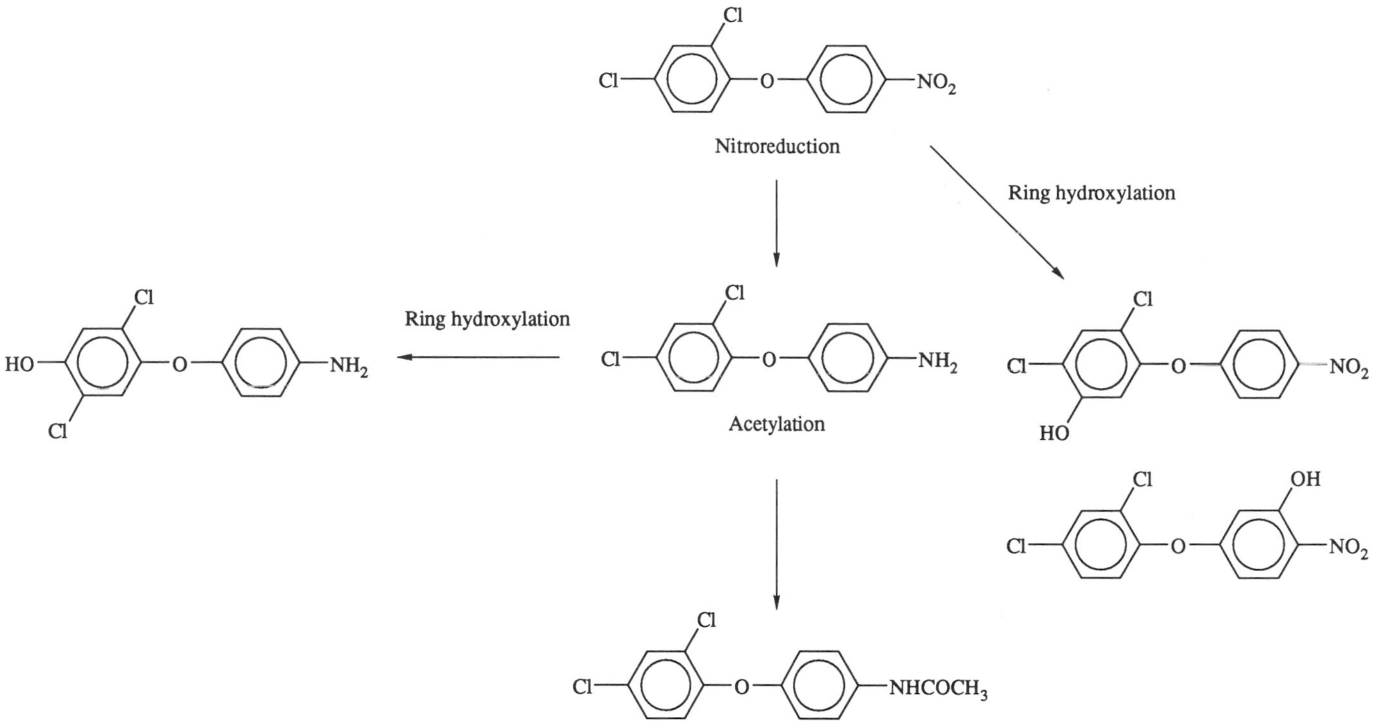

Figure 20.7   Metabolism of nitrofen.

Physical and Chemical Properties   Nitrofen has the empirical formula $C_{12}H_7Cl_2NO_3$ and a molecular weight of 284.1. It is crystalline and has a melting point of 70–71°C. The vapor pressure at 40°C is 8×10^{-6} mm Hg. It is slightly soluble in water (0.7–1.2 mg/liter at 22°C) but is more soluble in acetone, methanol, and xylene.

Use   Nitrofen was first produced commercially in the United States in 1963. It is made by the reaction of 1-chloro-4-nitrobenzene with a salt of 2,4-dichlorophenol. Its use is primarily as a pre- and postemergence herbicide in agricultural applications. It is thought that nitrofen produces its phytotoxic effects by competing with ADP to inhibit energy transfer in the ATP synthase reaction (Lambert *et al.*, 1979).

20.13.1.2 Toxicity to Laboratory Animals

Basic Findings   Nitrofen exhibited very low acute toxicity when administered to a number of mammalian species by a variety of routes. Upon acute exposure to these doses, animals exhibited mainly neurological and respiratory signs of toxicity. Nitrofen has tested positive for mutagenicity in a number of bacterial systems, and chronic administration of doses of 470 mg/kg/day or greater increased the incidence of hepatic tumors. However, the developing rather than adult animal appears to be especially sensitive to nitrofen. The administration of nitrofen during pregnancy at dosages two to three orders of magnitude below the LD 50 has been shown to cause a number of developmental alterations in the newborn pups. The anomalies consisted of diaphragmatic hernias, heart and lung defects, effects on

the development and secretion of the Harderian glands, hydronephrosis, and effects on the thyroid and gonads. Of these, hydronephrosis seems to be the most sensitive to prenatal exposure. As little as 0.3 mg/kg/day given orally to pregnant rats during days 6–15 of gestation has been shown to produce this lesion in the newborn animals (Costlow *et al.*, 1981). Neonatal deaths appear after repeated maternal doses of 3 mg/kg/day and higher. These findings have drawn attention to nitrofen as a potent teratogen. Recent reviews that emphasize the teratogenic aspects of this compound include those by Hurt *et al.* (1983) and the International Agency for Research on Cancer (IARC) (1983).

Absorption, Distribution, Metabolism, and Excretion
Hunt *et al.* (1977) performed a study in which 40 mg/kg of ^{14}C-labeled nitrofen was orally administered to a male sheep. Blood levels peaked at 19 hr with a plateau at 11–31 hr. By 99 hr, 76.2% of the administered radioactivity was recovered in the excreta, with 39 and 37.2% in the urine and feces, respectively. The animal was killed at 100 hr. The fat contained the highest level of radioactivity, which was approximately 7- to 23-fold higher than that in any of the other tissues examined. Of the radioactivity present in feces, 30% was as the parent compound. The predominant metabolites present in urine and feces were 2,4-dichlorophenyl-4-aminophenyl ether, 2,4-dichloro-5-hydroxyphenyl-4-nitrophenyl ether, 2,4-dichlorophenol, 2-chlorophenyl-4-nitrophenyl ether, and sulfate, glucuronide, and glycine conjugates.

A cow fed a diet containing 5 ppm radiolabeled nitrofen

showed only trace levels of radioactivity present in samples of urine, feces, and milk. These levels were 1.7, 1.4, and 0.15 ppm, respectively. A fat sample contained a level of 1.06 ppm, of which 25% was as nitrofen (Roser and Adler, 1971).

A few studies examining the pharmacokinetics of nitrofen in adult rats have been reported (Adler *et al.*, 1970/1971; Steiger-walt *et al.*, 1980). In general, these results agree with those found in the sheep. The rate of metabolism and elimination is rapid, with nearly all of the radiolabeled material (nitrofen plus metabolites) being eliminated within 48–92 hr after the last administered dose. Feces appear to be the predominant route of elimination, containing approximately three- to fivefold more total radioactivity than urine. All of the radioactivity in urine is as metabolites, whereas up to half of the radioactivity present in feces is as nitrofen itself. The principal metabolites were hy-droxylated nitrofen; its amino, acetamido, and proprionamido derivatives; and formamido and acetamido nitrofen. These ap-peared in approximately equal amounts. The levels of radioac-tivity found in fat were 4- to 10-fold higher than in other tissues.

Of particular interest is a study performed by Costlow and Manson (1983) in which the distribution of radiolabeled nitro-fen was examined in pregnant animals. Pregnant rats were or-ally administered a [^{14}C]nitrofen dose of 120 mg/kg on day 11 of gestation, and dams were killed 2–60 hr later. In the maternal blood, the peak concentration of radioactivity occurred 7–9 hr after dosing. Concentrations in the maternal fat were greater than 1000 ppm, and other tissues had concentrations of 9 ppm or less. Fetal blood levels were highest at 4–6 hr, and tissue con-centrations were as high as 50 ppm. Analysis of extracts of the embryoplacental tissues and maternal blood and liver showed the presence of the parent nitrofen plus aminonitrofen, aceta-midonitrofen, and two hydroxylated derivatives. When the em-bryo alone, i.e. without placental tissue, was examined, only the parent compound could be found. Similar levels of nitrofen in both the maternal and fetal tissues suggested that the embryo is more susceptible than the mother to this compound. Further-more, the embryo appears to be a deep compartment for the accumulation of nitrofen (Brown and Manson, 1986).

Toxicity in Adult Animals   Nitrofen had been shown to be only slightly toxic to a number of different mammalian species by the oral, dermal, and inhalation routes. LD 50 values range from 450 to >5000 mg/kg. Intoxication is characterized by decreased levels of activity, depression, and respiratory dis-tress. At lethal doses, tremors, and convulsions precede death within 2–8 days after treatment (Ivanova, 1967; Ambrose *et al.*, 1971; Shardina, 1972; Kimbrough *et al.*, 1974).

In subchronic exposure studies, significant effects on tissue and body weights were observed only at very high levels (>500 ppm) of nitrofen in the diet. The only significant pathologic effect reported was in rats fed diets containing 12,500 and 50,000 ppm. The liver from these animals showed edema, pe-ripheral localization of glycogen granules, and cytoplasmic and nuclear swelling (Ambrose *et al.*, 1971; NCI, 1978b, 1979).

Ambrose *et al.* (1971) observed no significant effects other than decreased body weight and increased relative weights of liver and kidney in rats receiving nitrofen in the diet at levels up to 1000 ppm for 97 weeks. A study conducted by the National Cancer Institute observed significant increases in the incidence of hepatocellular carcinomas in both male and female mice and of hemangiosarcomas in male mice following 78-week con-sumption of diets containing up to 4696 mg nitrofen/kg (NCI, 1978b). A similar study using 6000 mg nitrofen/kg diet demon-strated an increased incidence of hepatocellular carcinomas in both male and female mice (NCI, 1979). Female Osborne-Men-del rats consuming a diet containing an average level of 3627 mg nitrofen/kg also showed an increased incidence of adenocar-cinoma of the pancreas (NCI, 1978b). No increased tumor inci-dence was observed in Fisher 344 rats fed diets containing up to 6000 mg nitrofen/kg (NCI, 1979). However, it should be noted that relatively impure technical grade nitrofen was used in these studies. An increased incidence of hepatocellular carcinomas was observed in B6C3F1 mice fed nitrofen at concentrations of 4700 and 6000 ppm for up to 78 days (Robens, 1980).

Mutagenesis and Carcinogenicity   The results on the muta-genic capabilities of nitrofen appear to be equivocal. In initial studies, the mutagenic activity, as assessed in bacterial systems, varied between investigators and between different lots of tech-nical product (Hurt *et al.*, 1983). More recent results suggest that nitrofen itself is weakly or not mutagenic. A chemical impurity, bis(4-nitrophenyl) ether, has high mutagenic activity (Seiler, 1983), and certain metabolites may also be mutagenic (Draper and Casida, 1983; Miyauchi *et al.*, 1983; Hurt *et al.*, 1983). Nitrofen produced no evidence of morphological trans-formation in the 3T3 mammalian cell transformation assay (Lit-ton Bionetics, Inc., 1979).

As summarized by the Public Health Service (1985), nitrofen has been found to be carcinogenic in animals; liver cancers were noted in mice of both sexes and cancers of the pancreas were observed in female rats (see Table 4.1). However, the oncogenic potential of other compounds in this class has not been docu-mented.

Reproductive and Prenatal Toxicity   In 1971 Ambrose *et al.* first noted that prenatal exposure of rats to nitrofen at a level in the maternal diet of 100 ppm or more elicited neonatal mortality. These data were subsequently confirmed by Kimbrough *et al.* (1974) and Stone and Manson (1981), the latter study utilizing dosages of 20–50 mg/kg/day from days 8 to 18 of pregnancy. Pups exposed *in utero* developed signs of respiratory distress immediately after delivery, became cyanotic, and died within 1 hr after birth. Microscopic examination of the lungs revealed an abnormal appearance of type II cells and lack of expansion of the air sacs. Extensive fibrosis and proliferation of the alveolar epithelium was observed in lungs of 10–14-day-old pups that survived the *in utero* exposure. Day 11 of gestation was the most sensitive day for the induction of neonatal mortality, and 116 mg/kg to the dam was the LD 50 for the neonate. Although cardiac malformations and diaphragmatic hernias appeared to be the leading causes of death in these animals (Costlow and Manson, 1981), studies by Lau *et al.* (1986) suggest that other physiological factors such as improper delivery and cellular utilization of oxygen may be involved. Whatever the primary event may be, it is clear that respiratory distress and altered lung function are significant events leading to death in the neonates (Raub *et al.*, 1983).

Other serious, but not necessarily lethal, malformations occur in neonatal animals exposed *in utero* to nitrofen. These include hydronephrosis, apparent microphthalmia resulting from alterations of the Harderian glands, hydrocephaly, thyroid abnormalities, and hyperactivity (Gray *et al.*, 1982; Kavlock *et al.*, 1982; Kavlock and Gray, 1983; Gray *et al.*, 1983; Costlow *et al.*, 1981; Francis, 1986). In one study, nitrofen was administered dermally to pregnant rats on days 6–15 of gestation at dose levels of 0, 0.3, 0.6, 1.2, and 12.0 mg/kg/day. At these doses no maternal toxicity occurred. At 12 mg/kg, neonatal survival was decreased and animals that died had a high incidence of diaphragmatic hernias. Survivors showed increased occurrence of diaphragmatic hernias, missing or reduced Harderian glands, and slight to severe hydronephrosis. The incidence of hydronephrosis was increased at dosages of 0.3 mg/kg/day and higher. The no-observable-effect level was estimated to be 0.28 mg/kg in males and 0.17 mg/kg in females, based on a linear exprapolation model (Costlow and Manson, 1983). Similar results were reported in mice by Ostby *et al.* (1985) and in rats by Gray *et al.* (1983). The latter investigators also demonstrated that the developmental alterations were produced solely by prenatal exposure, as cross-fostered pups exposed to nitrofen in the milk alone were unaffected. Strain differences exist in the pattern of malformations produced by prenatal exposure. Sprague-Dawley rats had a higher incidence of diaphragm and lung anomalies than the Long-Evans hooded strain. Conversely, the Long-Evans rats had greater frequency of kidney malformations (Kang *et al.*, 1986). Hamsters appeared to be less susceptible to the *in utero* effects of nitrofen exposure. Effect on the Harderian glands, gonads, and kidneys were reported with a minimum effect level of 100 mg/kg and a maximum no-observed-effect level of 50 mg/kg/day (Gray *et al.*, 1982). No developmental anomalies were detected in rabbits at doses of 5 and 20 mg/kg/day during days 6–15 of gestation. At a dosage of 80 mg/kg/day, embryolethality was increased slightly (Siou, 1979).

Ambrose *et al.* (1971) conducted a three-generation reproductive study in which weanling male and female rats were given diets containing 0, 10, 100, or 1000 ppm nitrofen. Animals were mated after 11 weeks of feeding in each generation. At the highest dose, there was an increased incidence of stillbirths and nearly total pup mortality. In the 100 ppm group, the number of stillbirths was increased in the offspring of the F_0 generation. No other effects were observed at this level, and no alterations were observed in any generation at the 10 ppm level.

Similar results were reported by Kimbrough *et al.* (1974) for dietary levels of 0, 20, 100, and 500 ppm nitrofen. Feeding of male rats with nitrofen at levels up to 2500 ppm in the diet 13 weeks prior to mating produced no significant effects on fertility, gestation, litter size, or weight of the pups, despite significant effects on body and tissue weights of the adult males (O'Hara *et al.*, 1983).

Several lines of evidence have indicated that nitrofen exerts its teratogenic effect by alterations in thyroid hormone status (Manson *et al.*, 1984; Manson, 1984; Gray and Kavlock, 1983). Nitrofen has a stereochemical structure similar to that of thyroxine. A metabolite of nitrofen, 4-hydroxy-2,5-dichloro-4'-aminodiphenyl ether, has been found to cross-react with antibody for 3,5,3'-triiodo L-thyronine (T_3) in radioimmunoassays (Manson *et al.*, 1984). Serum levels of thyroid-stimulating hormone are significantly depressed in thyroidectomized rats and euthyroid rats exposed to nitrofen on day 11 of pregnancy. In addition, the amount of thyroid-stimulating hormone released after thyrotropin-releasing hormone challenge is depressed with nitrofen exposure. Administration of thyroxine on days 2–22 of pregnancy to thyroidectomized rats also exposed to nitrofen resulted in a 70% decrease in the frequency of malformed fetuses compared to nitrofen exposure alone. It has been postulated that nitrofen itself or a derivative may have thyroid hormone activity (Manson, 1986).

20.13.1.3 Toxicity to Humans

Nitrofen has been reported to have irritating effects on the skin and eyes in occupationally exposed subjects [Imaizumi *et al.*, 1972; Suga, 1972; Hanada *et al.*, 1977; Tsyrkunov, 1979; California Department of Food and Agriculture (CDFA), 1980].

There has only been one reported incident in which significant toxicity has resulted from exposure to nitrofen. The case involved a 37-year-old man whose occupation involved recycling barrels from various sources for use in local canneries. His job was to remove the tops from the barrels, pour out the contents, use a torch to cut the barrels, and "flame" the barrels in a furnace containing no exhaust stack. On the day of the incident, the barrels being worked on were marked as having contained TOK (nitrofen). The man initially complained of transient upper respiratory tract irritation, headaches, vertigo, abdominal pain, diarrhea, and vomiting. Three days after the onset of symptoms the patient complained of decreased appetite, occasional nausea, and intermittent diarrhea. All other vital signs and blood analysis were normal. Symptoms resolved gradually within a week (Shusterman, 1985).

The exposure potential of food consumers, applicators, and field workers has been reviewed by Hurt *et al.* (1983) and Putnam *et al.* (1983). Provided adequate care is taken by workers in the application of nitrofen, the potential for significant exposure appears to be negligible.

Treatment of Poisoning   Treatment is symptomatic.

Table 20.6
Acute Oral Toxicity of Dinitroanilines

Generic name	Trade name	Rat oral LD 50[a,b] (mg/kg)
benefin	Benfluralin®, Balan®	>10,000
dinitramine	Cobex®	3,700
ethalfluralin	Sonalan®	>10,000
isopropalin	Paarlan®	>5,000
oryzalin	Surflan®, Ryzelan®	>10,000
pendimethalin	Prowl®, Stomp®, Herbadox®	1,150
trifluralin	Treflan®	>10,000

[a]Herbicide Handbook, 1983.
[b]Farm Chemicals Handbook, 1987.

20.14 DINITROANILINES

As a class of herbicides, the dinitroanilines represent compounds of low acute toxicity. Subchronic studies, too, generally show the materials to be of low toxicity. The dinitroanilines are generally highly lipid-soluble. Several of the compounds are shown in Table 20.6.

Human poisoning by dinitroaniline formulations is infrequent. Expected symptoms are related to the effects of solvents and other formulants. Symptomatic treatment would be recommended in cases of human poisoning.

20.15 NITRILES

It has been stated that some of these compounds act as uncouplers of oxidative phosphorylation in plants, but there apparently is no clear evidence that they do so in mammals. It is also entirely conceivable that nitriles might inhibit cytochrome oxidase, but again clear evidence appears to be lacking. Under the circumstances, it is uncertain whether they have a single common mechanism of action. The herbicidal nitriles are essentially substituted phenols or they are metabolized to them (see Section 20.12); often the substitutions include a halogen in addition to the cyano group. Some representative members of this class are bromoxynil (ANSI, BSI, ISO, WSSA) (oral LD 50 in the rat, 260 mg/kg), chloroxynil (ISO) (oral LD 50 in the rat, 757 mg/kg), and diphenatril (oral LD 50 in the rat, 3500 mg/kg). Dichlobenil and ioxynil are considered in detail in Sections 20.15.1 and 20.15.2, respectively. See Fig. 20.8.

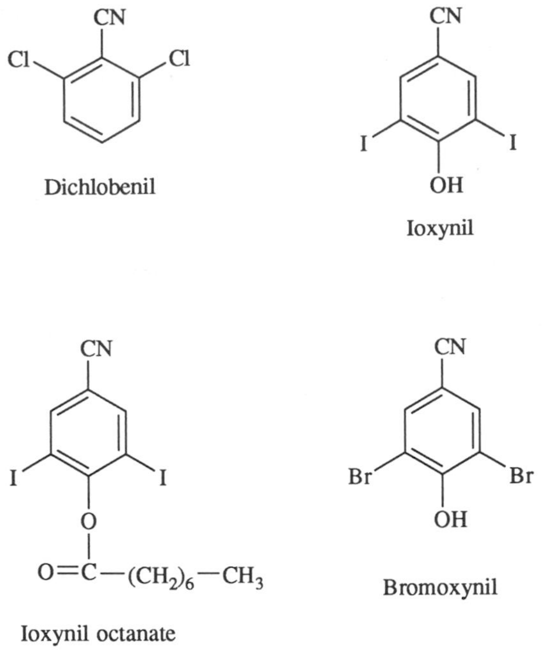

20.15.1 DICHLOBENIL

20.15.1.1 Identity, Properties, and Uses

Chemical Name Dichlobenil is 2,6-dichlorobenzonitrile.

Figure 20.8 Nitrile herbicides.

Structure See Fig. 20.8.

Synonyms The common name dichlobenil (ANSI, BSI, CSA, ISO, WSSA) is in general use. Other names are 2,6-dichlorobenzonitrile and DCB. Trade names include Casoron®, Decabane®, Dyclomec®, Niagara 5006®, Norosac®, and Prefix® D. Code designations include H-133 and NIA-5966. The CAS registry number is 1194-65-6.

Physical and Chemical Properties Dichlobenil has the empirical formula $C_7H_3Cl_2N$ and a molecular weight of 172.01. It is a white to off-white crystalline solid with an aromatic odor and a melting point of 145–146°C. The technical product is at least 94% pure. The vapor pressure of dichlobenil is 5.5×10^{-4} mm Hg at 20°C. The solubility of dichlobenil in water is 25 ppm at 20°C, and it is only slightly soluble (5–10 ppm) in most organic solvents. The compound is stable to heat and acids but is hydrolyzed by alkali. It is noncorrosive and is compatible with other herbicides.

History, Formulations, and Uses Dichlobenil was introduced in 1960 by Philips-Duphar B. V. Dichlobenil is a powerful inhibitor of germination and of actively dividing meristems and acts primarily on growing points and root tips. It is used to control annual and perennial weeds in the seedling stages and many of them in more advanced stages. It can be used as a selective weed killer, both pre- and postemergence, as an aquatic weed killer, and for total weed killing. Available formulations include a 45% wettable powder and granules in concentrations ranging from 2 to 20%. Dichlobenil is also formulated as granules in combination with dalapon, bromacil, and simazine.

20.15.1.2 Toxicity to Laboratory Animals

Basic Findings   Dichlobenil is a compound of moderate acute oral toxicity in the rabbit and guinea pig (LD 50 values of 270 and 501 mg/kg, respectively) and low toxicity in the rat and mouse (LD 50 values of 3160 and 2056–2162 mg/kg, respectively). The difference probably is not due mainly to absorption because the LD 50 by intraperitoneal injection in the mouse is 603 mg/kg (Beste, 1983).

In rats, 12-week feeding tests produced an increase in liver weight at a dietary level of 100 ppm and an increase in the weight of the kidneys also at 200 ppm. Rabbits showed an increase in liver weight associated with a dietary level of 500 ppm for 12 weeks. A no-effect level in short-term tests in rats, rabbits, and pigs was 50 ppm, corresponding to a dosage of 2.5 mg/kg/day in the rat. In fact, no toxic effect was observed in rats at a dietary level of 100 ppm for 2 years, suggesting that there was a gradual adaptation in this species to the effect of dichlobenil in the liver (Van Genderen and Van Esch, 1968).

The acute dermal LD 50 in albino rabbits is 1350 mg/kg; dichlobenil was applied to rabbit skin for 21 days at levels as high as 500 mg/kg/day. The no-effect level was 100 mg/kg/day (Beste, 1983).

Absorption, Distribution, Metabolism, and Excretion   Studies with [^{14}C]dichlobenil showed that more of it was absorbed by rabbits than by rats. Rats formed a higher proportion of 2,6-dichloro-3-hydroxybenzonitrile, whereas rats formed about equal proportions of this and of the 4-hydroxy analog. Both rats and rabbits conjugated metabolites with sulfate, and rabbits conjugated them with glucuronic acid also. Unchanged dichlobenil was not found in the urine but was found in the feces. Some metabolites remained unidentified. However, hydrolysis of the nitrile group was insignificant (Wit and Van Genderen, 1966a).

The metabolites just mentioned are, like other chlorophenols, uncouplers of oxidative phorphorylation (Wit and Van Genderen, 1966b). Because hydroxylation of dichlorobenil presumably occurs in the liver, this uncoupling may explain the liver injury.

Biochemical Effects   In rabbits there was a striking correlation between high serum levels of sorbitol dehydrogenase and death. In normal rabbits the enzyme activity varied from 0.07 to 1.4 and averaged 0.5 μmol/ml/hr. Rabbits that died had serum enzyme levels of ≥10 with an average of 52 μmol/ml/hr. In fatally poisoned rabbits the enzyme activity remained normal for about 10 hr and then shot up rapidly during the last few hours of life (Van Genderen and Van Esch, 1968).

20.15.1.3 Toxicity to Humans

Six men engaged in mixing or bagging dichlobenil developed dermatitis within 1 week to 5 months after first exposure (Deeken, 1974). Although the condition involved comedones and was spoken of as chloracne, no cysts were observed, and judging from the description and one photograph, the dermatitis was not severe. The possibility that this mild condition may have been associated with a contaminant does not seem to have been explored.

Treatment of Poisoning   During 10 years of experience in factories, laboratories, and commercial use, no intoxication with dichlobenil was documented. In case of ingestion, gastric lavage and symptomatic therapy are recommended (Beste, 1983).

20.15.2 IOXYNIL

20.15.2.1 Identity, Properties, and Uses

Chemical Name   4-Hydroxy-3,5-diiodobenzonitrile.

Structure   See Fig. 20.8.

Synonyms   Ioxynil (ANSI, BSI, ISO, WSSA) is the common name in use except in parts of Europe, where the trade name Toxynil® is used as a nonproprietary name. Trade names for ioxynil include Actril®, Actrilawn® (sodium salt), Bantrol®, Certol®, Iotril®, Mate®, Oxytril® (a mixture of ioxynil and bromoxynil), Totril®, and Toxynil®. Code designations include ACP 63-303, MB 8873, and MB 11461 (ioxynil octanoate). The CAS registry number is 1698-83-4.

Physical and Chemical Properties   Ioxynil has the empirical formula $C_7H_3I_2NO$ and a molecular weight of 370.9. It is a colorless, odorless solid that melts at 209°C and sublimes at about 140°C at 0.1 mm Hg. The technical product is a cream-colored powder with a faint phenolic odor and a melting point of 200°C. The solubility of ioxynil in water at 25°C is 130 ppm, but the alkali salts are water soluble. Ioxynil is soluble in acetone, methanol, and tetrahydrofuran. The esters with higher fatty acids (e.g., octanoic acid) are soluble in petroleum oils.

History, Formulations, and Uses   Ioxynil was discovered by Am Chem Products in 1960 and introduced in England in 1963. It is a herbicide used to control broadleaf weeds. Formulations include aqueous concentrates of the alkali metal salts, water-soluble amines, oil-soluble amines, and emulsifiable concentrates of the octanoate ester. Actril C® is a mixture of potassium salts of ioxynil and mecoprop (total 300 gm/liter). It is sold in combination with several products; these include 2,4-D, mecoprop, bromoxynil, dichloroprop, and isoproturon.

20.15.2.2 Toxicity to Laboratory Animals

Basic Findings The LD 50 values for ioxynil are shown in Table 20.7. Bromoxynil is nearly equitoxic to ioxynil in the same species (Carpenter *et al.*, 1964). Ioxynil octanoate was found to have oral and dermal LD 50 values in the rat of 130 and >500 mg/kg, respectively.

Dogs tolerated the administration of 4.5 mg/kg/day of ioxynil octanoate daily for 3 months without detectable adverse effects (Beste, 1983). Rats tolerated either bromoxynil or ioxynil for 3 months at a level of 110 ppm (about 5.4 mg/kg/day) without observed effects (Hayes, 1982).

Mutagenicity Ioxynil was not mutagenic in bacterial systems, either with or without metabolic activation (Torracca *et al.*, 1976).

20.15.2.3 Toxicity to Humans

Accidental and Intentional Poisoning A 54-year-old man who had undergone total gastrectomy swallowed a small amount of an unknown fluid, which he had stored with his homemade wine. He died 45 min later en route to the hospital. Chemical analysis involving infrared and nuclear magnetic resonance spectroscopy and ultraviolet spectrophotometry established that the remaining material was ioxynil at a concentration of 11.3%. It was estimated that the victim had swallowed 2000–3000 mg. Ioxynil was measured in the serum by thin-layer chromatography at a concentration of 13.2 ppm, and its identity was confirmed by infrared spectroscopy. Alcohol also was present at a concentration of 0.135%. Autopsy revealed hyperemia of all organs, edema of the lungs, and edema of the brain with an occipital cone (Smysl *et al.*, 1977). It may be noted that the estimated dosage (<43 mg/kg) was less than the LD 50 values for animals, but the investigators cautioned that the course may have been influenced by gastrectomy and by alcohol.

Four men who worked in the same plant manufacturing bromoxynil and ioxynil became ill, one during the summer of 1974 and the others in 1975. The onset was insidious in each instance. They suffered from inordinate sweating and thirst. Some suffered fever, headache, dizziness, vomiting, asthenia, weight loss, and/or myalgia of the legs. The two who had myalgia had transitory elevation of creatinine phosphokinase (CPK), lactate

Table 20.7
Approximate LD 50 Values of Ioxynil

Species	Route	LD 50 (mg/kg)	Reference
Rat	oral	110	Carpenter *et al.* (1964)
Rat	dermal	210	Beste (1983)
Mouse	oral	200	Carpenter *et al.* (1964)
Rabbit	oral	160	Carpenter *et al.* (1964)
Guinea pig	oral	76	Carpenter *et al.* (1964)
Dog	oral	>100	Carpenter *et al.* (1964)
Cat	oral	75	Carpenter *et al.* (1964)

dehydrogenase (LDH), aldolase, and SGOT, but a muscle biopsy on one of them showed nothing abnormal. All four men recovered promptly when separated from exposure. The occurrence of poisoning in a factory that had operated for several years without trouble was explained by an important increase in the volume of production. No further cases were observed after the ventilation was increased, hours of work were shortened, and personal hygiene was improved (Conso *et al.*, 1977). The illnesses were attributed to uncoupling of oxidative phosphorylation on the basis of similar symptomatology and a report (Wain, 1963) that the compounds have this action in plant tissues. It must be pointed out, however, that these illnesses were more gradual in onset and milder in clinical course than some seen in persons exposed to pentachlorophenol or to dinitrophenols.

Treatment of Poisoning Treatment is symptomatic.

20.16 QUATERNARY NITROGEN COMPOUNDS

So far, the only quaternary nitrogen compounds used as herbicides are bipyridinium compounds. Judged by oral LD 50 values in the rat, they are compounds of moderate toxicity. The value for paraquat, the more toxic example of the class, is 100 mg/kg. However, the frequent irreversibility of the unique injury produced by paraquat, the fact that many species, including humans, may be more susceptible than the rat to this injury, and, finally, the large number of human fatalities have directed much attention to this extremely valuable herbicide.

More detailed information on the mammalian toxicology of paraquat and related compounds than can be covered here may be found in a book edited by Autor (1977).

20.16.1 PARAQUAT

20.16.1.1 Identity, Properties, and Uses

Chemical Name Paraquat is 1,1'-dimethyl-4,4-bipyridyldiylium ion, also known as the 1,1'-dimethyl-4,4-bipyridinium ion.

Structure See Fig. 20.8.

Synonyms The common name paraquat (ANSI, BSI, ISO, JMAF, WSSA) is in general use, except in Germany. Trade names for paraquat dichloride include Crisquat®, Dextrone®, Dexuron®, Esgram®, Goldquat 276, Gramoxone®, Herbaxon®, Osaquat Super®, and Sweep®. Mixtures of paraquat with various residual herbicides are sold under the names Dexuron®, Gramonol®, Gramron®, Para-Col®, Pathclear®, Tota-Col®, and Weedol®. Code designations for the material are PP-148 and PP-910. Paraquat usually is formulated as the dichloride, for which the CAS registry number is 1910-42-5. The CAS registry number for the bipyridyldiylium ion is 4685-14-7 and for the dimethyl sulfate is 2074-50-2.

Physical and Chemical Properties The empirical formula of the cation is $C_{12}H_{14}N_2$ and it has a molecular weight of 186.3; the dichloride is $C_{12}H_{14}Cl_2N_2$ with a molecular weight of 257.2. Both the dichloride and dimethanosulfate are white crystalline solids. The latter is deliquescent. The dichloride forms colorless crystals that decompose at 300°C. It is insoluble in hydrocarbons, slightly soluble in the lower alcohols, and very soluble in water. Paraquat dimethyl sulfate has similar properties. Both compounds are stable in acid and neutral aqueous solutions but not in alkaline solutions.

History, Formulations, and Uses The first report of the herbicidal activity of paraquat salts was by R. C. Brian in 1958. Their properties were reviewed by A. Calderbank in 1968. Paraquat is a quick-acting herbicide that destroys green plant tissue by contact action and some translocation. It is used as a plant desiccant for preharvest of cotton and potatoes. It also has been suggested for control of aquatic weeds. Paraquat is rapidly and tightly bound by the soil. Soil-bound paraquat is not available to the plant. Treated water may be used for furrow irrigation of sensitive crops but not for overhead irrigation. Paraquat is formulated as an aqueous solution with surface-active agents.

20.16.1.2 Toxicity to Laboratory Animals

Symptomatology Individual animals of the same species show an unusually large variation in the time from dosing to death following identical dosage. In rats this interval varies from 2 to 12 days, with some tendency for the deaths to be concentrated in an early and a late peak (Clark et al., 1966). Rats and mice that die promptly often do so after hyperexcitability, severe and varied ataxia, convulsions, or a combination of them. Rats and mice that survive for several days show signs of increasing respiratory difficulty and usually die of respiratory failure. Sick rabbits tend to die suddenly with little warning except failure to eat or drink (Clark et al., 1966).

When rats were weighed daily following a single oral or intravenous dose at a rate that would kill some but not all of them, it was found that those that were minimally affected lost weight only briefly and then began gradually to regain, whereas those that were severely affected continued to lose weight. Weights of the two groups were statistically different after the first day following oral administration and on all days following intravenous administration. Weight loss appeared to be the result of lesser intake of food. Whether as the result of less absorption following oral administration or of greater excretion or sequestration regardless of the route of administration, minimally affected rats contained less paraquat in their lungs, kidneys, and stomach during days 1–8 than did severely affected ones, including those that died (Sharp et al., 1972).

Irritation and Sensitization A single application of a 0.29% aqueous solution of paraquat does not injure the rabbit's eye. More concentrated solutions produce progressively greater injury consisting of delayed mild inflammation of the conjunctiva and nictitating membrane. The injury develops gradually within

12 hr and lasts 48–96 hr (Clark et al., 1966). The instillation of 3.01–48.4 mg of paraquat ion contained in 0.2 ml of water into the eyes of rabbits produced the expected eye injury and a good dosage response, ranging from about 10 on the Draize sale following 3.01 mg to about 75 following 24.2 mg. A dose of 48.4 mg ($\geq$16 mg/kg) was fatal in all rabbits that received it (Snow and Wei, 1973). The authors expressed surprise at the fatal outcome. It shows that absorption of paraquat from the eye is about as efficient as absorption from the peritoneal cavity, a relationship that is not astonishing. These observations may be relevant to many species, especially since the rabbit is considered relatively resistant to paraquat toxicity (Dikshith et al., 1979).

Repeated dermal application to the rabbit apparently leads to little or no irritation if the skin is not covered. When the skin was covered by an occlusive dressing, a dosage of 1.56 mg ion/kg/day produced some skin injury, and a dosage of 5.0 mg ion/kg/day produced reddening and sloughing of the superficial layers. Under these conditions, absorption was promoted and toxicity increased.

Although 99.1% of paraquat applied to the skin of rabbits can be removed by washing with water, the animals still develop ulceration of the tongue if they are allowed to lick the washed site. The ulceration interferes with feeding. If licking is completely prevented by restraint and if the site is not covered, rabbits tolerate a single application of 480 mg/kg measured in terms of the ion. By contrast, a single application of 240 mg/kg is fatal within 72 hr when applied beneath an occlusive dressing that promotes excoriation. In a similar way, the 20-dose dermal LD 50 was 24 mg/kg or about 4.5 mg/kg in rabbits, depending on whether the application site was bare or covered (McElligott, 1972).

Dosage Response The various salts of paraquat are equally toxic when expressed on the basis of paraquat ion (Clark et al., 1966). The compound is highly toxic (LD 50, 3–19 mg/kg) by the intraperitoneal route. The lesser toxicity by the oral route may reflect microbial degradation, poor absorption by that route, or an altered distribution within the tissues. Cats and guinea pigs are more susceptible than rats and chickens (see Table 20.8). There is some evidence that young animals are more susceptible than older ones (Clark et al., 1966). The Siv strain of rat is distinctly less susceptible than the Sprague–Dawley strain (Cegla et al., 1975).

Kimbrough and Gaines (1970) found that the acute dermal LD 50 is 80 mg/kg in male rats and 90 mg/kg in females. The fact that the compound is more toxic to rats dermally than when given by mouth probably reflects poor intestinal absorption and perhaps greater degradation of the compound in the intestine than on the skin.

Barabas et al. (1968) reported that, during an observation period of 72 hr, mice dosed with approximately the LD 50 of paraquat showed greater survival in the dark and decreased survival in continuous light when compared to controls kept under natural daylight with darkness at night. The authors suggested that light may facilitate the cycle, enhancing the

Table 20.8
Acute Toxicity of Paraquat Ion

Species	Route	LD 50 (mg/kg)	Reference
Rat, F	oral	112	Clark *et al.* (1966)
Rat, F	oral	150	Clark *et al.* (1966)
Rat, M	oral	100	Gaines (1969)
Rat, F	oral	110	Gaines (1969)
Rat	oral	126	Murray and Gibson (1972)
Rat, M	dermal	80	Gaines (1969)
Rat, F	dermal	90	Gaines (1969)
Rat, F	intraperitoneal	19	Clark *et al.* (1966)
Mouse	oral	98	Tsunenari *et al.* (1976)
Guinea pig, M	oral	30	Clark *et al.* (1966)
Guinea pig	oral	22	Murray and Gibson (1972)
Guinea pig, F	intraperitoneal	3	Clark *et al.* (1966)
Rabbit	dermal	236	Clark *et al.* (1966)
Cat, F	oral	35	Clark *et al.* (1966)
Monkey	oral	50	Murray and Gibson (1972)
Chicken, F	oral	262	Clark *et al.* (1966)

formation of the superoxide radical often considered responsible for much of the observed toxicity.

In tests on the same strain in the same laboratory, the 1-dose and 90-dose oral LD 50 values in female rats were 110 and 21 mg/kg, respectively, giving a chronicity index of 5.2 (Kimbrough and Gaines, 1970). This is a remarkably low value in view of the chronic, fibrotic nature of the characteristic morphologic lesion. This ability to withstand a moderate daily dosage has been observed in other laboratories, although the exact dosage withstood has varied from one laboratory to another. Rats were killed in 27–57 days by a dietary level of 250 ppm (about 12.5 mg/kg/day). Females appeared more susceptible and died earlier. Both sexes tolerated 100 ppm (about 5 mg/kg/day) for many months (Clark *et al.*, 1966) or 125 ppm for life (Howe and Wright, 1965). Dogs were unaffected by a dietary level of 50 ppm (about 0.9 mg/kg/day) for 2 years (Howe and Wright, 1965). Results reported by Luty *et al.* (1978) were consistent; mice that received 0.1 of an LD 50 by stomach tube daily for 3 months developed pathology, and some died, whereas those that received 0.02 or 0.01 LD 50 daily were unaffected.

Tolerance in the strict sense was developed in mice by starting them on paraquat in their drinking water at 50 ppm and increasing the concentration by 50 ppm every 3 weeks. A maximal concentration of 700 ppm was reached in 9 months. This schedule produced a mortality of only 25%. Although most of the mice survived, light and electron microscopy revealed pathology of the lungs (Niden and Khurana, 1976).

When animals were exposed to aerosols of known particle-size range, particles measuring 3 μm were most retained by rats because larger ones usually did not reach the alveolus and smaller ones tended to escape. Using aerosols in which approximately half of the weight of material consisted of particles near the 3-μm size, rats were readily killed by a concentration of 1.3

mg/m³ or higher, and the lethal concentration–time (CT) product was 240–330 mg min/m³ in different experiments. After a single 6-hr exposure, no deaths were observed at concentrations of 0.75 mg/m³, even though the CT value was 270 mg min/m³ and 0.1 mg/m³ was a no-effect level, producing no ill effect regardless of the number of 6-hr daily exposures.

Rats remained well during exposure, but later respiration became more rapid and shallow and terminally labored; they became pale and cold and showed piloerection. Death usually occurred in 1–4 days but was sometimes later, the observed limit being 11 days. Nearly all rats that showed marked effects died. Microscopic examination showed that the lungs were congested with diffuse edema accentuated around bronchi and vessels. There was alveolar hemorrhage and an increase in polymorphonuclear lymphocytes and histiocytes, especially around the bronchi and vessels. Proliferation of neither fibroblasts nor epithelium was observed. Changes in other organs were minimal. The susceptibility of guinea pigs and male mice to acute exposure was about the same as that of male and female rats. Female mice were less affected. Female rabbits were unaffected by a concentration lethal to rats, and no toxic sign was seen in a dog exposed to five times the CT product lethal for rats (Gage, 1968).

For about the same concentrations in air, Bainova *et al.* (1972) reported less toxicity and a different distribution of effects. The size of aerosol was not specified but presumably was larger. Effects were greater in the upper respiratory tract. In studies of rabbits, Seidenfeld *et al.* (1978) confirmed that a single exposure to a concentrated aerosol could be fatal, whereas repeated exposures to less concentrated ones were tolerated without effect.

Absorption In the rat, absorption from the gastrointestinal tract is incomplete. In studies with ^{14}C-labeled paraquat dimethosulfate in which recovery of the compound varied from 92 to 105%, 69–86% of the compound was found in the feces following oral administration but only 14–16% was found following subcutaneous administration. An even larger proportion (93–96%) appeared in the feces after oral administration of paraquat dichloride (Daniel and Gage, 1966). Since excretion of paraquat is largely complete in 2 days, the prolonged course of poisoning by the compound is not considered to be the result of prolonged absorption.

Absorption of the compound from the gastrointestinal tract of cattle also is poor. Excluding the feces, only about 0.27% of radioactive paraquat could be accounted for (Stevens and Walley, 1966).

Whereas gastrointestinal absorption certainly is incomplete, it is not "slow," as sometimes is stated. In fact, the highest serum values of [^{14}C]paraquat were reached in 0.5–1 hr in rats, guinea pigs, and monkeys (Murray and Gibson, 1974). Absorption is incomplete but rapid in dogs also, reaching a peak plasma concentration in 75 min after a small oral dose in 200 ml of water. Six hours after oral administration at rates of 0.12, 2, and 5 mg/kg, absorption reached 46–66%, 22–38%, and 25–28%, respectively. Within the same period, 70–90% of the amount predicted by a model to be absorbed was, in fact, recovered in the urine. Propantheline (15 mg, iv) administered 15 min before an oral dose of paraquat delayed the peak plasma concentration by 3–6 hr, indicating that the stomach is not a major site of absorption in the dog. The dosage relationship of paraquat absorption suggests facilitated absorption, perhaps in the small intestine. The absorption of diquat is less complete, does not reach an early peak in the plasma, and may be entirely by passive diffusion (Bennett et al., 1976).

Distribution and Storage   A detailed study of [^{14}C]paraquat in rats following intravenous administration showed that concentrations decreased rapidly at first and then more slowly in all tissues examined. However, the time at which the rates changed and the half-lives during the second phase differed from one tissue to the other. The rapid phase of decline in the lung ended within 20 min, and subsequent loss was extremely slow, with the result that the lung had a concentration of paraquat higher than that in any other tissue from the fourth hour through the eighth day, after which muscle levels tended to be higher (Sharp et al., 1972). The fact that paraquat tends to reach higher and more prolonged levels in the lungs of rats has been confirmed (Ilett et al., 1974).

Following an oral dosage of 126 mg/kg to rats, the lung concentration of paraquat rose from 5 to 14 ppm between 4 and 32 hr, while the plasma concentration remained constant at about 1 ppm (Murray and Gibson, 1974; Rose et al., 1974). This pattern has been confirmed for the lung but excluded for other organs except the kidney, in which the concentration tends to remain high throughout (Rose et al., 1976a; Rose and Smith, 1977). Following intraperitoneal injection into rats, as much as a twofold variation in the concentration of paraquat was found in different parts of the same lung (O'Neill et al., 1977). Clearly, such a difference would help to account for the variation in histology sometimes observed.

Results in mice were similar. Following intravenous injection, the compound was rapidly distributed throughout most of the tissues, except the brain and spinal cord. Localization in liver and cartilage was soon evident. However, more rapid excretion from these and most other tissues resulted in selective retention in the lung and skeletal muscle 24 hr after injection, and this retention persisted (Litchfield et al., 1973).

Paraquat is preferentially localized in the lungs of rabbits, even though this species does not show any histopathological or biochemical signs of lung damage. It is true that the compound is cleared from the rabbit lung faster than from the rat lung (Ilett et al., 1974).

When sheep were given paraquat intraperitoneally at a rate of 4–5 mg/kg, the peak plasma levels were 9–12 ppm; plasma levels declined until none could be detected (<0.5 ppm) 8 hr after administration. Concentrations in lung lymph from the same animals reached peaks of 11–16 ppm at an average of 30 min after the plasma peak of each animal, and thereafter the lymph level remained higher than the plasma level, paraquat being still detectable in lung lymph collected 23 hr after injection (Hasegawa and Gorin, 1977).

No subcellular localization of paraquat in the lungs of rats or rabbits was found, and the compound is not covalently bound to tissue macromolecules (Ilett et al., 1974; Van Osten and Gibson, 1975; Oskarsson and Tjaelve, 1976). This is not necessarily inconsistent with the report that paraquat is bound in vitro to nucleic acids and acid mucopolysaccharides but that the binding is greatly reduced by moderate concentrations of salt (Conning et al., 1969).

There was no tendency for paraquat to accumulate in any tissue of rats maintained for 8 weeks on dietary levels as high as 250 ppm in terms of the ion. After 7 days on uncontaminated food, the paraquat was undetectable (<0.1 ppm) in all tissues (Litchfield et al., 1973).

The concentrations of paraquat in the lungs of rats were 8–33 times higher than those for diquat for at least the first 10 days after intravenous injection at the same rate (20 mg/kg). The same was true to a lesser extent of muscle, where the factor of difference was 2- to 16-fold (Sharp et al., 1972). The striking difference in the affinity of the lung for the two compounds has been confirmed (Rose et al., 1974).

Metabolism   Daniel and Gage (1966) found that analysis of excreta by colorimetric and radiometric methods gave excellent agreement and accounted for an average of 100% of the dose following subcutaneous administration of paraquat. The colorimetric method failed to detect 0.5–5.1% of the excreted material following oral administration. In other tests, a much higher proportion of the material in the feces was metabolized. Paraquat could be recovered quantitatively when it was incubated with boiled cecal contents, but much was lost during incubation with fresh contents. The authors concluded that metabolism of paraquat in the rat is confined to the intestinal lumen and caused by microbiological degradation.

Chromatography of urine from rats following oral administration of [^{14}C]paraquat gave no evidence of a metabolite. In other studies, no radioactivity was recovered in expired air or flatus (Murray and Gibson, 1974). These studies are evidence against microbial metabolism of paraquat to carbon dioxide, but may not exclude the possibility of a microbial metabolite with different solubilities from those of paraquat.

Microbial degradation of paraquat apparently has not been studied in cattle. However, inability to detect metabolites in the milk constitutes some evidence against significant metabolism in this species (Stevens and Walley, 1966).

The fact that instillation of paraquat into lung or muscle produces characteristic lesions offers strong evidence but not proof that the compound itself and not a metabolite is responsible for the injury. It has been shown that rats not only survive an intravenous dosage of 3.0 mg/kg but develop no gross or microscopic pathology of the lung. However, instillation of a few drops of dilute paraquat into the lung at a total body rate of 0.05 mg/kg produces fibrosis and epithelial proliferation restricted to the area of deposit. Injection into muscle at a total body dose of 0.8 mg/kg also produces a local fibrosis without systemic illness (Kimbrough and Gaines, 1970). Another indication of the small dosage required for lung injury is the finding that the lethal concentration of a 5-μm aerosol in the air is 3–4 mg/m³ (Matthew *et al.*, 1971).

Excretion   Early studies indicated that, following subcutaneous injection of paraquat dimethosulfate in the rat, 73–96% of a single dose was recovered from the urine and all of the remainder from the feces. Slightly over 90% of the excretion occurred during the first day. Following oral administration much of the compound was unabsorbed and appeared in the feces. From 6 to 23% was recovered from the urine but none from the bile. In rats, excretion is essentially complete 2 days after a single dose. Occasionally, a small amount was found in the urine on the third day and, in the presence of constipation, might appear in the feces as late as the fourth day (Daniel and Gage, 1966).

There appears to be important disagreement between early and later reports on the excretion of paraquat in the rat. The difference cannot be explained simply by improved methodology, for the early report of Daniel and Gage (1966) was based on measurement of radioactivity from [¹⁴C]paraquat, and approximately 100% of the dose was accounted for. Whatever the reason, recent studies (while confirming incomplete absorption after oral administration) have suggested a less regular pattern of excretion as well as continuing excretion often at a low level for many days. This is consistent with the finding of rapid initial loss of paraquat from blood and tissues followed by a prolonged slow loss.

Working with groups of orally dosed rats, Murray and Gibson (1974) reported a progressive increase in the cumulative proportion of the administered dose that was recovered in the urine up to 128 hr when 18.4% had been accounted for. After that, the proportion recovered was actually much less, perhaps reflecting the lesser absorption of an oral dose of paraquat by those that survive it, as discussed under Symptomatology above.

Following a single oral dose, monkeys excreted 8.9, 3.0, 1.4, and 0.7% of the total amount in the urine on days 1, 2, 3, and 4, respectively. During days 5–21, daily excretion varied from 0.1 to 0.3% of the total dose. The pattern for fecal excretion was similar, but late fecal excretion was slightly greater than late urinary excretion. The total recovery in urine plus feces in 21 days was 71% (Murray and Gibson, 1974). The fact that fecal excretion continued so long must indicate some true excretion by this route, in addition to the early passage of unabsorbed compound.

In cattle, only about 0.26% of a single oral dose was recovered from the urine and only 0.01% from the milk. The material in the milk was apparently unchanged paraquat. The maximal level in the milk was reached on the day after dosing (Stevens and Walley, 1966).

Paraquat is found at an average concentration of 0.74 ppm in the urine of dogs on a dietary level of 50 ppm for 27 months, a regimen without effect on their growth or behavior (Swan, 1969). Dogs reabsorb, probably in the proximal tubules, from 15 to 65% of the paraquat filtered by the kidney. Clearance is independent of plasma concentration in the range of 10–150

ppm and in most experiments varied with urine flow rates, suggesting that passive diffusion is responsible for reabsorption (Ferguson, 1971).

Paraquat is excreted unchanged in the bile of rats, guinea pigs, and rabbits, but the amount is less than 10% of the dose (Hughes *et al.*, 1973).

Biochemical Effects   The biochemical lesion in paraquat poisoning appears to be excessive production of superoxide in response to cyclic reduction–oxidation of the compound in the tissues. However, when incubated with liver or lung microsomes and suitable cofactors, both paraquat and diquat stimulated superoxide, hydrogen peroxide, and lipid peroxide production, and diquat was the more active of the two compounds (Talcott *et al.*, 1977). Therefore, although this mechanism is generally accepted in connection with lung injury, the process apparently involves preferential distribution in some tissues (Rose and Smith, 1977). This preferential distribution is necessary to account for (*a*) differences between the clinical action of paraquat on the lung and those of diquat and some other related herbicides that have the same basic action and (*b*) marked species differences that exist in the organ specificity of paraquat. In other words, the specificity of paraquat for the lung is unexplained by the mere formation of a free radical *in vitro*, either as regards different organs or as regards paraquat compared with diquat and morfamquat (Baldwin *et al.*, 1975).

The contrast is usually drawn between diquat, which does not cause significant lung injury, and paraquat, which causes spectacular lung injury in several species and tends to be thought of as unique. The fact is, however, that benzyl viologen (a compound in which one hydrogen in each methyl group of paraquat is substituted by a benzene ring) causes lung injury in mice when injected intraperitoneally at a rate of 10 mg/kg (Greenberg and Eisenberg, 1977). This injury apparently is similar to that caused by paraquat and some other viologens (Ross and Krieger, 1978). Thus a really satisfactory explanation must explain the contrast between the clinical effects of paraquat and some other viologens and those of diquat and morfamquat.

Regardless of the theoretical details, the practical point is clear that oxygen enhances the toxicity of paraquat or, perhaps more basically, paraquat enhances the toxicity of oxygen. Rats injected intravenously with paraquat with a rate of 27 mg/kg survived an average of 3 days in air but one of 20 of them kept in oxygen died within 22 hr. Saline-injected control rats survived when exposed to oxygen for the same period, although the lesions produced by paraquat are similar to those produced by sufficient exposure to oxygen or ozone alone (Fisher *et al.*, 1973; Roujeau *et al.*, 1973; Smith and Heath, 1974b; Bus and Gibson, 1975; Witschi *et al.*, 1977; Pratt *et al.*, 1979). In fact, rats poisoned by paraquat and kept in 10% oxygen had significantly lower mortality than controls kept in room air (Rhodes, 1974). These findings are consistent with the fact that rats made oxygen-tolerant by exposure to 85% oxygen for 7 days are also somewhat tolerant to paraquat (Bus *et al.*, 1976).

The absorption of paraquat by the lung is not increased by high oxygen tensions (Kehrer *et al.*, 1979; Montgomery *et al.*,

1979b). However, low oxygen tensions do inhibit uptake of paraquat by the lung, at least *in vitro* (Montgomery *et al.*, 1979a).

The toxic interaction between oxygen and paraquat extends to other organisms, notably *Escherichia coli*, in which the biochemical relationship has been studied in intricate detail (Hassan and Fridovich, 1978; Fridovich and Hassan, 1979).

The weight of experimental evidence suggests that the toxicity of paraquat involves lipid peroxidation catalyzed by singlet oxygen. Transition metal catalysis is reported to be integral to the generation of the active oxygen species (Aust *et al.*, 1985). The attack is thought to be on the polyunsaturated lipids of cell membranes. It was reported by Bus *et al.* (1974) that (*a*) anaerobic reduction of paraquat by mouse lung microsomes to form a free radical was inhibited by antibody to NADPH–cytochrome-*c* reductase, and the degree of inhibition corresponded to the *in vitro* dose of antibody; (*b*) paraquat, even at $10^{-6} M$, did induce lipid peroxidation *in vitro;* and (*c*) this lipid peroxidation was reduced by 20 μM superoxide dismutase. The same authors (Bus *et al.*, 1975a,b; Cagen and Gibson, 1977) showed that the toxicity of paraquat to mice was enhanced (and liver injury was increased) if their diet prior to exposure was deficient in selenium or in vitamin E or if they were pretreated with diethyl maleate. Supplementation of the deficient diets reduced the toxicity of paraquat to normal, but high levels of selenium or vitamin E did not offer any added protection. Diethyl maleate depletes reduced glutathione (GSH) and thus interferes with the function of GSH peroxidase, an enzyme that serves to detoxify lipid hydroperoxides. Although results were not consistent, administration of GSH prior to paraquat exposure appeared to reduce the toxic effects (Matkovics *et al.*, 1980b). Insofar as the work of Bus and his colleagues involved vitamin E, it confirmed earlier work showing that this vitamin is protective against poisoning by paraquat (Conning *et al.*, 1969) and oxygen (Mengal and Kann, 1966). The relation of selenium to paraquat poisoning has been confirmed (Omaye *et al.*, 1978).

Changes in the concentrations of enzymes involved in peroxide metabolism have been reported in paraquat studies. The time-dependent (Szabo *et al.*, 1980) and dose-dependent (Matkovics *et al.*, 1980a) effects of paraquat administration to mice on superoxide dismutase, catalase, and peroxidase support the free radical mechanism proposed for the compound. Similar studies in guinea pigs (Barabas *et al.*, 1982a,b) reported that effects on superoxide dismutase, catalase, peroxidase, and lipid peroxidation were dose-dependent. Finally, coadministration of catalase and superoxide dismutase appeared to reduce paraquat toxicity while horseradish peroxidase appeared to enhance the toxicity (Matkovics *et al.*, 1983).

The probable toxic mechanism in animals is basically similar to the mechanism considered responsible for the death of plants (Mees, 1960; Dodge, 1972).

Quite aside from its appropriateness for explaining lung injury by paraquat, some investigators have expressed reservations about the superoxide–lipid peroxidation theory as a basic explanation for injury to various tissues by dipyridylium herbicides generally (Ilett *et al.*, 1974; Rose *et al.*, 1976d). There certainly are some results that appear inconsistent with the theory. For example, Talcott *et al.* (1977) and Shu *et al.* (1979) found in mice that either administration of N,N'-diphenyl-*p*-phenylenediamine or a fat-free diet virtually abolished the stimulation of lung microsomal lipid peroxidation by paraquat (tested *in vitro*) but had little effect on the lethal effect of paraquat *in vivo*. Although not all *in vitro* findings appear consistent, it seems inescapable that some abnormality of oxidation is the biochemical lesion in paraquat toxicity. On the basis of further *in vitro* studies, Talcott *et al.* (1979) discussed the possibility of lipid peroxidation independent of superoxide and peroxide. Smith *et al.* (1979) suggested that the primary mechanism of paraquat toxicity involves the extreme oxidation of NADPH, thus inhibiting vital physiological processes and rendering the cell susceptible to attack from hyperoxides. However, Witschi *et al.* (1977) questioned whether the depletion of NADPH, which they demonstrated, is related to cell injury, partly because paraquat (and diquat also) does not prevent synthesis of NADPH. Kurisaki (1985) has suggested that lipid peroxidation may not be the primary mechanism of paraquat toxicity; his suggestion is based on the observation that malondialdehyde concentrations were increased in human lungs, but not in rat lungs, by poisoning.

Finally, Kornburst and Mavis (1980) presented results which they interpreted as proof that paraquat does not cause peroxidation of lung lipids and that the decrease of palmitate in paraquat-damaged lungs is consistent with inhibition of fatty acid synthesis as an early event in the pathogenesis of paraquat toxicity.

It is, of course, well known that paraquat produces striking lung injury in many species, whereas diquat, which also forms a free radical, produces little or no injury to the lung. The difference is consistent with the fact that paraquat tends to accumulate in the lungs, whereas diquat does not (see Distribution and Storage). However, it is impossible by studies on poisoned animals to exclude the logical possibility that accumulation is secondary to injury. This possibility was excluded by the finding that when rat lung slices were incubated in media containing 10^{-5}–$10^{-3} M$ [^{14}C]diquat, absorption was complete within 30 min and the concentration in the slices remained constant between 30 and 120 min of incubation, whereas in a comparable situation, lung slices continued to accumulate [^{14}C]paraquat in a linear fashion between 30 and 240 min of incubation, with the result that the final concentration was higher for paraquat than for diquat. When either rotenone or a combination of KCN plus iodoacetate was added to the medium after lung slices had taken up some paraquat, no further accumulation occurred. This inhibition is an indication that the continuing uptake of paraquat is energy dependent (Rose *et al.*, 1974).

Lung tissues of some other species, including human (Rose *et al.*, 1975), dog, monkey, and rabbit (Rose *et al.*, 1976a), also accumulate paraquat (but not diquat) *in vitro*.

Rat brain slices concentrated paraquat (but not diquat) from the medium but not to the same degree as did lung slices. The process was energy dependent. Other organs examined, including the kidney, showed little or no ability to accumulate either paraquat or diquat *in vitro* (Rose *et al.*, 1976a). *In vivo*, erythrocyte takes up paraquat rapidly when it is injected intravenously in solutions of low toxicity but take it up relatively slowly from solutions of higher toxicity or following oral, intraperitoneal, or subcutaneous administration. Absorption by hemolyzed erythrocytes is more rapid than absorption by intact erythrocytes. Melanin also accumulates paraquat (Oskarsson and Tjaelve, 1976).

Kidney slices of mice, unlike those of rats, accumulate paraquat; this is inhibited by metabolic inhibitors or the absence of oxygen, indicating energy dependence (Ecker *et al.*, 1975a).

The accumulation of paraquat by slices of rat lung *in vitro* was inhibited by rat plasma, and the inhibition was proportional to the concentration of the plasma in the solution. An ultrafiltrate of plasma was effective, indicating that the inhibitor had a low molecular weight. A number of endogenous amines, including norepinephrine, 5-hydroxytryptamine, and histamine, as well as several drugs, including imipramine, propranolol, burimamide, and betazole, reduced paraquat uptake by lung slices. It was pointed out that interference of this kind does not imply that the interfering substance is accumulated or has the same site of action. It was hoped that study of interference might lead to a therapeutic advance (Rose *et al.*, 1976b). No speculation was offered on how accumulation is possible *in vivo* in the presence of plasma.

There are many differences in the uptake of paraquat and of 5-hydroxytryptamine; it has been concluded that they occur in different cell types (Smith *et al.*, 1976) and, specifically, that type I and type II alveolar cells are responsible for the energy-dependent uptake of paraquat (Rose and Smith, 1977).

One line of effort to explain the peculiar susceptibility of the lung of some species has centered on pulmonary surfactant because that material is peculiar to the lung and critical to its function. This effort apparently never has been extended to the question of how paraquat could interfere with the action of surfactant in some species but not in others to which surfactant is equally critical. Study of surfactant has been essentially independent of the study of superoxide and lipid peroxidation, although the two lines of study might be related if—as remains to be proved—surfactant is more susceptible than some components in the cell membrane to lipid peroxidation.

Most studies of the effect of paraquat on surfactant have involved intact animals and have failed to distinguish loss of production from loss of function (perhaps leading to failure of standard lung washing techniques). However, one study showed that a concentration of paraquat that did not change the surface tension when incubated with a saline solution did change the surface tension when incubated with a surfactant preparation, and this effect was accentuated by oxygen in excess of atmospheric level (Bedwell and Anderson, 1974).

Manktelow (1967) showed there is a loss of pulmonary surfactant in mice poisoned by paraquat, and a somewhat similar lack of surfactant is associated with the pulmonary dysfunction and peculiar morphological change seen in the lungs of newborn babies with respiratory distress syndrome. The physiological similarity of these conditions and their etiological dissimilarity have been emphasized by Robertson (1973). Fisher *et al.* (1973) also reported a reduction of alveolar surfactant 3 days after a single injection of paraquat at a rate of 27 mg/kg. This change and the decrease in saturated lecithins were considered to be an important cause of the atelectasis and abnormal pulmonary function that were present also. In a study made 1 day after subcutaneous injection at the rate of 35 mg/kg, lung homogenates contained approximately 30% less total lecithin, and lung washings contained 75% less total lecithin but 400% as much protein as in controls. It was considered that paraquat interferes with phospholipid metabolism in the alveolar epithelium and thus promotes alveolar collapse (Malmqvist *et al.*, 1973).

After 6 but not after 2 days following oral administration of paraquat to rats, there was a large increase in the proportion of arachidonic acid and a small increase in the cholesterol ester fraction of the lungs. The changes can be attributed chiefly to an increase in macrophages, which, however, differ in lipid composition from peritoneal macrophages (Fletcher and Wyatt, 1970).

Subcutaneous injection of paraquat at a rate of 35 mg/kg caused rats to develop respiratory distress in 12–24 hr; this became severe 2–3 days after injection and began to subside after the fourth day. The surface-active properties of alveolar washings from such rats became markedly abnormal within 2 hr after injection and deteriorated progressively. The phospholipid content of the washings did not differ significantly from that of the controls. The onset of symptoms corresponded with the appearance of atelectasis, and this too reached its maximum 2–3 days after injection. Other pathology was similar to that described by others (Robertson *et al.*, 1970).

In another study, it was found that deterioration of surfactant activity was accompanied by an increase in phospholipid concentration in lung washings. This was interpreted as showing that part of the phospholipid in poisoned animals is inactive (Kuncova *et al.*, 1979).

A careful chemical and physiological study of rats following an intravenous dosage of 27 mg/kg led to the conclusion that lung edema occurred as early as changes in surfactant or lung mechanical properties could be detected (Fisher *et al.*, 1975). Actually, the loss of surfactant must be a secondary effect in paraquat poisoning, although not in all chemically induced pulmonary edema (Roujeau *et al.*, 1973). The material is produced in the lamellar bodies of the granular pneumocytes (Schaefer *et al.*, 1964). As discussed under Pathology, these cells usually show pathologic change only after changes in other alveolar cells are well advanced. Furthermore, Fletcher and Wyatt (1972) showed that the administration of paraquat dichloride to rats by stomach tube at a rate of 125 mg/kg did not influence the degree to which intravenously injected [3H]palmitic acid was incorporated into dipalmitoyl lecithin (DPL) (a major constituent of lung surfactant) in their lungs or the rate at which the radioactivity was lost from DPL. This was true whether the radioactive palmitic acid was injected 5, 24, 48, or 144 hr after the single dose of paraquat. Finally, rats fed paraquat at a dietary level of 200–300 ppm develop pulmonary fibrosis without an intervening stage of severe lung hemorrhage and edema, and in these rats no change in the surface properties of lung washings can be seen. It must be concluded that the biochemical action of paraquat is not connected with the phospholipid metabolism of the lungs.

Paraquat stimulates the pentose phosphate pathway of glucose metabolism (Rose *et al.,* 1976c; Abrams *et al.,* 1976; O'Neill *et al.,* 1977) and decreases the NADPH/NADP ratio (Fabregat *et al.,* 1985). However, diquat does the same thing. *In vitro,* a lower concentration of diquat caused comparable stimulation. *In vivo,* at the same molar dosage, diquat caused as much activation or more. Under these circumstances, and because only paraquat produces lung damage, there can be no simple relationship between the stimulation of the pentose phosphate pathway and the production of lung damage (Rose *et al.,* 1976c).

Paraquat causes various other disorders of metabolism and appears to increase the response of the adrenal cortex to ACTH (Rose *et al.,* 1974; Witschi, 1973; Witschi and Kacew, 1974). Paraquat produces serum protein and glycoprotein changes in rabbits following oral subchronic (12-week) administration (Barabas *et al.,* 1981). In mice, it causes reduced serum triglycerides and hypothermia (Barabas *et al.,* 1982c). These changes are presumed to be secondary, and there is no evidence they are not. Furthermore, many parameters such as lung RNA, protein synthesis, and several enzymes remain normal (Witschi, 1973; Witschi and Kacew, 1974).

A sufficient concentration of paraquat inhibits acetylcholinesterase *in vitro* (Brown and Maling, 1975) but there is no evidence that this has any bearing on ordinary poisoning.

Oral administration of paraquat to rats at a rate of 126 mg/kg caused an increase in protein synthesis and a decrease in the synthesis of DNA and RNA in several organs, and the timing correlated with histological changes (Van Osten and Gibson, 1975). There was no reason to suppose that these biochemical changes were any more primary than the histological ones.

A study in hamsters offered no evidence that hypersensitivity to paraquat is an important factor in the production of lung injury (Butler, 1973, 1975).

At normal body temperature, paraquat interfered with the excretion of bromosulfophthalein, but not with excretion of indocyanine green, by the rat liver (Cagen and Gibson, 1974; Cagen *et al.,* 1976). Why the two dyes behave differently is not really known.

Following oral administration of paraquat at the rate of 250 mg/kg, the lungs were damaged in 3–5 days in such a way that the rate of absorption of intratracheally administered drugs was increased 1.4- to 2.8-fold, as indicated by assay for unabsorbed compound. Function returned to near normal in 15 days (Gardiner and Schanker, 1976).

Intravenous injection of paraquat increased collagen synthesis as measured by radioactive hydroxyproline determinations on hydrolysates of lung slices incubated with labeled proline (Greenberg and Last, 1977).The ratio of type I to type III collagen remains normal following stimulation of collagen formation by paraquat or ozone (Reiser *et al.,* 1979). Collagen and perhaps basement membranes are increased in the kidneys of poisoned rats (Kuttan *et al.,* 1979), but presumably to a smaller degree than in the lung.

Thymidine incorporation into lung DNA was significantly decreased 1 day after rats were poisoned by paraquat but increased during the proliferative phase of lung injury. As might be expected, diquat did not increase thymidine incorporation (Smith and Rose, 1977).

Effects on Organs and Tissues   Paraquat did not significantly increase the rate of preimplantation zygote losses or postimplantation early fetal deaths in female mice mated to treated males. However, paraquat caused a marked reduction of pregnancy rates in females mated to males with sperm that had been treated in the postmeiotic late spermatid stage. Thus, according to this test, the compound interferes with fertility although it is not mutagenic (Pasi *et al.,* 1974; Pasi and Embree, 1975). Later work confirmed the lack of mutagenicity but failed to confirm the antifertility effect (Anderson *et al.,* 1976).

A study of bone marrow cells of mice that had received a respiratory dosage estimated at 0.25 mg/kg indicated an absence of mutagenic effect (Selypes *et al.,* 1978).

Paraquat at concentrations as low as 10^{-6} *M in vitro* caused irreversible damage within 30 min to rat alveolar or peritoneal macrophages. Concentrations of 10^{-5} *M* or less did not reduce the viability of mouse fibroblasts but did interfere with cloning (Styles, 1974).

An intratracheal dosage of only 0.5 mg/kg caused an approximate doubling of respiratory rate, and the functional residual lung volume increased significantly. Both parameters returned to normal following bilateral, cervical vagotomy. Histologically, the injury consisted of focal distribution of typical lesions (Vizek *et al.,* 1976).

Although kidney damage early in the course of paraquat poisoning in animals is unlikely to be noticed clinically, it was easily demonstrated by kidney function tests. The injury seems to be confirmed to the proximal tubules (Ecker *et al.,* 1975b).

Effects on Reproduction   A standard three-generation reproduction test was carried out in rats maintained on dietary levels of 100, 30, and 0 ppm. No effect of paraquat on food intake, growth, fertility, fecundity, or neonatal morbidity and mortality was observed. No teratogenesis or other change in gross or histological morphology was seen, except for a slight increase in the incidence of renal hydropic degeneration in 3- to 4-week-old young receiving 100 ppm (about 10 mg/kg/day for this age group). Pregnant and young animals did not appear more susceptible than adults [Food and Agriculture Organization/World Health Organization (FAO/WHO), 1973].

Rats injected intraperitoneally with paraquat on the sixth day of gestation showed a higher incidence of malformations of the costal cartilages. However, this effect was not dosage-related on the sixth day and was not observed when the single injection was on days 7–14 (Khera and Whitta, 1970).

When mice were injected intraperitoneally with paraquat on days 8–16 of gestation at a rate of 3.35 mg/kg/day, most of the dams were killed, and the resorption rate among fetuses of the surviving dams increased to 22%. Paraquat did not significantly increase the incidence of gross, soft tissue, or skeletal anomalies in mice, although intraperitoneal injection at a rate of 1.6 mg/kg/day or gavage at a rate of 20 mg/kg/day did slightly delay ossification. When a single dose of paraquat was injected into rats intravenously at a rate of 15 mg/kg on any one of several days of gestation, 17% of the dams were killed, and the rate of dead and resorbing fetuses in the others was 7.6%. When [14C]paraquat was administered to mice either intraperitoneally or orally on day 11 of gestation, the concentration reaching the embryo was low, and it reached equilibrium with the maternal serum after 2 hr. Considerably higher levels were reached in the maternal lungs and very much higher levels in maternal liver and kidney. Paraquat showed a far greater tendency to accumulate in the fetal lung when administered on day 21 instead of day 16 of gestation (Bus *et al.*, 1975c).

Paraquat administered in drinking water at concentrations of 50 and 100 ppm to mice beginning on day 8 of gestation and to the young until 42 days after birth did not influence postnatal growth rate of survivors; 100 but not 50 ppm increased postnatal mortality. Both concentrations sensitized mice to oxygen toxicity (Bus and Gibson, 1975).

Pathology   Paraquat injures the lungs more than other organs. The form of the lung lesions following sufficient dosage depends mainly on the interval from first exposure to examination. If death occurs rapidly, the lungs are grossly congested, tend to be plum-colored, and often sink in water. If death is delayed sufficiently, hemorrhage and edema are no longer evident, but consolidation, scarring, and in some instances honeycombing are evident. The lungs may be gray rather than plum-colored; they sink in water (Clark *et al.*, 1966).

Microscopic examinations of the lung of rats that died in 5–6 days after a single oral dose revealed predominantly pulmonary edema, congestion, and intraalveolar hemorrhage. In rats that survived a single dose for 10 days or more, fibrosis predominated, but multinuclear cells, epithelial proliferation, and squamous metaplasia were observed also. Extensive diffuse fibrosis occurred in the lungs of almost all rats that died following repeated doses. Less frequent findings in these rats included intraalveolar hemorrhage, multinucleated epithelial cells, proliferation of the epithelium, and periarteritis. Rats that survived repeated doses at about the 90-dose LD 50 level showed areas of circumscribed fibrosis ranging up to 1–2 cm in diameter (Kimbrough and Gaines, 1970). Similar results were reported by L. L. Smith *et al.* (1974), who emphasized intraalveolar fibrosis.

Studies with the electron microscope revealed no change in the rat lung 1 hr after a single oral dose of 400 mg/kg. Four hours after such a dose, the membranous pneumocytes showed intracellular edema and an increased prominence of collagen, elastin, and glycogen; there was no change in the granular pneumocytes. Forty-eight hours after a dose of only 150 mg/kg, the membranous granulocytes showed a marked increase of glycogen, and collagen had so increased that it disrupted the cellular membrane; the mitochondria were reduced in size and dark. By this time, the granular pneumocytes also showed changes including much lighter cytoplasm with loss of reticular endothelium, a marked reduction in the number of mitochondria, and

shrinkage of the lamellar bodies (Kimbrough and Gaines, 1970). Similar findings have been reported by others (Vijeyaratnam and Corin, 1971; Smith and Heath, 1974b).

Different observers have reported different orders of injury. There are conflicting reports that the earliest injury involves the membranous pneumatocytes, the granular pneumatocytes, or the lung capillary endothelium. It is not clear whether capillary endothelial cells and the two types of pneumatocytes are affected almost simultaneously, as suggested by a report by Robertson *et al.* (1976), or whether the reported differences depend on experimental variables or even on the attention of the investigators. In any event, Smith (1971) examined the lungs of rats that received paraquat intravenously every 14 days for up to 112 days. The first lesion seen in rats killed between days 15 and 60 consisted of cytoplasmic edema in granular pneumatocytes. This was followed by disintegration of alveolar epithelium and inflammation of alveolar walls. Large numbers of mesenchymal cells infiltrated the alveolar walls and spaces at 67 days. The appearance of pump fibroblasts dominated the picture between 70 and 98 days, and by 100 days large areas were occupied by loose fibrous matter with alveolar spaces obliterated. The two rats killed on day 112 contained, in addition to the loose fibrosis, areas of compact intestinal fibrosis, patent alveoli, alveolar macrophages, and granular pneumatocytes continuously lining the alveoli. Similar findings were reported following a single larger dose of paraquat. Initial injury to granular pneumatocytes and later injury to membranous pneumatocytes were reported also by Thurlbeck and Thurlbeck (1976).

It seems that P. Smith *et al.* (1974) have reported the ultimate in resistance of the capillary endothelium, specifically, complete destruction of the alveolar epithelium with the alveolar capillaries still essentially normal. The resulting ultrastructural picture was one of isolated, intact capillaries interspersed with fibroblasts, ground substance, and collagen. Emphasis was placed on intraalveolar fibrosis.

By contrast, Brooks (1971) reported that focal swelling and blebbing of capillary endothelial cells and their loosening from the underlying basal membrane were the earliest lesion in mice whose water contained 50–300 ppm paraquat. He did not observe endothelial cell membrane breakage or loss of integrity of cell junctions. Erythrocyte and platelet aggregations in capillaries and small veins, interseptal edema, and damage to some type I pneumatocytes were other early effects.

In most rats, the microscopic lesion involves proliferation of cells that at first appears as more or less typical fibroblasts arising from the adventitia of the vessels and the fibrous tissue around the bronchi. This proliferation begins as early as the third day after dosing and at that time is accompanied by edema fluid in many alveoli, perivascular and peribronchial edema, and the presence of polymorphonuclear lymphocytes, mononuclears, macrophages, and occasionally large numbers of eosinophils or a few giant cells. In animals that survive longer, the proliferating cells lose the appearance of fibroblasts, but proliferation continues and mitoses are very numerous. The mesenchymal cells extend into the alveolar walls, and hypertrophy of the epithelial cells of the alveoli contributes to thickening of the septa. In a smaller proportion of rats, epithelial hypertrophy and proliferation of either the alveolar cells, the terminal bronchial epithelium, or both predominate over the fibrosis. Thus, in a series of animals, the histological pictures were very diverse (Clark *et al.*, 1966).

The liver and kidney of poisoned rats occasionally show focal necrosis. The adrenals are congested. The thymus and spleen sometimes show lympholysis. The testis may show degenerative changes.

Pathologic changes generally similar to those in the rat occur in the dog (Clark *et al.*, 1966) and in the monkey (Schwartz and Silverman, 1976).

Clark *et al.* (1966) found changes in mice similar to those they observed in rats, except that polymorphonuclear leukocytes were more prominent in and around blood vessels, around bronchi, in the alveolar wall, and in the alveoli. Manktelow (1967) found neither inflammatory lesions nor fibrosis in mice that died rapidly following a large intravenous dose. He did find intense congestion, collapse of alveoli, and dilatation of alveolar ducts and terminal bronchioles. Some of the mouse lungs showed eosinophilic, periodic acid–Schiff (PAS) positive hyaline membranes considered identical to those seen in some cases of respiratory distress syndrome of infants.

Findings in rabbits apparently differ from those in other species (Clark *et al.*, 1966; Butler and Kleinerman, 1971; Ilett *et al.*, 1974). Clark *et al.* (1966) found that pulmonary proliferation was less marked than in other species, but the lungs were generally congested. The changes in other organs of rabbits were similar to those seen in corresponding organs of other species, except that rabbits were subject to glossitis and esophagitis, sometimes progressing to ulceration. Butler and Kleinerman (1971) confirmed the absence of delayed pulmonary changes in rabbits that received intraperitoneal dosages of 25 mg/kg or more. They did find atrophy of the thymus and minimal renal tubular changes in animals found dead within 4 days of administration or killed soon thereafter. The changes failed to explain the cause of death. Oral administration of paraquat to rabbits (11 mg/kg/day for 30 days) was reported to produce alveolar edema as well as proliferation of fibrous and epithelial cells (Dikshith *et al.*, 1979). Lung damage can be produced in rabbits by intrabronchial paraquat (Zavala and Rhodes, 1978).

The lung changes so characteristic of paraquat injury in mammals apparently are lacking in turkeys, in which oral administration produces extensive gastroenteritis and dermal application produces severe emaciation with pathology confined mainly to the skin (Smalley, 1973).

Pathology caused by repeated doses of paraquat is confined largely to the lung, and it is similar to that in animals that suffer delayed death following a single dose (Bainova, 1969; Kimbrough and Gaines, 1970). A thorough study of this matter involved female rats receiving a dietary level of 500 ppm that resulted in a dosage of 20.4 mg/kg/day early in the study when their food intake was reduced and later a dosage of about 29 mg/kg/day. This dosage was slightly greater than that found earlier in the same laboratory to be a 90-day LD 50, and a few animals did die in the course of the study. The lungs were normal by all means of examination in rats killed 1 and 3 weeks after feeding began. By the fifth week, some animals remained normal, some showed only changes detectable by electron microscopy, and one showed several areas of consolidation in the lung on gross examination. This range of individual variation was found also after 7 and after 11 weeks of exposure. The authors considered that vacuolization and degeneration of the membranous pneumatocytes was the primary change induced by paraquat. This change was followed by an increase of collagen and reticulum in the basement membranes, proliferation of granular pneumatocytes, swelling of endothelial cells, proliferation of fibroblasts, and an increase of macrophages. A well-developed lesion showed areas where the alveoli were completely obliterated or filled with noncellular material, either in the form of a lattice reminiscent of surfactant or in the form of whorls similar to those constituting the lamellar bodies of the granular pneumatocytes (Kimbrough and Linder, 1973). On the basis of these findings, it seems possible that the surfactant was not deficient but excessive and perhaps defective.

Whether because of a different route and schedule or for other reasons, fibrosis was far more prominent in rats that received paraquat intraperitoneally at the rate of 10 mg/kg (as ion) on days 1, 23, 39, 60, 86, and 106 of an experiment. Emphasis was placed on intraalveolar fibrosis but some instances of compact interstitial fibrosis were reported (P. Smith *et al.*, 1974). In some instances, the distinction between these two forms of fibrosis seemed questionable.

Induction of smooth endoplasmic reticulum and other changes possibly similar to those produced in rodent liver cells by chlorinated hydrocarbon insecticides have been reported in cells of the proximal convoluted tubules of mice receiving paraquat in their drinking water (Fowler and Brooks, 1971).

In seeking a rodent model of interstitial pulmonary disease free of spontaneous infection, Butler (1975) found that, in the hamster, single doses of paraquat were unsatisfactory, but a dependable model could be obtained by suitable repeated doses. Single doses, depending on their rates, tended to be harmless or to produce acute, often fatal lesions. All of the animals that received subcutaneous injections at the rate of 6 mg/kg/week for 4 or 8 weeks developed more interstitial inflammation and fibrosis, and the process involved 15% or more of the lung in nearly half of them and nearly 40% of the lung in a few. These animals receiving multiple small doses soon showed reduced intake of food and water and progressive weight loss, but they showed little respiratory distress, sometimes began to improve clinically before the series of injections was complete, and survived after the last injection until killed for study.

Another approach to developing a model for diffuse interstitial pulmonary fibrosis involved stepwise increases in the oral intake of paraquat by mice (Niden and Khurana, 1976).

Most of the foregoing concerned nonrespiratory exposure to paraquat, whether acute or repeated. When hamsters were exposed for 4 hr or less to an aerosol of unmeasured particle size and unmeasured air concentration, examination of the lungs within 24 hr revealed a sparing of the alveolar epithelium but extensive damage of the airway epithelium all the way down to the respiratory bronchioles. Damage was greatest to the secretory and ciliated cells. Remaining cells spread out to cover the basal lamina following extrusion of some cells (Kilburn et al., 1974).

The apparent difference in the reaction of the rabbit may be simply a difference in dosage at the tissue level. In any event, rabbits repeatedly exposed to a paraquat aerosol formed by an "ultrasonic nebulizer" showed focal interstitial fibrosis and other findings characteristic of paraquat injury (Seidenfeld et al., 1977).

Paraquat potentiates the toxicity of oxygen or ozone, and the lesions they produce are similar, as discussed under Biochemical Effects. However, the lesions may follow a different time course if different oxidants are administered separately. For example when ozone was administered to rats at a concentration of 1 ppm for 24 hr, the lung lesions appeared promptly but resolved within 7–14 days. By contrast, the lesions caused by paraquat at an intraperitoneal dosage of 20 mg/kg first became evident by 7–14 days, and they persisted (Montgomery et al., 1979b). The difference in the timing of effects is partly or perhaps entirely secondary to the difference in the persistence of the compounds in the lung.

Treatment of Poisoning in Animals   A number of absorbents have been tested to determine their ability to prevent gastrointestinal absorption of paraquat. Most were ineffective, but bentonite and fuller's earth prevented deaths due to paraquat in rats and reduced absorption in cats. Both were more effective than gastric lavage. Both clays were recommended for treatment of patients, but fuller's earth was considered preferable. It can be used as a 30% suspension, whereas bentonite swells in water and can be used only as a 6–7% suspension. Fuller's earth may be effective against diquat and related compounds (Clark, 1971). Apparently unaware of the earlier works, Staiff et al. (1973) screened 25 materials, including charcoal but not including bentonite or fuller's earth. They found Amberlite CG-120 ion exchange resin to be the most active material tested in vitro. However, Clark (1971) found Amberlite ineffective in vivo. Gandréault et al. (1985) found charcoal to be effective in binding paraquat in the presence of magnesium citrate.

The nature of the complexes formed by paraquat and diquat with the bentonite has been studied spectrophotometrically (Haque et al., 1970).

It was possible to protect all of 10 rats in which treatment was delayed 4 hr after stomach tube administration of a dose of paraquat that killed 27 of 29 control rats within 8 days. Even when treatment was delayed until 10 hr after administration of the poison, only 2 of 10 rats died within 5 days, and there was no further mortality in any group within a 14-day period of observation. The treatment was confined to evacuation of the gastrointestinal tract by gastric lavage, castor oil, and magnesium sulfate and by adsorption by bentonite of paraquat not already evacuated. Dosing with bentonite and castor oil was repeated three more times at intervals of 2–3 hr. Analytical studies showed that, in spite of the realistic delay in treatment, the concentrations of paraquat in the plasma and in the lungs of treated rats were kept very much lower than corresponding values in controls (P. Smith et al. (1974).

In an in vitro test of hemoperfusion, it was shown that activated charcoal and especially a cation exchange resin (Zerolit 225 SRC21) were effective in removing paraquat from bovine blood. When hemoperfusion was carried out on dogs that had been injected intravenously with paraquat, plasma clearance values remained consistently high with the exchange resin but were lower and more variable with activated charcoal. After hemoperfusion with exchange resin was discontinued, it took 90 min for the concentration of paraquat in plasma to increase to control values, but this took only 30 min after charcoal (Maini and Winchester, 1975). In a study in intact dogs, hemoperfusion with coated charcoal within 3 hr after oral administration of paraquat at a rate of 10 mg/kg removed 16% of the dose. Additional delay led to lesser recovery, but eight of nine dogs perfused within 12 hr survived, whereas those perfused at 18 hr and also unperfused control dogs all died (Widdop et al., 1977). Some further discussion of hemoperfusion is given in Section 8.2.2.3.

Continued exposure of mice to hypoxia for 7 days after they had received an intraperitoneal injection of paraquat reduced mortality compared to that of similarly poisoned control mice kept in room air. When mice were first placed in the hypoxic atmosphere, the oxygen concentration was 14%, and it was reduced stepwise to 10% in 48 hr. Mortality did not increase significantly among the treated mice when they were removed from the hypoxic atmosphere after 7 days and kept in room air for an additional 2 or 3 weeks for observation. However, when hypoxia was interrupted for only a few brief periods during the first 54 hr after injection, there was no therapeutic benefit from the profound but intermittent hypoxia. Some of the mice became acutely tachypneic when the chamber was opened, and part of these reactors died within a few minutes (Rhodes et al., 1976).

Because it has become second nature for physicians to give dyspneic patients supplementary oxygen, there is a real question whether hypoxic treatment of patients would ever be carried out consistently.

A variety of expectorants, of which ammonium chloride and potassium iodide apparently were most effective, reduced the loss of pulmonary surfactant, decreased pulmonary resistance, and increased pulmonary compliance in rats previously injected with paraquat (Cambar and Aviado, 1970). Apparently, the effect of expectorants on survival in paraquat poisoning has not been explored.

Mortality from paraquat was somewhat reduced among rats that received repeated subcutaneous doses of d,l-propranolol, a β-adrenergic receptor blocking agent. These agents blocked uptake of paraquat by rat lung slices in vitro and it was suggested that they may do the same thing in vivo (Maling et al., 1975). However, in a further study, no relationship was found between the effect of any of several drugs on paraquat mortality and its effects on paraquat uptake by lung slices in vitro (Maling et al., 1976).

Some rats pretreated for 5 days with aspirin, indomethacin,

or hydrocortisone survived for 48 hr following intraperitoneal injection of paraquat at a rate of 29 mg/kg, whereas controls all die within that period. The drugs changed the activity of lung cytosolic superoxide dismutase, glutathione peroxidase, glutathione reductase, and total nonprotein sulfhydryls. The results were interpreted as evidence that oxygen and lipid peroxidation have roles in lung damage produced by paraquat (Reddy *et al.*, 1976). Szabo *et al.* (1986) observed that treatment with reduced glutathione (GSH), D-penicillamine, or cysteine increased survival of mice 72 hr after dosing. Equimolar dosing led to the following order of activity: cysteine > D-penicillamine > GSH.

Intermittent exogenous superoxide dismutase was without value to mice poisoned by paraquat (Rhodes and Patterson, 1977) but was said to prolong survival (Autor, 1974) or even to decrease mortality in rats (Wasserman and Block, 1978). The reason for the difference is not apparent. In a separate study, Matkovics *et al.* (1983) observed that simultaneous treatment with catalase or superoxide dismutase reduced mortality at 96 hr from paraquat intoxication, while horseradish peroxidase appeared to exacerbate the lethality of the dose.

Daily doses of ascorbic acid (15 mg/mouse) decreased mortality from paraquat (Barabase and Suveges, 1978), as suggested by earlier biochemical studies (Mason *et al.*, 1977) and supported by later biochemical studies (Matkovics *et al.*, 1980b; Barabase *et al.*, 1986).

20.16.1.3 Toxicity to Humans

Experimental Exposure   Few studies have been conducted to evaluate absorption of paraquat in humans. The absorption of paraquat from the hand, leg, and forearm was determined for a 24-hr period (Wester *et al.*, 1984); a zero-order absorption rate of 0.03 mg/cm^2/day was estimated. The authors concluded that paraquat can be absorbed through human skin, but only minimally.

Accidental and Intentional Poisoning   A number of accidents and suicides with paraquat demonstrate that its effects in humans usually are very similar to those in rats and the majority of other experimental animals (Bronkhorst *et al.*, 1968; Campbell, 1968; Lloyd, 1969; Bony *et al.*, 1971; Brzeski *et al.*, 1971; Grundies *et al.*, 1971; Wanic *et al.*, 1971; Araki *et al.*, 1972; Castaing *et al.*, 1972; Moriyama *et al.*, 1972, 1973; Okada *et al.*, 1972; Conso *et al.*, 1973; Caultier *et al.*, 1973; Hearn, 1973; Nakamura *et al.*, 1973; Almog and Siegelbaum, 1974; Grabensee, 1974; Kusic *et al.*, 1974; Gulic *et al.*, 1975; Lareng *et al.*, 1975; von Butenandt *et al.*, 1975; Fairshter *et al.*, 1976; Funke *et al.*, 1976; Konno *et al.*, 1976; Schlatter, 1976; Tsunenari *et al.*, 1976; Hanawa *et al.*, 1977; Klaff *et al.*, 1977; Takeuchi *et al.*, 1977; Wakabayashi *et al.*, 1977; Bier and Osborne, 1978; Pickersgill *et al.*, 1978; Robin *et al.*, 1978; Takekawa *et al.*, 1978; Vucinovic, 1978; Cravey, 1979; Hayakawa *et al.*, 1979; Isoda, 1979; Yoneda *et al.*, 1979; Matsumoto, 1985; Schultek and Markwalder, 1985; Tashiro *et al.*, 1985; Addo and Poon-King, 1986; Imamura *et al.*, 1986; and other references listed below). By 1971, a world total of 124 deaths caused by

paraquat were known to the manufacturers (Anonymous, 1971) and, by 1972, 142 were known (Chao, 1972). By 1977, the number of fatalities was 564 (Harley *et al.*, 1977).

The National Poisons Information Service, United Kingdom (Whitehead *et al.*, 1984), in cooperation with the manufacturer, has reported that the number of animal fatalities remained static from 1977 through 1983. They reported that in the United Kingdom the number of fatal accidental poisonings accounts for less than 5% of the total cases. The rest of the cases (95%) are associated with deliberate intent. Preliminary indications in the United Kingdom suggest that the emetic included in the formulation since 1979 is further reducing the number of illnesses following accidental ingestion.

In Ireland during the period between June 1967 and May 1977, mortality was 73% in 77 cases of intentional poisoning; 42% in accidental cases, and 100% in 19 cases of unknown cause (Fitzgerald *et al.*, 1978).

Howe and Wright (1965) mentioned without further description a case in which death with convulsions came within hours after a "massive" dose. Malone *et al.* (1971) reported that most of the 19 cases they reviewed died within the first 2 or 3 days, only 2 of 19 surviving 10 and 13 days, respectively. In eight suicides recorded by Chao (1972) death occurred in 9–48 hr after ingestion; in fact, large dosages and early death are characteristic of suicides with paraquat (Hargraeve *et al.*, 1969; Harrison *et al.*, 1972; Nienhaus and Ehrenfeld, 1971; Nagi, 1970; Hofmann and Frohberg, 1972; Yamashita *et al.*, 1974). Sun-Leung Lee *et al.* (1985) reviewed 20 cases of paraquat poisoning. They reported that early deaths were due to direct drug toxicity (renal, hepatic, etc.) or complications such as sepsis, while later death was due to respiratory failure. It thus appears that large doses lead to early death, while intermediate doses may result in reversal of many symptoms and death occurs from respiratory distress.

In typical accidental poisoning (moderate doses), the interval between ingestion and death may be as long as 26 days (Grabensee *et al.*, 1971), 30 days (Weston *et al.*, 1972), or even 102 days (Ohkubo *et al.*, 1979). In a case that was not typical, death, which was not directly related to poisoning, occurred after 46 days (Beebeejaun *et al.*, 1971). In a second atypical case recovery occurred even though the course was protracted. It was 20 days after ingestion that pharyngitis and erosion of the tongue became severe enough to make the patient seek medical aid. Recovery was complete, and the patient was released after 40 days of hospitalization (Uetake *et al.*, 1972). However, the findings were so unusual that the presence of unrecognized factors must be considered. Poder *et al.* (1985) reported a case of accidental exposure in a 5-year-old male that resulted in a unilateral pulmonary lesion that markedly regressed, showing nearly complete recovery after 1 year.

With the exception of the cases involving rapid death, the symptomatology and progress of the reported fatal cases were remarkably similar regardless of the route of absorption—oral, dermal, subcutaneous, or intravenous. In all instances, there were early signs of gastrointestinal irritation followed by more or less prominent signs of dysfunction of the liver, kidneys, and heart. Following ingestion, ulceration of the mouth and pharynx is common. In some instances, there were signs of diffuse damage to the central nervous system. All of these signs either failed to progress to a threatening degree or even regressed. In the meantime there was a gradual onset and progression of respiratory difficulty, ultimately leading to death. In general, the disease in humans, as compared with that in animals, seems to involve slightly greater emphasis on organs other than the lung. The difference may depend more on the quality of observation than on the nature of the disease. Although it is impossible to state that the dysfunction of other organs in humans does not contribute to pulmonary dysfunction, lung injury is unquestionably the usual cause of death.

Most of the features of poisoning by paraquat are illustrated by a case reported by Almog and Tal (1967) involving suicide by subcutaneous injection of the compound. The dosage was said to be 1 ml of 20% paraquat dimethanosulfate. The patient, a 30-year-old male with a history of schizophrenia, reported to the hospital a few hours after the injection because he had already vomited and passed loose bloody stools. Obviously, the action of paraquat on the gastrointestinal tract does not depend exclusively on the presence of unabsorbed poison in the lumen. The admission physical examination was normal and the patient felt well for the first 2 days. Two days after admission there was right facial paralysis, absence of abdominal reflexes on the right, and a positive Oppenheim's sign on the left. All of these signs disappeared by the fifth day. However, on the third day after admission, the patient complained of anorexia and chest pain, and his temperature rose to 39°C. He was not dyspneic, but X-ray examination showed a slight infiltration of the right lung base. After 5 days he again improved and had neither pain nor fever, but his radiological changes persisted. Jaundice appeared on the eighth day; the liver was felt 6 cm below the rib margin, and the area was tender. These findings in turn disappeared by day 11, and the patient felt well for the next 3 days. On day 14 he developed dyspnea and tachycardia. X-ray examination showed areas of opacity in both lungs and a shift of the mediastinum to the left. He became oxygen dependent, grew steadily worse, and died of severe respiratory difficulty on day 18.

Some other systemic cases have shown tachycardia, electrocardiographic evidence of conduction defect, and myocarditis. Some also showed greater evidence of renal damage (Bullivant, 1966; Oreopoulos et al., 1968; Vaziri et al., 1979; Yagi et al., 1977). In a rare case reported by McKean (1968), there was severe involvement of the kidneys and lesser involvement of the heart and liver but no evidence of any lung disease. The patient, an 11-year-old boy, survived.

Ingestion may produce severe irritation of the mouth, pharynx, esophagus, and stomach. It may be followed by ulceration of the mouth and perforation of the esophagus. There is often recurrent vomiting. Postmortem examination of a 49-year-old male who drank seven to eight times an expected lethal dose of paraquat identified numerous raised plaques of necrotic mucosa throughout the colon (Imamura et al., 1986). The authors suggested that the pseudomembranous colitis may have been the result of vessel injury by paraquat.

A 3-year-old boy who spilled paraquat on his clothing suffered a first-degree burn on the anterior aspect of his thigh and raised erythematous areas on the backs of his hands. He had no oral lesions and developed no systemic findings (McDonagh and Martin, 1970). However, slightly erythematous spots up to 10 mm in diameter have been reported in at least two patients thought to have ingested paraquat (Uetake et al., 1972). There are a few other records of local effects associated with accidental exposure. Perhaps the narrowest escape was that of a 2.5-year-old child who suffered only swollen lips after sucking the neck of a paraquat container (Great Britain Ministry of Agriculture, Fisheries and Food, 1972). There have been a number of fatal poisonings following dermal absorption. They are discussed under Use Experience, although some were the result of gross carelessness or a gross accident associated with occupation.

It is generally assumed that patients who survive systemic poisoning by paraquat have received no injury to their lungs and that they recover completely. This view is not necessarily inconsistent with the fact (discussed under Treatment of Poisoning) that some persons live in spite of signs or symptoms referable to the respiratory tract—but perhaps only the upper tract. At least one case (Anderson, 1970) appears to show that fibrosis of the lung may be limited and does not exclude survival. X rays were normal on the second and fourth days of poisoning that was treated very promptly so that symptomatology was limited to sore throat and "laryngitis." However, 18 months later, when the asymptomatic man was examined routinely in connection with a new job, both X-ray and lung function studies were slightly abnormal and consistent with persistent, mild pulmonary fibrosis. Specifically, the X ray showed a "chronic bronchitis" pattern, and the function tests revealed a slightly reduced forced expiratory volume and a reduced carbon monoxide diffusing capacity. The tests were repeated over a 10-month period without any evidence of change.

A study of 13 patients who had survived at least 1 year after acute poisoning showed that two children and five nonsmoking adults had no clinical, radiological, or functional signs of pulmonary disease, whereas four smokers had mild pulmonary dysfunction and two others had pronounced arterial hypoxemia. The last two had histories of respiratory disability prior to poisoning, but one of them displayed new and persistent pulmonary infiltrates indicating permanent lung damage attributed to paraquat (Fitzgerald et al., 1979).

Use Experience   When paraquat was applied by tractor-mounted, low-boom sprayers or to low-growing vegetation by means of a properly operating, pressurized hand sprayer, the highest measured dermal exposure rate was 3.4 mg/person/hr. Practically all the dermal contamination was found on the hands. Respiratory exposure usually was not detectable but was as high as 0.002 mg/hr in one sample (Staiff et al., 1975). The exposure situation may be quite different, especially when high-growing vegetation is treated.

Mild irritation of the skin and eyes occurred in about half of the men who were employed full-time in spraying weeds with a knapsack sprayer. In spite of some systemic absorption, demonstrated by urinary excretion of unchanged paraquat in the urine, such spraying for 6 days/week for 12 weeks did not produce systemic illness or lung changes detectable by X-ray (Swan, 1969).

Workers exposed to a fine mist of paraquat have suffered nosebleeds (Howe and Wright, 1965; Swan, 1969). It is also reported that exposure to spray mists may cause skin irritation, irritation and inflammation of the mouth and upper respiratory tract, cough, chest pain, asthmatic attacks, frontal headache, vomiting, and pain and swelling of the joints (Howe and Wright, 1965) and, on rare occasions, contact dermatitis (Botella *et al.,* 1985). Injury to the nails, especially of the index, middle, and ring fingers on the right hand, may follow exposure to concentrations or leakage of dilute spray from a defective sprayer valve. The injury may take the form of white bands, but loss of surface, transverse ridging, gross deformity of the nail plate, and loss of nails may occur. These injuries have not been accompanied by systemic illness, and nail growth returned to normal after exposure stopped (Samman and Johnston, 1969; Hearn and Keir, 1971; Baran, 1974). Similar complaints without long-term effects on the skin, mucous membranes, or general health have been described among formulators exposed for several years (Howard, 1978b).

In a series of 121 cases in Ireland, 12 patients claimed at the time of hospitalization that their illness was the result of normal agricultural use. Actually, the more serious cases had deviated grossly from label instructions. However, there were three instances of minor ill effect when the instructions seemed to have been followed explicitly, and paraquat was detected in the urine of two of these individuals (Fitzgerald *et al.,* 1977a).

Severe injury of a farmer's eye was caused by a splash while he was adding an equal mixture of paraquat and diquat to water. Under the circumstances, there was no way to estimate the concentration of herbicide in the droplets entering the eye. The man noticed slight irritation at the time and washed the eye with water. Mild irritation recurred gradually, and on the third day he consulted his family doctor. One week later the eye became considerably worse and he was hospitalized. Examination showed extensive loss of bulbar and tarsal conjunctiva, as well as loss of part of the corneal epithelium. The denuded area was clean. There was a minimal anterior uveitis. Healing did not begin until 14 days after the accident but was essentially complete in 11 additional days. During recovery, it was necessary repeatedly to separate the opposing conjunctival surfaces to avoid adhesions (Cant and Lewis, 1968). Other severe cases have involved paraquat alone at concentrations ranging from 0.24 to 24%; healing required 3–5 weeks (Tane *et al.,* 1974; Mikuni and Suzuki, 1976). A case that in one sense was more severe than any other was atypical in that the patient had little discomfort immediately after his eye was splashed with paraquat. He noticed some reduction in visual acuity 7 days later but did not go to an ophthalmologist until 4 weeks after injury. By that time

the eye was white and capable only of perceiving light. A circular, 5-mm corneal opacity was evident, as well as some peripheral infiltration and fluorescein staining. The peripheral lesions cleared in 2 weeks with conservative treatment, but the corneal lesion remained stable. Six months after injury, a 6-mm penetrating keratoplasty was done. The corneal disc showed that the epithelium had reformed but was thickened in the middle, where Bowman's layer was missing (Joyce, 1969). Recovery was no more rapid (2–10 weeks) in other cases of paraquat conjunctivitis in which the degree of injury apparently was less (Joyce, 1969; Guardascione and Mazzella di Bosco, 1969; Fujita, 1973a,b, 1975; Oishi, 1975). Uchida (1975) attributed part of the injury to the eye to acidic erosion, but probably without sufficient evidence. Other cases of severe eye injury associate with splashes were reported by Watanabe *et al.* (1979).

Swan (1968) pointed out that, whereas bipyridyls produce more injury to the eye in humans than in experimental animals, the damage (unlike that caused by alkali) is mainly superficial and, given prompt and adequate treatment to control infection and prevent the formation of adhesions between denuded bulbar and palpebral surfaces, the prospects of full and complete recovery are excellent.

Not unlike the eye injury insofar as epithelial erosion is concerned was a "vaccination" with paraquat. A 30-year-old man received superficial scratches above and below both knees while spraying spiny grass and other weeds. Six days later he consulted a physician because of marked inflammation of some of the scratches. The vesiculation developed to resemble primary vaccination. The concentration of paraquat in the urine was only 0.01 ppm and there were no systemic symptoms. The lesions healed in 14–21 days, but marks were visible for some time afterward (Barber, 1971). Another case of severe burns without systemic illness was reported by Withers *et al.* (1979).

Several other cases show that dermal absorption of a dangerous dose of paraquat is possible. One of these began very much like the "vaccination" case. A 39-year-old woman who worked with paraquat in orchards was hospitalized because minor scratches on her arms and legs developed raised lesions exuding clear or bloody fluid. Other symptoms included headache, breathlessness, tightness of the chest, anorexia, and loss of weight. Biopsy of the ulcerated lesions showed necrosis of the epidermis and dermis. Pulmonary function studies revealed a moderate restrictive pulmonary defect. Within 14 days of topical dermal therapy, there was marked improvement, and the patient was sent home. Seventeen days later she was readmitted with new skin lesions plus dyspnea, cough, fever, nausea, and vomiting. Progressive deterioration included extensive coagulative necrosis of the skin down to the fat, hepatic and renal dysfunction, and respiratory failure. She died 12 days after second admission (Newhouse *et al.,* 1978).

A second case involved a 44-year-old man who failed to dilute paraquat sufficiently for spraying and then used an old sprayer that leaked material down his neck, back, and legs. Six days later he was hospitalized with respiratory difficulties, and he died 3 days later of renal and respiratory insufficiency. In addition to expected lesions in the lungs and kidneys, dry bloody necrosis was found in several areas of the neck and scrotum (Jaros, 1978). A third fatal case involved a 39-year-old farmer who fell from his bicycle and broke a bottle of paraquat he was carrying in his pocket so that the material spilled on his lower abdomen, perineum, and thighs (Waight, 1979). Other deaths have followed the misguided application of paraquat to kill body lice (Binns, 1976; Howard, 1978a). Other cases of fatal or nonfatal systemic poisoning by the dermal route have been reported (Levin et al., 1979).

Paraquat has been used to destroy marijuana in the hope of prevent its use as a drug. However, some of the sprayed crop was harvested and seized samples were shown to bear residues as high as 2264 ppm. This led to a great controversy regarding the possible effect of the residues on those who smoked the marijuana (Smith, 1978; Trux and Torrey, 1978). After 1976, the proportion of samples found positive declined gradually (Turner et al., 1978). In a study of samples seized between 1975 and January 1979 (mainly in 1978), paraquat was found in 33 of 910 seizures. In these positive samples, the concentration ranged from 10 to 461 ppm, with a median of 52 ppm (Anonymous, 1979). Using average residue values, it has been calculated that 0.00005–0.00025 mg of paraquat could be inhaled with the smoke of one marijuana cigarette. Physicians have differed on whether the complaint that marijuana smokers attributed to paraquat were valid or psychosomatic (Fairshter and Wilson, 1978; Cross and Last, 1978). This suggests that the complaints that have been made were not associated with physical abnormalities or functional loss.

Atypical Cases of Various Origins There have been few reports of systemic illness attributed to paraquat that do not fit the characteristic symptomatology closely. One report (de Larrard, 1969) must be recorded, even though, in the absence of adequate exposure, the atypical findings probably were unrelated to paraquat. Briefly, a 60-year-old man who had used paraquat one afternoon without recognized incident awoke next morning with vomiting and diarrhea. Around 11 a.m. he lost consciousness for 10 min and exhibited extreme cyanosis and muscle cramps. He was taken to the hospital, where he improved rapidly, although some tetanic spasm persisted for a time. The right hand remained contracted with the fingers in hyperflexion that he could not overcome unaided. His body was rigid, his vision blurred, and his ears hummed. However, he was able to speak. He was entirely well when released from hospital 3 days later.

A 40-year-old farm worker used paraquat for the first time, for only part of 1 day, and without any unusual exposure being recognized. One day later, he began to complain of weakness, infrequent urination, and wine-colored urine. He was agitated and had auditory hallucinations. The only history of possible significance involved the consumption of 1.5 liters of wine per day. In the hospital, he was found to have hepatomegaly, splenomegaly, an increase in serum transaminases, and traces of glucose in his urine. His recovery apparently was uneventful, but 9 months later he was considered to have chronic hepatitis

(Guardascione and Mazzella di Bosco, 1969). The absence of signs and symptoms typical of paraquat poisoning is noteworthy. No chemical tests were reported that would demonstrate the absorption of paraquat or rule out the presence of porphyria.

The absence of any characteristic sign of paraquat poisoning following the "suspected" ingestion of a maximum of 2.2 gm of paraquat (about 31 mg/kg) was attributed to early treatment (Slocombe et al., 1973) but, in spite of a screening test for urinary paraquat reported as positive, strongly suggests a lack of exposure.

A 59-year-old man attributed his persistent headaches to the pesticides he applied outdoors. Following application of paraquat, he complained of headache, ocular hyperemia, pain in the throat, and cough followed by amnesia, hallucinations, and neurosis. He showed chronic bronchitis on X-ray, some disturbance of lung function, and loss of sensation in the right extremities (Nakabayashi et al., 1975).

Idiopathic diffuse interstitial fibrosis of the lung, sometimes called Hamman–Rich syndrome, is a rare, chronic, usually progressive and fatal disease of insidious onset and unknown cause ordinarily observed in adults but occasionally in infants and children. The condition lasts from 1 month to many years. It usually involves right-sided heart failure and (besides interstitial fibrosis) also alveolar capillary block and infiltration of lung issues by lymphocytes, plasma cells, and occasionally eosinophils. The pathology that accompanies fibrosis is, therefore, strikingly different from that in paraquat poisoning. The condition was first recognized during the 1930s (Hamman and Rich, 1944; Rubin and Lubliner, 1957). Finberg (1974) raised the question of whether this syndrome might be caused by paraquat; apparently the only evidence was his "clinical hunch."

Dosage Response An oral dosage exceeding 300 mg/kg was fatal within 23 hr (Guyon et al., 1975).

Apparently the smallest dose leading to death was 1 gm ingested by a 23-year-old woman (FAO/WHO, 1973), indicating a dosage of about 16.7 mg/kg. This is consistent with the view (Binnie, 1975) that anything over 5 ml of 20% solution (about 14 mg/kg) is likely to be fatal. In one instance, a man ingested "only a mouthful of [20%] liquid, most of which was said to have been rejected immediately" (Bullivant, 1966). A mouthful is about 50 ml. Therefore, if the patient's account was accurate, he may have swallowed about 20 ml, or a dosage of about 57 mg/kg. The dose was fatal in 15 days. Many other fatal dosages apparently were larger. Solfrank et al. (1977) expressed the view that 3000 mg of paraquat (about 43 mg/kg) was the largest dose allowing a chance for survival. However, there are exceptions to all such rules. Thus a 40-year-old man survived a dose estimated as 7200 mg (Mayama et al., 1979).

Perhaps as a result of vigorous treatment, a man survived the ingestion of 45 gm of a 5% solution (estimated 32 mg/kg) (Kerr et al., 1968). With treatment, a boy survived taking a "mouthful" of paraquat solution; although he spat it out at once, the dose was sufficient to cause ulceration of the tip of his tongue, involvement of his kidneys and heart, and probable involvement of his liver (McKean, 1968). Another boy survived a similar dose followed promptly by vomiting; he, too, suffered ulceration of the mouth, and he excreted paraquat in his urine but there were no systemic symptoms (Greig, cited by Matthew *et al.*, 1968).

Even the ingestion of what was thought to be a few drops of 24% paraquat dichloride in about 150 ml of water (equivalent to approximately 1 mg/kg) led to a white coating on the tongue, pharyngeal pain, and hoarseness that caused the patient to enter hospital 20 days after ingestion. Laboratory study showed increased blood urea nitrogen (BUN), SGOT, and SGPT, as well as an increase in white blood cell count, presumably in response to the erosion of mucous membranes. There was occult blood in the feces. After 2 weeks, slightly elevated erythematous spots appeared on the face, arms, and trunk. The patient recovered completely and was discharged after 40 days in the hospital (Uetake *et al.*, 1972). The case was unique because of the protected course in the absence of detectable injury to the lungs.

A subcutaneous dosage of about 4 mg/kg was fatal in 18 days (Almog and Tal, 1967). A 24-year-old woman, who had attempted suicide repeatedly, injected herself intramuscularly with about 60 mg of a "commercial preparation" of paraquat. This produced little or no systemic effect. However, intravenous injection of 550–600 mg 30 days later led to death in 20 days (Harley *et al.*, 1977). If this was the usual 20% commercial formulation, the intramuscular and intravenous dosages were approximately 0.2 and 2 mg/kg, respectively.

The threshold limit value of 0.1 mg/m^3 indicates that occupational intake at a rate of 0.014 mg/kg/day is considered safe.

Storage in Blood   Except for a very brief period after ingestion, the concentration of paraquat in blood is less than that in the tissues, and it is also less than that in urine. Blood samples are necessary for calculating clearance. Tissue and urine samples are more likely to be positive and, therefore, sometimes better for establishing a diagnosis.

Blood levels ranging from 1.4 to 15 ppm were recorded in fatal cases (Hargraeve *et al.*, 1969; Spector *et al.*, 1978; Nakai *et al.*, 1979). Levels of 0.85 and 0.18 ppm were found in cases with recovery (Tompsett, 1970; Mahieu *et al.*, 1977).

The concentration of paraquat was measured in 79 patients, and the measurements were serial in 25 patients. A graph of the serial observations consisted of an early rapid phase and a late slow phase. The flexure between the two phases tended to fall between 10 and 15 hr after ingestion. The slopes of the first portion of the different curves were remarkably similar, although there may have been a tendency for the slope to be inversely proportional to initial concentration. At any given time (including the time of hospital admission) after ingestion, the concentrations for the patients who subsequently died usually exceeded those of the survivors. It was suggested that plasma levels were useful for assessing severity and for predicting outcome, and the authors suggested a curve to separate points associated with life from those associated with death. Loci on this curve were 2.0, 0.6, 0.16, and 0.10 ppm at 4, 6, 10, 16, and

24 hr, respectively. The results for only one survivor lay above the proposed curve, and no results associated with mortality lay below it (Proudfoot *et al.*, 1979). A curve that corresponds better with the pharmacodynamic results and might separate the living from the dead just as well in a large series is a straight line on semilogarithmic paper extending from 7.0 ppm at zero time to 0.1 ppm at 15 hr.

It must be noted that the degree of overlapping was far less for the plasma values for those who survived and for those who died than was true for corresponding urinary values, discussed in a later paragraph. Probably marked variation in urinary flow leads to variation in urinary excretion of paraquat. However, regardless of the reason, it seems clear that plasma values constitute the best basis for prognosis.

Storage in Other Tissues   In cases of fatal paraquat poisoning, the compound almost always can be demonstrated in tissues taken at autopsy. The following is a list of ranges of reported concentrations and, in parentheses, the total number of samples recorded, the number positive, and the mean of positive values where more than one was positive: (*a*) liver, 0.02–61.4 ppm (17, 16, 8.9 ppm); (*b*) kidney, 0.02–73.8 ppm (20, 19, 11.6 ppm); (*c*) lung, 0.02–73.8 ppm (8, 7, 20.2 ppm); (*d*) brain, 0.02–5.1 ppm (6, 5, 1.4 ppm); (*e*) spleen, 0.01–15.3 ppm (5, 5, 0.6 ppm); (*f*) fat, 0.01–1.8 ppm (5, 4, 0.6 ppm); (*g*) muscle, 0.4–0.83 ppm (2, 2, 0.6 ppm) (Campbell, 1968; Tompsett, 1970; Carson, 1972; Weston *et al.*, 1972; Tsunenari *et al.*, 1975; Sasaki *et al.*, 1975; Harley *et al.*, 1977; Prochnicka *et al.*, 1977; Fairshter *et al.*, 1979; Miura *et al.*, 1979; Nakai *et al.*, 1979). As might be expected, tissue levels tend to be higher in persons who die quickly and lower in those who die slowly (Carson, 1972).

In the case treated by lung transplant, the concentration in the lung removed at operation 7 days after ingestion was 8.5 ppm, compared to a concentration of 0.4 ppm in the blood at that time. Following death 20 days after ingestion, no paraquat was detected in either lung or in the kidneys, liver, spleen, bone, or brain (Matthew *et al.*, 1968).

Excretion   Measurement of paraquat in the urine is a way of estimating the minimal absorbed dose, and it has been much used for gauging the success of diuresis in removing the poison. Urinary excretion is likely to give a deceptively low estimate of the absorbed dose, because a substantial proportion of this dose is retained in the tissues and because animal studies show that true fecal excretion exists.

In the case treated by lung transplant, 204 mg of paraquat was recovered in the urine during the first 2 days and about 44 mg during the remainder of the illness. About 1 mg/day was recovered as late as day 16 after ingestion (Swan, 1969).

A correlation of survival with low early excretion of paraquat has been noted (Matthew *et al.*, 1971). Hayes (1982) plotted all available data on the concentration of paraquat in urine related to different times after ingestion for patients who survived and those who did not. It seemed possible to account for some but not all of the overlapping between fatal and nonfatal cases by the effect of very high urinary volume following forced fluids or by age, perhaps indicating a greater susceptibility of children. He concluded that the prognosis is good if the concentration of paraquat in the urine during the first 3 hr (and before diuresis) is not over 200 ppm and is progressively worse with higher values. However, he pointed out that the degree of overlapping between fatal and nonfatal cases was far less for plasma values than for corresponding urinary values, and he recommended that plasma values of paraquat (discussed earlier) be used for prognosis where possible.

Starting forced fluids several days after ingestion may promote both relatively high urinary concentrations and relatively high total daily excretion. For example, in an attempted suicide reported by Pasi and Hine (1971), the patient did not seek medical care until the third day, when his urinary volume was low; however, by maintaining urinary flow at 100–100 ml/hr the urinary concentration of paraquat reached a maximum of 40 ppm on day 11 after ingestion, and the patient survived.

The criterion of 200 ppm during the first 3 hr is consistent with the cutoff point suggested by Wright *et al.* (1978)—that is, excretion at a rate equal to or greater than 1 mg/hr 8 hr or more after ingestion. This statement is also consistent with, but not at all identical to, the advice of Swan (1970) to the effect that a level over 2 ppm 3 days after ingestion requires a guarded prognosis. The prognosis is good if the urinary concentration at 3 days does not exceed 1 ppm. Certainly, the physician should follow the advice of Goulding and his colleagues (1976) to treat at once every patient whose urine gives a positive result in the relatively simple test for paraquat and diquat that they proposed. If the test is sensitive to 1.0 ppm in clear urine as they state, then their advice is conservative as well as wise, and patients with a weak test in an early sample should have a real chance of survival.

During the first day the concentration of paraquat in the urine is decreased to half within about 4–6 hr, but the rate of change is much lower during subsequent days.

As in the rat, the critical period for action or fixation of the toxin in humans may be during the first day after ingestion, because after that urinary excretion of paraquat may be lower in fatal cases than it was initially in some nonfatal ones.

Men who applied an average of just under 2600 gallons of 1 : 40 paraquat solution with knapsack sprayers during a 12-week period excreted an average concentration of 0.04 ppm and had a peak value of 0.32 ppm in their urine. There was no rising trend as the operation continued. Most of the men continued to excrete paraquat at decreasing concentrations for a few days after spraying stopped. In one man, no residues were found on days 4–7 after spraying but residues were detected again in weekly samples taken from the second to the fifth weeks but not in later samples. In other spraying operations in which somewhat greater precautions were taken and many of the men wore rubber boats, the urinary concentrations averaged 0.006 ppm and the peak value was only 0.15 ppm (Swan, 1969).

These values, ranging up to 0.32 ppm in workers, are of a different order of magnitude from those observed within 24 hr of exposure in cases with systemic symptoms.

Other Laboratory Findings Following moderate dosages, pulmonary function tests are likely to be abnormal sooner than physical or X-ray findings. If performed early and serially, function tests may be of diagnostic value, but similar changes occur in pneumonia, pulmonary edema, pulmonary thromboembolism, and advanced degrees of the alveolar capillary block syndrome. Therefore the clinical state of the patient must be considered as well as the results of special tests. Often beginning between the fifth and sixth days in paraquat poisoning there is a restriction of the forced expiratory volume, the 1-sec forced expiratory volume, and the static lung volume as measured by helium dilution. These changes are followed by a drop in arterial oxygen tension and an increase in the gradient of alveolar to arterial tension. Finally, there is the development of a functional shunt by which a decreasing fraction of the blood passing through the lung is oxygenated (Cooke *et al.*, 1973).

Radiological changes in the lungs reflect poorly the severity of pulmonary lesions (Ramachamdran *et al.*, 1974).

In patients with subacute toxic reactions to paraquat (death in 11–14 days), the extent of lipid peroxidation, expressed as malondialdehyde, is higher than in controls or in patients who survived. Massive doses (death in 1–3 days) did not result in increased levels of malondialdehyde (Yasaka *et al.*, 1981, 1986).

Other findings, including those reflecting kidney failure and liver dysfunction, are nonspecific. Using the case reported by Almog and Tal (1967) as an example, laboratory findings at one time or another reflected dysfunction of the kidneys (some erythrocytes and leukocytes in the urine, blood urea up to 140 mg %) and liver (total serum bilirubin of 2.6 mg %, SGOT of 250 units, serum ammonia of 275 μg %, and leucine aminopeptidase of 264 units). In one or more other cases, the following tests gave abnormally high results: total serum bilirubin, serum alkaline phosphatase, thymol turbidity, serum nonprotein nitrogen, blood urea, serum SGOT and SGPT, and urinary albumin (Bullivant, 1966; McKean, 1968). Serum protein was decreased in one case but increased in another with a large increase in all globulin fractions (Bullivant, 1966; Matthew *et al.*, 1968).

Normochromic anemia developed rapidly in all five of the cases reported by Lautenschläger *et al.* (1974). This was accompanied by suppression of erythropoiesis in the bone marrow but little or no effect on other aspects of hemopoiesis. Maximal suppression of erythropoiesis occurred in 5–14 days and improved very little while poisoning persisted. However, the bone marrow had returned to normal in one patient who survived and was reexamined 6 months after poisoning. Important blood changes have been reported rarely in paraquat poisoning, but whether this is the result of limited examination or of real, unexplained differences between cases is not clear. Paraquat (1 mM) has been reported to cause *in vitro* hemolysis of human erythrocytes (Okahata, 1980), but hemolysis did not occur in the presence of added superoxide dismutase and histidine. Catalase and methionine did not affect the hemolysis rate. Interestingly, introduction of superoxide dismutase genetically into mouse L cells or human HeLa cells led to a greater resistance to paraquat (Elroy-Stein *et al.*, 1986).

Pathology The autopsy findings in poisoning by paraquat reflect the clinical course, being confined to tissue destruction in those who die in a day or two and involving more and more evidence of "repair" in those who survive longer.

An especially thorough study of an acute death is that of Nienhaus and Ehrenfeld (1971). In the lungs of a man who died 52 hr after ingestion, they found desquamation of alveolar epithelial cells and edematous endothelial cells of the capillaries with rupture of some capillaries, widespread capillary hemorrhage into some alveolar spaces, and leakage of edema fluid rich in protein into other spaces. In some areas, the alveolar basement membrane and supporting tissue had disintegrated. The arterioles and venules, as well as the terminal bronchioles, remained intact. Similar observations were reported by von der Hardt and Cardesa (1971) and by Poche (1974), who also noted a remarkable dilatation of some alveolar capillaries, presumably prior to hemorrhage. In acute deaths, the condition of the lungs at autopsy often is described simply as "pulmonary edema" (Harrison et al., 1972).

In the case detailed above representative of a prolonged course, there was no gross abnormality of the liver or kidneys at autopsy in spite of the clinical evidence of their dysfunction early in the illness. There was some swelling of periportal hepatic cells. The upper portion of the lungs was emphysematous and had intrapulmonary and subpleural hemorrhages. The lower portions were contracted and atelectatic bilaterally. Microscopic examination revealed that the epithelial cells of the alveoli were cuboidal, and there was marked proliferation of the epithelium of the terminal bronchioles, often partly or completely occluding the lumen of the prealveolar duct (Almog and Tal, 1967; Herczeg and Reif, 1968). Other outstanding descriptions are those of Borchard et al. (1974). Smith and Heath (1974a), Pariente et al. (1974), Okubo et al. (1975), Rebello and Mason (1978), and Dearden et al. (1978).

Fibrosis may be extensive in as little as 8 days (Lanzinger et al., 1969). Although emphasis usually is not placed on emphysema, it certainly can occur. Iff et al. (1971) recorded a honeycomb-like structure in the median and upper portions of lungs in which microscopic study showed that the normal structure had been destroyed. Similar lesions were figured by Thurlbeck and Thurlbeck (1976) and spoken of as "microcysts." Lareng et al. (1975) mentioned the simultaneous presence of lesions of different ages in the same person, but it is not clear that their concept of succeeding waves of involvement of the lung is justified.

Some cases combine the early and late types of lung findings and, in some, fibrosis is prominent. For example, Bullivant (1966) reported a case in which congestion and hemorrhage were prominent, and edema fluid in some alveoli contained much fibrin. However, much of the tissue was solid and airless from heavy proliferation of fibroblastic cells in the alveolar walls and elsewhere. In a few places, considerable proliferation of the epithelium of the terminal bronchi had led to small glandlike structures. Focal and diffuse polymorphonuclear, mononuclear, and eosinophilic infiltration and many macrophages accompanied the other changes in some areas.

In some cases the distribution of fibrosis is intraalveolar and not interstitial (Copland et al., 1974; Harley et al., 1977), but both distributions may occur in the same case (Toner et al., 1970; Borchard, 1974).

Multinucleated giant cells may be present in the alveolar wall (Fennelly et al., 1968).

Thus, the lung changes in humans are essentially identical to those described in animals, being characterized early by hemorrhage, edema, and hyaline membranes and later by interstitial proliferation of plump fibroblasts in diffuse and whorled patterns, proliferation of bronchiolar and alveolar epithelium, and infiltration by chronic inflammatory cells (Matthew et al., 1968; Lanzinger et al., 1969; Masterson and Roche, 1970a,b; McDonagh and Martin, 1970; Yamashita et al., 1974; Borchard, 1974). The progression of changes from loss of alveolar lining epithelium to severe fibrosis has been followed by biopsy and autopsy samples in the same case (Toner et al., 1970).

The findings in paraquat poisoning have considerable resemblance to those caused by excessive oxygen (Matthew et al., 1971).

Local findings such as ulcers of the mouth and pharynx are common. In two cases, perforation of the esophagus led to death from mediastinitis (Ackrill et al., 1978). Erosion of other epithelial surfaces, including the bladder, has been reported (Yamashita et al., 1974).

Reports of some cases have mentioned liver and kidney damage, including edema, hemorrhage, cellular degeneration, some infiltration by lymphocytes, or mitotic activity (Faure et al., 1973; Borchard et al., 1974). Some autopsies have revealed hemorrhage of the brain stem (Yamashita et al., 1974); hemorrhagic leukoencephalopathy accompanied by focal demyelination (Mukada et al., 1978); degeneration of peripheral nerve cells, axons, and medullary sheaths (Yamashita et al., 1974); myocardial degeneration (Masterson and Roche, 1970a,b; Nagi, 1970; Harrison et al., 1972); atrophy of the smooth muscles (Yamashita et al., 1974); diffuse or focal cortical necrosis of the adrenal (Nagi, 1970; Kodagoda et al., 1973; Yamashita et al., 1974; Fitzgerald et al., 1977b; Kuhara et al., 1977; Koike et al., 1978; Spector et al., 1978; Takahashi et al., 1978); hemorrhage of the spleen (Yamashita et al., 1974); multiple fibrin thrombi in vessels of various sizes (Adachi et al., 1978); other abnormal clotting (Nakamura et al., 1979); and edematous degeneration and necrosis of the epithelium of the pancreatic ducts (Takahashi et al., 1978).

Electron microscopic study of a renal biopsy permitted a detailed description of lesions of the convoluted tubules. The patient's main problem involved kidney function; respiratory dysfunction was minor, and recovery was complete (Bescol-Liversac et al., 1975).

A 22-year-old woman intentionally ingested a large dose of paraquat during her seventh month of pregnancy. The clinical course and autopsy of the mother were typical. The fetal heartbeat disappeared on day 13 of poisoning, and the dead fetus was delivered next day. The mother died 3 days later. Autopsy showed that the infant's lungs had expanded and were filled with debris of amniotic fluid, suggesting that the fetus had begun to breathe in response to hypoxia. No indication of paraquat poisoning was noted in the fetus (Takayama *et al.*, 1978).

Treatment of Poisoning   No specific treatment for paraquat poisoning is known.

Unfortunately, the value of many forms of nonspecific treatments remains questionable. The relative lack of symptoms and the low initial plasma and urinary concentrations of paraquat in some cases suggest (but cannot prove) that recovery would occur even without treatment. Certainly, no treatment or regimen has led to a dramatic reduction of the proportion of cases that progress to death. About all that can be said is that the harmful effects of oxygen therapy have been established by theory, animal experiments, and clinical experience. Any measure (e.g., vomiting, gastric lavage, gut lavage, and adsorbents; see Treatment of Poisoning in Animals in Section 20.16.1.2) that prevents some poison from being absorbed or any measure (e.g., forced diuresis, hemodialysis, peritoneal dialysis, or hemoperfusion; see Treatment of Poisoning in Animals in Section 20.16.1.2 and Therapeutic Procedures Requiring Evaluation in Section 8.2.2.3) that prevents some absorbed poison from reaching a critical site of action is a step in the right direction.

Although gut lavage is relatively new, it has been shown to be capable of removing a substantial amount of dipyridylium herbicide from the human intestine. It has been suggested that patients tolerate gut lavage better than thorough catharsis. Although there apparently has been no test to compare the efficiency of gut lavage and catharsis in clearing the intestine, it seems likely that gut lavage will be used more extensively in the future.

Gut lavage has been tested mainly in humans rather than animals and—in relation to pesticides—mainly in connection with dipyridylium herbicides. The method was first described by Hewitt *et al.* (1973) for minimizing bacterial contamination preliminary to surgery on the large intestine. The method was tolerated by healthy volunteers without great complaint, and a throughput of about 4 liters/hr could be obtained without incurring any water or salt imbalance in the blood. The solution containing sodium chloride (6.14 gm/liter), potassium chloride (0.75 gm/liter), and sodium bicarbonate (2.94 gm/liter) was introduced via stomach tube using a peristaltic pump. At a pumping rate of 75 ml/min, about 3.5–4 liters/hr passed through the intestine, while 0.5–1 liter/hr was absorbed. When this procedure was applied to a man who had ingested an unknown but probably large quantity of diquat 30 hr before admission, about 27 mg of the herbicide was recovered from 6900 ml of gut washings, but only about 0.2 mg from 980 ml of initial stomach washings and slightly over 1 mg through hemodialysis carried out simultaneously with the washing procedures (Okonek *et al.*, 1976). The fact that the patient died 17 hr after admission is hardly a reflection on the methods used to remove the poison, because he was already anuric when first seen.

Gut lavage has been used with fuller's earth or bentonite in the fluid. This probably is a good thing, but presence of the clay prevents measurement of the amount of herbicide removed.

Some authors have advocated the use of adsorbents, e.g., fuller's earth or bentonite, known to inactivate the herbicidal action of paraquat (Anonymous, 1968; McDonagh and Martin, 1970; Browne, 1971; Grabensee *et al.*, 1971; Greig and Streat, 1977). It could not be expected that this or any other treatment always would be successful. Records of failure include those of Iff *et al.* (1971), Malcolmson and Beesley (1975), Van Dijk *et al.* (1975), Fairshter *et al.* (1976), and Vale *et al.* (1977). On the contrary, there are records of other cases in which patients survived following treatment with adsorbents (Van Dijk *et al.*, 1975; Thomas *et al.*, 1977; Vale *et al.*, 1977). Evaluation of the practical value of adsorbents under real clinical conditions is incomplete.

In treating paraquat poisoning, probably most emphasis has been put on forced diuresis (McDonagh and Martin, 1970; Fennelly and Fitzgerald, 1971; Grabensee *et al.*, 1971; Fisher *et al.*, 1971; Hensel and Duerr, 1971; Almog and Siegelbaum, 1974; Butenant *et al.*, 1974). However, even this treatment can produce complications (Fennelly and Fitzgerald, 1971; Gardiner, 1972; Lewis, 1974).

When forced diuresis has been possible, it has been noted that the relative amount of paraquat that can be removed by dialysis is small and unrewarding (Fisher *et al.*, 1971; Hensel and Duerr, 1971; Mascie Taylor *et al.*, 1983). However, in cases of severe renal failure, dialysis seems clearly indicated, regardless of its rather limited ability to remove paraquat (Malone *et al.*, 1971; Eliahou *et al.*, 1973).

Based on clearance values in patients, hemoperfusion was found seven times more effective than hemodialysis (Solfrank *et al.*, 1977).

Replacement blood transfusion removed about 280 mg of paraquat in one case but without benefit to the patient (Mickleson and Fulton, 1971). Survival following plasmapheresis was reported in one case (Dearnaley and Martin, 1978), but the dosage of paraquat had been small.

Judging from general principles as well as from the success of L. L. Smith *et al.* (1974) in treating poisoned animals (see Section 20.16.1.2), emphasis ought to be placed on prompt evacuation of the gastrointestinal tract by gastric and gut lavage, using fuller's earth or bentonite for absorption of unabsorbed paraquat. Actual dosage of cathartics, if used, should be based on medical experience rather than on the animal experiments.

Because animals in oxygen are more sensitive to paraquat than are those in room air, patients should be given supplementary oxygen more as benediction than as a treatment. Fisher *et al.* (1971) considered that atelectasis due to altered alveolar surface forces may be a cause of hypoxemia in paraquat poisoning. Insofar as that is true, efforts to maintain lung inflation should help to avoid a need for increased oxygen tension.

Apparently, Lanzinger *et al.* (1969) were correct when they stated that no treatment had been effective once changes had occurred in the lungs. Since then, exceptions have been rare, and when they do occur there is no way absolutely to prove that the lung trouble is not secondary or in some other way qualitatively different from that in fatal cases. In any event, cases now have been reported in which survival occurred, even though poisoning was marked and there was no reason to suppose that the pulmonary changes were not a direct effect of paraquat. Contrary to Davidson and MacPherson (1972), there has been survival in cases in which there was radiographic indication of lung damage.

In one of these cases, the patient did not enter hospital until the sixth day, and vigorous treatment (prolonged forced diuresis and, somewhat later, brief peritoneal dialysis) was not begun until the eighth day after ingestion. The patient never complained of respiratory symptoms, but fine basal rales were heard from day 10 until day 21, and chest X-rays showed the gradual accumulation of small bilateral effusions between days 12 and 17. A small area of atelactasis or infiltrate appeared in the right upper lobe. The patient was discharged on day 22. When reexamined on day 139, the lung infiltrate, though present, showed further diminution (Fisher *et al.*, 1971). Matthew (1972) questioned whether the lung findings in this case were the same as those in genuine paraquat poisoning, but his objections were satisfactorily refuted by Fisher's response published on the same page.

In a second case (characterized by oliguria, increased BUN, jaundice, and fever), irritating cough and hemoptysis that developed on day 5 were still present on day 10 when X-ray first showed small, bilateral, pleural effusions and a soft shadow in the left lower lobe. Clinical improvement started about day 6, and recovery eventually was complete. Survival was attributed to prolonged hemodialysis (Eliahou *et al.*, 1973). A third case involved renal and cardiac findings as well as slightly abnormal pulmonary function tests and abnormal shadows on X rays of the lungs. Treatment was mainly by peritoneal dialysis (Jones and Owen-Lloyd, 1973). It must be pointed out that, in spite of X-ray and physical findings, the symptoms of respiratory distress in some of these cases seemed to involve the upper tract and that signs or symptoms characteristic of hypoxia were not reported. Furthermore, where measured, the rate of urinary excretion of paraquat was consistent with survival. However, in a fourth case, recovery occurred in spite of "typical pulmonary damage" and a urinary paraquat level of 68 ppm 52 hr after ingestion; the patient was treated by forced diuresis up to day 24, but no steroid and no oxygen were administered (Galloway and Petrie, 1972).

Other cases involving recovery in spite of signs and/or symptoms referable to the respiratory tract have been reported (Grabensee *et al.*, 1971; Pasi and Hine, 1971; Gardiner, 1972; Beevers and Rogers, 1973; Lewis, 1974; Lautenschläger *et al.*, 1974). Perhaps the most dramatic example involved a 32-year-old schizophrenic man who diluted between one-fourth and one-third cup of 20% paraquat with orange juice and drank it. In spite of severe inflammation of the tongue, palate, and pharynx, he did not inform his physician for 6 days. When admitted to hospital 7 days after ingestion, the patient was moderately dyspneic at rest. Chest X rays showed nonspecific consolidation in the left lower lung field, considered consistent with paraquat poisoning. Albuminaria and hematuria were present intermittently. Blood urea was 216 mg %, and creatinine was 10.5 mg %. A qualitative test for paraquat was negative. Initially, he was treated with prednisolone (100 mg daily) and a broad-spectrum antibiotic. However, his condition deteriorated. A chest film

taken on the sixth hospital day showed that the left lobe consolidation had greatly increased and the lateral aspect of the right lung was showing involvement, with overlying pleural reaction. The patient was very dyspneic at rest. His Po_2 fell to 50 mm Hg, and his Pco_2 remained stable at 36 mm Hg. Blood pH was 7.48. In spite of this, oxygen therapy was withheld deliberately. Because some features of the case were similar to those of massive pulmonary fibrosis and because of the possibility that a delayed immune response might contribute to the lung damage, the patient was started on azathioprine 50 mg four times daily. He also received potassium aminobenzoate as an antifibrotic measure. The immunosuppressant therapy was monitored and found effective. By hospital day 33 the appearance of the lungs on X ray had improved, especially on the right, and by hospital day 40 there was further resolution of the lesions. Concomitantly, the blood urea declined to 62 mg %, the creatinine dropped to 0.7 mg %, and the Po_2 steadily rose. There was progressive clinical improvement (Laithwaite, 1975, 1976).

Another case that must be included in this list of survivals is that reported by Beebeejaun *et al.* (1971), in which the patient died 46 days after ingestion but the death was not directly related to poisoning.

A wide range of other drugs has been suggested or actually used for treating paraquat poisoning. The use of vitamin C has been suggested by Halliwell (1976) on the basis of its demonstrated reaction with superoxide (Nashikimi, 1975), its ability to counteract the toxicity of hyperbaric oxygen (Jamieson and van der Brenk, 1964), and its recognized low toxicity in humans. It must be cautioned, however, that its action against hyperbaric oxygen is limited.

Drugs other than (*a*) vitamin C that have been used include (*b*) corticoids such as prednisone (prednisolone) or hydrocortisone (Bullivant, 1966; Kerr *et al.*, 1968; McKean, 1968; Matthew *et al.*, 1968; Douglas *et al.*, 1973) or beclamethasone, a corticosteroid used in the treatment of asthma (Anonymous, 1973); (*c*) d-propranolol as a possible competitor for paraquat on membranes of lung tissue, where it is thought to bind (Anonymous, 1973); (*d*) orgotenin to break down free radicals (Anonymous, 1973); (*e*) immunosuppressants such as azathioprine (Malcolmson and Beesley, 1975; Laithwaite, 1975, 1976), cyclophosphamide (Malone *et al.*, 1971; Douglas *et al.*, 1973), and bleomycin (Mahieu *et al.*, 1977); (*f*) heparin (5000 units intravenously every 4 hr) on the theory that disseminated intravascular coagulation may be a factor in poisoning (Harrison *et al.*, 1972); (*g*) various antibiotics used prophylactically; (*h*) superoxide dismutase, either intravenously or by aerosol (Fairshter *et al.*, 1976); and (*i*) vitamin E, which has had no effect on survival (Yasaka *et al.*, 1986).

Although antibiotics have been given "prophylactically" to many patients, there apparently is no account of a case complicated at any stage by infection. The fact is that, except under anaerobic conditions (Fisher and Williams, 1976), paraquat is antibacterial.

In at least two cases, transplantation of a lung was carried out. In one, the patient survived until 13 days after a transplant made 7 days after ingestion, but pathology considered entirely similar to that in the remaining lung was found in the transplanted one (Matthew *et al.*, 1968). In the second case, one lung transplantation was performed, but (as in the first case) the transplant was subsequently damaged by remaining blood levels of paraquat. An extracorporeal membrane oxygenator and charcoal hemoperfusions (19 days) maintained oxygenation and reduced blood paraquat levels to the undetectable range. A second lung transplantation was then performed. The patient developed a progressive, severe, toxic myopathy with inability to maintain respiration. Death occurred from a cerebrovascular accident 93 days after the initial lung transplant. The authors (Saunders *et al.*, 1985) proposed that the progressive toxic myopathy was due to the paraquat exposure but had not been observed previously because of the brief survival associated with most high exposures.

20.16.2 DIQUAT

20.16.2.1 Identity, Properties, and Uses

Chemical Name   Diquat is the 1,1'-ethylene-2,2'-bipyridylium ion.

Structure   See Fig. 20.9.

Synonyms   The common name diquat (BSI, ISO) is in general use, except in Germany and the USSR, which use the names deiquat and reglon, respectively. Trade names have included Aquacide®; the dibromides are called Reglone®, Reglox®, and Weedtrim D®. A code designation is FB/2. The CAS registry numbers are 231-36-7 for the free ion, 85-00-7 for the dibromide, and 6385-62-2 for the dibromide monohydrate.

Physical and Chemical Properties   The cation has the empirical formula $C_{12}H_{12}N_2$ and a molecular weight of 184.24. The dibromide is $C_{12}H_{12}Br_2N_2$ and has a molecular weight of 344.06. Technical diquat bromide is greater than 95% pure. It forms white to yellow crystals that decompose above 300°C. It has no measurable vapor pressure. The compound is slightly soluble in alcohols and hydroxylic solvents; it is practically insoluble in nonpolar organic solvents. Its solubility in water at 20°C is 70 gm/100 ml. Diquat is stable in acid and neutral solution but unstable under alkaline solutions.

History, Formulations, and Uses   Diquat dibromide was introduced in 1957 by ICI Ltd. It is a quick-acting contact herbicide and plant desiccant with some translocation properties and little residual activity. It is used to control floating and submerged weeds in water not to be used for humans or animals, for preharvest desiccation of various seed crops, and for postemergence control of weeds in cotton. Diquat is formulated as dust or as a 50% solution in water with nonionic surface-active agents or humerents, or both. It is available as water-soluble granules containing 2.5% diquat and 2.5% paraquat.

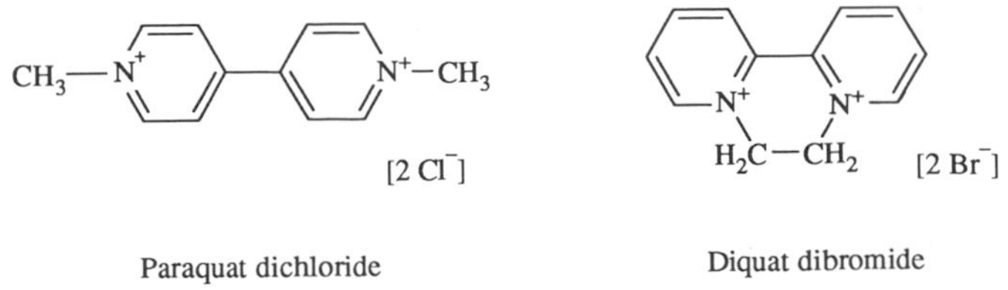

20.16.2.2 Toxicity to Laboratory Animals

Symptomatology   Rats receiving diquat in the LD 50 dosage range show few signs of illness for the first 24 hr. They then become lethargic, show slight pupillary dilatation and some respiratory distress, lose weight, become weaker, and die between 2 and 14 days after dosing. Abdominal distension may be present. Symptomatology is similar in the mouse, guinea pig, rabbit, dog, cow, and hen (Howe and Wright, 1965; Clark and Hurst, 1970). Even after subcutaneous injections, the rat shows no sign of illness for several hours. Pupillary dilatation then occurs to a far greater degree than after oral doses; the light reflex is abolished, and this condition persists until death. The rest of the course is similar to that after an oral dose, except that rats surviving 7 days or more often have greatly distended abdoments (Clark and Hurst, 1970). Diquat administered orally to rats at the LD 50 rate had an effect on the distribution of water within the body, and early deaths were associated with rapid fluid loss into the gastrointestinal tract. The effect of subcutaneous diquat on water distribution was delayed and was less pronounced (Crabtree *et al.*, 1977). The accumulation of fluid was caused mainly by increased production and not by reduced emptying time, although emptying time was delayed (Crabtree and Rose, 1978).

The accumulation of water in the lung (edema) and increased uptake of thymidine by lung DNA that occurred on the third day after a single oral administration of paraquat at the rate of 105 μmol/kg were not seen after an equal dosage of diquat (Smith and Rose, 1977).

A subcutaneous dose of diquat at four to five times the LD 50 level makes rats quiet in a few minutes and produces labored respiration within an hour. The animals die within a few hours in generalized convulsions (Clark and Hurst, 1970).

The effects of diquat and paraquat are much more similar following repeated doses than after one or a few doses. Diquat at a dosage of 4 mg/kg/day for 2 years produced no behavioral differences or change in general condition or mortality. There was no evidence of malignancy and no significant change in the liver, kidneys, and myocardium. However, this dosage caused swelling and desquamation of lung cells, thickening of the interalveolar septa, and hyperplasia of the peribronchial lymph tissues. A dosage of 2 mg/kg/day produced only relatively minor changes in the lungs (Bainova and Vlucheva, 1978).

A single dose of diquat is not irritating to the skin of rabbits. Repeated dermal doses cause mild redness, thickening, and scabbing (Howe and Wright, 1965; Clark and Hurst, 1970; Pirie and Ress, 1970).

Figure 20.9   Two bipyridal herbicides.

Dosage Responses The acute toxicity of diquat (see Table 20.9) is similar to that of paraquat. Except for the greater susceptibility of cattle, there is little species difference. Rats observed for a year after surviving a lethal dose of diquat remained well throughout the period (Clark and Hurst, 1970).

Rats are not killed by a dietary level of 1000 ppm for 2 years, but their food consumption and growth are reduced. A dietary level of 500 ppm (about 25 mg/kg/day) does not affect food intake, growth, blood or urinary findings, or pathology, except that of the eye. Cataracts show a clear dosage–response relationship, appearing earlier, more severely, and more frequently at higher dietary levels. At a level of 1000 ppm complete opacities appear in one or both lenses within 6 months. At 50 ppm, slight opacities appear in some animals in 12 months, but about three-fourths of these animals show no cataracts, even after a year. A dietary level of 10 ppm (about 0.5 mg/kg/day) does not produce cataracts in a 2-year test.

At higher dosage levels, development of cataract is followed by secondary changes, including anterior or posterior synechiae, hemorrhage into the vitreous humor, and detachment of the retina.

Prolonged exposure to diquat is necessary to produce cataracts. A single near-fatal dose is not effective. A dietary level of 50 ppm does not produce cataract within a year if the rats are transferred to a normal diet at the end of an 8-week feeding period.

Some forms of cataract respond to light, but not those caused by diquat. Ascorbic acid (20%) in the drinking water of rats receiving diquat in their diet does not influence development of cataract (Clark and Hurst, 1970).

Dogs tolerate a dosage of 15 mg/kg/day for 2 years without change in growth, blood and urinary findings, liver function, or

Table 20.9
Acute Toxicity of Diquat Ion

Species	Route	LD 50 (mg/kg)	Reference
Rat	oral	400	Howe and Wright (1965)
Rat, F	oral	231	Clark and Hurst (1970)
Rat, F	subcutaneous	11–20	Clark and Hurst (1970)
Mouse	oral	170	Howe and Wright (1965)
Mouse, M	oral	125	Clark and Hurst (1970)
Guinea pig	oral	100	Clark and Hurst (1970)
Rabbit	oral	190	Howe and Wright (1965)
Rabbit, F	oral	101	Clark and Hurst (1970)
Rabbit	dermal	500[a]	Howe and Wright (1965)
Rabbit	dermal	>400	Clark and Hurst (1970)
Dog	oral	>200	Howe and Wright (1965)
Dog, F	oral	100–200	Clark and Hurst (1970)
Cow	oral	30[a]	Howe and Wright (1965)
Cow	oral	30[a]	Clark and Hurst (1970)
Hen	oral	200–400	Clark and Hurst (1970)

[a]Approximate.

histology, except that of the eye. As in the rat, the cataracts show a definite dosage–response relationship. At 15 mg/kg/day, bilateral opacities appear in 10–11 months. Dogs tolerate 1.7 mg/kg/day for 4 years without developing cataracts (Clark and Hurst, 1970).

When rats, mice, and dogs were exposed to aerosols of carefully controlled particle size, lung irritation was found to be much less with diquat than with paraquat. Whereas 0.1 mg/m³ of respirable paraquat would not be excessive, this standard could be 0.5 mg/m³ for diquat (Gage, 1968). Somewhat less toxicity and major injury to the upper rather than the lower respiratory tract were found in connection with a similar range of concentrations (Bainova et al., 1972), presumably because of larger particle sizes.

Absorption, Distribution, Metabolism, and Excretion Absorption of orally administered radioactive diquat in rats was poor. Not over 6% was recovered in the urine, even though 88–98% appeared in the urine when the compound was given subcutaneously (Daniel and Gage, 1966).

When diquat was administered to dogs orally at the rate of 0.012 mg/kg, there was no definite plasma peak, and only about 10–20% was absorbed in 6 hr (Bennett et al., 1976).

Radioanalysis of the tissues of a calf killed 24 hr after oral dosing showed that little diquat or metabolite remained in any organ. A concentration of 0.20 ppm diquat equivalent was found in the liver and 0.66 ppm in the kidney. The lung contained only 0.03 ppm, no more than the blood serum. Much of this material was metabolized; in fact, no diquat ion (<0.01 ppm) was found in the kidney (Stevens and Walley, 1966). Another calf dosed orally at the rate of 8.3 mg/kg with bridge-labeled diquat dibromide had radioactivity reported as diquat ion as follows: kidney, 1.06 ppm; liver, 0.31; other organs (including lung, heart, pancreas, spleen, and testes), 0.02–0.05 ppm; and fat and muscle, about 0.01 (Howe and Wright, 1965).

Following intravenous administration, diquat and paraquat are distributed in a similar way in mice, except that paraquat but not diquat persists in lung and muscle. Diquat did not accumulate in rats at a dietary level of 25 ppm for 8 weeks (Litchfield et al., 1973).

Diquat apparently is not metabolized in the body. However, about 70% of it is metabolized in the intestine and a portion of the altered material amounting to 0.5–5.4% of the original dose is absorbed and excreted in the urine. The metabolism is promoted by fresh, but not heated, cecal contents (Daniel and Gage, 1966).

Following subcutaneous injection in rats, excretion of about 90% of the compound occurred in the urine on the first day and almost all of the remainder on the next day. Not more than 2% was found in the feces. No excretion was detected after the third day. A total of 90–98% of the dose was accounted for (Daniel and Gage, 1966).

Following oral administration in rats, most of the compound was unabsorbed and appeared in the feces. Only 4–6% was recovered in the urine in tests in which total recovery varied from 93 to 101%. Even after oral administration, urinary excretion was usually greatest on the first day (Daniel and Gage, 1966).

After oral dosing, 1.1–4.8% was recovered in the bile during the first 24 hr (Daniel and Gage, 1966).

In cattle 0.004–0.015% of an oral dose was recovered in the milk, chiefly in the form of two unidentified metabolites. Only 0.4–2.6%, also largely metabolized, was recovered in the urine (Stevens and Walley, 1966).

Biochemical Effects   The toxicity of diquat depends entirely on the cation; the various anions (dibromide, dichloride) contribute nothing to the injury (Clark and Hurst, 1970).

Diquat free radical can be formed by reaction of the compound with glutathione reductase. The inhibitory effect of superoxide dismutase in these reactions indicates that superoxide radicals are formed by the aerobic autoxidation of diquat free radicals, which in turn indicates that superoxide radicals can be formed in this way in tissues of intact animals (Stancliffe and Pirie, 1971).

When dipyridylium herbicides were incubated in homogenates of rat lung, kidney, and liver, specific rates for appearance of the radical decreased in the following order: morfamquat > diquat > paraquat. Carbon monoxide inhibited the rate of appearance of the diquat radical in all three homogenates but did not change radical formation from morfamquat or paraquat. On the basis of this and other findings, it was concluded that diquat is reduced by an electron-transferring agent different from that effective for the other two compounds (Baldwin *et al.*, 1975).

Many of the papers discussed in connection with the Biochemical Effects of paraquat (Section 20.16.1.2) are concerned with diquat also. In summary, it can be said that both compounds act by forming free radicals, but whereas there are many differences in the details of their biochemical effects, the reasons for the differences in their clinical effects remain obscure.

Plasma corticosteroid concentrations were significantly increased in rats within 15 min after an intraperitoneal or subcutaneous LD 50 dose, but were posponed about 1 hr after an equivalent oral dose. On the basis of extensive study, it was concluded that the increase in adrenal steroid synthesis was caused by increased response of the adrenal cortex to ACTH and by release of ACTH from the pituitary (Rose *et al.*, 1974; Crabtree and Rose, 1976).

Effects on Organs and Tissues   Diquat was not mutagenic when tested in the Ames test (Andersen *et al.*, 1972; Benigni *et al.*, 1979; Levin *et al.*, 1982). It was not mutagenic when tested in the mouse dominant lethal test (Pasi *et al.*, 1974), but fertility of males was reduced, regardless of the stage of spermatogenesis at treatment. The lack of a mutagenic effect was observed in other studies including chromosomal aberrations in mice (Selypes *et al.*, 1980) and recessive lethal tests in *Drosophila melanogaster*.

In contrast, positive effects in mutagenicity tests with diquat have been reported with gene conversion in *Saccharomyces cerevisiae* (Siebert and Lemperle, 1974), DNA repair in *Salmonella typhimurium*, and gene mutation in *Aspergillus nidulans* (Benigni *et al.*, 1979). Irrespective of the notorious insensitivity of the dominant lethal test, most of the mutagenicity data suggests that diquat is not mutagenic. Furthermore, diquat did not induce tumors in 2-year rat feeding studies at dietary levels of 720 ppm (Clark and Hurst, 1970).

The toxicity of diquat to mouse fibroblasts *in vitro* is approximately 10 times greater than that of paraquat (Styles, 1974).

As discussed under Symptomatology, rats killed by diquat may have greatly distended abdomens resulting from filling of the gastrointestinal tract by fluid. Following an oral dose at the LD 50 level, this distension reaches a maximum after 24 hr, when it amounts to approximately 14 ml per rat. Other tissues, especially blood, are dehydrated. The degree of water displacement is dosage related. Following subcutaneous injection, the increase in fluid in the gastrointestinal tract is delayed; severe changes are limited to fatally poisoned animals; and tissue water is significantly increased, not decreased. Just what bearing the redistribution of water has on toxicity is not clear, especially because tissue is dehydrated after a fatal oral dose but hydrated after a fatal subcutaneous dose (Crabtree *et al.*, 1977).

There is some indication that the early decrease in glomerular filtration rate and in the clearance of acidic compounds by the kidney is the result of change of hemodynamics secondary to fluid loss (Lock, 1979). Later toxic changes in the kidney tubules no doubt contribute to renal dysfunction.

Following intraperitoneal injection of radioactive diquat, radioactivity appears in the lens, as well as in other tissues. The ascorbic acid content of the lens and of the intraocular fluids falls during development of cataracts, but reduced glutathione of the lens remains high (Pirie and Rees, 1970; Pirie *et al.*, 1970).

Effects on Reproduction   A standard three-generation test in rats was carried out with diquat at dietary levels of 500, 250, and 0 ppm. The food intake of animals receiving 500 ppm (normally about 25 mg/kg/day in nonlactating adult rats but higher in others) was reduced, and they did not grow normally; however, their reproduction was unaffected. Specifically, fertility, period between mating and production of litters, mean litter size, number of stillborn, sex distribution, and congenital abnormalities were statistically indistinguishable from those of controls. Behavior was unaffected. Gross and microscopic pathology showed no difference from the controls, except for lens opacities. These were seen in animals receiving 500 ppm in 91, 106, and 124 days in the P, F_{1b}, and F_{2b} generations, respectively, and after about 280 days the lesion reached incidences of 55, 70, and 47% in the same generations. Thus, the time of onset and the incidence were not different in rats first exposed when they were 35 days old and those exposed during the intrauterine and neonatal periods. Rats on a dietary level of 250 ppm showed less than normal weight during part but not all of their lives and in only one generation. Their reproduction and other findings were normal (FAO/WHO, 1973).

When [^{14}C]diquat and [^{14}C]paraquat were injected separately intravenously into rats at the rate of 15 mg/kg on any one day from days 7–21 of gestation, more diquat than paraquat reached the fetuses, and diquat caused a correspondingly greater fetal mortality and resorption. The two compounds caused about equal mortality among the dams (Bus *et al.*, 1975c).

A single intraperitoneal injection of 7 mg/kg during days 6–14 of gestation produced a high incidence of reduced weight gain and retarded ossification in rats but no true teratogenesis. Repeated intraperitoneal injections of 0.5 mg/kg/day did not cause an increase in embryopathic effects (Khera and Whitta, 1970).

Pathology Rats killed by oral doses of diquat often show some dilatation of both the pupils and the intestines. Rats killed by the subcutaneous route show extreme mydriasis, gross distension of the cecum, and sometimes a reduction of the size of the spleen and thymus. The intestines of those killed within 24 hr after an oral dose often contain quantities of greenish-yellow or grass-green fluid due to the reduction of diquat by bacterial action. The same color can be produced by the action of fresh intestinal contents or of bacteria isolated therefrom. The color of the intestinal contents is gray-green or olive-green stained by bile pigments following subcutaneous administration (Clark and Hurst, 1970).

Accumulation of fluid in the stomach of rats following an oral dose of diquat at the LD 50 level was associated with erosion of the surface mucus-secreting layers of cells of the antrum of the stomach and some of the underlying glandular mucosa also. Less marked erosion of the mucosa plus focal vacuolation of parietal cells was seen in the fundus. Edema fluid was present in the interstitium as well as in the vacuoles, and this was not secondary to vascular changes (Pratt *et al.*, 1978). However, Crabtree *et al.* (1977) regarded the histological changes in the gastrointestinal tract as minimal and inadequate to explain the pooling of fluid in the tract.

The most important histopathological changes in cynomolgus monkeys following oral administration of diquat ion at rates of 100–400 mg/kg were necrosis of the epithelium and villi of the gastrointestinal tract and of the epithelium of the proximal and distal convoluted tubules of the kidneys; changes in the liver were minimal (Cobb and Grimshaw, 1979).

Opacities of the lens develop in rats maintained on a diet containing diquat at a concentration of 500–700 ppm (Pirie and Ress, 1970).

Significant vascular disorders; focal necrosis of brain ganglionic cells with associated glial proliferation; focal necrosis in the kidneys, liver, and myocardium; and, most interestingly, focal fibrosis of the lungs were reported in rats that received 0.02 LD 50 per day for 12 months or 0.1 LD 50 per day for 6 months (Pushkar', 1969). Apparently, these results have not been confirmed exactly. Bainova (1969) found no significant deviation in clinical and laboratory findings for rats that received 0.1 LD 50 twice a week for 4.5 months, but did report papillomatous growth of the bronchial epithelium in rats receiving 0.2 LD 50 doses (26 mg/kg/day). It may be that the differences in the long-term effects of diquat and paraquat on the lung are more quantitative than qualitative.

20.16.2.3 Toxicity to Humans

Experimental Exposure Although 61% of diquat injected intravenously was recovered in the urine, only about 0.3% was excreted following dermal application (Feldmann and Maibach, 1974).

Accidental and Intentional Poisoning There is less information about the toxicity of diquat to humans than about many other compounds because there have been fewer cases of human poisoning. Some examples are found in the literature [World Health Organization (WHO), 1984]. The initial course of a man who drank diquat with suicidal intent resembled that typical of paraquat: gastrointestinal symptoms, ulceration of the mucous membranes, acute renal failure, toxic liver damage, and respiratory difficulty. However, central nervous system effects apparently were more severe and certainly were the result of bleeding into the brain stem. Death was due to cardiac arrest on the sixth day. Autopsy revealed, in addition to the brain hemorrhage, inter- and intraalveolar exudation and hyaline membranes, but no proliferative or fibroplastic change (Schönborn *et al.*, 1971). Similar findings, with the exception of neurological involvement, were found in another case (Narita *et al.*, 1978).

A 53-year-old man accidentally swallowed less than a mouthful of diquat of unstated concentration. Nausea, emesis, and diarrhea were the first symptoms. Adsorbents were administered soon after poisoning. Despite forced fluids for 2 or 3 days, the patient developed oliguria and then anuria with consequent azotemia. He was treated by hemodialysis for 6–7 hr daily at 2- to 3-day intervals. During the second week, the patient developed bilateral pneumonia, which responded to antibiotic therapy. The patient was discharged in good condition on day 26 (Fel *et al.*, 1976). The pneumonia can be considered coincidental insofar as it was bacterial in origin and responded to antibiotics. In their discussion, the authors spoke of a pulmonary stage as typical of poisoning, but neither animal experiments nor the course of other human cases justifies this view.

In another instance, illness was limited to diarrhea and difficulty in swallowing associated with ulceration in the mouth. Forced diuresis was started a little over 56 hr after accidental ingestion; the average 24-hr urinary output during the first 10 days was 9739 ml. Thereafter, the diuresis diminished gradually during 6 days. Diquat was detected in the urine for 11 days after ingestion. No progression of illness was detected; the patient was discharged on day 22 in very good condition (Oreopolos and McEvoy, 1969).

Powell *et al.* (1983) describe a case involving a 2.5-year-old child who consumed a lethal dose of diquat. Renal, gastrointestinal, pulmonary, and CNS involvement resembled that seen in adults after ingestion of diquat. Hemoperfusion with cellulose-coated activated charcoal reduced plasma levels of diquat (Amberlite XAD-4 was ineffective), but sequestration of diquat in the tissue produced a rebound of the plasma concentrations after treatment. Mahieu *et al.* (1984) reported a case in which renal proximal tubule damage was estimated by plasma and urine diquat concentration.

Use Experience   Workers who have skin contact with concentrated diquat solutions may show a color change and softening of one or more fingernails. The injury is local and not symmetrical. In some instances, the nail was shed and was not regrown (Samman and Johnston, 1969).

Dust or mist of the compound has led to nosebleeds (Howe and Wright, 1965; Clark and Hurst, 1970). It is also reported that mists may cause skin irritation, irritation of the mouth and upper respiratory tract, cough, and chest pain. A case of severe eye injury caused by a mixture of paraquat and diquat is described under paraquat (Section 20.16.1.3). Concentrated solutions may delay the healing of superficial cuts on the hands and interfere with nail growth if they contact the base of the nail for a few minutes (Clark and Hurst, 1970).

Diquat is not known to have caused cataract in humans. This may be due to lack of sufficient exposure. However, the absence in poisoned people of signs commonly seen in animals (lethargy, pupillary dilatation, weight loss, and abdominal distension) may indicate a true species difference.

Atypical Cases of Various Origins   A 45-year-old man developed myalgia, intermittent periorbital headache, and cough productive of thick, red, jelly-like sputum. He was treated with tetracycline, but he became worse and entered the hospital 4 days after onset. At that time he had neck stiffness, cough, and a temperature of 40.5°C, and he was in a confused state. Both physical findings and X-ray indicated consolidation of certain lung areas. Over the next several days, these consolidations cleared while new ones appeared in other lung areas. The patient was started on ampicillin, but this was changed to erythromycin. He gradually became somewhat worse; his temperature increased. On the fourth hospital day, he developed a slight icterus, and a blotchy erythematous rash appeared on the left arm. At this point the possibility was considered that the illness might be caused by diquat, and treatment with prednisone (15 mg every 6 hr orally) was begun. By the next day crisis had occurred. The patient's temperature had dropped from 41.5° to 35°C; he was rational, and his rash had begun to clear. Within 2 days, the rash resolved, and the jaundice cleared; in 5 days chest roentgenograms were normal. The patient was able to recall that his pressurized hand sprayer had discharged a cloud of aerosol in his face when its nozzle became unclogged. The paper failed to record when this happened (Wood *et al.*, 1976). Although little is known of what effect diquat aerosol might have on people, the absence of any irritation of the eyes, face, or nasal mucosa and the presence of high fever make the diagnosis of diquat poisoning in this case very doubtful. Animal studies (Section 20.16.2.2) indicate that diquat is much less irritant than paraquat to the lungs. Affected animals become cold rather than developing a fever.

Dosage Response   Vanholder *et al.* (1981) reviewed 11 cases of diquat exposure and concluded that the lethal human dose is 6–12 gm of diquat dibromide. The threshold limit value of 0.5 mg/m^3 indicates that occupational intake of diquat at a rate of about 0.07 mg/kg/day is considered safe.

Laboratory Findings   Prior to death, concentrations of 1.15–1.85 ppm were found in the urine and 0.45–0.55 ppm were found in the blood. Following autopsy, concentrations of 0.11–1.19 ppm were found in different organs, the highest value being for the kidney (Schönborn *et al.*, 1971).

Pathology   In one case, autopsy revealed ulceration of the mouth and upper gastrointestinal tract and general necrosis of the renal tubules with relatively normal glomeruli. Numerous punctate hemorrhages were seen in the lungs and in the retroperitoneal lymph nodes (Narita *et al.*, 1978).

Treatment of Poisoning   Treatment of poisoning by diquat is the same as treatment of poisoning by paraquat (see Section 20.16.1.3). The following paragraph is concerned with treatment in a specific case of diquat poisoning.

A 43-year-old woman entered the hospital when she was already stuporous, anuric, and in a state of shock; areas of hemorrhagic necrosis were present on the mucosa of the mouth, throat, and esophagus. With suicidal intent she had swallowed an unknown quantity of diquat 3 days earlier and again 1 day earlier. Within the first 27 hr in hospital, two hemodialyses were carried out for 6.5 and 5 hr, respectively. At the end of the first period, the concentration of diquat in the blood was reduced to 30% of its starting value, but it dropped to only 60% in the second period. Clearance was calculated as 3.17 ml/min. However, the concentration in blood was low at all times, and only 0.84 mg of diquat was cleared, corresponding to only 0.7% of the 12 gm estimated to have been absorbed. It was concluded that hemodialysis is not an efficient way to eliminate diquat more than 1 day after injection. The patient died following prolonged cardiovascular collapse.

20.17 TRIAZINES AND TRIAZOLES

The triazines constitute the second largest group of herbicides sold in the United States (see Section 20.1). In fact atrazine in this class is the second largest-selling herbicide in the United States, with an annual application of 79 million pounds (National Research Council, 1987). Triazole products have found efficacious use not only as herbicides but also as fungicides (agriculturally and clinically) and as insecticides. The structures of four chlorotriazines—atrazine, cyanazine, propazine, and simazine—and the triazole amitrole are presented in Fig. 20.10. (These compounds will each be considered in greater detail.)

The chemical structures of the substituted *s*-triazine herbicides are centered about a common six-membered ring composed of three nitrogens and three carbons arranged symmetrically (i.e., alternating) about the ring. Substitutions occur in the 2, 4, and 6 positions; the most common substitutions in the 2 position are chlorine, methoxyl, and methylthio. In the 4 and 6 positions, amino substitutions are the most common. Triazoles are five-membered rings with two carbons and three nitrogens. The substitutions on the ring vary substantially within this class.

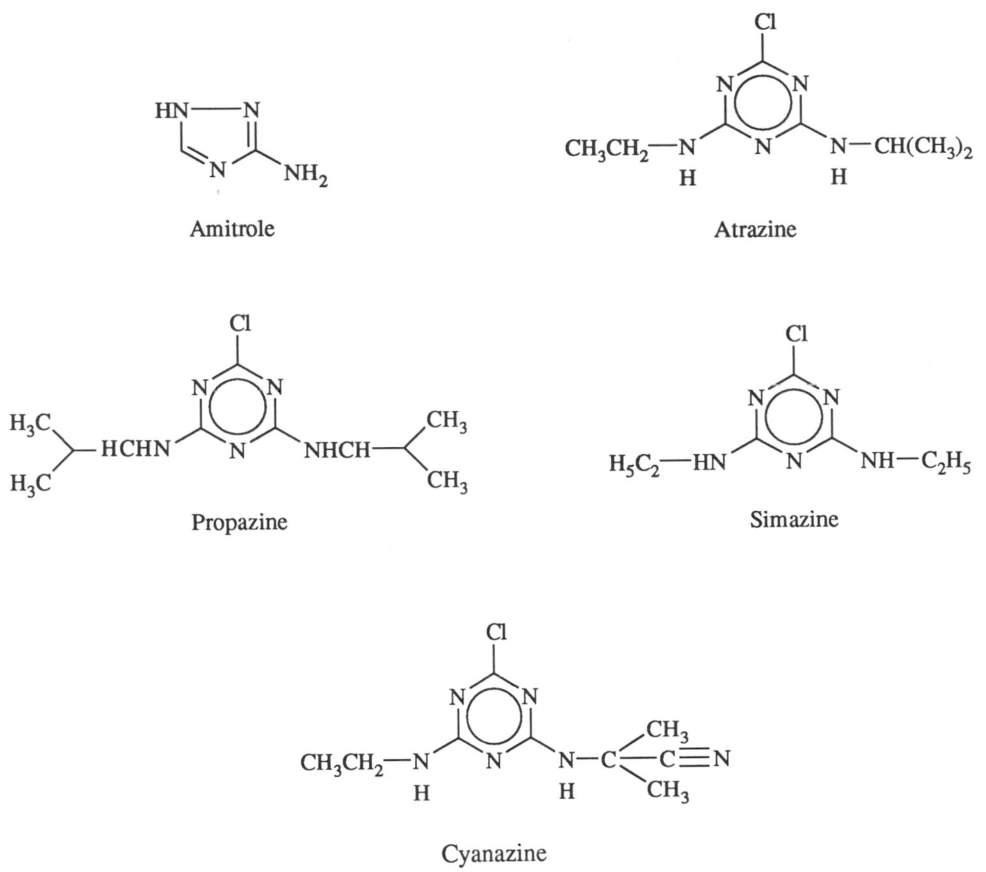

Figure 20.10 Selected triazole and triazine herbicides.

In addition to atrazine, cyanazine, propazine, and simazine, other important triazines include ametryn (ANSI, BSI, ISO, WSSA) (oral LD 50 in rat of 110–1750 mg/kg), atratone (BSI, ISO) (oral LD 50 in rat of 1465–2400 mg/kg), aziprotyne (BSI, ISO) or aziprotryn (WSSA) (oral LD 50 in rat of 3600–5800 mg/kg), desmetryn (ISO) or desmetryne (BSI, WSSA) (oral LD 50 in rat of 1390 mg/kg), methoprotryne (BSI, ISO) (discontinued in 1984; LD 50 > 5000 mg/kg), metribuzin (BSI, ISO, WSSA) (oral LD 50 of 1100–2300 mg/kg), prometon (ANSI, BSI, ISO, WSSA) (oral LD 50 in rat of 2980 mg/kg), prometryn (ANSI, ISO, WSSA) or prometryne (BSI) (oral LD 50 in rat of 3150–5235 mg/kg), simetryn (ISO, WSSA) or simetryne (BSI) (oral LD 50 in rat of 1830 mg/kg), terbutryn (ANSI, ISO, WSSA) or terbutryne (BSI) (oral LD 50 in rat of 2000–2980 mg/kg), and trietazine (ANSI, BSI, WSSA) (oral LD 50 in rat of 594–841 mg/kg).

20.17.1 ATRAZINE

20.17.1.1 Identity, Properties, and Uses

Chemical Name Atrazine is 2-chloro-4-ethylamino-6-isopropylamine-*s*-triazine (CAS) and 6-chloro-*N*-ethyl-*N*'-isopropyl-1,3,5-triazinediyl-2,4-diamine (IUPAC).

Structure See Fig. 20.7.

Synonyms The common name atrazine (ANSI, BSI, E-ISO, F-ISO, JMAF, WSSA) is in general use. Trade names include AAtre®, Actinite® PK, Aktikon® PK, Aktikon®, Aktinit® A, Aktinit® PK, Argezin®, Atranex®, Atrasine®, Atrataf®, Atratol®, Atrazinek®, Atrazin®, Atred®, Candex®, Cekuzina-T®, Chromozin®, Crisazine®, Cyazin®, Fenatrol®, Gesaprim®, Griffex®, Hungazin® PK, Hungazin®, Inakor®, Oleogesaprim®, Pitezin®, Primase®, Primatol® A, Vectal SC®, Weedex® A, Wonuk®, Zeazin®, and Zeazine®. A code designation is G-30027. The CAS registry number is 1912-24-9.

Physical and Chemical Properties Atrazine has the empirical formula $C_8H_{14}ClN_5$ and a molecular weight of 215.69. It forms colorless crystals with a melting point of 175–177°C and a vapor pressure of 3.0×10^{-7} mm Hg at 20°C. The solubility of atrazine in water is 30 mg/liter at 20°C; in methanol it is 18,000 mg/liter and in chloroform it is 52,000 mg/liter. Atrazine is stable in neutral, slightly acidic, or basic material, but it is hydrolyzed by alkali or mineral acids at higher temperatures. It has a slight sensitivity to natural light and extreme temperature. Atrazine has a good shelf life and residual activity.

History, Formulations, and Uses Atrazine was introduced in 1958 by J. R. Geigy S. A. It is a selective pre- and postemergence herbicide used on crops such as maize, sorghum, sugarcane, pineapples, and nursery conifers as well as in forestry conservation. Its mode of action is inhibition of the Hill reaction involved in the photosynthesis process (Gysin and Knuesli, 1960). It also is used for general weed control at higher rates and for selective control of pond weeds, especially submerged plants. Atrazine is available as 50 and 80% wettable powders and in a flowable formulation.

20.17.1.2 Toxicity to Laboratory Animals

Symptomatology   At lethal or near-lethal doses, rats showed excitation followed by depression with reduced respiratory rate, motor incoordination, clonic and sometimes tonic spasms, and hypothermia; they died within 12–24 hr after oral administration.

Irritation and Sensitization   Although atrazine has been reported as irritating to the eye (Gzhegotskiy *et al.*, 1977), the manufacturers of technical atrazine have found the material to be nonirritating to the rabbit eye and slightly irritating to the rabbit skin. Atrazine in a modified Buehler sensitization test in the guinea pig was found to be a sensitizer (CIBA-GEIGY, 1982b).

Response to Single Dose   Atrazine is a compound of low acute toxicity. Oral LD 50 values of approximately 1900–3000 mg/kg in rats have been reported (Worthing, 1987). The oral LD 50 values for mice and rabbits have been reported as 1750 and 750 mg/kg, respectively (Hartley and Kidd, 1983). Dermal LD 50 in rats and inhalation LC 50 (1 hr) were reported in excess of 3000 mg/kg and 700 mg/m³ (Worthing, 1987). In fact, the actual dermal LD 50 for rabbits has been reported as 7500 mt/kt (Reinhardt and Brittelli, 1981).

Response to Repeated Doses   In rats fed atrazine for 6 months, dietary levels of 100 and 500 ppm caused growth retardation, partly due to reduction in food intake. Histological examination revealed no lesions (Suschetet *et al.*, 1974).

Absorption, Distribution, Metabolism, and Excretion   *In vitro* study of the biotransformation of atrazine by rat liver fraction showed that dealkylation predominated over conjugation. The isopropyl group was more easily removed than the ethyl group. For atrazine and its metabolites that were studied, dealkylation and conjugation were accomplished by the microsomal and soluble fractions, respectively. No evidence for dechlorination of chloro-*s*-thiazines was observed (Dauterman and Muecke, 1974). The major metabolites in the rat appear to be mono- or di-*N*-dealkylated products; approximately 80% of a radiolabeled dose is eliminated in 72 hr (Bakke *et al.*, 1972).

In vivo, chickens remove the ethyl rather than the isopropyl group, and they also replace the chlorine with a hydroxyl group. Some atrazine and its metabolites continued to be excreted for 4 days after feeding of atrazine was stopped. More metabolites were identified in the tissues than in the urine. After atrazine had been fed at a dietary level of 100 ppm for 7 days, the highest

concentration of atrazine (38.8 ppm) was in abdominal fat, but the highest concentrations of hydroxyatrazine (16.2 ppm) and of deethylhydroxyatrazine (15.5 ppm) were in the liver (Foster and Khan, 1976; Khan and Foster, 1976).

Following oral administration, technical atrazine and its metabolites were detected in the urine of pigs for slightly over 24 hr. Gas chromatographic–mass spectrophotometric analysis showed conclusively that the parent compound was the main material excreted (Erickson *et al.*, 1979).

Mutagenesis   Atrazine has been examined in more than four dozen different mutagenicity studies, including studies designed to evaluate gene mutation and chromosomal aberrations, and other tests designed to look at interaction with DNA. Evaluation techniques have been employed which utilize plant, animal, and microbial systems. The weight of evidence ascertained from more than 50 studies reported in the literature as well as information found in the manufacturer's files indicates that atrazine alone or atrazine following mammalian activation is not mutagenic (CIBA-GEIGY, 1987).

Carcinogenesis   Atrazine was not tumorigenic when tested in two strains of mice receiving an oral exposure to 21.5 mg/kg/day from age 1 to 4 weeks followed by dietary administration of 82 mg/kg for an additional 17 months (Innes *et al.*, 1969). Despite these findings, the National Research Council (1987) indicated that the Environmental Protection Agency had received information that atrazine showed positive results for oncogenicity in animals. Mammary tumors were observed in rats after lifetime administration. This response was restricted to female Sprague–Dawley rats or mice of either sex.

Effects on Reproduction   Subcutaneous injection of atrazine at 800 mg/kg/day on days 3, 6, and 9 of gestation resulted in the death and resorption of some or all the pups in each litter of rats. Dosages as high as 200 mg/kg/day by this route did not affect the number of pups per litter or their weight at weaning. Dietary levels up to 1000 ppm (about 50 mg/kg/day) also were harmless (Peters and Cook, 1973).

A dosage of 30 mg/kg killed pregnant and nonpregnant ewes in 36–60 days; the embryos in some pregnant ones had been killed, but some fetuses appeared normal when the dam died. All ewes that received 15 mg/kg/day throughout pregnancy delivered normal lambs at term. These lambs were nursed by their mothers for 30 days while the ewes continued to receive atrazine, without any indication of poisoning of either (Binns and Johnson, 1970).

As shown by the Bionetics Study, atrazine caused no significant increase in anomalies in fetuses of three strains of mice after a maternal dosage of 46.4 mg/kg/day during days 6–14 of gestation (Mrak, 1969).

Pathology   Rats that died within 6 hr after oral administration at the rate of 3000 mg/kg showed lung edema with extensive hemorrhagic foci, cardiac dilation, and macroscopic hemorrhages in the liver and spleen. Rats that died during the second day following the same dosage showed hemorrhagic pneumonia, hemorrhage in other organs, and dystrophic changes of the kidney tubules (Molnar, 1971).

Of rats that received atrazine orally for 6 months at a rate of 20 mg/kg/day, 40% died with signs of respiratory distress and paralysis of the limbs. Incurrent bronchitis and peribronchitis were most likely the cause of the respiratory distress; capillary and pericapillary edema of the brain with dystrophy of cerebral and cerebellar cells may have been related to the paralysis (Nezefi, 1971). These findings contrast significantly with those of Suschetet *et al.* (1974), who found no pathology in rats that received about 25 mg/kg/day for 6 months, and they are totally inconsistent with the available data base for atrazine (Beste, 1983). It has been speculated that the difference in the response in Nezefi's work and that of others may depend on one or more contaminants in the more toxic formulation (Hayes, 1982).

20.17.1.3 Toxicity to Humans

Exposure and Use Experience There have been no substantiated cases of acute poisonings in humans from the ingestion of atrazine (CIBA-GEIGY, 1982b). The following are representative cases of eye and skin exposure incidents. While clearing a clogged vent hose in a tank car, an adult male was exposed to a formulation of atrazine containing 4 lb/gal when the valve suddenly gave under pressure, splashing the material on part of his body and face. He immediately rinsed his eyes with water and went to an ophthalmologist. The physician found a slight abrasion of his cornea and prescribed medication. Recovery was effected within a week.

In a second case, a farmer developed a skin rash on his face and swelling of the area around his eyes 5–6 hr after the use of an 80% wettable powder formulation of atrazine. When he visited his physician the next morning, the swelling had considerably decreased. The physician administered antihistamine; the swelling and dermatitis cleared up satisfactorily.

Atypical Cases of Various Origins A farmer, who had developed dermatitis of the hands and forearms from propachlor 1 year and also a few weeks earlier, sprayed atrazine and cleaned the clogged nozzles without protection. During the same afternoon he sprayed cyanazine. Before he had finished spraying, blisters began forming on his hands and forearms. The condition became so severe that he sought medical help during the night. When seen by the physician approximately 14 hr after onset, his hands were painful, swollen, red, and blistered. Hemorrhagic bullae were seen between the fingers. There were no other significant physical findings. Nine hours later the hands were more ecchymotic, and more vesicles were present. The condition, which was completely incapacitating, was photographed. Treatment included codeine and prednisone and soaking of the hands in 0.25% acetic acid. Tetracycline was administered prophylactically. Within 4 days the pain was gone and the swelling was slightly reduced. Ninety percent recovery of the hands and

forearms was achieved in 28 days (Schlicher and Beat, 1972). Several months later a patch test was done using 1:1000 dilution of a commercial atrazine formulation. Within 48 hr the reaction was strongly positive with clusters of tiny vesicles on an erythematous base (J. E. Schlicher, personal communication to W. J. Hayes, Jr., 1978). There can be no doubt that the dermatitis was caused by the atrazine formulation, which was contacted during the morning in great quantity. However, the fact that the farmer twice had experienced a vesicular dermatitis in response to propachlor and that one of these instances involved a granular formulation suggests a very unusual susceptibility to amides and, even in the absence of any test, suggests that ancillary materials in the spray contributed little to the dermatitis.

Treatment of Poisoning Treatment is entirely symptomatic.

20.17.2 CYANAZINE

20.17.2.1 Identity, Properties, and Uses

Chemical Name Cyanazine is 2-[[4-chloro-6-(ethylamino)-*s*-triazin-2-yl]amino]-2-methylpropionitrile (IUPAC) or [2-chloro-4-(1-cyano-1-methylethylamino)-6-ethylamino-*s*-triazine] (CAS).

Structure See Fig. 20.10.

Synonyms The common name cyanazine (BSI, ISO, WSSA) is in general use. Trade names include Bladex® and Fortrol®. Code designations include SD15418 and WL19805. The CAS registry number is 21725-46-2.

Physical and Chemical Properties Cyanazine has the empirical formula $C_9H_{13}ClN_6$ and a molecular weight of 240.7. It is a white crystalline solid that melts at 166.5–167°C and has a vapor pressure of 1.6×10^{-9} mm Hg at 20°C. The solubility of cyanazine in water at 25°C is 171 ppm; it is very soluble in chloroform, acetone, ethanol, and benzene. Cyanazine is stable to ultraviolet irradiation; the product is hydrolyzed at pH values lower than 5 or higher than 9.

History, Formulations, and Uses Cyanazine was introduced in 1971 by Shell Chemical Company. It is a pre- and postemergence herbicide for control of annual grasses and broadleaf weeds. Cyanazine is registered for use on corn, cotton, grain sorghum, and wheat fallow. It is available as a granular product, wettable powder, flowable concentrate, emulsifiable concentrate, and soluble concentrate. It is sold in combination with atrazine, alachlor, metolachlor, paraquat, and butylate.

20.17.2.2 Toxicity to Laboratory Animals

Symptomatology High doses of cyanazine produce depression and inactivity in laboratory animals (Beste, 1983).

Response to Single Dose   The oral LD 50 in rats is equal to 334 mg/kg and the dermal LD 50 in rabbits is <2000 mg/kg; an inhalation toxicity evaluation in rats with an 80% wettable powder revealed no mortality after 1 hr of exposure to 4.9 ml/liter (Beste, 1983). Worthing (1987) placed the oral LD 50 in rats at 182–380 mg/kg and defined the oral LD 50 in the mouse at 380 mg/kg; he also set the dermal LD 50 in rats at >1200 mg/kg.

Response to Repeated Doses   In 2-year feeding studies in rats and dogs, no toxicological effects were noted in either species at daily dietary levels up to and including 25 ppm cyanazine (Beste, 1983).

Absorption, Distribution, Metabolism, and Excretion
Worthing (1987) indicated that cyanazine is rapidly metabolized and eliminated from the body by rats and dogs (within 4 days). Indeed, Hutson *et al.* (1970) showed that after the oral administration of [^{14}C]cyanazine the material was absorbed and metabolized rapidly; about 40% of the administered dose was excreted in the urine and 47% in the feces. The primary pathway for metabolism of cyanazine in rats is *N*-deethylation to yield an amine. In addition, *N*-acetylcysteinyl derivatives were found in the urine. Dechlorination resulting in a 2-hydroxy triazine was noted, as well as the cyano group hydrolyzed to an amide and then further to a carboxyl analog. The 2-hydroxy compound was a major metabolite in the feces. The bile contained glutathione conjugates.

Mutagenicity   Mutagenicity studies covering the classes of gene mutation and chromosomal aberration as well as other tests have been completed and indicate that cyanazine is not mutagenic (Office of Pesticide Programs, 1984b).

Carcinogenicity   The oncogenic potential of cyanazine was evaluated in mice at feeding levels of 10, 25, and 1000 ppm; no oncogenic response was seen at any level (Office of Pesticide Programs, 1986).

Effects on Reproduction   In 1985 the Environmental Protection Agency initiated a special review of cyanazine based on head anomalies observed in fetuses taken from female Fisher 344 rats administered 25 mg/kg/day during gestational days 6–15 (Offices of Pesticides and Toxic Substances, 1985). A clear no-effect level of 10 mg/kg/day was established in this study. In another study in the Sprague–Dawley rat, no teratogenic effects or developmental effects were noted at the highest level tested, 30 mg/kg/day. In a second teratology study conducted with the Fisher 344 rats at levels of 5, 25, and 75 mg/kg/day, a no-observable-effect level was not established for maternal and developmental toxicity. Head anomalies were noted at 75 mg/kg/day. A teratology study in the New Zealand rabbit did not indicate any teratogenic potential; the no-observable-effect level was established at 1 mg/kg/day. Fetotoxicity was noted at 2 mg/kg/day. In another teratology study in New Zealand rab-

bits, malformations were noted at the highest dose tested, 4 mg/kg/day orally administered (Office of Pesticide Programs, 1987). In a rabbit teratology study in which doses were applied dermally at levels of 96, 283, 573, and 955 mg/kg, no teratogenic effects were noted at any level. However, some evidence of fetotoxicity was noted at the highest level; thus the no-observable-effect level for the study was set at 753 mg/kg. The question of the teratogenicity potential of cyanazine is still an open issue.

20.17.2.3 Toxicity to Humans

Use Experience   A case of severe, acute contact dermatitis in a farmer whose exposure included cyanazine is recorded in the Section 20.17.1.3 on atrazine. However, no similar case has been reported, and it was the view of Beste (1983) that no case of cyanazine overexposure is known.

Treatment of Poisoning   Treatment of poisoning with cyanazine would be symptomatic.

20.17.3 PROPAZINE

20.17.3.1 Identity, Properties, and Uses

Chemical Name   Propazine is 2-chloro-4,6-bis(isopropylamino)-*s*-triazine.

Structure   See Fig. 20.10.

Synonyms   The common name propazine (ANSI, BSI, ISO, WSSA) is in general use, except in Canada, Germany, and Sweden. Trade names include Gesamil®, Milogard®, Milo-Pro, Primatol® P, and Prozinex®. Code designations include G-30028. The CAS registry number is 139-40-2.

Physical and Chemical Properties   Propazine has the empirical formula $C_9H_{16}ClN_5$ and a molecular weight of 229.71. It forms colorless crystals that melt at 212–214°C and has a vapor pressure of 2.9×10^{-8} mm Hg at 20°C. The technical material is more than 95% pure. The solubility of propazine in water at 20°C is 8.6 ppm; it is difficultly soluble in organic solvents. It is stable in neutral, slightly acid, or alkaline media, but it is hydrolyzed by stronger acids and alkalis.

History, Formulations, and Uses   Propazine was introduced in 1960 by J. R. Geigy S. A. It is a preemergence herbicide for use on broad-leaved and grass weeds in millet and umbelliferous crops. It is available as 50 and 80% wettable powders as well as a 4 lb/gal emulsifiable concentrate and a 90% water-dispersible granule. It is sold in combination with metolachlor.

20.17.3.2 Toxicity to Laboratory Animals

Symptomatology   Propazine is a compound of low toxicity. Administration of single lethal or near-lethal doses of propazine to rats elicits hypoactivity, ruffled fur, muscular weakness, rhinitis, emaciation, diarrhea, and labored breathing (CIBA-GEIGY, 1982c).

Response to Single Dose   Dinerman and Lavrent'eva (1969) reported that the oral LD 50 of a sample of Swiss manufacture was 5000 mg/kg, but that a sample of Soviet manufacture was even less toxic (>7500 mg/kg). Propazine technical has an acute oral LD 50 in the rat of >7700 mg/kg. The dermal LD 50 in the rat is >3100 mg/kg, and the inhalation LC 50 for a 4-hr exposure is >1 mg/liter (CIBA-GEIGY, 1982c).

Irritation and Sensitization   Propazine technical is nonirritating to the rabbit eye and mildly irritating to the rabbit skin. Propazine was not found to have sensitizing properties in a standard guinea pig sensitization test (CIBA-GEIGY, 1982c).

No effect was noted following application of propazine to the skin of rabbits (Gzhegotskiy and Doloshitskiy, 1971).

Response to Repeated Doses   Tests run for 56 days revealed low toxicity and lack of accumulation in the tissues. Oral administration of propazine to rabbits at a rate of 500 mg/kg/day for 4 months affected the blood and liver, but some of the reported changes do not seem mutually consistent, and the toxicity of the sample must have been different from that studied by Dinerman and Lavrent'eva (1969). The condition was characterized by hypochromic, macrocytic anemia, leukopenia, some atrophy of lymph nodes, and hepatomegaly with focal necrosis and fatty degeneration. The anemia presumably was caused by the observed degeneration of the erythrocytes. Repair was indicated by marked reticulocytosis, but reported inhibition of myelopoiesis and decreased soluble protein, DNA, and RNA in the bone marrow were inconsistent with repair. Of great interest is the report that no lesions appeared in rabbits given the same dosage of propazine plus exogenous thymidine (Semencheva *et al.*, 1972).

Absorption, Distribution, Metabolism, and Excretion
When ring-labeled propazine was administered to rats by stomach tube at rates of 41–56 mg/kg, excretion of radioactive material was most rapid during the first 24 hr and decreased to trace amounts by 72 hr. At this time 65.8 and 23% had been recovered from the urine and feces, respectively. At 4 days, the tissue concentrations of related compounds expressed as propazine varied from 19.8 to 39.3 ppm, the lowest values involving the liver and lung. All of the tissue levels fell slowly, the corresponding range at 8 days being 13.0–30.3 ppm. Concentrations tended to be higher in the eviscerated carcass and especially in the skin. When rats were given propazine labeled in the 2 position of the isopropyl groups, total recovery of excreted radioactivity was the same as that for the ring-labeled compound, but about 50% of the dose was recovered from the expired air as $^{14}CO_2$, in contrast to no recovery from air with the ring-labeled compound. Ion exchange chromatography indicated at least 18 metabolites in the urine (Bakke *et al.*, 1967).

Very similar results were found in goats and sheep (Robbins *et al.*, 1968).

Carcinogenesis   In studies conducted in two strains of mice, propazine was not found to be tumorigenic (Innes *et al.*, 1969). CIBA-GEIGY (1982c) indicated that oral exposure in rats at an extremely high dose level has produced an increased incidence of benign neoplasia.

20.17.3.3 Toxicity to Humans

Use Experience   Yelizarov (1972) reported 124 cases of contact dermatitis among workers manufacturing propazine and simazine. Mild cases lasting 3 or 4 days involved pale pink erythema and slight edema. Serious cases lasting 7–10 days involved greater erythema and edema and also a vesiculopapular reaction that sometimes progressed to the production of bullae. Blagodatin *et al.* (1971) expressed the view that the initial and intermediate products in the synthesis of propazine were more likely than propazine itself to be a danger to workers.

Treatment of Poisoning   Treatment, if required, is entirely symptomatic.

20.17.4 SIMAZINE

20.17.4.1 Identity, Properties, and Uses

Chemical Name   Simazine is 2-chloro-4,6-bis(ethylamino)-*s*-triazine.

Structure   See Fig. 20.10.

Synonyms   The common name simazine (ANSI, BSI, ISO, WSSA) is in general use, except in Turkey. Trade names include Aquazinc®, Cekusan®, Gesatop®, Primatol/S®, Princep®, Simadex®, and Simanex®. Its code designation is G-27692. The CAS registry number is 122-34-9.

Physical and Chemical Properties   Simazine has the empirical formula $C_7H_{12}ClN_5$ and a molecular weight of 201.66. It is a white crystalline solid that melts at 225–227°C and has a vapor pressure of 6.1×10^{-9} mm Hg at 20°C. The solubility of simazine in water at 20–22°C is 5 ppm; in methanol it is 400 ppm, and in light petroleum it is 2 ppm. Simazine is stable in neutral and slightly basic or acidic media, but it is hydrolyzed by stronger acids and bases.

History, Formulations, and Uses   Simazine was introduced in 1956 by J. R. Geigy S. A. It is a preemergence herbicide used to control broad-leaved and grassy weeds in deep-rooted crops. It is also used on maize and shows promise for controlling submerged vegetation and algae. Simazine is available as 50 and 80% wettable powders as well as a water-dispersible granule containing 90% active ingredient.

20.17.4.2 Toxicity to Laboratory Animals

Symptomatology   Oral administration of 5000 mg/kg to rats produced drowsiness and irregular respiration.

Response to Single Dose   The oral LD 50 in the rat is >5000 mg/kg, and the acute dermal LD 50 in the rabbit is >10,000 mg/kg (Worthing, 1987). The inhalation LC 50 (4-hr) of simazine for rats is greater than 2 mg/liter (CIBA-GEIGY, 1982d).

For completely unknown reasons, sheep are much more susceptible to poisoning by simazine. Palmer and Radeleff (1964) reported this in connection with repeated administrations which were fatal after a total dose of 1400 mg/kg or more. However, Hapke (1968) showed that a single dose at a rate as low as 500 mg/kg could be fatal, but there was a considerable delay in onset. Death occurred within 6–16 days. Those that recovered were sick for 2–4 weeks. Signs included intake of less food but more water than usual, incoordination, tremor, and weakness, especially of the hindquarters. Cyanosis and clonic convulsions were seen in some sheep.

Irritation and Sensitization   Simazine technical is nonirritating to eyes or skin of rabbits (CIBA-GEIGY, 1982d).

Response to Repeated Doses   When rats were given simazine orally at the rate of 15 mg/kg/day, a few hepatocytes degenerated during the first 3 days, but the condition did not progress; instead, the liver adapted and the compound was metabolized (Oledzka-Slotwinska, 1974).

Mutagenicity   When injected into male *Drosophila melanogaster,* simazine increased the frequence of X-linked lethals, but it failed to do so when fed to larvae. Other tests for mutagenicity in this species were negative (Murnik and Nash, 1977).

Carcinogenicity   At the highest tolerated dose, Innes *et al.* (1969) found simazine not tumorigenic in mice. The compound was found to produce sarcoma at the site of subcutaneous injection in both rats and mice (Pliss and Zabezhinskiy, 1970), but this is not an appropriate route for testing. Simazine was found to be oncogenic in the rat at the highest feeding level tested, 100 ppm. Tumors were restricted to mammary tumors in female Sprague–Dawley rats (Office of Pesticide Programs, 1989).

20.17.4.3 Toxicity to Humans

Experimental Exposure   In a repeated patch insult test in 50 human subjects, the 80% wettable powder formulation of simazine was not found to be a primary irritant, fatiguing agent, or sensitizer (CIBA-GEIGY, 1982d).

Use Experience   After over 20 years of use, no substantiated cases of poisoning in humans from the ingestion of simazine have been reported. However, occasional transient skin erruptions have been reported from experimental or commercial use (CIBA-GEIGY, 1982d). In one such case, a 55-year-old male reported a skin rash with no itching 1 week after use of the 80% wettable powder of simazine. Within 2–3 days after the appearance of the rash, blistering occurred. He had previously used the product for years without incident. The report by Yelizarov (1972) of dermatitis among workers manufacturing simazine and propazine is discussed in Section 20.17.3.3.

Treatment of Poisoning   Treatment, if required, is entirely symptomatic.

20.17.5 AMITROLE

20.17.5.1 Identity, Properties, and Uses

Chemical Name   Amitrole is 3-amino-1,2,4-triazole.

Structure   See Figure 20.10.

Synonyms   The common name amitrole is approved by ANSI, BSI, ISO, and WSSA. The approved name aminotriazole (ATA, MAF) is accepted in France, Great Britain, New Zealand, and the USSR. An acronym for aminotriazole is ATA; the compound also has been known by the codes 3A-T and ENT-25445. Trade names include Amerol®, AminoTriazole Weed Kill 90, Amitrol T®, Amizol®, Azolan®, Azole®, Cytrol®, Diurol®, and Weedazol®. The CAS registry number is 61-82-5.

Physical and Chemical Properties   Amitrole has the empirical formula $C_2H_4N_4$ and a molecular weight of 84.08. It is a white, odorless crystalline powder with a bitter taste; its melting point is 157–159°C. The solubility of amitrole in water is 280 gm/liter at 25°C; in ethanol it is 260 gm/kg at 75°C. The compound is insoluble in nonpolar solvents.

History, Formulation, and Uses   Amitrole was introduced in 1954 by Amchem Products, Inc. It is used as a nonselective herbicide on fallow land. Its activity is enhanced by ammonium thiocyanate. Amitrole is available as a 50% water-soluble powder and as an equimolar mixture of 2 lb amitrole plus 1 lb 13 oz ammonium thiocyanate per gallon.

20.17.5.2 Toxicity to Laboratory Animals

Symptomatology   Poisoning of several species by amitrole is characterized by increased intestinal peristalsis, pulmonary edema, and hemorrhages in various organs. These effects are thought to reflect direct stimulation of smooth muscles of the gut and bronchi plus vascular paralysis (Hapke, 1967).

Response to Single Dose   Amitrole is a compound of very low acute toxicity. Hapke (1967) listed the oral LD 50 in mice as 11,000 mg/kg but noted that 4000 mg/kg was fatal to sheep. Gaines *et al.* (1973) found that the largest oral and dermal doses they tested in rats (4080 and 2500 mg/kg, respectively) caused no detectable toxicity. Beste (1983) reported an oral LD 50 of 24,600 mg/kg in rat and 15,000 mg/kg in mice.

Irritation and Sensitization Amitrole in the acid form produced mild irritation in the rabbit eye, which subsided by 48 hr (Beste, 1983).

Absorption, Distribution, Metabolism, and Excretion Absorption of amitrole from the gastrointestinal tract is rapid. The highest radioactivity in all tissue generally is reached in 1 hr, and the concentration begins to decline after 2–6 hrs (Fang *et al.*, 1964, 1966).

Following intravenous injection, [^{14}C]amitrole was distributed to many soft tissues of mice, notably the red pulp and germinal centers of the spleen, bone marrow, cortex of the thymus, germinal centers of the lymph nodes, liver, mucosa of the gastrointestinal tract, kidneys, and urinary bladder. It reached higher concentrations in the actively growing parts of transplanted tumors than in normal tissues (Tjälve, 1974).

When [^{14}C]amitrole was given to rats orally at a dosage of 50 mg/kg, most of the radioactivity that appeared in the urine during the first 24 hr was unmetabolized, but 3-amino-5-mercapto-1,2,4-triazole and 3-amino-1,2,4-triazolyl-(5)-mercapturic acid also were present (Grunow *et al.*, 1975).

The pattern of distribution of [^{14}C]amitrole in the fetus is similar to that in the adult, and what reaches the fetus is mainly in unmetabolized form (Tjälve, 1975).

When [^{14}C]amitrole was administered to rats by stomach tube at a rate of about 3 mg/kg, only insignificant traces of ^{14}C were found in the expired air during the first 3 days. During the first 24 hr, from 70.0 to 95.5% of the radioactivity was found in the urine, which contained two radioactive metabolites in addition to the parent compound. Radioactivity was detectable in the feces for 2 or 3 days in most rats but for 5 days in one; in 6 days, 2.0–2.1% of the dose was recovered from the feces of different rats. During the same period from 79.9 to 102.0% of the dose was recovered in the total excreta. The radioactivity remaining in the body at the end of 6 days varied from only 0.28 to 1.36% of the dose. Most of this activity was in the liver. In other rats killed at intervals during the first 24 hr, a metabolite was first detectable in the liver 1 hr after dosing; by 24 hr, this metabolite (which was not identified) constituted 100% of the radioactivity remaining in the liver (Fang *et al.*, 1964). Further study of excretion showed that an average of 85% of the dose was recovered in the excreta during the first 24 hr and 2.1% more during the second 24 hr. There was no significant difference in these percentages associated with dosages ranging from about 3 to 600 mg/kg; however, the proportion of metabolite in the urine decreased as the dosage increased (Fang *et al.*, 1966).

When metabolites of amitrole formed by bean plants were fed to rats, 96% of one of them was excreted within 48 hr, mainly in the urine and mainly unchanged. Another metabolite was excreted more slowly mainly in the feces; after 172 hr only 67–78% had been recovered from the excreta of different animals, and the remainder was accounted for fully in the tissues (Fang *et al.*, 1966).

Biochemical Effects At a dietary level of 1000 ppm, significant enlargement of the thyroid could be noted as early as the third day of feeding. At this high dosage level, the goiter did not regress within a 23-day observation period following 83 days of treatment. Also at this dosage level, amitrole interfered not only with the linking of iodine to tyrosine but also with the coupling of iodotyrosines to form iodothyronines (Mayberry, 1968). Feeding of amitrole to rats at dietary levels of 60 or 120 ppm for as little as 2 weeks caused enlargement of the thyroid and reduced uptake of radioiodine by this gland (Jukes and Shaffer, 1960).

Different investigators have reported different thresholds for an effect on iodine uptake, but the identity of factors leading to the difference remains unknown. Jukes and Shaffer (1960) found no significant reduction of uptake of radioactive iodine by rats at dietary levels of [^{14}C]amitrole as high as 30 ppm. On the contrary, Fregley (1968) found decreased uptake of radioactivity by the thyroid, decreased protein-bound iodine, and increased number of blood vessels per low-power microscope field at a dietary level of 10 ppm and found the first two of these changes at 2 ppm; at 0.25 and 0.50 ppm, no significant effect could be detected in 16 measures of thyroid activity.

Several investigations have shown that amitrole inhibits one or another microsomal enzyme of the liver (Matsushima and Weisburger, 1972; Langhans and Schimassek, 1974). However, it inhibits only the increase of cytochrome P-450 and not the proliferation of smooth endoplasmic reticulum induced by phenobarbital (Raisfeld *et al.*, 1970; Stenger and Johnson, 1972). Furthermore, there is a considerable sex and strain variation in the interaction (Levine, 1973). A strange relationship was demonstrated by Lotlikar *et al.* (1973): amitrole (1000 mg/kg/day for 9 days) increased both ring- and *N*-hydroxylated metabolites of AAF in the urine. Ligation of the bile duct also increased excretion of these metabolites. Although these results seem to imply that amitrole reduces biliary flow, direct study showed that bile flow really was increased by amitrole (Levine, 1973). Thus the change in the disposition of AAF metabolites remains completely unexplained.

Amitrole inhibits a number of other enzymes, including δ-aminolevulinic acid dehydratase (Baron and Tephley, 1969), peroxidase, and catalase.

Among other locations, inhibition of peroxidase was demonstrated in the endoplasmic reticulum of the rat thyroid. However, some enzyme activity persists even in large goiters (Strum and Karnovsky, 1971; Tsuda, 1975).

Inhibition of catalase by amitrole was reported early (Heim *et al.*, 1956). *In vivo* inhibition involves the liver and kidney but not the blood. *In vitro*, complete, irreversible, and relatively rapid inhibition of crystalline preparations of both liver and erythrocyte catalases occurred in the presence of low and constant concentrations of hydrogen peroxide. The difference observed *in vivo* depends on the different abilities of blood and liver to form hydrogen peroxide (Margoliash and Novogrodsky, 1958; Tephley *et al.*, 1961). Even a high dosage of amitrole does not cause complete inhibition of catalase *in vivo*, probably due to continuing synthesis of the enzyme (Nakamura and

Minakami, 1973, 1974; Teruya and Higashi, 1973). It seems unlikely that inhibition of catalase in the thyroid is responsible for inhibition of iodine uptake, for the latter effect occurs at dosages too low to affect catalase (Alexander, 1959a). The complex relation of thyroid peroxidase to inhibition of iodine uptake has been explored by Alexander (1959b).

Effects on Organs and Tissues   Amitrole, like other antithyroid compounds and like diets that are low in iodine, produces adenomatous changes in the thyroid glands of rats when fed continuously for long periods. Such changes are reversible if the antithyroid regime is discontinued. Not all antithyroid compounds are synthetic; some occur naturally in ordinary foods, as discussed in Section 21.12.1.2. Davis *et al.* (1983) and Bentley *et al.* (1985) found that effects on the kidney noted with amitrole administration were reversed by treatment with the thyroid hormone thyroxine (T_4), hence the premise that the antithyroid effect of amitrole goes beyond the thyroid gland.

Carcinogenicity   When amitrole was fed to rats at dietary levels of 0, 10, 50, and 100 ppm for 2 years, there was a dosage-related increase in adenomas of the thyroid. A few of the tumors in animals that had received 50 and 100 ppm were considered adenocarcinomas by some, but not all, pathologists. In another study, thyroid adenoma was produced by feeding amitrole at 500 ppm for 17 weeks; the thyroid returned to normal appearance in rats within 2 weeks after this treatment was stopped (Jukes and Shaffer, 1960). Innes *et al.* (1969) employed amitrole as a "positive control" in testing the carcinogenicity of various pesticides and industrial chemicals. At an initial dosage of 1000 mg/kg/day and later at a dietary level of 2192 ppm, it caused a substantial increase in the incidence of hepatomas and of carcinoma of the thyroid in mice. In another study, tiny nodules were noticed only occasionally in the livers of mice that received amitrole at a rate so high that most died, but nodules were confluent and the livers were large, irregular, and hard in mice that received amitrole at the same rate plus propylthiouracil (N. Sato *et al.*, 1974). Mori *et al.* (1985) found that hepatocellular tumors occurred rapidly in the NOD strain of mouse and were less predominant in the ICR and DS strains. Using light and electron microscopy, Reitze and Seitz (1985) further evaluated the process of hepatocellular tumorigenesis in mice treated with amitrole.

Hodge *et al.* (1966) used amitrole as one positive control to test the value of administering compounds subcutaneously or dermally to mice as a test of carcinogenicity. The results with this and the five other compounds studied were uniformly negative. It was concluded that such dermal tests are less sensitive than long-term feeding studies.

It is interesting that injections of amitrole significantly delayed the production of liver cancer in rats receiving 4-dimethylaminoazobenzene (Hoshino, 1960). Further, Sumi *et al.* (1985) found that amitrole reduced the incidence of hepatic tumor in animals receiving diethylstilbestrol and speculated that the effect was due to interference with metabolic activation of the hormone. On the other hand, amitrole increased the inci-

dence of thyroid tumors formed by exposure to *N*-bis(2-hydroxypropyl)nitrosamine (Hiasa *et al.*, 1982).

These and other studies have been reviewed by an expert group (WHO, 1974), and it was concluded that amitrole has induced thyroid and liver tumors in both rats and mice.

Steinhoff *et al.* (1983) reported a study with amitrole designed to evaluate the oncogenic potential of this product in Wistar rats, NMRI mice, and golden hamsters. The concentrations used for each species were 1, 10, and 100 ppm in the diet. At least 75 animals per sex per species were used in the treatment groups as well as the control groups. The 100 ppm feeding level was adequate to produce a clear biological response in all three species; however, pituitary and thyroid tumors were noted only in rats. The U.S. Environmental Protection Agency issued a special review of amitrole based on the oncogenic response in the thyroid, pituitary, and liver of laboratory animals (McDavit, 1986). The review is still in progress.

Mutagenicity   Amitrole was evaluated for gene mutation potential using intraperitoneally administered *Salmonella* as the genetic indicator. Amitrole was only weakly mutagenic when administered orally with an equimolar dose of sodium nitrite (Braun *et al.*, 1978). Further, amitrole did not increase mutation frequencies in tests involving two genera of bacteria, *Drosophila*, and human lymphocyte cell cultures (Sorsa and Gripenberg, 1976; Laamanen *et al.*, 1976; Meretoja *et al.*, 1976).

WHO (1974) reported additional negative results in *Salmonella* strains and yeast cells with amitrole as well as a negative response in a host-mediated assay. Further, no cytogenetic effects were observed in bone marrow cells from rats treated with amitrole at 2.5, 25, and 250 mg/kg/day for 5 days. Amitrole was tested in a cell transformation system utilizing Syrian hamster embryo cells in culture and found to induce gene mutations in this system (Tsutsui *et al.*, 1984).

Effects on Reproduction   In a two-generation study in rats, the number of pups per litter and their weight at weaning were reduced for dams fed 500 or 1000 ppm. Within a week after weaning, most of these pups died of a condition resumbling runt disease. Pups from dams fed 500 ppm had atrophic thymuses and spleens when they were killed for study 24–26 days after birth. Dietary levels of 25 and 100 ppm did not have a statistically significant effect on reproduction of either the P or F_1 generation, and no abnormality of the thymus or spleen was detected in the F_1 or F_2 pups. No anomalies were seen in pups following dietary intake of amitrole by the dam or, in another study, following administration of amitrole to dams by stomach tube on days 7–15 of pregnancy at dosages as high as 100 mg/kg/day (Gaines *et al.*, 1973). Both the marked retardation of development and the lack of anomalies have been observed in mice (Tjälve, 1975).

Pathology   Hyperplasia of the thyroid was seen in all rats fed dietary levels of 100 ppm or greater and in some, but not all, fed 25 ppm (about 1.2 mg/kg/day). The follicles were smaller but more numerous than normal, lined by high columnar epithelium, and filled with little colloid. Small adenomas were seen in some glands of rats fed 1000 ppm. Atrophy of the thymus and spleen was seen in the pups of dams fed dietary levels of 500 or 1000 ppm (Gaines *et al.*, 1973). Similar changes, sometime with invasion of surrounding tissues, have been confirmed in rats (Tsuda *et al.*, 1974) and mice (K. Sato *et al.*, 1974).

Goiter but no neoplastic change of the thyroid was seen in dogs treated for as much as 50 weeks; no gross or histological change was seen in the pituitary, adrenal, liver, or kidney of these animals (Hikosaka, 1975).

20.17.5.3 Toxicity to Humans

Accidental and Intentional Poisoning   In an attempted suicide, a 39-year-old woman ingested a mixture (see Section 20.11.1.3) that included amitrole, for which the dosage ingested was 20 mg/kg. She did not become ill, although unchanged amitrole at a concentration of 1000 ppm was isolated from the urine and identified (Geldmacher-von Mallinckrodt and Schmidt, 1970).

Use Experience   Amitrole generally has not been a source of difficulty to workers at the time they manufactured, formulated, or applied the compound. A question has been raised regarding the possibility that it increased the incidence of cancer. However, the number of cases involved is probably too small to justify any conclusion. Briefly, a study was made of railroad workers who had been exposed to one or more herbicides for a total of 46 days or more within the period from 1957 to 1971. During this period 45–50 metric tons of herbicides were used per year. Of a total of 324 workers, 143 had been exposed mainly to amitrole. The incidence of cancer among these 143 persons was 7 (each in a different organ), compared to 1.9 expected on the basis of national statistics adjusted for age and sex. In addition, there were 2 cancers of the lung, whereas 0.24 was expected. However, both patients with lung cancer had smoked, and the tumors were of different cell types (Sundell *et al.*, 1973; Axelson *et al.*, 1974). The lack of a similar report regarding persons heavily exposed to amitrole in its manufacture is noteworthy.

The Cranberry Crisis   Amitrole, then called aminotriazole, was the compound that gave rise to the U.S. cranberry crisis of 1959. The compound was duly registered for use on cranberries soon after harvest, a practice that led to no detectable residue in the crop produced the following year. However, in 1957 residues were detected on some lots of berries, doubtless as the result of preharvest application, and 1587 metric tons were withdrawn from the market by the FDA. Apparently, few growers misused the compound in 1958, and no seizures were made. In 1959 the compound again was misused, perhaps in response to a rumor that a tolerance for the compound on cranberries would be established. Actually, the application was refused on May 29, 1959, on the basis that tests run for the applicant by an independent laboratory showed that the compound is a possible carcinogen. At his press conference on November 9, 1959 (15 days before Thanksgiving, the one day of the year on which the eating of cranberries is traditional), Arthur S. Flemming, then Secretary of Health, Education, and Welfare, announced that part of the current crop was contaminated by a weed killer, aminotriazole, which he said caused cancer of the thyroid when it was contained in diets. On November 23, 1959, 3 days before the holiday, a plan was announced for certifying sufficient cranberries to meet the Thanksgiving demand (DuShane, 1959; Anonymous, 1959).

Growers no doubt learned to follow label directions more carefully. Many citizens learned for the first time of the existence of the Delaney Amendment. Some learned that a person would have to eat tons of contaminated cranberries in order to receive a dosage proportional to that necessary to produce thyroid tumors in rats. Some wondered why Mr. Flemming had chosen this particular way of enforcing the law. A news item in the *Journal of Agriculture and Food Chemistry* (Anonymous, 1959) hinted that an answer might appear in upcoming budget hearings or political conventions.

Some perspective on the matter should have been given by Astwood (1960), who pointed out that Swedish turnips naturally contain about 100 times as much antithyroid activity as do cranberries badly contaminated by amitrole.

Treatment of Poisoning   Treatment, if required, would be symptomatic.

20.18 OTHER HETEROCYLIC COMPOUNDS

In addition to bipyridinium compounds, triazines, and triazoles, there is a wide variety of heterocyclic herbicides. These include chloridazon, bromacil (ANSI, BSI, ISO, WSSA) (oral LD 50 in the rat of 5200 mg/kg), brompyrazon (BSI, ISO) (oral LD 50 in the rat of 6400 mg/kg), dazomet (BSI, ISO, WSSA) (oral LD 50 in the rat of 640 mg/kg), lenacil (ANSI, BSI, ISO, WSSA) (oral LD 50 in the rat of 11,000 mg/kg), maleic hydrazide (BSI, ISO) or MH (WSSA) (oral LD 50 in the rat of 6950 mg/kg), methazole (ANSI, BSI, ISO, WSSA) (oral LD 50 in the rat of 2501 mg/kg), and picloram (ANSI, BSI, ISO, WSSA) (oral LD 50 in the rat of 8200 mg/kg).

20.18.1 CHLORIDAZON

20.18.1.1 Identity, Properties, and Uses

Chemical Name   Chloridazon is 5-amino-4-chloro-2-phenyl-3(2*H*)-pyridazinone.

Structure   See Fig. 20.11.

Synonyms   The common name accepted by BSI, ISO, and WSSA is chloridazon. The common name pyrazone, used for the calcium salt of phenylbutazone, is still accepted by ANSI. JMAF uses the common name PCA. The common name

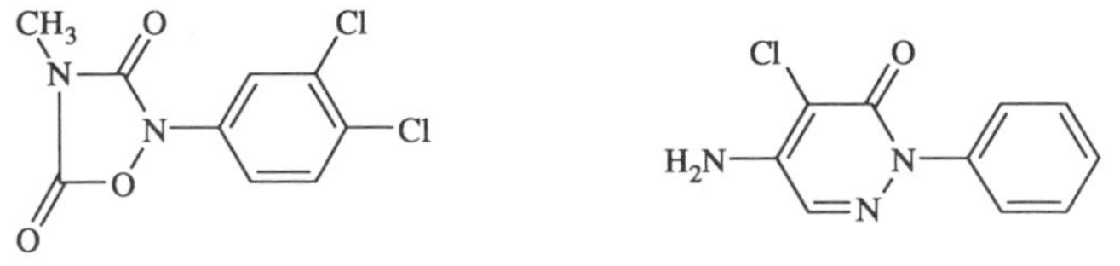

Methazole   Chloridazon

Figure 20.11 Other heterocyclic herbicides.

chlorazon has been used in the USSR. Trade names include Alicep® (discontinued), Burex®, Pyramin®, Pyrazone®, and Pyrazonyl®. The code designation is BAS-119H. The CAS registry number is 1698-60-8.

Physical and Chemical Properties Chloridazon has the empirical formula $C_{10}H_8ClN_3O$ and a molecular weight of 221.65. It is a pale yellowish odorless solid with a melting point of 205–206°C and a vapor pressure of 7.4×10^{-2} mm Hg. The solubility of chloridazon in water at 20°C is 400 ppm. Its solubility in acetone is 2.8%, in methanol 3.4%, and in benzene 0.075. It is stable and noncorrosive.

History, Formulations, and Uses Chloridazon was introduced in 1962 by Badische Anilin-Soda-Fabrik AG. It is a pre- and postemergence herbicide for use especially on beets. It is available as a wettable powder containing 65% technical chloridazon as well as a flowable at 430 gm/liter.

20.18.1.2 Toxicity to Laboratory Animals

Symptomatology Poisoning appeared in 15–25 min and was characterized by increased excitability, incoordination, tonic convulsions, and reduction of both blood pressure and body temperature. Death usually occurred within 1.5 hr.

Response to Single Dose Chloridazon is a compound of low toxicity. Oral LD 50 values of 3600, 2500, and 3200 mg/kg in rats, mice, and guinea pigs, respectively, were reported by Gzhegotskiy and Martyniuk (1968). The value of 2000 mg/kg reported for the rat by Gruzdev *et al.* (1969) is similar. The oral LD 50 in the rabbit is 1250 mg/kg (Beste, 1983).

Irritation and Sensitization A single illustration of 10% solution had no effect on the eyes of rabbits; slight hyperemia of the conjunctiva appeared on the sixth day of repeated application but cleared 4–5 days after exposure ceased.

Response to Repeated Doses Rats that had received doses of 600 mg/kg/day every other day for as much as 6 months often showed desquamation of the bronchi, purulent sputum, generalized foci of atelectasis, and small foci of diffuse hyperplasia (Gruzdev *et al.*, 1969). It was not clear whether the bronchopulmonary effects were due directly to chloridazon or were the primary result of infection in debilitated animals. In any event, the fact that animals can tolerate large repeated doses for

extended periods indicates a very low degree of cumulative effect.

20.18.1.3 Toxicity to Humans

Accidental Poisoning Recognized human injury associated with chloridazon really was caused by two precursors in its manufacture, namely 1-phenyl-4,5-dichloropyridazone-6 and mucochloric acid. Contact with these substances produced acute local irritation that gradually developed the character of a second-degree burn. Six to 10 days later, when the local changes were beginning to resolve, digestive disorders and slight liver enlargement appeared in those with more extensive local injuries. All of the patients had abnormal SGPT and LDH tests, and their blood proteins were abnormal for as much as 2 months. Photosensitization was also noted (Kolesar and Romancik, 1974).

Treatment of Poisoning Treatment, if required, is entirely symptomatic.

20.18.2 PICLORAM

20.18.2.1 Identity, Properties, and Uses

Chemical Name Picloram is 4-amino-3,5,6-trichloropicolinic acid.

Structure See Fig. 20.12.

Synonyms The common name picloram is approved by ANSI, BSI, and ISO, and WSSA. Trade names include Grazon® and Tordon®. The trade names Amdon®, Borolin®, and K-Pin® have been discontinued.

Physical and Chemical Properties Picloram has the empirical formula $C_6H_3Cl_3N_2O_2$ and a molecular weight of 241.5. Picloram is a white powder with a chlorine-like odor. Picloram is soluble in polar organic solvents (19,800 ppm in acetone) and relatively soluble in nonpolar organic and aqueous solutions (200 ppm in benzene and 430 ppm in water).

History, Formulations, and Uses Picloram was introduced by Dow Chemical Co. in 1971 for woody and broadleaf weed control in grasses and in 1976 for weed control in small grains. It is also used in utility rights-of-way. Picloram is sold under the trade name Tordon® as potassium or amine salts. It is available

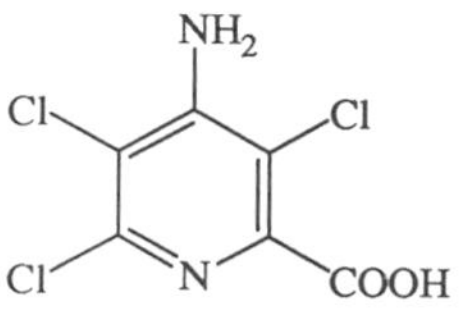

Figure 20.12 Picloram.

in granular and water-soluble liquid formulations. Tordon 101 and Tordon RTU mixtures also contain 2,4-D.

20.18.2.2 Toxicity to Laboratory Animals

Symptomatology J. E. Hayes *et al.* (1986) noted that Sprague-Dawley rats administered lethal doses (approximately 1 gm/kg) by oral gavage exhibited depression, prostration, ataxia, tremors, and convulsions preceding death.

Response to Single Dose The acute oral LD 50 for picloram in the rat is reported to be 8200 mg/kg. Other species show similar low toxicity. Mice (2000–4000 mg/kg), rabbits (2000 mg/kg), guinea pigs (3000 mg/kg), sheep (>1000 mg/kg), and cattle (>750 mg/kg) show the material to have low toxicity in several mammalian species. Dermal LD 50 studies in rabbits produced no mortality at 4000 mg/kg, the highest level tested (Sine and Meister, 1987).

Irritation and Sensitization Picloram is reported to cause mild dermal irritation and moderate ocular irritation without corneal involvement. It is not reported to be a sensitizer.

Effects on Organs and Tissues Repeated administration of picloram in the drinking water of Sprague-Dawley-derived rats at 600 and 1070 mg/kg/day for 9 days resulted in exacerbation of renal and hepatic lesions commonly noted in rats of this age (J. E. Hayes *et al.*, 1986). Dietary administration of picloram to Fischer rats at 2000 mg/kg for 52 weeks, 500 mg/kg for 13 weeks, or 200 mg/kg for 52 weeks resulted in liver lesions (Gorzinski *et al.*, 1987). These investigators noted that, regardless of the duration of exposure, liver effects characterized by increased weight, hypertrophy, and pallor in the centrilobular hepatocytes were noted in male and female rats.

Robens (1980) and Reuber (1981) reported that B6C3F1 mice and Fischer 344 rats administered picloram in bioassays sponsored by the National Cancer Institute developed target organ toxicity. Male rats fed either 7437 or 14,875 ppm for 2 years exhibited an increase in the incidence of testicular atrophy, polyarteritis, and chronic renal disease. Mice fed an average level of 2531 ppm were also noted to develop testicular atrophy.

Carcinogenicity B6F3C1 mice and Fischer 344 rats were fed picloram for 190 and 104 weeks, respectively (Reuber, 1981). Male and female rats administered an average level of 7437 and 14,875 ppm developed an increase in neoplasms of the endocrine organs. Pituitary tumors were induced in both sexes, as well as thyroid and mammary tumors in females and adrenal tumors in both sexes. Male mice fed an average level of 5062 ppm exhibited an increased incidence of tumors of the spleen.

Effects on Reproduction John-Greene *et al.* (1985) conducted a teratological investigation with picloram potassium salt in New Zealand rabbits. No evidence of embryotoxic or teratogenic response was observed in fetuses from dams administered doses of 40, 200, and 400 mg/kg/day between days 6 and 18 of gestation.

20.18.2.3 Toxicity to Humans

Experimental Exposure Picloram has been administered to six human volunteers at levels of both 0.5 and 5.0 mg/kg of body weight perorally and applied to the skin of one volunteer at the level of 2 mg/kg of body weight (Nolan *et al.*, 1984). This study, designed to evaluate the pharmacokinetics of picloram in humans, showed picloram to be rapidly absorbed from the gastrointestinal tract ($t_{\frac{1}{2}} \cong 20$ min) but only slowly absorbed through the skin (reported $t_{\frac{1}{2}} = 12$ hr). In this study, 78–98% of an oral dose but only 0.1–0.5% of the dermal dose was excreted in the urine. Subjects washed the exposed dermal areas 12–14 hr after exposure.

Blood levels and urinary excretion of picloram show the product to be rapidly excreted; the data fit a two-compartment open pharmacokinetic model with an initial phase in which most of the product is excreted with a $t_{\frac{1}{2}}$ of 37–104 min and a second phase with $t_{\frac{1}{2}}$ ranging from 4 to 57 hr. Over 90% of the oral doses were recovered as urinary unchanged picloram within 72 hr. Most of the dose was excreted within 6 hr (>75%).

No adverse effects were observed in this study; however, the volunteers indicated that the orally administered material tasted bitter.

Use Experience No report of any overexposure or accident involving picloram was found.

20.19 MISCELLANEOUS HERBICIDES

In addition to the structural configurations that are likely to confer phytotoxic properties and that already have been mentioned, there remain other miscellaneous configurations. The herbicide development process has not remained static but instead has selected the most efficacious products, both old and new, and discarded the remainder. It is, therefore, not possible to discuss comprehensively all of the available herbicides in use. It is hoped that the majority of these agents have been considered. Today, the market has become more discerning, looking not only at efficacy but also at safety—both mammalian and environmental. Many of the established herbicides address these concerns; many more are still in development.

REFERENCES

Abrams, R. M., Noteloritz, M., and Wilcox, C. J. (1976). Stimulation of the pentose cycle by paraquat in isolated perfused rat lungs. *Physiologist* **19**, 117.

Ackrill, P., Hasleton, P. S., and Ralston, A. J. (1978). Oesophageal perforation due to paraquat. *Br. Med. J.* **1,**1252–1253.

Adachi, H., Yokota, T., Fujihara, S., Nakamura, H., and Uchino, F. (1978). Two autopsy cases of paraquat poisoning. *Tokoku J. Exp. Med.* **125,**331–339.

Addo, E., and Poon-King, T. (1986). Leucocyte suppression in treatment of 72 patients with paraquat poisoning. *Lancet* **1,**1117–1120.

Adler, I. L., Wargo, J. P., Roser, R. L., and Allen, S. S. (1970/1971). "Material Balance and Metabolism Studies in the Rat." Rohm and Haas Report. Springhouse, Pennsylvania.

Aleksandrova, L. G., and Klisenko, M. A. (1978). Kinetics of the accumulation and elimination of thiocarbamine pesticides from warm-blooded animals. *Gig. Sanit.* **43**,101–103 (in Russian).

Aleksashina, Z. A., Buslovich, S. Yu., and Kolosovskaya, V. M. (1973). Embryotoxic effect of 2,4-D diethylamine salt. *Gig. Sanit.* **38**,100–101 (in Russian).

Aleksashina, Z. A., Buslovich, S. Yu., and Kolosovskaia, V. M. (1979). Characteristic features of embryotoxic effect of herbicides—derivatives of 2,4-dichlorophenoxyacetic acid. *Gig. Sanit.* **44**,40–71 (in Russian).

Alexander, N. M. (1959a). Antithyroid action of 3-amino-1,2,4-triazole. *J. Biol. Chem.* **234**,148–150.

Alexander, N. M. (1959b). Iodide peroxidase in rat thyroid and salivary glands and its inhibition by antithyroid compounds. *J. Biol. Chem.* **234**,1530–1533.

Alix, B., Courtadon, M., Jourde, M., Chone, A. F., and Jallut, H. (1974). Benign acute pericarditis caused by the inhalation of pesticides—a report of 2 observations. *Coeur Med. Interne* **13**,165–169 (in French).

Almog, C., and Siegelbaum, Y. (1974). Paraquat poisoning in Israel. *Harefuah* **89**,400–403 (in Hebrew).

Almog, C., and Tal, E. (1967). Death from paraquat after subcutaneous injection. *Br. Med. J.* **3**,721.

Ambrose, A. M., Larson, P. S., Borzelleca, J. F., Smith, R. B., and Hennigar, G. R. (1971). Toxicologic studies on 2,4-dichlorophenyl-*p*-nitrophenyl ether. *Toxicol. Appl. Pharmacol.* **19**,263–275.

Ambrose, A. M., Larson, P. M., Borzelleca, J. F., and Hennigar, G. R., Jr. (1972). Toxicologic studies on 3′,4′-dichloropropionanilide. *Toxicol. Appl. Pharmacol.* **23**,650–659.

Amirov, R. O., Alekperov, I. I., Shekhtman, B. A., Bashirov, A. A., Ter-Bagdasarova, I. K., Aslanova, A. T., Aleskerova, Sh. R., Tabuaeva, V. I., Novikova, N. I., and Lukoshkina, L. P. (1968). The health condition of workers producing the herbicide 2,4-D. *Tr. Azerb. Nauchno-Issled. Inst. Gig. Tr. Prof. Zabol.* **2**,128–132 (in Russian).

Andersen, K. J., Leighty, E. G., and Takahashi, M. T. (1972). Evaluation of herbicides for possible mutagenic properties. *J. Agric. Food Chem.* **20**,649–656.

Anderson, C. G. (1970). Paraquat and the lung. *Australas. Radiol.* **14**,409–411.

Anderson, D., McGregor, D. B., and Purchase, I. F. H. (1976). Dominant lethal studies with paraquat and diquat in male CD-1 mice. *Mutat. Res.* **40**,349–358.

Anderson, W. P. (1983). "Weed Science: Principles," 2nd ed. West Publishing Company, St. Paul, Minnesota.

Anina, I. A., Medved', I. L., and Proklina, T. L. (1975). Gonadotoxic action of pesticidal thiocarbamic acid derivatives. *Farmakol. Toksikol. (Moscow)* **38**,90–93 (in Russian).

Anonymous (1959). Cranberry crisis. *J. Agric. Food Chem.* **7**,807.

Anonymous (1968). Treating paraquat poisoning. *Pharmacol. J.* **201**,627.

Anonymous (1971). Paraquat poisoning. *Lancet* **1**,1018–1019.

Anonymous (1972). Fetotoxicity. *N. Z. Med. J.* **75**,304–305.

Anonymous (1973). Paraquat attacked. *Nature (London)* **245**,64.

Anonymous (1979). Paraquat contamination of marijuana—United States. *Morbid. Mortal. Wkly. Rep.* **28**,93–94.

Araki, S., Ushio, K., and Iwabuchi, T. (1972). A case history and autopsy findings in acute poisoning by the herbicide, Gramoxone. *J. Jpn. Accident Med. Assoc.* **20**,43–44 (in Japanese).

Ashton, F. M., and Crafts, A. S. (1973). "Mode of Action of Herbicides." Wiley, New York.

Assouly, M. (1951). Selective herbicides and growth regulators. Summary techniques. Pathological effects on man in the course of manufacture of the ester of 2,4-D. *Arch. Mal. Prof. Med. Trav. Secur. Soc.* **12**,26–30 (in French).

Astwood, D. B. (1960). Cranberries, turnips, and goiter. *JAMA, J. Am. Med. Assoc.* **172**,1319–1320.

Audus, L. J., ed. (1964). "The Physiology and Biochemistry of Herbicides." Academic Press, London.

Aust, S. D., Morehouse, L. A., and Thomas, C. E. (1985). Role of metals in oxygen radical reactions. *J. Free Radicals Biol. Med.* **1**(1),3–25.

Autor, A. P. (1974). Reduction of paraquat toxicity by superoxide dismutase. *Life Sci.* **14**,1309–1319.

Autor, A. P., ed. (1977). "Biochemical Mechanisms of Paraquat Toxicity." Academic Press, New York.

Axelson, O., Rehn, M., and Sundell, L. (1974). Exposure to herbicides—mortality and tumor incidence. An epidemiologic investigation of Swedish railroad workers. *Laekartidningen* **71**,2466–2470 (in Swedish).

Axelson, O., Sundell, L., Andersson, K., Edling, C., Hogstedt, C., and Kling, H. (1980). Herbicide exposure and tumor mortality. An updated epidemiologic investigation on Swedish railroad workers. *Scand. J. Work, Environ. Health* **6**,73–79 (in Swedish).

Baage, G., Cekanova, E., and Larsson, K. S. (1973). Teratogenic and embryotoxic effects of the herbicides di- and trichlorophenoxyacetic acids (2,4-D and 2,4,5-T). *Acta Pharmacol. Toxicol.* **32**,408–416.

Bainova, A. (1969). Chronic oral toxicity of dipyridil herbicides. *Khig. Zdraveopaz.* **12**,325–332 (in Bulgarian).

Bainova, A., and Vulcheva, V. S. (1978). Chronic action of diquat on lungs. *Dokl. Bolg. Akad. Nauk* **31**,1369–1372 (in Bulgarian).

Bainova, A., Zlateva, M., and Y'lcheva, V. (1972). Chronic inhalant toxicity of dipyridilium herbicides. *Khig. Zdraveopaz.* **15**,25–31.

Bakke, J. E., Robbins, J. D., and Feil, V. J. (1967). Metabolism of 2-chloro-4,6-bis(isopropylamino)-*s*-triazine (propazine) and 2-methoxy-4,4-bis(isopropylamino)-*s*-triazine (prometone) in the rat. Balance study and urinary metabolite separation. *J. Agric. Food Chem.* **15**,628–631.

Bakke, J. E., Larson, J. D., and Price, C. E. (1972). Metabolism of atrazine and 2-hydroxyatrazine by the rat. *J. Agric. Food Chem.* **20**,603–607.

Baldwin, R. C., Pasi, A., MacGregor, J. T., and Hine, C. H. (1975). The rates of radical formation from the dipyridylium herbicides paraquat, diquat, and morfamquat in homogenates of rat lung, kidney, and liver: An inhibitory effect of carbon monoxide. *Toxicol. Appl. Pharmacol.* **32**,298–304.

Bankowska, J., and Bojanowska, A. (1972). Detoxification of organophosphorus insecticides following enzymatic induction caused by urea herbicides. *Rocz. Panstw. Zakl. Hig.* **23**,487–494 (in Polish).

Bankowska, J., and Bojanowska, A. (1973a). Distribution of activity of demethylases in certain fractions of rat liver cells exposed previously to urea herbicides. *Rocz. Panstw. Zakl. Hig.* **24**,93–100 (in Polish).

Bankowska, J., and Bojanowska, A. (1973b). Ultrastructural changes of rat liver cells caused by certain herbicides. *Rocz. Panstw. Zakl. Hig.* **24**,371–376 (in Polish).

Barabas, K., and Suveges, G. (1978). The effect of reductant substances on the toxicity of paraquat. *Proc. Hung. Annu. Meet. Biochem.* **18**,95–96.

Barabas, K., Varga, Sz. I., and Matkovics, B. (1981). Serum protein and glycoprotein changes in chronic paraquat intoxication. *Gen. Pharmacol.* **12**,229–231.

Barabas, K., Szabo, L., Varga, Sz. I., Berencsi, G., Bartkowiak, A., and Matkovics, B. (1982a). Study of the effects of paraquat on the peroxide metabolism enzymes in guinea pig. *Gen. Pharmacol.* **13**,133–137.

Barabas, K., Matkovics, B., and Berencsi, G. (1982b). New considerations on the time-dependence of toxic changes caused by paraquat poisoning. *Gen. Pharmacol.* **14**,381–383.

Barabas, K., Szabo, L., Matkovics, B., Vigh, L., and Horvath, I. (1982c). Effects of ascorbic acid *in vivo* on the fatty acid composition of the tissues of mice treated with Gramoxone. *Gen. Pharmacol.* **17**,363–365.

Barabas, K., Szabo, L., Matkovics, B., and Varga, Sz. I. (1986). The effect of light on the toxicity of paraquat in the mouse. *Gen. Pharmacol.* **17**,359–362.

Baran, R. L. (1974). Nail damage caused by weed killers and insecticides. *Arch. Dermatol.* **110**,467.

Barber, P. J. (1971). Accidental vaccination with paraquat. *Br. Med. J.* **2**,768.

Baron, J., and Tephley, T. R. (1969). Effect of 3-amino-1,2,4-triazole on the stimulation of hepatic microsomal heme synthesis and induction of hepatic microsomal oxidases produced by phenobarbital. *Mol. Pharmacol.* **5**,10–20.

Bashirov, A. A. (1969). The state of health in workers manufacturing the herbicides, the amine salt and the butyl ester of 2,4-D acid. *Vrach. Delo* **10**,92–95 (in Russian).

Bashirov, A. A., and Ter-Bagadasarova, I. K. (1970). The state of the cardiovascular system in workers manufacturing the herbicides, the amine salt and butyl ester of 2,4-D—dichlorophenoxyacetic acid. *Azerb. Med. Zh.* **47**, 44–48.

Bates, M. N. (1977). The safety of the herbicide 2,4,5-T. *N. Z. Med. J.* **86**,35–36.

Beck, S. L. (1977). Postnatal detection of prenatal exposure to herbicides in mice using normally occurring variations in skeletal development. *Teratology* **15**,15A.

Becroft, D. M. O. (1977). The safety of the herbicide 2,4,5-T. *N. Z. Med. J.* **86**, 35.

Bedwell, W., and Anderson, W. H. (1974). Paraquat and oxygen effects on surfactant. *Clin. Res.* **22**,44A.

Beebeejaun, A. R., Beevers, G., and Rogers, W. N. (1971). Paraquat poisoning—prolonged excretion. *Clin. Toxicol.* **4**,397–407.

Beevers, D. G., and Rogers, W. N. (1973). Paraquat poisoning. *Clin. Toxicol.* **6**,503–505.

Belomyttseva, L. A. (1969). Clinical aspects of chronic poisoning with a herbicide consisting of the sodium salt of 2,4-dichlorophenoxyacetic acid (2,4-D). *Ref. Zh. Otd. Vyp. Farmakol. Khimioter. Sredstva. Toxsikol.* **10** (54),935 (in Russian).

Benigni, R., Bignami, M., Carere, A., Conti, G., Conti, L., Crebelli, R., Dogliotti, E., Gualandi, G., Novelleto, A., and Ortali, V. A. (1979). Mutational studies with diquat and paraquat *in vitro. Mutat. Res.* **68**,183–193.

Bennett, P. N., Davies, D. S., and Hawkesworth, G. M. (1976). *In vivo* absorption studies with paraquat and diquat in the dog. *Br. J. Pharmacol.* **58**,284P.

Bentley, A. G., Madsen, K. M., Davis, R. G., and Tisher, C. C. (1985). Response of the medullary thick ascending limb to hypothyroidism in the rat. *Am. J. Pathol.* **120**,215–221.

Berkley, M. C., and Magee, K. R. (1963). Neuropathy following exposure to a dimethylamine salt of 2,4-D. *Arch. Intern. Med.* **111**,351–352.

Berndt, W. O., and Koschier, F. (1973). *In vitro* uptake of 2,4-dichlorophenoxyacetic acid (2,4-D) and 2,4,5-trichlorophenoxyacetic acid (2,4,5-T) by renal cortical tissue of rabbits and rats. *Toxicol. Appl. Pharmacol.* **26**,559–570.

Berwick, P. (1970). 2,4-Dichlorophenoxyacetic acid poisoning in man: Some interesting clinical and laboratory findings. *JAMA, J. Am. Med. Assoc.* **214**, 1114–1117.

Bescol-Liversac, J., Paquelin A., and Guillam, C. (1975). Study of the ultrastructure of a kidney biopsy of a patient intoxicated with paraquat. *Eur. J. Toxicol. Environ. Hyg.* **8**,236–246 (in French).

Beste, C. E. (1983). "Herbicide Handbook of the Weed Science Society of America," 5th ed. Weed Sci. Soc. Am., Champaign, Illinois.

Bezuglyi, V. P., Fokina, K. V., Komarova L. I., Sivitskaia, I. I., Il'ina, V. I., and Gorskaia, N. Z. (1979). Clinical manifestations of long-term sequela of acute poisoning with 2,4-dichlorophenoxyacetic acid. *Gig. Tr. Prof. Zabol.* **3**,47–48 (in Russian).

Bier, R. K., and Osborne, I. J. T. (1978). Pulmonary changes in paraquat poisoning. *Radiology (Easton, Pa.)* **127**,308.

Binnie, G. A. C. (1975). Paraquat. *Lancet* **1**,169–170.

Binns, C. W. (1976). A deadly cure for lice—a case of paraquat poisoning. *Papua New Guinea Med. J.* **19**,105–107.

Binns, C. W., and Johnson, A. E. (1970). Chronic and teretogenic effects of 2,4-D (2,4-dichlorophenoxyacetic acid) and atrazine (2-chloro-4-ethylamino-6-isopropylamino-s-triazine) to sheep. *Proc. North Cent. Weed Control Conf.* **25**,100.

Bjerke, E. L., Herman, J. L., Miller, P. W., and Wetters, J. H. (1972). Residue study of phenoxy herbicides in milk and cream. *J. Agric. Food Chem.* **20**, 963–967.

Bjoerklund, N. E., and Erne, K. (1971). Phenoxy-acid-induced renal changes in the chicken. I. Ultrastructure. *Acta Vet. Scand.* **12**,243–256.

Blagodatin, V. M., Dorofeeva, E. D., Mel'nikova, K. V., and Elizarov, G. P. (1971). The hygienic characteristics of the working conditions and the state of health of the workers in the manufacture of some triazine herbicides. *Gig. Tr. Prof. Zabol.* **15**,45–47 (in Russian).

Boehme, C., and Ernst, W. (1965). The metabolism of urea-herbicides in the rat. 2. Diuron and linuron. *Food Cosmet. Toxicol.* **3**,797–802 (in German).

Boffey, P. M. (1971). Herbicides in Vietnam: AAAS study finds widespread devastation. *Science* **171**,43–47.

Bogen, A. (1979). Symptoms of Vietnam veterans exposed to Agent Orange. *JAMA, J. Am. Med. Assoc.* **242**,2391.

Bonderman, D. P., Mick, D. L., and Long, K. R. (1971). Occupational exposure to aldrin, 2,4-D and 2,4,5-T and its relationship to esterases. *Ind. Med. Surg.* **40**,(b),23–27.

Bony, D., Favarel-Garriques, J. C., Cledes, J., Cambeilh, J., and Castaing, R. (1971). Paraquat poisoning. *J. Eur. Toxicol.* **4**,406–411 (in French).

Borchard, F. (1974). Ultrastructural and light microscopic findings from three fatal cases of paraquat poisonings. *Pneumonologie* **150**,185–189 (in German).

Borchard, F., Grabensee, B., Jax, W., and Huth, F. (1974). Morphological findings in paraquat poisoning. *Klin. Wochenschr.* **52**,657–671 (in German).

Botella, R., Sastre, A., and Castells, A. (1985). Contact dermatitis to paraquat. *Contact Dermatitis* **13**(2),123–124.

Boyd, E. M., and Krupa, V. (1970). Protein-deficient diet and diuron toxicity. *J. Agric. Food Chem.* **18**,1104–1107.

Brandt, M. R. (1971). Herbatox poisoning: A brief review and report of a new case. *Ugeskr. Laeg.* **133**,500–503 (in Danish).

Braun, R., Schoeneich, J., and Ziebarth, D. (1978). *In vivo* formation of *N*-nitroso compounds and detection of their mutagenic activity in host-mediated assay. *Cancer Res.* **37**,4572–4579.

Brody, I. A. (1973). Myotonia induced by monocarboxylic aromatic acids. A possible mechanism. *Arch. Neurol. (Chicago)* **28**,243–246.

Bronkhorst, F. B., vanDall, J. M., and Tan, H. D. (1968). Fatal poisoning with paraquat (Gramoxone). *Ned. Tijdschr. Geneeskd.* **112**,310–313.

Brooks, R. E. (1971). Ultrastructure of lung lesions produced by ingested chemicals. I. Effect of the herbicide paraquat on mouse lung. *Lab. Invest.* **25**,536–545.

Brown, E. A. B., and Maling, H. M. (1975). The effects of paraquat and related herbicides on the acetylcholinesterase of rat lung. *Fed. Proc., Fed. Am. Soc. Exp. Brol.* **34**,226.

Brown, T. J., and Manson, J. M. (1986). Further characterization of the distribution and metabolism of nitrofen in the pregnant rat. *Teratology* **34**,129–139.

Browne, T. D. (1971). Treatment of paraquat ingestion. *Br. Med. J.* **3**,580.

Brzeski, Z., Krupa, A., and Czuczwar, Z. (1971). Fatal poisoning with Gramoxone—a dipyridyl herbicide. *Pol. Tyg. Lek.* **26**,1368–1369 (in Polish).

Bucher, L. R. (1946). Effects of 2,4-dichlorophenoxyacetic acid on experimental animals. *Proc. Soc. Exp. Biol. Med.* **63**,204–205.

Bullivant, C. M. (1966). Accidental poisoning by paraquat: Report of two cases in man. *Br. Med. J.* **1**,1272–1273.

Bus, J. S., and Gibson, J. E. (1975). Postnatal toxicity of chronically administered paraquat in mice and interactions with oxygen and bromobenzene. *Toxicol. Appl. Pharmacol.* **33**,461–470.

Bus, J. S., Aust, S. D., and Gibson, J. E. (1974). Superoxide and singlet oxygen-catalyzed lipid peroxidation as a possible mechanism for paraquat (methyl viologen) toxicity. *Biochem. Biophys. Res. Commun.* **58**,749–755.

Bus, J. S., Aust, S. D., and Gibson, J. E. (1975a). Lipid peroxidation: A possible mechanism for paraquat toxicity. *Res. Commun. Chem. Pathol. Pharmacol.* **11**,31–88.

Bus, J. S., Cagen, S. Z., Aust, S. D., and Gibson, J. E. (1975b). Lipid peroxidation: A possible mechanism for paraquat toxicity. *Toxicol. Appl. Pharmacol.* **33**,197–198.

Bus, J. S., Preache, M. M., Cagen, S. Z., Posner, H. S., Eliason, B. C., Sharp, C. W., and Gibson, J. E. (1975c). Fetal toxicity and distribution of paraquat and diquat in mice and rats. *Toxicol. Appl. Pharmacol.* **33**,450–460.

Bus, J. S., Cagen, S. Z., Olgaard, M., and Gibson, J. E. (1976). A mechanism of paraquat toxicity in mice and rats. *Toxicol. Appl. Pharmacol.* **35**,501–513.

Buselmaier, W., Roehrborn, G., and Propping, P. (1973). Comparative investigations on the mutagenicity of pesticides in mammalian test systems. *Mutat. Res.* **21**,25–26.

Buslovich, S. Yu., Voinova, I. V., and Mil'china, M. G. (1973). Distribution of herbicidal chloro-phenoxy-acids in the body of albino rats. *Gig. Tr. Prof. Zabol.* **17**,35–37 (in Russian).

Buslovich, S. Yu., Aleksashina, Z. A., and Kolosovskaya, V. M. (1979). Effect of phenobarbital on the embryotoxic effect of 2-methyl-4-chlorophenoxyacetic acid. *Farmakol. Toksikol. (Moscow)* **42**,167–170 (in Russian).

Butenandt, I., Mantel, K., and Fendel, H. (1974). Paraquat poisoning in children. *Fortschr. Med.* **92,**677–680.

Butler, C., II (1973). Modification of paraquat injury in hamsters. *Lab. Invest.* **28,**379.

Butler, C., II (1975). Pulmonary interstitial fibrosis from paraquat in the hamster. *Arch. Pathol.* **99,**503–507.

Butler, C., II, and Kleinerman, J. (1971). Paraquat in rabbit. *Br. J. Ind. Med.* **28,**67–71.

Cagen, S. Z., and Gibson, J. E. (1974). Effect of paraquat (methyl viologen) on plasma disappearance of sulfobromophthalein (BSP) and indocyanine green. *Pharmacologist* **16,**266.

Cagen, S. Z., and Gibson, J. E. (1977). Liver damage following paraquat in selenium-deficient and diethyl maleate-pretreated mice. *Toxicol. Appl. Pharmacol.* **40,**193–200.

Cagen, S. Z., Janoff, A. S., Bus, J. S., and Gibson, J. E. (1976). Effect of paraquat (methyl viologen) on liver function in mice. *J. Pharmacol. Exp. Ther.* **198,**222–228.

Cambar, P. J., and Aviado, D. M. (1970). Bronchopulmonary effects of paraquat and expectorants. *Arch. Environ. Health* **20,**488–494.

Campbell, S. (1968). Death from paraquat in a child. *Lancet* **1,**144.

Cant, J. S., and Lewis, D. R. H. (1968). Ocular damage due to paraquat and diquat. *Br. Med. J.* **2,**224.

Cappuccilli, E. (1985). Synthetic Organic Chemicals, 1985: Sect. XIII. U.S. Int. Trade Comm., U.S. Govt. Printing Office, Washington, D.C.

Carpenter, K., Cottrell, H. J., DeSilva, W. H., Heywood, B. J., Leeds, W. G., Rivett, K. F., and Soundy, M. L. (1964). Chemical and biological properties of two new herbicides—ioxynil and bromoxynil. *Weed Res.* **4,**175–195.

Carson, E. D. (1972). Fatal paraquat poisoning in Northern Ireland. *J. Forensic Sci. Soc.* **12,**437–443.

Casida, J. E., Kimmel, E. C., Ohkawa, H., and Ohkawa, R. (1975). Sulfoxidation of thiocarbamate herbicides and metabolism of thiocarbamate sulfoxides in living mice and liver enzyme systems. *Pestic. Biochem. Physiol.* **5,**1–11.

Castaing, R., Bony, D., Haglund, P., Cledes, J., Bourzai, M., and Cambeilh, J. (1972). Paraquat poisoning. *Bordeaux Med.* **5,**1577–1582.

Cegla, U. H., Kroidl, R. F., Kronberger, H., and Weber, H. (1975). An experimental animal model for lung fibrosis in the rat following paraquat injection. *Pneumonologie* **152,**65–74 (in German).

Ceppi, G. (1974). Letter. *Inquinamento* **16,**27–28.

Chang, H., Rip, J. W., and Cherry, J. H. (1974). Effects of phenoxyacetic acids on rat liver tissues. *J. Agric. Food Chem.* **22,**62–65.

Chao, T. C. (1972). Paraquat poisoning. *Ann. Acad. Med. Gedanensis* **1,**68–73.

Chow, A. Y. K., and Murphy, S. D. (1974). Propanil-induced methemoglobin formation in relation to its metabolism *in vitro. Toxicol. Appl. Pharmacol.* **29,**125–126.

Chow, A. Y. K., and Murphy, S. D. (1975). Propanil (3,4-dichloropropionanilide)-induced methemoglobin formation in relation to its metabolism *in vitro. Toxicol. Appl. Pharmacol.* **33,**14–20.

CIBA-GEIGY (1982a). "Dual® Herbicides," CIBA-GEIGY Toxicol. Data. Agric. Div., Dept. Toxicol., CIBA-GEIGY, Greensboro, North Carolina.

CIBA-GEIGY (1982b). "AAtrex® Herbicides," Toxicol. Data. Agric. Div., Dept. Toxicol., CIBA-GEIGY, Greensboro, North Carolina.

CIBA-GEIGY (1982c). "Milogard® Herbicides," Toxicol. Data. Agric. Div., Dept. Toxicol., CIBA-GEIGY, Greensboro, North Carolina.

CIBA-GEIGY (1982d). "Princep® Herbicides," Toxicol. Data. Agric. Div., Dept. Toxicol., CIBA-GEIGY, Greensboro, North Carolina.

CIBA-GEIGY (1984). "Dual® Herbicide," Tech. Bull. Agric. Div., CIBA-GEIGY, Greensboro, North Carolina.

CIBA-GEIGY (1987). "Review of Mutagenicity Data Base for Atrazine," Unpublished and published report (CIBA-GEIGY unpublished report).

Clark, D. E., and Palmer, J. S. (1971). Residual aspects of 2,4,5-T and an ester in sheep and cattle with observations on concomitant toxicological effects. *J. Agric. Food Chem.* **19,**761–764.

Clark, D. E., Young, J. E., Younger, R. L., Hunt, L. M., and McLaran, J. K. (1964). The fate of 2,4-dichlorophenoxyacetic acid in sheep. *J. Agric. Food Chem.* **12,**43–45.

Clark, D. G. (1971). Inhibition of the absorption of paraquat from the gastrointestinal tract by adsorbents. *Br. J. Ind. Med.* **28,**51–55.

Clark, D. G., and Hurst, E. W. (1970). The toxicity of diquat. *Br. J. Ind. Med.* **27,**51–55.

Clark, D. G., McElligott, T. F., and Hurst, E. W. (1966). The toxicity of paraquat. *Br. J. Ind. Med.* **23,**126–132.

Cobb, L. M., and Grimshaw, P. (1979). Acute toxicity of oral diquat (1,1′-ethylene-2,2′-bipyridinium) in cynomolgus monkeys. *Toxicol. Appl. Pharmacol.* **51,**277–282.

Coggon, D., and Acheson, E. D. (1982). Do phenoxy herbicides cause cancer in man? *Lancet* **1,**1057–1059.

Colburn, W. A. (1978). A model for the dose-dependent pharmacokinetics of chlorophenoxy acid herbicides in the rat: The effect of enterohepatic recycling. *J. Pharmacokinet. Biopharm.* **6,**417–426.

Collins, T. F. X., and Williams, C. H. (1971). Teratogenic studies with 2,4,5-T and 2,4-D in the hamster. *Bull. Environ. Contam. Toxicol.* **6,**559–567.

Conning, D. M., Fletcher, K., and Swan, A. A. B. (1969). Paraquat and related bipyridyls. *Br. Med. Bull.* **25,**245–249.

Conso, F., Guillam, C., and Bescol-Liversac, J. (1973). Intoxication by dimethylpyridylium. Presentation of electron microscopic images. *Med. Leg. Dommage Corpor.* **6,**420–422 (in French).

Conso, F., Neel, P., Pouzoulet, C., Efthymiou, M. L., Gervais, P., and Gaultier, M. (1977). Toxicity in man of halogen derivative of hydroxybenzonitrile (ioxynil, bromoxynil). *Arch. Mal. Prof. Med. Trav. Secur. Soc.* **38,**674–677 (in French).

Cooke, N. J., Flenley, D. C., and Matthew, H. (1973). Paraquat poisoning. Serial studies of lung function. *Q. J. Med.* [N. Sr.] **42,**683–692.

Copland, G. M., Kolin, A., and Shulman, H. S. (1974). Fatal pulmonary intraalveolar fibrosis after paraquat ingestion. *N. Engl. J. Med.* **291,**290–292.

Costlow, R. D., and Manson, J. M. (1981). The heart and diaphragm: Target organs in the neonatal death induced by nitrofen (2,4-dichlorophenyl-*p*-nitrophenyl ether). *Toxicology* **20,**209–227.

Costlow, R. D., and Manson, J. M. (1983). Distribution and metabolism of the teratogen nitrofen (2,4-dichloro-4′-nitro diphenyl ether in pregnant rats. *Toxicology* **26,**11–23.

Costlow, R. D., Hirsekorn, J. M., Stiratelli, R. G., O'Hara, B. P., Black, D. L., Kane, W. W., Burke, S. S., Smith, J. M., and Hayes, A. W. (1981). The effects on rat pups when nitrofen (4-(2,4-dichlorophenoxy) nitrobenzene) was applied dermally to the dam during organogenesis. *Toxicology* **28,**37–50.

Courtney, K. D. (1977). Prenatal effects of herbicides: Evaluation by the prenatal development index. *Q. J. Med.* [N. Sr.] **42,**683–692.

Courtney, K. D., and Moore, J. A. (1971). Teratology studies with 2,4,5-trichlorophenoxyacetic acid and 2,3,7,8-tetrachlorodibenzo-*p*-dioxin. *Toxicol. Appl. Pharmacol.* **20,**396.

Courtney, K. D., Gaylor, D. W., Hogan, M. D., Falk, H. L., Bates, R. R., and Mitchell, I. (1970). Teratogenic evaluation of 2,4,5-T. *Science* **168,**864–866.

Courtney, K. D., Ebron, M. T., and Tucker, A. W. (1977). Distribution of 2,4,5-trichlorophenoxyacetic acid in the mouse fetus. *Toxicol. Lett.* **1,**103–108.

Coutselinas, A., Kentarchou, R., and Boukis, D. (1977). Concentration levels of 2,4-D and 2,4,5-T in forensic material. *Forensic Sci.* **10,**203–204.

Crabtree, H. C., and Rose, M. S. (1976). Early effects of diquat on plasma corticosteroid concentrations in rats. *Biochem. Pharmacol.* **25,**2465–2468.

Crabtree, H. C., and Rose, M. S. (1978). Effect of diquat dichloride on gastric emptying and fluid accumulation in the rat stomach. *Toxicol. Appl. Pharmacol.* **45,**250–260.

Crabtree, H. C., Lock, E. A., and Rose, M. S. (1977). Effects of diquat on the gastrointestinal tract of rats. *Toxicol. Appl. Pharmacol.* **41,**585–595.

Crafts, A. S. (1961). "The Chemistry and Mode of Action of Herbicides." Wiley (Interscience), New York.

Cravey, R. H. (1979). Poisoning by paraquat. *Clin. Toxicol.* **14,**195–198.

Cross, C. E., and Last, J. A. (1978). Paraquat goes to pot. *Chest* **74,**358.

Curry, A. S. (1962). Twenty-one uncommon cases of poisoning. *Br. Med. J.* **1,**687–689.

Cutting, R. T., Phuoc, T. H., Ballo, J. M., Benenson, M. W., and Evans, C. H.

(1970). "Congenital Malformations, Hydatidiform Moles, and Stillbirths in the Republic of Vietnam, 1960–1969." U.S. Govt. Printing Office, Washington, D.C.

Daniel, J. W., and Gage, J. C. (1966). Absorption and excretion of diquat and paraquat in rats. *Br. J. Ind. Med.* **23,**133–136.

Danon, J. M., Karpati, G., Carpenter, S., and Wolfe, L. S. (1976). Experimental myotonic myopathy. *Neurology* **26,**384.

Dauterman, W. C., and Muecke, W. (1974). *In vitro* metabolism of atrazine by rat liver. *Pestic. Biochem. Physiol.* **4,**212–219.

Davidson, J. D., and MacPherson P. (1972). Pulmonary changes in paraquat poisoning. *Clin. Radiol.* **23,**18–25.

Davis, R. G., Madsen, K. M., Fregly, M. J., and Tisher, C. C. (1983). Kidney structure in hypothyroidism. *Am. J. Pathol.* **113,**41–49.

Dävring, L., and Hultgren, K. (1977). Cytogenic effects on *in vivo* bone-marrow cells of *Mus musculus* induced by a commercial 2,4,5-T ester product. *Hereditas* **85,**123–134.

Dearden, L. C., Fairshter, R. D., McRae, D. M., Smith, W. R., Glauser, F. L., and Wilson, A. F. (1978). Pulmonary ultrastructure of the late aspects of human paraquat poisoning. *Am. J. Pathol.* **93,**667–680.

Dearnaley, D. P., and Martin, M. F. R. (1978). Plasmapheresis for paraquat poisoning. *Lancet* **1,**162.

DeBaun, J. R., Bova, D. L., Finley, K. A., and Menn, J. J. (1978a). Metabolism of (ring ^{14}C) Ordham (molinate) in the rat. 1. Balance and tissue residue study. *J. Agric. Food Chem.* **26,**1096–1098.

DeBaun, J. R., Bova, D. L., Iseng, C. K., and Menn, J. J. (1978b). Metabolism of (ring ^{14}C) Ordham (molinate) in the rat. 2. Urinary metabolite identification. *J. Agric. Food Chem.* **26,**1098–1104.

Deeken, J. H. (1974). Chloracne induced by 2,6-dichlorobenzonitrile. *Arch. Dermatol.* **109,**245–246.

de Larrard, J. (1969). Intoxication by a quaternary ammonium agrochemical (Gramoxone). *Arch. Mal. Prof. Med. Trav. Secur. Soc.* **30,**421 (in French).

de Larrard, J., and Barbaste, M. (1969). Fatal suicidal poisoning due to 2,4-D. *Arch. Mal. Prof. Med. Trav. Secur. Soc.* **30,**434 (in French).

Delvo, H. W. (1987). "Inputs: Outlook and Situation Report, Economic Research Service," IOS-6. U.S. Department of Agriculture, Washington, D.C.

Dencker, L. (1976). Tissue localization of some teratogens at early and late gestation related to fetal effects. *Acta Pharmacol. Toxicol.* **39,**1–13.

Desi, I., and Sos, J. (1962). Central nervous injury by a chemical herbicide. *Acta Med. Acad. Sci. Hung.* **18,**429–433.

Dikshith, T. S. S., Datta, K. K., Raizada, R. B., and Kushwah, H. S. (1979). Effects of paraquat dichloride in male rabbits. *Indian J. Exp. Biol.* **17,**926–928.

Dinerman, A. A., and Lavrent'eva, N. A. (1969). The toxicity of the herbicides propazine and prometryn. *Gig. Sanit.* **34,**94–96 (in Russian).

Dmitriyev, V. I. (1974). Harmful effects of chemical substances used by the U.S. Army in Indochina. *Voen.-Med. Zh.* **1,**88–90 (in Russian).

Dodge, A. D. (1972). The mode of action of the bipyridylium herbicides, paraquat and diaquat. *Endeavour* **30,**130–135.

Dougherty, W. J., Coulston, F., and Goldberg, L. (1973). Non-teratogenicity of 2,4,5-trichlorophenoxyacetic acid in monkeys (*Macaca mulatta*). *Toxicol. Appl. Pharmacol.* **25,**442.

Dougherty, W. J., Herbst, M., and Coulston, F. (1975). The non-teratogenicity of 2,4,5-trichlorophenoxyacetic acid in the rhesus monkey (*Macaca mulatta*). *Bull. Environ. Contam. Toxicol.* **13,**477–482.

Douglas, J. F., McGeown, M. G., and McEvoy, J. (1973). The treatment of paraquat poisoning: Three cases of recovery. *Ulster Med. J.* **42,**209–212.

Dragsnes, L., Helgeland, K., and Jonsen, J. (1975). Effects of the herbicide 2,4,5-trichlorophenoxyacetic acid on growth and morphology of L 929 cells. *Acta Pharmacol. Toxicol.* **36,**97–102.

Draper, W. M., and Casida, J. E. (1983). Diphenyl ether herbicides: Mutagenic metabolites and photoproducts of nitrofen. *J. Agric. Food Chem.* **31,**227–231.

Draper, W. M., and Street, J. C. (1982). Applicator exposure to 2,4-D, dicamba and a dicamba isomer. *J. Environ. Sci. Health, Part B* **B17,**321–339.

Drill, V. A., and Hiratzka, T. (1953). Toxicity of 2,4-dichlorophenoxyacetic acid and 2,4,5-trichlorophenoxyacetic acid: A report on their acute and chronic toxicity in dogs. *Arch. Ind. Hyg. Occup. Med.* **7,**61–67.

Dudley, A. W., Jr., and Thapar, N. T. (1972). Fatal human ingestion of 2,4-D, a common herbicide. *Arch. Pathol.* **94,**270–275.

DuShane, G. (1959). Cranberry smash. *Science* **130,**1447.

Dux, E., Toth, I., Kiszely, G., Dux, L., and Joo, F. (1977). The possible cellular mechanism of 2,4-dichlorophenoxyacetic-induced myopathy. *FEBS Lett.* **82,**219–222.

Ebron, M., and Courtney, K. D. (1976). Difference in 2,4,5-T distribution in fetal mice and guinea pigs. *Toxicol. Appl. Pharmacol.* **37,**144–145.

Ecker, J. L., Gibson, J. E., and Hook, J. B. (1975a). *In vitro* analysis of the renal handling of paraquat. *Toxicol. Appl. Pharmacol.* **34,**170–177.

Ecker, J. L., Hook, J. B., and Gibson, J. E. (1975b). Nephrotoxicity of paraquat in mice. *Toxicol. Appl. Pharmacol.* **34,**178–186.

Editorial (1977). 2,4,5-T, spina bifida, and after. *N. Z. Med. J.* **86,**99–100.

Edson, E. F., and Sanderson, D. M. (1965). Toxicity of the herbicides, 2-methoxy-3,6-dichlorobenzoic acid (dicamba) and 2-methoxy-3,5,6-trichlorobenzoic acid (tricamba). *Food Cosmet. Toxicol.* **3,**299–304.

Eliahou, H. E., Almog, C., Gura, V., and Iaina, A. (1973). Treatment of paraquat poisoning by hemodialysis. *Isr. J. Med. Sci.* **9,**459–462.

Elo, H. A. (1976). Distribution and elimination of 2-methyl-4-chlorophenoxyacetic acid (MCPA) in male rats. *Acta Pharmacol. Toxicol.* **39,**58–64.

Elo, H. A., and Ylitalo, P. (1977). Substantial increase in the levels of chlorophenoxyacetic acids in the CNS of rats as a result of severe intoxication. *Acta Pharmacol. Toxicol.* **41,**280–284.

Elo, H. A., and Ylitalo, P. (1979). Distribution of 2-methyl-4-chlorophenoxyacetic acid and 2,4-dichlorophenoxyacetic acid in male rats: Evidence for the involvement of the central nervous system in their toxicity. *Toxicol. Appl. Pharmacol.* **51,**439–446.

Elo, H. A., Ylitalo, P., Kyottila, J., and Hervonen, H. (1982). Increase in the penetration of tracer compounds into the rat brain during 2-methyl-4-chlorophenoxyacetic acid (MCPA) intoxication. *Acta Pharmacol. Toxicol.* **50,** 104–107.

Elroy-Stein, O., Bernstein, Y., and Groner, Y. (1986). Overproduction of human Cu/Zn-superoxide dismutase in transfected cells: Extenuation of paraquat-mediated cytotoxicity and enhancement of lipid peroxidation. *EMBO J.* **5**(3),615–622.

Emerson, J. L., Thompson, D. J., Strebing, R. J., Gerbig, C. G., and Robinson, V. B. (1971). Teratogenic studies of 2,4,5-trichlorophenoxyacetic acid in the rat and rabbit. *Food Cosmet. Toxicol.* **9,**395–404.

Environmental Protection Agency (1986). Pesticide tolerances for metolachlor. *Fed. Regist.* **51,**25696–25697.

Erickson, M. D., Frank, C. W., and Morgan, D. P. (1979). Determination of *s*-triazine herbicide residues in urine. Studies of excretion and metabolism in swine as a model to human metabolism. *J. Agric. Food Chem.* **27,**743–746.

Erne, K. (1966). Studies on the analytical chemistry and toxicology of phenoxy herbicides. *Sven. Farm. Tidskr.* **70,**837–840 (in Swedish).

Fabregat, I., Vitorica, J., Satrustegui, J., and Machado, A. (1985). The pentose phosphate cycle is regulated by NADPH/NADP ratio in a rat liver. *Arch. Biochem. Biophys.* **236,**(1),110–118.

Faerber, G. I. (1962). The use of sodium trichloroacetate as a weed-killer. A report on its irritative effects on the upper respiratory system and the conjunctiva in municipal workers. *Med. Proc.* **8,**248–251.

Fairshter, R. D., and Wilson, A. F. (1978). Paraquat and marihuana. *Chest* **74,** 357.

Fairshter, R. D., Rosen, S. M., Smith, W. R., Glauser, F. L., McRae, D. M., and Wilson, A. F. (1976). Paraquat poisoning: New aspects of therapy. *Q. J. Med.* **45,**551–565.

Fairshter, R. D., Dabir-Vaziri, N., Smith, W. R., Glauser, F. L., and Wilson, A. F. (1979). Paraquat poisoning: An analytical and toxicologic study of three cases. *Toxicology* **12,**259–266.

Fang, S. C., George, M., and Yu, T. C. (1964). Metabolism of 3-amino-1,2,4-triazole-5-C^{14} by rats. *J. Agric. Food Chem.* **12,**219–223.

Fang, S. C., Khanna, S., and Rao, A. V. (1966). Further study on the metabolism of labeled 3-amino-1,2,4-triazole (ATA) an its plant metabolites in rats. *J. Agric. Food Chem.* **14,**262–265.

Fang, S. C., Montgomery, M. L., and Freed, V. H. (1972). The metabolism and distribution of 2,4,5-trichlorophenoxyacetic acid in female rats. *Toxicol. Appl. Pharmacol.* **22,**317–318.

Fang, S. C., Fallin, E., Montgomery, M. L., and Freed, V. H. (1973). The metabolism and distribution of 2,4,5-trichlorophenoxyacetic acid in female rats. *Toxicol. Appl. Pharmacol.* **24**,555–563.

Fassett, D. W. (1963). Organic acids, anhydrides, lactones, acid halides and amides, thioacids. In "Industrial Hygiene and Toxicology" (F. A. Patty, ed.), 2nd ed., pp. 1771–1837. Wiley (Interscience), New York.

Faure, J., Marka, C., Faure, H., Yacoub, M., and Cau, G. (1973). Histopathological and toxicology data from a poisoning death from paraquat. *Med. Leg. Dommage Corpor.* **6**,417–419 (in French).

Fedorova, L. M., Belova, R. S., Kovtunova, N. E., Kiriukhina, N. N., and Voichonok, H. G. (1977). Residue levels of chlorophenoxyacetic acids in the environment and in the human body. *Gig. Sanit.* **6**,101–103 (in Russian).

Fel, P., Zala, I., Szule, E., and Varga, L. (1976). Hemodialysis in diquat poisoning. *Orv. Hetil.* **117**,1773–1774 (in Hungarian).

Feldmann, R. J., and Maibach, H. I. (1974). Percutaneous penetration of some pesticides and herbicides in man. *Toxicol. Appl. Pharmacol.* **28**,126–132.

Fennelly, J. J., and Fitzgerald, M. X. (1971). Recovery from severe paraquat poisoning following forced diuresis and immunosuppressive therapy. *J. Ir. Med. Assoc.* **64**,69–71.

Fennelly, J. J., Gallagher, J. T., and Carroll, R. J. (1968). Paraquat poisoning in a pregnant woman. *Br. Med. J.* **3**,722–723.

Ferguson, D. M. (1971). Renal handling of paraquat. *Br. J. Pharmacol.* **42**, 636.

Fetisov, M. I. (1966). Problems of occupational hygiene in work with herbicides of 2,4-D group. *Gig. Sanit.* **31**,28–30.

Field, B., and Kerr, C. (1979). Herbicide use and incidence of neural tube defects. *Lancet* **1**,1341–1342.

Finberg, L. (1974). Interaction of the chemical environment with the infant and young child. *Pediatrics* **53**,831–837.

Fisher, H. K., and Williams, G. (1976). Paraquat is not bacteriostatic under anaerobic conditions. *Life Sci.* **19**,421–426.

Fisher, H. K., Humphries, M., and Bails, R. (1971). Paraquat poisoning. Recovery from renal and pulmonary damage. *Ann. Intern. Med.* **75**,731–736.

Fisher, H. K., Clements, J. A., and Wright, R. R. (1973). Enhancement of oxygen toxicity by the herbicide paraquat. *Am. Rev. Respir. Dis.* **107**,246–252.

Fisher, H. K., Clements, J. A., Tierney, D. F., and Wright, R. R. (1975). Pulmonary effects of paraquat in the first day after injection. *Am. J. Physiol.* **228**,1217–1223.

Fitzgerald, G. R., Barniville, G., Black, J., Silke, B., Carmody, M., and O'Dwyer, W. F. (1977a). Occupational paraquat poisoning. *Q. J. Med.* **46**, 561–562.

Fitzgerald, G. R., Barniville, G., FitzPatrick, P., Edwards, A., Silke, B., Carmody, M., and O'Dwyer, W. F. (1977b). Adrenal abnormalities in paraquat poisoning. An indication for corticosteroid therapy? *Ir. J. Med. Sci.* **146**,421–423.

Fitzgerald, G. R., Barniville, G., Flanagan, M., Silke, B., Carmody, M., and O'Dwyer, W. F. (1978). The changing pattern of paraquat poisoning: An epidemiologic study. *J. Ir. Med. Assoc.* **71**,103–108.

Fitzgerald, G. R., Barniville, G., Gibney, R. T. N., and Fitzgerald, M. X. (1979). Clinical, radiological, and pulmonary function assessment in 13 long-term survivors of paraquat poisoning. *Thorax* **34**,414–415.

Fjeldstad, P., and Wannag, A. (1977). Human urinary excretion of the herbicide 2-methyl-4-chlorophenoxyacetic acid. *Scand. J. Work Environ. Health* **3**, 100–103.

Fletcher, K., and Wyatt, I. (1970). The composition of lung lipids after poisoning with paraquat. *Br. J. Exp. Pathol.* **51**,604–610.

Fletcher, K., and Wyatt, I. (1972). The action of paraquat on the incorporation of palmitic acid into dipalmitoyl lecithin in mouse lungs. *Br. J. Exp. Pathol.* **53**,225–230.

Food and Agriculture Organization/World Health Organization (FAO/WHO) (1973). "1972 Evaluations of Some Pesticide Residues in Food." Monograph prepared by the Joint Meeting of the FAO Working Party of Experts on Pesticide Residues and the WHO Expert Committee on Pesticide Residues that met in Rome from 20 to 28 November 1972 (WHO Pestic. Residues Ser., No. 2. World Health Organ., Geneva.

Foster, T. S., and Khan, S. U. (1976). Metabolism of atrazine by the chicken. *J. Agric. Food Chem.* **24**,566–570.

Fowler, B. L., and Brooks, R. E. (1971). Effects of the herbicide paraquat on the ultrastructure of mouse kidney. *Am. J. Pathol.* **63**,505–512.

Francis, B. M. (1986). Teratogenicity of bifenox and nitrofen in rodents. *J. Environ. Sci. Health, Part B* **B21**,303–317.

Frank, R., Campbell, R. A., and Sirons, G. J. (1985). Forestry workers involved in aerial application of 2,4-dichlorophenoxyacetic acid (2,4-D): Exposure and urinary excretion. *Arch. Environ. Contam. Toxicol.* **14**,427–435.

Fraser, A. D., Isner, A. F., and Perry, R. A. (1984). Toxicologic studies in a fatal overdose of 2,4-D, mecoprop, and dicamba. *J. Forensic Sci.* **29**,1237–1244.

Fregley, M. J. (1968). Effect of aminotriazole on thyroid function in the rat. *Toxicol. Appl. Pharmacol.* **13**,272–286.

Fridovich, I., and Hassan, H. M. (1979). Paraquat and the exacerbation of oxygen toxicity. *Trends Biochem. Sci.* **4**,113–115.

Frohberg, H. (1974). Investigations on the embryotoxic effect of 2,4,5-T in NMRI-mice. *Naunyn-Schmiedeberg's Arch. Pharmacol.* **282**,R22.

Fujita, K. (1973a). Cases of chemical burn of corona by a herbicide, 1,1'-dimethyl-4,4'-bipyridinium dichloride (paraquat dichloride). *J. Jpn. Assoc. Rural Med.* **22**,194–195 (in Japanese).

Fujita, K. (1973b). Ocular chemical burn by a herbicide, paraquat dichloride. *Clin. Ophthalmol.* **27**,1399–1401 (in Japanese).

Fujita, K. (1975). Keratitis and conjunctivitis due to pesticides. *J. Jpn. Assoc. Rural Med.* **24**,16–18 (in Japanese).

Fujita, K., Fujita, H., and Funazaki, Z. (1975). Chromosomal abnormality caused by 2,4,5-T. *J. Jpn. Assoc. Rural Med.* **24**,77–79 (in Japanese).

Funazaki, Z. (1971). Herbicides and deformities in Vietnam. *Jpn. J. Public Health Nurse* **27**,54–55 (in Japanese).

Funazaki, Z. (1972). Teratogenicity of 2,4,5-T. *Biotech.* **3**,464–470 (in Japanese).

Funke, K., Goehler, G., Futh, U., and Lignitz, E. (1976). The clinical prognosis, therapy and morphology of a paraquat poisoning. *Dtsch. Gesundheitswes.* **31**,2143–2145 (in German).

Gage, J. C. (1968). Toxicity of paraquat and diquat aerosols generated by a size-selective cyclone: Effect of particle size distribution. *Br. J. Ind. Med.* **25**, 304–314.

Gaines, T. B. (1969). Acute toxicity of pesticides. *Toxicol. Appl. Pharmacol.* **14**,515–534.

Gaines, T. B., Kimbrough, R. D., and Linder, R. E. (1973). The toxicity of amitrole in the rat. *Toxicol. Appl. Pharmacol.* **26**,118–129.

Gaines, T. B., Holson, J. F., Jr., Nelson, C. J., and Schumacher, H. J. (1975). Analysis of strain differences in sensitivity and reproducibility of results in assessing 2,4,5-T teratogenicity in mice. *Toxicol. Appl. Pharmacol.* **33**, 174–175.

Gale, T. F., and Ferm, V. H. (1973). Effects of the herbicides 2,4,5-T and pyrazon on embryogenesis in the hamster. *Anat. Rec.* **175**,503.

Galloway, D. B., and Petrie, J. C. (1972). Recovery from severe paraquat poisoning. *Postgrad. Med. J.* **48**,684–686.

Gamble, W. (1975). Mechanism of action of hypolipidemic and herbicidal aryloxy acids. *J. Theor. Biol.* **54**,181–190.

Gamble, W., Olson, R. J., and Trumble, T. E. (1974). Action of aryloxy acids on cholesterol and fatty acid biosynthesis by rat liver homogenates. *Fed. Proc., Fed. Am. Soc. Exp. Biol.* **33**,1499.

Gandréault, P., Friedman, P. A., and Lovejoy, F. H., Jr. (1985). Efficacy of activated charcoal and magnesium citrate in the treatment of oral paraquat intoxication. *Ann. Emerg. Med.* **14**,(2),123–125.

Gardiner, A. J. S. (1972). Pulmonary edema in paraquat poisoning. *Thorax* **27**, 132–135.

Gardiner, T. H., and Schanker, L. S. (1976). Effect of paraquat induced lung damage on permeability of rat lung to drugs. *Proc. Soc. Exp. Biol. Med.* **151**,288–292.

Gaultier, M., Bescol-Liversac, J., Frejaville, J. P., Leclerc, J. P., Guillam, C., and Rodde, M. T. (1973). Clinical, anatomical, and experimental study of intoxication with paraquat. Ultrastructural lesions. *Sem. Hop.* **49**,1972–1987 (in French).

Gehring, P. J., Kramer, C. G., Schwetz, B. A., Rose, J. Q., and Rowe, V. K.

(1973). The fate of 2,4,5-trichlorophenoxyacetic acid (2,4,5-T) following oral administration to man. *Toxicol. Appl. Pharmacol.* **26,**352–361.

Geldmacher-von Mallinckrodt, M., and Lautenbach, L. (1966). Two poisoning deaths (suicides) with chlorinated phenoxy acid (2,4-D and MCPA). *Arch. Toxikol.* **21,**261–278 (in German).

Geldmacher-von Mallinckrodt, M., and Schmidt, H. P. (1970). The toxicity and metabolism of aminotriazole in man. *Arch. Toxikol.* **27,**13–18 (in German).

Geldmacher-von Mallinckrodt, M., and Schüssler, F. (1971). The metabolism and toxicity of 1-(3,4-dichlorophenyl)-3,3-dimethyl urea (diuron) by man. *Arch. Toxikol.* **27,**187–192 (in German).

Georgian, L., Moraru, I., and Draghicescu, T. (1983). Cytogenic effects of alachlor and mancozeb. *Mutation Research,* **116,**341–348.

Goldstein, N. P., Jones, P. H., and Brown, J. R. (1959). Peripheral neuropathy after exposure to an ester of dichlorophenoxyacetic acid. *JAMA, J. Am. Med. Assoc.* **171,**1306–1309.

Golovan', D. I. (1970). Experimental basis for the permissible level of dianate and 2,3,6-trichlorobenzoic acid in reservoirs. *Gig. Sanit.* **35,**14–17 (in Russian).

Gorshkov, A. I. (1971). Hygienic evaluation of chlorocholine chloride (CCC) and of its combination with 2,4-D amine salt. *Gig. Sanit.* **36,**33–36 (in Russian).

Gorzinski, S. J., Johnson, K. A., Campbell, R. A., and Landry, T. D. (1987). Dietary toxicity of picloram herbicide in rats. *J. Toxicol. Environ. Health* **20,**367–377.

Goulding, R., Volans, G. N., Crome, P., and Widdop, B. (1976). Paraquat poisoning. *Br. Med. J.* **1,**42.

Grabensee, B. (1974). Clinical profile of paraquat poisoning. *Pneumonologie* **150,**173–179 (in German).

Grabensee, B., Veltmann, G., Muertz, R., and Borchard, F. (1971). Paraquat poisoning. *Dtsch. Med. Wochenschr.* **96,**498–506 (in German).

Gray, L. E., Jr., and Kavlock, R. J. (1983). The effects of the herbicide 2,4-dichlorophenyl-*p*-nitrophenyl ether (NIT) on serum thyroid hormones in adult female mice. *Toxicol. Lett.* **15,**231–235.

Gray, L. E., Jr., Kavlock, R. J., Chernoff, N., Ferrell, J., McLamb, J., and Ostby, J. (1982). Prenatal exposure to the herbicide 2,4-dichlorophenyl-*p*-nitrophenyl ether destroys the rodent Harderian gland. *Science* **215,**293–294.

Gray, L. E., Jr., Kavlock, R. J., Chernoff, N., Ostby, J., and Ferrell, J. (1983). Postnatal developmental alterations following prenatal exposure to the herbicide 2,4-dichlorophenyl-*p*-nitrophenyl ether: A dose response evaluation in the mouse. *Toxicol. Appl. Pharmacol.* **67,**1–44.

Great Britain Ministry of Agriculture, Fisheries and Food (1972). Report on the use of poisonous substances in agriculture and on the working of the Agriculture (Poisonous Substances) Regulations during 1972. An excerpt appeared in the *WHO Inf. Circ. Toxic. Pestic. Man* **VBC/TOX/74,**13 (1974).

Greenberg, D. B., and Last, J. A. (1977). Collagen biosynthesis by lung slices from rats administered paraquat, a fibrotic agent. *Chest* **72,**400.

Greenberg, S. R., and Eisenberg, G. M. (1977). The pulmonary effects of benzyl-viologen in Swiss mice. *Environ. Pollut.* **12,**255–259.

Greig, D., and Streat, S. (1977). Intentional paraquat poisoning: Case report. *N. Z. Med. J.* **88,**12–13.

Grundies, H., Kolmar, D., and Bennhold, I. (1971). Paraquat intoxication: A case report with particular reference to hemodialysis. *Dtsch. Med. Wochenschr.* **26,**588–589 (in German).

Grunow, W., Altmann, H. J., and Boehme, C. (1975). The metabolism of 3-amino-1,2,4-triazole in rats. *Arch. Toxikol.* **34,**315–324 (in German).

Grunow, W., and Boehme, C. (1974). The metabolism of 2,4,5-T and 2,4-D by rats and mice. *Arch. Toxicol.* **32,**217–225 (in German).

Grunow, W., Boehme, C., and Budczies, B. (1971). Renal metabolism of 2,4,5-T by rats. *Food Cosmet. Toxicol.* **9,**667–670 (in German).

Gruzdev, A. I., Nevskaia, T. L., and Prokopchuk, V. S. (1969). Toxicological characteristics of the new herbicide Pyramin. *Farmakol. Toksikol. (Moscow)* **32,**333–336 (in Russian).

Guardascione, V., and Mazzella di Bosco, M. (1969). Contribution to the knowledge of occupational intoxication with paraquat, dipyridilium herbicide. *Folia Med. (Napes)* **52,**728–738 (in Italian).

Gulic, F., Hojs, M., and Rogl, F. (1975). A case of paraquat poisoning. *Arh. Hig. Rada Toksikol.* **26,**227–232 (in Serbo-Croatian).

Gurd, M. R., Harmer, G. L. M., and Lessel, B. (1965). Acute toxicity and 7-month feeding studies with mecoprop and MCPA. *Food Cosmet. Toxicol.* **3,**883–885.

Gutenmann, W. H., and Lisk, D. J. (1975). A feeding study with diphenylamine in a dairy cow. *Bull. Environ. Contam. Toxicol.* **13,**177–180.

Guyon, F., Bismuth, C., Leclerc, J. P., and Dauchy, F. (1975). Severe intoxication with paraquat followed by death in less than 24 hours. Toxicological and clinical anatomy studies. *J. Eur. Toxicol.* **7,**182–187.

Gysin, H., and Knuesli, E. (1960). Chemistry and herbicidal properties of triazine derivatives. *In* "Advances in Pest Control Research" (R. Metcalf, ed.), Wiley (Interscience), New York.

Gzhegotskiy, M. I., and Doloshitskiy, S. L. (1971). Skin absorption effects of herbicides. *Vrach. Delo* **11,**133–134 (in Russian).

Gzhegotskiy, M. I., and Martyniuk, V. Z. (1968). Toxicological and hygienic evaluation of the new chlorine-containing herbicide Pyramin. *Vrach. Delo* **8,**112–116 (in Russian).

Gzhegotskiy, M. I., Shkliaruk, L. V., and Dychok, L. A. (1977). Toxicological characteristics of the herbicide Zeazin. *Vrach. Delo* **5,**133–136 (in Russian).

Hall, S. M. (1972). Effects on pregnant rats and their progeny of adequate or low protein diets containing 2,4,5-trichlorophenoxyacetic acid (2,4,5-T) or *p,p*′-DDT. *Fed. Proc., Fed. Am. Soc. Exp. Biol.* **31,**726.

Halliwell, B. (1976). Ascorbic acid and paraquat toxicity. *Lancet* **2,**854.

Hamman, L., and Rich, A. R. (1944). Acute diffuse interstitial fibrosis of the lungs. *Bull. Johns Hopkins Hosp.* **74,**177–212.

Hamner, C. L., and Tukey, H. B. (1974). The herbicidal action of 2,4-dichlorophenoxyacetic and 2,4,5-trichlorophenoxyacetic acid on bindweed. *Science* **100,**154–155.

Hanada, K., Kameda, T., Suzuki, Y., Kayashi, S., Ohobi, A., and Sugaya, H. (1977). An investigation of patch test dermatitis. Part IV. A comparison between farmers and non-farmers. *Akita J. Rural Med.* **23.**

Hanawa, M., Fujisawa, M., Akimoto, Y., Oishi, M., Kobayashi, H., Osuji, H., Nishida, S., Kitahara, K., and Otani, T. (1977). An autopsy record of interstitial pneumonia due to acute intoxication by paraquat dichloride. *J. Jpn. Soc. Int. Med.* **66,**1597–1598 (in Japanese).

Hanify, J. A., Metcalf, P., Nobbs, C. L., and Worsley, K. J. (1981). Aerial spraying of 2,4,5-T and human birth malformations: An epidemiological investigation. *Science* **212,**349–357.

Hansen, W. H., Quaife, M. L., Habermann, R. T., and Fitzhugh, O. G. (1971). Chronic toxicity of 2,4-dichlorophenoxyacetic acid in rats and dogs. *Toxicol. Appl. Pharmacol.* **20,**122–129.

Hapke, H. J. (1967). The toxicity of aminotriazol for domestic animals. *Zentralbl. Veterinaer med.* **14,**469–486 (in German).

Hapke, H. J. (1968). Studies on the toxicology of the weedkiller Simazin. *Berl. Munch. Tieraerztl. Wochenschr.* **81,**301–303 (in German).

Haque, R., Lilley, S., and Coshow, W. (1970). Mechanism of adsorption of diquat and paraquat on montmorillonite surface. *J. Colloid Interface Sci.* **33,**187–188.

Hardell, L., and Sandström, A. (1978). Malignant mesenchymal soft-tissue tumors and exposure to phenoxy acids or chlorophenols. A case control study. *Laekartidningen* **75,**3535–3536 (in Swedish).

Hardell, L., and Sandström, A. (1979). Case-control study: Soft-tissue sarcomas and exposure to phenoxyacetic acids or chlorophenols. *Br. J. Cancer* **39,**711–717.

Hargreave, T. B., Gresham, Y. A., and Karayannupoulos, S. (1969). Paraquat poisoning. *Postgrad. Med. J.* **45,**633–635.

Harley, J. B., Grinspan, S., and Root, R. K. (1977). Paraquat suicide in a young woman: Results of therapy directed against the superoxide radical. *Yale J. Biol. Med.* **50,**481–488.

Harrison, L. C., Dortimer, A. C., and Murphy, D. S. (1972). Fatalities due to the weedkiller paraquat. *Med. J. Aust.* **2,**774–777.

Hartley, D., and Kidd, H. (1983). "The Agrochemicals Handbook." Royal Society of Chemistry, Unwin Bros. Ltd., Surrey, U.K.

Hasegawa, G., and Gorin, A. B. (1977). Clearance of paraquat from plasma and lung lymph in sheep. *Am. Rev. Respir. Dis.* **115,**220.

Hassan, H. M., and Fridovich, I. (1978). Superoxide radical and the oxygen enhancement of the toxicity of paraquat in *Escherichia coli. J. Biol. Chem.* **253,**8143–8148.

Hattula, M. L., Elo, H., Sorvari, T. E., Teunauen, H., and Arstila, A. (1977). Acute and subchronic toxicity of 2-methyl-4-chlorophenoxyacetic acid (MCPA) in male rats. I. Light microscopy and tissue concentrations of MCPA. *Bull. Environ. Contam. Toxicol.* **18,**152–158.

Hayakawa, Y., Kikuoka, M., Nakamura, T., Fujiwara, Y., Ueda, S., Uchiyama, T., Okayasu, D., Amaki, T., Ariga, H., and Sakurai, I. (1979). An autopsy case from intoxication due to paraquat. *J. Jpn. Soc. Int. Med.* **68,**313 (in Japanese).

Hayes, J. E., Condie, L. W., and Borzelleca, J. F. (1986). Acute, 14-day repeated dosing, and 90-day subchronic toxicity studies of potassium picloram. *Fundam. Appl. Toxicol.* **7,**464–470.

Hayes, W. J., Jr. (1975). "Toxicology of Pesticides." Williams & Wilkins, Baltimore, Maryland.

Hayes, W. J., Jr. (1982). Chapter 11. Herbicides. *In* "Pesticides Studied in Man," pp. 520–567. Williams & Wilkins, Baltimore, Maryland.

Hearn, C. E. D. (1973). A review of agricultural pesticide incidents in man in England and Wales, 1952–1971. *Br. J. Ind. Med.* **30,**253–258.

Hearn, C. E. D., and Keir, W. (1971). Nail damage in spray operators exposed to paraquat. *Br. J. Ind. Med.* **28,**399–403.

Heene, R. (1968). Electron microscopic findings in experimental 2,4-dichlorophenoxyacetate (2,4-D) myopathy in mammals. The development of early changes in myopathies. *Dtsch. Z. Nervenheilkd.* **193,**265–278 (in German).

Heene, R. (1975). Experimental myopathies and muscular dystrophy. Studies in the formal pathogenesis of the myopathy of 2,4-dichlorophenoxyacetate. *Schriftenr. Neurol., Neurol. Ser.* **16,**1–97 (in German).

Heim, W. G., Appleman, D., and Pyfrom, H. T. (1956). Effects of 3-amino-1,2,4-triazole (AT) on catalase and other compounds. *Am. J. Physiol.* **186,**19–23.

Hensel, G., and Duerr, F. (1971). Dialysis treatment in a case of paraquat poisoning. *Med. Welt* **22,**1790–1794.

Herczeg, E., and Reif, A. (1968). Lung damage in victim of paraquat poisoning. *Zentralbl. Allg. Pathol. Pathol. Anat.* **111,**325–328 (in German).

Hessl, S. M., and Berman, C. (1982). Severe neuropathy after exposure to monosodium methyl arsonate. *J. Toxicol. Clin. Toxicol.* **19**(3),281–287.

Hewitt, J., Rigby, J., Reeve, J., and Cox, A. G. (1973). Whole gut irrigation in preparation for large bowel surgery. *Lancet* **2,**337–340.

Hiasa, Y., Ohshima, M., Kitahori, Y., Yuasa, T., Fujita, T., and Iwata, C. (1982). Promoting effects of 3-amino-1,2,4-triazole on the development of thyroid tumors in rats treated with *N*-bis(2-hydroxypropyl) nitrosamine. *Carcinogenesis (London)* **3,**381–384.

Highman, B., Gaines, T. B., and Schumacher, H. J. (1976). Sequential histopathologic, hematologic, and blood chemistry changes induced in mice by a technical and a purified preparation of 2,4,5-trichlorophenoxyacetic acid. *J. Toxicol. Environ. Health* **1,**469–484.

Highman, B., Gaines, T. B., and Schumacher, H. J. (1977). Retarded development of fetal renal alkaline phosphatase in mice given 2,4,5-trichlorophenoxyacetic acid. *J. Toxicol. Environ. Health* **2,**1007–1018.

Highman, B., Wordinger, R. J., and Schumacher, H. J. (1979). Use of the periodic acid Schiff stain to grade retarded fetal renal development in mice. *Toxicol. Lett.* **4,**61–69.

Hikosaka, T. (1975). Clinicopathological study on the effect of 3-amino-1,2,4-triazole on dog thyroid. *J. Nagoya City Univ. Med. Assoc.* **26,**99–111 (in Japanese).

Hill, E. V., and Carlisle, H. (1947). Toxicity of 2,4-dichlorophenoxyacetic acid for experimental animals. *J. Ind. Hyg. Toxicol.* **29,**85–95.

Hoar, S. K., Blair, A., Holmes, F. F., Boysen, C. D., Robel, R. J., Hoover, R., and Fraumeni, J. F. (1986). Agricultural herbicide use and risk of lymphoma and soft tissue sarcoma. *JAMA, J. Am. Med. Assoc.* **256**(9),1141–1147.

Hodge, H. C., Elliott, A. M., Downs, W. L., Ashton, J. K., and Salerno, L. L. (1966). Tests on mice for evaluating carcinogenicity. *Toxicol. Appl. Pharmacol.* **9,**583–596.

Hodge, H. C., Downs, W. L., Panner, B. S., Smith, D. W., Maynard, E. A., Clayton, J. W., Jr., and Rhodes, R. C. (1967). Oral toxicity and metabolism of diuron (*N*-(3,4-dichlorophenyl)-*N,N*-dimethylurea) in rats and dogs. *Food Cosmet. Toxicol.* **5,**513–531.

Hodogaya Chemical Co., Ltd. (1986). "Short Review of Herbicides, 1986," 5th ed. Zenkoku Noson Kyoiki Kyokai Publishing Co., Ltd., Tokyo.

Hofmann, A., and Frohberg, H. (1972). Paraquat poisoning in Germany. *Dtsch. Med. Wochenschr.* **97,**1200–1303 (in German).

Hook, J. B., Bailie, M. D., Jonnson, J. T., and Gehring, P. J. (1974). *In vitro* analysis and transport of 2,4,5-trichlorophenoxyacetic acid by rat and dog kidney. *Food Cosmet. Toxicol.* **12,**209–218.

Hook, J. B., Cardona, R., Osborn, J. L., and Bailie, M. D. (1976). The renal handling of 2,4,5-trichlorophenoxyacetic acid (2,4,5-T) in the dog. *Food Cosmet. Toxicol.* **14,**19–23.

Hoshino, M. (1960). Effect of 3-amino-1,2,4-triazole on the experimental production of liver cancer. *Nature (London)* **186,**174–175.

House, W. B., Goodson, L. H., Gadberry, H. M., and Dockter, K. W. (1967). "Assessment of Ecological Effects of Extensive or Repeated Use of Herbicides: Final Report," AD 824 314. U.S. Department of Defense, Washington, D.C. Available from Clearinghouse for Federal Scientific and Technical Information, Springfield, Virginia.

Howard, J. K. (1978a). Dermal exposure to paraquat. *Lancet* **1,**1100.

Howard, J. K. (1978b). A clinical survey of paraquat formulation workers. *Br. J. Ind. Med.* **36,**220–223.

Howe, D. J. T., and Wright, N. (1965). The toxicity of paraquat and diquat. *Proc. Conf. N.Z. Weed Pest Control Conf., 18th,* pp. 105–114. New Zealand Weed and Pest Control, Wellington, New Zealand.

Huep, W. W., and Hesselman, J. (1979). Severe, acute erosive—hemorrhagic gastroduodenitis after spraying Banvel M. *Dtsch. Med. Wochenschr.* **104,** 525 (in German).

Hughes, D. W. D. (1962). Acquired aplastic anemia in childhood. A review of 22 cases. *Med. J. Aust.* **2,**251–259.

Hughes, R. D., Milburn, P., and Williams, R. T. (1973). Biliary excretion of some diquaternary ammonium cations in the rat, guinea pig and rabbit. *Biochem. J.* **136,**979–984.

Hunt, L. M., Chamberlain, W. F., Gilbert, B. N., Hopkins, D. E., and Gingrich, A. R. (1977). Absorption, excretion, and metabolism of nitrofen by a sheep. *J. Agric. Food Chem.* **25,**1062–1065.

Hurt, S. S. B., Smith, J. M., and Hayes, A. W. (1983). Nitrofen: A review and perspective. *Toxicology* **29,**1–37.

Hutson, D. H., Hoadley, E. C., Griffiths, M. H., and Donninger, C. (1970). Mercapturic-acid formation in the metabolism of 2-chloro-4-ethylamino-6-1-methyl-1-cyanoethylamino-*s*-triazine in the rat. *J. Agric. Food Chem.* **18,**507–512.

Iff, H. W., Brewos, R. A. L., Mallick, N. P., Mawer, G. E., Orr, W. McN., and Stern, M. A. (1971). Paraquat poisoning. *Schweiz. Med. Wochenschr.* **101,** 84–88 (in German).

Ilett, K. F., Stripp, B., Menard, R. H., Reid, W. D., and Gillette, J. R. (1974). Studies on the mechanism of the lung toxicity of paraquat: Comparison of tissue distribution and some biochemical parameters in rats and rabbits. *Toxicol. Appl. Pharmacol.* **28,**216–226.

Imaizumi, K., Atsumi, A., Tanifuji, Y., Ishikawa, I., and Hoshi, H. (1972). Clinical observation of ophthalmic disturbance due to agricultural chemicals. *Nippon Ganka Kiyo* **22,**154–156 (in Japanese).

Imamura, T., Tsuruta, J., Kambara, T., and Maki, S. (1986). Pseudomembranous colitis in a patient of paraquat intoxication. *Acta Pathol. Jpn.* **36** (2),309–316.

Innes, J. R. M., Ulland, B. M., Valerio, M. G., Petrucelli, L., Fishbein, L., Hart, E. R., Pallotta, A. J., Bates, R. R., Falk, H. L., Gart, J. J., Klein, M., Mitchell, I., and Peters, J. (1969). Bioassay of pesticides and industrial chemicals for tumorigenicity in mice: A preliminary note. *J. Natl. Cancer Inst. (U.S.)* **42,**1101–1114.

International Agency for Research on Cancer (IARC) (1977). "Monographs on the Evaluation of Carcinogenic Risk of Chemicals to Man," Vol. 15. Int. Agency Res. Cancer, Lyon, France.

Isoda, N. (1979). A death case of intoxication due to paraquat dichloride. *Jpn. J. Rural Med.* **28,**85–86 (in Japanese).

Ivanova, T. P. (1967). The maximum permissible concentration of nitrophen in the air of the working zone. *Hyg. Sanit.* **32,**20–26.

Jamieson, D., and van der Brenk, H. A. S. (1964). The effects of antioxidants on high pressure oxygen toxicity. *Biochem. Pharmacol.* **13,**159–164.

Jaros, F. (1978). Acute percutaneous paraquat poisoning. *Lancet* **1,**275.

Jenssen, D., and Renberg, L. (1976). Distribution and cytogenic test of 2,4-D and 2,4,5-T phenoxyacetic acids in mouse blood tissues. *Chem.-Biol. Interact.* **14,**291–299.

John-Greene, J. A., Ouellette, J. H., and Jeffries, T. K. (1985). Teratological evaluation of picloram potassium salt in rabbits. *Food Chem. Toxicol.* **23,** 753–756.

Johnson, H. R. M., and Koumides, O. (1965). A further case of MCPA poisoning. *Br. Med. J.* **2,**625–630.

Jones, D. I. R., Knight, A. G., and Smith, A. J. (1967). Attempted suicide with herbicide containing MCPA. *Arch. Environ. Health* **14,**363–366.

Jones, G. R., and Owen-Lloyd P. (1973). Recovery from poisoning by 20% paraquat. *Br. J. Clin. Pract.* **27,**69–70.

Joyce, M. (1969). Ocular damage caused by paraquat. *Br. J. Ophthalmol.* **53,** 688–690.

Jukes, T. H., and Shaffer, C. B. (1960). Antithyroid effects of aminotriazole. *Science* **132,**296.

Jung, H. D., and Wolf, F. (1977). Contact dermatitis through use of the herbicide Selest 100 in forestry. *Dtsch. Gesundheitswes.* **32,**1464–1467 (in German).

Jung, H. D., Hruloy, K., Gossing, H., and Haubenstock, A. (1983). Acute dinoseb poisoning. *Inn. Med.* (Stuttgart) **10,**219–224 (in German).

Kang, Y. J., Zolna, L., and Manson, J. M. (1986). Strain differences in response of Sprague-Dawley and Long Evans hooded rats to the teratogen nitrofen. *Teratology* **34,**213–223.

Karlsmark, T., Weismann, K., and Pock-Steen, B. (1982). Allergic contact dermatitis following use of sodium methyldithiocarbamate (Metam-Na) for eradicating roots. *Ugeskr. Laeg.* **144,**1782–1783.

Kaskevich, L. M., and Soboleva, L. P. (1978). A case of acute poisoning by 2,4-D (late sequelae). *Gig. Tr. Prof. Zabol.* **10,**49–50.

Kavlock, R. J., and Gray, J. A. (1983). Postnatal evaluation of morphological and functional effects of prenatal exposure to nitrofen in the Long Evans rat. *J. Toxicol. Environ. Health* **11,**679–690.

Kavlock, R. J., Chernoff, N., Rogers, E., Whitehouse, D., Carver, B., Gray, J., and Robinson, K. (1982). An analysis of fetotoxicity using biochemical endpoints of organ differentiation. *Teratology* **26,**183–194.

Kay, J. H., Palazzolo, R. J., and Calandra, J. C. (1965). Subacute dermal toxicity of 2,4-D. *Arch. Environ. Health* **11,**648–651.

Kaye, C. I., Rao, S., and Simpson, S. J. (1985). Evaluation of chromosomal damage in males exposed to Agent Orange and their families. *J. Graviofac. Genet. Dev. Biol.* **5,**259–265.

Kearney, P. C., and Kaufman, D. D., eds. (1976). "Herbicides: Chemistry, Degradation, and Mode of Action," 2 vols. Dekker, New York.

Kehrer, J. P., Haschek, W., and Witschi, H. P. (1979). Peracute toxicity of paraquat and diquat in 100% oxygen. *Toxicol. Appl. Pharmacol.* **48,** A59.

Kerr, F., Patel, A. R., Scott, P. D. R., and Tompsett, S. L. (1968). Paraquat poisoning treated by forced diuresis. *Br. Med. J.* **3,**290–291.

Khan, S. U., and Foster, T. S. (1976). Residues of atrazine (2-chloro-4-ethylamino-6-isopropylamino-s-triazine) and its metabolites in chicken tissues. *J. Agric. Food Chem.* **24,**768–771.

Khanna, S., and Fang, S. C. (1966). Metabolism of C14-labeled 2,4-dichlorophenoxyacetic acid in rats. *J. Agric. Food Chem.* **14,**500–503.

Khera, K. S., and McKinley, W. P. (1972). Pre- and postnatal studies on 2,4,5-trichlorophenoxyacetic acid, 2,4,5-trichlorophenoxyacetic acid and their derivatives in rats. *Toxicol. Appl. Pharmacol.* **22,**14–28.

Khera, K. S., and Whitta, L. L. (1970). Embryopathic effects of diquat and paraquat in rats. *In* "Pesticides Symposia" (W. B. Deichmann, ed.). Halos and Associates, Miami, Florida.

Khera, K. S., Whalen, C., Trivett, G., and Angers, G. (1979). Teratogenicity studies on pesticidal formulations of dimethoate, diuron and lindane in rats. *Bull. Environ. Contam. Toxicol.* **22,**522–529.

Khibin, L. S., Taitsel', L. A., and Slatov, I. V. (1968). Clinical aspects of acute Dicotex-40 poisoning. *Gig. Tr. Prof. Zabol.* **12,**52–54 (in Russian).

Kilburn, K. H., Hudson, A. R., Halprin, G. M., McKenzie, W. N., and Merchant, J. A. (1974). Two patterns for bronchial damage from inhaled materials. *Chest* **65,** Suppl.,61S–62S.

Kimbrough, R. D. (1980). Human health effects of selected pesticides, chloroaniline derivatives. *J. Environ. Sci. Health* **15,**977–992.

Kimbrough, R. D., and Gaines, T. B. (1970). Toxicity of paraquat to rats and its effect on rat lungs. *Toxicol. Appl. Pharmacol.* **17,**679–690.

Kimbrough, R. D., and Linder, R. E. (1973). The ultrastructure of the paraquat lung lesion in the rat. *Environ. Res.* **6,**265–273.

Kimbrough, R. D., Gaines, T. B., and Linder, R. E. (1974). 2,4-Dichlorophenyl-p-nitrophenyl ether (TOK). Effects on the lung maturation of rat fetus. *Arch. Environ. Health* **28,**316–320.

Kinoshita, F. K., and DuBois, K. P. (1970). Induction of hepatic microsomal enzymes by Herban, diuron and other substituted urea herbicides. *Toxicol. Appl. Pharmacol.* **17,**406–417.

Klaff, L. S., Levin, P. J., Potgeiter, P. D., Losman, L. G., Nochomorits, L. E., and Ferguson, A. D. (1977). Treatment of paraquat poisoning with the membrane oxygenator. *S. Afr. Med. J.* **51,**203–205.

Kociba, R. J., Keyes, D. J., Lisowe, R. W., Kalnins, R. P., Dittenber, D. D., Wade, C. E., Gorzinski, S. J., Mahle, N. H., and Schwetz, B. A. (1979). Results of a two-year chronic toxicity and oncogenic study of rats ingesting diets containing 2,4,5-trichlorophenoxyacetic acid (2,4,5-T). *Food Cosmet. Toxicol.* **17,**205–221.

Kodagoda, N., Jayewardene, R. P., and Attygalle, D. (1973). Poisoning with paraquat. *Forensic Sci.* **2,**107–111.

Kohli, J. D., Khanna, R. N., Gupta, B. N., Dhar, M. M., Tandon, J. S., and Sircar, K. P. (1974a). Absorption and excretion of 2,4,5-trichlorophenoxyacetic acid in man. *Arch. Int. Pharmocodyn. Ther.* **210,**250–255.

Kohli, J. D., Khanna, R. N., Gupta, B. N., Dhar, M. M., Tandon, J. S., and Sircar, K. P. (1974b). Absorption and excretion of 2,4-dichlorophenoxyacetic acid in man. *Xenobiotica* **4,**97–100.

Koike, M., Ninomura, N., Yamanaka, A., and Takahashi, A. (1978). Histopathological study on pulmonary lesions in the case of intoxication due to paraquat dichloride. *Trans. Soc. Pathol. Jpn.* **67,**272–273 (in Japanese).

Kolesar, D., and Romancik, V. (1974). Clinical and laboratory findings in acute injury by precursors of the herbicide Burex. *Bratisl. Lik. Listy* **64,**132–140 (in Slovakian).

Kolny, H., and Kita, K. (1978). Intoxication with Aminopielik D. *Med. Pr.* **29,** 61–63 (in Polish).

Kolmodin, B., and Erne, K. (1979). Estimation of occupational exposure to phenoxy acids (2,4-D and 2,4,5-T). *Eur. Soc. Toxicol.* **21,**45.

Konno, J., Hongu, M., Oizumi, K., Arimichi, F., Hayashi, I., Koyozawa, A., Arai, H., and Saito, S. (1976). Experimental pulmonary fibrosis of rats. *J. Jpn. Soc. Intern. Med.* **65,**602–603 (in Japanese).

Konstantinova, T. K. (1964). Experiments on the effects of 2,4,5-T butyl ester on pregnant animals and on the development of their offspring. *Gig. Sanit.* **39,**101–102 (in Russian).

Konstantinova, T. K. (1976). Studies of the conditions of carbohydrate and phosphate metabolism in heart muscle following chronic intoxication with pesticide mixtures. *Gig. Tr. Prof. Zabol.* **8,**15–19 (in Russian).

Konstantinova, T. K., Efimenko, L. P., and Antonenko, T. A. (1975). Embryotropic effects of decomposition products of herbicides based on 2,4-D. *Gig. Sanit.* **11,**102–105.

Kornbrust, D. J., and Mavis, R. D. (1980). The effect of paraquat on microsomal lipid peroxidation *in vitro* and *in vivo. Toxicol. Appl. Pharmacol.* **53,** 323–332.

Koschier, F. J., and Acara, M. (1978). Renal tubular transport of 2,4,5-trichlorophenoxyacetate (2,4,5-T). *Pharmacologist* **20,**222.

Koschier, F. J., and Berndt, W. O. (1977). Evaluation of acute and short-term administration of 2,4,5-trichlorophenoxyacetate with respect to renal proximal tubular transport. *Food Cosmet. Toxicol.* **15,**297–301.

Koschier, F. J., Hong, S. K., and Berndt, W. O. (1979). Serum protein and renal tissue binding of 2,4,5-trichlorophenoxyacetic acid. *Toxicol. Appl. Pharmacol.* **49,**237–244.

Koshakji, R. P., Ahmed, M. A., Harbison, R. D., and Bush, M. T. (1978). The metabolism and distribution of 2,4,5-trichlorophenoxyacetic acid in pregnant mice. *Toxicol. Appl. Pharmacol.* **45,**241.

Kuhara, H., Wakabayashi, T., Kishimoto, H., Hayashi, K., Suchi, T., and Matsunaga, T. (1977). Report of five autopsies performed in deaths from intoxication by paraquat dichloride. *J. Jpn. Assoc. Rural Med.* **26,**647–656 (in Japanese).

Kuncova, M., Kunc, L., Soldan, F., and Holusa, R. (1979). Lung surface tension and morphology in rats after paraquat poisoning. *Prac. Lek.* **31,** 126–131 (in Czech).

Kurisaki, E. (1985). Lipid peroxidation in human paraquat poisoning. *J. Toxicol. Sci.* **10,**(1),29–33.

Kusic, R., Raicevic, B., Spasic, P., Cosic, V., and Matunovic, A. (1974). Clinical and histopathological data on paraquat poisoning. *Vojnosanit. Pregl.* **31,**397–399 (in Serbo-Croatian).

Kuttan, R., Spall, R., Sipes, I. G., Meezan, E., and Brendel, K. (1979). Effect of paraquat treatment on rat kidney basement membranes. *Toxicol. Appl. Pharmacol.* **48,**A177.

Laamanen, I., Sorsa, M., Bamford, D., Gripenberg, U., and Meretoja, T. (1976). Mutagenicity and toxicity of amitrole. I. *Drosophila* tests. *Mutat. Res.* **40,**185–190.

Laithwaite, J. A. (1975). Paraquat poisoning treated with immunosuppressants and potassium aminobenzoate. *Br. Med. J.* **1,**266–267.

Laithwaite, J. A. (1976). Paraquat poisoning. *Br. J. Clin. Pract.* **30,**71–73.

Lambert, R., Kunert, J. J., and Boger, P. (1979). On the phytotoxic mode of action of nitrofen. *Pestic. Biochem. Physiol.* **II,**267.

Langhans, W., and Schimassek, H. (1974). Prevention of halothane induced changes in rat liver enzymes by 3-amino-1,2,4-triazole. *Biochem. Pharmacol.* **23,**403–409.

Lanzinger, G., Ritz, E., Franz, H. E., Kuhn, H. M., and Klein, H. (1969). Acut interstitial pulmonary fibrosis in paraquat poisoning: Clinical anatomical observation of a case with fatal outcome. *Muench. Med. Wochenschr.* **111,** 944–949 (in German).

Lareng, L., Fabre, J., Cathala, B., Fabre-Planques, M., Voigt, J. J., and Counillon, F. (1975). Intoxication deaths from paraquat. *Councours Med.* **97,** 680–687 (in French).

Lau, C., Cameron, A. M., Irsula, O., and Robinson, K. S. (1986). Effects of prenatal nitrofen exposure on cardiac structure and function in the rat. *Toxicol. Appl. Pharmacol.* **86,**22–32.

Lautenschläger, J., Grabensee, B., and Poettgen, W. (1974). Paraquat intoxications and isolated aplastic anemia. *Dtsch. Med. Wochenschr.* **99,**2348–2351 (in German).

Leng, M. L. (1972). Residues in milk and meat and safety to livestock from the use of phenoxy herbicides in pasture and rangeland. *Down Earth* **28,** 12–20.

Levin, D. E., Hollstein, M., Christman, M. F., Schwiers, E. A., and Ames, B. N. (1982). A new *Salmonella* tester strain (TA 102) with AT base pairs at the site of mutation detects oxidative mutagens. *Proc. Natl. Acad. Sci. U.S.A.* **79,**7445–7449.

Levin, P. J., Klaff, L. J., Rose, A. G., and Ferguson, A. D. (1979). Pulmonary effects of contact exposure: A clinical and experimental study. *Thorax* **34,** 150–160.

Levine, W. G. (1973). Effect of phenobarbital and 3-amino-1,2,4-triazole on the metabolism and biliary excretion of 3,4-benzpyrene in the rat. *Life Sci.* **13,** 723–732.

Lewis, T. D. (1974). Paraquat overdose. *Med. J. Aust.* **2,**814–815.

Linder, R. E., Scotti, T. M., Svendsgaard, D. J., McElroy, W. K., and Curley, A. (1982). Testicular effects of dinoseb in rats. *Arch. Environ. Contam. Toxicol.* **11,**475–485.

Lindquist, N. G. (1974). An autoradiographic study on the distribution of the herbicide 4-chloro-2-methyl phenoxyacetic acid in pregnant mice. *Toxicol. Appl. Pharmacol.* **30,**227–237.

Lindquist, N. G., and Ullberg, S. (1971). Distribution of the herbicides 2,4,5-T and 2,4-D in pregnant mice. Accumulation in yolk sac epithelium. *Experientia* **27,**1439–1441.

Litchfield, M. H., Daniel, J. W., and Longshaw, S. (1973). The tissue distribution of the bipyridylium herbicides diquat and paraquat in rats and mice. *Toxicology* **1,**155–165.

Litton Bionetics, Inc. (1979). "Tok® Technical, Lot 8910: Mammalian Cell Transformation Assay," LBI Rep. Litton Bionetics, Inc., Maryland.

Lloyd, E. L. (1969). Recovery after taking Weedol. *Br. Med. J.* **2,**189.

Lock, E. A. (1979). The effect of paraquat and diquat on renal function in the rat. *Toxicol. Appl. Pharmacol.* **48,**327–336.

Loktionov, V. N., Budarkov, V. A., and Kuznetsova, N. V. (1973). Toxicological characterization of dichlorophenoxyacetic acid derivatives. *Veterinariya (Moscow)* **5,**107–109 (in Russian).

Lotlikar, P. D., Wasserman, M. B., and Luha, L. (1973). Effect of 3-amino-1,2,4-triazole pretreatment on *N*- and ring-hydroxylation of 2-acetylaminofluorene by the rat. *Proc. Soc. Exp. Biol. Med.* **144,**445–449.

Luty, S., Latuszynska, J., Cisak, E., and Przylepa, E. (1978). Effect of paraquat on the internal organs in mice. *Bromatol. Chem. Toksykol.* **11,**23–29 (in Polish).

Lynge, E. (1985). A follow-up study of cancer incidence among workers in manufacture of phenoxy herbicides in Denmark. *Br. J. Cancer* **52,**259–270.

Magnusson, J., Ramel, C., and Eriksson, A. (1977). Mutagenic effects of chlorinated phenoxyacetic acids on *Drosophila melanogaster*. *Hereditas* **87,**121–123.

Mahieu, P., Hassaun, A., Fautsch, G., Lauwerijs, R., and Tremouroux, J. (1977). Paraquat poisoning. Survival without pulmonary insufficiency after early Bleomycin treatment. *Acta Pharmacol. Toxicol.* **41,**246–248.

Mahieu, P., Bonduelle, Y., Bernard, A., De Cabooter, M., Gala, M., Hassoun, A., Koenig, J., and Lauwerys, R. (1984). Acute diquat intoxication. Interest of its repeated determination in urine and the evaluation of renal proximal tubule integrity. *J. Toxicol., Clin. Toxicol.* **22,**363–369.

Maibach, H. I. (1986). Irritation, sensitization, photoirritation and photosensitization assays with a glyphosate herbicide. *Contact Dermatitis* **15,**152–156.

Maini, R., and Winchester, J. F. (1975). Removal of paraquat from blood by haemoperfusion over sorbent materials. *Br. Med. J.* **3,**281–282.

Majumdar, S. K., and Golia, J. (1974). Mutation test of 2,4,5-trichlorophenoxyacetic acid on *Drosophila melanogaster*. *Can. J. Genet. Cytol.* **16,**465–466.

Majumdar, S. K., and Hall, R. C. (1973). Cytogenic effects of 2,4,5-T on *in vivo* bone marrow cells of Mongolian gerbils. *J. Hered.* **64,**213–216.

Malcolmson, E., and Beesley, J. (1975). Unsuccessful immunosuppressant treatment of paraquat poisoning. *Br. Med. J.* **3,**650–651.

Maling, H. M., Saul, W., Williams, M. A., and Brown, E. A. B. (1975). Propranolol treatment of experimental paraquat poisoning in rats. *Fed. Proc., Fed. Am. Soc. Exp. Biol.* **34,**226.

Maling, H. M., Saul, W., Williams, M. A., Brown, E. A., and Gillette, J. P. (1976). The relation of the potentiation of paraquat 48-hr mortality in rats and mice by 1-isoproterenol to its effects on renal clearance of paraquat. *Pharmacologist* **18,**244.

Malmqvist, E., Grossmann, G., Ivemark, B., and Robertson, B. (1973). Pulmonary phospholipids and surface properties of alveolar wash in experimental paraquat poisoning. *Scand. J. Respir. Dis.* **54,**206–214.

Malone, J. D. G., Carmody, M., Keogh, B., and O'Dwyer, W. F. (1971). Paraquat poisoning—a review of nineteen cases. *J. Ir. Med. Assoc.* **64,**59–68.

Manktelow, B. W. (1967). The loss of pulmonary surfactant in paraquat poisoning: A model for the study of the respiratory distress syndrome. *Br. J. Exp. Pathol.* **43,**366–369.

Manson, J. M. (1984). Mechanism of environmental agents by class associated with adverse female reproductive outcome. *Prog. Clin. Biol. Res.* **160,**237–248.

Manson, J. M. (1986). Mechanism of nitrofen teratogenesis. *Environ. Health Perspect.* **70,**137–147.

Manson, J. M., Brown, T., and Baldwin, D. M. (1984). Teratogenicity of nitrofen (2,4-dichloro-4'-nitrophenyl ether) and its effects on thyroid function in the rat. *Toxicol. Appl. Pharmacol.* **73,**332–335.

Margoliash, E., and Novogrodsky, A. (1958). A study of the inhibition of catalase by 3-amino-1,2,4-triazole. *Biochem. J.* **68,**468–475.

Markosyan, V. Ye. (1973). Toxicity of the 3-nitro-4-hydroxybenzyl ester of 2,4-dichlorophenoxyacetic acid. *Zh. Eksp. Klin. Med.* **13,**35–37 (in Russian).

Mascie Taylor, B. H., Thompson, J., and Davison, A. M. (1983). Haemoperfusion ineffective for paraquat removal in life-threatening poisoning. *Lancet* **1,**1376–1377.

Mason, R. P., Peterson, F. J., Holtzman, J. L., and Callaghan, J. T. (1977). Ascorbic acid destruction of the O_2 generated by nitrofurantoin and paraquat free radicals. *Pharmacologist* **19,**192.

Masterson, J. G., and Roche, W. J. (1970a). Another paraquat fatality. *Br. Med. J.* **2**,482.

Masterson, J. G., and Roche, W. J. (1970b). Fatal paraquat poisoning. *J. Ir. Med. Assoc.* **63**,261–264.

Matkovics, B., Szabo, L., Varga, Sz. I., Novak, R., Barabase, K., and Berencsi, G. (1980a). *In vivo* effects on paraquat on some oxidative enzymes of mice. *Gen. Pharmacol.* **11**,267–270.

Matkovics, B., Barabas, K., Szabo, L., and Berencsi, G. (1980b). *In vivo* study of the mechanism of protective effects of ascorbic acid and reduced glutathione in paraquat poisoning. *Gen. Pharmacol.* **11**,455–461.

Matkovics, B., Barabas, K., Szabo, L., Varga, I., and Berencsi, G. (1983). Screening of antidotes for paraquat detoxication. *In* "Oxy Radicals and Their Scavenger Systems, Proceedings of the Third International Conference on Superoxide and Superoxide Dismutase" (G. Cohen and R. A. Greenwald, eds.). Am. Elsevier, New York.

Matsushima, T., and Weisburger, J. H. (1972). Effect of carbon monoxide or of 3-aminotriazole on *C*- and *N*-hydroxylation of the carcinogen *N*-2-fluorenylacetamide by liver microsomes of hamsters pretreated with 3-methylcholanthrene. *Xenobiotica* **2**,423–430.

Matsumoto, K. (1985). A study of paraquat lung. *Japn. J. Clin. Radiol.* **30** (9),991–996.

Matthew, H. (1972). Paraquat poisoning. *Clin. Toxicol.* **5**,581–582.

Matthew, H., Logan, A., Woodruff, M. F. A., and Heard, B. (1968). Paraquat poisoning—lung transplantation. *Br. Med. J.* **3**,759–763.

Matthew, H., Wright, N., Robson, J. S., Flenley, D. C., Brown, S. S., Heard, B. E., Housley, E., Swan, A. A. B., Kennedy, W. P. U., Donald, K. W., McHardy, G. J. R., and Prescott, L. F. (1971). Paraquat poisoning: Clinopathological conference. *Scott. Med. J.* **16**,407–421.

Mayama, S., Haneda, T., Shimazu, W., Sato, H., Makino, E., Yajima, T., Kumakura, M., Obata, H., and Hattori, T. (1979). A case of acute intoxication due to paraquat dichloride. *J. Jpn. Soc. Int. Med.* **68**,559–560 (in Japanese).

Mayberry, W. E. (1968). Antithyroid effects of 3-amino-1,2,4-triazole. *Proc. Soc. Exp. Biol. Med.* **129**,551–556.

McDavit, M. (1986). Decision and emergency order suspending the registration of all pesticide products containing dinoseb. *Fed. Regist.* **51**,36634–36635.

McDonagh, B. J., and Martin, J. (1970). Paraquat poisoning in children. *Arch. Dis. Child.* **45**,452–427.

McElligott, T. F. (1972). The dermal toxicity of paraquat: Differences due to techniques of application. *Toxicol. Appl. Pharmacol.* **21**,361–368.

McKean, W. I. (1968). Recovery from paraquat poisoning. *Br. Med. J.* **3**,292.

Mees, G. C. (1960). Experiments on the herbicidal action of 1,1′-ethylene-2-2′-dipyridylium dibromide. *Ann. Appl. Biol.* **48**,601–612.

Mehlman, M., Shapiro, R. E., and Blumenthal, H. (1976). "New Concepts in Safety Evaluation," Part 1, p. 218. Hemisphere Publishing, Washington, D.C.

Mengal, C. E., and Kann, H. E. (1966). Effect of *in vivo* hyperoxia on erythrocytes. III. *In vivo* peroxidation of erythrocyte lipid. *J. Clin. Invest.* **45**, 1150–1158.

Meretoja, T., Gripenberg, U., Bamford, D., Laamanen, I., and Sorsa, M. (1976). Mutagenicity and toxicity of amitrole. II. Human lymphocyte culture tests. *Mutat. Res.* **40**,191–196.

Meselson, M. S., Westing, A. H., and Constable, J. D. (1972). Herbicide Assessment Commission for the American Association for the Advancement of Science: Background material relevant to presentations at the 1970 annual meeting of the AAAS. U.S. Congressional Record, Vol. 118, Part 6, March 3, 1972, pp. 6807–6813.

Mickleson, K. N. P., and Fulton, D. B. (1971). Paraquat poisoning treated by a replacement blood transfusion: Case report. *N. Z. Med. J.* **74**,26–27.

Mikuni, I., and Suzuki, A. (1976). A case of ocular corrosion by a herbicide, paraquat dichloride. *Jpn. Rev. Clin. Ophthalmol.* **70**,395–398 (in Japanese).

Minakawa, O., Ishii, S., and Konno, H. (1978). Analytical method of residue of molinate, a herbicide in paddy field, and actions of molinate to living bodies. *Jpn. J. Public Health* **25**,645–651 (in Japanese).

Mitchell, J. W., Hodgson, R. E., and Gaetjens, C. F. (1946). Tolerance of farm animals to feed containing 2,4-dichlorophenoxyacetic acid. *J. Anim. Sci.* **5**, 226.

Miura, H., Omori, S., and Yamakawa, M. (1978). Are chlorinated phenols capable of inducing hepatic porphyria? *Jpn. J. Ind. Health* **20**,162–173.

Miura, O., Sasaki, S., Kagaya, S., Watabe, K., and Sugaya, H. (1979). Concentration of paraquat in the organs, blood and urine of the dead persons due to intoxication by paraquat in 1978. *J. Jpn. Soc. Rural Med.* **28**,470–471 (in Japanese).

Miyauchi, M., Haga, M., Takou, Y., and Uematsu, T. (1983). Mutagenic activity of chlorinated 4-nitrobiphenyl ethers and their nitroso- and aminoderivatives. *Chem.-Biol. Interact.* **44**,133–141.

Molnar, V. (1971). Symptomatology and pathomorphology of experimental poisoning with atrazine. *Rev. Med. HSE* **17**,271–274 (in Portugese).

Monarca, G., and Di Vitto, G. (1961). On acute poisoning by a weed killer (2,4-dichlorophenoxyacetic acid). A clinical contribution. *Folia Med. (Napoli)* **44**,480–485.

Monsanto (1985). "1986 Crop Chemical Sample Label Guide." Monsanto Company, St. Louis, Missouri.

Montgomery, M. R., Wyatt, I., and Smith, L. (1979a). Oxygen effects on active uptake and metabolism in rat lung slices. *Toxicol. Appl. Pharmacol.* **48**, A79.

Montgomery, M. R., Casey, P. J., Valls, A. A., Cosio, M. G., and Niewoehner, D. E. (1979b). Biochemical and morphological correlation of oxidant-induced pulmonary injury: Low dose exposure to paraquat, oxygen, and ozone. *Arch. Environ. Health* **34**,396–401.

Moore, J. A. (1973). Characterization and interpretation of kidney anomalies associated with 2,3,7,8-tetrachlorodibenzo-*p*-dioxin (TCDD). *Teratology* **7**,A24.

Moore, J. A., and Courtney, K. D. (1971). Teratology studies with the trichlorophenoxyacid herbicides, 2,4,5-T and silvex. *Teratology* **4**,236.

Morgan, D. P. (1982). "Recognition and Management of Pesticide Poisonings," 3rd ed. U.S. Govt. Printing Office, Washington, D.C.

Mori, S., Takeuchi, Y., Toyama, M., Makino, S., Ohhara, T., Tochino, Y., and Hayashi, Y. (1985). Amitrole: Strain differences in morphological response of the liver following subchronic administration to mice. *Toxicol. Lett.* **29**, 145–152.

Moriyama, I., Ichikawa, H., and Ide, H. (1972). Death after accidental ingestion of Gramoxone resulting in fibrosis of the lung. *J. Jpn. Assoc. Rural Med.* **21**,244–245 (in Japanese).

Moriyama, I., Ide, H., Ichikawa, H., and Hikosaka, R. (1973). A death by acute pulmonary fibrosis after swallowing Gramoxone by mistake. *Jpn. J. Thorac. Dis.* **11**,316 (in Japanese).

Morse, D. L., and Baker, E. L. (1979). Propanil-chloracne and methomyl toxicity in workers of a pesticide manufacturing plant. *Clin. Toxicol.* **15**,13–21.

Mrak, E. M. (1969). "Report of the Secretary's Commission on Pesticides and Their Relationship to Environmental Health," p. 673. U.S. Department of Health, Education and Welfare, Washington, D.C.

Mukada, T., Sasano, N., and Sato, K. (1978). Autopsy findings in a case of acute paraquat poisoning with extensive cerebral purpura. *Tohoku J. Exp. Med.* **125**,253–263.

Mullison, W. R. (1986). "An Interim Report Summarizing 2,4-D Toxicological Research Sponsored by the Industry Task Force on 2,4-D Research Data and a Brief Review of 2,4-D Environmental Effects." Industry Task Force on 2,4-D Research Data, Washington, D.C.

Murnik, M. R., and Nash, C. L. (1977). Mutagenicity in the triazine herbicides atrazine, cyanazine, and simazine in *Drosophila melanogaster. J. Toxicol. Environ. Health* **3**,691–697.

Murphy, S. D. (1986). Toxic Effects of Pesticides, Chapter 18. *In* "Casarett and Doull's Toxicology: The Basic Science of Poisons" (C. D. Klassen, M. O. Amdur, and J. Doull, eds.), 3rd ed., pp. 519–581. Macmillan, New York.

Murray, R. E., and Gibson, J. E. (1972). Comparative study of paraquat intoxication in rats, guinea pigs, and monkeys. *Exp. Mol. Pathol.* **17**,317–325.

Murray, R. E., and Gibson, J. E. (1974). Paraquat disposition in rats, guinea pigs and monkeys. *Toxicol. Appl. Pharmacol.* **27**,283–291.

Nagi, A. J. (1970). Paraquat and adrenal cortical necrosis. *Br. Med. J.* **2**,669.

Nakabayashi, H., Aga, N., and Hara, I. (1975). Two cases of paraquat poisoning—a case of occupational poisoning in a 59-year-old man and of suicide by a 24-year-old woman. *Ind. Med.* **17,**53.

Nakai, K., Abo, K., Inata, J., Takezawa, H., Konishi, T., Okuda, K., and Nakano, T. (1979). Autopsy case of a patient intoxicated by paraquat dichloride. *J. Jpn. Soc. Intern. Med.* **68,**423 (in Japanese).

Nakamura, A., and Minakami, S. (1973). Turnover of hepatic catalase modified by aminotriazole. *J. Biochem. (Tokyo)* **74,**683–689.

Nakamura, A., and Minakami, S. (1974). Synthesis of catalase in liver slices from aminotriazole-pretreated rats. *J. Biochem. (Tokyo)* **75,**1373–1375.

Nakamura, I., Maeda, M., Mori, M., Miki, S., and Teranishi, Y. (1973). A case of intoxidation due to paraquat dichloride. *J. Jpn. Soc. Intern. Med.* **62,**1394.

Nakamura, M., Kumanomido, Y., Kobuchi, K., Kajitani, T., Nagano, H., Mizushima, M., Kamioka, K., and Ito, J. (1979). An autopsy on a child intoxicated by paraquat-dichloride. *J. Pediatr. Pract.* **42,**293–297.

Narita, S., Motojuku, H., Sato, J., and Mori, H. (1978). Autopsy in acute suicidal poisoning with diquat dibromide. *Jpn. J. Rural Med.* **27,**454–455 (in Japanese).

Nashikimi, M. (1975). Oxidation of ascorbic acid with superoxide anion generated by the xanthine–xanthine oxidase system. *Biochem. Res. Commun.* **63,** 463–468.

Nater, J. P., and Grosfeld, J. C. M. (1979). Allergic contact dermatitis from Betanol (phenmedipham). *Contact Dermatitis* **5,**59–60.

National Cancer Institute (NCI) (1978a). "Bioassay of Sulfallate for Possible Carcinogenicity," Tech. Rep. Ser. No. 115, DHEW Publ. No. (NIH) 78-1370. Natl. Cancer Inst., Bethesda, Maryland.

National Cancer Institute (NCI) (1978b). "Bioassay of Nitrofen for Possible Carcinogenicity," Tech. Rep. Ser. No. 26, DHEW Publ. No. (NIH) 78-826. Natl. Cancer Inst., Washington, D.C.

National Cancer Institute (NCI) (1979). "Bioassay of Nitrofen for Possible Carcinogenicity," Tech. Rep. Ser. No. 184, DHEW Publ. No. (NIH) 79-1740. Natl. Cancer Inst., Washington, D.C.

National Health and Medical Research Council (1978). Report of the ad-hoc working party of council on the use and safety of 2,4,5-T. *Med. J. Aust.* **2,** Spec. Suppl. No. 3,2–3.

National Research Committee on the Effects of Herbicides in Vietnam (1974). "The Effects of Herbicides in South Vietnam." Div. Biol. Sci., Assembly Life Sci., National Research Council, National Academy of Sciences, Washington, D.C.

National Research Council (1987). "Regulating Pesticides in Food: The Delaney Paradox." National Academy Press, Washington, D.C.

Nelson, B. (1969). Herbicides: Order on 2,4,5-T issued at unusually high level. *Science* **166,**977–979.

Nelson, C. J., Holson, J. F., Green, H. G., and Gaylor, D. W. (1979). Retrospective study of the relationship between agricultural use of 2,4,5-T and cleft palate occurrence in Arkansas. *Teratology* **19,**377–384.

Neubert, D., and Dillman, I. (1972). Embryotoxic effects in mice treated with 2,4,5-trichlorophenoxyacetic acid and 2,3,7,8-tetrachlorodibenzo-*p*-dioxin. *Naunyn-Schmiedeberg's Arch. Pharmacol.* **272,**243–264.

Newhouse, M., McEvoy, D., and Rosenthal, D. (1978). Percutaneous paraquat adsorption. *Arch. Dermatol.* **114,**1516–1519.

Nezefi, T. A. (1971). Morphological alterations in the organs of white rats during chronic treatment with atrazine. *Zdravookhr. Turkm.* **15,**9–12.

Nicolau, G. Y. (1983). Circadian rhythms of RNA, DNA, and protein in the rat thyroid, adrenal and testis in chronic pesticide exposure. II. Effects of the herbicides aminotriazole and alachlor. *Endocrinologie (Bucharest)* **21,**105–112.

Niden, A. H., and Khurana, M. M. L. (1976). An animal model for diffuse interstitial pulmonary fibrosis—chronic low dose paraquat ingestion. *Fed. Proc., Fed. Am. Soc. Exp. Biol.* **35,**631.

Nielsen, K., Kaempe, B., and Jensen-Holm, J. (1965). Fatal poisoning in man by 2,4-dichlorophenoxyacetic acid (2,4-D): Determination of the agent in forensic materials. *Acta Pharmacol. Toxicol.* **22,**224–234.

Nienhaus, H., and Ehrenfeld, M. (1971). Pathogenesis of lung disease in paraquat poisoning. *Beitr. Pathol.* **142,**244–267 (in German).

Nolan, R. J., Freshour, N. L., Kastl, P. E., and Saunders, J. H. (1984). Pharma-

cokinetics of picloram in male volunteers. *Toxicol. Appl. Pharmacol.* **76,** 264–269.

Office of Pesticide Programs (1984a). "Alachlor; Position Document 1." U.S. Environ. Prot. Agency, Washington, D.C.

Office of Pesticide Programs (1984b). "Guidance for the Reregistration of Pesticide Products Containing Alachlor as the Active Ingredient." U.S. Environ. Prot. Agency, Washington, D.C.

Office of Pesticide Programs (1986). "Alachlor; Special Review Technical Support Document." U.S. Environ. Prot. Agency, Washington, D.C.

Office of Pesticide Programs (1987). "Cyanazine: Special Review Technical Support Document." Office of Pesticides and Toxic Substances. U.S. Environ. Prot. Agency, Washington, D.C.

Office of Pesticides and Toxic Substances (1985). "Cyanazine Special Review Position Document 1." U.S. Environ. Prot. Agency, Washington, D.C.

Office of Pesticides and Toxic Substances (1989). Peer Review of Simagene. U.S. Environ. Prot. Agency, Washington, D.C.

O'Hara, G. P., Chan, P. K., Harris, J. C., Burke, S. S., Smith, J. M., and Hayes, A. W. (1983). The effect of nitrofen (4-(2,4-dichlorophenoxy)nitrobenzene) on the reproductive performance of male rats. *Toxicology* **28,**332–333.

Ohkubo, T., Takeda, K., Okano, T., Shigeizumi, Y., Oikawa, M., Toyohara, T., Hayashi, S., Hirata, M., Komatsuda, H., Sugaya, H., Sasaki, S., and Watanuki, T. (1979). A case of death due to paraquat intoxication. *J. Jpn. Soc. Rural Med.* **28,**472–473 (in Japanese).

Oishi, S. (1975). A case of ocular injury by paraquat dichloride. *Jpn. J. Ind. Health* **17,**522 (in Japanese).

Okada, H., Kamata, T., Nakagawa, A., and Hirakawa, S. (1972). A case of acute intoxication due to paraquat-dichloride. *Jpn. J. Thorac. Dis.* **10,**673 (in Japanese).

Okahata, S. (1980). Mechanism of methyl viologen induced hemolysis. *Hiroshima J. Med. Sci.* **29**(2),49–54.

Okonek, S., Hofmann, A., and Henningsen, B. (1976). Efficacy of gut lavage, hemodialysis, and hemoperfusion in the therapy of paraquat or diquat intoxication. *Arch. Toxicol.* **36,**43–51.

Okubo, S., Kanazawa, Y., Tachikawa, H., Hayashi, S., Komatsuda, H., Hirata, M., and Watanuku, T. (1975). Findings in two autopsies performed after fatal acute paraquat dichloride poisoning. *J. Jpn. Assoc. Rural Med.* **24,**460–461 (in Japanese).

Oledzka-Slotwinska, H. (1974). Effect of simazine on hepatocyte ultrastructure and the activity of certain hydrolase. *Bull. Assoc. Anat.* **58,**445–446 (in French).

Olorunsogo, O. O., and Bababunmi, E. A. (1980). Inhibition of succinatelinking reduction of pyridine nucleotide in rat liver mitochondria *in vivo* by *N*-(phosphonomethyl) glycine. *Toxicol. Lett.* **7,**149–152.

Olson, R. J., Trumble, T. E., and Gamble, W. (1974). Alterations in cholesterol and fatty acid synthesis in rat liver homogenates by aryloxy acids. *Biochem. J.* **142,**445–448.

Omaye, S. T., Reddy, K. A., and Cross, C. E. (1978). Enhanced lung toxicity of paraquat in selenium-deficient rats. *Toxicol. Appl. Pharmacol.* **43,**237–247.

O'Neill, J. J., Engelbrecht, F. M., and Wilson, A. G. E. (1977). Paraquat uptake and distribution by rat lungs. *Am. Rev. Respir. Dis.* **115,**A234.

Oreopoulos, D. G., and McEvoy, J. (1969). Diquat poisoning. *Postgrad. Med. J.* **45,**635–637.

Oreopoulos, D. G., Soyannowo, M. A. O., Sinniah, R., Fenton, S. S. A., McGeown, M. G., and Bruce, J. H. (1968). Acute renal failure in case of paraquat poisoning. *Br. Med. J.* **1,**749–750.

Oshima, H., and Imai, M. (1976). On the mammalian toxicity of a phenoxyacetic acid type herbicide. Part 2. Subacute toxicity of 2-methyl-4-chlorophenoxy acetanilide. *Jpn. J. Ind. Health* **18,**51 (in Japanese).

Oshima, H., Imai, M., and Kawagishi, T. (1974). On the toxicity of *n*-butyl and allyl-2-methyl-4-chlorophenoxyacetate, two herbicidal MCP esters. *Mie Med. Sci.* **17,**95–100 (in Japanese).

Oskarsson, A., and Tjaelve, H. (1976). High uptake in the erythrocytes and the spleen of the quaternary dipyridylium salt paraquat injected intravenously in hypotonic solutions. *Acta Pharmacol. Toxicol.* **39,**481–499.

Ostby, J. S., Gray, L. E., Kavlock, R. J., and Ferrell, J. M. (1985). The postnatal effects of prenatal exposure to low doses of nitrofen (2,4-dichlorophenyl-p-nitrophenyl ether) in Sprague-Dawley rats. *Toxicology* **34,** 285–297.

Osterloh, J., Lotti, M., and Pond, S. M. (1983). Toxicologic studies in a fatal overdose of 2,4-D, MCPP and chlorpyrifos. *J. Anal. Toxicol.* **7,** 125–129.

Paggiaro, P. L., Martino, E., and Mariotti, S. (1974). A case of 2,4-dichlorophenoxyacetic acid (2,4-D) intoxication. *Med. Lav.* **65,**128–135.

Palmer, J. S., and Radeleff, R. D. (1964). The toxicologic effects of certain fungicides and herbicides on sheep and cattle. *Ann. N. Y. Acad. Sci.* **111,** 729–736.

Palva, H. L. A., Koivisto, O., and Palva, I. P. (1975). Aplastic anemia after exposure to a weed killer, 2-methyl-4-chlorophenoxyacetic acid. *Acta Haematol.* **53,**105–108.

Pariente, R., Bismuth, C., Legrand, M., and Gauthier, M. (1974). Data on cause from the ultrastructural study in two cases of human poisoning by paraquat. *Rev. Fr. Mal. Respir.* **2,**968–977 (in French).

Park, J., Darrien, I., and Prescott, L. F. (1977). Pharmacokinetic studies and severe intoxication with 2,4-D and mecoprop. *Proc. Eur. Soc. Toxicol.* **18,** 154–155.

Pasi, A., and Embree, J. W., Jr. (1975). Further comments on the assessment of the mutagenic properties of diquat and paraquat in the murine dominant lethal test. *Mutat. Res.* **31,**123–125.

Pasi, A., and Hine, C. H. (1971). Paraquat poisoning. *Proc. West. Pharmacol. Soc.* **14,**169–172.

Pasi, A., Embree, J. W., Jr., Eisenlord, G. H., and Hine, C. H. (1974). Assessment of the mutagenic properties of diquat and paraquat in the murine dominant lethal test. *Mutat. Res.* **26,**171–175.

Pearce, N. E., Smith, A. H., Howard, J. K., Sheppard, R. A., Giles, H. J., and Teague, C. A. (1986). Norr Hodgkin's lymphoma and exposure to phenoxy herbicides, chlorophenols, fencing work and meat work employment: A case-control study. *Br. J. Ind. Med.* **43,**75–83.

Pearn, J. H. (1985). Herbicides and congenital malformations: A review for the pediatrician. *Aust. Paediatr. J.* **21,**237–242.

Peoples, S. A., Maddy, K. T., Peifer, W. R., and Edmiston, S. (1979). Occupational exposure to pesticides containing organoarsenicals in California. *Vet. Hum. Toxicol.* **21**(6),417–421.

Peters, J. W., and Cook, R. M. (1973). Effects of atrazine on reproduction in rats. *Bull. Environ. Contam. Toxicol.* **9,**301–304.

Pickersgill, J., Robin, E. D., Theodore, J., Raffin, T. A., Laman, P. D., and Simon, L. M. (1978). Paraquat ingestion and pulmonary injury. *West. J. Med.* **128,**26–34.

Pilinskaya, M. A. (1974). Cytogenic effect of the herbicide 2,4-D on human and animal chromosomes. *Tsitol. Genet.* **8,**202–206 (in Russian).

Piper, W. N., Rose, J. Q., and Gehring, P. J. (1972). Metabolism of 2,4,5-trichlorophenoxyacetic acid (2,4,5-T) in rats. *Toxicol. Appl. Pharmacol.* **22,**317.

Piper, W. N., Rose, J. Q., Leng, M. L., and Gehring, P. J. (1973). The fate of 2,4,5-trichlorophenoxyacetic acid (2,4,5-T) following oral administration to rats and dogs. *Toxicol. Appl. Pharmacol.* **26,**339–351.

Pirie, A., and Rees, J. R. (1970). Diquat cataract in the rat. *Exp. Eye Res.* **9,** 198–203.

Pirie, A., Rees, J. R., and Holberg, N. J. (1970). Diquat cataract: Formation of the free radical and its reaction with constituents of the eye. *Exp. Eye Res.* **9,** 204–218.

Pliss, G. B., and Zabezhinskiy, M. A. (1970). Carcinogenicity of symmetric triazine derivatives. *Vopr. Onkol.* **16,**82–85 (in Russian).

Poche, R. (1974). Pathogenesis of paraquat lung. *Pneumonologie* **150,**181–184 (in German).

Poder, G., Oszvald, P., Hegy, L., Mezei, G., and Schmidt, Z. (1985). Complete recovery from paraquat poisoning causing severe unilateral pulmonary lesion. *Acta Paediatr. Hung.* **26**(1),53–54.

Popham, R. D., and Davies, D. M. (1964). A case of MCPA poisoning. *Br. Med. J.* **1,**677–678.

Powell, D., Pond, S. M., Allen, T. B., and Portale, A. A. (1983). Hemoperfusion in a child who ingested diquat and died from pontine infarction and hemorrhage. *J. Toxicol. Clin. Toxicol.* **20,**405–420.

Pratt, I., Crabtree, H. C., and Rose, M. S. (1978). The effect of diaquat dichloride on the histology and ultrastructure of rat stomach. *Toxicol. Appl. Pharmacol.* **45,**259.

Pratt, I., Keeling, P. L., and Smith, L. L. (1979). The effect of high concentrations of oxygen on the toxicity of paraquat and diquat in rats. *Toxicol. Appl. Pharmacol.* **48,**A59.

Prescott, L. F., Park, J., and Darrien, L. (1979). Treatment of severe 2,4-D and mecoprop intoxication with alkaline diuresis. *Br. J. Clin. Pharmacol.* **7,** 111–116.

Prochnicka, B., Kwiecien-Glowacka, E., and Bialka, J. (1977). A case of fatal intoxication with paraquat. *Prezegl. Lek.* **34,**511–512 (in Polish).

Proudfoot, A. T., Steward, M. S., Levitt, T., and Widdop, B. (1979). Paraquat poisoning: Significance of plasma-paraquat concentrations. *Lancet* **2,**330–332.

Public Health Service (1985). Nitrofen. *In* "Fourth Annual Report on Carcinogens Summary 1958," NTP 85-002. U.S. Dept. of Health and Human Services, Washington, D.C.

Pushkar', M. S. (1969). Morphological changes in the organism under the action of the herbicide Reglon (diquat). *Vrach. Delo* **9,**92–96 (in Russian).

Putnam, A. R., Willis, M. D., Binning, L. K., and Boldt, P. F. (1983). Exposure of pesticide applicators to nitrofen: Influence of formulation, handling systems, and protective garments. *J. Agric. Food Chem.* **31,**645–650.

Raisfeld, I. H., Bacchin, P., Hutterer, F., and Schaffner, F. (1970). The effect of 3-amino-1,2,4-triazole on the phenobarbital-induced formation of hepatic microsomal membranes. *Mol. Pharmacol.* **6,**231–239.

Ramachamdran, S., Rajapakse, C. N. A., and Perera, M. V. F. (1974). Further observations on paraquat poisoning. *Forensic Sci.* **4,**257–266.

Rasanen, L., Hattula, M. L., and Arstila, A. U. (1977). The mutagenicity of MCPA and its soil metabolites, chlorinated phenols, catechols and some widely used slimicides in Finland. *Bull. Environ. Contam. Toxicol.* **18,** 565–571.

Rashid, K. A., Babish, J. G., and Mumma, R. O. (1984). Potential of 2,4-dichlorophenoxyacetic acid conjugates as promutagens in the *Salmonella*/microsome mutagenicity test. *J. Environ. Sci. Health* **19,**689–701.

Raub, J. A., Mercer, R. R., and Kavlock, R. J. (1983). Effects of prenatal nitrofen exposure on postnatal lung function in the rat. *Prog. Clin. Biol. Res.* **140,**119–134.

Rebello, G., and Mason, J. D. (1978). Pulmonary histological appearances in fatal paraquat poisoning. *Histopathology* **2,**53–66.

Rebrin, V. G., and Aleksandrova, L. G. (1971). Toxicohygienic characteristics of the new herbicide Ronit. *Vrach. Delo* **12,**118–121 (in Russian).

Reddy, K., Omaye, S., Chiu, M., Litov, R., Hasegawa, G., and Cross, C. (1976). Effect of aspirin (ASA), indomethacin (IND) and hydrocortisone (HYC) pretreatments on selected aspects of rat lung metabolism before and after paraquat administration. *Am. Rev. Respir. Dis.* **113,**102.

Reinhardt, C. F., and Brittelli, M. R. (1981). Heterocyclic and miscellaneous nitrogen compounds. *In* "Patty's Industrial Hygiene and Toxicology," (G. D. Clayton and F. E. Clayton, eds.), Chapter 38. Wiley (Interscience), New York.

Reiser, K. M., Greenberg, D. B., and Last, J. A. (1979). Type I/type III collagen ratios in lungs of rats with experimental pulmonary fibrosis. *Fed. Proc., Fed. Am. Soc. Exp. Biol.* **38,**817.

Reitze, H. K., and Seitz, K. A. (1985). Light and electron microscopical changes in the livers of mice following treatment with aminotriazole. *Exp. Pathol.* **27,**17–31.

Reuber, M. D. (1981). Carcinogenicity of picloram. *J. Toxicol. Environ. Health* **7,**207–222.

Rhodes, M. L. (1974). Hypoxic protection in paraquat poisoning: A model for respiratory distress syndrome. *Chest* **66,**341–342.

Rhodes, M. L., and Patterson, C. E. (1977). Effect of exogenous superoxide dismutase on paraquat toxicity. *Clin. Res.* **25,**592A.

Rhodes, M. L., Zavala, D. C., and Brown, D. (1976). Hypoxic protection in paraquat poisoning. *Lab Invest.* **35,**496–500.

Rip, J. W., and Cherry, J. H. (1976). Liver enlargement induced by the herbicide

2,4,5-trichlorophenoxyacetic acid (2,4,5-T). *J. Agric. Food Chem.* **24,** 245–250.

Rivers, J. B., Yauger, W. L., Jr., and Klemmer, H. W. (1970). Simultaneous gas chromatographic determination of 2,4-D and dicamba in human blood and urine. *J. Chromatogr.* **50,** 334–337.

Robbins, J. D., Bakke, J. E., and Feil, V. J. (1968). Metabolism of 2-chloro-4,6-bis(isopropylamino)-*s*-triazine(propazine-^{14}C) in milk goat and sheep. *J. Agric. Food Chem.* **16,** 698–700.

Robens, J. F. (1980). Carcinogenicity studies of selected herbicides. *Vet. Hum. Toxicol.* **22,** 328–334.

Robertson, B. (1973). Paraquat poisoning as an experimental model of the idiopathic respiratory distress syndrome. *Bull. Physio-Pathol. Respir.* **9,** 1433–1452.

Robertson, B., Enhoerning, G., Ivemark, B., Ma'mqvist, E., and Modee, J. (1970). Paraquat-induced derangement of pulmonary surfactant in the rat. *Acta Paediatr. Scand., Suppl.* **2065,** 37–39.

Robertson, B., Grossmann, G., and Ivemark, B. (1976). The alveolar lining layer in experimental paraquat poisoning. *Acta Pathol. Microbiol. Scand., Sect. A* **84A,** 40–46.

Robin, E. D., Raffin, T. A., Pickersgill, J., Theodore, J., Laman, P. D., and Simon, L. M. (1978). Paraquat ingestion and pulmonary injury. *West. J. Med.* **128,** 26–34.

Robinson, B. D. (1979). "Safety Aspects of 2,4,5-T Herbicides," Technote No. 5/79, pp. 1–5. Department of Agriculture and Fisheries of South Australia, Adelaide, Australia.

Roll, R. (1971). Study of the teratogenic effects of 2,4,5-T in the mouse. *Food Cosmet. Toxicol.* **9,** 671–676 (in German).

Roll, R. (1973). Toxicological evaluation of special organochlorinated compounds. *Environ. Qual. Saf.* **2,** 117–124.

Rose, H. A., and Rose, S. P. R. (1972). Chemical spraying as reported by refugees from S. Vietnam. *Science* **177,** 710–712.

Rose, M. S., and Smith, L. L. (1977). Tissue uptake of paraquat and diquat. *Gen. Pharmacol.* **8,** 173–176.

Rose, M. S., Smith, L. L., and Wyatt, I. (1974). Evidence for energy-dependent accumulation of paraquat into rat lung. *Nature (London)* **252,** 314–315.

Rose, M. S., Smith, L. L., and Wyatt, I. (1975). The accumulation of paraquat by the lung and the relevance of this to the treatment of paraquat poisoning. *Toxicol. Appl. Pharmacol.* **33,** 136.

Rose, M. S., Lock, E. H., Smith, L. L., and Wyatt, I. (1976a). Paraquat accumulation: Tissue and species specificity. *Biochem. Pharmacol.* **25,** 419–423.

Rose, M. S., Smith, L. L., and Wyatt, I. (1976b). Inhibition of paraquat accumulation in rat lung slices by a component of rat plasma and a variety of drugs and endogenous amines. *Biochem. Pharmacol.* **25,** 1769–1772.

Rose, M. S., Smith, L. L., and Wyatt, I. (1976c). The relevance of pentose phosphate pathway stimulation in rat lung to the mechanism of paraquat toxicity. *Biochem. Pharmacol.* **33,** 136.

Rose, M. S., Smith, L. L., and Wyatt, I. (1976d). The relevance of free radical formation in rat lung to the mechanism of paraquat toxicity. *Toxicol. Appl. Pharmacol.* **37,** 105.

Roser, R. L., and Adler, I. L. (1971). "The Nature of Aged Residues of Tok." Rohm and Haas Report. Springhouse, Pennsylvania.

Ross, J. G., and Krieger, R. I. (1978). Toxicity of paraquat and other selected viologens in rats. *Toxicol. Appl. Pharmacol.* **45,** 233–234.

Roujeau, J., Pfister, A., and Nogues, C. (1973). Histogenic conclusions concerning diffuse interstitial fibrosis. *Sem. Hop.* **49,** 1995–1999 (in French).

Rowe, V. K., and Hymas, T. A. (1954). Summary of toxicological information on 2,4-D and 2,4,5-T type herbicides and an evaluation of the hazards to livestock associated with their use. *Am. J. Vet. Res.* **15,** 622–629.

Rubin, E. H., and Lubliner, R. (1957). The Hamman-Rich syndrome: Review of the literature and analysis of 15 cases. *Medicine (Baltimore)* **36,** 397–463.

St. John, L. E., Jr., and Lisk, D. J. (1969). Metabolism of Banvel-D herbicide in a dairy cow. *J. Dairy Sci.* **52,** 392–393.

Samman, P. D., and Johnston, E. N. M. (1969). Nail damage associated with handling of paraquat and diquat. *Br. Med. J.* **1,** 818–819.

Sanderson, C. A., and Rogers, L. J. (1981). 2,4,5-Trichlorophenoxyacetic acid causes behavioral effects in chickens at environmentally relevant doses. *Science* **211,** 593–595.

Sare, W. M. (1972). The weedicide 2,4-D as a cause of headaches and diplopia. *N. Z. Med. J.* **75,** 173–174.

Sare, W. M. (1979). 2,4,5-T and the problems of toxicity. *Med. J. Aust.* **1,** 526.

Sare, W. M., and Forbes, P. I. (1972). Possible dysmorphogenic effects of an agricultural chemical: 2,4,5-T. *N. Z. Med. J.* **75,** 37–38.

Sare, W. M., and Forbes, P. I. (1977). The herbicide 2,4,5-T and its possible dysmorphogenic effect. *N. Z. Med. J.* **85,** 439.

Sasaki, S., Sugaya, H., Kagaya, S., Watanabe, K., and Miura, O. (1975). Determination of paraquat dichloride in human tissues. *J. Jpn. Assoc. Rural Med.* **24,** 456–457 (in Japanese).

Sato, K., Yagawa, K., and Nishio, Y. (1974). Morphological study of the thyroid gland of mouse given 3-amino-1,2,4-triazole and/or propylthiouracil for long periods. *Trans. Soc. Pathol. Jpn.* **63,** 185 (in Japanese).

Sato, N., Yakawa, K., Nishio, Y., and Uemura, K. (1974). The alteration of mouse liver by long-term administration of 3-amino-1,2,4-triazole and propylthiouracil. *Proc. Jpn. Cancer Assoc.* **33,** 49 (in Japanese).

Sauerhoff, M. W., Braun, W. H., Blau, G. E., and Behring, P. J. (1976a). The dose-dependent pharmacokinetic profile of 2,4,5-trichlorophenoxyacetic acid following intravenous administration to rats. *Toxicol. Appl. Pharmacol.* **36,** 491–501.

Sauerhoff, M. W., Braun, W. H., and Gehring, P. J. (1976b). The dose-dependent pharmacokinetic profile of 2(2,4,5-trichlorophenoxy) propionic acid (silvex) following intravenous administration to rats. *Toxicol. Appl. Pharmacol.* **37,** 95.

Sauerhoff, M. W., Braun, W. H., and LeBeau, J. E. (1977a). Dose-dependent pharmacokinetic profile of silvex following intravenous administration in rats. *J. Toxicol. Environ. Health* **2,** 605–618.

Sauerhoff, M. W., Chenoweth, M. B., Karbowiski, R. J., Braun, W. H., Ramsey, J. C., Gehring, P. J., and Blau, G. E. (1977b). Fate of silvex following oral administration to humans. *J. Toxicol. Environ. Health* **3,** 941–952.

Sauerhoff, M. W., Braun, W. H., Blau, G. E., and Gehring, P. J. (1977c). The fate of 2,4-dichlorophenoxyacetic acid (2,4-D) following oral administration to man. *Toxicol. Appl. Pharmacol.* **37,** 136–137.

Saunders, N. R., Alpert, H. M., and Cooper, J. D. (1985). Sequential bilateral lung transplantation for paraquat poisoning. A case report. *J. Thorac. Cardiovasc. Surg.* **89**(5), 734–742.

Schaefer, K. E., Avery, M. E., and Bensch, K. (1964). Time course of changes in surface tension and morphology of alveolar epithelial cells in CO_2-induced hyaline membrane disease. *J. Clin. Invest.* **43,** 2080–2093.

Schlatter, I. (1976). Poisoning with the herbicide paraquat. *Schweiz. Rundsch. Med./Prax.* **65,** 837–842 (in German).

Schlicher, J. E., and Beat, V. B. (1972). Dermatitis resulting from herbicide use—a case study. *J. Iowa Med. Soc.* **62,** 419–420.

Schönborn, H., Schuster, H. P., and Koessling, F. K. (1971). Clinical profile and morphology of acute oral diquat intoxication (Reglone). *Arch. Toxikol.* **27,** 204–216 (in German).

Schultek, T., and Markwalder, C. (1985). Acute paraquat intoxication: Pathomorphological change. *Z. Rechtsmed.* **94,** (4), 317–324 (in German).

Schwartz, L. W., and Silverman, S. (1976). Paraquat induced pulmonary damage in nonhuman primates. A morphological study. *Am. Rev. Respir. Dis.* **113,** 108.

Schwetz, B. A., Sparschu, G. L., and Gehring, P. J. (1971). The effect of 2,4-dichlorophenoxyacetic acid (2,4-D) and esters of 2,4-D on rat embryonal, foetal and neonatal growth and development. *Food Cosmet. Toxicol.* **9,** 801–807.

Seabury, J. H. (1963). Toxicity of 2,4-dichlorophenoxyacetic acid for man and dog. *Arch. Environ. Health* **7,** 202–209.

Seidenfeld, J., Wycoff, D., Zavala, D., and Richerson, H. (1977). Paraquat lung injury in rabbits. *Clin. Res.* **25,** 423A.

Seidenfeld, J., Wycoff, D., Zavala, D., and Richerson, H. (1978). Paraquat lung injury in rabbits. *Br. J. Ind. Med.* **35,** 245–257.

Seiler, J. P. (1983). Chemical impurity as the possible cause of nitrofen mutagenicity. *Carcinogenesis (London)* **6,** 1811–1813.

Selypes, A., Nehez, M., Paldy, A., Nagymajtenyi, L., and Berencsi, Gy. (1978). Study of *in vivo* cytogenic effect of paraquat in mice. *Egeszsegtudomany* **22,** 277–280.

Selypes, A., Nagymajtenyi, L., and Berencsi, G. (1980). Mutagenic and embryotoxic effects of paraquat and diquat. *Bull. Environ. Contam. Toxicol.* **25,**513–517.

Semencheva, E. M., Rodionov, G. A., Duznetsova, L. I., and Bebeshko, V. G. (1972). Action mechanims of propazine—a compound of the symmetrical triazine group—on the organism. *Byull. Eksp. Biol. Med.* **73,**47–51 (in Russian).

Senczuk, W., and Pogorzelska, H. (1975). The course of excretion of 2,4-dichlorophenoxyacetic acid with urine. *Rocz. Panstw. Zakl. Hig.* **26,**217–222 (in Polish).

Shafik, M. T., Sullivan, H. C., and Enos, H. F. (1971). A method for determination of low levels of exposure to 2,4-D and 2,4,5-T. *Int. J. Environ. Anal. Chem.* **1,**25–33.

Shardina, R. A. (1972). Hygienic and toxicological assessment of nitrofen in water reservoirs. *Med. Zh. Uzb.* **5,**26–28.

Sharp, C. W., Ottolenghi, A., and Posner, H. S. (1972). Correlation of paraquat toxicity with tissue concentrations and weight loss of the rat. *Toxicol. Appl. Pharmacol.* **22,**241–251.

Shu, H., Talcott, R. E., Rice, S. A., and Wei, E. T. (1979). Lipid peroxidation and paraquat toxicity. *Biochem. Pharmacol.* **28,**327–331.

Shusterman, D. (1985). Problem-solving techniques in occupational medicine. *J. Family Pract.* **21,**195–199.

Siebert, D., and Lemperle, E. (1974). Genetic effects of herbicides: Induction of mitotic gene conversion in *Saccharomyces cerevisiae*. *Mutat. Res.* **22,**111–120.

Sine, C., and Meister, R. T. (1987). "Farm Chemical Handbook '87." Meister Publ. Co., Willoughby, Ohio.

Singleton, S. D., and Murphy, S. D. (1973). Propanil (3,4-dichloropropionanilide)-induced methemoglobin formation in mice in relation to acylamidase activity. *Toxicol. Appl. Pharmacol.* **25,**20–29.

Siou, G. (1979). "Study on the Effect of Tok on the Prenatal and Postnatal Development of the Rabbit." Laboratoire d'Histopathologie CERTI, Versailles, France (in French).

Sjöden, P. O., and Söderberg, U. (1972). Sex-dependent effects of prenatal 2,4,5-trichlorophenoxy-acetic acid on rats' open field behavior. *Physiol. Behav.* **9,**357–360.

Sjöden, P. O., Archer, T., and Söderberg, U. (1977). Effects of 2,4,5-trichlorophenoxyacetic acid (2,4,5-T) on radioiodine distribution in rats. *Bull. Environ. Contam. Toxicol.* **17,**670–678.

Slocombe, G., Thorn, P. E., Toohill, J., and Wood, J. (1973). A case of paraquat poisoning. *Nurs. Times* **69,**111–112.

Smalley, H. E. (1973). Toxicity and hazard of the herbicide, paraquat, in turkeys. *Poult. Sci.* **52,**1625–1628.

Smith, A. H. (1979). "Seasonal Analysis of Oregon Data on Spontaneous Abortions and 2,4,5-T Spraying," Annu. Conf. N. Z. Branch, ANZSERCH, Dunedin.

Smith, A. H., Pearce, N. E., Fisher, D. O., Giles, H. J., Teague, C. A., and Howard, J. K. (1984). Soft tissue sarcoma and exposure to phenoxy herbicides and chlorophenols in New Zealand. *JNCI, J. Natl. Cancer Inst.* **73,** 1111–1117.

Smith, F. A., Schwetz, B. A., Murray, F. J., Crawford, A. A., John, J. A., Kociba, R. J., and Humiston, C. G. (1978). Three-generation reproduction study of rats ingesting 2,4,5-trichlorophenoxyacetic acid in the diet. *Toxicol. Appl. Pharmacol.* **45,**293.

Smith, L. L., and Rose, M. S. (1977). A comparison of the effects of paraquat and diquat on the water content of rat lung and the incorporation of thymidine into lung DNA. *Toxicology* **8,**223–230.

Smith, L. L., Wright, A., Wyatt, I., and Rose, M. S. (1974). Effective treatment for paraquat poisoning in rats and its relevance to treatment of paraquat poisoning in man. *Br. Med. J.* **4,**569–571.

Smith, L. L., Lock, E. A., and Rose, M. S. (1976). The relationship between 5-hydroxytryptamine and paraquat accumulation into rat lung. *Biochem. Pharmacol.* **25,**2485–2487.

Smith, L. L., Rose, M. S., and Wyatt, I. (1979). The pathology and biochemistry of paraquat. *Ciba Found. Symp.* **65,**321–341.

Smith, P. (1971). A light- and electron-microscope study of the pulmonary lesions induced in rats by paraquat. *J. Pathol.* **104**(3),P vii.

Smith, P., and Heath, D. (1974a). Paraquat lung: A reappraisal. *Thorax* **29,** 643–653.

Smith, P., and Heath, D. (1974b). The ultrastructure and time sequence of the early stages of paraquat lung in rats. *J. Pathol.* **114,**177–184.

Smith, P., Heath, D., and Kay, J. M. (1974). The pathogenesis and structure of paraquat-induced pulmonary fibrosis in rats. *J. Pathol.* **114,**57–67.

Smith, R. J. (1978). Poisoned pot becomes burning issue in high places. *Science* **200,**417–418.

Smysl, B., Smyslova, O., and Kostik, A. (1977). Acute fatal ioxynil poisoning. *Arch. Toxicol.* **37,**241–245 (in German).

Snow, J., and Wei, E. (1973). Ocular toxicity of paraquat. *Bull. Environ. Contam. Toxicol.* **9,**163–168.

Sokolik, I. Yu. (1973). The effect of 2,4,5-trichlorophenoxyacetic acid and its butyl ester on rat embryogenesis. *Byull. Eksp. Biol. Med.* **76,**90–92 (in Russian).

Solfrank, G., Mathes, G., Clarman, M., and Beyer, K. H. (1977). Haemoperfusion through activated charcoal in paraquat intoxication. *Acta Pharmacol. Toxicol.* **41,**91–101.

Sorsa, M., and Gripenberg, U. (1976). Organization of a mutagenicity test system combining instructive purposes: Testing for mutagenic effects of the herbicide "amitrole." *Mutat. Res.* **38,**132.

Sparschu, G. L., Dunn, F. L., Lisowe, R. W., and Rowe, V. K. (1971). Study on the effects of high levels of 2,4,5-trichlorophenoxyacetic acid on foetal development in the rat. *Food Cosmet. Toxicol.* **9,**527–530.

Spector, D., Whorton, D., Zachary, J., and Slavin, R. (1978). Fatal paraquat poisoning: Tissue concentrations and implications for treatment. *Johns Hopkins Med. J.* **142,**110–113.

Spencer, F., and Sing, T. L. (1982). Reproductivity toxicity in pseudopregnant and pregnant rat following postimplantational exposure. Effects of the herbicide dinoseb. *Pestic. Biochem. Physiol.* **18,**150–157.

Spencer, M. C. (1966). Herbicide dermatitis. *JAMA, J. Am. Med. Assoc.* **198,** 169–170.

Staiff, D. C., Irle, G. K., and Felsenstein, W. C. (1973). Screening of various adsorbents for protection against paraquat poisoning. *Bull. Environ. Contam. Toxicol.* **10,**193–199.

Staiff, D. C., Comer, S. W., Armstrong, J. F., and Wolfe, H. R. (1975). Exposure to the herbicide paraquat. *Bull. Environ. Contam. Toxicol.* **14,** 334–340.

Stancliffe, T. C., and Pirie, A. (1971). The production of superoxide radicals in reactions of the herbicide diquat. *FEBS Lett.* **17,**297–299.

Steigerwalt, R. B., Godfrey, W. J., and Deckert, F. W. (1980). "Tok Comparative Metabolism Study." Rohm and Haas Report. Springhouse, Pennsylvania.

Steinhoff, D., Weber, H., Mohr, U., and Boehme, K. (1983). Evaluation of amitrole (aminotriazole) for potential carcinogenicity in orally dosed rats, mice and golden hamsters. *Toxicol. Appl. Pharmacol.* **69,**161–169.

Stenger, R. J., and Johnson, E. A. (1972). Modifying effect of 3-amino-1,2,4-triazole on phenobarbital-induced changes in rat liver. *Exp. Mol. Pathol.* **16,** 147–157.

Stevens, J. T., Hall, L. L., Farmer, J. D., DiPasquale, L. C., Chernoff, N., and Durham, W. F. (1977). Disposition of ^{14}C and/or ^{14}As-cacodylic acid in rats after intravenous, intratracheal, or peroral administration. *Environ. Health Perspect.* **19,**151–157.

Stevens, M. A., and Walley, J. K. (1966). Tissue and milk residues arising from the ingestion of single doses of diquat and paraquat by cattle. *J. Sci. Food Agric.* **17,**472–475.

Stone, L. C., and Manson, J. M. (1981). Effects of the herbicide 2,4-dichlorophenyl-p-nitrophenyl ether (nitrofen) on fetal lung development in rats. *Toxicology* **20,**195–207.

Strum, J. M., and Karnovsky, M. J. (1971). Amino-triazole goiter: Fine structure and localization of thyroid peroxidase activity. *Lab. Invest.* **24,**1–12.

Styles, J. A. (1974). Studies on the effects of paraquat and diquat on cells in culture. Viability of macrophages and fibroblasts incubated with paraquat and diquat. *Br. J. Exp. Pathol.* **55,**71–77.

Suga, K. (1972). Environmental pollution and eye damage. *Jpn. Rev. Clin. Ophthalmol.* **66,**537–539 (in Japanese).

Sumi, C., Yokoro, K., and Matsushima, R. (1985). Inhibition by 3-amino-1*H*-1,2,4-triazole of hepatic tumorigenesis induced by diethylstilbestrol alone or combined with *N*-nitrosobutyl urea in WF rats. *JNCI, J. Natl. Cancer Inst.* **74,** 1329–1334.

Sundell, L., Rehn, M., and Axelson, O. (1973). An epidemiological study concerning herbicides. *Arh. Hig. Rada Toksikol.* **24,**375–380.

Sun-Leung Lee, Shu-chuen Lau, Kwok-Ting, *et al.* (1985). The effects of paraquat on the respiratory system. *Chin. Med. J.* **35**(3),192–198.

Suschetet, M., Leclerc, J., Lhuissier, M., and Loisel, W. (1974). The toxicity and nutritional effects for the rat of two herbicides: Picloram (4-amino-3,5,6-trichloropicolinic acid) and atrazine (2-chloro-4-ethylamino-6-isopropylamino-*s*-triazine). *Ann. Nutr. Aliment.* **28,**29–47.

Swan, A. A. B. (1968). Ocular damage due to paraquat and diquat. *Br. Med. J.* **2,**624.

Swan, A. A. B. (1969). Exposure of spray operators to paraquat. *Br. J. Ind. Med.* **26,**322–329.

Swan, A. A. B. (1970). Modern toxicological dangers. *In* "Sixth Symposium on Advanced Medicine" (J. D. H. Slater, ed.). Pitman, London.

Szabo, L., Barabas, K., Matkovics, B., and Berencsi, G. (1980). Time-dependence of paraquat poisoning. *Gen. Pharmacol.* **11,**573–574.

Szabo, L., Matkovics, B., Barabas, K., and Oroszlan, G. (1986). Properties of enzymes. 27. Effects of various thiols on paraquat toxicity. *Comp. Biochem. Physiol. [C]* **83C,**149–153.

Takahashi, T., Yammamoto, K., Sawai, T., Okubo, T., Mukoda, J., Minagawa, N., and Sugaya, H. (1978). Examination of 5 cases of autopsies of paraquat dichloride intoxications, especially lesions of parenchymatous organs. *Trans. Soc. Pathol. Jpn.* **67,**138–139 (in Japanese).

Takayama, K., Takeuchi, K., Suga, E., Iwabuchi, K., and Tomichi, N. (1978). A case of autopsy on paraquat dichloride intoxication. *Trans. Soc. Pathol. Jpn.* **63,**139 (in Japanese).

Takekawa, T., Oda, S., Kaku, K., Shiomura, K., Sasai, K., Unoki, T., Matsumoto, N., and Miwa, S. (1978). An autopsy record of a man intoxicated by paraquat-dichloride. *Yamaguchi Med. J.* **27,**351 (in Japanese).

Takeuchi, S., Kameda, N., Sato, T., and Kasukawa, R. (1977). A case of necropsy on acute intoxication due to paraquat dichloride. *Fukushima Med. J.* **27,**494 (in Japanese).

Talcott, R. E., Shu H., and Wei, E. T. (1977). Lipid peroxidation and paraquat toxicity. *Fed. Proc., Fed. Am. Soc. Exp. Biol.* **36,**998.

Talcott, R. E., Shu H., and Wei, E. T. (1979). Dissociation of microsomal oxygen reduction and lipid peroxidation with the electron acceptors, paraquat and menadione. *Biochem. Pharmacol.* **28,**665–671.

Tane, S., Muromoto, M., and Kouno, E. (1974). Treatment of the ocular disturbance due to splashing of paraquat concentrate into a farmer's eye. *St. Marianna Med. Coll. J.* **2,**78–82 (in Japanese).

Tashiro, T., Kuroda, Y., Goto, Y. *et al.* (1985). An autopsy case of paraquat poisoning: Correlation of paraquat toxicity with tissue concentration. *Jpn. J. Thorac. Dis.* **23**(5), 623–628.

Telegina, K. A., and Bikbulatove, L. I. (1970). State of the skin in persons in contact with Methoxone during its industrial production. *Vestn. Dermatol. Venerol.* **44,**76–79 (in Russian).

Tephley, T. R., Mannering, G. J., and Parks, R. E., Jr. (1961). Studies on the mechanism of inhibition of liver and erythrocyte catalase activity by 3-amino-1,2,4-triazole (AT). *J. Pharmacol. Exp. Ther.* **134,**77–82.

Teruya, A., and Higashi, T. (1973). Differential effect of 3-amino-1,2,4-triazole on multiple forms of rat liver catalase. *Chem. Pharm. Bull.* **21,**840–845.

Thomas, P. D., Thomas, D., Yuk-Luen, C., and Clarkson, A. R. (1977). Paraquat poisoning is not necessarily fatal. *Med. J. Aust.* **2,**564–565.

Thurlbeck, W. M., and Thurlbeck, S. M. (1976). Pulmonary effects of paraquat poisoning. *Chest* **69,**276–280.

Timonen, T. T., and Palva, I. P. (1980). Acute leukaemia after exposure to a weed killer, 2-methyl-4-chlorphenoxyacetic acid. *Acta Haematol.* **63,**170–171.

Tjälve, H. (1974). Accumulation of labelled aminotriazole in some transplanted tumours in mice. *Br. J. Cancer* **30,**136–141.

Tjälve, H. (1975). Fetal uptake and embryogenic effects of aminotriazole in mice. *Arch. Toxicol.* **33,**41–48.

Todd, R. L. (1962). A case of 2,4-D intoxication. *J. Iowa Med. Soc.* **52,**663–664.

Tompsett, S. L. (1970). Paraquat poisoning. *Acta Pharmacol. Toxicol.* **28,**346–358.

Toner, P. G., Vetters, J. M., Spilig, W. G. S., and Harland, W. A. (1970). Fine structure of the lung lesion in a case of paraquat poisoning. *J. Pathol.* **102,**182–185.

Ton That, T., Tran Thi, A., Nguyen Dang, T., Pham Hoang, P., Nguyen Nhu, B., Ton That, B., Hoang Van, S., and Do Kim, S. (1973). Primary cancer of the liver in Viet-nam. *Chirurgie* **99,**427–436 (in French).

Torracca, A. M., Cardamone, G. C., Ortali, V., Carere, A., Raschetti, R., and Ricciardi, G. (1976). Mutagenicity of pesticides as pure compounds and after metabolic activation with rat liver microsomes. *Atti Assoc. Genet. Ital.* **21,**28–29.

Trux, J., and Torrey, L. (1978). Poison pot probe. *New Sci.* **78,**242.

Tsapko, V. G. (1966). On the possible harmful action of the herbicide 2,4-D on agricultural workers. *Gig. Sanit.* **31,**79–80 (in Russian).

Tsuda, H. (1975). Studies on the effects of 3-amino-1,2,4-triazole in rat thyroids. *J. Nagoya City Univ. Med. Assoc.* **62,**87–94 (in Japanese).

Tsuda, H., Hirse, M., Fukushima, A., and Takahashi, M. (1974). Changes in the thyroid gland of rats given 3-amino-1,2,4-triazole. Part 2. Changes following long-term administration. *Trans. Soc. Pathol. Jpn.* **63,**186 (in Japanese).

Tsunenari, S., Muto, H., Inour, S., Sasaki, S., Sugita, H., and Kanda, M. (1975). Forensic toxicological studies of a herbicide, Gramoxone. *Jpn. J. Leg. Med.* **29,**88–102 (in Japanese).

Tsunenari, S., Kita, G., Obo, S., and Ogata, Y. (1976). Forensic toxicological studies on the herbicide paraquat. *Jpn. J. Leg. Med.* **29,**236–237 (in Japanese).

Tsutsui, T., Moizumi, H., and Barnett, J. C. (1984). Amitrole-induced cell transformation and gene mutations in Syrian hamster embryo cells in culture. *Mutat. Res.* **140,**205–207.

Tsyrkunov, L. P. (1979). Chemical dermatosis due to exposure to nitrophen. *Gig. Tr. Prof. Zabol.* **7,**48 (in Romanian).

Turkula, T. E., and Jalal, S. M. (1985). Increased rates of sister chromatid exchanges induced by the herbicide 2,4-D. *J. Hered.* **76,**213–214.

Turner, C. E., Elsohly, M. A., Cheng, F. P., and Torres, L. M. (1978). Marijuana and paraquat. *JAMA, J. Am. Med. Assoc.* **240,**857.

Turner, D. J. (1977). "The Safety of the Herbicides 2,4-D and 2,4,5-T," For. Comm. Bull. No. 57. H. M. Stationery Office, London.

Tye, R., and Engel, D. (1967). Distribution and excretion of dicamba by rats as determined by radiotracer technique. *J. Agric. Food Chem.* **15,**837–840.

Uchida, A. (1975). A case of corneoconjunctival erosion by Gramoxon, paraquat dichloride. *Jpn. J. Clin. Ophthalmol.* **69,**778–779 (in Japanese).

Uetake, S., Yamada, K., Seta, K., Shirojura, T., Maekawa, T., Shigitani, R., Ogura, H., Satane, B., and Toyoda, O. (1972). A case of Gramoxone intoxication. *J. Jpn. Soc. Intern. Med.* **61,**1435–1436 (in Japanese).

Unger, T. M., Kliethermes, J., Van Goethem, D., and Short, R. D. (1981). Teratology and postnatal studies in rats of the propylene glycol butyl ester and isooctyl esters of 2,4-dichlorophenoxyacetic acid. *U.S. NTIS, PB Rep.* **PB 81–191,**140.

U.S. Senate (1970). "Effects of 2,4,5-T on Man and the Environment" (Hearings before the Subcommittee on Energy, Natural Resources, and the Environment of the Committee on Commerce, United States Senate), Ser. 91–60. U.S. Govt. Printing Office, Washington, D.C.

Vainio, H., Linnairmaa, K., Kahonen, M., Nichels, J., Hietanen, E., Marniemi, J., and Peltonen, P. (1983). Hyperlipidemia and peroxisome proliferation induced by phenoxyacetic acid herbicides in rats. *Biochem. Pharmacol.* **32,**2775–2779.

Vale, J. A., Crome, P., Volans, G. N., Widdop, B., and Goulding, R. (1977). The treatment of paraquat poisoning using oral sorbents and charcoal hemoperfusion. *Acta Pharmacol. Toxicol.* **41,**109–117.

Van Dijk, A., Maes, R. A. A., and Drost, R. H. (1975). Paraquat poisoning in man. *Arch. Toxicol.* **34,**129–136.

Van Genderen, H., and Van Esch, G. J. (1968). Toxicology of the herbicide dichlobenil (2,6-dichlorobenzonitrile) and its main metabolites. *Food Cosmet. Toxicol.* **5,**261–269.

Vanholder, R., Colardyn, F., De Reuck, J., Praet, M., Lameire, N., and Ringoir, S. (1981). Diquat intoxication: Report of two cases and review of the literature. *Am. J. Med.* **70,**1267–1271.

Van Osten, G. K., and Gibson, J. E. (1975). Effect of paraquat on the biosynthesis of doexyribonucleic acid and protein in the rat. *Food Cosmet. Toxicol.* **13**,47–54.

van Overbeek, J. (1964). Survey of mechanisms of herbicide action. *In* "The Physiology and Biochemistry of Herbicides" (L. J. Audus, ed.), pp. 387–400. Academic Press, London.

Vaziri, N. D., Ness, R. L., Fairshter, R. D., Smith, W. R., and Rosen, S. M. (1979). Nephrotoxicity of paraquat in man. *Arch. Intern. Med.* **139**,172–174.

Verschuuren, H. G., Kroes, R., and Den Tonkelaar, E. M. (1975). Short-term oral and dermal toxicity of MCPA and MCPP. *Toxicology* **3**,349–359.

Vigfusson, N. V., and Vyse, E. R. (1980). The effect of the pesticides, Dexon, Captan and Roundup, on sister-chromatid exchanges in human lymphocytes *in vitro. Mutat. Res.* **79**,53–57.

Vijeyaratnam, G. S., and Corin, B. (1971). Experimental paraquat poisoning: A histological and electron-optical study of the changes in the lung. *J. Pathol.* **103**,123–129.

Vizek, M., Holusa, R., and Palecek, F. (1976). Lung function in acute paraquat intoxication. *Physiol. Bohemoslov.* **24**,559–564 (in Russian).

Vogel, E., and Chandler, J. L. R. (1974). Mutagenicity testing of cyclamate and some pesticides in *Drosophila melanogaster. Experientia* **30**,621–623.

Von Butenandt, I., Mantel, K., and Fendel, H. (1975). Intoxication with paraquat in 2 children. *Clin. Med.* **82**,16.

von der Hardt, H., and Cardesa, A. (1971). The early histopathological changes in paraquat intoxication. *Klin. Wochenschr.* **49**,544–550 (in German).

Voytenko, G. A., and Medved', I. L. (1973). Effect of some thiocarbamates on reproductive function. *Gig. Sanit.* **38**,111–114 (in Russian).

Vucinovic, B. (1978). Four cases of poisoning with paraquat. *Arh. Hig. Rada Toksikol.* **29**,261–265 (in Serbo-Croatian).

Wagner, S. L. (1983). "Clinical Toxicology of Agricultural Chemicals." Noyes Data Corporation, Park Ridge, New Jersey.

Waight, J. J. J. (1979). Fatal percutaneous paraquat poisoning. *JAMA, J. Am. Med. Assoc.* **242**,272.

Wain, R. L. (1963). 3,5-Dihalogeno-4-hydroxybenzonitriles: New herbicides with molluscicidal activity. *Nature (London)* **200**,28.

Wakabayashi, T., Chihara, M., Nishimoto, M., Kuroda, T., and Shiaku, Y. (1977). A therapeutic experience in the ICU on a patient acutely intoxicated with a herbicide, paraquat dichloride. *J. Med. Assoc. Okayama* **89**,1389 (in Japanese).

Walker, E. M., Gadsden, R. H., Atkins, L. M., and Gale, G. R. (1972). Some effects of 2,4-D and 2,4,5-T on Ehrlich ascites tumor cells *in vivo* and *in vitro. Ind. Med. Surg.* **41**,22–27.

Wanic, W., Marciniak, J., Sikorshi, M., and Dabrowski, H. (1971). In case of lethal poisoning with Gramoxone. *Pol. Tyg. Lek.* **26**,1166–1168 (in Polish).

Wasserman, B., and Bock, E. R. (1978). Prevention of acute paraquat toxicity in rats by superoxide dismutase. *Aviat. Space Environ. Med.* **49**,805–809.

Watanabe, I., Sakai, H., Toyama, K., Ueno, M., and Watanabe, M. (1979). Ocular impairment due to paraquat-dichloride. *Jpn. Rev. Clin. Ophthalmol.* **73**,660.

Wester, R. C., Maibach, H. O., Bucks, D. A. W., and Auferer, M. B. (1984). *In vivo* percutaneous absorption of paraquat from hand, leg, and forearm of humans. *J. Toxicol. Environ. Health* **14**,(5–6),759–762.

Weston, J. T., Liebow, A. A., Dixon, M. G., and Rich, T. H. (1972). Untoward effects of oxogenous inhalants on the lung. *J. Forensic Sci.* **17**,199–279.

Whitehead, A. P., Volans, G. N., and Hart, T. B. (1984). Toxicovigilance for pesticides: Paraquat poisoning in the United Kingdom. *J. Toxicol. Med.* **4** (1),51–53.

Whitehead, C. C., and Pettigrew, R. J. (1972). The subacute toxicity of 2,4-dichlorophenoxyacetic acid and 2,4,5-trichlorophenoxyacetic acid to chicks. *Toxicol. Appl. Pharmacol.* **21**,348–354.

Widdop, B., Medd, R. K., and Braithwaite, R. A. (1977). Charcoal hemoperfusion in the treatment of paraquat poisoning. *Proc. Eur. Soc. Toxicol.* **18**, 156–159.

Wiklund, K., and Holm, L. E. (1986). Soft tissue sarcoma risk in Swedish agricultural and forestry workers. *JNCI, J. Natl. Cancer Inst.* **76**,229–234.

Wilson, J. G., Boutwell, R. K., David, D. E., Dost, F. N., Hayes, W. J., Jr., Kalter, H., Loomis, T. A., Schulert, A., Sterling, T. D., and Bowen, D. L.

(1971). "Report of the Advisory Committee on 2,4,5-T to the Administrator of the Environmental Protection Agency," unpublished report. U.S. Environ. Prot. Agency, Washington, D.C.

Wit, J. G., and Van Genderen, H. (1966a). Metabolism of the herbicide 2,6-dichlorobenzonitrile in rabbits and rats. *Biochem. J.* **101**,698–706.

Wit, J. G., and Van Genderen, H. (1966b). The monophenolic metabolites of the herbicide 2,6-dichlorobenzonitrile in animals as uncouplers of oxidative phosphorylation. *Biochem. J.* **101**,707–710.

Withers, E. H., Madden, J. J., and Lynch, J. B. (1979). Pancreatitis as a complication of anticholinesterase insecticide intoxication. *Ann. Surg.* **189**, 199–204.

Witschi, H. P. (1973). The biochemical pathology of rat lung after acute paraquat poisoning. *Toxicol. Appl. Pharmacol.* **25**,485–486.

Witschi, H. P., and Kacew, S. (1974). Studies on the pathological biochemistry of lung parenchyma in acute paraquat poisoning. *Med. Biol.* **52**,104–110.

Witschi, H. P., Kacew, S., Hirai, K., and Cote, M. G. (1977). *In vivo* oxidation of reduced nicotinamide-adenine dinucleotide phosphate by paraquat and diquat in rat lung. *Chem.-Biol. Interact.* **19**,143–160.

Wood, T. E., Edgar, H., and Salcedo, J. (1976). Recovery from inhalation of diquat aerosol. *Chest* **70**,774–775.

Woodard, G., Lange, S. W., Nelson, K. W., and Calvery, H. O. (1941). The acute oral toxicity of acetic chloroacetic, dichloroacetic, and trichloroacetic acids. *J. Ind. Hyg. Toxicol.* **23**,78–82.

World Health Organization (WHO) (1974). World Health Organization International Agency for Research on Cancer. "IARC Monographs on the Evaluation of Carcinogenic Risk of Chemicals to Man," Vol. 7. Int. Agency Res. Cancer, Lyon, France.

World Health Organization (WHO) (1984). "Paraquat and Diquat: Environmental Health Criteria 39." World Health Organ., Geneva.

Worthing, C. R., ed. (1987). "The Pesticide Manual: A World Compendium," 8th ed. Br. Crop Prot. Counc., Thornton Heath, U.K.

Wright, N., Yeoman, W. B., and Hale, K. A. (1978). Assessment of severity of paraquat poisoning. *Br. Med. J.* **2**,396.

Yagi, F., Kanafuki, Y., Manabe, K., Ise, H., and Imakawa, O. (1977). A case report of acute intoxication due to paraquat-dichloride. *J. Jpn. Assoc. Rural Med.* **26**,330–331 (in Japanese).

Yamashita, K., Aoyama, S., Ikuta, S., Miyake, T., and Arima, K. (1974). A case of acute intoxication and autopsy, due to paraquat-dichloride: Comment on comparison between the injury by insecticide and herbicide. *J. Jpn. Assoc. Rural Med.* **23**,27–38 (in Japanese).

Yasaka, T., Ohya, I., Matsumoto, J., Shiramizu, T., and Sasaguri, Y. (1981). Acceleration of lipid peroxidation in human paraquat poisoning. *Arch. Intern. Med.* **141**(9)1169–1171.

Yasaka, T., Okudaira, K., Fujito, H., and Shiramizu, T. (1986). Further studies of lipid peroxidation in human paraquat poisoning. *Arch. Intern. Med.* **146** (4),681–685.

Yeary, R. A. (1986). Urinary excretion of 2,4-D in commercial lawn specialists. *Appl. Ind. Hyg.* **1**,119–121.

Yefimenko, L. P. (1974). Materials for assessing the gonadotrophic and mutagenic action of the herbicide, 2,4,5-T butyl ester. *Gig. Tr. Prof. Zabol.* **18**, 24–27.

Yelizarov, G. P. (1972). Occupational skin diseases caused by simazine and propazine. *Vestn. Dermatol. Venerol.* **46**,27–29 (in Russian).

Yoneda, S., Sawada, Y., Kaimasu, I., Ochaia, K., Hino, Y., Miyake, M., and Kuga, M. (1979). Autopsy report on a man intoxicated by paraquat. *J. Jpn. Soc. Intern. Med.* **33**,777 (in Japanese).

Young, J. F., and Haley, T. J. (1977). Pharmacokinetic study of a patient intoxicated with 2,4-dichlorophenoxyacetic acid and 2-methoxy-3,6-dichlorobenzoic acid. *Clin. Toxicol.* **11**,489–500.

Zakharov, G. G., Shevchenko, A. M., Zub, G. A., and Pershai, L. K. (1968). The clinical aspects and prevention of intoxication with the herbicide Dicotex. *Zdravookhr. Beloruss.* **14**,17–21 (in Russian).

Zavala, D. C., and Rhodes, M. L. (1978). An effect of paraquat on the lungs of rabbits: Its implications in smoking contaminated marihuana. *Chest* **74**, 418–420.

Zetterberg, G. (1978). Mutagenicity of chlorinated phenoxyacetic acids in *Saccharomyces cerevisiae. Mutat. Res.* **53**,285–286.

Zetterberg, G. (1979). Mechanism of the lethal and mutagenic effects of phenoxyacetic acids in *Saccharomyces cerevisiae*. *Mutat. Res.* **60,**291–300.

Zetterberg, G., Busk, L., Elovson, R., Starce-Nordenhammer, I., and Ryttman, H. (1977). The influence of pH on the effects of 2,4-D (2,4-di-chlorophenoxyacetic acid, Na salt) on *Saccharomyces cerevisiae* and *Salmonella typhimurium*. *Mutat. Res.* **42,**3–18.

Zielinski, W. L., and Fishbein, L. (1967). Gas chromatographic measurements of disappearance rates of 2,4-D and 2,4,5-T acids and 2,4-D esters in mice. *J. Agric. Food Chem.* **15,**841–844.

chapter 21

Fungicides
and Related Compounds

I. Ralph Edwards, Donald G. Ferry,
and Wayne A. Temple

University of Otago, New Zealand

21.1 INTRODUCTION

The fungi differ so greatly from other forms of life that it is now common practice to treat them as a separate kingdom, just as animals and plants constitute separate kingdoms. Because they are distinct not only in form but also in physiology, fungi may be combatted successfully by compounds that have only extremely low toxicities to other organisms, notably mammals. This fact accounts for the generally good safety record of fungicides. Of course, the distinctiveness of the fungi does not exclude their susceptibility to compounds such as alkyl mercury that are highly toxic to most forms of life, nor does it exclude the possibility that certain compounds will injure pathogenic fungi by one chemical mechanism and injure humans or useful animals by a totally different mechanism, such as allergic sensitization.

With the exception of organic sulfur compounds, the classification used in the remainder of this chapter has most of the same broad outlines and many of the details to be found in books dealing with the same range of compounds from the standpoint of the control of fungi (Torgeson, 1969; Lukens, 1971). The distinctions made in the following classifications are chemical ones, with fewer pharmacological implications than are now possible in connection with insecticides or rodenticides. Furthermore, active groups apparently have been recombined more by those who have designed fungicides than by the designers of other pesticides, with the possible exception of herbicides. The result is that the classification of fungicides might be viewed more as a web than as a list. For example, chlorine substitutions, quinone structure, heterocyclic nitrogen structure, and other active groups may be found in some compounds assigned to groups whose names do not imply the presence of these structures.

The organic sulfur compounds have not been considered together as a single group because they seem completely heterogeneous from the standpoint of mammalian toxicology. As a matter of fact, it is not at all clear whether sulfur *per se* contributes to the fungicidal action of organic sulfur compounds. This is totally different from the situation with organic copper compounds that clearly produce copper poisoning in both fungi and mammals.

21.2 INORGANIC AND ORGANOMETAL FUNGICIDES

In addition to elementary sulfur and lime sulfur, a variety of organometallic compounds, especially those of chromium, copper, zinc, cadmium, and mercury, are used as fungicides. Some of them are discussed in Chapter 12. The range of toxicity is tremendous. The acute toxicity of elementary sulfur is low, and it has no known cumulative effect. At the opposite extreme, the alkyl mercury compounds are highly toxic; the effects of small doses are cumulative, and the illness that results either from a single dose or from repeated doses may be chronic and severe.

21.3 ANTIBIOTICS AND BOTANICALS

At least one antibiotic, griseofulvin, is used not only as an agricultural fungicide but also as a systemic drug to combat fungal infection in humans. Another, streptomycin, used almost exclusively against bacteria in human medicine, is used against both bacteria and fungi that attack crops. Finally, some antibiotics used against crop pests have found no place in medicine.

The antifungal antibiotics are not a homogeneous group. They range from such relatively simple compounds as penicillamine (α-amino-β-methyl-β-mercaptobutyric acid) to complex, extensively substituted, multiring compounds. As might be expected of chemically heterogeneous compounds, the toxicity of these antifungal compounds varies widely. For example, the oral LD 50 of blasticidin-S in rats is 16 mg/kg, whereas that of validamycin A is >20,000 mg/kg. The toxicity of streptomycin lies somewhere between these values; the usual therapeutic (intramuscular) dosage in humans is 15–25 mg/kg/day.

The effects of the different compounds also vary greatly in their seriousness and chronicity. For example, streptomycin causes eighth-nerve damage fairly often and can cause aplastic anemia and other serious conditions, whereas blasticidin-S, which has a much greater acute toxicity, has produced conjunctivitis, dermatitis, and other reversible effects that are mainly, if not exclusively, irritative in origin.

The toxicity of the antibiotics important in agriculture and known to have been studied in humans in this connection are discussed in Chapter 13. In addition, fungicides used as drugs are discussed in textbooks of pharmacology and in the AMA Drug Evaluations [American Medical Association (AMA), 1986].

Although not yet of economic importance, some components of green plants are fungicidal. Some of these belong to the same chemical classes as have been exploited in connection with synthetic fungicides. They include ketones, aldehydes, carboxylic acids, lactones, coumarins, phenolic compounds, hydroxystilbenes, tannins, quinones, tropolones, amino acids, alkaloids, benzoxazolinones, sulfoxides, isothiocyanates, and others. Finally, there are two compounds with one or more triple bonds that are fungicidal at concentrations in the range of 0.25–4 ppm (Fawcett and Spencer, in Torgeson, 1969).

21.4 ALIPHATIC AND ALICYCLIC FUNGICIDES

A number of aliphatic and alicyclic compounds are fungicides. They include cationic, anionic, and nonionic compounds, many of them chemically simple. Some, especially the nonionic compounds, have substitutions of chlorine, cyanate, or both. Few are powerful fungicides, but some have very important practical uses depending on special properties. For example, because of its high vapor pressure, formaldehyde may be used as a soil disinfectant. By contrast, the low toxicity of sorbic acid permits its use for food preservation. Other aliphatic and alicyclic fungicides include dodine (ANSI, BSI, ISO), propionic acid, dehydroacetic acid, chloropicrin, methyl bromide, allyl alcohol, and propylene oxide. Of these, chloropicrin and methyl bromide are discussed in Sections 14.7.3 and 14.7.1, respectively.

21.5 CHLOROALKYL THIO FUNGICIDES

The chloroalkyl thio compounds are also spoken of as the R-SCCl compounds. Some authors treat the group as a subdivision of nitrogen heterocyclic compounds. However, nitrogen attachment of the —$SCCl_3$ group is not required for fungitoxic action. Many S—$SCCl_3$, C—$SCCl_3$, and O—$SCCl_3$ compounds are fungicides. Some fungicides based on —$SCCl_3$ contain no nitrogen in the molecule (e.g., trichloromethylthio-3,4-dichlorobenzene sulfonate). Furthermore, at least one chlorine may be replaced by another halogen (e.g., —$SCCl_2F$) or the alkyl chain may be longer (e.g., $SCCl_2$—$CHCl_2$).

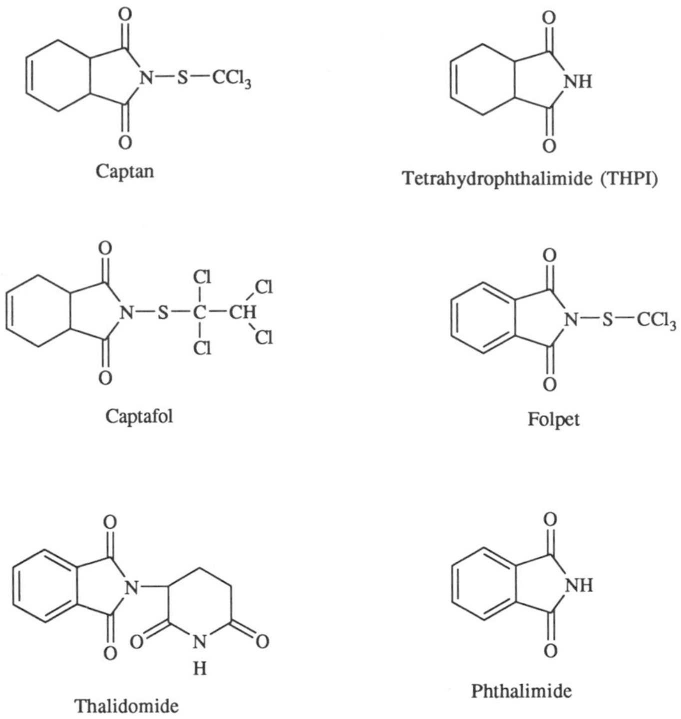

Figure 21.1 Three choloralkyl thio fungicides (captan, catafol, and folpet), two metabolites, and thalidomide.

Effects on Reproduction Because of the similarity or, in the case of folpet, identity of the double ring moiety of some of the chloroalkyl thio fungicides to the corresponding portion of the thalidomide molecule (see Fig. 21.1), it was to be expected that there would be a very thorough investigation of the possible teratogenic effects of these fungicides and their metabolites. Such studies have been carried out in several species, including rabbits and monkeys, in which it formerly had been shown that thalidomide produces effects similar to those it produced in human babies. The results for the fungicides were negative in all mammalian species, although concurrent positive controls with thalidomide were positive. This strongly suggests that the teratogenic effects of thalidomide in mammals depend on the glutarimide part of its molecule, which is entirely lacking in the fungicides, or on the configuration of the entire molecule (see Sections 21.5.1.2 and 21.5.2.2).

21.5.1 CAPTAN

21.5.1.1 Identity, Properties, and Uses

Chemical Name 3A,4,7,7A-Tetrahydro-2-(trichloromethylthio)-1H-isoindole-1,3-(2H)-dione.

Structure See Fig. 21.1

Synonyms The common name captan (BSI,ISO) is in general use. It is also known as captane (France), captano (Italy), Orthocide®, Orthocide 406®, and Vancide 89®. A code designation is SR-406. The CAS registry number is 133-06-2.

Physical and Chemical Properties Captan has the empirical formula $C_9H_8Cl_3NO_2S$ and a molecular weight of 300.57. It forms white crystals with a melting point of 178°C and a vapor pressure of $<1 \times 10^{-5}$ mm Hg at 25°C. Captan's solubility at room temperature in water is less than 0.5 ppm, and it is insoluble in petroleum oils. It is stable, except under alkaline conditions, and is compatible with most other pesticides.

History, Formulations, and Uses Captan was introduced in 1949 by the Standard Oil Development Company. The fungicide captan is used mainly for foliage protection and is nonphytotoxic.

21.5.1.2 Toxicity to Laboratory Animals

Most investigators have found that captan has a low oral toxicity to laboratory animals. In the rat, LD 50 values of 12,600 and >17,000 mg/kg have been found (Boyd and Krijnen, 1968; Urbanek-Karlowska, 1975). On the contrary, Vashakidze *et al.* (1973) reported a value of 2650 mg/kg in the rat but of only 38 mg/kg in the mouse. The latter value is smaller than that Innes *et al.* (1969) administered by gavage to infant mice that survived not only treatment at a rate of 215 mg/kg but a subsequent 13 months of dietary intake at a rate of 560 ppm. This suggests that the formulation used by Vashakidze and his colleagues may have contained a toxic impurity. Stevens *et al.* (1978) reported oral LD 50 values of 7840 and 7000 mg/kg for male and female mice, respectively, and corresponding intraperitoneal values of 518 and 462 mg/kg. Milled captan had approximate LD 50 values of 142 and 310 mg/kg for male and female mice and was much more toxic than the coarser dust of the commercial product.

Sheep and, to a lesser degree, cattle are specifically susceptible to captan. Some sheep were killed by a single dose at the rate of 250 mg/kg, and a heifer was poisoned by three doses and killed by six doses at the same rate. For sheep, the tolerated and lethal levels are close. Sheep were unaffected by 100 doses at the rate of 50 mg/kg/day, and they survived with only moderate poisoning 72 doses at 100 mg/kg/day or 38 doses at 200 mg/kg/day. Signs of toxicity included depression and anorexia (Palmer, 1963a; Palmer and Radeleff, 1964).

A dietary level of 10,000 ppm for 54 weeks produced marked growth depression in both male and female rats. Female rats fed 5000 ppm for 2 years also showed growth retardation but males did not. Female rats fed 1000 ppm for 2 years (about 50 mg/kg/day) showed growth depression during the last 16 weeks of the 104-week study. At autopsy, testicular atrophy was found in some animals fed 10,000 ppm. Otherwise, the organ weights, hematology, and gross and histological morphology (including incidence of tumors) were not significantly different from those of controls [unpublished reports, cited by the Food and Agricultural Organization/World Health Organization (FAO/WHO), 1970]. The late effects seen in female rats at 1000 ppm may not have been related to captan because in other studies, illness caused by captan has occurred in the first 43 days or not at all.

The most thorough study of the effect of repeated doses of captan given by stomach tube to rats is that by Boyd and Carsky (1971). The 100-day LD 50 was 916 mg/kg/day or 7.3% of the 1-dose LD 50 that Boyd found to be 12,500 mg/kg. Ignoring the difference that might be introduced by using gavage rather than feeding, these results indicate a chronicity index of 13.65. Whereas this is a moderately high index, it is only fair to observe that the 100-day LD 50 indicates a low toxicity of repeated doses of captan. In the 100-day test, signs of toxicity were most marked during the first 3 weeks. They included weight loss, decreased food intake, increased water intake, diarrhea, hypothermia, and prostration. Illness subsided in survivors after they had received captan for 22–42 days. From day 43 to day 100, while still receiving captan, the rats actually ate slightly more than the controls but not enough to permit their catching up with the body weight of the controls. During the last 57 days, the captan-treated rats showed polydipsia, diuresis, and a slight fever. Samples studied by Zhorzholiani (1972) were substantially more toxic; dosages of 530 and 27 mg/kg/day were fatal to 50% or more rats and mice, respectively, within 60 days. No-effect levels in the two species were 53 and 6.9 mg/kg/day.

In spite of the low acute toxicity of captan, repeated administration by stomach tube at the rate of 1000 mg/kg/day killed all guinea pigs within 10–12 days. A dosage of 100 mg/kg/day for 7 or especially for 21 days caused a variety of enzymatic shifts in the epithelial cells of the stomach but apparently was without effect on the health of the animals (Krolikowska-Prasal, 1974).

Dogs that received oral doses at the rate of 300 mg/kg/day for 48 weeks following 18 weeks at lower rates showed a slight increase of liver and kidney weights. This increase was not present in dogs that received 100 mg/kg/day. In both groups of dogs, there was no clinical illness and no change in hematology, clinical laboratory findings, or gross or historical morphology (unpublished reports, cited by FAO/WHO, 1970).

Absorption, Distribution, Metabolism, and Excretion Following an oral dose of [^{35}S]captan to rats at a rate of 143 or 390 mg/kg, at least 60% was absorbed inasmuch as it was accounted for in the urine. Within the first 24 hr, more than 90% was excreted in the urine and feces, and almost all the rest was excreted during the next 2 days. Only 0.01–0.05% of the radioactivity was deposited in the organs in the form of metabolites or of moieties incorporated into normal body constituents (Seidler *et al.*, 1971). Similar results were found by Engst and Raab (1973), who were unable to detect unchanged captan or the split-off side chain in the blood of rats; they did identify tetrahydrophthalimide and tetrahydrophthalic acid for a short time until they were excreted.

When captan tagged with ^{14}C in the trichloromethyl group was administered to rats orally, activity was recovered as follows: 51.8% in the urine, 22.8% in the expired air, 15.9% in the feces, and 0.6% in the tissues. Urinary metabolites of orally administered captan marked in this way included (*a*) thiazolidine-2-thione-4-carboxylic acid, (*b*) a salt of dithiobis(methanesulfonic acid), and (*c*) the disulfide monoxide derivative of dithiobis(methanesulfonic acid). The latter two derivatives were not detected in the urine of rats that received captan intraperitoneally. This and other evidence indicated that degradation in the gastrointestinal tract plays a major role in the metabolism of captan. The metabolite in (a) above was found in radioactive form in the urine of rats that had received non-radioactive captan plus [^{14}C]glutathione. The metabolite in (b) was radioactive in the urine of rats that had received nonradioactive captan or thiophosgene plus sodium [^{35}S]sulfite. The metabolism of captan seems to involve evolution of thiophosgene. This is detoxified by at least three mechanisms: oxidation and/or hydrolysis to carbon dioxide, reaction with cystine to form metabolite (a), and reaction with sulfite to produce metabolite (b) (DeBaun et al., 1974).

The rapid excretion of [^{35}S]captan was further documented by Couch et al. (1977).

Biochemical Effects   Large dosages of captan must be administered repeatedly in order to produce any detectable effect on liver enzymes. Several enzymes were altered by seven doses at the rate of 1000 mg/kg/day but not at the rate of 100 mg/kg/day (Krolikowska-Prasal, 1973).

In vitro, captan caused rapid swelling of rat liver mitochondria. Both biochemical and electron microscopic evidence supported the belief that this is the result of a breakdown of the permeability barriers of the inner membrane. This reaction with membranes may be more important than interaction with specific enzymes (Nelson, 1971b). Treatment of human erythrocytes in buffered saline with 0.5 μM captan caused rapid loss of intracellular potassium. This effect was prevented when the same molar concentration of glutathione was added to the cells before the addition of captan. Permeability was altered by reaction of captan with sulfhydryl and amino groups of the proteins of the cell membrane (Kumar et al., 1975). Even the ability of captan to induce mutations in bacteria was nullified by L-cysteine (Moriya et al., 1976) or by rat or human blood or serum (Ficsor et al., 1977).

The inhibition of mitochondrial function produced by captan *in vitro* is nonspecific, involving several sites. The inhibition involves an uncoupling of oxidative phosphorylation (Nelson, 1971a), but the mode of death of animals killed by the compound indicates that this is not the dominant mode of action.

Effect on Organs and Tissues   Most investigators have found captan mutagenic when brought into direct contact with susceptible cells, but many believe it is not mutagenic in intact higher animals, except perhaps at dosage levels encountered only in suicides.

The rate of mutation was increased in bacteria exposed directly to captan, and the number of chromosome breaks was increased in mammalian cells grown *in vitro* in the presence of captan (Legator et al., 1969). Similar results in some but not all bacteria either with or without the presence of liver microsomes has been reported (Ficsor and Nii, 1970; Propping et al., 1973; Seiler, 1973; Herbold and Buselmaier, 1976).

In certain *Escherichia coli* strains, the increased mutation was influenced by excision repair (Clarke, 1971; Bridges et al., 1972).

Results of host-mediated tests with captan have been contradictory. Buselmaier et al. (1972) reported positive findings with a subcutaneous dosage of 500 mg/kg administered three times at hourly intervals for a total of 1500 mg/kg. In another study, indicator organisms recovered from the peritoneal cavity of rats previously gavaged with captan for 14 days at a rate of 125 or 250 mg/kg/day showed no increase in the number of revertants following *in vitro* incubation. A similar negative result was obtained following thalidomide at 500 or 1000 mg/kg/day (Kennedy et al., 1975a).

The presence of captan in the culture medium permitted chromosomal division without division in cells derived from a Chinese hamster (Sutou and Tokuyama, 1974). There is no indication that this has any more clinical significance than the similar action of the drug colchicine.

Captan demonstrated mutagenic ability in the forward mutation system but not in the reverse mutation system of the slime mold *Neurospora crassa* (Malling and DeSerres, 1970). It induced only a weak apparent induction of gene conversion in the ascomycete *Saccharomyces cerevisiae* (Siebert et al., 1970).

Captan was not mutagenic in fruit flies (*Drosophila* sp.), whether administered at tolerated or at toxic dosage levels. This was true of separate tests involving sex-limited recessive lethals, dominant lethals, or translocation (Mollet, 1973; Kramers and Knaap, 1973). Captan also failed to produce somatic mutations and recombinations in somatic cells of *Drosophila* (Mollet and Wurgler, 1974). It is thought that the negative results of different laboratories for *Drosophila* may be due to detoxication of captan before it can reach cells that otherwise might be sensitive. However, some of the tests involved injection of the compound into the hemocele of the flies.

Captan (9 mg/kg/day intraperitoneally and 500–600 mg/kg/day orally) did not increase the incidence of dominant lethals in mice (Epstein and Shafner, 1968; Shirasu et al., 1978; Tezuka et al., 1978).

Male mice received a single intraperitoneal dose of captan (either 3 or 6 mg/kg) or thalidomide (500 or 1000 mg/kg) and then were mated at weekly intervals in a dominant lethal test. There was no increase in early embryonic death due to either treatment (Kennedy et al., 1975a). A similar result was found by Jorgenson et al. (1976). However, when captan was administered for 5 days to male rats and mice at intraperitoneal dosages of 2.5, 5.0, and 10.0 mg/kg/day and at oral dosages of 50, 100 and 200 mg/kg/day, evidence of dominant lethal effects was found. Captan had negligible effects on the number of litters produced or on the total number of implants per pregnancy but did increase the mean number of early fetal deaths in both species, and the response was dosage-related. In rats, a mutagenic effect was questionable at 5.0 mg/kg/day (ip) and nonexistent at 2.5 mg/kg/day (ip); 50 mg/kg/day was considered a no-effect oral level. In mice an intraperitoneal dosage of 2.5 mg/kg/day and an oral dosage of 50 mg/kg/day were no-effect levels (Collins, 1972a).

Captan caused no increase of chromosomal aberrations in the bone marrow of rats that received single oral doses at rates as high as 2000 mg/kg or repeated oral doses at rates as high as 800 mg/kg/day for 5 days. There was a tendency for the chromosomes to be sticky, and mitosis was inhibited. Results were also negative for human diploid fibroblasts at *in vitro* concentrations as high as 4 ppm (Shirasu *et al.*, 1978; Tezuka *et al.*, 1978).

The mutagenic effects of captan and related fungicides were reviewed by Bridges (1975), who concluded that their use should be reevaluated and the use of nonmutagenic substitutes with similar low toxicity should be promoted. It seems probable that no such substitutes are known. Furthermore, a more general review of mutagenicity (Legator and Zimmering, 1975) reached the conclusion that captan may be an example of an active mutagen that is detoxicated by the intact host, a conclusion supported by the work of Moriya *et al.* (1978a).

Captan was not tumorigenic in two strains of mice that received it at the highest tolerated level (Innes *et al.*, 1969). However, in another study, mice that received dietary levels of 8000 or 16,000 ppm for 80 weeks showed a significant increase of adenomatous polyps and of polypoid carcinoma of the duodenum. No statistically significant increase of any neoplasm was found in rats on dietary levels of 2225 or 6050 ppm for 80 weeks [National Cancer Institute (NCI), 1977].

An impressive reduction of the rate of development of Ehrlich ascites tumor cells was reported by Steckerl and Turner (1965) in mice injected intraperitoneally with captan for 14 days at a rate of 150 mg/kg/day; the survival time of treated mice was more than doubled. The protective effect of captan was confirmed repeatedly by Gale *et al.* (1971), although the lives of their mice were prolonged by much shorter intervals. The protective effect of whatever intensity may be related to inhibition of synthesis of RNA in the tumor cells, which was demonstrated *in vivo* as well as *in vitro* by Gale and his colleagues using [^{14}C]purines and [^{14}C]formate.

In weanling rats, captan administered at a dietary concentration of 100 mg/kg for 3 weeks depressed lymphocyte count and relative thymus weight, while the serum IgG level was significantly increased. However, more detailed immune function studies showed that captan administered at a level of 2000 mg/kg virtually did not alter immune parameters (Vos and Krajne, 1983).

Effects on Reproduction A study on pseudopregnant and pregnant rats demonstrated a reduction in uterine weight, particularly affecting the endometrium, occurring in a dose-dependent fashion up to 10,000 ppm. Fetal survival was similarly reduced to 17% when captan was fed at a 10% dietary level. Variations in toxicity to other organs were also noted, with the spleen and kidney being affected more than the adrenal, and in particular there was no effect on ovarian weight or tissue (Spencer, 1984). These findings would be consistent with difficulties in implantation leading to abortion at high levels but they support the studies described below which suggest lack of teratogenicity.

In a three-generation study, rats reproduced normally when maintained on captan at a dietary level of 1000 ppm (about 50 mg/kg/day for most adults but substantially more for weanlings and lactating females). Fertility and litter sizes were normal; the incidence of stillbirths was less than 5%; the growth and survival of the young at all stages were normal, and the pups were free of anomalies (Kennedy *et al.*, 1968). On the contrary, thresholds for nonspecific gonadal injury of 10 and 5 mg/kg/day in male and female rats, respectively, and of 4 and 1 mg/kg/day in mice have been reported (Zhorzholiani, 1971).

Captan revealed no sign of significant embryotoxicity when administered by stomach tube to New Zealand White rabbits on days 7–12 inclusive of pregnancy at the rate of 80 mg/kg/day (Fabro *et al.*, 1965).

In another study captan was found to be nonteratogenic in rats, hamsters, and two strains of rabbits. The rabbits were chosen because they were particularly sensitive to the teratogenic action of thalidomide. The dosages used were 50, 100, and 250 mg/kg/day on days 6–15 of gestation and 500, 1000, and 2000 mg/kg/day on days 8–10 of gestation in rats; 125, 250, 500 and 1000 mg/kg/day throughout pregnancy in hamsters; and 18.75, 37.5, and 75.0 mg/kg/day on days 6–16 or 18 of gestation in rabbits. The higher dosages were not without harmful effects. In rats a dosage of 2000 mg/kg/day caused weight loss in the dams and slight failure of growth in the fetuses (4.5 gm compared with 4.8 gm in the controls). Malformations of the young were not characteristic of thalidomide, and (except for dosages of 1000 mg/kg and greater in rats) their incidence was not greater than in the controls. The incidence of malformations in the young of rats receiving 1000 and 2000 mg/kg/day was 5.1 and 3.3%, respectively, and therefore not dosage related (Kennedy *et al.*, 1968).

A different result in rabbits was reported briefly from another laboratory (McLaughlin *et al.*, 1969). One malformed individual was recognized among the young of six does that had received 37.5 mg/kg/day; nine malformed individuals were found among the young of nine does that had received 75 mg/kg/day, but apparently all the young from mothers that had received 150 mg/kg/day were normal. Because the deformities were not typical of thalidomide, the response was not proportional to dosage, and the number of deformed rabbits was small, the results are difficult to interpret. Other reports of reduced viability, retarded sexual development, and disturbances in the estrous cycle in rats (Vashakidze *et al.*, 1973) may have been associated with impurities in formulations of unusual acute toxicity. In a test of "reproductive fitness," male mice were given captan by stomach tube for 5 days at rates of 50 and 100 mg/kg/day and then bred to untreated females. The resulting young were not treated but were bred twice to produce F_{2a} and F_{2b} pups. Considering all generations, there was no statistical difference between the controls and the 50 mg/kg/day series in the fertility index or the survival index. The F_1 females showed a statistically significant reduction of the viability index from 99 to 96%, but this index for F_1 males and the F_{2a} and F_{2b} females was indistinguishable from that of the corresponding control generation. The weaning index of the experimental mice was indistinguishable from that of the controls except for the F_{2a} females, whose survival of 99% was statistically *better* than that of the controls. In connection with the 150 mg/kg/day dosage, the average weight of the pups at weaning was statistically less for F_1 females (9.8 gm) than for the controls (10.0 gm), but the weights were indistinguishable for F_3 pups. The differences were greater in connection with a dosage of 100 mg/kg/day but were statistically insignificant for the fertility index and the weaning index. The viability index was significantly low in one of six comparisons (92 versus 98% for F_1 females and their controls). Only the survival index was changed substantially, the average for all generations of both sexes being 75.7%, compared with 85% for the controls (Collins, 1972c).

Change of route did not change the results; captan was nonteratogenic when given by the oral, subcutaneous, or respiratory routes (Courtney *et al.*, 1978).

Hamsters were more susceptible to the teratogenic effects of several compounds when given a single massive dose on day 7 or 8 of gestation than when given repeated doses, even though, strangely enough, the daily dose that was repeated was as large as or larger than the single dose. This anomalous result was explained only in part by higher maternal and fetal mortality caused by repeated administration. Captan was possibly teratogenic at an oral dosage of 300 mg/kg and certainly teratogenic at single dosages of 750 mg/kg or more (Robens, 1970).

Captan was not teratogenic in dogs. The bitches received dietary levels of 0, 30, or 60 ppm during gestation, giving a dosage of about 1.38 mg/kg/day at the highest level. After the pups were born, some mothers were continued on their original diet and some that had received captan were given control feed. Both the adults and the pups were normal clinically and in gross and histological morphology (Kennedy *et al.*, 1975b).

Captan was administered to pregnant rhesus monkeys at dosages of 10, 25, and 75 mg/kg/day and to stump-tailed macaques at dosages of 10 and 75 mg/kg/day during days 21–24 or 34 of gestation. The highest dosage was given from day 21 through 34. Thalidomide at a dosage of 5 or 10 mg/kg/day was administered for a slightly shorter period as a positive control. Captan produced no abortions, no anomalies in the young, and no injury of the mothers. Typical deformities and numerous abortions were produced by thalidomide in both kinds of subhuman primate (Vondruska *et al.*, 1971).

Factors Influencing Toxicity   As discussed elsewhere (Section 2.4.11.2), the effect of very severe protein deficiency increases the susceptibility of rats far more to captan than to any other pesticide investigated. The mechanism of this dramatic action is unknown. To be sure, reduced activity of liver microsomal enzymes has been proposed as a reason for the increased susceptibility of protein-deficient animals to foreign chemicals, but there is no critical evidence linking this explanation to the great difference in the response to different chemicals. Another possibility is that the striking effect of severe protein deficiency on poisoning by captan may reflect a specific deficiency of

cysteine and/or gluthathione. As discussed under Biochemical Effects, deficiency of these compounds is known to permit mutagenic action of captan. Fortunately, protein deficiency is not likely to be a practical problem in connection with the toxicity of captan because the difference was hardly measurable if protein intake was as much as 35% of normal; toxicity was increased about 25 times if protein intake was 13% of normal and increased 2100 times if protein intake was zero (Boyd and Krijnen, 1968; Krijnen and Boyd, 1970). Very similar results were reported by Urbanek-Karlowska, 1975).

Pathology   Repeated gavage with captan produced marked irritation and inflammatory reaction of the gastrointestinal tract to the point of ulceration. Many organs showed capillary congestion, and some showed venous thrombosis; some, notably the testis, showed degenerative changes. All of the pathology was much less marked in animals killed for study after 100 days of dosing than in those that died in 21 days or less while receiving the same dosages (Boyd and Carsky, 1971).

21.5.1.3   Toxicity to Humans

Experimental Exposure   Sensitivity to captan was demonstrated among volunteers following application of the compound to their backs (Jordan and King, 1977).

Therapeutic Use   Noting that captan was well tolerated by applicators, Simeray (1966) used it to treat 250 cases of tinea versicolor. The treatment was well tolerated by the patients, and the relapse rate was only 2% within less than 2 years and only 3.5% within 4 years. The dermatitis usually cleared in about 3 days. Whereas eight treatments probably were sufficient, 15 daily treatments were recommended. Captan was applied in the form of lanolin-Vaseline® or polyethylene glycol salves or as a water suspension. The last was the best tolerated; toxic effects (urticaria or eczema) were seen in 5, 50, and 0.6%, respectively, of the patients treated with the different formulations. Withdrawal of treatment was necessary in only one case. Captan was also successful in treating many other forms of fungal dermatitis, but the number of cases of any one kind was too small to permit clear evaluation.

Use Experience   Use experience usually has been good. Two cases involving skin reactions have been reported. In one case on 18-year-old gardener was sufficiently sensitive that he reacted to treated plants as well as to the formulation. Inhalation and skin test established that captan was the factor in the formulation to which the patient reacted. Recovery was prompt after exposure was stopped (Croy, 1973). In the other, a 73-year-old retired fruit grower exhibited persistent erythema, itching, and desquamation of the face and backs of hands. The condition was exacerbated when he was close to spraying operations using captan. He also suffered from attendant photodermatitis. Epicutaneous testing revealed reactions to both captan and thiram. Light testing confirmed the photosensitivity, which was considered to be caused by his antihypertensive medication with agents known to cause photodermatitis reactions (Dooms-Goossens *et al.*, 1986). The rarity of reactions under practical conditions stands in contrast to the report of a high rate of reactivity to 1% captan applied as a patch test among patients in a dermatitis clinic (Rudner, 1977).

A study of chromosomes in workers employed in a captan factory failed to reveal any damage (Durham and Williams, 1972).

Exposure of workers to captan has been reported in three field studies. The extent of potential dermal absorption was assessed in a group of 10 strawberry harvesters by measurement of the amount trapped on gauze pads and cotton gloves. The captan had been applied 4 days prior to the study. The average dermal exposure was found to be 39 mg/hr with a range of 13–51 mg/hr (Zweig *et al.*, 1983). Contact exposure was also evaluated in workers handling seed potatoes which had been dusted with captan. Estimates were made for potential dermal and inhalational exposure. The values for dermal exposure ranged from 0.33 mg/hr for observers to 15 mg/hr for persons who filled the dusting machine. Respiratory exposure was much less, ranging from 0.03 to 1.7 mg/hr for the same workers (Stevens and Davis, 1981). Dermal and inhalational exposure to captan for commercial apple growers using aeroblast sprayers was determined. The data indicated that the amount available for absorption by the inhalational route was minimal compared with that via the dermal route. The maximum amount available for absorption was calculated to be 2.2 mg/hr (McJilton *et al.*, 1983). The calculated total daily body doses for the strawberry harvesters and the two most exposed groups of potato workers were 4.5, 1.9 and 0.9 mg/kg/day. These values exceed the acceptable occupational intake of 0.7 mg/kg/day mentioned below. However, it must be emphasized that the extent of dermal absorption is not known and the above values must be considered as a maximum intake.

Dosage Response The threshold limit value of 5 mg/m^3 indicates that occupational intake at a rate of 0.7 mg/kg/day is considered safe.

Treatment of Poisoning If treatment were required it would have to be symptomatic.

21.5.2 CAPTAFOL

21.5.2.1 Identity, Properties, and Uses

Chemical Name 3*a*,4,7,7*a*-Tetrahydro-2-[(1,1,2,2-tetrachloroethyl)thio]-1*H*-isoindole-1,3(2*H*)-dione.

Structure See Fig. 21.1.

Synonyms Captafol is the common name approved by ANSI, BSI, and ISO. Difolatan is the name approved by JMAF. Trade names for the compound include Folci®, Sabsoir®, and Sulfenimede®. The CAS registry number is 2425-06-1.

Physical and Chemical Properties The empirical formula for captafol is $C_{10}H_9Cl_4NO_2S$ and it has a molecular weight of 249.09. Captafol is a white crystalline solid melting at 160–161°C. Its vapor pressure is negligible at room temperature. Captafol is practically insoluble in water and slightly soluble in most organic solvents. It is stable except under strongly alkaline conditions; it slowly decomposes at its melting point.

History, Formulations and Uses Captafol was introduced by the Chevron Chemical Company in 1961 under the trade name Difolatan®. Formulations of captafol include Ortho Difolatan 80W® wettable powder (800 gm active ingredients per kilogram) and Ortho Difolatan 4® flowable liquid suspension (4 lb active ingredients per U.S. gallon). Captafol is used for control of foliage and fruit diseases of tomatoes, potato blight, coffee berry disease, and tapping panel disease of *Hevea*. It also is used by the lumber and timber industries to reduce wood rot fungi in logs and wood products.

21.5.2.2 Toxicity to Experimental Animals

Basic Finding Captafol is a compound of low toxicity. The oral LD 50 in the rat varies from 2500 to 6200 mg/kg, depending on whether it is presented as an oil solution or aqueous suspension. The dermal LD 50 in rabbits is 15,400 mg/kg.

Rats that received captafol at dietary levels of 1500 and 5000 ppm did not grow normally, their livers were enlarged, and mortality was increased at the higher level. At autopsy, these rats showed vacuolization of liver cells and infiltration by mononuclear cells, whereas the kidneys showed many giant cells with large irregular nuclei and other changes of the proximal and distal tubules. At a dietary level of 500 ppm the liver was enlarged at 12 months in both sexes, and this was true of males fed 250 ppm; however, at the end of 2 years, no difference of liver weight was present and no histological changes were present. The incidence of tumors was not increased at any dosage.

Dogs that received captafol at 300 or 100 mg/kg/day suffered frequent vomiting and diarrhea during the first 4 weeks, and they were slightly anaemic and deficient in growth during a 2-year study. Dogs at dosages of 30 mg/kg/day or greater developed both absolute and relative increase of the weights of the liver and kidneys; however, their hematology and liver function tests were normal. A dosage of 10 mg/kg/day was a no-effect level (unpublished reports, cited by FAO/WHO, 1970).

Because simple enlargement of the liver can be adaptive in the rat and because of the results in the three-generation study mentioned below, 25 mg/kg/day may be taken as a nonharmful effect level in the rat.

Absorption, Distribution, Metabolism, and Excretion When rats, dogs and monkeys were fed [^{14}C]captafol, almost 80% was excreted within 36 hr, mainly in the urine and none via expired carbon dioxide. Most of the small amount in the feces was unmetabolized and probably unabsorbed. No unchanged captafol was detected in the blood, tissues, or urine. The major single metabolite, tetrahydrophthalimide, was detected in blood, feces, and urine, but most of the activity in the blood and urine was in the form of more soluble metabolites. No captafol epoxide was detectable (unpublished report, cited by FAO/WHO, 1970).

Effects on Organs and Tissues Captafol was given to male rats intraperitoneally at rates of 2.5, 5.0 and 10.0 mg/kg/day or orally at 50, 100 and 200 mg/kg/day for 5 days, and then the animals were bred for the following 10 weeks in a dominant lethal test. Neither fertility nor mean total implants were affected. Mean early deaths per pregnancy were consistently higher than those of the controls, regardless of route of administration. The percentage of litters with two or more early deaths per litter showed statistically significant increases after treatment at the higher dosages. An oral dosage of 50 mg/kg/day was considered a no-effect level (Collins, 1972b).

Male mice were given a single intraperitoneal injection of captafol (1.5 or 3.0 mg/kg) and a dominant lethal test was carried out. There was no increase in early embryonic death among conceptuses of females mated to treated males. A similar result was obtained in rats after the males were dosed orally for 14 days at rates of 125 or 250 mg/kg/day. Indicator microorganisms recovered from the peritoneal cavity of treated male rats showed no increase in reversion rate. Thus, captafol was not mutagenic at the dosages tested in any of these systems (Kennedy *et al.*, 1975a).

Effects on Reproduction In a three-generation study in rats, there was a slight reduction in the weight of pups at weaning when the dams had been fed captafol at a dietary level of 1000 ppm, and the difference was statistically significant in the F_{1a}, F_{1b}, F_{3a}, and F_{3b} animals but not in the F_{2a} and F_{2b} animals. There was no other abnormality at this dietary level and no abnormalities of any kind at lower dosage levels (Kennedy *et al.*, 1968).

When captafol was administered to two strains of rabbits at dosages ranging from 37.5 to 150 mg/kg/day from day 6 through 16 of gestation or to rats at dosages of 100 and 500 mg/kg/day from day 6 through 15, no evidence of teratogenicity was found (Kennedy *et al.*, 1968). Furthermore, captafol was not teratogenic when administered to rhesus monkeys at dosages of 6.25, 12.5 and 25.0 mg/kg/day during days 22–32 of gestation (Vondruska *et al.*, 1971) (see also Section 21.5).

21.5.2.3 Toxicity to Humans

Experimental Exposure Breakdown products may contribute to the skin irritation associated with captafol. Twenty-three fractions were separated from an ether extract of the thermal decomposition products. Six of the 23 materials produced irritation when patch-tested on volunteers. The most active compound was isolated as a yellowish, scaly crystalline solid melting at 109–110°C, but it was not identified (Arimatsu, 1970).

Use Experience Surveys in Kumamoto Prefecture in Japan revealed a high incidence of skin irritation among farmers using captafol in tangerine orchards. The number of cases and the incidence reported varied somewhat in different accounts, but the following are representative: 442 cases (31.4% of exposed persons) in 1966; 572 cases (40.5%) in 1967; 442 cases (31.1%) in 1968; and 332 cases (24.6%) in 1969. The eruption appeared in 1–3 days after exposure and usually disappeared within a week. The irritation usually took the form of an erythematous dermatitis of the eyelids with local edema; it often was phototoxic in type and varied from slight to severe (Takamatsu *et al.*, 1968; Arimatsu, 1970). Rashes caused by captafol have been reported from other localities (Takamatsu *et al.*, 1968; Matsushita *et al.*, 1979). Itching may be present, and the irritation usually is localized to the conjunctiva or to skin areas with direct contact (Imaizumi *et al.*, 1972; Kasai and Sugimoto, 1973; Itoh, 1978). Reaction may be severe and may include dermatitis, conjunctivitis, stomatitis, and painful bronchitis (Verhagen, 1974).

Many persons who complained of skin rash following exposure to captafol and who were selected for special study were found to have systemic as well as dermal disorders. Hypertension occurred especially in persons with marked edema. Other findings, which also usually paralleled the degree of dermatitis, included protein and urobilinogen in the urine, depression of liver function, anemia, and depression of cholinesterase activity (Watanabe, 1971).

The sudden appearance of wheezing and of vesiculation and edema of the face and hands of a welder was attributed to contact with bags of the material in the course of maintenance work for a company that distributed the compound. Subsequent exposures led to recurrences. Patch tests were positive (Groundwater, 1977).

Patch tests to captafol were also positive in two laboratory chemists who had previously worked with the chemical. In one case the chemist had not handled captafol for several years but had exhibited skin irritation toward the end of that period. In the second case there was no previous evidence of sensitivity but when contact resumed after an interval of several months the chemist developed a rash on the neck and cheeks (Brown, 1984).

Dosage Response Apparently, dermatitis caused by captafol always has been associated with substantial exposure, but it is unclear just how extensive the exposure of susceptible persons must be in order to cause the disorder. The rarity of difficulty in industrial situations indicates that the threshold limit value of 0.1 mg/m³ (implying occupational intake not exceeding 0.014 mg/kg/day) may be sufficiently low to prevent dermatitis as well as systemic illness.

Treatment of Poisoning Treatment is symptomatic.

21.6 PHENOLS AND PHENOLIC ESTERS

The toxicology of phenolic compounds is considered in Chapter 18. Among the phenols used as fungicides are most of the

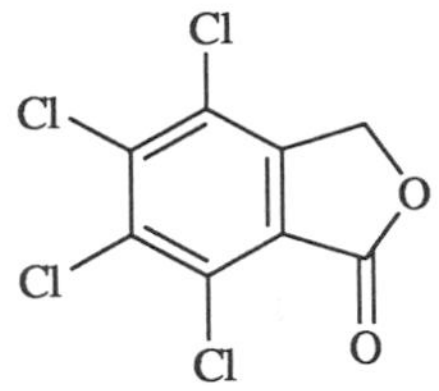

Figure 21.2 Tetrachlorophthalide

dinitrophenols, pentachlorophenol, trichlorophenol, chloroneb, dichlorophen, etoxyquin, o-phenylphenol, and 8-quininol.

21.7 QUINONES AND RELATED FUNGICIDES

A number of quinones and related compounds, many of them with chlorine or cyanide substitutions, are fungicides. In addition to tetrachlorophthalide, which is discussed below, examples include chloranil (ICPC), dichlone (BASI, ISO), and dithianon (BSI, JMAF, ISO). The oral LD 50 values of these four compounds in rats range from 1015 to 20,000, with a geometric mean of about 3200 mg/kg.

21.7.1 TETRACHLOROPHTHALIDE

21.7.1.1 Identity, Properties, and Uses

Chemical Name The chemical name for tetrachlorophthalide is 4,5,6,7-tetrachlorophthalide.

Structure See Fig. 21.2

Synonyms Tetrachlorophthalide is the name in general use. The compound also is known as phthalide and as Rabcide®. The CAS registry number is 27355-22-2.

Physical and Chemical Properties The empirical formula for tetrachlorophthalide is $C_8H_2Cl_4O_2$, and the molecular weight is 271.90. It is slightly soluble in water.

History, Formulations, and Uses Tetrachlorophthalide was first introduced in Japan in 1968. Its use is for control of rice blast.

21.7.1.2 Toxicity to Laboratory Animals

LD 50 values for 4,5,6,7-tetrachlorophthalide are >10,000 mg/kg orally in the rat and mouse, 9780 and >15,000 mg/kg intraperitoneally in male and female rats, respectively, and >10,000 mg/kg intraperitoneally in the mouse. The compound is not irritating to the skin and eyes (Ishida and Nambu, 1975). A dietary level of 50,000 ppm for 2 years inhibited growth of rats

and mice and altered the result of the SGPT test; numerous other laboratory tests including hematology remained normal. When killed, animals that had received this dietary level showed fatty degeneration and necrosis of liver cells as well as turbidity and swelling of renal tubular cells. A dietary level of 10,000 ppm produced minimal toxicity, and 2000 ppm was tolerated (Abe *et al.*, 1974; Ishida and Nambu, 1975).

The compound was not teratogenic in rodents (Ishida and Nambu, 1975). Identified metabolites included tetrachlorophthalic acid, trichlorophthalic acids, and an open ring form. There was no significant accumulation of the parent compound or its metabolites (Ishida and Nambu, 1975).

21.7.1.3 Toxicity to Humans

Two cases of keratitis and conjunctivitis associated with tetrachlorophthalide have been reported. Recovery was without sequelae (Fujita, 1975).

Treatment is symptomatic.

21.8 ANILINO AND NITROBENZENOID FUNGICIDES

The compounds discussed below (dicloran, quintozene, and 1-chloro-2,4-dinitrobenzene, shown in Fig. 21.3) are typical of the anilino and nitrobenzenoid compounds used as fungicides. Some of this general group have an amine or a nitro substitution on a benzene ring, and some have both substitutions on the same ring. Some, but not all, are chlorinated. A few have other substitutions, notably sulfur. Similar compounds find wide use in industry for completely different purposes. They are toxicologically similar in that they tend to produce methemoglobinemia as the initial and frequently the only injury. The rate at which methemoglobin appears in the blood and the ratio between moles of hemoglobin converted to methemoglobin per mole of compound depend on the compound. The molecular ratio for aniline is about 2.5, whereas that for *p*-dinitrobenzene lies somewhere between 55 and 198 (Bodansky, 1951). Species differ in their sensitivity, the cat being most sensitive. In the cat, a single subcutaneous dose of the common industrial chemical aniline at the rate of only 10 mg/kg is sufficient to convert over one-third of the hemoglobin to methemoglobin. Other effects, inherent toxicity, vapor pressure, and fat solubility are, of course, determined by the total molecule and may vary not only for different substitutions but even for different isomers of the same compound. Because of the general characteristic of the group, the ability of some of the fungicides to form methemoglobin has been investigated. Although they do form this inactive hemoglobin, they are not efficient at doing so. Apparently, methemoglobinemia has not been a problem in persons working with the fungicides.

The oral LD 50 values of the anilino and nitrobenzenoid fungicides in rats range from 425 to 8000 with an average near 3500 mg/kg.

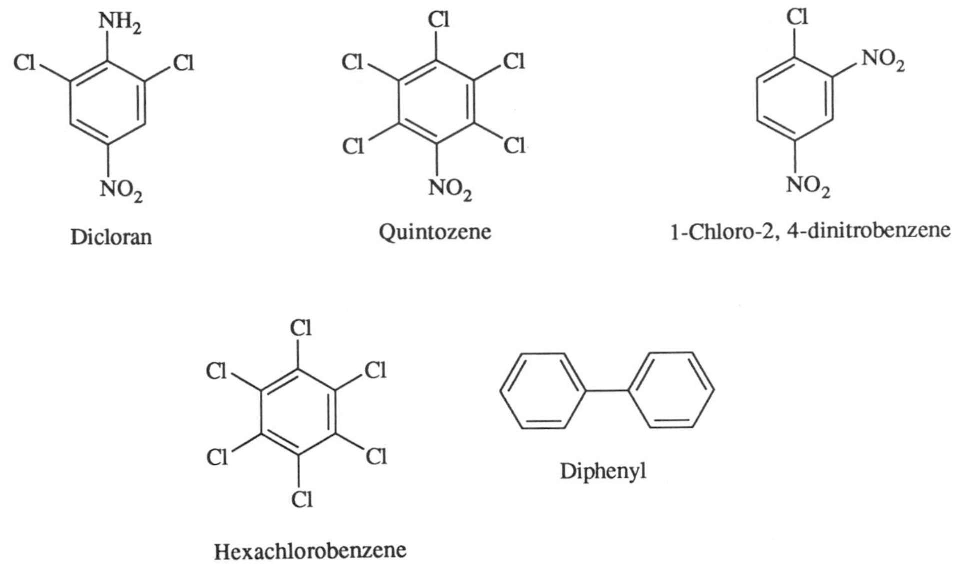

Dicloran   Quintozene   1-Chloro-2, 4-dinitrobenzene

Hexachlorobenzene   Diphenyl

Figure 21.3   Some anilino, nitrobenzoid, and other aromatic fungicides.

21.8.1 DICLORAN

21.8.1.1 Identity, Properties, and Uses

Chemical Name   Dicloran is the common name of 2,6-dichloro-4-nitroaniline.

Structure   See Fig. 21.3.

Synonyms   The common name dicloran (BSI, JMAF) is in general use. A possibility for confusion arises from the fact that Dichloran has been used as a trade name for a completely unrelated compound, and dichloran has been used extensively as a common name for the compound under discussion. The acronym DCNA also has been used. Trade names include Allisan®, Botran®, and Ditranil®. Code designations are AL-50 and U-2,069. The CAS registry number is 99-30-9.

Physical and Chemical Properties   Dicloran has the empirical formula $C_6H_4Cl_2N_2O_2$ and a molecular weight of 207.02. It is an odorless, yellow, crystalline solid with a melting point of 195°C and a vapor pressure of 1.2×10^{-6} mm Hg at 20°C. It is practically insoluble in water and moderately soluble in polar organic solvents. Dicloran is stable to hydrolysis and to oxidation and is compatible with other pesticides.

History, Formulations, and Uses   The Boots Company Limited first introduced dicloran in 1959 under the trade name Allisan®. The main formulations are wettable powders containing 500 or 750 gm of active ingredient per kilogram, dusts (40–80 gm of active ingredient per kilogram), and flowable powder (500 gm of active ingredient per kilogram). Dicloran is a protectant fungicide; it has little effect on spore germination but causes hyphal distortion. It is effective against a wide range of fungal pathogens.

21.8.1.2 Toxicity to Laboratory Animals

Basic Findings   Dicloran has a low toxicity in the rat, the oral LD 50 being 8000 mg/kg. Some mortality occurred following repeated intake at the rate of 1000 mg/kg/day, but 400 mg/kg/day was well tolerated during a 3-month study. Monkeys are much more susceptible to dicloran. Oral administration at a rate of 160 mg/kg/day was fatal to them in less than 3 months (Serrone et al., 1967).

Although a dietary level of 3000 ppm for 2 years did not increase mortality of rats, it did reduce their final body weight to about 75% of that of controls. A dietary level of 100 ppm did not affect weight significantly and produced no histological change (Johnston et al., 1968). Dietary levels as high as 1000 ppm (about 50 mg/kg/day) for 2 years were without harmful effect on rats (FAO/WHO, 1975).

Dogs fed dicloran at a rate of 192 mg/kg/day died after 49–53 days (Earl et al., 1971). The general health of others was not affected by 48 mg/kg/day for 2 years but this level caused corneal opacities, as discussed below (Bernstein et al., 1970). In another study, one dog receiving a dietary level of 3000 ppm (equivalent to about 21 mg/kg/day) died after 74 weeks but without weight loss (Johnston et al., 1968).

Absorption, Distribution, Metabolism, and Excretion   Dicloran is well absorbed.

Rats fed dicloran excrete a trace of the unchanged compound plus 3,5-dichloro-4-aminophenol and 2,6-dichloro-p-phenylenediamine. This apparently represents two routes of metabolism, as interconversion of the two metabolites could not be demonstrated. In rats given [14C]dicloran, 70% of the activity in the first 24-hr urine represented the phenol, 2.4% represented the other metabolite, and the remainder was in the form of unidentified materials (Maté et al., 1967; Gallo et al., 1976).

Rats given [14C]dicloran at rates of 5 or 10 mg/rat (about 20 or 40 mg/kg) excreted 70 and 77%, respectively, in the urine within 24 hr following intraperitoneal and oral intake; by 48 hr, the corresponding values were 80 and 90%. Only about 1% was excreted in the feces, and this was less than one-fifth of the amount excreted in the bile (Maté *et al.*, 1967). Similar results were found in another laboratory (unpublished results, cited by FAO/WHO, 1975).

Biochemical Effects   Either single or repeated oral doses of dicloran produced significant enlargement of the liver and induction of liver microsomal enzymes in the rat but not in the monkey (Serrone *et al.*, 1967). Some dogs on dietary levels of 3000 ppm (about 21 mg/kg/day) showed increases in serum transaminases (Johnston *et al.*, 1968).

The biochemical effects of dicloran were thoroughly studied by Bachmann *et al.* (1971) and Gallo *et al.* (1972, 1976). Briefly, doses given by stomach tube at rates of 10 to 1500 mg/kg stimulated liver microsomal enzymes of rats. At 1000 mg/kg this stimulation was maximal and about 3-fold. Dosages over 500 mg/kg decreased succinate oxidation without uncoupling of oxidative phosphorylation. This appears related to different degrees of injury to the mitochondria, which have been described and figured in detail. However, dicloran and 3,5-dichloro-4-aminophenol, one of its metabolites, but not 2,6-dichloro-*p*-phenylenediamine, another metabolite, uncoupled oxidative phosphorylation *in vitro* at concentrations not much greater than that at which 2,4-dinitrophenol is active.

Unlike 4-nitroaniline, dicloran does not cause methemoglobinemia (FAO/WHO, 1975).

Effects on Organs and Tissues   Dogs provided with outdoor runs developed corneal opacities within about 55 days when fed dicloran at the rate of 48 mg/kg/day and several weeks later at a dosage of 24 mg/kg/day. No abnormalities could be detected with a slit lamp at lower dosage levels, but a few lipid droplets could be seen in histological sections from animals fed 6 mg/kg/day. No effect under any condition was observed in dogs receiving 0.75 mg/kg/day. Whereas corneal opacities developed in dogs with access to outdoor runs, they did not develop in dogs receiving 48 mg/kg/day or more but kept in the dark or indoors where lighting by fluorescent bulbs provided up to 25 footcandles of illumination or in others with access to outdoor runs but with their eyelids sutured shut. Opacities did not occur in dogs kept in the dark during treatment, even though they were put in the light as soon as dosing was stopped. Pretreatment of animals for 55 days in the dark did not hasten the onset of opacities when they were placed in the light and dosing was continued. The eye damage was dosage-dependent. The lesion remained unchanged for as much as 1 year after administration of dicloran stopped.

Gross examination of affected eyes showed an oval, hazy area corresponding to the intrapalpebral fissure, that is, the part that had been exposed to light. Diffuse stippling of the entire cornea could be demonstrated by special equipment. Opacity of the lens began as an abnormal prominence of the normal Y-suture just under the surface. Then the fibers vertical to this

suture became more visible, resulting in a feathery appearance. Finally, the central, anterior, subcapsular area became hazy and eventually plaque-like. No further progression occurred in spite of continued dosing. Histological examination of damaged corneas revealed small droplets of an unidentified substance associated with the superficial corneal stromal cell nuclei. (An orange discoloration of the urine also occurred.) These droplets tended to coalesce toward the apex of the cornea, producing the oval opacity seen macroscopically. Edema and inflammation were lacking. The corneal epithelium was uninvolved. The normal condition of the epithelium was confirmed by electron microscopy. This examination revealed that the lipid droplets were lamellar vacuolated inclusion bodies within large histiocytes. There was some irregularity of the collagen lamellae in the anterior portion of the stroma. Daily direct application of a dicloran dust or of 5% solution to the eyes of dogs for 3 months had no effect on the cornea or the conjunctiva. However, central corneal lesions were produced within several weeks by placing 20–30 mg of dicloran powder every day into the inferior cul-de-sac of the eye (Bernstein *et al.*, 1970; Earl *et al.*, 1971).

At the higher dosage levels, some dogs showed Heinz bodies in their erythrocytes and an increased proportion of reticulocytes.

Pigs failed to develop eye lesions or any clinical evidence of toxicity when dicloran was administered at a rate of 48 mg/kg/day for 267 days or 192 mg/kg/day for 62 days. Some of these animals did show the blood changes seen in dogs (Earl *et al.*, 1971).

Dicloran was not tumorigenic when fed to two strains of mice at the highest tolerated rate (Innes *et al.*, 1969) or when fed to rats for 2 years at dietary levels as great as 3000 ppm (Johnston *et al.*, 1968).

Effects on Reproduction   A three-generation study of reproduction in rats at a dietary level of 100 ppm (about 5 mg/kg/day in most adults but higher in weanlings and in lactating dams) revealed no adverse effect on the number of pups per litter, the number of litters per group, stillbirth rates, mean weight at birth and weaning, and survival of pups after weaning (Johnston *et al.*, 1968).

Dicloran fed to rabbits at dietary levels of 100 and 1000 ppm from day 8 to 16 of gestation was not teratogenic (FAO/WHO, 1975).

Pathology   Structural changes have been observed in both the liver and kidney of rats and monkeys by both light and electron microscopy. Centrilobular fatty infiltration of the liver was seen in monkey liver. Swelling of mitochondria, with distortion of the cristae, was observed in electron micrographs of the liver and kidney (Serrone *et al.*, 1967). Liver changes also occur in dogs on high dosage levels (Johnston *et al.*, 1968).

21.8.1.3 Toxicity to Humans

Experimental Exposure   In a double-blind study, 20 men received dicloran at a rate of 10 mg/man/day for 90 days, and 10 others served as controls. This dosage of about 0.14 mg/kg/day produced no clinical effect and no detectable effect on hemotology, liver function, or kidney function measured periodically throughout the test (unpublished results, cited by FAO/WHO, 1975).

Within 7 days after oral administration of [^{14}C]dicloran to three men, 75% of the dose was accounted for in the urine and 32% in the feces. During the first 36 hr, the apparent half-life was 9.26 hr, and 73% of the urinary excretion occurred during this time. Excretion then continued at an apparent half-life of 27.4 hr (Eberts, 1965).

Use Experience Study of occupationally exposed men revealed no evidence of ocular opacities such as have been produced in dogs, and no other injury was detected (FAO/WHO, 1975).

Laboratory Findings Using electron-capture gas chromatography, a material reported as dicloran was found in the blood and urine of a pilot who used 6% dicloran dust and of four formulators engaged in manufacturing this dust from 75% wettable powder. There was a general correspondence between exposure and analytical results. The two formulators with direct exposure had higher levels than the two with indirect exposure. However, both blood and urinary levels persisted for several days so that they did not reflect daily exposure precisely. Whereas urinary levels tended to decrease during a weekend, blood levels remained stable. The highest blood level measured was 0.0184 ppm, and the highest urinary level was 0.0473 ppm. There was no evidence of toxicity (Edmundson *et al.*, 1967). Although the infrared spectrogram of the material extracted from blood and urine was considered identical to that of dicloran, no comparison with metabolites was made. Thus the real identity of the extracted material remains uncertain, although it was clearly related to dicloran.

Treatment of Poisoning If treatment were required, it would have to be symptomatic.

21.8.2 QUINTOZENE

21.8.2.1 Identity, Properties, and Uses

Chemical Name Quintozene is the common name for pentachloronitrobenzene.

Structure See Fig. 21.3.

Synonyms The common name quintozene (BSI, ISO) is in general use, but the compound also is known as quintozène (France), terrachlor (Turkey), PKhNB (USSR), and PCNB (JMAF), and the chemical name often is used as a common name. Trade names include Avicol®, Botrilex®, Brassicol®, Folosan®, Terraclor®, Tilcarex®, and Tritisan®. The CAS registry number is 82-68-8.

Physical and Chemical Properties The empirical formula for quintozene is $C_6Cl_5NO_2$ and it has a molecular weight of 295.36. Quintozene forms colorless needles from alcohol and platelets from carbon disulfide. The boiling point is 328°C, the melting point is 146°C, density is 1.718, and vapor pressure is 133×10^{-4} mm Hg at 25°C. Quintozene is soluble in benzenes, carbon disulfide, and chloroform and soluble to about 2% in ethanol at 25°C. It is practically insoluble in water. Quintozene has a high stability in soil and is compatible with all pesticides at pH 7 or less.

History, Formulations, and Uses Quintozene was introduced in the late 1930s by I. G. Farbenindustrie AG. It is a fungicide used for seed and soil treatment.

21.8.2.2 Toxicity to Laboratory Animals

Basic Findings The oral LD 50 values for quintozene in rats are 1710 and 1650 mg/kg in males and females, respectively. The corresponding value for the rabbit is about 800 mg/kg. In the dog, no deaths were produced by the highest feasible dosage (2500 mg/kg) (Finnegan *et al.*, 1958).

No rabbits were killed by a single dermal dosage of 4000 mg/kg, the highest level tested. Neither skin irritation nor signs of intoxication were observed (Borzelleca *et al.*, 1971).

A dietary level of 5000 ppm reduced growth and survival of both sexes of rats within 3 months, and growth was suppressed in males at 2500 ppm. The relative weight of the liver was increased in both sexes at 635 ppm and higher and at 63.5 ppm in males. When rats were fed quintozene for 2 years, weight gain was reduced in females at dietary levels as low as 100 ppm, but this depression was little, if any, greater at 2500 ppm and was not observed in males (Finnegan *et al.*, 1958). In dogs fed quintozene for 1 year, there was no adverse effect on growth or survival at the highest dietary level tested (1000 ppm or about 20 mg/kg/day). Some liver cells of dogs receiving only 25 ppm showed enlargement and pale-staining cytoplasm, but these effects did not increase with dosage and their significance is unknown (Finnegan *et al.*, 1958).

A moderate degree of cholestatic hepatosis with secondary bile nephrosis was found in dogs fed quintozene at a dietary level of 1080 ppm and to a minimal degree in those fed 180 ppm. The lesion was reversible. A dietary level of 30 ppm (about 0.6 mg/kg/day) was the highest level tested that produced no effect (Borzelleca *et al.*, 1971).

Absorption, Distribution, Metabolism, and Excretion Quintozene was not stored in the tissues of rats fed as much as 500 ppm, dogs fed as much as 1080 ppm, or a cow fed as much as 1000 ppm. Pentachloroaniline and methyl pentachlorophenyl sulfide, metabolites of quintozene, were found in the tissues of all three species. In addition, hexachlorobenzene and pentachlorobenzene, contaminants of technical quintozene, were found. The metabolism of quintozene itself is rapid; that of its contaminants is slow (Kuchar *et al.*, 1969; Borzelleca *et al.*,

1971). Quintozene is either undetectable in the rat fetus (Villeneuve and Khera, 1975) or present in low concentration (<0.2 ppm) soon after a large dose (Courtney *et al.*, 1976).

There is general agreement that pentachloroaniline is a metabolite of quintozene (Betts *et al.*, 1955; Kuchar *et al.*, 1969). In addition, methyl pentachlorophenyl sulfide has been isolated and identified by mass spectrometry by Kuchar *et al.* (1969), and N-acetyl-S-pentachlorophenylcysteine has been reported as a metabolite by Betts *et al.* (1955).

When [^{14}C]quintozene was administered to rats by mouth, 89.8% of the activity was recovered in the feces and a small proportion in the urine; residues were not detected in the tissues (Korte *et al.*, 1978). Only slightly lower elimination in the feces has been reported by others (Betts *et al.*, 1955). Whereas fecal excretion has been viewed as unabsorbed material, the importance of enterohepatic circulation in the metabolism of quintozene is not yet clear.

In the monkey, quintozene was absorbed very rapidly from the gastrointestinal tract and transported to the liver mainly by the hepatic portal vein. It was rapidly metabolized and excreted in the bile. High concentrations of ^{14}C were found in the gallbladder, cecal wall, mesenteric fat, and thymus of monkeys that had received labelled compound orally. As in the rat, the main metabolite was pentachloroaniline; other important metabolites were pentachlorophenol, pentachlorobenzene, pentachlorothioanisole, and bis-methyl-tetrachlorobenzene (Koegel *et al.*, 1978, 1979b). Excretion was slow, being only 50% complete in 4 days. Following daily feeding, storage equilibrium was reached in 30–40 days (Koegel *et al.*, 1979a).

Effects on Organs and Tissues Oral administration of quintozene to cats at the rate of 1600 mg/kg caused some formation of methemoglobin that was maximal at 24 hr (10.99%) and only slightly decreased at 48 hr. The occurrence of Heinz bodies in erythrocytes was increased 10-fold. Intravenous administration of methylene blue at a rate of 2 mg/kg caused a sharp drop in the concentration of methemoglobin within 1 hr (Schumann and Borzelleca, 1978).

Quintozene produced papillomas of the skin of mice to which it was applied twice a week for 12 weeks followed by croton oil for 20 weeks (Searle, 1966). The incidence of liver tumors was increased in mice that received a maximal tolerated dosage of quintozene [464 mg/kg/day by gavage from day 7 to 28 of age and 1206 ppm (about 150 mg/kg/day) until sacrifice at 78 weeks] (Innes *et al.*, 1969) or under slightly different conditions (Haseman and Hoel, 1979).

The observed mutagenicity of quintozene in *Escherichia coli* is influenced by excision repair (Clarke, 1971). On the contrary, no significant increase in mutation rates was observed following subcutaneous injection of the compound into mice (Buselmaier *et al.*, 1973) and tests for dominant lethal effect in mice were negative (Jorgenson *et al.*, 1976).

Effects on Reproduction In a three-generation reproduction study, quintozene produced no adverse effect when administered to rats at dietary levels as high as 500 ppm (about 25 mg/kg/day for most adults but higher for weanlings and lactating females) (Borzelleca *et al.*, 1971).

No effect on reproduction was observed in rats that received quintozene orally on days 6–15 of gestation at rates of 8, 20, 50, and 125 mg/kg/day. Parameters included the number and position of implantations, incidence of dead or resorbed fetuses, viable litter size, fetal sex ratios, birth weights, and the presence of visceral and skeletal malformations in fetuses removed on day 20 of gestation (Jordan *et al.*, 1975). Similar negative results were found in rats by other investigators even at 200 mg/kg (Khera and Villeneuve, 1975). When mice received the compound from day 7 to 11 of gestation at the much higher oral rate of 500 mg/kg/day, unilateral agenesis of the kidney occurred about twice as often in the fetuses of treated dams of one strain as in those of controls, and cleft palate was increased in two strains. However, the sample of quintozene contained 11% hexachlorobenzene, which tended to produce the same effect when administered alone. Even the contaminated quintozene was not teratogenic in rats. Purified quintozene (<20 ppm hexachlorobenzene) did not produce kidney malformations but did produce a few cleft palates. It was concluded that the teratogenic activity of contaminated quintozene probably was due to hexachlorobenzene. Tetrachloronitrobenzene, another contaminant, and pentachloroaniline, a metabolite, were not teratogenic in rats or mice (Courtney *et al.*, 1976).

Pathology No hematological changes were seen in rats fed high dietary levels of quintozene, and histological change was limited to fine vacuolization of liver cell cytoplasm at 5000 ppm. Changes in the dog also were confined to the liver (Finnegan *et al.*, 1958).

21.8.2.3 Toxicity to Humans

Experimental Exposure When quintozene 75% wettable powder was held beneath an airtight patch on the right forearm of 50 volunteers for 48 hr, there was no sign or symptom of irritation in any subject. When the same test was repeated 2 weeks later on the left arm of the same subjects, 4 of the 50 showed positive reactions when the patch was removed, and 9 others developed delayed reactions within 8 hr to several days. The immediate and delayed reactions included erythema and itching and, in some subjects, edema and the formation of small vesicles. The reactions reached a peak in a few days and then subsided gradually. Scaling of the skin accompanied subsidence (Finnegan *et al.*, 1958).

Use Experience Although the severe test in volunteers indicated that sensitization might occur, in practice it apparently has not been reported.

Splashing of quintozene into the eyes led to a case of conjunctivitis with corneal injury. Recovery was somewhat slower than with other irritants except paraquat but was eventually complete and without sequelae (Fujita, 1975).

Treatment of Poisoning   If treatment were needed, it would have to be symptomatic.

21.8.3 1-CHLORODINITROBENZENE

21.8.3.1 Identity, Properties, and Uses

Chemical Name   1-Chlorodinitrobenzene is 1-chloro-2,4-dinitrobenzene.

Structure   See Fig. 21.3.

Synonyms   1-Chlorodinitrobenzene is the name in common use for this compound. Other names in use are dinitrochlorobenzol and DNCB. The CAS registry number is 97-00-7.

Physical and Chemical Properties   1-Chlorodinitrobenzene has the empirical formula $C_6H_3ClN_2O_4$ and a molecular weight of 202.56. It forms yellow crystals with a density of about 1.7, a melting point of 52–54°C, and a boiling point of 315°C. It is soluble in hot alcohol, ether, benzene, and CS_2; slightly soluble in cold alcohol; and practically insoluble in water.

History, Formulations, and Uses   1-Chlorodinitrobenzene is used for slime control and as a reagent for the detection and determination of nicotinic acid, nicotinamide, and other compounds.

21.8.3.2 Toxicity to Laboratory Animals

According to Smyth *et al.* (1962), the oral LD 50 of chlorodinitrobenzene in rats is 1070 mg/kg, but the dermal LD 50 in rabbits is only 130 mg/kg. Others have found the compound somewhat more toxic (LD 50 values in rats of 640 and 280 mg/kg by oral and intraperitoneal routes, respectively) (Sziza and Magos, 1959), but the difference may have been due to impurities in the more toxic preparation.

The compound is irritating to the skin of rabbits and highly irritating to their eyes.

21.8.3.3 Toxicity to Humans

Dermatitis caused by 1-chloro-2,4-dinitrobenzene has been observed in workers who used the compound to control algae and other organisms in the coolant water of air-conditioning systems. The eruption caused by this compound is characterized by erythema, vesicles, and itching and thus resembles the effect of poison ivy. The reaction probably is allergic in all instances. In one case, the characteristic changes appeared 2 weeks after the fungicide was splashed on the skin; however, when the same man was reexposed 20 days later, blistering and weeping developed within 24 hr. In other cases, the first recognized eruption appeared within 2–3 hr after exposure. Sensitized persons reacted to patch tests with dilutions as low as 1 : 1,000,000 (Adams *et al.*, 1971).

The isomers of chlorodinitrobenzene are used in the manufacture of dyes, in other dye intermediates, and in the explosive roburite. The commercial product is usually a mixture of the six possible isomers. The material is of little importance as a systemic poison but is very active as a sensitizer, causing contact dermatitis in 60–80% of those who have even the slightest contact with it. The condition may vary from a few itching vesicles to a generalized exfoliative dermatitis (Hamblin, 1963).

Treatment is symptomatic.

21.9 OTHER AROMATIC HYDROCARBONS

In addition to phenolic, anilino, and nitrobenzenoid compounds and in addition to diphenyl and hexachlorobenzene, which are discussed below, a number of substituted or unsubstituted, mononuclear or polynuclear aromatic compounds are fungicidal. Many are substituted with chlorine or cyanate groups, or both, on the same ring. However, some unsubstituted aromatic compounds, especially biphenyl, are active. Some aromatic acids, notably benzoic and salicylic acids and their esters, are fungicides.

All are compounds of low acute toxicity. Hexachlorobenzene is highly cumulative in its effects and is more active than any other compound now known in causing porphyria. It seems unlikely that less chlorinated or completely unsubstituted aromatic hydrocarbon fungicides would be so cumulative. Just what feature of hexachlorobenzene makes it so porphyrigenic is unknown, and therefore it is uncertain what effect a similar compound such as chlorthalonil (ANSI, BSI, ISO) would have if eaten repeatedly.

21.9.1 HEXACHLOROBENZENE

21.9.1.1 Identity, Properties, and Uses

Chemical Name   Hexachlorobenzene.

Structure   See Fig. 21.3.

Synonyms   The compound should not be confused with benzene hexachloride (see γ-hexachlorocyclohexane, lindane). Hexachlorobenzene was deemed by BSI and ISO not to need a common name. Some other names for this compound are perchlorobenzene, Julin's carbon chloride, and HCB. Trade names include Anti-Carie®, Bent-cure®, and Bent-no-more®. The CAS registry number is 118-74-1.

Physical and Chemical Properties   The empirical formula for hexachlorobenzene is C_6Cl_6, and the molecular weight is 284.80. It forms colorless crystals with a melting point of 226°C and a vapor pressure of 1089×10^{-5} mm Hg at 20°C. It is soluble in hot benzene but practically insoluble in water and in cold ethanol.

History, Formulations, and Uses   Hexachlorobenzene was introduced by H. Yersin *et al.* in 1945 for seed treatment, especially for control of bunt of wheat. It is usually formulated as a dust with or without other seed protectants. There are several sources of hexachlorobenzene in the environment other than its direct use as a fungicide. It may be a contaminant of some other useful compounds, including the fungicides quintozene (BSI, ISO) and tecnazine (BSI, ISO) and the herbicide chlorthal-dimethyl (BSI, ISO). Hexachlorobenzene also is a waste formed in the synthesis of some chlorinated solvents, including perchlorethylene. Storage of hexachlorobenzene in people has been traced to ordinary application of chlorthal-dimethyl and to exposure to industrial waste, as well as to the illegal use of hexachlorobenzene-treated seed as feed for animals that subsequently contribute to human food.

21.9.1.2 Toxicity to Laboratory Animals

Basic Findings   A single dose of hexachlorobenzene has a low toxicity, but even rather small repeated doses are toxic.

It was shown in an early study of chlorobenzenes that rats tolerate a single subcutaneous dose as great as 500 mg/kg without detectable injury, including liver injury (Cameron *et al.,* 1937). Oral LD 50 values of 3500, 4000, 2600, and 1700 mg/kg in the rat, mouse, rabbit, and cat, respectively, were reported by Savitakii (1964).

The most prominent effects in rodents involve the nervous system. The animals become lethargic but hyperresponsive, and develop weakness or even paralysis (DeMatteis *et al.,* 1961; Haeger-Aronsen, 1964; Ockner and Schmid, 1961). Clonic contractions and convulsions occasionally are seen, the latter especially in infant rats suckled by mothers fed the compound, regardless of whether the young were exposed during the fetal period (DeMatteis *et al.,* 1961).

In addition to effects on the nervous system, there may be loss of weight, oliguria, and constipation.

Ninety-five percent of female rats and 30% of males died within 4 months when fed hexachlorobenzene at a dietary level of 1000 ppm; the first death occurred 30 days after feeding started. Mortality was lower at 500 ppm, and all rats survived 100 ppm (about 5 mg/kg/day). Rats receiving 500 or 1000 ppm showed tremor, hyperexcitability, and skin eruptions; those receiving 100 ppm remained clinically well, but the females showed decreased hemoglobin and hematocrit values and the males had increased liver weights. At the higher levels of intake, there were increases in both the absolute and relative weights of the liver, spleen, kidneys, and lungs (Kimbrough and Linder, 1974). In another study, rats survived an oral dosage of 50 mg/kg every other day for 53 weeks without differing from the controls in body weight, but the liver, spleen, kidney, and adrenal showed relative increases in weight. At the end of a 38-week period during which no hexachlorobenzene was administered, the organs of the treated animals were normal in weight, but the porphyrin content of the liver had increased, whereas that of the urine had decreased almost to normal (Koss *et al.,* 1978).

Rabbits developed porphyria and later died when fed a dietary level of 5000 ppm (DeMatteis *et al.,* 1961).

Similar results were observed in pigs. Those that received 50 mg/kg/day developed signs of porphyria and died before a 90-day toxicity test was complete. Illness was not observed at 5 mg/kg/day or lower dosages, but excretions of coproporphyrin and induction of liver microsomal enzymes were found even at 0.5 mg/kg/day. The fungicide was detectable in blood and tissues at a dosage of 0.5 mg/kg/day. It was also detectable in blood and tissues at a dosage of 0.05 mg/kg/day, which was otherwise a no-effect level (Den Tonkelaar *et al.,* 1978). Similar results were reported by Hansen *et al.* (1977).

Monkeys were somewhat less susceptible, surviving gastric intubation at a rate of 128 mg/kg/day for 60 days. However, dosages as low as 8 mg/kg/day produced loss of appetite and weight loss, and, near the end of the feeding period, monkeys that had received 64 or 128 mg/kg/day showed lethargy, muscular weakness, and/or severe tremors. Clinical laboratory findings and later pathology indicated liver and kidney damage (Knauf and Hobson, 1979). A dosage of 0.11 mg/animal/day produced storage in adult monkeys but did not produce any detectable harmful effect (Rozman *et al.,* 1978).

When three monkeys with nursing young were given hexachlorobenzene by gavage at a rate of 64 mg/kg/day for 22, 38, and 60 days, the concentration of the compound in the milk was high, and two of the infants died. They showed only mild degenerative changes including vacuolation of the proximal tubules of the kidney and centrilobular hypertrophy and fatty change of the liver. The concentration of the compound was higher in the serum of the young than in that of their mothers (Iatropoulos *et al.,* 1978).

Although experiments suitable for calculating an exact chronicity index for hexachlorobenzene have not been done, it is evident that this index is high (approximately 70).

A careful study of toxicity, enzyme induction, and porphyria was carried out using technical hexachlorobenzene and the purest sample available. The technical material contained 200 ppm decachlorobiphenyl and 4 ppm octachlorodibenzofuran but undetectable amounts (<0.5 ppm) of other chlorinated dibenzofurans or dibenzo-*p*-dioxins. The pure sample contained 0.5 ppm decachlorobiphenyl but no other detectable contaminants. At a dietary level of 100 ppm, rats usually showed greater hypertrophy and proliferation of the endothelial cells of the smaller pulmonary blood vessels if fed technical rather than pure hexachlorobenzene. The effect was not seen at 30 ppm, and there was no difference in the degree of effect among rats receiving technical or pure compound at a dietary level of 300 ppm. The porphyria, cutaneous lesions, hyperexcitability, changes in liver enzymes, and morphological changes in the liver were identical at the same dietary level, regardless of whether the technical or pure material was fed. Thus the effects of the technical product were due to the major constituent and not to contaminants (Goldstein *et al.,* 1978). However, it is not certain that this conclusion applies to all lots of hexachlorobenzene. There is ample evidence that samples vary considerably but not enough information to define the full range of variation. In a study of three other samples of unstated origin, pentachlorobenzene was the major contaminant in each instance, the concentrations varying from 200 to 81,000 ppm. All three samples contained decachlorobiphenyl, two contained octachlorobiphenyl, and one contained nonachlorobiphenyl. A number of other contaminants were identified by mass spectrometry. Of particular interest were octachlorodibenzofuran in all samples (0.35–58.3 ppm) and octachlorodibenzo-*p*-dioxin in two samples (0.05–211.9 ppm) (Villanueva *et al.*, 1974).

Absorption, Distribution, Metabolism, and Excretion
When [^{14}C]hexachlorobenzene was administered orally to rats, absorption was about 80% from an oil solution but only 6% from an aqueous suspension (Koss and Koransky, 1975). In both rats and monkeys absorption of the compound is mainly by way of the lymph (Rozman *et al.*, 1979a).

Sheep fed hexachlorobenzene stored the compound in their fat at equilibrium concentrations about 7–9 times greater than those in their feed. Concentrations in the blood corresponded to those in the fat but were about 1000 times less. The half-life varied from 10 to 18 weeks depending on dosage. Sheep with a maximal concentration of 75 ppm in their fat following a dietary level of 10 ppm remained entirely well, but growth was reduced in those with a maximal tissue level of 650 ppm following a dietary level of 100 ppm (Avrahami and Steele, 1972a).

Results in chickens were similar to those in sheep with three exceptions: a dietary level of 100 ppm had no apparent effect on the health of chickens, the hatchability of eggs, or the health of chicks produced from them; storage in chicken fat was 20–31 times higher than the dietary level (probably reflecting the high feed consumption of chickens); and storage, although greater at greater dietary levels, was less efficient at higher levels (indicating relatively more effective metabolism at higher dosage levels). Equilibrium of storage was reached after 1–2 months of feeding (Avrahami and Steele, 1972b,c).

Storage equilibrium in the rat is reached before 104 days (Kuiper-Goodman *et al.*, 1975, 1977) or about 63 days (Koss *et al.*, 1978).

Although hexachlorobenzene is transmitted to the fetus via the placenta, almost all of the compound present in young rats just before weaning is acquired through the milk, as demonstrated by cross-fostering experiments (Mendoza *et al.*, 1977, 1978).

There is a marked species difference in the distribution of hexachlorobenzene to red cells and plasma; *in vivo,* the concentration of the radioactive compound is about six times greater in the whole blood than in the plasma of rats but about equal in blood and plasma of monkeys. *In vitro,* the compound is bound to the red cells of rats, mice, and rabbits, but there is little or no binding to the cells of human, monkey, pig, cow, horse, donkey, sheep, goat, dog, guinea pig, hamster, turkey, or chicken. In the rat, the binding is rapid and firm; the compound can be removed by toluene extraction but not by dialysis or by repeated washing with saline (Yang, 1975).

Susceptibility to poisoning by hexachlorobenzene shows little relation to its storage. Female rats are more susceptible but store only as much as males. Guinea pigs are more susceptible

than rats but store less (Villeneuve and Newsome, 1975). In animals of the same species, on the contrary, symptomatology may be more directly related to tissue levels than to dosage *per se.* Thus, Knauf and Hobson (1979) found that in a study lasting only 60 days, a very thin monkey receiving 64 mg/kg/day developed more severe neurological symptoms and higher tissue levels than a fat monkey receiving 128 mg/kg/day. The concentrations of hexachlorobenzene in the fat and brain of the thin monkey were 540 and 108 ppm, respectively; the corresponding values in the fat monkey were 215 and 19 ppm.

In rats, hexachlorobenzene is metabolized to pentachlorophenol (Lui and Sweeney, 1975; Mehendale *et al.*, 1975; Rozman *et al.*, 1975; Engst *et al.*, 1976), pentachlorobenzene, tetrachlorobenzene, and some unidentified compounds (Mehendale *et al.*, 1975; Rozman *et al.*, 1975; Engst *et al.*, 1976). More recently, some tetrachlorophenol and traces of trichlorophenol were detected, partly in the form of glucuronides (Engst *et al.*, 1976; Renner and Schuster, 1977). A number of sulfur-containing metabolites have been identified, including tetra- and pentachlorobenzenethiol, methylthiopentachlorobenzene, 1,4-bis(methylthio)-2,3,4,6-tetrachlorobenzene, methylthiotetrachlorobenzenethiol, tetrachlorobenzenedithiol (Jansson and Bergman, 1978), and *N*-acetyl-*S*-(pentachlorophenyl)-cysteine (Renner and Schuster, 1978a,b). Pentachlorothiophenol and pentachlorothioanisole have been isolated from the liver but not the excreta of animals treated with hexachlorobenzene, and the further metabolism has been investigated (Koss *et al.*, 1979). The metabolism of pentachlorobenzene has been studied in the monkey (Rozman *et al.*, 1979b).

The major metabolites of hexachlorobenzene in monkeys are the same as the major metabolites in rats. When these animals received a small, daily dosage for 11 or more months, 59% of the daily intake could be accounted for by excretion during the last 10 days of the experiment, but it was uncertain whether a steady rate had been achieved (Rozman *et al.*, 1977).

Within 7 days after a single dose of [^{14}C]hexachlorobenzene, 16% was excreted in the feces, less than 1% in the urine, and 70% was measured in the tissues of male rats (Mehendale *et al.*, 1975). Very similar proportions (17.1 and 1.8%) were recovered in the feces and urine of a monkey (Yang and Pittman, 1975). In other experiments, recoveries in feces and urine during 40 days were 28.9–35.0% and 30.3–36.1%, respectively, in rats and 9.8–28% and 12.4–29.9%, respectively, in monkeys (Rozman *et al.*, 1975). Presumably, the higher proportion of excretion was explained by the longer period of collection of samples. Whether this same factor and/or the small dosage (0.4–0.6 mg/kg in rats and 0.5 mg/kg in monkeys) accounted for the relatively higher proportion recovered in the urine is not clear.

Much of the unchanged compound as well as metabolites recovered from the feces represent true excretion. Within 2 weeks, after a single intraperitoneal dose to rats at the rate of 4 mg/kg, 34% of the radioactivity was recovered in the feces and only 5% in the urine (Koss and Koransky, 1975).

The half-life of hexachlorobenzene following a single small

dose was 3–4 months in rats and 2.5–3 years in Rhesus monkeys (Rozman *et al.*, 1975). The extreme tenacity of storage in monkeys has been emphasized by Yang *et al.* (1978).

During the phase of slow excretion after dosage had been stopped, the half-life for loss of hexachlorobenzene from the tissues of rats was 4–5 months (Koss *et al.*, 1978).

Biochemical Effects: Porphyria   General background information on human porphyrias (including several hereditary conditions and the more common porphyria cutanea tarda, which is not known to be hereditary) has been reviewed (see Section 2.4.17.2). Hexachlorobenzene has produced porphyria in all species studied (Schmid, 1960; Kantemir *et al.*, 1960; Ockner and Schmid, 1961; DeMatteis *et al.*, 1961; Gajdos and Gajdos-Török, 1961a,b,c; Haeger-Aronsen, 1964). The details of the disorder differ greatly from one species to another. The spectrum of porphyrins excreted by rabbits is most like that in humans (DeMatteis *et al.*, 1961; Haeger-Aronsen, 1964).

In spite of some differences in the proportion of isomers (San Martin de Viale *et al.*, 1970), porphyria produced in experimental animals by hexachlorobenzene shows a biochemical resemblance to naturally occurring porphyria cutanea tarda. Several investigators (Taljaard *et al.*, 1971; Tschudy and Bonkowsky, 1972; Stonard, 1974; Elder, 1974) have concluded that porphyria produced by hexachlorobenzene is a suitable model for studying symptomatic porphyria. The paper by Elder involved detailed study of porphyrins from patients with that condition. In spite of the report that the condition in the rabbit is a better model, most studies have been made in rats.

Although the term "porphyria cutanea tarda" sometimes was used in reference to poisoning by hexachlorobenzene, the term should be reserved for cases without clearly established hereditary defect and without demonstrable exposure to a clear-cut porphyrigen.

Actually, there is a familial tendency to this condition and many of the patients arc alcoholics. However, no hereditary pattern has been established, and alcohol is a weak porphyrigen at worst (Waldenström and Haeger-Aronsen, 1963).

It is of particular interest that, if the dosage of rats is discontinued soon after peak values of porphyrin excretion are reached, the disturbance of porphyrin metabolism is reversed rapidly, whereas two or three additional weeks of feeding lead to an apparently irreversible porphyric state (Ockner and Schmid, 1961; Pearson and Malkinson, 1965).

Iron metabolism constitutes one of the links between porphyria cutanea tarda and the porphyria caused by hexachlorobenzene, and it is one of several factors known to influence the toxic process. In a comprehensive study of 100 patients with the spontaneous disease, the only abnormality, other than porphyria itself, present in all patients was hepatic siderosis. However, not all persons with siderosis suffered from porphyria; the difference may lie in the greater reduction of uroporphyrinogen decarboxylase in those who develop clinical disease (Joubert *et al.*, 1973). The importance of this enzyme is suggested by the

fact that its activity is partially reduced in siderotics without symptomatic porphyria, and the higher carboxylated porphyrins are relatively more abundant in their livers than in normal livers (Joubert *et al.*, 1973).

Iron differs quantitatively but also qualitatively in porphyria cutanea tarda; chloroquine affected urinary excretion of iron and biochemical and clinical remission in patients with this disease but did not influence iron excretion in other people with siderosis (Joubert *et al.*, 1973). Similar results were found in rats made porphyric by hexachlorobenzene. Chloroquine decreased the excess production of porphyrins even in rats that continued to receive the fungicide (Vizcthum *et al.*, 1979).

On the contrary, hexachlorobenzene profoundly affects iron distribution in the liver, and porphyrin accumulation in the liver is related to this change (Joubert *et al.*, 1973). Some studies have shown that hexachlorobenzene causes an increase in iron content of the liver, and others have shown that it causes a decrease. The reason for the opposite results is not known (Doyle *et al.*, 1979). That the changes in the distribution of iron, zinc, copper, manganese, and perhaps other metals reflect the state of porphyria and depend on the degree and duration of exposure to hexachlorobenzene does not seem to have been explored systematically.

A number of experiments have demonstrated that iron loading can hasten the onset and increase the intensity of porphyria caused by hexachlorobenzene in rats (Taljaard *et al.*, 1971, 1972; Shanley *et al.*, 1972). In a typical study, the iron was administered as iron/dextran in five intraperitoneal doses totaling 50 mg/rat during the course of 10–14 days; starting 14 days after completion of this treatment, some of the rats as well as other rats that had received no supplementary iron were placed on diets containing 3000 ppm hexachlorobenzene (Louw *et al.*, 1977). The potentiating action of iron on porphyria is preceded and presumably caused by further inhibition of uroporphyrinogen decarboxylase, further induction of δ-aminolevulinic acid synthetase, and decrease (but not elimination) of the induction of liver microsomal enzymes, all of which are caused by hexachlorobenzene. The increase in total porphyrins is accompanied by a relative increase in the higher carboxylated ones, that is, 7- and 8-carboxyl porphyrins. Degenerative changes in the liver may be seen before onset of porphyria, so that liver damage must be regarded as the cause of porphyria rather than the reverse.

Other factors known to influence the porphyria produced by hexachlorobenzene include sex hormones, some other steroids, alcohol, and caloric intake. Ultraviolet light influences the development of dermal lesions and also survival.

Porphyrins are increased in the female rat at a dosage level of hexachlorobenzene similar to that which produces human poisoning. The concentration of porphyrins in the liver of rats receiving a dietary level of 80 ppm (about 3.9 mg/kg/day) were 202 and 0.12 nmol/gm in females and males, respectively (Grant *et al.*, 1974a,b). At a higher dietary level (2500 ppm) porphyria occurred in only 5 weeks in female rats, 10 weeks in males, and 7 weeks in castrate males (Sweeney and Jones,

1976). The greater susceptibility of the female rat to porphyria has been confirmed (Kuiper-Goodman *et al.*, 1977).

Removal of the testes of males increased and removal of the ovaries of females decreased the concentration of porphyrins in the liver compared to those in intact animals receiving the same dietary level of 100 ppm. At 500 ppm, the gonadectomy appeared to be masked (Grant *et al.*, 1975).

When female rats received the same dietary level for 2 weeks before mating and thereafter, the concentrations of porphyrins in the liver were about the same in male and female pups killed at the age of 18 days (Mendoza *et al.*, 1975).

Estrogen, progesterone, and androgen had little effect on porphyrin metabolism in normal rats, but they had marked effects on rats in "latent porphyria" as a result of receiving hexachlorobenzene at a dietary level of 2000 ppm three times per week. Either 5 mg of estradiol alone or in combination with 150 mg of 17 α-hydroxyprogesterone or 50 mg of testosterone provoked severe porphyria (Ippen *et al.*, 1972b). Similar results were reported by Zawirska and Dzik (1977). Alcohol has an effect opposite to that of iron. Rats and mice receiving the same dietary level of hexachlorobenzene (2000 ppm) developed porphyria later and somewhat less severely if they drank concurrently a 5% solution of alcohol as their only source of water. This relationship did not hold when the intake of hexachlorobenzene was intermittent (Ippen *et al.*, 1972a). Whether the therapeutic effect of alcohol contributed to the relative resistance of grown people to porphyria caused by hexachlorobenzene is entirely speculative.

Porphyria is produced by hexachlorobenzene and not by any of its metabolites that have been studied in this regard or by certain other chlorobenzenes not recognized as metabolites (Carlson, 1977; Goerz *et al.*, 1978).

The distribution of porphyrins in different tissues and even the penetration of these compounds into the cell nucleus have been investigated by fluorescence microscopy and by direct and indirect immunofluorescence (Szabo *et al.*, 1973a,b).

When the intake of hexachlorobenzene was held constant but intake of a balanced ration was restricted to half the normal intake, the resulting tissue levels of the fungicide were higher, induction of liver microsomal enzymes was greater, and (when the dosage was about 5 mg/kg/day) liver enlargement occurred (Villeneuve *et al.*, 1977).

Hexachlorobenzene usually produced no irritation or sensitization in nonirradiated rodents. DeMatteis *et al.* (1961) and some others observed excoriation of the shoulder area of rats after they were excreting porphyrins in high concentration; however, the investigators thought these lesions might be the result of scratching rather than a direct manifestation of porphyria. Gajdos and Gajdos-Török (1961a,c) produced a cutaneous syndrome in rats characterized by poor quality and brownish discoloration of the hair and eruptions on the head, back, and feet. At least in some of the studies, the dietary level was extremely high (20,000 ppm) and the relation of these lesions to those observed in humans is unknown.

DeMatteis *et al.* (1961) were unable to produce skin changes in porphyric rats by acute exposure to ultraviolet light. However, Pearson and Malkinson (1965) consistently produced characteristic skin lesions by exposing plucked or shaved female rats to long-wave ultraviolet irradiation after porphyria was well established. The dietary level (2000 ppm) of hexachlorobenzene they used permitted unirradiated rats to survive for long periods. However, if an area of 25 cm² or larger was plucked or shaved at the beginning of the exposure period, most of the animals died in 3–14 days. Prolonged exposure to the same ultraviolet irradiation had no effect on porphyric rats fully covered with hair or on normal rats that were plucked or shaved repeatedly. When the ultraviolet bulbs in the cages were replaced by daylight bulbs, there was no injury to plucked or shaved porphyric rats.

The lesions developed by porphyric rats exposed to long-wave ultraviolet light included erosions and blisters in response to gentle friction and (in those that survived irradiation) a delayed regrowth of hair. Histologically, there were degenerative changes of the epidermis and follicles demonstrable by both light and electron microscopy. The blisters were in the corium just below the epidermal basement membrane or slightly deeper, and they showed a similarity to those found in human porphyria cutanea tarda. Porphyrins were shown by fluorescence microscopy to be selectively concentrated in the rat epidermis and follicular epithelium, although some diffuse fluorescence was visible in the corium also. This distribution is similar to that seen in patients with photosensitive hepatic porphyria. A rapid method of monitoring the development of porphyria was to observe the rats' teeth in Wood's light.

Similar results were reported by Burnett and Pathak (1964), who emphasized that, whereas radiation had no effect on excretion of porphyrins in normal rats, it tended to increase excretion and decrease tissue levels in rats rendered porphyric by hexachlorobenzene.

The pharmacokinetics of porphyrins in rats poisoned by hexachlorobenzene is not entirely clear, partly because not all parameters have been measured by all investigators. According to some (Mehendale *et al.*, 1975), urinary coproporphyrin levels more than doubled by the fourth day of treatment and remained relatively constant thereafter; however, the entire study lasted only 7 days and the animals remained healthy. On the contrary, Taljaard *et al.* (1972) found no substantial increase in urinary excretion of porphyrins by rats until day 55 of feeding hexachlorobenzene at a dietary level of 3000 ppm. The interval could be shortened to 33 days by simultaneous administration of iron/dextran. In either instance, the increase of uroporphyrin and coproporphyrin was sudden (Taljaard *et al.*, 1972). In another study, a sudden increase in urinary porphyrins (in this instance after day 40 of feeding 2000 ppm) was seen following a sudden, secondary increase in cytochrome P-450 and some microsomal enzymes after day 30 of treatment (Lissner *et al.*, 1975; Kreig *et al.*, 1977). In yet another study, the delayed appearance of porphyria was accompanied by a progressive fall in uroporphyrinogen decarboxylase activity, and the porphyria was considered a result of this enzyme inhibition. Iron accumulation in the liver was not noted (Elder *et al.*, 1976).

The disturbance of porphyrin metabolism associated with

poisoning by hexachlorobenzene is so complex that no claim can be made that its mechanism is understood. On the other hand, it seems unlikely that inhibition of uroporphyrinogen decarboxylase (Taljaard et al., 1971; Rios de Molina et al., 1975; Elder et al., 1976; San Martin de Viale et al., 1977; Louw et al., 1977) and stimulation of δ-aminolevulinic acid synthetase activity (Stonard, 1974; Taljaard et al., 1972; Louw et al., 1977) do not make an important contribution to the condition. Special evidence for the importance of the decarboxylase is the parallelism between the susceptibility of the forms of it in different tissues to inhibition and the susceptibility of the porphyrins in the same tissues to change under the influence of hexachlorobenzene (San Martin de Viale et al., 1977). Other investigators (N. Simon et al., 1978) have questioned whether there is any direct relationship between δ-aminolevulinic acid synthetase activity and the level of porphyrin excretion.

Whereas the decarboxylase is inhibited and the synthetase is stimulated, the degrees and times of onset of the two actions tend to be similar under any given set of experimental conditions (Louw et al., 1977).

A different approach to understanding the action of hexachlorobenzene involves physical chemistry. Because the porphyrin ring and the hexachlorobenzene molecule are very similar in size, flatness, and polarizability, there could be considerable van der Waals interaction between them, and it has been suggested that their similarity might be the basis for interference by the fungicide in heme synthesis (Pedersen and Carlson, 1975).

Biochemical Effects: Microsomal Enzymes The ability of hexachlorobenzene to induce microsomal enzymes of the liver is fully established (Turner and Green, 1974; Carlson and Tardiff, 1976). The compound stimulates not only its own metabolism, as evidenced by less efficient storage at higher dosages, but also that of dieldrin. Dieldrin storage was half that observed in control animals when hexachlorobenzene residues in body fat were approximately 330 ppm (Avrahami and Gernert, 1972). The induction of paraoxon dealkylation activity (measured in vitro) was significantly increased in rats by feeding them hexachlorobenzene for 2 weeks at a dietary level of 2 ppm; liver weight, microsomal protein, and P-450 were not affected by 2 ppm but were increased by 10 ppm (Iverson, 1976). The fungicide also induced enzymes that metabolize a number of other pesticides (Mendoza et al., 1976). On the contrary, the enzymes induced by phenobarbital in animals with stored hexachlorobenzene did not cause a detectable increase in the loss of this fungicide in rats (Villeneuve et al., 1974a) or in cattle (Hembry et al., 1975). The presence of a qualitative difference in the enzyme-inducing activity of these two compounds has been confirmed (Stonard and Nenov, 1974). Later, Stonard (1975), following a detailed study, concluded that hexachlorobenzene represented a new class of inducers with some features of both classical types. Less convincing was the suggestion (Stonard and Greig, 1976) that there is a connection between this pattern of induction and the production of porphyria.

That porphyria and the induction of microsomal enzymes are

different and, to a considerable extent, opposite processes is emphasized by their relationships in male and female rats. As already noted, female rats are more susceptible than males to porphyria, illness, and death caused by repeated doses of hexachlorobenzene. By contrast, cytochrome P-450 and several liver enzymes were increased in males receiving dietary levels of 40 ppm or more but were not increased in females at dietary levels as high as 160 ppm for 274 days (Grant et al., 1974a,b). However, induction must have been more extensive than the in vitro tests showed, for the pharmacological actions of pentobarbital and zoxazolamine were shortened in both males and females fed 20 ppm or more. In a related study it was shown that enlargement of the liver in the male was mainly due to an increase in smooth endoplasmic reticulum. Microsomal enzyme induction reached a maximum in 6 weeks, and activity was still elevated 8 weeks after feeding was discontinued. Within a period of only 12 weeks, 26% of female rats receiving 32 mg/kg/day died, but no males died at this dosage level (Kuiper-Goodman et al., 1974, 1975). The greater susceptibility of the female rat presumably is at least partially the result of lesser response of her liver microsomal enzymes.

Although induction of microsomal enzymes and porphyria are largely separate, there is some interaction. Cytochrome P-450 induced by hexachlorobenzene showed a greater admixture of hemoproteins than it did without induction or when induced by some other compounds (Blekkenhorst et al., 1978).

In lambs, some liver microsomal enzymes were induced by hexachlorobenzene at a dietary level of 1.0 ppm but not at a level of 0.1 ppm. Even 1.0 ppm did not produce any detectable harmful effect during 90 days of exposure (Mull et al., 1978).

Under test conditions where no microsomal enzyme activity was detectable in the skin of control rats, such activity was induced within 70 days, but not within 10 days by hexachlorobenzene at a dietary rate of 500 ppm. In the induced rats, the skin activity was 100 times less than that in the liver, and it was qualitatively different also (Goerz et al., 1979).

Effects on Organs and Tissues Dominant lethal studies of hexachlorobenzene in rats were negative (Khera, 1974; G. S. Simon et al., 1978, 1979).

Treatment of rats with the fungicide induced microsomal enzymes in their livers in a dosage-responsive way so that, when bacteria were incubated with 2,4-diaminoanisole plus a liver preparation in vitro, their mutation rate was increased compared to that of bacteria incubated with the same compound and with control liver (Dybing and Aune, 1977).

When hamsters received hexachlorobenzene for their lifetime, the proportions of animals with one or more tumors were 10, 56, 75, and 92% in those receiving dietary levels of 0, 50, 100, and 200 ppm (about 0, 4, 8, and 16 mg/kg/day), respectively. Only the highest dosage caused some reduction in life span evident at 70 weeks but not at 50 weeks. There was also a dosage-related increase in animals with more than one tumor. The kinds of tumors significantly increased included alveolar adenomas of the thyroid, hepatomas, and hemangioendotheliomas of the liver and spleen (Cabral et al., 1977). Results in mice have been inconsistent. Shirai *et al.* (1978) reported negative results. Cabral *et al.* (1978, 1979) found an increase in hepatomas in mice on dietary levels of 200 and 100 ppm but not in those receiving 50 ppm. The tumors did not metastasize.

Mice that had received hexachlorobenzene at a dietary level of 167 ppm for 6 weeks showed only about half the normal peak response of splenic Ab plaque-forming cells in response to sheep red blood cells, but there was no delay in the response. Serum IgA levels were reduced in treated mice (Loose *et al.*, 1977). These changes were reflected in the animals' 32-fold increased susceptibility to endotoxin and their 31% reduction in survival after a standard inoculation of malaria (Loose *et al.*, 1978a,b). On the contrary, cell-mediated immunity in mice was enhanced (Silkworth and Loose, 1978). Results reported in rats were entirely different—that is, stimulation of the humoral response and no effect on cell-mediated immunity (Vos *et al.*, 1979). Whether the difference depends on species or on some other variable is unclear.

Effects on Reproduction   At least in some circumstances, young rats are in greater danger from hexachlorobenzene during lactation than during gestation. Pups that had survived the fetal period died in convulsions 7 to 8 days after birth to a dam receiving the fungicide; foster pups that were substituted died within 3–4 days, and later the dam died (DeMatteis *et al.*, 1961; Grant *et al.*, 1977).

In a four-generation study, the higher dietary levels were toxic to the P-generation females; 50 and 20% of them died while eating 640 and 320 ppm, respectively, and all of the pups produced by survivors died within 5 days of birth. When the maternal dietary level was 160 ppm, only 55% of pups survived 5 days after birth, and of those that did live 5 days, those alive at weaning dropped from 30% for the F_{1a} and F_{1b} generations to 0% for the F_{2a} and F_{2b} generations. At 80 ppm, the proportion of pups alive at 5 days that survived at weaning dropped from 93% in the F_{1a} to 40% in the F_{3b} generation. Fertility, survival to 5 days, and survival to weaning were only slightly affected at a dietary level of 40 ppm, questionably affected at 20 ppm, and not affected at 10 ppm. No gross abnormalities were observed in the pups at any dosage level (Grant *et al.*, 1977).

When rabbits received hexachlorobenzene from day 1 to 28 of gestation, the concentration of the compound in the fetuses at term corresponded to dosage. Fetal liver concentrations were higher but brain concentrations were lower than corresponding maternal values. At the highest maternal dosage tested (10 mg/kg/day) the compound did not affect the health of the dams or the fetuses (Villeneuve *et al.*, 1974b,c). The concentration of hexachlorobenzene in cows and their newborn calves was the same (Henbry *et al.*, 1975).

Dosages of 80 or 120 mg/kg/day during 4 or more days of pregnancy were toxic to female rats and reduced the weight of their fetuses. These and lower dosages produced some increase in the incidence of a 14th rib but no significant toxic or teratogenic effect (Khera, 1974). The same lack of effect was obtained in another study of rats, but mice showed a cleft palate

in one litter and some kidney malformations following a maternal dosage of 100 mg/kg/day on days 7–16 of pregnancy (Courtney *et al.*, 1976).

A dosage of 4 mg/kg/day reduced estrogen levels in four female monkeys and blocked ovulation in one of them. It did not change luteinizing and follicle-stimulating hormones (Mueller *et al.*, 1978a).

Pathology   Closely related to the laboratory findings is the finding of fluorescence in the liver and bones of animals that survive more than a few weeks of dosing. Some investigators found the fluorescence confined to the bone shaft (Ockner and Schmid, 1961), but others have seen it in the marrow also (Campbell, 1963). Fluorescence of the liver and gastrointestinal tract was observed in rats receiving dietary levels of 1000 and 500 ppm but not in those receiving 100 ppm for 4 months (Kimbrough and Linder, 1974).

In spite of the prominence of neurological signs, pathology has not been found in the nervous system of rats, either centrally or peripherally (Campbell, 1963; DeMatteis *et al.*, 1961).

The most striking changes are in the liver. After 5–9 weeks of dosing at a dietary rate of 2000 ppm, rats showed marked enlargement of the liver (13 gm), and of the liver cells, especially centrilobularly. Further dosing caused the liver to shrink gradually to a normal or slightly subnormal size. The cells were atrophic, and there was focal necrosis, but cirrhosis was not seen. There was some deposit of iron in the liver (Campbell, 1963). Histologically, hepatocytes of the rat enlarge and the endoplasmic reticulum increases. At a dietary level of 2000 ppm, laminated inclusions were detected by the end of the third week. Another interesting structure observed was protrusion of the cytoplasm of hepatocytes through spaces of Disse into sinusoidal lamina (Medline *et al.*, 1973). The inclusions resemble those produced in rat hepatocytes by DDT but are less compact. Laminated inclusions were observed in hepatocytes of rats fed dietary levels of hexachlorobenzene as low as 100 ppm for 4 months (Kimbrough and Linder, 1974). Multinucleated hepatocytes, sometimes with clefts but never with detectable foreign bodies, were seen in many female rats fed 500 or 1000 ppm and in a few males fed 1000 ppm. Focal necrosis, inflammatory cells in the sinusoids, and interstitial fibrosis also were more common in females, in contrast to cytoplasmic inclusions, which were more common in males (Kimbrough and Linder, 1974). Minor differences in descriptions by other investigators (Iwanow *et al.*, 1973; Kuiper-Goodman *et al.*, 1977) appear to be explained by differences in dosage or other experimental conditions. The apparent presence of porphyrins in red cells within certain organs and the occurrence of a pigment (possibly a lipofuscin) in the kidneys is not clear.

Pathology is not confined to the liver. Some rats maintained on a dietary level of only 100 ppm for 4 months showed hyperplasia of the zona fasciculata of the adrenal plus increased macrophages and fibrosis of the lungs. Rats fed 500 or 1000 ppm showed these same changes more frequently and also showed fibrosis of the heart and hemorrhage, edema, and inflammation of the lung. Adrenal hyperplasia, fibrosis of the heart, and all of the lung lesions except increased macrophages were more common in females (Kimbrough and Linder, 1974).

In female rhesus monkeys gavaged for 60 days, liver changes consisted of cloudy swelling, fatty degeneration, centrilobular hepatocellular hypertrophy, bile duct proliferation, bile casts, and hemosiderosis. Other changes included thymic cortical atrophy, vacuolization of the proximal renal tubules, thickening of the ovarian germinal epithelium, and a change from 0.01 to 0.44 in the ratio of corpora lutea to primary ovarian follicles. All of these changes showed a dosage–response relationship, being moderate or marked following 128 mg/kg/day, slight or absent after 8 mg/kg/day, and of intermediate intensity after 32 and 64 mg/kg/day (Iatropoulos *et al.*, 1976). A male monkey that had received [^{14}C]hexachlorobenzene (10 ppm) in its food for 540 days showed thymic cortical atrophy and degenerative changes in the cerebellum and kidney but no detectable radioactivity in any tissue (Mueller *et al.*, 1978b).

Treatment of Poisoning in Animals Gajdos and Gajdos-Török (1961b,c) found that hexachlorobenzene at a dietary level of 20,000 ppm produced cutaneous lesions as well as other signs of intoxication in rats. When some of these rats were given intramuscular injections of 20 mg of adenosine-5-monophosphoric acid per rat daily after illness had begun and while exposure to the fungicide was continued, most showed healing of skin lesions, recovery of lost weight, practical disappearance of neurological signs, decrease in excretion of porphyrins, and reduction of liver injury. Some treated rats died in spite of visible improvement in skin lesions and the condition of the fur. Controls that received the fungicide but no treatment showed a gradual progression of the disease.

An entirely different approach involved use of mineral oil. Following either a single intraperitoneal dose (50 mg/kg) of hexachlorobenzene or after feeding it at a dietary level of 1.5 ppm for 7 days, elimination was promoted in a striking but brief way by mineral oil administered by gavage (10 ml/kg/day or 8% in the diet) (Richter *et al.*, 1977).

21.9.1.3 Toxicity to Humans

Accidental and Intentional Poisoning From 1955 through 1959 a disease, previously unknown in the area, appeared commonly in three southeastern provinces of Turkey. The people called it "the new disease" or "black sore" (Wray *et al.*, 1962). The illness was characterized by blistering and epidermolysis of the skin, especially of the hands and face. The skin was unusually sensitive both to light and to minor mechanical trauma. The blisters broke easily, formed crusts, healed poorly, and often became infected. If the blisters healed, they were replaced by pigmented scars containing microcysts about 1 mm in diameter, and contractures were common in areas where tissue loss had occurred. Scarring also led to permanent alopecia or corneal opacity. In some patients, the infection involved deeper tissues with suppurative arthritis and osteomyelitis, especially of the

fingers (Cam and Nigogosyn, 1963). The infection apparently was superimposed on another lesion of the joints, for eventually over half of 376 patients developed swelling and spindling of the fingers. X-ray examination of 18 patients showed osteoporosis restricted to the phalanges, the metacarpal and carpal bones, and the distal metaphysis and epiphysis of both the ulna and the radius and to the corresponding bones of the lower extremities. Interphalangeal arthritis leading to a narrowing of the joint spaces was striking and somewhat reminiscent of rheumatoid arthritis. Erosion of the terminal phalanges was seen in two cases. The joint changes persisted at the last examination 1–2 years after clinical signs and abnormal excretion of porphyrins disappeared (Doğramaci *et al.*, 1962c).

Many patients had increased pigmentation of the skin (but not the mucosae) most noticeable on the face and hands but also involving other parts of the body. In addition, a layer of fine dark hair often appeared around the eyes and chin and on the extremities, and occasionally over the entire body. The combination of atrophic hands, dark pigmentation, and a fine covering of hair was spoken of as "monkey disease" by the peasants (Cam, 1959; Cam and Nigogosyn, 1963; Schmid, 1960).

Signs of systemic disease included hepatomegaly in the majority of hospitalized patients. The liver edge was firm, sharp, and tender. The thyroid was enlarged in over 30% of cases but there was no indication of increased function. Subnormal temperature, anorexia, weight loss, and muscle atrophy were common. Suppuration was accompanied by enlargement of regional lymph nodes. Even in early stages of the disease, the urine of all patients was port wine red or darker in color. No erythrodontia, no neurological or mental disturbances, and no typical abdominal crises such as those seen in some forms of porphyria were observed (Cam, 1959; Cam and Nigogosyn, 1963; Schmid, 1960). However, some patients did complain of bouts of abdominal pain (Doğramaci *et al.*, 1962b; Peters *et al.*, 1966).

It was noticed very early that the disease ran a seasonal course, all signs tending to be worse in summer and improved in winter. Persons who were affected in 1955 or 1956 usually had relapses each summer, at least through 1959. After the cause was discovered and dosage stopped, many of the patients recovered but in some the disease continued at least for many months after intake stopped. Many persons were seriously disfigured. The mortality was 10% (Peters *et al.*, 1966).

The disease was essentially confined to rural areas when it first appeared, but in later years it also occurred in towns. It was not confined to a single ethnic group but occurred among Turks, Kurds, and Armenians. In some instances almost entire large families were sick. However, not all persons known to have ingested hexachlorobenzene became sick. Based on a study of 348 hospitalized cases, Cam and Nigogosyn (1963) found the condition predominantly in males (76%) and in children 4–14 years of age (81%). However, some adults, including a few over 50 years of age, were affected. The cutoff at 4 years was not due to any immunity of infants and young children, but merely to the fact that poisoning had different characteristics among them, as discussed below.

When he had seen only four cases, Cam (1957) quite reasonably supposed that the disease just described was congenital porphyria. However, the explosive occurrence of a large number of cases of porphyria among different ethnic groups in an area where porphyria previously was unknown suggested that the cause was a toxic substance, not a genetically determined metabolic disorder, and Cam (1958) showed that hexachlorobenzene was the cause. It was found that the disease occurred almost exclusively in persons who admitted eating wheat distributed by the government, not for food but for seed. Before 1954 seed treated with mercury had been used. A small amount of seed treated with hexachlorobenzene was distributed in 1954 and much more in 1955 and subsequent years until distribution was stopped. A few cases were observed in 1955, and a great many were seen in 1956 and later. The relationship between chemical and disease was reported in 1958, and the government discontinued use of this fungicide during 1959. New cases gradually ceased to appear, and none was seen by 1963 (Cam and Nigogosyan, 1963).

Details of how the grain was distributed and how it happened to be misused were given by Wray *et al.* (1962). It was estimated by Cam and Nigogosyan (1963) that their 348 hospitalized patients had ingested hexachlorobenzene at the rate of approximately 50–200 mg/person/day for relatively long periods before dermal lesions became apparent. This intake corresponds to the commercially recommended rate of application of hexachlorobenzene to wheat but not to the rate of application reported by Wray *et al.* (1962).

In the same areas where hexachlorobenzene produced the disease just described in children and adults, it produced a disease called "pembe yara" or pink sore in at least one adult but chiefly in infants of mothers who had eaten contaminated bread. The mortality rate of about 95% almost eliminated children between 2 and 5 years of age in many villages in the years between 1955 and 1960. Thus, the number of children surviving to have the porphyric form of the disease was greatly reduced. Although no abnormal excretion of porphyrins was observed in the infants, hexachlorobenzene was demonstrated by gas chromatography in the milk of their mothers (Peters *et al.*, 1966).

The disease in infants occurred at all times of the year but was most frequent in summer. It began with diarrhea, fever, and pink or skin-colored papules on the back of the hands and fingers, on the wrists, and sometimes on the feet and legs, especially the knees. Later the skin lesions formed plaques and rings of different color and texture, imperfectly reminiscent of a great many different kinds of dermatitis. The mucosa of the mouth often had white spots. X-ray examination revealed an infiltration of the lungs. Subcutaneous abscesses developed in some cases. The infants lost so much weight that the skin hung in folds. They were so dehydrated they were too weak to cry. The liver was always hypertrophied. There was severe hypochronic anemia but a leukocytosis. Some infants were saved through removal from breast feeding and attention to supportive care. Resolution of the skin lesion and improvement of general health often required 1–2 months (Cam, 1960).

Twenty years after the outbreak in Turkey, 32 of the approx-

imately 4000 patients were reexamined. Their average age was 29.5 years, indicating that many of them were children during the outbreak. The 32 were selected because local physicians knew that they were not recovered fully. Examination of this group revealed hyperpigmentation in 53%, hirsutism in 41%, scarring of the hands and face in 50%, pinched faces in 53%, rhagades in 22%, fragile skin of the hands and face in 12.5%, enlarged liver in 9%, small hands with sclerodermoid thickening and shortening of the distal phalanx and painless arthritis in 44%, and enlarged thyroid in 38%. Porphyrins still were elevated significantly in five subjects. As shown in Table 21.1, hexachlorobenzene levels, with the exception of one sample of milk, were not high compared with those in other population groups (Cripps *et al.*, 1980). Whereas this study showed that porphyria could persist for 20 years after ingestion of hexachlorobenzene, it failed to show how often persistence occurred.

Use Experience   Hexachlorobenzene is mentioned in some texts on occupational health but only to the effect that it is the least toxic of the chlorobenzenes. Apparently it has led to no difficulty among persons who manufactured or formulated it.

Atypical Cases of Various Origins   A case that was entirely typical in its clinical manifestations was atypical in that the illness was attributed without explanation to the patient's work as a farmer (Mazzei and Mazzei, 1972, 1973). There can be no doubt that the compound was absorbed, for it was found in substantial concentration in the patient's blood. In the account, hexachlorobenzene was referred to as an insecticide associated with dieldrin and BHC. This confusion invites the speculation that the patient had used hexachlorobenzene in a very unconventional way and does not exclude the possibility that the patient had eaten the residues of the fungicide.

Dosage Response   It was estimated that intake of hexachlorobenzene by those who ate it over a prolonged period in Turkey was 50–200 mg/person/day (Cam and Nigogosyan, 1963). Because illness of the "black sore" type was most common in persons 4–14 years old, and because the larger people can be assumed to have eaten more, the dosage may be calculated in the range of 2.6–4.1 mg/kg/day.

Laboratory Findings   It is unfortunate that few measurements of hexachlorobenzene were made in a tissue or fluid from anyone poisoned by it in Turkey. The compound was measured in poisoned agricultural workers, and it has been detected in the general populations of some but not all countries where analyses were carried out.

Values reported for the worker and for several groups of people with different degrees of exposure are shown in Table 21.1.

In a group of 20 sprayers, absorption of measurable quantities was explained by the fact that exposure to hexachlorobenzene as a contaminant of the herbicide chlorthal-dimethyl (BSI, ISO) was greater than the usual exposure associated with prepar-

Table 21.1
Storage and Excretion of Hexachlorobenzene by People

Samples Kind	Number	Population	Continent and country	Year	Positive (%)	Concentration (ppm) Range	Mean	Reference
Fat			Europe					
	60	gp[a]	Belgium	1977			1.36	Dejonckheera et al. (1978)
	29	gp, men		1977	100		0.98	Van Haver et al. (1978)
	44	gp, women		1977	100		0.96	Van Haver et al. (1978)
	20	gp	Germany				6.3	Acker and Schulte (1970)
		gp				0.08–5.5	2.9	Acker and Schulte (1974)
		gp				1.2–21	6.4	Acker and Schulte (1974)
	10	gp	Norway	1976?	100	0.03–0.19[b]		Bjorseth et al. (1977)
	90	gp		1975–1976	100	0.08–0.29[c]		Brevik and Bjerk (1978)
	64	gp	Poland	1976–1977	44	0.097		Syrowatka et al. (1978)
	100	gp		1977–1978	?	0.06–0.48		Syrowatka et al. (1979)
	12	rural gp	Spain	1977	100		0.84	Pozo Lora et al. (1978)
	28	urban gp		1977	100		1.08	Pozo Lora et al. (1978)
			Asia					
	241	gp	Japan			0.003–0.77	0.08	Curley et al. (1973)
	1	patient	Turkey			0.21		Cripps et al. (1980)
			Oceania					
	75	gp[a]	Australia		100	tr–8.2	1.25	Brady and Siyali (1972)
	38	gp	New Guinea		63	0.0–2.8	0.26	Brady and Siyali (1972)
Liver			Europe					
	10	gp	Norway	1976?	100	0.11–0.23[b]	0.15[b]	Bjorseth et al. (1977)
Blood or serum			North America					
	20	sprayers	United States	1973?	95	0.0–0.310	0.040	Burns et al. (1974)
	86	"bystanders"			99	0.0–0.023	0.0036	Burns and Miller (1975)
	43	gp			95	0.0–0.002	0.0005	Burns and Miller (1975)
			South America					
	1	worker	Argentina		100	0.383[d]	0.040	Zeman et al. (1971); Mazzei and Mazzei (1973)
			Europe					
	98	gp, boys	Germany	1975	100	0.0026–0.0779	0.022	Richter and Schmid (1976)
	96	gp, girls		1975	100		0.017	Richter and Schmid (1976)
			Asia					
	8	patients	Turkey		50	0.003–0.018		Cripps et al. (1980)
			Oceania					
	185	exposed	Australia		100	0.0–0.095	0.0220	Siyali (1972)
	52	gp			100	0.0–0.095	0.0220	Siyali (1972)
	47	gp		1973	100	0.001–0.179	0.0599	Siyali and Ouw (1973)
	29	exposed[e]		1973	100	0.005–0.168	0.0571	Siyali and Ouw (1973)
Milk			Europe					
	43	gp	Germany				0.153	Acker and Schulte (1970)
	44	gp	Norway	1975–1976	100	0.003–0.009[c]		Brevik and Bjerk (1978)
			Asia					
	1	patient	Turkey			0.7		Cripps et al. (1980)
			Oceania					
	39	rural gp	Australia	1970	100	0.005–0.17	0.031[f]	Newton and Greene (1972)
	28	urban gp		1970	100	0.002–0.33	0.040[f]	Newton and Greene (1972)
	45	gp		1972	100	0.002–0.079	0.016	Siyali (1973)

[a] gp, General population.
[b] Lipid basis.
[c] Range of mean values for different groups.
[d] This level dropped to 0.268 ppm in a year, when symptomatic recovery occurred.
[e] Occupationally exposed to pesticides but not necessarily to hexachlorobenzene.
[f] Geometric mean.

ing or planting seed protected by hexachlorobenzene itself (Burns *et al.*, 1974). Burns and Miller (1975) showed that the persons (called "by-standers" in the table) who lived along a road on which industrial waste containing hexachlorobenzene was hauled had higher concentrations of the compound than did controls. Persons working in the plant from which the contaminated wastes were removed had plasma levels of hexachlorobenzene ranging from 0.014 to 0.233 ppm.

In at least one instance, storage of the compounds in persons of the general populations was traced to the feeding of treated grain to chickens that subsequently were used as human food (Brady and Siyali, 1972; Siyali, 1972).

In several instances, however, there was no evidence that use of the compound as a pesticide was the cause of observed storage. The compound is used in organic synthesis, as a plasticizer, and as a flame retardant in plastics, and it might enter the environment as an industrial waste.

Richter and Schmid (1976) analyzed the whole blood of 194 children. Every sample contained detectable hexachlorobenzene. Substantial concentrations began to appear 9–10 months after birth, and the concentrations increased rapidly at first and then more gradually, tending toward a limiting value of 0.022 ppm for boys and 0.017 ppm for girls. The rate of increase in concentration was inversely proportional to the square of age in years.

Finally, Steinwandter and Bruene (1977), having noted that the amounts of hexachlorobenzene in the environment in Germany far exceeded those directly dispersed for agricultural purposes, examined six specimens of preserved human fat. In samples collected in 1930 or earlier, the concentrations were low and erratic; specifically, the values for individual samples were below the limit of detection (<0.001 ppm in 1896, 0.232 ppm in 1900, 0.0043 in 1920, 0.0064 in 1923, and >0.001 in 1927 and 1930). The values for 15 samples collected during 1973 and 1974 ranged from 3.5 to 15 ppm. No samples were available for the period 1931–1972 that would permit identification of the transition period (Steinwandter and Bruene, 1977). The authors were aware that some microorganisms are capable of synthesizing polychlorinated benzenes, but they interpreted their data as indicating that hexachlorobenzene is not formed in this way. Whether this hypothesis can be considered disproved, and especially whether the small measured concentrations can be ignored as due to contamination of some samples, is questionable. After all, if the true concentration of some samples is low, one would expect undetectable levels in other samples.

As already mentioned, the urine of persons poisoned by hexachlorobenzene is port wine or darker in color. Ether–acid extracts of it give a red fluorescence with ultraviolet light. The concentrations of porphyrins in the urine and feces in this condition are shown in Table 2.12 summarized from various authors (Cam and Nigogosyan, 1973; Watson, 1960) and converted to standard units. It may be seen that the pattern of porphyrin excretion differs from one disorder of porphyrin metabolism to another. It is interesting that the concentrations of protoporphyrin and coproporphyrin in the feces of a patient who had been poisoned by hexachlorobenzene but had been clinically well for

2 years were about the same as those in other patients who were sick. Also, there was wide, persistent variation in porphyrin excretion by patients who seemed about equally sick (Peters *et al.*, 1966).

Treatment with 100–150 mg of secobarbital (a drug that causes exacerbation of pyrroloporphyria and protocoproporphyria) produced no clinical change or change in porphyrin excretion in patients poisoned by hexachlorobenzene (Doğramaci *et al.*, 1963).

Pathology   The pathology of poisoning by hexachlorobenzene includes, of course, all the dermal lesions seen in the living patient. It may include enlargement of the liver, thyroid, and lymph nodes. Liver biopsies showed a precirrhotic condition with slight focal necrosis, infiltration with monocytes and some polymorphonuclear granulocytes, increase in connective tissue in the portal spaces, and some regeneration of lobules. A diffuse red fluorescence was seen in the parenchyma of fresh-frozen sections (Doğramaci *et al.*, 1962a).

Treatment of Poisoning   When a large number of cases were available, no useful treatment was found except symptomatic care and avoidance of sunlight. After the number of cases was sharply reduced, seven patients were treated with the calcium disodium salt of ethylenediaminetetraacetic acid (EDTA). Some received 1.5 gm intravenously for 5 days. All were given oral doses ranging from 0.5 to 1.5 gm daily for as much as 52 weeks. As had proved true earlier in some other forms of porphyria treated with chelating agents, the patients showed definite improvement. Skin lesions cleared and pigmentation and hirsutism were reduced over a period of months, even though exposure to the sun was not restricted. The patients gained weight and felt stronger. One patient relapsed 10 months after treatment was stopped, but symptoms disappeared promptly on resumption of the drug. As might have been expected, the treatment led to a marked, somewhat temporary increase in urinary excretion of zinc, copper, and lead. The results of analysis of urinary and fecal porphyrins were interpreted as showing an initial stimulation of excretion followed by a decline to near-normal limits after 9 months of treatment (Peters *et al.*, 1966). The supposed stimulation of porphyrin excretion is difficult to evaluate because apparently the levels were not measured for a significant interval before treatment began. It is certainly true that for some patients the values reported during the first few months of treatment were much higher than those reported by others for untreated patients. The gradual decrease in excretion over a period of months was convincing, but in the absence of controls it may have been no greater than would have occurred spontaneously. A most interesting fact was that some patients never showed very high levels of porphyrin excretion, even though they seemed just as sick as others who did have sustained high levels of excretion.

The reason for the apparent value of calcium disodium EDTA in the treatment of poisoning by hexachlorobenzene is unknown. However, Chu and Chu (1970) found that *in vitro* zinc ions are required for hexachlorobenzene to metabolize δ-aminolevulinic acid to a porphyrin pattern similar to that found in patients. This suggests that EDTA may act in patients by influencing the distribution of zinc and/or other metals and not by a more direct action on porphyria.

Apparently, adenosine-5-monophosphoric acid has never been used in treating patients poisoned by hexachlorobenzene. It is of value for treating this kind of poisoning in rats and for treating certain other forms of porphyria in humans (Gajdos and Gajdos-Török, 1961c).

Because hexachlorobenzene and its metabolites undergo true fecal excretion, it seems probable that the total rate of excretion could be increased by cholestyramine, activated charcoal, or some other nonabsorbable chemisorbant or adsorbant (see Section 15.2.5.1).

21.9.2 DIPHENYL

21.9.2.1 Identity, Properties, and Uses

Chemical Name 1,1′-Biphenyl.

Structure See Fig. 21.3.

Synonyms The common name diphenyl is in general use. Other names have included bibenzene, biphenyl, difenile, and phenylbenzene. The CAS registry number is 92-52-4.

Physical and Chemical Properties Diphenyl has the empirical formula $C_{12}H_{10}$ and a molecular weight of 154.22. It forms colorless leaflets with a density of 1.041, a melting point of 70.5°C, and a boiling point of 256.1°C. It is considered dangerous if the vapor concentrations become greater than 5 mg/m³. Diphenyl is soluble in most organic solvent, but it is practically insoluble in water.

History, Formulations, and Uses Diphenyl was introduced by B. B. Ramsey in 1944 to inhibit the mycelial growth and spore formation of citrus fruit rots.

21.9.2.2 Toxicity to Laboratory Animals

Basic Findings Diphenyl is a compound of low acute toxicity. Deichmann *et al.* (1947) reported oral LD 50 values of 2410 and 3280 mg/kg in the rabbit and rat, respectively. The animals showed increased respiratory rate, lacrimation, loss of appetite and weight, muscular weakness, respiratory distress, and death in coma. Some animals showed mild paralysis of the hind legs and mild asphyxial convulsions. The signs of illness appeared mild until coma developed with little warning. The interval from gavage to death varied from 2 to 18 days.

In a 2-year feeding test, the growth rate of both males and females was reduced and their mortality was increased at dietary levels of 10,000 and 5000 ppm. A paired feeding study showed that the decrease in growth was due to decreased food intake. There was no clear dosage-related change in organ weights. The same was true of hemoglobin, but it tended to be reduced at the higher dietary levels. Dietary levels of 1000 and above influenced the excretion of urinary solids, indicating altered kidney function. There was no effect at dietary levels of 500 ppm (about 25 mg/kg/day) or at 50 or 10 ppm (Ambrose *et al.*, 1960).

The highest dietary level, that is, 1000 ppm (about 20 mg/kg/day), proved to be a no-effect level in a 1-year feeding test in dogs. Weight gains, hematology, liver and kidney function tests, and histology were normal (unpublished report, cited by Lehman, 1965).

When monkeys were fed diphenyl at dietary levels of 0, 100, 1000, and 10,000 ppm for 1 year, those with the highest intake showed an increase in relative liver weight. Weight gain, hematology, and blood urea nitrogen were normal. A dietary level of 1000 ppm (about 20 mg/kg/day) was considered a no-effect level (unpublished report, cited by Lehman, 1965).

Dermal applications of diphenyl to rabbits at a rate of 500 mg/kg/day for 20 or more days produced weight loss and the death of one animal after eight applications, but no skin lesion (Deichmann *et al.*, 1947).

Skin application of a 23% solution in oil twice a week for 7 months produced local inflammatory changes in mice but no tumors (unpublished reports, cited by FAO/WHO, 1967).

When the shaved backs of rats were painted with a dilute solution of diphenyl, the animals lost some weight and some skin irritation appeared in 15 days (Hanada, 1975). A maximum of 62 respiratory exposures of animals to diphenyl dust for 7 hr/day at an average concentration of 5 mg/m³ was fatal to some mice. A similar exposure to 40 mg/m³ was fatal to some rats, but rabbits showed no signs of illness when exposed 64 times to 300 mg/m³ (Deichmann *et al.*, 1947).

Absorption, Distribution, Metabolism, and Excretion The main metabolic product of diphenyl in dogs, rats, and rabbits is 4-hydroxydiphenyl. This and other hydroxylation products are excreted in the urine partly as sulfates and glucuronides (Klingenberg, 1891; Stroud, 1940; Deichmann *et al.*, 1947; West *et al.*, 1956). Later, small amounts of three other metabolites were identified, namely, 4,4′-dihydroxydiphenyl, 3,4-dihydroxydiphenyl, and diphenylmercapturic acid (West *et al.*, 1956). Some species including hamsters excrete 2-hydroxydiphenyl (Bridges and Burke, 1971).

In vitro, 4-hydroxylation of diphenyl by liver microsomal enzymes obtained from 12 species including humans has been demonstrated. Of the species tested, only preparations from mice, hamsters, coypus, cats, frogs, rats, and young rabbits caused 2-hydroxylation (Creaven and Williams, 1963; Creaven *et al.*, 1965). Appropriate induction of enzymes permits *in vitro* formation of 3-hydroxybiphenyl also (Billings and McMahon, 1976). Metabolites produced *in vivo* either with or without prior induction of microsomal enzymes are 2-, 3-, and 4-hydroxybiphenyl and 3,4-dihydroxybiphenyl (Halpaap *et al.*, 1978).

In a study in which [¹⁴C]diphenyl was administered to rats orally at a rate of 100 mg/kg, 75.8 and 5.8% were recovered from the urine and feces, respectively, within 24 hr. This recovery increased to a total of 84.8 and 7.3% within 96 hr. Only trace amounts of $^{14}CO_2$ were detected in the expired air, and only 0.6% of the dose was found still present in the rats 96 hr after oral administration, the total recovery being 92.7% (Meyer *et al.*, 1976).

The growth of rats whose diet contained only 6% protein was stopped at once when diphenyl was added at a concentration of 10,000 ppm. However, growth did not stop when either L-cysteine (0.12%) or DL-methionine (0.15%) was added to the diet along with diphenyl. It was concluded that these amino acids were used preferentially as a primary source of sulfur for the conjugation and detoxication of diphenyl; supplementation of the diet permitted both detoxication and growth. However, the relationship was complex, for the sulfur was not adequately accounted for in conjugated metabolites that were recovered (West, 1940; West and Jefferson, 1942).

Biochemical Effects In hamsters, the relative rates of 4- and 2-hydroxylation were 25 : 1 in controls, 70 : 1 in animals pretreated with phenobarbital, but only 2.5 : 1 in those pretreated with 3-methylcholanthrene (Bridges and Burke, 1971). Stimulation of diphenyl 2-hydroxylation but not of 4-hydroxylation was produced in hepatic microsomal preparations from both rats and hamsters by several carcinogens but not by phenobarbital or several other compounds. It was concluded that enhanced diphenyl 4-hydroxylation, but not enhanced diphenyl 2-hydroxylation, requires the synthesis of new microsomal enzymes (McPherson *et al.*, 1975).

Effects on Reproduction In a one-generation test, dietary levels of 1000 and 5000 ppm fed to male and female rats for 11–60 days before mating had no effect on fertility, lactation, viability, or the number of pups per litter brought to weaning (Lehman, 1965). In a three-generation test, fertility of females, size of litters, and growth of the young rats were reduced at a dietary level of 10,000 ppm; however, these effects did not increase in succeeding generations. The reproduction record of rats receiving 100 and 1000 ppm (that is, up to 50 mg/kg/day with higher rates for lactating females and weaned pups) was indistinguishable from that of controls (Ambrose *et al.*, 1960).

Effects on Organs and Tissues Diphenyl was not tumorigenic to mice that received the highest tolerated dosage (64 mg/kg/day) for their lifetime (Innes *et al.*, 1969). This confirmed earlier negative results commented on by Lehman (1965).

Rats ingesting diets containing 5000 ppm diphenyl developed within about 60 days focal dilatations of kidney tubules. When feeding at this level was continued a total of 165 days and the rats were then returned to uncontaminated feed for 60 days, the kidney lesions were found to have healed with scarring. Polyuria proved a more sensitive criterion of renal effect. At a dietary level of 10,000 ppm, polyuria started after 4 days. The rate reached a maximum of about six times normal on about day 20, after which it remained relatively constant until feeding of diphenyl was stopped; the urinary output then returned to nearly normal within 30 days. No evidence of polyuria or histological

damage was observed from a dietary level of 1000 ppm for 120 days (Booth *et al.*, 1961).

Pathology A single fatal oral dose produced albuminous and, to a lesser degree, fatty hepatocellular degeneration as well as severe nephrotic changes. Slight to severe degenerative changes may be present in the myocardium. Congestion and edema of the lungs occur regularly but may represent terminal changes (Deichmann *et al.*, 1947).

21.9.2.3 Toxicity to Humans

Experimental Exposure During a period of 13 weeks a volunteer took without any adverse effect a total of 435 mg of diphenyl divided into nine doses of which the largest was 100 mg (about 1.4 mg/kg (Farkas, 1939).

Use Experience Use experience with diphenyl involves astonishing contrasts. In most instances, apparently including all use as a pesticide *per se,* this experience has been good. In a few instances involving the manufacture of diphenyl-impregnated paper, the results ranged from poor to disastrous. There seems to be no reason to suppose that any factor other than a very great difference in dosage contributed to the difference.

A 32-year-old man who had worked for 11 years in a mill that had diphenyl-impregnated paper among its products began to complain of fatigue, abdominal pain, headache, irritability, sleep disturbances, and loss of memory during the summer of 1969. He visited two physicians during the autumn but he was not diagnosed and he continued to work until November, 4 days before he entered hospital. By that time he was somnolent, icteric, and had severe ascites and massive edema; 6.8 liters of ascites fluid were removed on one occasion and 3.7 liters on another. He became progressively worse and died about a month later following a large hematemesis. At autopsy, the liver showed necrosis of most cells but there were cirrhotic areas as well. The kidneys showed severe nephrosis, and the heart muscle was degenerated. The brain was edematous, and there was degeneration of ganglion cells. The bone marrow was hyperactive.

Some workers in the paper mill had complained in 1959 about the strong odor and of irritation of the throat and eyes. Measurement showed that the average concentration of diphenyl in the air of different parts of the mill at that time ranged from 4.4 to 128 mg/m³. Minor improvements were made in ventilation, but no more measurements were made until January 1970, when the range was 0.6–123 mg/m³. (As early as 1947 and on the basis of animal studies, Deichmann *et al.* concluded that an air concentration of 5 mg/m³ should be considered dangerous for prolonged human exposure.)

The duties of the man who had died involved dermal exposure to diphenyl as well as extensive respiratory exposure to vapor and dust. Because his use of alcohol and his exposure to solvents had been completely inadequate to explain his illness, poisoning by diphenyl remained as the only reasonable explanation. This conclusion led to medical examination of one stockkeeper and one paper cutter in addition to all of the 31 men involved in impregnating paper with diphenyl. The most common complaints were headache, diffuse pain, nausea, indigestion, and numbness and aching of the limbs. Eight men were sick enough to require extensive examination including liver biopsy in hospital. Ten persons had some elevation of the SGOT or similar tests; three hospitalized patients had hepatic cellular changes. The neurological aspects of some of these cases led to special neurophysiological study of 1 woman and 23 men with occupational exposure to diphenyl. Fifteen persons had one or more pathological result. Ten men showed nonspecific electroencephalographic (EEG) abnormalities compatible with generalized cerebral involvement; the abnormalities persisted on reexamination 1 and 2 years later. Nine persons had electromyographic (EMG) abnormalities, and seven showed fibrillations in some muscles. One subject showed a long rhythmic series of fasciculations similar to the spontaneous activity described in infantile spinal muscular atrophy. Nerve conduction velocity, especially that of slower motor fibers, was reduced in several cases. The electroneuromyographic changes also persisted on reexamination (Hakkinen *et al.*, 1973; Seppalainen and Hakkinen, 1975). Although the findings reported among the 33 workers examined were impressive, it must be observed that they did not lead to spontaneous complaints. The workers were examined because the death of a fellow worker had been attributed to diphenyl. The massiveness of their exposure and the fact that abnormalities were found in such a high proportion of the workers leave no doubt that many of them were affected by diphenyl. The same epidemiological reasoning does not apply to the one man who died. His entire illness may have been caused by diphenyl, but there is no way to exclude the possibility that some other factor contributed to his exceptional course.

Apparently similar but far less severe poisoning also occurred among workers in another paper mill. Some of them suffered transient nausea, vomiting, and bronchitis (Weil *et al.*, 1965).

Dosage Response   The air levels that led to illnesses were as high as 128 mg/m³, implying potential dosages as high as 18 mg/kg/day. The experimental finding that a volunteer tolerated 1.4 mg/kg without adverse effect is consistent with the threshold limit value of 1.5 mg/m³, indicating that occupational intake at a rate of 0.2 mg/kg/day is considered safe.

21.9.3 CHLOROTHALONIL

21.9.3.1 Identity, Properties, and Uses

Chemical Name   Chlorothalonil is tetrachloroisophthalonitrile.

Structure   See Fig. 21.3.

Synonyms   Chlorothalonil (BSI, ISO, ANSI) is the common name in use. The compound is also known as TPN (JMAF). Trade names include Bravo®, Daconil®, Exotherm®, Forturf®, Nopocide®, and Termil®. The CAS registry number is 1897-45-6.

Physical and Chemical Properties   The empirical formula for chlorothalonil is $C_8Cl_4N_2$ and it has a molecular weight of 265.9. It forms odorless, colorless crystals with a melting point of 250–251°C, boiling point of 350°C, and vapor pressure of 9.7×10^{-3} mm Hg at 40°C. Chlorothalonil is soluble at 25°C in butanone, dimethylformamide, dimethyl sulfoxide, acetone (20 gm/kg), cyclohexanone (30 gm/kg), kerosene (<10 gm/kg), and xylene (80 gm/kg) and is only slightly soluble in water (0.6 mg/kg). The technical grade (approximately 98% pure) has a slightly pungent odor. Chlorothalonil is thermally stable under normal storage conditions and is stable to alkaline and acid aqueous solutions and to ultraviolet light.

History, Formulations, and Uses   Chlorothalonil was introduced in 1965 by Diamond Shamrock Co. It is used in agriculture, horticulture, and the timber industry as a fungicide and preservative. Its formulations include "Bravo W-75" and "Daconil® 2787W-75 Fungicide," wettable powder (750 gm active ingredient per kilogram) and "Bravo 500" and "Daconil Flowable," suspension concentrate (500 gm/liter).

21.9.3.2 Toxicity to Laboratory Animals

The acute toxicity of chlorothalonil by the oral and dermal routes was found to be low, but it was high by the respiratory route. The rat oral LD 50 was 10,000 mg/kg, the rat inhalation LD 50 was 4.7 mg/kg, and the rabbit acute percutaneous LD 50 was 10,000 mg/kg. In 2-year feeding trials, no ill effect was observed in rats fed chlorothalonil at 60 ppm in the diet and in dogs given chlorothalonil at a dietary level of 120 ppm. At higher dietary levels given to rats and dogs, histological examination suggested a toxicological problem associated with the kidney [World Health Organization (WHO), 1975]. Cutaneous irritation studies with New Zealand White rabbits demonstrated the influence of solvent vehicle on the degree of primary dermal irritation. Chlorothalonil, 0.1% in saline, did not cause a significant increase in irritation. Petrolatum alone produced a mild degree of irritation, but when chlorothalonil was included the index doubled. Acetone was nonirritant but there was a considerable increase with chlorothalonil added (Flannigan and Tucker, 1985). A further study in rabbits using a cumulative irritation assay confirmed the irritant properties of 0.1% chlorothalonil in acetone and produced evidence that 0.01% chlorothalonil caused mild irritation below the threshold for clinical problems (Flannigan *et al.*, 1986).

Chlorothalonil is rapidly excreted primarily unchanged. A metabolite, the 4-hydroxy compound, is more acutely toxic, with an oral LD 50 in male rats of 332 mg/kg, and is more persistent than the parent molecules (WHO, 1975). In studies done at maternally toxic levels of chlorothalonil there were no effects on reproduction but there was some evidence of growth retardation in the pups. The results of mutagenicity and teratogenicity tests were negative within the parameters of the defined studies (Vettorazzi, 1977).

21.9.3.3 Toxicity to Humans

Use Experience   Although it appears to have been known as early as 1978 that occupational exposure to chlorothalonil could cause contact dermatitis in humans (Johnsson *et al.*, 1983), the first published reports appeared in 1980. A 55-year-old cabinetmaker acquired a dermatitis on his hands which gradually spread to his arms and sometimes also to his face after 9 months of handling a wood preservative containing chlorothalonil. The patient gave a positive patch test to a solution of 0.01% of chlorothalonil in acetone and a marked reaction to a 1% solution. In contrast, patch tests on groups of controls showed no reaction at 0.01% in 10 people, a positive reaction in 2 of 10 controls at 0.1%, and toxic skin reactions in the two persons tested with a 1% solution. The dermatitis disappeared when the cabinetmaker was away from work for 3 weeks but reappeared when he returned, possibly due to contact with wood dust produced by sandpapering (Bach and Pedersen, 1980). A similar report described skin reactions, especially periorbital, in three people after a similar type of work (Spindelreier and Deichmann, 1980). In what was described as an epidemic of contact dermatitis in a Norwegian wooden-ware factory, 14 of 20 workers had skin complaints which were attributed to chlorothalonil. Seven out of these 14 subjects had positive patch test reactions to a solution of 0.01% chlorothalonil in acetone, compared with only 1 of 14 controls (Johnsson *et al.*, 1983). Allergic contact dermatitis from chlorothalonil has been described in vegetable growers (Horinchi and Ando, 1980) and in horticulture workers (Bruynzeel and van Ketel, 1986).

Treatment of Poisoning   Treatment is symptomatic.

21.10 QUATERNARY NITROGEN FUNGICIDES

A number of quaternary nitrogen compounds are fungicides. A few are large, flat, multiring structures. However, there is no evidence that they behave in plants like the quaternary nitrogen herbicides; more important, there is no evidence that they behave in mammals like the herbicide paraquat (see Section 20.16.1).

Examples of quaternary nitrogen fungicides include benzalkonium chloride and phenacridane chloride. These compounds are used mainly as disinfectants and sanitizers. Their oral LD 50 values in rats are usually in the range of 230 to 1,250 mg/kg.

21.11 HYDRAZINES, HYDROZONES, AND DIAZO FUNGICIDES

Most compounds in this group are moderately toxic, as evidenced by oral LD 50 values in the rat ranging from 60 to 130 mg/kg. Examples include benquinox (ISO), drazoxolon (BSI, ISO), and fenaminosulf (BSI, ISO).

21.12 DITHIOCARBAMATES

21.12.1 INTRODUCTION

21.12.1.1 Classification and Metabolism

Classification   Most dithiocarbamate pesticides are used as fungicides: a few are used as herbicides; at least one, methamsodium, has important use as a nematocide. The chemical structures of the major subgroups and of some individual compounds are shown in Table 21.2. As may be seen, the division into subgroups is based on the character of the substitution for one or both hydrogens on each nitrogen. An important advantage of this classification is that it separates compounds capable of being metabolized to ethylene thiourea (ethylenebisdithiocarbamates) from compounds incapable of forming this compound. The reason that this may be important for human safety is discussed in a following section. Whereas ethylene thiourea may have no special importance for fungi, it is interesting that some consistent differences in fungicidal action of the two groups of fungicides can be recognized, according to Thorn and Ludwig (1962), in whose excellent book the basic chemistry and the applications of a wide range of dithiocarbamates are discussed in detail.

Metabolism   Apparently, the metabolism of no dithiocarbamate has been studied in sufficient detail. However, valuable insight can be gained by pooling information from all sources. Much of what we know comes from studies of disulfiram, a drug extensively used for treating alcoholism (see Fig. 21.4).

The metal or comparable moiety of each ethylenebisdithiocarbamate is lost in metabolism so that identifiable, nonmetal metabolites of the different compounds are identical (Truhaut *et al.*, 1973). This was illustrated by a study of [^{54}Mn]maneb which showed that no manganese complex was absorbed from the gastrointestinal tract of rats, whereas when [^{14}C]maneb was administered in the same way, about 50% of the activity appeared in the urine and 1% appeared in the expired air. Simultaneous administration of Fe(III), Zn(II), and Cu(II) significantly reduced the urinary excretion of ^{14}C. It was concluded that cations occurring naturally in food may influence the proportion of ethylenebisdithiocarbamate residues absorbed, especially at low dosage levels (Brocker and Schlatter, 1979). Nonmetal metabolites of ethylenebisdithiocarbamates that have been isolated are shown in Fig. 21.5. An extensive study of the degradation products of maneb, zineb, and nabam (Engst *et al.*, 1971) revealed nothing that would indicate a different mode of action, although the fraction rich in ethylenebisthiuram monosulfide was more toxic than the parent compounds (LD 50 values of 580 and 1570 mg/kg in mice and rats, respectively).

The initial metabolites of these ethylenebisdithiocarbamates are different from the initial metabolites of dimethyldithiocarbamates (compare Figs. 21.4 and 21.5). It appears that carbon disulfide and its metabolites are the only compounds common to the metabolism of all dithiocarbamate fungicides. It may be that this fact, rather than the nature of the compounds themselves,

Table 21.2
Identity of Some Fungicidal and One Herbicidal Dithiocarbamate

Name	Structural formula	R
Methyldithiocarbamates		
methan-sodium	$R{-}S{-}\overset{\overset{S}{\|}}{C}{-}\overset{\overset{H}{}}{N}\diagdown_{CH_3}$	Na^+
Dimethyldithiocarbamates		
DDC		Na^+
ferbam	$R{-}\left[{-}S{-}\overset{\overset{S}{\|}}{C}{-}N\diagup^{CH_3}_{\diagdown CH_3}\right]_n$	Fe^{3+}
thiram[b]		$S{-}C(S){-}N{-}(CH_3)_2$
ziram		Zn^{2+}
Diethyldithiocarbamate		Cl
sulfallate	$R{-}S{-}\overset{\overset{S}{\|}}{C}{-}N\diagup^{C_2H_5}_{\diagdown C_2H_5}$	$-CH{-}C{=}CH_2$
Ethylenebisdithiocarbamates[a]		
anobam		$(NH_4)_2$
maneb	$R\diagdown^{S{-}\overset{\overset{S}{\|}}{C}{-}\overset{\overset{H}{\|}}{N}{-}CH_2}_{S{-}\overset{\overset{S}{\|}}{C}{-}\overset{\overset{H}{\|}}{N}{-}CH_2}$	Mn
nabam[c]		$(Na)_2$
zineb[c]		Zn

[a]In addition to the compounds shown, there are several linear polymers such as metiram and mancozeb based on the same structure.

[b]Disulfiram is the ethyl analog.

[c]Compound is a polymer in which the ethylenebisdithiocarbamate moiety alternates with the divalent metal.

determines the similarity of the action of the materials both in fungi and in mammals. Of course, the properties of the fungicides themselves control their stability on treated plants, their absorption through living membranes, and (insofar as they persist) their distribution to specific reaction sites. The similarity of the toxic properties of different kinds of dithiocarbamates suggests the relative unimportance of the metals and of the other initial metabolites involved. Conversely, this similarity suggests the importance of the common metabolite, carbon disulfide, and of its metabolites. In fact, the similarity of poisoning by various dithiocarbamates and poisoning by carbon disulfide has been noted (Kane, 1970; Rainey and Neal, 1975). What has been said applies to the entire syndrome of acute poisoning by dithiocarbamates, to the results of their interaction with alcohol, and to most of the clinically evident effects of repeated exposure to dithiocarbamates; it does not apply to the antithyroid effects, which are not produced in humans or animals by carbon disulfide.

Table 21.3 records compounds that have been demonstrated to produce carbon disulfide under various conditions. Clearly, a high proportion of a dose of a dithiocarbamate may be metabolized to this compound. The portion of it that is exhaled presumably has not undergone reaction with tissue constituents, but exhalation is clear evidence for exposure of the tissues to this compound.

It has been claimed that thiourea is a major metabolite of carbon disulfide (Pergal *et al.*, 1972b). Since thiourea is an antithyroid substance, it might explain the tendency of different classes of dithiocarbamates to affect the thyroid. However, evidence for the identity of thiourea as a metabolite of carbon disulfide is weak and how such a conversion could occur is obscure. Thiourea cannot be considered a satisfactory explanation of the antithyroid effects of dithiocarbamates.

Hunter and Neal (1974) showed that ethylene thiourea is metabolized *in vivo* and *in vitro* to ethylene urea with the release of a highly reactive form of atomic sulfur. This reactive form of sulfur appears to bind to the macromolecules in the liver (the only organ studied) and bring about a decrease in the activity of some enzymes located in the endoplasmic reticulum. These workers postulated that the metabolic release and binding of atomic sulfur in the thyroid gland may be the cause of the decrease in iodination of tyrosine and the resultant thyroid dysfunction seen on exposure to this compound.

21.12.1.2 Toxicity

General Considerations All the dithiocarbamates are of moderate to extremely low acute toxicity. The oral LD 50 values of the compounds shown in Table 21.2 range from 285 to 7500 and average >2523 mg/kg. Relatively high proportions of the

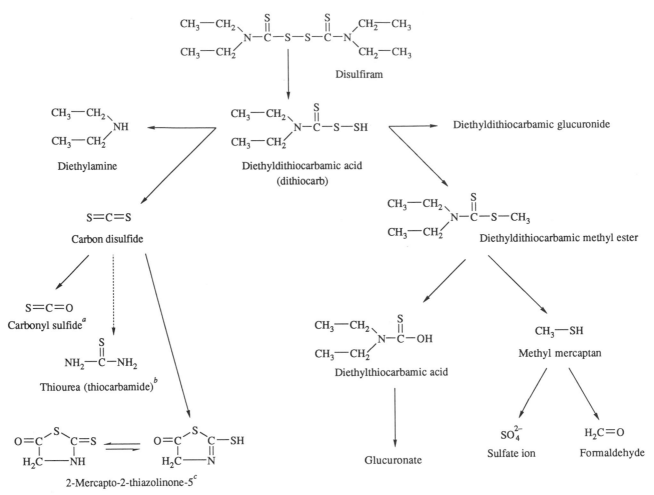

Figure 21.4   Metabolic pathways of disulfiram according to Gessner and Jakubowski (1972) and others, including (a) Dalvi et al. (1974), (b) Pergal et al. (1972b), and (c) Pergal et al. (1972a).

less toxic ones are eliminated unmetabolized in the feces. Regardless of the underlying mechanism, the net acute toxicity is increased greatly by alcohol.

A single dose of a dithiocarbamate can affect the thyroid, and repeated doses of some cause goiters.

Because they are metabolized to ethylene thiourea, the ethylenebisdithiocarbamates are suspected of being carcinogens.

Interaction with Alcohol   Disulfiram (Antabuse®) is the only dithiocarbamate that is used therapeutically to produce intolerance to alcohol. Use of disulfiram for this purpose was introduced by Hald and Jacobsen (1948a; Hald et al., 1948). The pharmacology was reported in a series of papers in a single issue of Acta Pharmacologica et Toxicologica, of which one by Hald, Jacobsen, and Larsen (1948) was the first. When several related compounds were investigated, thiram was found more effective in producing the "alcohol effect," but it was rejected because of its greater toxicity (Hald et al., 1952; Freundt and Netz, 1977). Repeated doses of disulfiram are employed but interaction with alcohol can occur following a single dose of the drug.

The interaction of thiuram compounds with alcohol has been confirmed in a study which examined structure–activity relationships (de Torres et al., 1983). Acetaldehyde production was measured in alcohol-dosed rats that had been given some dithiocarbamates and other nitrogen–carbon–sulfur compounds. The fungicides thiram and ziram all produced a comparable elevation in acetaldehyde concentrations but those obtained after zineb were less. Tetramethylthiuram monosulfide, a rubber accelerator, was more effective than any of the compounds evaluated, while the pesticide ANIT and the synthetic organic rodenticide ANTU failed to increase the blood acetaldehyde concentration. Calcium cyanide (Temposil®), which is used therapeutically for the treatment of alcoholism, was less active than thiram.

Following any given level of alcohol intake after treatment with disulfiram, the concentration of acetaldehyde in the blood is greatly and proportionally increased. The illness that treated persons develop if they drink, formerly was attributed to the high blood level of acetaldehyde (Hald and Jacobsen, 1948b; Asmussen et al., 1948). However, there has been a growing tendency to attribute the illness to some changes in the metabolism of disulfiram. As pointed out by Strömme (1965), the fact that ethanol lowers the rate at which diethyldithiocarbamate is conjugated with glucuronic acid offers a possible explanation because, at the very least, it would lead to the presence of a higher concentration of free diethyldithiocarbamic acid and per-

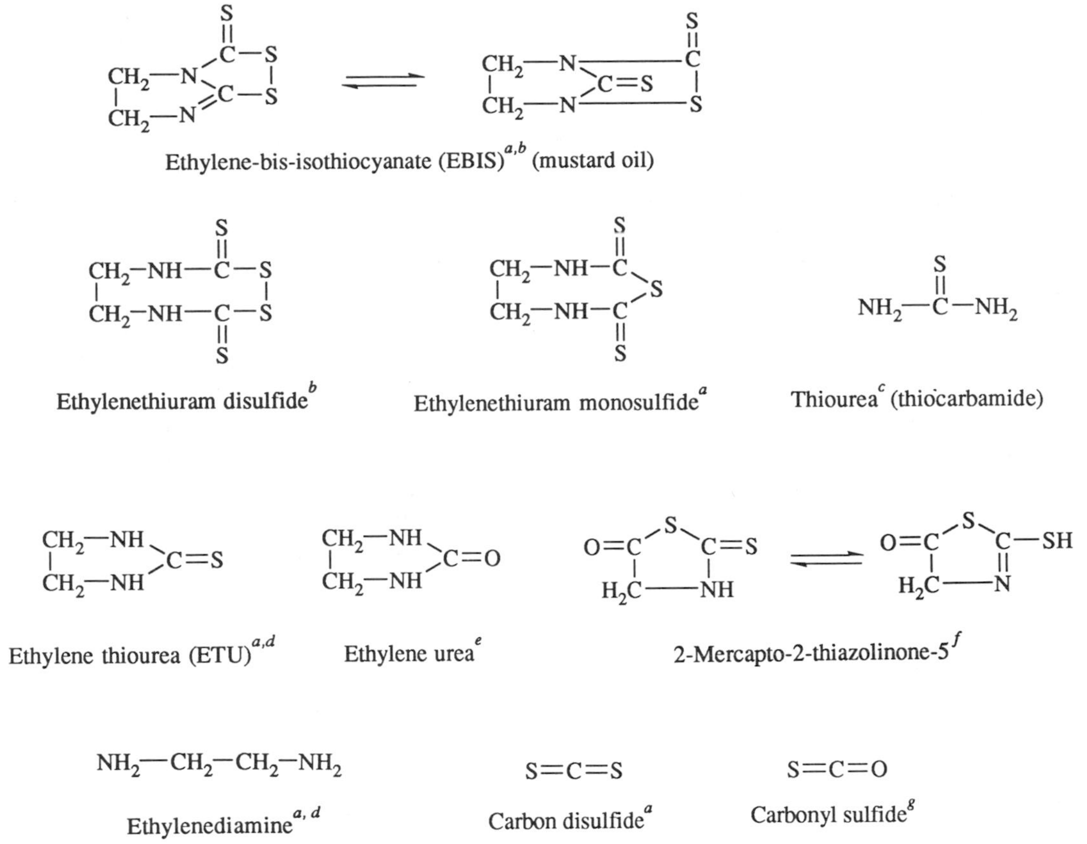

Ethylene-bis-isothiocyanate (EBIS)[a,b] (mustard oil)

Ethylenethiuram disulfide[b]   Ethylenethiuram monosulfide[a]   Thiourea[c] (thiocarbamide)

Ethylene thiourea (ETU)[a,d]   Ethylene urea[e]   2-Mercapto-2-thiazolinone-5[f]

$NH_2—CH_2—CH_2—NH_2$ $S=C=S$ $S=C=O$

Ethylenediamine[a,d]   Carbon disulfide[a]   Carbonyl sulfide[g]

Figure 21.5 Metabolites of diethylenedithiocarbamates as reported by (a) Truhaut *et al.* (1973), (b) Engst *et al.* (1971), (c) Pergal *et al.* (1972b), (d) Seidler *et al.* (1970), (e) Hunter and Neal (1974), (f) Pergal *et al.* (1972a), and (g) Dalvi *et al.* (1974).

Table 21.3
Compounds Demonstrated to Produce Carbon Disulfide under Different Conditions

Compound	Species and system	Proportion recovered as CS_2 (%)	Reference
disulfiram	human, *in vivo*, breath	46–53	Merlevede and Casier (1961)
sodium diethyl-dithio-car-bamate	human, *in vivo*, breath	28–82	Merlevede and Casier (1961)
zineb	rat, *in vivo*, breath	NM[a]	Truhaut *et al.* (1973)
disulfiram	rat, liver homogenate	NM	Johnston and Prickett (1952)
disulfiram	rat, *in vivo*, breath	NM	Johnston and Prickett (1952)
disulfiram	rat, *in vivo*, breath	2	Strömme (1965)
thiram	rat, *in vivo*, blood	0.003	Melson and Weigelt (1967)

[a]Identified but not measured.

haps to the production of more carbon disulfide. Aversion to alcohol has been noted in men with occupational exposure to carbon disulfide (Novak *et al.*, 1969; Mihail *et al.*, 1970). Arguing against the importance of CS_2 in this regard is the finding of Merlevede and Casier (1961) that the percentage of disulfiram expired as CS_2 usually was not changed following administration of alcohol; however, when a change did occur it was a slight increase, as expected. Later experiments in anesthetized dogs led Casier and Merlevede (1962) to conclude that neither acetaldehyde nor carbon disulfide or any other metabolite of disulfiram was responsible for the acute toxic effects seen after the administration of disulfiram and alcohol. Instead, they concluded that the illness was caused by a compound formed either *in vitro* or *in vivo* by interaction of disulfiram and alcohol. The compound was crystallized. It was speculated that it might be a quaternary nitrogen compound, but no evidence was presented and it was administered as a suspension. Signs of poisoning, including apnea for 30 sec and a fall of blood pressure amounting to 20–30 mm Hg, were considered typical following an intravenous dosage of only 3 mg/kg. Higher dosages produced more persistent effects and often a greater fall in blood pressure.

In rare cases, disulfiram apparently can cause hepatotoxicity even when alcohol presumably is not involved. Potentiation by alcohol is difficult to disprove in such cases because only alcoholics receive the drug in the first place. In any event, Ranek and

Andreasen (1977) cited three cases from the literature and reported six others. Jaundice and other signs of liver disease started 3–25 weeks after administration of the drug began. In five of the cases there was only circumstantial evidence for a causal relationship because the patients died. However, in one case hepatitis due to disulfiram was confirmed by a challenge test.

It is interesting that one or more compounds in some mushrooms produce, in combination with alcohol, a condition similar to that produced by disulfiram and alcohol (Reynolds and Lowe, 1965).

Jakivarto (1950) reported that intravenous iron preparations quickly reverse the symptoms of the disulfiram–alcohol interaction, especially if given immediately after the alcohol is consumed. He used "Ferroscorbin," a Finnish product, administering 100 mg of ascorbic acid and 45.6 mg of ferrous chloride in 10 ml of distilled water. Whether intravenous iron is of use in treating poisoning by a dithiocarbamate not complicated by alcohol apparently has not been explored.

Antithyroid Effects Animal studies of maneb (Bankowska *et al.*, 1970), zineb (Bankowska *et al.*, 1970; Lessel and Cliffe, 1961), mancozeb (Larson, 1965), thiram (Griepentrog, 1962), and disulfiram (Christensen and Wase, 1954) have shown that the smallest dosage producing any clearly measurable effect usually affects the thyroid alone or the thyroid and other organs, depending on experimental conditions. In these studies, the useful criteria of effect have been reduction of uptake of radioactive iodine (Christensen and Wase, 1954; Bankowska *et al.*, 1970) and hypertrophy of the gland (Bankowska *et al.*, 1970; Christensen and Wase, 1954; Griepentrog, 1962; Larson, 1965). Protein-bound iodine and metabolic rate have been measured but were not sensitive criteria (Larson, 1965).

The effect of dithiocarbamates on iodine uptake by the thyroid is prompt. For example, marked reduction of iodine uptake was present when first measured 24 hr after a large dose of either maneb or zineb (Ivanova *et al.*, 1967). Reversal of early changes in the thyroid also is prompt. For example, slight hyperplasia caused by a dietary level of 1000 ppm zineb was reversed when animals were first examined 2 weeks after feeding was discontinued (Lessel and Cliffe, 1961).

There is a strong suggestion, if not proof, that some dithiocarbamates are much more active than others as antithyroid compounds. For example, Hodge *et al.* (1956) considered zineb to be clearly goitrogenic but questioned whether ziram affected the thyroid because the few changes they saw in rats treated with ziram were not dosage-related. They speculated that the difference might be related to the presence of hydrogen on each nitrogen of zineb, possibly permitting enolization and the formation of active —SH groups. However, the primary amines as a group do not seem any more active antithyroid compounds than the secondary amines.

Teratogenicity Several dithiocarbamates including maneb and zineb are teratogenic in rats. As discussed in Section 21.12.4.2, simultaneous administration of zinc acetate was capable of reducing the incidence of malformations caused by a large dosage of maneb, and the improvement increased with increasing dosage of zinc. However, because ethylenethiourea is teratogenic and also is a metabolite of ethylenebisdithiocarbamates including maneb, the effect of zinc acetate on the teratogenic action of ethylenethiourea was tested. No protective effect was found, and the zinc content of the maternal plasma and the conceptus was not changed when zinc acetate was fed to rats at a zinc concentration of 444 ppm (about 22 mg/kg/day) during days 11–14 of pregnancy (Khera and Shah, 1979). It is unclear what bearing these experiments have on the mechanism of teratogenicity of dithiocarbamates. Khera and Shah (1979) pointed out that the mechanism of action of zinc is unproved and may be due to local action in the gastrointestinal tract and not to overcoming a hypothetical deficiency of zinc in the maternal and/or fetal tissues. Finally, the possibility has not been excluded that the teratogenic actions of ethylenebisdithiocarbamate and ethylenethiourea are different, although they cause similar types of anomalies.

Carcinogenicity The suspicion that dithiocarbamates are carcinogenic involves two concerns: tumors arising in hyperplastic thyroid tissue as a result of hormonal imbalance and tumors of the liver and to a lesser degree other tissues. Ethylenethiourea at a dosage of 215 mg/kg/day was tumorogenic in mice (Innes *et al.*, 1969). Whereas emphasis has been placed on this metabolite as a basis for the possible carcinogenicity of compounds capable of forming it, dithiocarbamates incapable of forming it have been found tumorigenic; they include selenium diethyldithiocarbamate (Innes *et al.*, 1969) and potassium bis (2-hydroxyethyl)dithiocarbamate (Innes *et al.*, 1969).

Two mechanisms might be offered to explain the possible carcinogenicity of dithiocarbamates, including those that are not capable of forming ethylenethiourea. One mechanism depends on the carcinogenic action of thiourea. Fitzhugh and Nelson (1948) found liver tumors in 14 of 29 rats surviving a 2-year toxicity test. It will be recalled, however, that doubt has been expressed that thiourea is a metabolite of dithiocarbamates; even if it is a metabolite, there would remain a question of whether it reaches a critical dosage level. Another mechanism of possible carcinogenicity of dithiocarbamates is suggested by an observation of Eisenbrand *et al.* (1974). When ziram and nitrite solutions were introduced into the stomachs of rats, an average of 0.126 mg of dimethylnitrosamine was detectable within 15 min; this constituted about 0.9% of the theoretical yield. However, as noted in Section 21.12.2.2, thiram was not found tumorigenic by direct test.

As pointed out by a working group on the evaluation of the carcinogenic risk of chemicals to humans (WHO, 1974), the induction of thyroid tumors by antithyroid substances is a result of suppression of the rate of synthesis of thyroxine, leading to a hormonal imbalance. The group also considered that there is need to elucidate both the biological and morphological nature of tumors resulting from antithyroid substances in order to evaluate the carcinogenic risk arising from exposure to them.

Obviously, the absorption of dithiocarbamates by workers should not be as great as that of alcoholics who wish to break their habit. It does add perspective, however, to note that the usual dosage of disulfiram is 500 mg/person/day (about 7 mg/kg/day) for 2 weeks followed by 125–500 mg/person/day for months to years, depending on the individual.

Another perspective is offered by the finding that disulfiram at dietary levels of 200, 1000, and 5000 ppm, maneb at 5000 ppm, bis(ethylxanthogen) at 1000 and 5000 ppm, and sodium diethyldithiocarbamate at 300, 1500, and 7500 ppm for 17 weeks inhibited the development of bowel tumors that otherwise would have been induced in female mice by 16 weekly subcutaneous injections of 1,2-dimethylhydrazine at the rate of 0.4 mg/mouse. Injections of the carcinogen were started 1 week after the experimental diets began and stopped when the diets stopped. Where multiple levels of the dithio compounds were used, a definite dosage response was demonstrated. All the effective compounds were capable of metabolism to carbon disulfide, and chlorpropham, a carbamate that contains no sulfur, was not effective. Similar but somewhat less striking effects were obtained when azoxymethane was used as the carcinogen. It was thought likely that the dithio compounds inhibit the metabolism of 1,2-dimethylhydrazine at more than one oxidative step (Wattenberg *et al.*, 1977).

Other matters that must be considered in evaluating occupational or environmental exposure to dithiocarbamates are the natural occurrence of antithyroid compounds in food and the use of antithyroid compounds as drugs. Although the occurrence of antithyroid compounds in foods, especially such foods as cabbage, turnip, and rutabaga, is well recognized (Van Etten and Wolff, 1973), quantitative information that would permit a meaningful comparison between exposure from this source and likely exposure from dithiocarbamate fungicides appears to be lacking.

There is no hesitation in giving therapeutically effective doses of antithyroid drugs to patients with hyperthyroidism. While acknowledging that such people would not be treated if they were not sick in the first place, the incidence of tumors among them following therapy offers some indication of this particular danger of the drugs. Among 35,613 people treated for hyperthyroidism, malignant tumors of the thyroid were found at some time following treatment in 0.323% of 1238 treated with drugs, 0.460% of the 11,732 treated by surgery, and 0.129% of the 21,714 treated by radiation. However, none of the tumors in the drug patients were considered anaplastic, and there were no tumor-related deaths in this group. By contrast, the death rate among those judged to have malignant tumors of the thyroid was 7.4% for those treated earlier by surgery and 21% for those treated earlier by radiation (Dobyns *et al.*, 1974). Because of the complexity of the factors involved, no claim for statistical significance of the results can be made. However, the data contained nothing to suggest a serious danger of malignancy following treatment with antithyroid drugs.

Implications for Human Health It is clear that under practical conditions the greatest danger of dithiocarbamates to workers is associated with the potentiating action of these compounds and alcohol. A less serious but more common effect of some formulations has been dermatitis and/or irritation of mucous membranes (Bilancia, 1964; Shelley, 1964; Laborie *et al.*, 1964; Gunther, 1970). However, this is not sufficiently common or severe to interfere seriously with use of the materials.

A rare but serious danger that presumably might result from any one of the compounds was illustrated by the sulfhemoglobinemia and acute hemolytic anemia caused by zineb in a person with glucose-6-phosphate dehydrogenase deficiency and hypocatalasemia (Pinkhas *et al.*, 1963).

Reports of goiter and of other conditions not so clearly related to dithiocarbamates among workers exposed to thiram in the USSR (see Section 21.12.2.3) suggest either massive exposure or the presence of a highly toxic contaminant, or both. In other areas, the safety record of the dithiocarbamates is good.

21.12.2 THIRAM

21.12.2.1 Identity, Properties, and Uses

Chemical Name Thiram is tetramethylthiuram disulfide.

Structure See Table 21.2.

Synonyms The common name thiram (BSI, ISO) is in general use. In Japan the name used is thiuram, and in the Soviet Union the name is TMTD. Other nonproprietary names have included TMT and TMTDS. Trade names include Arasan®, Fernasan®, Nomersan®, Pomarsol®, Puralin®, Rezifilm®, Spotrete®, Tersan®, Thiosan®, Thiuramyl®, Thiurad®, Thiuram®, Thylate®, Tiuramyl®, Tuads®, and Tulisan®. The CAS registry number is 137-26-8.

Physical and Chemical Properties Thiram has the empirical formula $C_6H_{12}N_2S_4$ and a molecular weight of 240.44. It forms colorless crystals with a density of 1.29 at 20°C and a melting point of 155–156°C. Its solubility in water at room temperature is about 30 ppm. It is slightly soluble in ethanol and diethyl ether; it is soluble in acetone and chloroform.

History, Formulations, and Uses Thiram was introduced by E.I. du Pont de Nemours and Company, Inc. in 1931. It is formulated as wettable powder with up to 800 gm of active ingredient per kilogram. Dusts are used for seed treatment; the compound also is used in mixtures with other fungicides.

21.12.2.2 Toxicity to Laboratory Animals

As shown in Table 21.4, thiram is a compound of low acute toxicity. In rats and mice, large dosages of thiram caused ataxia and hyperactivity followed by inactivity, loss of muscular tone, labored breathing, and clonic convulsions. Most animals died within 2–7 days, but some died during the second week (Lee *et al.*, 1978).

A dietary level of 2500 ppm was fatal to all rats within 17 weeks; levels of 1000 ppm (about 49 mg/kg/day) did not increase mortality in a 2-year feeding test but did produce weakness, ataxia, and varying degrees of paralysis of the hind legs. A

Table 21.4
Single-Dose LD 50 for Thiram

Species	Route	LD 50 (mg/kg)	Reference
Rat	oral	865	Lehman (1951, 1952)
Rat, M	oral	640	Gaines (1969)
Rat, F	oral	620	Gaines (1969)
Rat, M	oral	4000	Lee *et al.* (1978)
Rat, F	oral	1900	Lee *et al.* (1978)
Rat, M	dermal	>2000	Gaines (1969)
Rat, F	dermal	>2000	Gaines (1969)
Mouse	oral	1500–2000	Kirchheim (1951)
Mouse, M	oral	4000	Lee *et al.* (1978)
Mouse, F	oral	3800	Lee *et al.* (1978)
Mouse	intraperitoneal	250	Hald *et al.* (1952)
Sheep	oral	225	Antsiferov *et al.* (1973)

few animals on a dietary level of 300 ppm developed the same symptoms. A dietary level of 100 ppm (about 4.9 mg/kg/day) was a no-effect level (Lehman, 1951, 1952, 1965). Similar results were reported by Lee *et al.* (1978). In a study lasting 80 weeks, paralysis and atrophy of the hind legs was seen in some female rats receiving 67 mg/kg/day. Patches of alopecia occurred in some male and female rats receiving 52–67 mg/kg/day and in a few receiving 20–26 mg/kg/day. Except for a very mild depression in growth of both sexes and a mild fatty infiltration of the pancreas in females, dosages of 5 mg/kg/day in males and 6 mg/kg/day in females were no-effect levels.

Lehman (1965) recorded a 1-year study in dogs showing that a dietary level of 200 ppm (about 4 mg/kg/day) was a no-effect level.

Allergic sensitization of guinea pigs by the subcutaneous and tracheal routes but not by the oral route has been reported (Brusilovskiy and Fialkovskiy, 1973a,b).

Tibial dyschondroplasia (TD) has been observed in broiler chickens administered thiram (Vargas *et al.*, 1983). In another investigation thiram was administered at dietary levels of 0, 30, and 60 ppm for a period of 6 weeks to day-old single-comb white leghorn chicks. Although these chicks are normally resistant to TD, the birds exhibited skeletal changes as early as 2 weeks of age. The highest incidence (67%) occurred in 6-week-old birds fed 60 ppm thiram in the diet (Veltmann *et al.*, 1985; Veltmann and Linton, 1986).

Absorption, Distribution, Metabolism, and Excretion
Rats were administered thiram intraperitoneally. The formation of carbon disulfide from thiram appeared to be dosage dependent. Increasing the dose from 15 to 30 mg/kg resulted in a 10-fold increase in the amount of CS_2 in the expired air. When the dose was increased four times to 60 mg/kg the CS_2 production was 40 times more than that at 15 mg/kg. In addition, it appears that the liver microsomal enzyme system is involved in the metabolism of thiram to CS_2. Although phenobarbitone treatment did not significantly increase the formation of CS_2, administration of the enzyme inhibitor SKF 525A significantly re-

duced the amount of carbon disulfide produced. It was concluded that CS_2 produced from thiram contributes to its toxicity to the liver (Dalvi and Deoras, 1986).

Biochemical Effects Thiram inhibits the conversion of [^{14}C]dopamine to [^{14}C]noradrenaline in the heart and adrenal of the rat and hamster (Lippmann and Lloyd, 1971).

Oral dosages of thiram ranging from 5 to 200 mg/kg caused a decrease in liver DNA and soluble liver protein and an increase in liver RNA. These shifts were prevented by concomitant treatment with thymidine (Sedokur, 1971). It had been reported earlier (Gal and Greenberg, 1954) that several B vitamins and ascorbic acid counteract the inhibition of alcohol metabolism and thus minimize the increase in acetaldehyde in the blood of animals given disulfiram followed by ethanol. The inhibition of microsomal enzymes has been confirmed (Zemaitis and Greene, 1979). At dosages of 0.05 LD 50 per day for 6 days or 0.02 LD 50 per day for 4 months, thiram inhibited liver microsomal enzymes of rats, as evidenced by increased hexabarbital sleeping time, but it also caused an increase in liver weight (Kolycheva *et al.*, 1973; Nadzhimutdinoz *et al.*, 1974).

Treatment of rats with thiram at a dose of 60 mg/kg caused a significant loss of cytochrome P-450 and benzphentamine *N*-demethylase activity in microsomal preparations but an elevation in the levels of serum sorbitol dehydrogenase and serum glutamic-oxalacetic transaminase, indicating probable liver damage (Dalvi and Deoras, 1986).

Effects on Organs and Tissues Unlike carbaryl, an insecticidal carbamate, thiram produced leukopenia, thrombocytopenia, suppression of hematopoiesis, and slowing of blood coagulation in rabbits when administered at a rate of 0.1 LD 50 per day for 15 days (Karpenko, 1971). A reduction of adrenal cortex functional reserve also has been reported (Dyadicheva, 1971). Repeated administration of thiram at a rate of 0.5 but not at a rate of 0.1 mg/kg/day interfered with phagocytosis and other aspects of immunity (Perelygin *et al.*, 1971). If these changes were confirmed, their relationship to suppression of thyroid function would remain obscure.

Tertiary amines, including thiram, can be nitrosated *in vitro* in the presence of nitrite under conditions that resemble those in the stomach (Egert and Greim, 1976). Whether this has any significance related to cancer in humans is uncertain; in 1970 the average dietary intake of all dithiocarbamates in the United States was <0.001 mg/person/day.

Thiram was found mutagenic to some microorganisms but not others. It was considered that the *N*-dimethyl group is necessary for mutagenic action of dithiocarbamates (Moriya *et al.*, 1978a; Zdzienicka *et al.*, 1979).

It is considered that inhibition of enzymes involved in the protection against oxygen species accounts for the mutagenicity of dithiocarbamates. The mutagenicity of thiram was enhanced by the addition of a microsomal enzyme system and by oxygen. Furthermore, thiram potentiated the mutagenic action of menadione, a substance that produces superoxide radicals in microsomes (Rannug and Rannug, 1984).

When administered to mice at the highest tolerated level, thiram was not carcinogenic (Innes *et al.*, 1969). Lee *et al.* (1978) found that thiram did not alter the occurrence or latent period of spontaneous tumors seen in control rats. This was consistent with the earlier finding of Lehman (1965) that dietary levels of 2500 ppm or less for 2 years caused no difference in the incidence of tumors. An expert group (WHO, 1976) regarded the available information as inconclusive but provided no substantial evidence to justify a positive conclusion.

The ataxia and paralysis of the hind legs reported by Lehman (1951, 1952, 1965) in rats poisoned by thiram was confirmed and shown to be associated with chromatolysis and pyknosis of neurons in the ventral horns of the lower lumbar region and with degeneration of the axons and demyelination of the sciatic nerve (Lee and Peters, 1976).

Effects on Reproduction   A dietary level of 100 ppm (about 4.9 mg/kg/day in adults) was a no-effect level in a three-generation reproduction study in rats (Lehman, 1965).

It has been reported that exposure of female rats to thiram in the air at a concentration of 3.8 mg/m³ 6 hr/day, 5 days/week, for 4.5 months reduced their rate of conception, their fertility, and the weight of the fetuses they produced (Davydova, 1973).

Oral administration of 30 mg of thiram per mouse to two strains of mice (about 1200 mg/kg/day) on days 6–17 of gestation produced, in addition to increased resorption of embryos and retarded fetal development, cleft palate, wavy ribs, curved long bones of the legs, and micrognathia. There was a clear dosage response. The ineffective dosage was approximately 250 mg/kg/day (Roll, 1971).

Both the severity and incidence of malformations caused by thiram were reduced by simultaneous administration of L-cysteine at a rate of 10 mg/animal/day (Matthiaschk, 1973).

Another study in mice included gametogenesis and the peri- and postnatal periods as well as organogenesis. A dosage of 132 mg/kg/day for 13 weeks produced infertility in males and a dosage of 96 mg/kg for 14 days delayed the estrous cycle in females. A maternal dosage of 40 mg/kg/day on days 6–15 of gestation reduced maternal weight gain and fetal body weight. Litter size was decreased at a dosage of 136 mg/kg/day or higher. Some mice died when given thiram at a rate of 300 mg/kg/day on days 6–14 of gestation, but development was not affected in the survivors. There was an increase in anomalies among both rats and mice at high dosages that injured the dams, but there was no pattern of well-defined anomalies, and the changes observed were considered the result of depressed growth. The administration of thiram to rats at a dietary level of 1000 ppm from gestation day 16 through postpartum day 21 reduced the growth and survival of pups; however, the pups remained healthy if transferred to control dams at birth, whereas control pups were injured when suckled by treated dams. Thiram interfered with reproduction only at dosage levels that produced toxicity in the adult (Short *et al.*, 1976; Vasilos *et al.*, 1978).

In hamsters, thiram was teratogenic but the very closely related drug disulfiram was not. Defects included exencephaly, spina bifida, fused ribs, and abnormalities of the legs, heart, great vessels, and kidneys. The proportion of abnormal fetuses was increased about four times at a maternal dosage of 125 mg/kg, the lowest dosage studied (Robens, 1969). The author pointed out that the dosages employed were at least 1000 times what people would receive from the levels permitted in food and even more extreme compared with what actually occurs in food.

Behavioral Effects   Possible interactions between thiram and some drugs acting on the central nervous system were investigated in rats by using behavioral methods. Potentiation was found after combined treatment with thiram and promethazine (Phenergan®) and after thiram and meprobamate (Equanil®). For trihexyphenidyl (Artane®) an additive interaction was observed (Fenyvesi *et al.*, 1985).

Pathology   Rounded calcified masses were found in the basal ganglia of the cerebellum of rats killed by a dietary level of 2500 ppm or kept on 1000 ppm (or in one of a group of rats on 300 ppm) for 2 years (Lehman, 1965). This unusual pathology apparently has not been explained, but for practical purposes tissue damage in animals killed by thiram is not diagnostic. Diagnosis must be based on chemical analysis (Antsiferov *et al.*, 1974).

21.12.2.3 Toxicity to Humans

Therapeutic Use   Percival (1942) reported the successful, nonirritating use of thiram for treating human scabies. Use of the compound as a sun screen or as a bactericide either applied directly to the skin or incorporated into soap has also been mentioned (Shelley, 1964).

Accidental and Intentional Poisoning   The basis for the interaction of dithiocarbamates with alcohol is discussed in Section 21.12.1.2. Examples of this systemic illness precipitated by thiram have been noted (Mihail *et al.*, 1970; Kaskevich and Bezuglyy, 1973b). In a typical instance, a 38-year-old floriculturist who had used thiram at his greenhouses previously without untoward effect became ill following application of about 1 kg each of thiram and captan dust on a very hot night. Although he protected his mouth during the operation, he was wearing only a shirt and short pants. He consumed only about half a liter of beer before going to bed. Following a restless night, he arose with gastric pains, nausea, vomiting, hyperirritability, a fine tremor of the fingers and tongue, blood pressure of 150/85 mm Hg, slight fever, and moderate lymphopenia. He was admitted to hospital, where he remained for 3 days (Reinl, 1966).

A much more severe case followed exposure to thiram for only 10 min in the process of mixing it with water, but the whisky ingested the evening before presumably contained more alcohol than is present in 0.5 liter of beer. In any event, in addition to the gastrointestinal upset, headache, and weakness that caused the patient to enter hospital 6 hr after exposure to thiram, the patient was found to have albumin, urobilinogen, and numerous casts in his urine and increased transaminase activity in his serum. On the fourth day, liver enlargement and severe ulceration of the oral cavity appeared. Both the liver enlargement and the ulceration persisted for 3 weeks despite symptomatic treatment (Krupa *et al.*, 1971). Ulceration of the mouth apparently has not been reported in otherwise similar cases; whether in this case it was a direct result of herpes (perhaps predisposed by poisoning) or was a direct but unexplained result of poisoning is not clear.

The interaction between a dithiocarbamate and alcohol has such a resemblance to severe poisoning by a dithiocarbamate alone that it is difficult to distinguish the two when neither the exact dosage of dithiocarbamate nor the involvement of alcohol is known. An example appears to be a case reported by Marcinkowski and Manikowski (1973). A man became ill and died 4 days after treating seed with thiram. He had done this work for 10 hr, and he had mixed the fungicide and seed with a spade rather than with a machine made for the purpose. It is clear that he received a substantial exposure, but whether he received enough thiram to produce death without exposure to alcohol is unclear.

The interaction of dithiocarbamates with alcohol can produce not only systemic illness but also dermatitis, and both of these reactions occur in everyone who is sufficiently exposed. By contrast, thiram without alcohol can produce contact dermatitis but only in a few susceptible people. The alcohol-related dermatitis is a transient affair occurring soon after ingestion of alcohol. The less frequent contact dermatitis is much more protracted and can persist as long as exposure to thiram continues. Oddly enough, there is an example of both kinds of dermatitis, each involving only the relatively slight exposure that golf players and bowlers receive in playing on thiram-treated greens.

In one of these examples, a man developed urticaria of the face and hands on three Sundays on which he bowled a few games on a green that had been treated with thiram. The condition was diagnosed as contact dermatitis on the basis of history and of a positive patch test. However, it was noted that the man had a few beers to drink each day he was exposed to the fungicidal residue (Gunther, 1970).

In the other example, a man suffered dermatitis for 3 years but only during the season when he played golf. During the first winters, the condition regressed completely, but after the third season of play the dermatitis persisted during the winter and then became progressively worse. When seen in August, the dermatitis was a severe, chronic, fissured, erythematous, and scaling eruption of the hands, forearms, neck, face, and legs, and there were numerous patches of eczematous change on the chest. The condition was traced to thiram used on golf greens, and the relationship was confirmed by patch test. The dermatitis cleared within 6 months after the patient avoided thiram completely (Shelley, 1964).

Use Experience A review of the literature (Shelley, 1964) showed that thiram has been (and in some instances still is) used as a catalytic accelerator in the vulcanization of rubber and for other purposes. One of the first reports of dermatitis associated with thiram involved rubber workers (Schwartz and Tulipan, 1933). At least a few cases have been associated with all the other uses, and instances of cross-sensitization to different products or to analogs of thiram (notably disulfiram) have been recorded.

Contact dermatitis to thiram is not common. In a study of 309 dermatologic patients who used for 2 weeks or more a soap containing the compound, only eight had any difficulty. There was reason to think that seven of these reactions were due to the soap rather than the bactericide. Only one positive reaction to thiram was seen when 214 people were patch-tested with it (Baer and Rosenthal, 1954). On the contrary, among 229 patients who had sought help in a dermatology clinic as a result of reactions to shoes or rubber, 7.97% gave positive patch tests to thiram (Baer *et al.*, 1973). A review of thiram in comparison with a wide range of other compounds reveals that it is an example of a borderline allergen, requiring repeated exposure before sensitizing potential appears (Kligman, 1967).

A case involving hand eczema following repeated exposure to rubber gloves has been reported. A surgical assistant who developed delayed-type contact dermatitis from rubber gloves showed positive patch tests to thiram. After several weeks holiday the dermatitis had healed, but shortly after starting operations again the original condition reoccurred (van Ketel, 1984). In a more detailed study the same author examined cross-sensitization between some dithiocarbamates in patients and surgical staff with proven allergy to thiram compounds. The reactions to the dithiocarbamate compounds were compared to those obtained with hypoallergenic and dithiocarbamate-containing surgical gloves. Although the results were equivocal, it appears that cross-sensitization to dithiocarbamates in thiram-allergic subjects has to be regarded as possible, and these people are advised to wear nonreacting rubber or PVC gloves (van Ketel and van den Berg, 1984). In view of possible cross-reactivity, this recommendation has particular significance for pesticide workers handling dithiocarbamates.

With the important exception of alcohol intolerance and the occasional occurrence of dermatitis, which is less serious, use experience with thiram has been good. Exceptions involve reports from the USSR of a sympathetic vascular, asthenic syndrome and many other complaints in as many as 50% of workers who were exposed to the compound (Khomenko and Kazakevich, 1973; Lyubchenko *et al.*, 1973; Sivitskaya, 1974; Yurchenko *et al.*, 1976) and of abnormalities of external respiration in persons with polyneuropathy or other nervous troubles attributed to pesticides (Doroscuk, 1974). Other investigators have emphasized liver injury (Kaskevich, 1975). Such findings are difficult to interpret because the same syndromes were reported in connection with compounds such as chlorinated hydrocarbon insecticides that are chemically and toxicologically unrelated. It is tempting to speculate that the syndromes may depend on a contaminant or other unrecognized factors. More readily understood as an effect of thiram were the reports of goiters in workers involved with thiram-treated seed (Cherpak *et al.*, 1971; D'yachuk, 1972; Kaskevich and Bezuglyy, 1973a). The same workers had numerous other complaints and findings. Concentrations of thiram in workroom air averaged $0.2–5.0 \, mg/m^3$ and were as high as $12.5 \, mg/m^3$ (D'yachuk, 1972). In another study the concentrations ranged from 0.03 to $3.2 \, mg/m^3$ (Kaskevich and Bezuglyy, 1973a).

Dosage Response Little information is available on dosages of thiram that have led to illness in humans. A guide can be estimated from disulfiram, for which the maintenance dosage to discourage alcoholism is 3.6 mg/kg/day. The threshold limit value of $5 \, mg/m^3$ for thiram indicates that occupational intake at the rate of 0.7 mg/kg/day is considered safe. This value may have to be modified for individuals who have become sensitized to thiram and related compounds. Oral administration of thiram (20 mg/day) for 2 days to a woman with a history of allergic dermatitis resulted in recurrence of the symptoms. The authors suggested that her eczema, which occurred at atypical sites remote from possible dermal contact, may have been caused by a dietary factor, noting that these compounds are used as antifermentive agents in food (Goitre et al., 1981).

Laboratory Findings The xanthurenic acid level in the urine of workers exposed to thiram was reported to be 38.5–59.6 mg/day, compared to 20–25 mg/day in controls (Sedokur and Luk'yanchuk, 1976).

Treatment of Poisoning Treatment is entirely symptomatic.

21.12.3 ZIRAM

21.12.3.1 Identity, Properties, and Uses

Chemical Name Ziram is zinc dimethyldithiocarbamate.

Structure See Table 21.2.

Synonyms The common name ziram (BSI, ISO, JMAF) is in general use except in West Germany, where it is regarded as a trademark. Trade names include Corozate®, Fuclasin®, Fuklasin®, Karbam White®, Mathasan®, Milbam®, Nibam®, Zimate®, and Zirberk®. The CAS registry number is 137-30-4.

Physical and Chemical Properties Ziram has the empirical formula $C_6H_{12}N_2S_4Zn$ and a molecular weight of 305.82. It is a white, odorless powder with a melting point of 250°C. It has a negligible vapor pressure at room temperature. The density at 23°C is 1.66. The solubility of ziram in water is 65 ppm at 25°C. It is slightly soluble in ethanol and diethyl ether and moderately soluble in acetone. It is soluble in dilute alkali, chloroform, and carbon disulfide. Ziram is stable under normal conditions but is decomposed by acids; it is compatible with other pesticides except copper and mercury compounds.

History, Formulations, and Uses Ziram was introduced in the early 1930s by E.I. du Pont de Nemours and Company, Inc. It is available as a 76% wettable powder. It is a protective fungicide for use on fruit and vegetable crops.

Table 21.5
Single-Dose LD 50 for Ziram

Species	Route	LD 50 (mg/kg)	Reference
Rat, F	oral	1400	Hodge et al. (1952)
Rat, M	intraperitoneal	23	Hodge et al. (1952)
Rat, F	intraperitoneal	33	Hodge et al. (1952)
Mouse	intraperitoneal	17	Kligman and Rosensweig (1948)
Mouse, M	intraperitoneal	73	Hodge et al. (1952)
Rabbit	oral	400	Brieger and Hodes (1949)
	intraperitoneal	5–50	Hodge et al. (1952)

21.12.3.2 Toxicity to Laboratory Animals

Basic Findings As shown in Table 21.5, ziram is a compound of moderate to low acute oral toxicity. The fact that the intraperitoneal toxicity is substantially greater suggests that absorption of an oral dose is relatively slow and/or incomplete.

Following intraperitoneal injection of ziram at an approximately LD 50 rate, animals show no reaction during the first hour; later they become stuporous and die in coma. Survivors appear entirely normal within 24 or 48 hr (Hodge et al., 1952).

Rats survived dietary levels of 5000 and 2500 ppm for a month, but growth was retarded and there was slight anemia. Growth retardation at 500 ppm was slight but possibly significant. At 100 ppm, growth equaled or surpassed that of controls. There were no significant histological changes in the thyroid or in other organs when the animals were killed for examination (Hodge et al., 1952). Later, Hodge et al. (1956) in a 2-year experiment confirmed that growth was retarded in rats fed 2500 ppm (about 125 mg/kg/day) even though their life span was normal. A dietary level of 250 did not interfere with growth. Rats that had received the compound at the rate of 2500 for about 2 months or more showed an abnormal reflex; when picked up by the tail, they did not thrust their hind legs out like normal rats but instead clasped the hind feet or crossed and stiffened their hind legs. Histological study of the rats after 2 years of feeding showed no significant changes with the possible exception of atrophy of the testis and hypertrophy of the thyroid. However, the intensity of these changes did not correspond to dosage, and both may occur in controls, although they did not in this particular experiment. Based largely on the experiments just reviewed, Lehman (1965) considered a dietary level of 250 ppm (about 12.5 mg/kg/day) to be the no-effect level for ziram in the rat.

Convulsions occurred in dogs fed ziram at a rate of 25 mg/kg/day, and some died after being dosed for 5–9 months. Symptomatology, hematology, urinalysis, organ weights, and histology were normal in dogs fed 5.0 or 0.5 mg/kg/day for 1 year (Hodge et al., 1956).

When placed in the conjunctival sac of rabbits, ziram was moderately irritating, whereas DDC, feram, and the corresponding calcium compounds were not (Kligman and Rosensweig, 1948). This indicates that the irritation was caused by the zinc and not by the dimethyldithiocarbamate moiety.

Absorption, Distribution, Metabolism, and Excretion
Rats that had received ziram at a dietary level of 2500 ppm for 2 years had a concentration of about 4 ppm of the compound in the liver. Thus an animal that received about 30 mg/day for 2 years had at most only 0.03 mg of the substance in its liver. On the contrary, the concentration of zinc stored in bone increased in an almost linear fashion corresponding to the logarithm of the concentration of ziram in the diet, the means increasing from 180 to 300 ppm zinc in bone ash in animals maintained for 2 years on diets containing 0 and 2500 ppm ziram, respectively. Thus, ziram is not stored but the zinc metabolized from it is stored to a slight degree (Hodge *et al.*, 1956).

Following oral administration of [^{35}S]ziram, rats eliminated a portion in the feces (largely in chloroform-soluble form) but by far the majority was excreted in the urine as water-soluble metabolites. After 24 hr only small concentrations, mainly in water-soluble form, remained in the tissues (Izmirova and Marinov, 1972). In addition to ziram, five chloroform-soluble metabolites and five water-soluble metabolites were distinguished by paper chromatography. In the feces, 57% of the chloroform-soluble activity was unchanged ziram. The five chloroform-soluble metabolites were found in the gastric contents, among other locations (Izmirova, 1972), suggesting but certainly not proving that part of the breakdown of ziram occurs before absorption.

The metabolism of dimethyldithiocarbamate fungicides is discussed in Section 13.12.1.1. In studies of ziram in rats, Vekshtein and Khitsenko (1971) confirmed the production of dimethyldithiocarbamic acid, dimethylamine, and carbon disulfide, and they reported two compounds that lacked zinc but contained four methyl groups that other investigators have not found.

Effects on Organs and Tissues A number of immunological changes were reported to appear and disappear at varying intervals in female rats that received oral doses of ziram for 9 months at a rate of 2.5 mg/kg/day (Shtenberg *et al.*, 1972).

Ziram is not tumorigenic (Hodge *et al.*, 1956; Innes *et al.*, 1969). Although an expert committee (WHO, 1976) cited no substantial evidence to the contrary, they considered the question still open.

Effects on Reproduction Rats that received ziram at a dosage of 50 mg/kg/day for 2 months or more became relatively sterile; some fetuses that were conceived were resorbed and some that were born had abnormal tails. A dosage level of 10 mg/kg/day produced no significant effect on reproduction (Ryazanova, 1967a).

21.12.3.3 Toxicity to Humans

Use Experience Use experience with ziram has been good with certain exceptions in the USSR. Enikeev (1968) pointed out that the material is a vulcanizing agent as well as a fungicide and considered aerosols of it in the workplace to constitute its principal danger. Injury consisted of irritation of the skin, nose,

throat, and eyes; gastritis; reduced hemoglobin; and vegetodystonia. Similar difficulties were described in several collective-farm workers who used a 70% formulation of ziram to treat seed. Several women had to be hospitalized for 2–4 days; they were considered recovered in 25 days. Some other workers lost as much as 3 days of work (Chernov, 1968). The method of treating the seed was not stated. On the contrary, apparently less severe irritation of the skin and upper respiratory tract was encountered in a factory where the concentration of ziram in the air ranged from 0.77 to 3.7 mg/m^3 (Martson' and Pilinskaya, 1971).

Possible inhibition of cholinesterase and changes in the bioelectric activity of the muscles during voluntary motion were reported in studies of workers (Komarova and Zotkina, 1971).

Abnormal chromosomes or chromatids were reported in 5.9% of cultured lymphocytes of workers with 3–5 years of occupational exposure to ziram, compared to 0.75% abnormalities in similar cells from controls. The concentration of ziram in the storage and packing areas of the workplace averaged 1.95 and 3.7 mg/m^3 but reached 71.3 mg/m^3 in isolated cases; prior to 1965 it had been much higher (Pilinskaya, 1970). The same author (Pilinskaya, 1971) later reported a dosage-related increase in chromosomal aberrations in cultured human lymphocytes at concentrations of 0.06, 0.015, and 0.003 ppm, but no effect at 0.0006 ppm. The changes in these *in vitro* experiments were mainly in chromosome 2. At a concentration of 0.003 ppm, the changes were quantitatively similar to those in persons with occupational exposure. The blood levels of ziram or its metabolites in such persons were not stated.

Pathology The ingestion of 0.5 liter of ziram solution was fatal within a few hours. Findings included focal necrosis of the mucosa of the small intestine, congestion and microscopic edema of many organs, diapedetic hemorrhages, focal atelectases, acute emphysema, and desquamation of alveolar and bronchial epithelium (Buklan, 1974). Apparently, there was no record of the concentration of the solution or of whether the patient had consumed alcohol. The pathology was, of course, nonspecific.

Treatment of Poisoning Treatment of poisoning by ziram is symptomatic.

21.12.4 MANEB

21.12.4.1 Identity, Properties, and Uses

Chemical Name Maneb is manganese 1,2-ethanediyl-bis(carbamodithioate).

Structure See Table 21.2.

Synonyms The common name maneb (BSI, ISO JMAF) is in general use. Another nonproprietary name is MEB. Trade names include Dithane M-22® and Manzate®. The CAS registry number is 12427-38-2.

Physical and Chemical Properties Maneb has the empirical formula $C_4H_6MnN_4S_4$ and a molecular weight of 265.29. It is a yellow crystalline solid that decomposes before melting. It is moderately soluble in water and insoluble in most organic solvents. Maneb is stable under normal storage conditions, but it decomposes rapidly on exposure to moisture or to acids.

History, Formulations, and Uses Maneb was introduced in 1950 by E.I. du Pont de Nemours and Company, Inc. It usually is formulated as a wettable powder (800 gm of active ingredient per kilogram). Maneb is a protective fungicide effective against many foliar blights, particularly of potato and tomato.

21.12.4.2 Toxicity to Laboratory Animals

Basic Findings Maneb has a low acute oral toxicity, the LD 50 in rats being 6750 mg/kg (FAO/WHO, 1968). Later studies indicated values of 8000 mg/kg for rats and mice of both sexes. Following a single large dose, rats and mice showed ataxia and hyperactivity followed by inactivity, loss of muscular tone, and alopecia. Most deaths occurred within 1–2 days (Lee *et al.*, 1978).

Rats that received 1500 mg/kg/day orally for 10 days showed weight loss, weakness of the hind legs, and increased mortality. When intake was prolonged for 90 days, mortality reached 80% in rats fed 10,000 ppm in their food (<500 mg/kg/day). In a 2-year study, mortality was increased at a dietary level of 2500 ppm, but this also impaired food consumption and growth and increased the relative weight of the liver. A level of 1250 ppm also produced some depression of growth and an increase in the relative weight of the liver. Rats tolerated dietary levels of 250 ppm (about 12.5 mg/kg/day) for 2 years (FAO/WHO, 1965, 1968).

Dogs fed maneb at a rate of 200 mg/kg/day developed flaccid paraplegia and were moribund within 3–7 months. Those receiving 75 mg/kg/day for 1 year showed persistent anorexia and weight loss, and 20 mg/kg/day produced similar but less severe effects. Toxic signs included tremors, weakness, gastrointestinal disturbances, and depression of reflexes, of coordination, and of tone of the hind legs. There was also evidence of impaired kidney function at dosages of 75 and 200 mg/kg/day. A dosage of 2 mg/kg/day produced no detectable effect (FAO/WHO, 1965).

A single respiratory exposure at a concentration of 700 mg/m³ or repeated exposure at 300 mg/m³ is toxic; the thresholds are 15 and 4.7 mg/m³ for single and repeated exposures. No embryotoxic effect was seen in rats exposed to concentrations of 30 mg/m³ or less (Matokhnyuk, 1971).

Absorption, Distribution, Metabolism, and Excretion When rats received [^{14}C]maneb by stomach tube at rates of 333–390 mg/kg, nearly 55% of the dose administered was excreted in the form of metabolites in the feces and urine within 5 days. The feces and urine contained ethylenediamine, ethylenebis-thiuram monosulfide, ethylenebis thiourea, and other unidentified metabolites (Seidler *et al.*, 1970). When [^{14}C]maneb was administered to mice by stomach tube, the proportions of the dose recovered in the feces and urine within 48 hr at one dosage level were 91.0 and 9.0%, respectively, and were 92.7 and 7.3% at the other dosage. No activity was recovered as $^{14}CO_2$. Of the smaller proportion in the urine, the part present as ethylene thiourea was 15.8 and 7.8% in the two studies. Most of the urinary metabolites were more polar than ethylene thiourea (Jordan and Neal, 1979).

Maneb was not found in the tissues of rats fed dietary levels as high as 2500 ppm for 2 years or in the tissues of dogs that received 75 mg/kg/day for 1 year (FAO/WHO, 1968).

Effects on Organs and Tissues Gross and microscopic changes in the thyroid gland, reduced uptake of radioactive iodine, and slightly reduced respiratory activity of liver mitochondria were observed in rats fed maneb at a concentration of 5000 ppm for 6 weeks. These and other parameters were normal in those fed 500 ppm (Bankowska *et al.*, 1970). Similar results were reported by others in rats fed 5000 ppm or more. At levels of 10,000 and 30,000 ppm, diffuse sclerosis accompanied proliferative changes of the thyroid (Kusevitskiy *et al.*, 1970). Rats receiving the same dosage levels (perhaps the same animals) showed morphological evidence of injury to the testes and ovaries (Kirlich, 1970). Whether the same degree of thyroid deficiency produced in another way would be associated with the same degree of gonadal damage apparently was not explored.

Morphological details of the effect of 30 large doses of maneb on the rat thyroid were reported by Ivanova-Tchemishanska *et al.* (1971). The decrease in thyroglobulin was demonstrated by electrophoresis of thyroid tissue of rats treated with maneb or ethylene thiourea (Sobotka, 1971).

Male rats that had inhaled maneb for 4 months at concentrations of 2 and 100 mg/m³ showed changes in the activity of lactate dehydrogenase isoenzymes of the testis, some being increased and others decreased (Izmirova *et al.*, 1969).

Using an unusually thorough protocol for studying the effects on rats of a dietary level of 150 ppm for 90 days (about 7.4 mg/kg/day), Seidler *et al.*, (1975) found that thyroxine levels were affected more strongly than triiodothyronine levels. Ethylene thiourea at the same dietary level produced the same reaction, but more strongly. The changes indicated interference with thyroxine storage or metabolism and interference with the oxidation of iodine and with hormone synthesis. The high thyroid quotient was indicative of stimulation of the thyroid gland, probably by thyrotropin. Part of the maneb was excreted unchanged in the feces before it could be metabolized to ethylene thiourea. Any direct reaction of maneb or its metabolites with iodine under physiological conditions was considered impossible.

In contrast, single doses of maneb (20–200 mg/kg, ip) to rats significantly decreased the cold-induced endogenous thyroid stimulating hormone (TSH) response. It had no effect on TSH secretion after administration of thyrotropin releasing hormone (TRH) or on serum levels of triiodothyronine and thyroxine. It is suggested that maneb inhibits rat TSH secretion at the hypothalamic or pituitary level by inhibition of dopamine β-hydroxylase (Laisi *et al.*, 1985).

Dosages of 300 mg/kg/day or greater but not dosages of 150

mg/kg/day or less produced ataxia and paralysis in rats. These effects occurred earlier and much more frequently in females. The neuropathy tended to resolve if dosing was stopped, whether or not the rats had become paralyzed (Rosenstein *et al.*, 1978).

Maneb was not tumorigenic when tested in two strains of mice at the highest tolerated level (Innes *et al.*, 1969). A second study in mice (Balin, 1970) revealed a significant increase in lung adenomas in one strain but not in another. Maneb administered orally to rats at 500 mg/kg once a week for 6 months induced adenoma of the lungs. The tumors mainly were subpleural in location and papillary in form. Even so, an expert committee considered the available data inadequate for evaluating the carcinogenicity of maneb (WHO, 1976).

Effects on Reproduction In a standard three-generation test at dietary levels of 0, 125, and 250 ppm, no effect was seen on fertility, gestation, viability, lactation, or litter size, and no gross or histological abnormalities were found in animals selected for study from the F_3 generation (FAO/WHO, 1968). The highest dietary level tested is equivalent to about 12.5 mg/kg/day for most adults but is higher for pups and lactating females.

When maneb was given to rats by stomach tube every other day during pregnancy at a rate of 50 mg/kg, the incidence of resorption, stillbirth, and nonviable young were doubled. Fertility was decreased in both males and females when they were fed maneb for 1 month and then 1.5 months later mated to animals on control diet. Normal function returned after 3.5 months (Marston', 1969). The statistical significance of these findings is unclear, but they are consistent with a report by Shtenberg *et al.* (1969) for rats dosed for 11 or 12 months. In those receiving 30 mg/kg/day, fertility was reduced and there was a high rate of stillbirths and neonatal deaths. Fertility was reduced at a dosage of 10 mg/kg/day; no dysfunction was reported at 5 mg/kg/day.

When maneb was administered to pregnant rats by stomach tube on either day 11 or 13 of organogenesis, congenital anomalies were produced by dosages of 1000, 2000, and 3000 mg/kg, and their frequency and severity were dosage-related. The anomalies were diverse and, at the highest dosage level, massive. The maximal dosage at which no teratogenic effect was observed was 500 mg/kg on either day 11 or 13. It was concluded that any hazard to normal development of the human embryo as a result of present levels of exposure to maneb in agriculture is unlikely (Petrova-Vergieva and Ivanova-Tchemishanska, 1973). At a maternal oral dosage of 770 mg/kg on day 11 of pregnancy, maneb dependably produced malformations in 100% of surviving rat pups. Simultaneous administration of zinc acetate at a dosage of 15 mg/kg did not decrease the incidence of deformity, but dosages of 30 and 60 mg/kg reduced the incidence to 64 and 11%, respectively. It was speculated that the mechanism of the teratogenicity of maneb is related to zinc deficiency (Larsson *et al.*, 1976).

Maneb was not teratogenic in mice (Larsson *et al.*, 1976).

Pathology Rats that received maneb by stomach tube for as long as 4 months at rates of 100 and 500 mg/kg/day showed proliferative changes of the epithelium of the thyroid, focal necrosis and other changes of the liver, but no change of the central nervous system (Balin, 1969). Nodular goiter was seen in rats fed maneb at a dietary level of 2500 ppm for 2 years (FAO/WHO, 1965).

Dogs that had received an oral dosage of 200 mg/kg/day for 3 or more months until they were moribund revealed spinal cord damage but no effect on the thyroid gland (FAO/WHO, 1965).

21.12.4.3 Toxicity to Humans

Use Experience Use experience has been good, but a few cases have occurred. A 55-year-old foreman of Japanese descent had used the compound for several years without difficulty. Following 1 week of spraying in 1958 he developed a marked, vesicular skin reaction resembling poison oak dermatitis. The reaction was confined to the face, neck, and hands and disappeared following administration of triamcinolone (Hayes, 1982).

Among certain citrus growers in Japan, the incidence of skin disease ranged from 38 to 61% in different years. Patch tests indicated that, of compounds thought to cause this disease, maneb caused the greatest primary irritation (Arimatsu *et al.*, 1978; Shiaku *et al.*, 1979). This conclusion seems contradictory to the conclusion reached earlier by Arimatsu *et al.* (1976) to the effect that dermatitis caused by dithiocarbamate fungicides is of the allergic type. Dermatitis has not been restricted to persons of Japanese ancestry; cases have been reported from the Netherlands (Nater *et al.*, 1979).

A case of dermatitis involving nonoccupational exposure has been reported in a female whose husband had stored maneb near their washer and dryer (Adams and Manchester, 1982).

Atypical Cases of Various Origins A 42-year-old man sprayed Manzidan®, a combination of maneb and zineb, on a cucumber plantation on two occasions during a week. After the first application behavioral changes appeared, which were exacerbated on the second occasion with loss of consciousness, convulsions, right hemiparesis, and diffuse slow rhythm in the EEG. Both behavioral and central nervous system (CNS) symptomatology disappeared after a few days. In view of the previous history of the patient, the sudden appearance and spontaneous disappearance of the symptoms, as well as an apparent dosage–response relationship, the authors concluded that maneb and zineb were the cause of the illness (Israeli *et al.*, 1983).

Treatment of Poisoning Treatment is symptomatic.

21.12.5 ZINEB

21.12.5.1 Identity, Properties, and Uses

Chemical Name Zineb is zinc ethylenebisdithiocarbamate.

Structure See Table 21.2.

Synonyms Zineb (BSI, ISO, JMAF) is the common name in use except for West Germany. Trade names include Dithane

Z-78®, Lodacol®, and Parzat®. The CAS registry number is 12122-67-7.

Physical and Chemical Properties The empirical formula for zineb is $C_4H_6N_2S_4Zn$, and it has a molecular weight of 275.75. It is a light-colored powder that decomposes before melting. Its vapor pressure at room temperature is negligible. Its solubility in water at room temperature is about 10 ppm. It is unstable to light, heat, and moisture.

History, Formulations, and Uses Zineb was introduced by the Rohm and Haas Company and by E.I. du Pont de Nemours and Company. It is a fungicide used for foliage protection and is nonphytotoxic except to zinc-sensitive varieties. It is formulated as wettable powder (70 and 75%) or as dust.

21.12.5.2 Toxicity to Experimental Animals

Basic Findings Zineb has a very low acute toxicity. Oral LD 50 values of >5200 mg/kg (Smith et al., 1953), 4400 mg/kg (Ivanova et al., 1966), and >5000 mg/kg (Gaines, 1969) have been reported in the rat; the dermal LD 50 in the same species is too high to measure (>2500 mg/kg) (Gaines, 1969). Lee et al., (1978) reported oral LD 50 values of 8200 and 8900 mg/kg for male and female rats and corresponding values of 7600 and 7000 mg/kg in mice. Following a large dose, the rats and mice showed ataxia and hyperactivity followed by inactivity, loss of muscular tone, and alopecia. Most deaths occurred within 1–2 days. The compound is not significantly irritating to the mucosa of the rabbit eye (Smith et al., 1953).

A dietary level of 500 ppm (the lowest concentration fed, equivalent to about 24.5 mg/kg/day) produced a statistically significant increase in the weight of the thyroid in rats fed for 30 days. However, a dietary level of 10,000 ppm for the same period was required to produce an abnormal degree of thyroid hyperplasia as judged by microscopic sections, and even then the change was not present in all animals.

In a 2-year study a dietary level of 10,000 ppm increased mortality of female rats; the results were equivocal at 5000 ppm, but neither level increased the mortality of males. A level of 10,000 ppm diminished growth and caused some kidney pathology in both sexes. The thyroid changes were essentially similar to those seen in the 30-day study. Other findings including those of hematological studies were normal (Smith et al., 1953).

Dietary levels up to 10,000 ppm for 1 year did not affect the survival, growth, or hematological findings in dogs. A level of 10,000 ppm did increase the weight of the thyroid gland and cause microscopically detectable hyperplasia. Other histological findings were normal at all feeding levels. Dietary levels of 2000 ppm (about 42 mg/kg/day) or less produced no detectable effect on the thyroid (Smith et al., 1953).

Sheep were killed within 3 weeks by oral doses of zineb at a rate of 500 mg/kg. Injury of the liver and kidney was evident at autopsy but may have been conditioned by intercurrent infection. Other sheep showed no adverse effect from dosages of 100 or 250 mg/kg/day for 19 weeks (Palmer, 1963b).

Absorption, Distribution, Metabolism, and Excretion
Smith et al. (1953) concluded that only 11–17% of an oral dose of zineb is absorbed from the gastrointestinal tract of the rat. Some additional material may be absorbed following breakdown in the intestine. At different dietary levels 68.5–74.9% of the ingested material was recovered unchanged in the feces. For metabolism see Section 21.12.1.1.

Biochemical Effects Dietary levels of zineb as low as 60 ppm (but not 15 ppm) for 4 weeks caused a reduction of some but not all hepatic microsomal oxygenases in rats (Pelissier et al., 1976). An essentially identical result was obtained by the same group of investigators (Lowy et al., 1977) using a more sensitive statistical approach. According to the most sensitive parameter (inhibition of aniline hydroxylase) the calculated least effective dosage was 74 ± 15 ppm. The corresponding calculated no-effect level with a confidence limit of 95% was 2 ± 0.3 ppm.

Five isoenzymes of lactate dehydrogenase were unaffected in the testes of rats that had inhaled zineb for 4 months at a concentration of 100 mg/m³ (Izmirova et al., 1969).

Prior exposure of intact animals to zineb slightly reduced the ability of rat liver microsomes to metabolize aflatoxin B but increased this activity in mouse liver microsomes (Decloitre and Hamon, 1979).

Effects on Organs and Tissues The mean lethal concentration (LC 50) of zineb for certain human cells in culture was 1976 ppm; low concentrations did not decrease mitosis or cause cell degeneration (Shpirt, 1973). For Chinese hamster ovary cells the LC 50 was 6×10^{-6} M (about 1.65 ppm) (Hodgson and Lee, 1977). The reason for the great difference in reported dosage effect is unknown.

Kiryushin (1975) reported that six daily oral doses of zineb at 1/15 of the LD 50 level caused gaps and chromatid breaks in bone marrow cells, but a 10-day intermission was sufficient for return to a normal chromosome picture.

In two strains of mice, the maximal tolerated dosage of zineb for life was not tumorigenic (Innes et al., 1969). In another study, oral dosages of 3500 mg/kg/week for 6 weeks caused one strain of mice to develop within 3 months more lung adenomas than were found in controls but caused no increase in a second strain. In the first strain, a dosage of 1750 mg/kg/week caused no significant increase in tumors (Chernov and Khitsenko, 1969).

There was no significant change in the incidence or kind of tumors in control rats and those fed different dietary levels of zineb up to 10,000 ppm (Smith et al., 1953). In another study in which oral doses were given to rats twice weekly at a rate of 285 mg/kg for as much as 22 months, there was not a statistically significant difference in the incidences of tumors between the treated rats and the controls (Andrianova and Alekseev, 1970).

Of 48 rats that received subcutaneous implantation of a paraffin pellet containing zineb at a dosage of 20 mg/kg, only six survived for 22 months; of these, four had tumors (one hepatoma, one fibrosarcoma, one spindle-cell sarcoma, and one rhabdomyosarcoma), compared with one fibrosarcoma among 46 controls that received no paraffin pellet (Andrianova and Alekseev, 1970). Although the difference was statistically significant, the lack of a proper control leaves the biological significance of the study in doubt.

A single intraperitoneal injection of mice with 4 mg of zineb (about 160 mg/kg) during the second half of pregnancy led to abortion in many instances and to weak young in other instances; of 38 young that survived the neonatal period, 18 died within 4 months. The remaining 20 were killed at 4 months, and 30% of them showed lung adenomas as well as preadenomas (Kvitnitskaya and Kolesnichenko, 1971).

It is clear that low dosages of zineb are not carcinogenic. Even for the high dosages that have been used, the IARC working group (WHO, 1976) concluded that the available data did not allow an evaluation of the carcinogenicity of the compound.

Oral doses of zineb at the rate of 125 mg/kg/day for 6 months retarded development of the splenic follicles in young rats, but 12.5 mg/kg/day produced negligible changes (Dinoyeva, 1974).

In male rats, a massive dosage (1000 mg/kg/day for 30 days) produced no illness but increased the weight and cellularity of the thyroid, increased the weight of the pituitary, and led to seminal tubular necrosis and giant cell formation without change in the weight of the testes (Raizada *et al.*, 1979).

Single doses of zineb (70–500 mg/kg, ip) significantly decreased TSH levels after cold induced endogenous and exogenous TRH. As found with maneb, administration of zineb did not significantly alter triiodothyronine and thyroxine levels in serum. The authors proposed that the action of zineb was at the hypothalamic or pituitary level, possibly by inhibition of dopamine β-hydroxylase (Laisi *et al.*, 1985).

Effects on Reproduction Two intraperitoneal doses of 8 mg (about 320 mg/kg/day) administered to mice during the last half of pregnancy produced abortion or stillbirth in most instances; three or more doses reduced living young to zero (Kvitnitskaya and Kolesnichenko, 1971).

A single oral dose of zineb at the rate of 8000 mg/kg on day 11 of gestation produced numerous terata in rats, as did four doses at the rate of 2000 mg/kg on days 10–13. Nineteen doses at the rate of 1000 mg/kg/day on days 2–20 produced no fetal anomalies (Petrova-Vergieva and Ivanova-Tchemishanska, 1971, 1973).

In a more realistic study, it was found that oral doses of zineb at a rate of 100 mg/kg/day for 2 months or more produced sterility, resorption of fetuses, and anomalous tails in newborn rats. However, 50 mg/kg/day for 6 months did not produce any significant changes compared with a control group (Ryazanova, 1967b).

21.12.5.3 Toxicity to Humans

Experimental Exposure Of 50 subjects patch-tested with zineb, 49 showed no reaction following initial application or reapplication to the opposite forearm 14 days later. One subject developed a small, papular eruption that persisted about a week following both applications, indicating primary irritation rather than sensitization (Smith *et al.*, 1953).

Use Experience Zorin (1970) reported 86 cases of dermatitis among people working in tobacco fields that had been sprayed with zineb 2–15 days earlier. Teen-age youngsters and young women were most susceptible. The condition lasted 5–15 days and involved hyperemia, vesicular rash, and edema. Skin tests carried out on former patients were positive in most instances. Nishiyama (1974) also mentioned skin irritation but found that applicators were exposed to only a very small fraction of the dangerous dose and following exposure showed no change in any of a wide range of clinical laboratory tests.

Two cases of dermatitis shown by skin tests to be caused by zineb were described by Jung (1976). At least one of the cases was considered to be due to sensitization following repeated contact over a period of several weeks. However, in a zineb factory the incidence of contact dermatitis was reduced from 21.4 to 3.25% by reducing leaks in the equipment and by stricter compliance with safety rules (Tomashivskiy, 1975). Thus various kinds of dermatitis can be reduced by minimizing exposure whether sensitization is involved or not.

A change in liver mixed-function oxidase as measured by urinary metabolites of an oral dose of aminopyrine was reported in all workers exposed to zineb (Popov, 1977).

Pilinskaya (1974) reported an increase in the frequency of aberrant metaphases in lymphocytes cultured from workers who had been manufacturing zineb for 1–10 months. The report was inconsistent regarding chromosomal aberrations. The author (Pilinskaya, 1976) suggested that the effects could be avoided by keeping exposure below the maximal allowable concentration.

Moderate anemia and other blood changes were reported in 150 female workers exposed to zineb in a chemical plant. The incidence of toxicosis during pregnancy was higher than in controls, and it was concluded that pregnant females should not be exposed to zineb (Neyko *et al.*, 1974). The statistical validity of the findings is open to question in view of the limited number of pregnancies involved.

The respiration of 41 male workers was measured after they had manufactured zineb for 1 and 6 months, respectively. Changes were reported in respiratory rate, minute volume, reserve coefficient, and oxygen consumption. Although oxygen consumption was greater in the workers, it was concluded that exposure to zineb may reduce the bronchial passage (Gerasimchuk *et al.*, 1975).

Atypical Cases of Various Origins Sulfhemoglobinemia associated with Heinz body formation and acute hemolytic anemia followed the exposure to zineb of a 32-year-old farmer who, on a hereditary basis, had low glucose-6-phosphate dehydrogenase activity, low and unstable reduced glutathione, and catalase activity only about 6–7% of normal. His only exposure resulted from working and eating breakfast in a field that had been sprayed with zineb during the early hours of the same morning. He began to feel unwell about noon and was hospitalized the same day. On the next day he became semicomatose, and his condition became critical on the fourth day, when his hemoglobin had dropped to 4.7% and his red cell count was only 1.7 million/mm^3. The patient responded to transfusion with blood and packed red cells. Three months later, when the patient was clinically normal, it was shown that zineb decreased the concentration of reduced glutathione in red blood cells from him and from other persons with the same enzymatic defect (Pinkhas *et al.*, 1963).

Allergic symptoms (sore throat, globus sensation, pain when swallowing, nausea, fever, and anxiety) occurred in a 43-year-old woman 2 hr after she began work in a field treated earlier with zineb. Forty-eight hours later the patient developed a dangerous edema of the laryngeal opening. The patient recovered following specialized treatment (Schubel and Linss, 1971).

A case involving behavioral and CNS effects after exposure to zineb and maneb has been reported (Section 21.12.4.3.).

Treatment of Poisoning   Treatment is symptomatic.

21.12.6 MANCOZEB

21.12.6.1 Identity, Properties, and Uses

Chemical Name   Mancozeb is manganese ethylenebis-(dithiocarbamate) (polymeric) complex with zinc salt. The ISO definition is a "complex of zinc and maneb containing 20% of manganese and 2.55% of zinc, the salt present being stated (for instance, mancozeb chloride)."

Structure   See Table 21.2.

Synonyms   Mancozeb (BSI, ISO) is the common name in use. Manzeb (JHAF) is also used. A trade name for the compound is Dithane M-45®. The CAS registry number is 8018-01-7.

Physical and Chemical Properties   Mancozeb is a grayish-yellow powder which decomposes without melting. The flash point (Tag open cup) is 137.8°C. Mancozeb is practically insoluble in water and most organic solvents. It is stable under normal storage conditions but is decomposed at high temperatures by moisture and by acid.

History, Formulations, and Uses   Mancozeb was introduced by Rohm & Haas Co. It is effective against a wide range of fungal diseases. It is used in combination with zineb against a range of foliage fungal diseases. Formulations include Dithane M-45®, Dithane 945® wettable powder (>800 gm mancozeb per kilogram), and Karamate® (mancozeb and zineb).

21.12.6.2 Toxicity to Laboratory Animals

Basic Findings   Mancozeb has a very low acute toxicity. The rat oral LD 50 value is 8000 mg/kg. In a long-term study in rats fed mancozeb in the diet at 100 ppm, there were no toxicological effects. In a 2-year feeding study on the dog a lower I uptake was observed in the 100 and 1000 ppm dietary groups after 24 months, but not at 6 and 12 months; the 25 ppm group did not differ from the controls (FAO/WHO, 1968). Male rats exposed to mancozeb at a concentration of 100 mg/m³ for 10 days (6 hr/day) over a 2-week period had a significant depression of

average body weight gain (Lu and Kennedy, 1986). In a three-generation rat reproduction study with mancozeb at a dietary level of 1000 ppm there was reduced fertility but no indication of embryotoxic or teratogenic effects (Vettorazzi, 1977).

Primigravida Charles River cesarean-derived rats were exposed to mancozeb by inhalation at doses of 1–890 mg/m³ for 6 hr/day from day 6 through 15 of gestation. Dams were killed 1 day prior to natural delivery and the fetuses examined for any anomalies. At doses above 55 mg/m³ the dams exhibited decreased body weight gain and hind limb weakness. At 110 mg/m³ and above there was evidence of breathing difficulties and various other signs of toxicity, which became more pronounced at higher doses. Death or termination *in extremis* increased significantly at doses above 110 mg/m³ to a rate of 30/37 at 890 mg/m³. There was a significant incidence of embryofetal toxicity at concentrations of 55 mg/m³ and above. This toxicity occurred only at concentrations toxic to the dam (Lu and Kennedy 1986).

21.12.6.3 Toxicity to Humans

Use Experience   In a study of plant workers engaged in manufacturing mancozeb, 54 employees exposed to varying levels of the fungicide were examined. Tests included physical examinations, hematology (including protein-bound iodine), and urinalysis. No abnormalities that could be related to mancozeb were encountered, except for dermatitis in a few sensitive subjects (WHO, 1988).

A 61-year-old vineyard worker developed a rash on the forearm as well as inflammation of the eyelids on three occasions after handling seedlings which had been treated with mancozeb. The patient was patch-tested with a 0.002% solution of both zineb and mancozeb. The results were positive, while tests in three controls were negative. Two potato planters, who developed dermatitis after handling seed potatoes treated with mancozeb powder, also gave positive patch tests with a 0.1% solution of mancozeb (Kleibl and Rackova, 1980).

In an unusual case, a 68-year-old agricultural worker developed a pellagra-like dermatitis on the face, neck, exposed part of the chest, forearms, and back of hands after working in a vineyard which had been sprayed with fungicides including mancozeb. Of particular interest was that the dermatitis appeared on vitiliginous areas. Patch test showed sensitization to mancozeb, maneb, and thiram (Lisi and Caraffini, 1985).

Treatment of Poisoning   Treatment is symptomatic.

21.13 NITROGEN HETEROCYCLIC FUNGICIDES NOT OTHERWISE CLASSIFIED

A large number of fungicides are nitrogen heterocyclic compounds that do not belong to any of the groups already discussed and never have been subdivided into smaller groups that are toxicologically meaningful. In addition, some compounds such as thiophanate-methyl (see below) that are converted to nitrogen heterocyclic compounds are classified here. The compounds vary from such relatively simple structures as Omadine® (1-hydroxy-2-pyridinethione) to others with sulfur as well as nitrogen in a ring and/or with as many as three rings. The toxicities also vary widely from one compound to another. Like benomyl and thiabendazole, which are discussed below, most of these compounds are of moderate to low toxicity with oral LD 50 values in the rat of 500 mg/kg or much higher. A striking exception is triamiphos (BSI, ISO), an organic phosphorus compound with an LD 50 value of 20 mg/kg. It seems likely that the toxicity of this exceptional compound depends on the phosphorylation of acetylcholine in mammals but depends on the heterocyclic nitrogen-leaving group in fungi.

21.13.1 BENOMYL

21.13.1.1 Identity, Properties, and Uses

Chemical Name Benomyl is methyl 1-(butylcarbamoyl)benzimidazol-2-ylcarbamate.

Structure See Fig. 21.6.

Synonyms The common name benomyl (ANSI, BSI, ISO, JMAF) is in general use. A trade name for the compound is Benlate®, and a code designation is F-1,991. The CAS registry number is 17804-35-2.

Physical and Chemical Properties Benomyl has the empirical formula $C_{14}H_{18}N_4O_3$ and a molecular weight of 290.36. It is a white crystalline solid with a faint acrid odor. It decomposes before melting and is nonvolatile at room temperature. Benomyl is soluble in chloroform but less soluble in other common organic solvents and oils. Its solubility in water at pH 7 and 20°C is 3.8 ppm.

History, Formulations, and Uses Benomyl was introduced by E.I. du Pont de Nemours and Company, Inc. in 1967. It is a protective and eradicant fungicide with systemic activity, effective against a wide range of fungi affecting fruits, nuts, vegetables, turf, and field crops. Its formulations include Benlate® fungicide, wettable powder (500 gm active ingredient per kilogram), and Benlate T® seed treatment (300 gm benomyl plus 300 gm thiram per kilogram).

21.13.1.2 Toxicity to Laboratory Animals

Basic Findings The oral LD 50 of benomyl in rats is >10,000 mg/kg (Shtenberg and Torchinskiy, 1972; Sherman et al., 1975). A sample studied by Strohmayer et al. (1975) was somewhat more toxic (LD 50 of about 10,000 mg/kg). The acute skin absorption LD 50 for the rabbit is >10,000 mg/kg. The acute inhalation LC 50 is >2000 mg/m³ (4-hr exposure) with a no-effect level in the range 100–410 mg/m³. In the dog the corresponding LC 50 value is >825 mg/m³ with a no-effect level in the range 325–825 mg/m³. In addition, 15 4-hr inhalation exposures at the equivalent of 100 mg/m³ over a period of 3 weeks

produced no clinical or histopathological evidence of cumulative effects [American Conference of Governmental Industrial Hygienists (ACGIH), 1980].

In 2-year chronic toxicity feeding studies the no-effect levels in the diet were found to be 2500 ppm for rats and 500 ppm for dogs (Gardiner et al., 1974).

According to Matsushita et al. (1977), benomyl produces little irritation of the skin of rats but does produce sensitization. Dermal application to guinea pigs of aqueous suspensions containing up to 25% benomyl resulted in negligible irritation. Similarly, instillation into the eyes of rabbits of 10 mg of dry 50% powder or 0.1 ml of 10% suspension in mineral oil caused only temporary mild conjunctival irritation (ACGIH, 1980).

Absorption, Distribution, Metabolism, and Excretion It may be that benomyl is broken down in the intestine or is merely poorly absorbed; sera from rats receiving it intraperitoneally were as cytotoxic as sera from animals receiving its metabolite that is also a fungicide, called carbendazim (BSI, ISO), but only one-tenth as toxic when the compounds were administered orally (Styles and Garner, 1974). The possibility of breakdown in the intestine is emphasized by the fact that there is a reversible conversion of benomyl to carbendazim plus n-butylisocyanate in a variety of solvents and the equilibrium constants have been determined (Chiba and Cherniak, 1978).

One hour following oral administration of [¹⁴C]benomyl at a rate of 900 mg/kg, 68% of the activity in the blood was in the form of a metabolite (carbendazim) and less than 15% was present as parent compound (Sherman et al., 1975).

Enzyme preparations from liver, other organs, blood of mice, rabbits, and sheep and from rumen fluid of sheep produced some or all of the metabolites excreted by these species and also 1-butylcarbomyl-2-aminobenzimidazole. Hydroxylation depended on microsomal enzymes and was inhibited by SKF 525A in vitro (Douch, 1973).

In the rat the major excreted metabolite of both benomyl and carbendazim is 5-hydroxy-2-benzimidazolecarbamate (5-HBC), which is present in the urine of rats as glucuronide and/or sulfate conjugates (Gardiner et al., 1968). Cows produce a 5-HBC and also 4-hydroxy-2-benzimidazolecarbamate (4-HBC) (Gardiner et al., 1974). Mice, rabbits, and sheep excreted 5-HBC and also 5-hydroxy-2-aminobenzimidazole (5-HAB), in both free and conjugated forms. In addition, they excreted carbendazim and 2-aminobenzimidazole unconjugated (Douch, 1973).

When rats received by stomach tube either [¹⁴C]benomyl or its metabolite [¹⁴C]carbendazim after having received the same but nonradioactive compound in their diet for 12 days, 78.9% of the activity was excreted in the urine and 8.7% in the feces within 24 hr, making a total of 87.6% of the dose. A total of 91.8% of the activity was accounted for in 72 hr, of which 99.5% was in the excreta. Over 99% of the activity was found in the urine and feces of a rat given [¹⁴C]carbendazim, and in this instance a total of 100.4% of the dose was accounted for. No activity was found in exhaled carbon dioxide in either experiment. In a pretreated dog, >99% of the activity from [¹⁴C]benomyl was excreted in 72 hr, but in this species most of the excretion was by the feces (Gardiner et al., 1974). Mice excreted >94% of ingested benomyl within 96 hr. In mice, rabbits, and sheep, about 20% of the dose was excreted in conjugated form. In these three species, urine contained 44–71% and feces 21–46% of the excreted metabolites (Douch, 1973).

Metabolism of the butylcarbamoyl group of benomyl was studied in rats that received the fungicide by stomach tube. The side chain was tagged with ^{14}C at the carboxyl carbon and with ^{3}H on the first butyl carbon. Most of the excretion occurred within the first 24 hr. Within that period 38.4–42.9% of the ^{14}C was recovered from different animals as expired CO_2, and 39.4–46.0% was recovered from the urine. During the same period, 55–69% of the tritium was recovered in the urine. Smaller proportions of both ^{14}C and ^{3}H were found in the feces. Identified metabolites of the side chain included S-(n-butylcarbomyl) cysteine, S-(n-butylcarbomyl)-N-acetylcysteine, and probably the N-glucuronide of butylamine (Axness and Fleeker, 1979).

Residue data on rat and dog tissues after 2-year feeding studies demonstrated that benomyl and its metabolites do not accumulate in animal tissues (Gardiner et al., 1974).

Biochemical Effects   Benomyl itself has little or no effect on cholinesterase. Under certain conditions, benomyl breaks down to produce carbendazim (BSI, ISO) and butyl isocyanate, of which the former is completely inactive against the enzyme but the latter is an irreversible inhibitor comparable in potency to active organic phosphorus compounds (Krupka, 1974). There is no evidence, however, that the mammalian toxicity of benomyl depends on cholinesterase inhibition caused by the isocyanate metabolite.

Effects on Organs and Tissues   Benomyl at a concentration of 5 ppm caused forward but not back mutation in the mold *Fusarium;* it caused no chromosomal changes in the roots of onions (Dassenoy and Meyer, 1973). Benomyl produced negative results in tests using *Salmonella* and *Streptomyces* (Carere et al., 1978).

Kappas et al. (1976) showed that benomyl produced mutations in certain strains of bacteria but not in those proficient in repair of DNA. They speculated that the compound was incorporated into and later removed from the DNA of all strains. They suggested that benomyl might be a new type of mutagen that acts not by misincorporation during normal replication of DNA but by imperfect repair of gaps it has caused in newly synthesized DNA. However, in other very thorough studies covering a wide range of concentrations of benomyl and carbendazim and including repair-deficient strains of bacteria, no indication of mutagenicity was found (Ficsor et al., 1978).

In *Aspergillus,* benomyl did not cause point mutation or crossing-over but did cause a high incidence of nondisjunction (Bignami et al., 1977). Whether nondisjunction was the basis of the instability of *Aspergillus* diploids exposed to 0.25–0.50 ppm as observed by Hastie (1970) is unclear, but Hastie gave evidence that benomyl does not cause point mutations.

Benomyl produced some micronuclei in the bone marrow of mice, apparently by interference with spindle formation. The effect occurred when the concentration of carbendazim in the serum reached 12 ppm even for a short interval but did not occur at continuous concentrations of 8 ppm. It was concluded that this dosage relationship excluded the possibility of genetic hazard from nonoccupational exposure to benomyl (Seiler, 1976).

Benomyl at the highest dietary level tested (2500 ppm) induced no dominant lethal mutation in rats (Sherman et al., 1975). At dosages as high as 500 mg/kg/day, the compound had no effect on the structure of the chromosomes of adult rats but did increase the rate of aberrations in fetal rats (Ruzicska et al., 1976).

An increased incidence of lymphosarcoma was observed in female but not in male mice that received benomyl by stomach tube twice a week at the rate of 500 mg/kg/day plus a constant supply of drinking water containing 500 ppm sodium nitrite. Under similar conditions, carbendazim produced a similar increase in female mice and a smaller increase in males. Rapid nitrosation of intragastrically administered benomyl was demonstrated *in vitro* (Borzsonyi et al., 1976). What bearing the results for such large dosages of the fungicides and of nitrites have on the practical hazard of the fungicides is obscure.

Effects on Reproduction   In a three-generation test in rats, the highest dietary level tested (2500 ppm, equivalent to a dosage of about 125 mg/kg/day) produced no difference in reproduction or lactation compared to the controls. No pathological change was found in weanling pups of the F_{3b} generation (Sherman et al., 1975).

When benomyl was administered to rats by intubation during the first 20 days of pregnancy at dosages of 500, 250, and 125 mg/kg/day, the corresponding incidence of fetal anomalies ranged from 100 to 9.6%. Anomalies included encephalocele, hydrocephalus, microphthalmia, and anophthalmia. The teratogenic effects were always associated with death and were considered the cause of death (Shtenberg and Torchinskiy, 1972). Similar anomalies were reported by Kavlock et al. (1982) in the offspring of Wistar rats given benomyl at doses of 15.6, 31.2, 62.5, and 125 mg/kg on days 7–16 of gestation. Common malformations observed in the offspring taken from the dams given the highest dose included encephalocele, hydrocephaly, clefts of the lip or jaw, gastroschisis, and fused vertebrae. The average fetal body weight of rats from mothers given doses of 31.2 mg/kg or greater was significantly less than that of controls. An unexpected result reported by Torchinskiy (1973) was the lessening of teratogenicity in the young of rats fed only 10% protein for 1 month before conception and during pregnancy as compared with those fed 19 or 35% protein. This observation has been confirmed in Sprague–Dawley rats given benomyl at 31.2 mg/kg on days 7–16 or 7–21 of gestation when on a diet containing either 24% or 8% casein. In all groups there was an increased incidence of anomalies when benomyl was given for the longer period (Zeman et al., 1986).

Benomyl at dietary levels as high as 5000 ppm (about 250 mg/kg/day) from day 6 through 15 of gestation did not affect embryonal development or the outcome of pregnancy (Sherman *et al.*, 1975). Another study at dietary doses up to 505 mg/kg/day also failed to produce a teratogenic response, but maternal weight and average fetal body weight were adversely affected (Kavlock *et al.*, 1982).

Benomyl given to CD-1 mice by gavage at doses of 50, 100, or 200 mg/kg/day on days 7–17 of gestation affected embryonic development. A variety of congenital malformations were noted in offspring from mice given 100 or 200 mg/kg/day (Kavlock *et al.*, 1982).

21.13.1.3 Toxicity to Humans

Use Experience A contact dermatitis occurred in women of Japanese origin who worked in warm, moist greenhouses where benomyl had been used. The eruption appeared on the back of the hands, on the forearms, and sometimes on other areas not covered by clothing. It consisted of redness and edema and cleared during about 3 weeks of both topical and systemic treatment. The eruption occurred only after a second spraying of benomyl, and it was not observed in Japanese men or in women of Mexican ancestry who were doing similar work. Patch tests with benomyl were positive in patients but negative in controls with the exception of one Japanese who received ultraviolet irradiation after exposure to benomyl (Savitt, 1972). If exposure is continued, the dermatitis may persist (van Ketel, 1977) but apparently without progression. Other investigators (Arimatsu *et al.*, 1976, 1978; Nomura and Wakatsuki, 1976; Nomura *et al.*, 1976) also have reported dermatitis in persons exposed to benomyl. Nomura and Wakatsuki (1976) noted that morbidity associated with benomyl was much less than that associated with some other fungicides, notably thiophanate-methyl. However, Arimatsu *et al.* (1976) reported that patch tests were more often positive with benomyl than with thiophanate-methyl.

It may be significant that many of the reports of dermatitis associated with benomyl involve Japanese, whether in Japan or elsewhere. Both Savitt (1972) and Arimatsu *et al.* (1976) reported a higher incidence in women than in men.

No change was detected in chromosomes of blood cells cultured from workers exposed to benomyl (Ruzicska *et al.*, 1976).

Dosage Response Patch tests indicate that susceptible persons respond to low concentrations of benomyl. The threshold limit value of 10 mg/m^3 indicates that occupational intake of about 1.4 mg/kg/day is considered safe for persons not sensitized to the compound.

Treatment of Poisoning Treatment is symptomatic.

21.13.2 THIABENDAZOLE

21.13.2.1 Identity, Properties, and Uses

Chemical Name Thiabendazole is 2-(thiazol-4-yl)benzimidazole.

Structure See Fig. 21.6.

Synonyms The common name thiabendazole (BSI, ISO, JMAF) is in general use. The recommended international nonproprietary name for the compound as a drug is tiabendazole, but thiabendazole is used for the drug also. Trade names for the compound are Bovizol®, Eprofil®, Equizole®, Lombristop®, Mertect®, Mintezol®, Minzolum®, Nemapan®, Omnizole®, Polival®, Storite®, Tecto®, Thiaben®, Thibenzole®, and Top Form Wormer®. A code designation is MK-360. The CAS registry number is 148-79-8.

Physical and Chemical Properties Thiabendazole has the empirical formula $C_{10}H_7N_3S$ and a molecular weight of 201.26. It is a white odorless powder with a melting point of 304–305°C. Its solubility in water is dependent on pH. Thiabendazole is stable under normal conditions to light, hydrolysis, and heat.

History, Formulations, and Uses Thiabendazole has been in use since 1962 as an anthelmintic. It was introduced as an agricultural fungicide by Merck and Company, Inc., in 1968. Its formulations include wettable powders (400, 600, and 900 gm active ingredient per kilogram), flowable suspensions (450 gm active ingredient per liter), and fumigation tablets (7 gm active ingredient).

21.13.2.2 Toxicity to Laboratory Animals

Basic Findings Acute oral LD 50 values in rats, mice, and rabbits are 3100, 3600, and >3800 mg/kg, respectively (Robinson *et al.*, 1965). Gladenko (1971) reported greater (but still small) toxicity in mice, the oral LD 50 being 1395 mg/kg. Dosages as high as 825 mg/kg did not cause any pathological change. Some animals that had received the compound somewhat above the LD 50 level showed fatty degeneration of the liver, a decrease in the number of malpighian bodies in the spleen, and a diffuse desquamation and necrosis of the intestinal epithelium.

At toxic dose levels, rats show weight loss, ataxia, and narcosis. Single oral doses of 200 mg/kg or more caused delayed vomiting in most dogs, and this interfered with determining an oral LD 50 in this species. Moderately rapid intravenous injection of thiabendazole hydrochloride also produced vomiting in dogs, but some tolerated very slow infusion at rates as high as 80 mg/kg. This dosage may be compared to intravenous LD 50 values of the hydrochloride in rats and mice of 180 and 160 mg/kg, respectively. The oral LD 50 values of the hydrochloride in rats and mice are 3600 and 2400 mg/kg, respectively, not greatly different from those of thiabendazole itself (Robinson *et al.*, 1964). This indicates that the dog is little or no more susceptible to poisoning by thiabendazole than rodents are, but vomiting, probably of central origin, would tend to limit absorption and even intake of the compound in the dog.

Application of 50% thiabendazole base in cold cream to the shaved skin of rabbits caused no sign of irritation even where

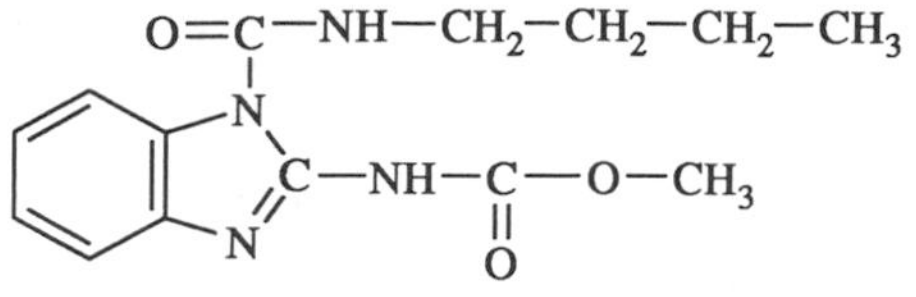

Figure 21.6 Some nitrogen heterocyclic fungicides not otherwise classified. Note that both benomyl and thiophanate-methyl are metabolized to carbendazim.

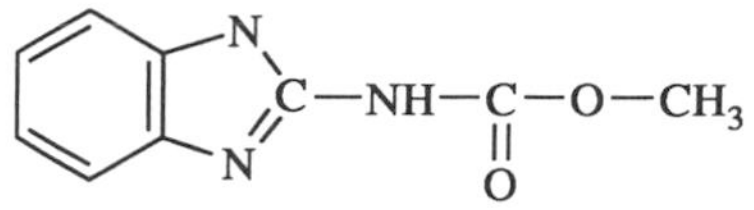

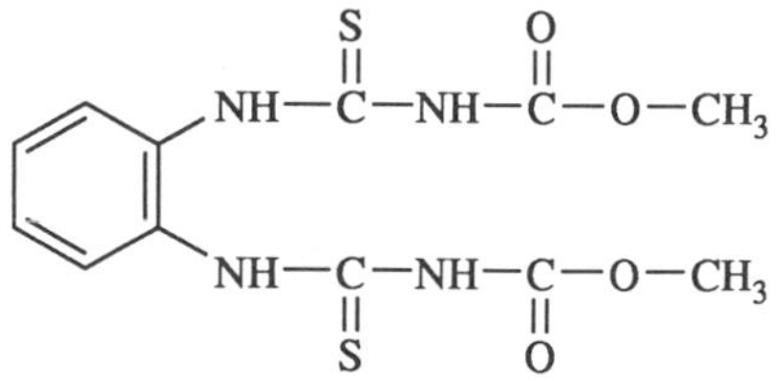

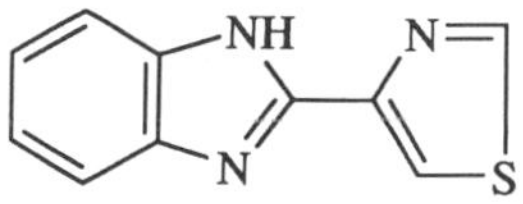

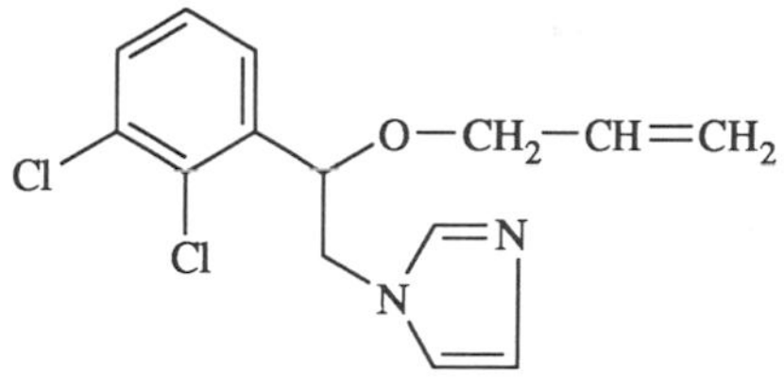

irradiated by ultraviolet light. Ophthalmic ointment (4%) or saline suspension (10%) was not irritating to the eyes of rabbits (Robinson *et al.,* 1965).

When rats were given thiabendazole by gavage at a rate of 1200 mg/kg/day, all died within a few days, usually in coma. At 800 mg/kg/day there was 30% mortality within 30 days and a marked retardation of growth of the survivors. At 400 mg/kg/day there was a moderate suppression of growth, especially in males, but there was no effect at 100 mg/kg/day. The result was similar in a 180-day study; 400 mg/kg/day by gavage caused moderate failure of growth, but no other sign of injury. Dosages of 200 mg/kg/day or less had little or no effect on growth even in males. Mice and rats grew at an essentially normal rate at a dietary level of 1000 ppm (about 50 mg/kg/day), but higher dietary levels led to retardation of growth.

None of the dogs treated orally at rates of 20, 100, or 200 mg/kg/day for 2 years or more died. Except for occasional vomiting during the early phases of the study, there were no outward signs of toxicity. Weight was essentially maintained. However, most dogs at a dosage of 100 mg/kg/day developed a normocytic, normochromic anemia (4.75 million cells/mm³ in the controls), from which they recovered by the end of the study. At 200 mg/kg/day a slightly greater depression of erythrocyte count occurred and persisted until the end of the study. Other laboratory findings for the dogs were normal (Robinson *et al.,* 1965).

Studies of cattle, sheep, goats, swine, horses, and several species of zoo animals are consistent with the conclusion that therapeutic doses of thiabendazole offer a wide margin of safety (Robinson *et al.,* 1969).

Absorption, Distribution, Metabolism, and Excretion   Absorption of [^{14}C]thiabendazole was slower in rats and dogs than in humans, perhaps because larger dosages were given to the animals. In any event, rats reached their highest levels of activity in the serum in the 2-, 3-, 4-, and, in one instance, 6-hr samples. Dogs reached maximal activity in the 2-hr sample. Subsequently, excretion was nearly as rapid in dogs as in humans, but it was distinctly slower in rats, which had serum levels of thiabendazole equivalent ranging from 2.7 to 5.4 ppm on day 8. This is significant because the highest level reached by any rat was 24 ppm, not much more than the highest found in humans. The fraction of the dose recovered in rats was 92% following a dosage of 25 mg/kg but only 79% following a dosage of 100 mg/kg. In dogs, total recovery varied from 55 to 104% at a dosage of 50 mg/kg. Fecal excretion accounted for an average of 28% in rats and 47% in dogs.

Identified metabolites in animals were similar to those in humans (Tocco *et al.,* 1966).

Having shown that thiabendazole is active *in vitro* against a number of pathogenic and saprophytic fungi, Robinson *et al.* (1964) speculated that the compound might be valuable for treating ocular infections due to fungus. When [^{14}C]thiabendazole was applied to the eyes of rabbits in the form of 1 and 4% ointments and a 4% suspension, a level of about 52 ppm was reached in the corneal tissue with progressively lower concentrations in the anterior chamber fluid, lens, vitreous humor, and plasma. Maximal concentration in the cornea was reached in about 1 hr. When the drug was removed from the eye, radioactivity in the tissues of the eye decreased rapidly within a 4-hr period of observation but remained essentially stable in the plasma, liver, and kidney while increasing in the urine (Robinson *et al.*, 1966).

Biochemical Effects Appropriate tests with large dosages of thiabendazole in anesthetized animals demonstrated that it lacks atropine-like adrenergic blocking or ganglionic blocking properties. It did not disturb the electrocardiogram (Robinson *et al.*, 1965).

Pathology Hemosiderosis was found throughout much of the reticuloendothelial system of rats and dogs that had received substantial dosages of thiabendazole. This was the only finding in dogs. Even in rats it was not accompanied by increased serum or ordinary bilirubin. Rats did show a reduction of active bone marrow not exceeding 20–30%. A similar depression of bone marrow occurs in starved rats, and that associated with thiabendazole may have been due to inanition and not directly to the compound. The bone marrow returns to normal when thiabendazole (or starvation) is discontinued (Robinson *et al.*, 1965).

21.13.2.3 Toxicity to Humans

Experimental Exposure When 1000 mg of [^{14}C]thiabendazole was given orally to each of four men, peak plasma concentrations of 13–18 ppm were found within 1 hr, in three subjects the concentrations were distinctly lower within another hour, and in all subjects they fell to zero or almost zero within 48 hr. More than 40% of the dose was excreted within 4 hr and approximately 80% within the first 24 hr. Less than 1% of the dose was excreted as unchanged thiabendazole or unconjugated 5-hydroxythiobendazole. Most of the dose was detected in the urine as the glucuronide (25%) and the sulfate ester (13%) of 5-hydroxythiabendazole. Fecal excretion accounted for 4–9% of the administered dose. The total amount accounted for in the excreta varied from 87 to 101% (Tocco *et al.*, 1966).

Therapeutic Use Papers constituting a symposium published in 1969 as Supplement 2 (pages 533–708) of Volume 27 of Texas Reports on Biology and Medicine contain hundreds of references to the literature and many original observations on the therapeutic value and side effects of thiabendazole as an anthelmintic in humans and animals. Little additional information has been added since 1969. Suffice it to say that thiabendazole is now considered the drug of choice in the treatment of *Strongyloides stercoralis* infestation in humans and also of cutaneous larva migrans caused by *Anchylostoma braziliense*. Thiabendazole is active against pinworm (*Enterobius vermicularis*), hookworms

(*A. duodenale* and *Necator americanus*), and roundworms (*Ascaris lumbricoides*), but less so than other available preparations. This drug also appears active against developing and migrating (but not encysted) larvae of *Trichinella spiralis*, against the guinea worm (*Dracunculus medinensis*), and against intraocular toxocariasis. In some parts of the world thiabendazole has been used to treat scabies (AMA, 1986).

The more common side effects are dizziness, anorexia, nausea, and vomiting. Diarrhea, fever, epigastric distress, flushing, chills, angiedema, itching, rash, body odor, lethargy, and headache occur less frequently. Tinnitus, hypotension, fainting, numbness, hyperglycemia, changes in liver function, and xanthopsia have been reported. These reactions are brief and appear to be dosage-related. However, the drug should be used cautiously in patients with impaired liver or kidney function (AMA, 1986).

The recommended dosage of thiabendazole for most forms of helminthiasis is 50 mg/kg/day in two divided doses and repeated for a variable number of days depending on the species of worm involved. In most instances, the total daily dose should not exceed 3000 mg, but a dosage of 100 mg/kg/day for 3 days has been used against guinea worm (AMA, 1986).

Treatment of Poisoning If required, treatment would have to be symptomatic.

21.13.3 THIOPHANATE-METHYL

21.13.3.1 Identity, Properties, and Uses

Chemical Name 1,2-Di(3-methoxycarbonyl-2-thioureido) benzene.

Structure See Fig. 21.6.

Synonyms Thiophanate-methyl (ANSI, BSI, ISO, JMAF) is in general use. Trade names include Cercobin® methyl, Cycosin®, Mildothane®, Tedion V-18®, and Topsin® methyl. A code designation is NF-44. The CAS registry number is 23564-05-8.

Physical and Chemical Properties The empirical formula for thiophanate-methyl is $C_{12}H_{14}N_4O_4S_2$ and it has a molecular weight of 342.42. It is a stable colorless crystalline solid. It melts at 172°C with decomposition. Thiophanate-methyl is slightly soluble in most organic solvents and has very low solubility in water.

History, Formulations, and Uses Thiophanate-methyl was introduced by Nippon Soda Company, Limited in 1970–1971 as a replacement for thiophanate. It is effective against a wide range of fungal diseases. Formulations include wettable powder (200 gm active ingredient/kg), emulsifiable concentrate (80 gm active ingredient/liter), and an emulsifiable concentrate containing dicofol plus tetradifon.

Table 21.6
Single-Dose LD 50 for Thiophanate-Methyl

Species	Route	LD 50 (mg/kg)	Reference
Rat, M	oral	7500	Hashimoto *et al.* (1972a)
Rat, F	oral	6640	Hashimoto *et al.* (1972a)
Rat, M	intraperitoneal	1640	Hashimoto *et al.* (1972a)
Rat, F	intraperitoneal	1140	Hashimoto *et al.* (1972a)
Mouse, M	oral	3510	Hashimoto *et al.* (1972a)
Mouse, F	oral	3400	Hashimoto *et al.* (1972a)
Mouse, M	intraperitoneal	790	Hashimoto *et al.* (1972a)
Mouse, F	intraperitoneal	1110	Hashimoto *et al.* (1972a)
Guinea pig, M	oral	3640	Hashimoto *et al.* (1972a)
Guinea pig, F	oral	6700	Hashimoto *et al.* (1972a)
Rabbit, M	oral	2270	Hashimoto *et al.* (1972a)
Rabbit, F	oral	2250	Hashimoto *et al.* (1972a)
Dog, M	oral	4000[a]	Hashimoto *et al.* (1972a)
Dog, F	oral	4000[a]	Hashimoto *et al.* (1972a)

[a]Minimal lethal dose.

21.13.3.2 Toxicity to Experimental Animals

Basic Findings The acute oral toxicity of thiophanate-methyl is shown in Table 21.6. The dermal LD 50 values for rats, mice, guinea pigs, rabbits, and dogs were all >10,000 mg/kg. Single exposures of mice for 30, 60, or 120 min to an aerosol of 70% wettable powder under dynamic conditions at a nominal concentration of 100,000 mg/m^3 caused lacrimation, salivation, and nasal exudation within 5–6 min after exposure began. For a few days after exposure the mice wheezed, and a crust was present around their eyes. However, they recovered completely and showed no change in growth compared to controls (Hashimoto *et al.*, 1972a).

Large oral doses caused tremor beginning 1–2 hr later; the animals became sensitive to touch and had tonic or clonic convulsions. Rabbits and dogs showed a slight decrease in respiratory rate, lethargy, loss of tone of the abdominal muscles, discharge from the eyes, and mydriasis prior to death (Hashimoto *et al.*, 1972a).

Contrary to experience with dermatitis in humans, thiophanate-methyl produced less sensitization in rats than benomyl produced (Matsushita *et al.*, 1977).

When mice were fed thiophanate-methyl for 6 months, there was a slight retardation of growth in those receiving 8000 ppm, and, when killed, these rats had slight enlargement of the liver with enlargement of some liver cells. The no-effect level was 1600 ppm (about 250 mg/kg/day). Similar results were obtained in rats; the no-effect level of 1600 ppm in this species corresponds to about 78 mg/kg/day (Noguchi, 1972).

A 2-year study in rats showed that a dietary level of 640 ppm caused a slight reduction in growth in both male and female rats and a slight increase in the relative weight of the kidneys in males. There was no indication of increased thyroid or liver weight such as had been seen in an earlier, briefer study; how-

ever, at the end of 2 years there was some enlargement of thyroid epithelial cells, especially in the males. Food consumption, survival, behavior, laboratory findings, and, with the exception of the thyroid, gross and microscopic morphology did not differ from those of the controls. A dietary level of 160 ppm (about 8 mg/kg/day) was a no-effect level (FAO/WHO, 1974).

In a 2-year study in mice, males on a dietary level of 640 ppm showed a slight retardation in growth, but females grew normally. A dietary level of 160 ppm (about 20 mg/kg/day) was a no-effect level. Even at the highest dosage there was no effect on survival, laboratory findings, incidence of tumors, or histology (FAO/WHO, 1974).

When dogs were fed capsules of thiophanate-methyl 7 days a week for 2 years, those receiving 250 mg/kg/day showed a marginal effect on thyroid weight; those that received 10 mg/kg/day or less showed no effect. Even the highest dosage did not affect survival or the gross or microscopic morphology of any tissue other than the thyroid (FAO/WHO, 1974).

Repeated dermal application of a 10% concentration to rabbits caused slight erythema, but this disappeared a few days after the last treatment. A 1% suspension was not irritating. Even the 10% suspension produced no clinical effect and no change in histology of the tissues. Studies in guinea pigs with repeated sensitizing injections and a delayed challenge dose indicated that thiophanate-methyl produced no primary irritation and only slight sensitization. The compound showed no phototoxic property (Hashimoto *et al.*, 1972a).

Absorption, Distribution, Metabolism, and Excretion Thiophanate-methyl is converted under suitable environmental conditions (including exposure to water) to a derivative identical to the fungicide carbendazim, and thiophate is converted to the corresponding ethyl ester. These methyl and ethyl esters of benzimidazole carbamic acid probably are the active fungicides (Selling *et al.*, 1970). These findings were confirmed and extended by Vonk and Sijpesteijn (1971) and by Fuchs *et al.* (1972).

Studies in mice with four radioactive forms of the molecule (^{14}C in the ring or as the thiourea carbon or the methyl carbon and ^{35}S) showed that the C=S bond was cleaved to a great extent prior to absorption from the gastrointestinal tract. Some of the methyl carbon apparently is metabolized to carbon dioxide. The major urinary metabolites are carbendazim and its 6-hydroxy derivative; these are excreted as *O*- or *N*-glucuronides. A compound in which the two =S's of thiophanate-methyl are replaced by =O's is a minor metabolite. Some other metabolites detectable by thin-layer chromatography of radioactive material remain unidentified (Noguchi, 1972).

Nearly all thiophanate-methyl is eliminated from the body in 24 hr; that left in the tissues after 24 hr is largely eliminated within 96 hr (Noguchi, 1972).

Pharmacological Effects When an anesthetized rabbit was given a fatal, intravenous dose of thiophanate-methyl (100 mg/kg) the blood pressure rapidly fell to zero, there was a gradual disturbance of the electrocardiogram (ECG), and then cessation of respiration was observed. The heart continued in ventricular flutter and ventricular fibrillation for some time after respiration stopped. However, intravenous dosages as high as 30 mg/kg produced only a temporary fall in blood pressure followed by a persistent rise of 20 mm Hg and persistent bradycardia with no remarkable change in ECG or respiration. These and other pharmacological studies (Hashimoto *et al.*, 1972b) far too extensive to review here failed to identify the mode of action.

Effects on Organs and Tissues Rabbits that received a single oral dose of thiophanate-methyl at the rate of 0.1 the LD 50 or 16 daily doses of 0.01 the LD 50 showed an increase of reticulocytes and of erythrocytes containing basophilic spots (Nakamura *et al.*, 1977).

Host-mediated assay and *in vitro* and *in vivo* cytogenic studies in rats and a dominant lethal test in mice were negative for mutagenic effect (Noguchi, 1972; Makita *et al.*, 1973).

Effects on Reproduction In a three-generation reproduction study, rats were fed dietary levels of 0, 40, 160, and 640 ppm. Even the highest dosage had no effect on reproduction, but 640 ppm reduced growth. The no-effect level was 160 ppm (about 8 mg/kg/day in most adults but much higher in weanlings and lactating females) (FAO/WHO, 1974).

Mice received thiophanate-methyl at oral dosages of 40, 200, 500, and 1000 mg/kg/day from day 1 to day 15 of gestation. The highest dosage caused a small reduction in the number of living fetuses (9.70/litter compared to 10.90/litter for the controls). Other groups receiving 500 mg/kg/day or less presented no differences from controls in implantation sites or number of dead fetuses. There was no significant difference in the number of malformed fetuses in any treated group compared with the controls (Makita *et al.*, 1973).

21.13.3.3 Toxicity to Humans

Use Experience Among men who treated citrus with thiophanate-methyl as well as emulsified sulfur and calcium polysulfide in Kumamoto Perfecture, the incidence of dermatitis is 30.3, 48.2, and 52.8% in 1972, 1973, and 1974, respectively. The corresponding values for women were 32.3, 56.3, and 64.8%. The areas affected were the abdomen, back, and waist. Symptoms included itching, redness, swelling, dryness, and sometimes sensitized dermatitis. Symptoms frequently appeared 1 week after first exposure. The ocular mucosa was congested. The incidence of positive patch tests was only about 5%. Medical examination revealed some abnormalities of hemoglobin (Nomura *et al.*, 1976; Nomura and Wakatsuki, 1976; Arimatsu *et al.*, 1976, 1978).

Treatment of Poisoning Treatment is symptomatic.

21.13.4 IMAZALIL

21.13.4.1 Identity, Properties, and Uses

Chemical Name Imazalil is allyl 1-(2,4-dichlorophenyl)-2-imidazol-1-yl ethyl ether.

Structure See Figure 21.6.

Synonyms Imazalil (BSI, ISO, ANSI) is the common name in use. Chloramizol is the name approved by the Republic of South Africa. As a drug, the compound is known as enilconazole. Trade names for the compound include Fungaflor® and Imaverol®. A code designation is R23979 for the base, R27180 for the hydrogen sulfate salt, and R18531 for the imazalil nitrate salt. The CAS registry numbers are 35554-44-0 base, 33586-66-2 nitrate (1 : 1), and 60534-80-7 sulfate (1 : 1).

Physical and Chemical Properties Imazalil has the empirical formula $C_{14}H_{14}Cl_2N_2O$ and a molecular weight of 297.2. It is a slightly yellowish to brownish oil. Imazalil is slightly soluble in water and freely soluble in organic acids. It is chemically stable at room temperature in the absence of light and stable at temperatures less than about 285°C. Imazalil hydrogen sulfate is an almost colorless to beige-colored powder, freely soluble in water and alcohols and slightly soluble in apolar organic solvents.

History, Foundations, and Uses Imazalil was introduced in 1969 by Janssen Pharmaceutical. Its formulations include emulsifiable concentrates containing 200, 500, or 700 gm of active ingredient per liter, and soluble powder (750 gm base per kilogram). Various other liquid and solid formulations occur in which imazalil is combined with other pesticides. A 10% solution of imazalil is available for veterinary use as an antimycotic. Imazalil is a systemic fungicide effective against a wide range of fungi affecting fruit, ornamentals, and vegetables. It is used as a seed treatment for the control of cereal diseases.

21.13.4.2 Toxicity to Laboratory Animals

The acute oral LD 50 values were 343 and 227 mg/kg in male and female Wistar rats, respectively. At the tested doses, varying degrees of symptoms such as ataxia, piloerection, hypotonia, and tremors were noted. In mongrel dogs the LD 50 was >640 mg/kg and no symptoms other than vomiting were observed (Thienpont *et al.*, 1981).

In chronic dosing, toxicity also appears minimal. Wistar rats given imazalil in the diet at levels up to 800 ppm (80 mg/kg/day) showed no mortality, clinical symptoms, or change in body weight, biochemistry, or hematology. After autopsy, gross pathology showed no abnormal findings apart from a marginal increase in the weight of some organs at 12 and 24 months at the 80 mg/kg dose. Histopathology showed slight overmodifications for the same dosage.

Twenty-four pure-bred beagle dogs given doses up to 20 mg/kg daily for 24 months showed a decreased appetite and an increase in liver glycogen and fat similar to that observed in the rat. All clinical and hematological tests were normal, and, apart from a slight change in serum calcium and alkaline phosphatase, all biochemical values were within the normal range.

In six New Zealand White rabbits a single drop of 98% imazalil into the conjunctival sac caused a moderate but transient eye irritation, whereas 0.1 ml of 1000 and 2000 ppm formulations for 7 days did not produce any eye irritation.

Dermal irritation studies were performed on New Zealand White rabbits at doses of 40, 160, and 640 mg/kg. At 640 mg/kg a slight erythema was observed 24 hr after dosing and lasted 7 days. Skin reactions were not observed at the other doses.

Imazalil was found to be not mutagenic as determined by the Ames test at doses up to 30 mg and the dominant lethal test at doses up to 160 mg/kg. Studies in rats and mice demonstrated no adverse effect on mortality or on tumor incidence or type at dietary doses up to 40 mg/kg/day for 24 months.

No effect was observed on fertility in rats given doses up to 80 mg/kg daily for 60 days to males and 14 days before and throughout gestation to females. Teratogenic effects were not observed in the offspring of Wistar rats that were fed imazalil in the diet which provided doses of about 5, 20, and 80 mg/kg from day 6 through day 15 of pregnancy. Similarly, there was no evidence of teratogenic effect on fetuses of New Zealand White rabbits gavaged at doses of 0.63 and 2.5 mg/kg/day from day 6 through day 18 of pregnancy. There was evidence of maternal toxicity with an attendant reduction in the survival rate of pups. Pregnant Wistar rats were given imazalil in the diet from day 16 of gestation and continued throughout the 3-week lactation period. At the highest dose of 80 mg/kg some maternal toxicity was evident, with 25% mortality. Continuous administration of the fungicide at levels of 50, 200, and 800 ppm in food (approximately 2.5, 9.8, and 39 mg/kg/day) did not affect the reproductive capacity of three consecutive generations of Wistar rats (Thienpont *et al.*, 1981).

21.13.4.3 Toxicity to Humans

Therapeutic Use Imazalil has been used in the therapy of human alternariosis, an uncommon infection. A 51-year-old white woman had a chronic fungal infection due to *Alternaria alternata*. Her disease involved the palate, nose, and sinuses and had been unresponsive to conventional therapy. Imazalil was applied topically to accessible areas in lubricating jelly or polyethylene glycol-400, in increasing concentrations until 5% was given. At this dose the patient experienced a local "burning" sensation. Oral administration was initiated and increased to 1200 mg/day for 6 months. A total of 170 gm of drug was given. The drug was tolerated without evident toxicity, though an unpleasant taste and nausea at doses above 800 mg were limiting. The infection was arrested but not eradicated.

Serum imazalil concentrations were determined by bioassay. Concentrations were not detectable at oral doses <200 mg. For the other doses peak concentrations occurred 1–2 hr after the dose. Peak serum concentrations of imazalil exceeded 4 ppm at the 1200 mg dose. The elimination half-life appeared to be about 2 hr, and there was no evidence of accumulation or altered clearance after 1 month of treatment. Hematological and biochemical tests and the ECG before, during, and after therapy were all within normal values (Stiller and Stevens, 1986).

Use Experience A 43-year-old female developed an acute eczematous contact dermatitis of the right hand and forearm 2 weeks after treatment of a dermatophytic skin infection with imazalil. After imazalil treatment was discontinued, the condition resolved. Patch tests showed allergy to several imizadole derivatives including imazalil (van Hecke and De Vos, 1983).

Treatment of Poisoning Treatment is symptomatic.

REFERENCES

Abe, E., Kurosawa, K., Sasaki, K., Shimazaki, K., Yanagisawa, T., and Matsushima, S. (1974). Studies on the toxicity of Rabcide (phthalide). On the acute and chronic toxicity of phthalide to rat and mouse. *Annu. Rep. Jpn. Inst. Rural Med.* **3**, 216–250 (in Japancsc).

Acker, L., and Schulte, E. (1970). On the occurrence of chlorinated biphenyls and hexachlorobenzene and related chlorinated hydrocarbon insecticides in human milk and fatty tissue. *Naturwissenshaften* **57**, 497 (in German).

Acker, L., and Schulte, E. (1974). Organochlorine compounds in human fat. *Naturwissenschaften* **61**, 32 (in German).

Adams, R. M., and Manchester, R. D. (1982). *Contact Dermatitis* **8**, 271–272.

Adams, R. M., Zimmerman, M. C., Bartlett, J. B., and Preston, J. R. (1971). 1-Chloro-2,4-dinitrobenzene as an algicide: Report of four cases of contact dermatitis. *Arch. Dermatol.* **103**, 191–193.

Ambrose, A. M., Booth, A. N., DeEds, F., and Cox, A. J., Jr. (1960). A toxicological study of biphenyl, a citrus fungistat. *Food Res.* **25**, 328–336.

American Conference of Governmental Industrial Hygenists (ACGIH) (1980). "Documentation of the Threshold Limit Values." 4th ed., p. 37. Am. Conf. Govt. Ind. Hyg., Cincinnati, Ohio.

American Medical Association (AMA) (1986). "AMA Drug Evaluations," 4th ed. Am. Med. Assoc., Chicago, Illinois.

Andrianova, M. M., and Alekseev, I. V. (1970). On the carcinogenic properties of the pesticides sevine, maneb, ciram and cineb. *Vopr. Pitan.* **29**, 71–74 (in Russian).

Antsiferov, S. D., Zhavoronkov, N. I., Akulov, A. V., and Yevdokimov, S. M. (1973). Toxic action of tetramethylthiuram disulfide on sheep. *Veterinariia* **7**, 90–91 (in Russian).

Antsiferov, S. D., Zhavoronkov, N. I., and Yevdokimov, S. M. (1974). Diagnosis of animal poisoning by thiram. *Veterinariia* **8**, 104–105 (in Russian).

Arimatsu, N. (1970). Study on the skin hazards caused by fungicide "Difolatan." *Kumamoto Igakkai Zasshi* **44**, 692–721 (in Japanese).

Arimatsu, N., Misumi, J., Ueda A., Matsushita, T., and Nomura, S. (1976). Skin injuries among fungicide applicators in citrus orchards. *J. Jpn. Assoc. Rural Med.* **25**, 342–343 (in Japanese).

Arimatsu, N., Furushiro, Y., Misumi, J., Ueda, A., and Nomura, S. (1978). Results of investigation on the impairment of applicators of colorants and antiseptics on citrus fruits. *J. Jpn. Assoc. Rural Med.* **24**, 723–733 (in Japanese).

Asmussen, E., Hald, J., and Larsen, V. (1948). The pharmacological action of acetaldehyde in the human organism. *Acta Pharmacol. Toxicol.* **4**, 311–320.

Avrahami, M., and Gernert, I. L. (1972). Hexachlorobenzene antagonism to dieldrin storage in adipose tissue of female rats. *N. Z. J. Agric. Res.* **15**, 783–787.

Avrahami, M., and Steele, R. T. (1972a). Hexachlorobenzene. I. Accumulation and elimination of HCB in sheep after oral dosing. *N. Z. J. Agric. Res.* **15**, 476–481.

Avrahami, M., and Steele, R. T. (1972b). Hexachlorobenzene. II. Residues in laying pullets fed HCB in their diet and the effects on egg production, egg hatchability and on chickens. *N. Z. J. Agric. Res.* **15**, 482–488.

Avrahami, M., and Steele, R. T. (1972c). Hexachlorobenzene. III. The effects of feeding HCB to growing chickens. *N. Z. J. Agric. Res.* **15**, 489–494.

Axness, M. E., and Fleeker, J. R. (1979). Metabolism of the butylcarbamoyl moiety of benomyl in rat. *Pestic. Biochem. Physiol.* **11**, 1–12.

Bach, B., and Pedersen, N. B. (1980). Contact dermatitis from a wood preservative containing tetrachloroisophthalonitrite. *Contact Dermatitis* **6**, 142.

Bachmann, E., Goldberg, L., and Thibodeau, L. (1971). Aspects of the determination of biphenyl hydroxylase activity in liver homogenates III. Influence of administration of 2,6-dichloro-4-nitroaniline to rats. *Exp. Mol. Pathol.* **14,** 306–326.

Baer, R. L., and Rosenthal, S. A. (1954). The germicidal action on human skin of soap containing tetramethylthiurium disulfide. *J. Invest. Dermatol.* **23,** 193–211.

Baer, R. L., Ramsey, D., and Biondi, E. (1973). The most common allergens. *Arch. Dermatol.* **108,** 74–78.

Balin, P. N. (1969). Pathologicomorphological changes in the organism occurring under the chronic action of the pesticide maneb. *Vrach. Delo* **10,** 95–99 (in Russian).

Balin, P. N. (1970). Experimental data on the blastomogenic activity of the fungicide, maneb. *Vrach. Delo* **4,** 21–24 (in Russian).

Bankowska, J., Bojanowska, A., Komorowska-Malewska, W., Krawcynski, K., Majle, T., Syrowatka, T., and Wiakrowska, B. (1970). Study of the effect of zineb and maneb on thyroid function and some related enzymatic systems. *Rocz. Panstw. Zakl. Hig.* **21,** 117–127 (in Polish).

Bernstein, H. N., Curtis, J., Earl, F. L., and Kuwabara, T. (1970). Phototoxic corneal and lens opacities in dogs receiving a fungicide, 2,6-dichloro-4-nitroaniline. *Arch. Ophthalmol. (Chicago)* **83,** 336–348.

Betts, J. J., James, S. P., and Thorpe, W. V. (1955). The metabolism of pentachloronitrobenzene and 2 : 3 : 4 : 6-tetrachloronitrobenzene and the formation of mercapturic acids in the rabbit. *Biochem. J.* **61,** 611–617.

Bignami, M., Aulicino, F., Velcich, A., Carere, A., and Morpurgo, G. (1977). Mutagenic and recombinogenic action of pesticides in *Aspergillus nidulans*. *Mutat. Res.* **46,** 395–402.

Bilancia, A. (1964). Erythroderm from zinc dithiocarbamate in an agricultural worker. *Arch. Ital. Dermatol. Venerol. Sessuol.* **33,** 33–42 (in Italian).

Billings, R. E., and McMahon, R. E. (1976). Liver microsomal hydroxylation of biphenyl to 3-hydroxybiphenyl. *Pharmacologist* **18,** 155.

Bjorseth, A., Lunde, G., and Dybing, E. (1977). Residues of persistent chlorinated hydrocarbons in human tissues as studied by neutron activation analysis and gas chromatography. *Bull. Environ. Contam. Toxicol.* **18,** 581–587.

Blekkenhorst, G. H., Eales, L., and Pimstone, N. R. (1978). The nature of hepatic cytochrome P-450 induced in hexachlorobenzene-fed rats. *Clin. Sci. Mol. Med.* **55,** 461–469.

Bodansky, O. (1951). Methemoglobinemia and methemoglobin-producing compounds. *Pharmacol. Rev.* **3,** 144–196.

Booth, A. N., Ambrose, A. M., DeEds, F., and Cox, A. J., Jr. (1961). The reversible nephrotoxic effects of biphenyl. *Toxicol. Appl. Pharmacol.* **3,** 560–567.

Borzelleca, J. F., Larson, P. S., Crawford, E. M., Hennigar, G. R., Jr., Kuchar, E. J., and Klein, H. H. (1971). Toxicologic and metabolic studies on pentachloronitrobenzene. *Toxicol. Appl. Pharmacol.* **18,** 522–534.

Borzsonyi, M., Pinter, A., Nadasdi, L., and Csik, M. (1976). The carcinogenic effects on *N*-nitroso compounds produced *in vivo* in mice from benzimidazole carbamate-containing pesticides. *Magy. Onkol.* **20,** 89–93 (in Hungarian).

Boyd, E., and Carsky, E. (1971). The 100-day LD 50 index of captan. *Acta Pharmacol. Toxicol.* **29,** 226–240.

Boyd, E., and Krijnen, C. J. (1968). Toxicity of captan and protein-deficient diet. *J. Clin. Pharmacol.* **8,** 225–234.

Brady, M. N., and Siyali, D. S. (1972). Hexachlorobenzene in human body fat. *Med. J. Aust.* **1,** 158–160.

Brevik, E. M., and Bjerk, J. E. (1978). Organochlorine compounds in Norwegian human fat and milk. *Acta Pharmacol. Toxicol.* **43,** 59–63.

Bridges, B. A. (1975). The mutagenicity of captan and related fungicides. *Mutat. Res.* **32,** 3–34.

Bridges, B. A., Mottershead, R. P., Rothwell, M. A., and Green, M. H. L. (1972). Repair-deficient bacterial strains suitable for mutagenicity screening: Tests with the fungicide captan. *Chem.-Biol. Interact.* **5,** 77–84.

Bridges, J. W., and Burke, M. D. (1971). Factors affecting the *in vitro* interaction of biphenyl with P-450 in the hamster. *Chem.-Biol. Interact.* **3,** 314–315.

Brieger, H., and Hodes, W. A. (1949). Toxicity of dithiocarbamates and the hazards of exposure to these compounds. *Proc. Int. Congr. Ind. Med. 9th, 1948,* pp. 598–602.

Brocker, E. R., and Schlatter, C. (1979). Influence of some cations on the intestinal absorption of maneb. *J. Agric. Food Chem.* **27,** 303–306.

Brown, R. (1984). Contact sensitivity to difolatan (captafol). *Contact Dermatitis* **10,** 181–182.

Brusilovskiy, Y. S., and Fialkovskiy, A. M. (1973a). Experimental study of the effect of thiram administration on various allergic reactions. *Gig. Tr. Prof. Zabol.* **17,** 52–54 (in Russian).

Brusilovskiy, Y. S., and Fialkovskiy, A. M. (1973b). Experimental study of the dermato-allergic effect of thiram. *Vestn. Dermatol. Venerol.* **47,** 28–31 (in Russian).

Bruynzeel, D. P., and van Ketel, W. G. (1986). Contact dermatitis due to chlorothalonil in floriculture. *Contact Dermatitis* **14,** 67–68.

Buklan, A. I. (1974). Acute poisoning with ziram. *Sud.-Med. Ekspert.* **17,** 51 (in Russian).

Burnett, J. W., and Pathak, M. A. (1964). Effects of light upon porphyrin metabolism of rats. *Arch. Dermatol.* **89,** 257–266.

Burns, J. E., and Miller, F. M. (1975). Hexachlorobenzene contamination: Its effects in a Louisiana population. *Arch. Environ. Health* **30,** 44–48.

Burns, J. E., Miller, F. M., Gomes, E. D., and Albert, R. A. (1974). Hexachlorobenzene exposure from contaminated DCPA in vegetable spraymen. *Arch. Environ. Health* **29,** 192–194.

Buselmaier, W., Röhrborn, G., and Propping, P. (1972). Host-mediated and dominant lethal mutagenicity tests of pesticides in mice. *Biol. Zentralbl.* **91,** 311–325 (in German).

Buselmaier, W., Röhrborn, G., and Propping, P. (1973). Comparative investigations on the mutagenicity of pesticides in mammalian test systems. *Mutat. Res.* **21,** 25–26.

Cabral, J. R. P., Shubik, P., Mollner, T., and Raitano, F. (1977). Carcinogenic activity of hexachlorobenzene in hamsters. *Nature (London)* **269,** 510–511.

Cabral, J. R. P., Mollner, T., Raitano, F., and Shubik, P. (1978). Carcinogenesis study in mice with hexachlorobenzene. *Toxicol. Appl. Pharmacol.* **45,** 323.

Cabral, J. R. P., Mollner, T., Raitano, F., and Shubik, P. (1979). Carcinogenesis of hexachlorobenzene in mice. *Int. J. Cancer* **23,** 47–51.

Cam, C. (1957). Four cases of congenital porphyria. *Nester* **1,** 2.

Cam, C. (1958). Cases of skin porphyria related to hexachlorobenzene intoxication. *Saglik Derg.* **32,** 215–216.

Cam, C. (1959). Cutaneous porphyria related to intoxication. *Dirim (Istanbul)* **34,** 11–15.

Cam, C. (1960). A new epidemic dermatosis for children. *Ann. Dermatol. Syphiligr.* **87,** 393–397 (in French).

Cam, C., and Nigogosyan, G. (1963). Acquired toxic porphyria cutanea tarda due to hexachlorobenzene. *JAMA J. Am. Med. Assoc.* **183,** 88–91.

Cameron, G. R., Thomas, J. C., Ashmore, S. A., Buchan, J. L., Warren, E. H., and McKenny Hughes, A. W. (1937). The toxicity of certain chlorine derivatives of benzene, with special reference to *o*-dichlorobenzene. *J. Pathol. Bacteriol.* **44,** 281–295.

Campbell, J. A. H. (1963). Pathological aspects of hexachlorobenzene feeding in rats. *S. Afr. J. Lab. Clin. Med.* **9,** 203–206.

Carere, A., Ortali, V. A., Cardamone, G., Torracca, A. M., and Raschetti, R. (1978). Microbiological mutagenicity studies of pesticides *in vitro*. *Mutat. Res.* **57,** 277–286.

Carlson, G. P. (1977). Chlorinated benzene induction of hepatic porphyria. *Experientia* **33,** 1627–1629.

Carlson, G. P., and Tardiff, R. G. (1976). Effect of chlorinated benzenes on the metabolism of foreign organic compounds. *Toxicol. Appl. Pharmacol.* **36,** 383–394.

Casier, H., and Merlevede, E. (1962). On the mechanism of the disulfiram–ethanol intoxication symptoms. *Arch. Int. Pharmacodyn. Ther.* **134,** 165–176.

Chernov, O. V. (1968). A case of occupational poisoning with the dimethyldithiocarbamate of zinc (ziram). *Gig. Tr. Prof. Zabol.* **12,** 35–37 (in Russian).

Chernov, O. V., and Khitsenko, I. I. (1969). Blastomogenic properties of some derivatives of dithiocarbamic acid. *Vopr. Onkol.* **15,** 71–74 (in Russian).

Cherpak, V. V., Bezuglyy, V. P., and Kaskevich, L. M. (1971). Sanitary and hygienic characteristics of working with tetramethylthiuramdisulfide (TMTD). *Vrach. Delo* **10,** 136–139 (in Russian).

Chiba, M., and Cherniak, E. A. (1978). Kinetic study of reversible conversion of methyl 1-(butylcarbamoyl)-2-benzimidazole carbamate (benomyl) to methyl 2-benzimidazole carbamate (MBC) and *n*-butyl isocyanate (BIC) in organic solvents. *J. Agric. Food Chem.* **26**, 573–576.

Christensen, J., and Wase, A. (1954). Tetraethylthiuram disulfide and thyroid activity. *Fed. Proc. Fed. Am. Soc. Exp. Biol.* **13**, 343.

Chu, T. C., and Chu, E. J. H. (1970). Effect of various additives on porphyrin synthesis. *Biochim. Biophys. Acta* **215**, 377–392.

Clarke, C. H. (1971). The mutagenic specificities of pentachloronitrobenzene and captan, two environmental mutagens. *Mutat. Res.* **11**, 247–248.

Collins, T. F. X. (1972a). Dominant lethal assay. I. Captan. *Food Cosmet. Toxicol.* **10**, 353–361.

Collins, T. F. X. (1972b). Dominant lethal assay. II. Folpet and difolatan. *Food Cosmet. Toxicol.* **10**, 363–371.

Collins, T. F. X. (1972c). Effect of captan and triethylenemelamine (TEM) on reproductive fitness of DBA/2J mice. *Toxicol. Appl. Pharmacol.* **23**, 277–287.

Couch, R. C., Siegel, M. R., and Dorough, H. W. (1977). Fate of captan and folpet in rats and their effects on isolated liver nuclei. *Pestic. Biochem. Physiol.* **7**, 547–558.

Courtney, K. D., Copeland, M. F., and Robbins, A. (1976). The effects of pentachloronitrobenzene, hexachlorobenzene and related compounds on fetal development. *Toxicol. Appl. Pharmacol.* **35**, 239–256.

Courtney, K. D., Andrews, J. E., and Stevens, J. T. (1978). Inhalation teratology studies with captan and folpet. *Toxicol. Appl. Pharmacol.* **47**, 292.

Creaven, P. J., and Williams, R. T. (1963). Post-mortem survival of aromatic hydroxylating activity in liver. *Biochem. J.* **87**, 19.

Creaven, P. J., Parke, D. V., and Williams, R. T. (1965). A fluorimetric study of the hydroxylation of biphenyl *in vitro* by liver preparations of various species. *Biochem. J.* **96**, 879–885.

Cripps, D. J., Gocmen, A., and Peters, H. A. (1980). Porphyria turcica. Twenty years after hexachlorobenzene intoxication. *Arch. Dermatol.* **116**, 46–50.

Croy, I. (1973). A case of urticaria involving a captan-derived antimycotic. *Z. Gesamte Hyg. Ihre Grenzgeb.* **19**, 710–711 (in German).

Curley, A., Burse, V. W., Jennings, R. W., and Villaneuva, E. C. (1973). Chlorinated hydrocarbon pesticides and related compounds in adipose tissue from people of Japan. *Nature (London)* **242**, 338–340.

Dalvi, R. R., and Deoras, D. P. (1986). Metabolism of a dithiocarbamate fungicide thiram to carbon disulfide in the rat and its hepatotoxic implications. *Acta Pharmacol. Toxicol.* **58**, 38–42.

Dalvi, R. R., Poore, R. E., and Neal, R. A. (1974). Studies of the metabolism of carbon disulfide by rat liver microsomes. *Life Sci.* **14**, 1785–1796.

Dassenoy, B., and Meyer, J. A. (1973). Mutagenic effect of benomyl on *Fusarium oxysporum*. *Mutat. Res.* **21**, 119–120.

Davydova, T. B. (1973). The effect of inhaled tetramethylthiuram disulfide (thiram) on the estrous cycle and the reproductive function of animals. *Gig. Sanit.* **38**, 101–110 (in Russian).

DeBaun, J. R., Miaullis, J. B., Knarr, J., Mihailovski, A., and Menn, J. J. (1974). The fate of *N*-trichloro^{14}C methylthio-4-cyclohexane-1,2-dicarboximide (^{14}C captan) in the rat. *Xenobiotica* **4**, 101–110.

Decloitre, F., and Hamon, G. (1979). Effect of two pesticides, lindane and zineb, on aflatoxic B$_1$ mutagenesis mediated by rat- and mouse-liver microsomes. *Mutat. Res.* **64**, 130–131.

Deichmann, W. B., Kitzmiller, K. V., Dierker, M., and Witherup, S. (1947). Observations on the effects of diphenyl, *o* and *p*-nitrophenyl and dihydroxyoctachlorodiphenyl upon experimental animals. *J. Ind. Hyg. Toxicol.* **29**, 1–13.

Dejonckheere, W., Steurbaut, W., Verstraeten, R., and Kips, R. H. (1978). Residues of organochlorine pesticides in human fat in Belgium. *Toxicol. Eur. Res.* **1**, 93–98.

DeMatteis, F., Prior, B. E., and Rimington, C. (1961). Nervous and biochemical disturbances following hexachlorobenzene intoxication. *Nature (London)* **191**, 363–366.

Den Tonkelaar, E. M., Verschurren, H. G., Bankovska, J., De Vries, T., Kroes, R., and van Esch, G. J. (1978). Hexachlorobenzene toxicity in pigs. *Toxicol. Appl. Pharmacol.* **43**, 137–145.

de Torres, G. G., Romer, K. G., Torres Alanis, O., and Freundt, K. J. (1983). Blood acetaldehyde levels in alcohol-dosed rats after treatment with ANIT, ANTU, dithiocarbamate derivatives, or cyanamide. *Drug Chem. Toxicol.* **6**, 317–328.

Dinoyeva, S. K. (1974). Dynamics of the changes in immunological structures of lymphatic follicles in spleen during pesticide poisoning. *Gig. Sanit.* **39**, 85–87 (in Russian).

Dobyns, B. M., Sheline, G. E., Workman, J. B., Thompkins, E. A., McConahey, W. M., and Becker, D. V. (1974). Malignant and benign neoplasms of the thyroid in patients treated for hyperthyroidism: A report of the co-operative thyrotoxicosis therapy follow-up study. *J. Clin. Endocrinol. Metab.* **38**, 976–998.

Doğramaci, I., Tinaztepe, B., and Gunalp, A. (1962a). Condition of the liver in patients with toxic cutaneous porphyria. *Turk. J. Pediatr.* **4**, 103–107.

Doğramaci, I., Wray, J. D., Ergene, T., Sezer, V., and Muftu, Y. (1962b). Porphyria turcica: A survey of 592 cases of cutaneous porphyria seen in southeastern Turkey. *Turk. J. Pediatr.* **4**, 138–148.

Doğramaci, I., Kenanoglu, A., Muftu, Y., Ergene, T., and Wray, J. D. (1962c). Bone and joint changes in patients with porphyria turcica: A clinical and roentgenologic study. *Turk. J. Pediatr.* **4**, 149–156.

Doğramaci, I., Ozand, P., Muftu, Y., and Ergene, T. (1963). The effect of barbiturates in porphyria turcica. *Turk. J. Pediatr.* **5**, 1–9.

Dooms-Goossens, A. E., Debusschere, K. M., Gevers, D. M., Dupre, K. M., Degreef, H. J., Loncke, J. P., and Snauwaert, J. E. (1986). Contact dermatitis caused by airborne agents. *J. Am. Acad. Dermatol.* **15**, 1–9.

Doroscuk, V. P. (1974). The external respiration in nervous conditions following exposure to certain pesticides. *Gig. Tr. Prof. Zabol.* **18**, 45–46 (in Russian).

Douch, P. G. C. (1973). The metabolism of benomyl fungicide in mammals. *Xenobiotica* **3**, 367–380.

Doyle, J. J., Clark, D. E., and Norman, J. D. (1979). Effects of dietary hexachlorobenzene on distribution of some trace metals in rat tissues. *Bull. Environ. Contam. Toxicol.* **21**, 225–229.

Duggan, R. E., and Corneiliussen, P. E. (1972). Dietary intake of pesticide chemicals in the United States (III), June 1968–April 1970. *Pestic. Monit. J.* **5**, 331–341.

Durham, W. F., and Williams, C. H. (1972). Mutagenic, teratogenic, and carcinogenic properties of pesticides. *Annu. Rev. Entomol.* **17**, 123–148.

D'yachuk, I. A. (1972). Hygienic assessment of the working conditions in seed treatment facilities. *Gig. Tr. Prof. Zabol.* **16**, 45–47 (in Russian).

Dyadicheva, T. V. (1971). Functional condition of the thyroid and of the adrenal cortex in chronic treatment with carbamate pesticides. *Vrach. Delo* **2**, 120–123 (in Russian).

Dybing, E., and Aune, T. (1977). Hexachlorobenzene induction of 2,4-diaminoanisole mutagenicity *in vitro*. *Acta Pharmacol. Toxicol.* **40**, 575–583.

Earl, F. L., Curtis, J. M., Bernstein, H. N., and Smalley, H. E. (1971). Ocular effects in dogs and pigs treated with dichloran (2,6-dichloro-4-nitroaniline). *Food Cosmet. Toxicol.* **9**, 819–828.

Eberts, F. S., Jr. (1965). Fate of Botran (2,6-dichloro-4-nitroaniline) in rat and man. Botran Symposium, Augusta, Mich. *Pesticides* **68**, 1123, 1968.

Edmundson, W. F., Freal, J. J., and Davies, J. E. (1967). Identification and measurement of dichloran in the blood and urine of man. *Environ. Res.* **1**, 240–246.

Egert, G., and Greim, H. (1976). Formation of dimethylnitrosamine from Chloroxuron, Cycluron, Dimefox and Thiram in the presence of nitrite. *Mutat. Res.* **38**, 136–137.

Eisenbrand, G., Ungerer, O., and Preussmann, R. (1974). Rapid formation of carcinogenic *N*-nitrosamines by interaction of nitrite with fungicides derived from dithiocarbamic acid *in vitro* under simulated gastric conditions and *in vivo* in the rat stomach. *Food Cosmet. Toxicol.* **12**, 229–232.

Elder, G. H. (1974). The metabolism of porphyrins of the isocoproporphyrin series. *Enzyme* **17**, 61–68.

Elder, G. H., Evans, J. O., and Matlin, S. A. (1976). The effect of the porphyrogenic compound, hexachlorobenzene, on the activity of hepatic uroporphyrinogen decarboxylase in the rat. *Clin. Sci. Mol. Med.* **51**, 71–80.

Engst, R., and Raab, M. (1973). The metabolism of phthalimide-derived fungicides in food—chemistry and toxicology. *Nahrung* **17**, 731–738 (in German).

Engst, R., Schnaak, W., and Lewerenz, H. J. (1971). Metabolic studies of the fungicides ethylene-bis-dithiocarbamate, maneb, zineb and nabam. V. The toxicology of the metabolites. *Z. Lebensm.-Unters.-Forsch.* **146**, 91–97 (in German).

Engst, R., Macholz, R. M., and Kujawa, M. (1976). The metabolism of hexachlorobenzene (HCB) in rats. *Bull. Environ. Contam. Toxicol.* **16**, 248–252.

Enikeev, V. Kh. (1968). Problems of work hygiene in the production of ziram. *Gig. Tr. Prof. Zabol.* **12**, 12–16 (in Russian).

Epstein, S. S., and Shafner, H. (1968). Chemical mutagens in the human environment. *Nature (London)* **219**, 385–387.

Fabro, S., Smith, R. L., and Williams, R. T. (1965). Embryotoxic activity of some pesticides and drugs related to phthalamide. *Food Cosmet. Toxicol.* **3**, 587–590.

Farkas, A. (1939). Control of wastage of citrus fruit by impregnated wrappers, on a commercial scale. *Hadar* **12**, 227–231.

Fenyvesi, G., Botos, M., and Ivan, J. (1985). Pesticide–drug interaction in rats. *Arch. Toxicol., Suppl.* **8**, 269–271.

Ficsor, G., and Nii, G. M. (1970). Captan-induced reversions of bacteria. *Newsl. Environ. Mutagen. Soc.* **3**, 38.

Ficsor, G., Bordas, S., Wade, S. M., Muthiani, E., Wertz, G. F., and Zimmer, D. M. (1977). Mammalian host- and fluid-mediated mutagenicity assays of captan and streptozotocin in *Salmonella typhimurium*. *Mutat. Res.* **48**, 1–16.

Ficsor, G., Bordas, S., and Stewart, S. J. (1978). Mutagenicity testing of benomyl, methyl-2-benzimidazole carbamate, streptozotocin and *N*-methyl-*N'*-nitro-*N*-nitrosoguanidine in *Salmonella typhimurium in vitro* and in rodent host-mediated assays. *Mutat. Res.* **51**, 151–164.

Finnegan, J. K., Larson, P. S., Smith, R. B., Jr., Haag, H. B., and Hennigar, G. R. (1958). Acute and chronic toxicity studies on pentachlorobenzene. *Arch. Int. Pharmacodyn. Ther.* **114**, 38–52.

Fitzhugh, O. G., and Nelson, A. A. (1948). Liver tumors in rats fed thiourea or thioacetamide. *Science* **108**, 626–628.

Flannigan, S. A., and Tucker, S. B. (1985). Influence of the vehicle on irritant contact dermatitis. *Contact Dermatitis* **12**, 177–178.

Flannigan, S. A., Tucker, S. B., and Calderon, V. (1986). Irritant dermatitis from tetrachloroisophthalonitrile. *Contact Dermatitis* **14**, 258–259.

Food and Agriculture Organization/World Health Organization (FAO/WHO) (1965). "Evaluation of the Toxicity of Pesticide Residues in Food" Monograph prepared by the Joint Meeting of the FAO Committee on Pesticides in Agriculture and the WHO Expert Committee on Pesticide Residues, which met in Rome, 15–22 March 1965. (WHO/Food Add./27.65). World Health Organ., Geneva.

Food and Agriculture Organization/World Health Organization (FAO/WHO) (1967). "Evaluation of Some Pesticide Residues in Food." Monograph prepared by the Joint Meeting of the FAO Working Party and the WHO Expert Committee on Pesticide Residues, which met in Geneva, 14–21 November 1966 (WHO/Food Add./67.32). World Health Organ., Geneva.

Food and Agriculture Organization/World Health Organization (FAO/WHO) (1968). "1967 Evaluations of Some Pesticide Residues in Food." Monograph prepared by the Joint Meeting of the FAO Working Party of Experts and the WHO Expert Committee on Pesticide Residues, which met in Rome, 4–11 December, 1967 (WHO/Food Add./68.30). World Health Organ., Geneva.

Food and Agriculture Organization/World Health Organization (FAO/WHO) (1970). "1969 Evaluations of Some Pesticide Residues in Food." Monograph prepared by the Joint Meeting of the FAO Working Party of Experts and the WHO Expert Group on Pesticide Residues, which met in Rome, 8–15 December 1969 (WHO/Food Add./70.38). World Health Organ., Geneva.

Food and Agriculture Organization/World Health Organization (FAO/WHO) (1974). "1973 Evaluations of Some Pesticide Residues in Food." Monograph presented by the Joint Meeting of the FAO Working Party of Experts on Pesticide Residues and the WHO Expert Committee on Pesticide Residues that met in Geneva, 26 November to 5 December 1973 (WHO Pestic. Residues Ser., No. 3). World Health Organ., Geneva.

Food and Agriculture Organization/World Health Organization (FAO/WHO) (1975). "1974 Evaluation of Some Pesticide Residues in Food." Monograph prepared by the Joint Meeting of the FAO Working Party of Experts on Pesticide Residues and the WHO Expert Committee on Pesticide Residues that met in Rome, 2 to 11 December 1974 (WHO Pestic. Residues Ser., No. 4). World Health Organ., Geneva.

Freundt, K. J., and Netz, H. (1977). Behaviour of blood acetaldehyde in alcohol-treated rats following administration of thiurams. *Arzneim.-Forsch.* **27**, 105 (in German).

Fuchs, A., Van Den Berg, G. A., and Davidse, L. C. (1972). A comparison of benomyl and thiophanates with respect to some chemical and systemic fungitoxic characteristics. *Pestic. Biochem. Physiol.* **2**, 191–205.

Fujita, K. (1975). Keratitis and conjunctivitis due to pesticides. *J. Jpn. Assoc. Rural Med.* **24**, 16–18 (in Japanese).

Gaines, T. B. (1969). Acute toxicity of pesticides. *Toxicol. Appl. Pharmacol.* **14**, 515–534.

Gajdos, A., and Gajdos-Török, M. (1961a). Experimental porphyria observed in rats after hexachlorobenzene intoxication. *Rev. Fr. Etud. Clin. Biol.* **6**, 549–552 (in French).

Gajdos, A., and Gajdos-Török, M. (1961b). Therapeutic action of adenosine-5-monophosphoric acid upon experimental porphyria of the white rat due to intoxication by hexachlorobenzene. *Rev. Fr. Etud. Clin. Biol.* **6**, 553–559 (in French).

Gajdos, A., and Gajdos-Török, M. (1961c). The therapeutic effect of adenosine-5-monophosphoric acid in porphyria. *Lancet* **2**, 175–177.

Gal, E. M., and Greenberg, D. M. (1954). Non-specific reversal by vitamins of inhibition of ethanol oxidation by Antabuse (tetraethylthiuram disulfide) in the rat. *Proc. Soc. Exp. Biol. Med.* **85**, 252–254.

Gale, G. R., Smith, A. B., Atkins, L. M., Walker, E. M., Jr., and Gadsden, R. H. (1971). Pharmacology of captan: Biochemical effects with special reference to macromolecular synthesis. *Toxicol. Appl. Pharmacol.* **18**, 426–441.

Gallo, M. A., Bachmann, E., and Golberg, L. (1972). Effects of 2,6-dichloro-4-nitroaniline and its metabolites on rat liver mitochondria. *Toxicol. Appl. Pharmacol.* **22**, 311.

Gallo, M. A., Bachmann, E., and Golberg, L. (1976). Mitochondrial effects of 2,6-dichloro-4-nitroaniline and its metabolites. *Toxicol. Appl. Pharmacol.* **35**, 51–61.

Gardiner, J. A., Brantley, R. K., and Sherman, H. (1968). Isolation and identification of a metabolite of methyl 1-(butylcarbamoyl)-2-benzimidazolecarbamate in rat urine. *J. Agric. Food Chem.* **16**, 1050–1052.

Gardiner, J. A., Kirland, J. J., Klopping, H. L., and Sherman, H. (1974). Fate of benomyl in animals. *J. Agric. Food Chem.* **22**, 118–126.

Gerasimchuk, A. S., Neyko, Y. M., Banenko, N. A., and Denisyuk, V. G. (1975). Functional state of the external respiratory apparatus in workers in contact with zineb. *Vrach. Delo* **1**, 125–127 (in Russian).

Gessner, T., and Jakubowski, M. (1972). Diethyldithiocarbamic acid methyl ester. A metabolite of disulfiram. *Biochem. Pharmacol.* **21**, 219–230.

Gladenko, V. I. (1971). Study of the toxicity of thiabendazole. *Farmakol. Toksikol. (Moscow)* **34**, 483–485 (in Russian).

Goerz, G., Vizethum, W., Bolsen, K., and Kreig, T. (1978). Porphyria in the rat caused by hexachlorobenzene (HCB). The influence of HCB-metabolites on the formation of haemoglobin. *Arch. Dermatol. Res.* **263**, 189–196 (in German).

Goerz, G., Vizethum, W., and Tsambaos, D. (1979). Cutaneous cytochrome P-450 activity during hexachlorobenzene induced experimental porphyria in rats. *Arch. Dermatol. Res.* **265**, 111–114.

Goitre, M., Bedello, P. G., and Cane, D. (1981). Allergic dermatitis and oral challenge to tetramethylthiuram disulphide. *Contact Dermatitis* **7**, 272–273.

Goldstein, J. A., Friesen, M., Scotti, T. M., Hickman, P., Haas, J. R., and Bergman, H. (1978). Assessment of the contribution of chlorinated dibenzo-*p*-dioxins and dibenzofurans to hexachlorobenzene-induced toxicity, porphyria, changes in mixed function oxygenases, and histopathological changes. *Toxicol. Appl. Pharmacol.* **46**, 633–649.

Grant, D. L., Iverson, F., Hatina, G. V., and Villeneuve, D. C. (1974a). Effects of hexachlorobenzene on liver porphyrin levels and microsomal enzymes in the rat. *Toxicol. Appl. Pharmacol.* **29**, 101.

Grant, D. L., Iverson, F., Hatina, G. V., and Villeneuve, D. C. (1974b). Effects of hexachlorobenzene on liver porphyrin levels and microsomal enzymes in the rat. *Environ. Physiol. Biochem.* **4**, 159–165.

Grant, D. L., Shields, J. B., and Villeneuve, D. C. (1975). Chemical (HCB) porphyria: Effect of removal of sex organs in the rat. *Bull. Environ. Contam. Toxicol.* **14**, 422–425.

Grant, D. L., Phillips, W. E. J., and Hatina, G. V. (1977). Effect of hexachlorobenzene on reproduction in the rat. *Arch. Environ. Contam. Toxicol.* **5**, 207–216.

Griepentrog, F. (1962). Tumor-like changes in the thyroid gland in chronic toxicological animal experiments with thiurams. *Beitr. Pathol. Anat. Allg. Pathol.* **126**, 243–255 (in German).

Groundwater, J. R. (1977). Difolatan dermatitis in a welder; non-agricultural exposure. *Contact Dermatitis* **3**, 104.

Gunther, L. W. (1970). Tetramethylthiuram disulphide (T.M.T.D.) and bowls. *Med. J. Aust.* **1**, 1177.

Haeger-Aronsen, B. (1964). Experimental disturbance of porphyrin metabolism and of liver catalase activity in guinea pigs and rabbits. *Acta Pharmacol. Toxicol.* **21**, 105–115.

Hakkinen, I., Hernberg, S., Siltanen, E., Seppalainen, A. M., Karli, P., and Vikkula, E. (1973). Diphenyl poisoning in fruit paper production. A new health hazard. *Arch. Environ. Health* **26**, 70–74.

Hald, J., and Jacobsen, E. (1948a). A drug sensitising the organism to ethyl alcohol. *Lancet* **255**, 1001–1004.

Hald, J., and Jacobsen, E. (1948b). The formation of acetaldehyde in the organism after ingestion of Antabuse (tetraethylthiuram disulphide) and alcohol. *Acta Pharmacol. Toxicol.* **4**, 305–310.

Hald, J., Jacobsen, E., and Larsen, V. (1948). The sensitizing effect of tetraethylthiuram disulphide (Antabuse) to ethyl alcohol. *Acta Pharmacol. Toxicol.* **4**, 285–296.

Hald, J., Jacobsen, E., and Larsen, V. (1952). The Antabuse effect of some compounds related to Antabuse and cyanamide. *Acta Pharmacol. Toxicol.* **8**, 329–337.

Halpaap, K., Horning, E. C., and Horning, M. G. (1978). Effects of β-naphthoflavone and phenobarbital pretreatment on the metabolism of biphenyl in the rat. *Fed. Proc., Fed. Am. Soc. Exp. Biol.* **37**, 465.

Hamblin, D. O. (1963). Aromatic nitro and amino compounds. *In* "Industrial Hygiene and Toxicology" (F. A. Patty, ed.), Chapter 46. Wiley (Interscience), New York.

Hanada, S. (1975). Studies on diphenyl and o-phenylphenol as food additives from the public viewpoint. Part I. Fungicidal activity. . *Nagoya City Univ. Med. Assoc.* **26**, 78–86. (in Japanese).

Hansen, L. G., Wilson, D. W., Byerly, C. S., Sundlof, S. F., and Dorn, S. B. (1977). Effects and residues of dietary hexachlorobenzene in growing swine. *J. Toxicol. Environ. Health* **2**, 557–567.

Haseman, J. K., and Hoel, D. G. (1979). Statistical design of toxicity assays: Role of genetic structure of test animal population. *J. Toxicol. Environ. Health* **5**, 89–101.

Hashimoto, Y., Makita, T., Ohnuma, N., and Noguchi, T. (1972a). Acute toxicity studies on dimethyl 4,4'-o-phenylene bis(3-thioallopha nate), thiophanatemethyl fungicide. *Toxicol. Appl. Pharmacol.* **23**, 606–615.

Hashimoto, Y., Mori, T., Ohnuma, N., and Noguchi, T. (1972b). Some pharmacologic properties of a new fungicide thiophanate-methyl. *Toxicol. Appl. Pharmacol.* **23**, 616–622.

Hastie, A. C. (1970). Benlate-induced instability of *Aspergillus* diploids. *Nature (London)* **226**, 771.

Hayes, W. J., Jr. (1975). "Toxicology of Pesticides." Williams & Wilkins, Baltimore, Maryland.

Henbry, F. G., Smart, L. I., Binder, T. D., and Dixon, J. M. (1975). Hexachlorobenzene decontamination of beef cattle. *J. Anim. Sci.* **41**, 269.

Herbold, B., and Buselmaier, W. (1976). Induction of point mutations by different chemical mechanisms in the liver microsomal assay. *Mutat. Res.* **40**, 73–84.

Hodge, H. C., Maynard, E. A., Downs, W. L., Blanchet, H. J., and Jones, C. K. (1952). Acute and short-term oral toxicity of tests of ferric dimethyldithiocarbamate (ferbam) and zinc dimethyldithiocarbamate (ziram). *J. Am. Pharm. Assoc., Sci. Ed.* **41**, 662–665.

Hodge, H. C., Maynard, E. A., Downs, W. L., Coye, R. D., and Steadman, L. T.

(1956). Chronic oral toxicity of ferric dimethyldithiocarbamate (ferbam) and zinc dimethyldithiocarbamate (ziram). *J. Pharmacol. Exp. Ther.* **118**, 174–181.

Hodgson, J. R., and Lee, C. C. (1977). Cytotoxicity studies on dithiocarbamate fungicides. *Toxicol. Appl. Pharmacol.* **40**, 19–22.

Horinchi, Y., and Ando, K. (1980). Contact dermatitis due to pesticides for agricultural use. *Jpn. J. Dermatol.* **90**, 289.

Hunter, A., and Neal, R. A. (1974). Response of the hepatic mixed function oxidase enzyme system to thionosulfur-containing compounds. *Pharmacologist* **16**, 239.

Iatropoulos, M. J., Hobson, W., Knauf, V., and Adams, H. P. (1976). Morphological effects of hexachlorobenzene toxicity in female rhesus monkeys. *Toxicol. Appl. Pharmacol.* **37**, 433–444.

Iatropoulos, M. J., Bailey, J., Adams, H. P., Coulston, F., and Hobson, W. (1978). Response of nursing infant rhesus to Clophen A-30 or hexachlorobenzene given to their lactating mothers. *Environ. Res.* **16**, 38–47.

Imaizumi, K., Atsumi, K., Tanifuji, Y., Ishikawa, Y., and Hoshi, H. (1972). Clinical observations of ophthalmic disturbances due to agricultural chemicals. *Folia Opthalmol. Jpn.* **22**, 154–156 (in Japanese).

Innes, J. R. M., Ulland, B. M., Valerio, M. G., Petrucelli, L., Fishbein, L., Hart, E. R., Pallotta, A. J., Bates, R. R., Falk, H. L., Gart, J. J., Klein, M., Mitchell, I., and Peters, J. (1969). Bioassay of pesticides and industrial chemicals for tumorigenicity in mice: A preliminary note. *J. Natl. Cancer Inst. (U.S.)* **42**, 1101–1114.

Ippen, H., Huettenhain, S., and Aust, D. (1972a). Clinical experimental studies on the genesis of porphyria. II. Experimental porphyria in hexachlorobenzene-treated rats: Effects of ethyl alcohol. *Arch. Dermatol. Forsch.* **245**, 191–202 (in German).

Ippen, H., Aust, D., and Goetz, G. (1972b). Clinical and experimental studies on the development of porphyria. III. Effects of some steroid hormones on latent hexachlorobenzene porphyria in the rat. *Arch. Dermatol. Forsch.* **245**, 305–317 (in German).

Ishida, M., and Nambu, K. (1975). Phthalide (Rabcide). *J. Pestic. Sci.* **3**, 10–26.

Israeli, R., Sculsky, M., and Tiberin, P. (1983). Acute intoxication due to exposure to maneb and zineb. A case with behavioral and central nervous system changes. *Scand. J. Work Environ. Health* **9**, 47–51.

Itoh, S. (1978). Acute and chronic ocular impairments due to agricultural pesticides. *Jpn. Rev. Clin. Ophthalmol.* **72**, 94–95 (in Japanese).

Ivanova, L., Dimov, G., and Mosheva, N. (1966). Experimental foundation of the maximally admitted concentration of Cineb in the air of working places. *Hig. Zdraveopaz.* **9**, 483–491.

Ivanova, L., Sheytanov, M., and Hosheva-Ismirova, N. (1967). Changes in the functional state of the thyroid gland upon acute intoxication with certain dithiocarbamates—zineb and maneb. *C.R. Acad. Bulg. Sci.* **20**, 1011–1013.

Ivanova-Tchemischanska, L., Markov, D. V., and Dashev, G. (1971). Light and electron microscopic observations on rat thyroid after administration of some dithiocarbamates. *Environ. Res.* **4**, 201–212.

Iverson, F. (1976). Induction of paraoxon dealkylation by hexachlorobenzene (HCB) and mirex. *J. Agric. Food Chem.* **24**, 1238–1246.

Iwanow, E., Hiebarowa, M., Krustev, L., Dimitrov, P., Orbetzova, V., Nenov, P., Kirjakov, A., and Tsontscheva, A. (1973). Biochemical and histomorphological changes in experimental hexachlorobenzene porphyria. *Acta Hepato-Gastroenterol.* **20**, 39–48 (in German).

Izmirova, N. (1972). A study of the water-soluble and chloroform-soluble metabolites of S-ziram by means of paper chromatography. *Eksp. Med. Morfol.* **11**, 240–243 (in Bulgarian).

Izmirova, N., and Marinov, V. (1972). Distribution and excretion of S-ziram and metabolic products in 24 hours following oral administration of the preparation to female rats. *Eksp. Med. Morfol.* **11**, 152–156 (in Bulgarian).

Izmirova, N., Ismirov, I., and Ivanova, L. (1969). The effect of zineb and maneb on the isoenzymes of lactate dehydrogenase in the testes of rats. *C.R. Acad. Bulg. Sci.* **22**, 225–227.

Jansson, B., and Bergman, A. (1978). Sulphur-containing derivatives of hexachlorobenzene (HCB) metabolites in the rat. *Chemosphere* **7**, 257–268.

Johnsson, M., Buhagen, M., Leira, H. L., and Solvang, S. (1983). Fungicide-induced contact dermatitis. *Contact Dermatitis* **9**, 285–288.

Johnston, D. C., and Prickett, C. S. (1952). The production of carbon disulfide from tetraethylthiuram disulfide (Antabuse) by rat liver. *Biochim. Biophys. Acta* **9,** 219–220.

Johnston, G., Woodard, G., and Cronin, M. T. I. (1968). Safety evaluation of Botram (2,6-dichloro-4-nitroaniline) in laboratory animals. *Toxicol. Appl. Pharmacol.* **12,** 314–315.

Jokivarto, E. (1950). Effect of iron preparations on "Antabuse"–alcohol toxicosis. *Q. J. Stud. Alcohol* **11,** 183–189.

Jordan, L. W., and Neal, R. A. (1979). Examination of the *in vivo* metabolism of maneb and zineb to ethylenethiourea (ETU) in mice. *Bull. Environ. Contam. Toxicol.* **22,** 271–277.

Jordan, R. L., Sperling, F., Klein, H. H., and Borzelleca, J. F. (1975). A study of the potential teratogenic effects of pentachloronitrobenzene in rats. *Toxicol. Appl. Pharmacol.* **33,** 222–230.

Jordan, W. P., and King, S. E. (1977). Delayed hypersensitivity in females. The development of allergic contact dermatitis in females during the comparison of two predictive patch tests. *Contact Dermatitis* **3,** 19–26.

Jorgenson, T. A., Rushbrook, C. J., and Newell, G. W. (1976). *In vivo* mutagenesis investigations of ten commercial pesticides. *Toxicol. Appl. Pharmacol.* **37,** 109.

Joubert, S. M., Taljaard, J. J. F., and Shanley, B. C. (1973). Aetiological relationship between hepatic siderosis and symptomatic porphyria cutanea tarda: Evidence based on work in Durban. *Enzyme* **16,** 305–313.

Jung, H. D. (1976). Occupational dermatitis caused by Bercema zineb 80 (zinc-ethylene-1,2-bisdithiocarbamate) in agriculture. *Dtsch. Gesundheitswes.* **31,** 573–576 (in German).

Kane, F. J., Jr. (1970). Carbon disulfide intoxication from overdosage of disulfiram. *Am. J. Psychiatry* **127,** 690–694.

Kantemir, I., Giner, S., and Kayaalp, O. (1960). Investigations with hexachlorobenzene and organic mercury compounds. *Turk. Hij. Deneysel. Biyol. Derg.* **20,** 19–30.

Kappas, A., Green, M. H. L., Bridges, B. A., Rogers, A. M., and Muriel, W. J. (1976). Benomyl—a novel type of base analogue mutagen? *Mutat. Res.* **40,** 379–382.

Karpenko, V. N. (1971). A study on hemopoiesis and blood coagulation in carbamate pesticide poisoning. *Vrach. Delo* **1,** 130–133 (in Russian).

Kasai, T., and Sugimoto, T. (1973). Studies on dermatitis caused by difolatan. *Jpn. Ind. Hyg. Soc. Proc.* **46,** 122–123 (in Japanese).

Kaskevich, L. M. (1975). Rheohepatography in the diagnosis of toxicochemical lesions of the liver in persons dealing with tetramethylthiuram disulfide (TMTD). *Gig. Tr. Prof. Zabol.* **6,** 16–19 (in Russian).

Kaskevich, L. M., and Bezuglyy, V. P. (1973a). The health status of subjects exposed occupationally to tetramethylthiuram disulfide (TMTD) in seed control laboratories and seed dressing plants. *Gig. Tr. Prof. Zabol.* **17,** 49–51 (in Russian).

Kaskevich, L. M., and Bezuglyy, V. P. (1973b). Clinical aspects of chronic thiram poisoning. *Vrach. Delo* **6,** 128–130 (in Russian).

Kavlock, R. J., Chernoff, N., Gray, L. E., Gray, J. A., and Whitehouse, D. (1982). Teratogenic effects of benomyl in the Wistar rat and the CD-1 mouse, with emphasis on the route of administration. *Toxicol. Appl. Pharmacol.* **62,** 44–54.

Kennedy, G., Fancher, O. E., and Calandra, J. C. (1968). An investigation of the teratogenic potential of captan, folpet and difolatan. *Toxicol. Appl. Pharmacol.* **13,** 420–430.

Kennedy, G. L., Jr., Arnold, D. W., and Keplinger, M. L. (1975a). Mutagenicity studies with captan, captafol, folpet and thalidomide. *Food Cosmet. Toxicol.* **13,** 55–61.

Kennedy, G. L., Jr., Fancher, O. E., and Calandra, J. C. (1975b). Nonteratogenicity of captan in beagles. *Teratology* **11,** 223–226.

Khera, K. S. (1974). Hexachlorobenzene: Teratogenicity and dominant lethal studies in rats. *Toxicol. Appl. Pharmacol.* **29,** 109.

Khera, K. S., and Shah, B. G. (1979). Failure of zinc acetate to reduce ethylenethiourea induced anomalies in rats. *Toxicol. Appl. Pharmacol.* **48,** 229–235.

Khera, K. S., and Villeneuve, D. C. (1975). Teratogenicity studies on halogenated benzenes (pentachloro-, pentachloronitro-, and hexabromo-) in rats. *Toxicology* **5,** 117–122.

Khomenko, N. R., and Kazakevich, R. L. (1973). Abnormalities of the knee reflex in chronic BHC and thiram poisoning. *Gig. Tr. Prof. Zabol.* **17,** 56–57 (in Russian).

Kimbrough, R. D., and Linder, R. E. (1974). The toxicity of technical hexachlorobenzene in the Sherman strain rat. A preliminary study. *Res. Commun. Chem. Pathol. Pharmacol.* **8,** 653–664.

Kirlich, A. E. (1970). Effect of maneb on testes and ovaries. *Veterinaria (Moscow)* **46,** 93–94 (in Russian).

Kiryushin, V. A. (1975). Mutagenic action of various pesticides in case of their successive entry into the body of albino rats. *Gig. Sanit.* **9,** 43–46 (in Russian).

Kleibl, K., and Rackova, M. (1980). Cutaneous allergic reactions to dithiocarbamates. *Contact Dermatitis* **6,** 348–349.

Kligman, A. M. (1967). Sensitization testing by human assay. *Drug Cosmet. Ind.* **100,** 46–48.

Kligman, A. M., and Rosensweig, W. (1948). Studies with new fungistatic agents. II. For treatment of superficial mycoses. *J. Invest. Dermatol.* **10,** 59–68.

Klingenberg, K. (1891). Studies on the oxidation of aromatic substance in animals. *Jahresber. Fortschr. Tierchem.* **21,** 57–58 (in German).

Knauf, V., and Hobson, W. (1979). Hexachlorobenzene ingestion by female rhesus monkeys: Tissue distribution and clinical symptomatology. *Bull. Environ. Contam. Toxicol.* **21,** 243–248.

Koegel, W., Iatropoulos, M. J., Mueller, W. F., Coulston, F., and Korte, F. (1978). Metabolism, body distribution and histopathology of pentachloronitrobenzene in rhesus monkeys. *Toxicol. Appl. Pharmacol.* **45,** 283.

Koegel, W., Mueller, W. F., Coulston, F., and Korte, F. (1979a). Uptake, body distribution, storage and excretion of pentachloronitrobenzene ^{14}C in rhesus monkeys. *Chemosphere* **8,** 89–95.

Koegel, W., Mueller, W. F., Coulston, F., and Korte, F. (1979b). Biotransformation of pentachloronitrobenzene ^{14}C in rhesus monkeys after single and chronic oral administration. *Chemosphere* **8,** 97–105.

Kolycheva, S. S., Nadzhimutdinov, K. N., and Murzabekov, Sh. M. (1973). Peculiarities of the effect of tetramethylthiuram disulfide on the action of hexenal and corazole in animals of various ages. *Sov. Zdravookhr. Kirg.* **6,** 57–59 (in Russian).

Komarova, A. A., and Zotkina, V. P. (1971). Application of electromyography and of certain parameters of acetylocholine metabolism for the evaluation of the condition of workers engaged in the manufacture of ziram. *Gig. Tr. Prof. Zabol.* **15,** 17–20 (in Russian).

Korte, F., Freitag, D., Geyer, H., Klein, W., Kraus, A. G., and Lahaniatis, E. (1978). A concept for establishing ecotoxicologic priority lists for chemicals. *Chemosphere* **7,** 79–102.

Koss, G., and Koransky, W. (1975). Studies on the toxicology of hexachlorobenzene. I. Pharmacokinetics. *Arch. Toxicol.* **34,** 203–212.

Koss, G., Seubert, S., Seubert, A., Koransky, W., and Ippen, H. (1978). Studies on the toxicology of hexachlorobenzene. III. Observations in a long-term experiment. *Arch. Toxicol.* **40,** 285–294.

Koss, G., Koransky, W., and Steinbach, K. (1979). Studies on the toxicology of hexachlorobenzene. IV. Sulphur-containing metabolites. *Arch. Toxicol.* **42,** 19–31.

Kramers, P. G. N., and Knaap, A. G. A. C. (1973). Mutagenicity tests with captan and folpet in *Drosophila melanogaster. Mutat. Res.* **21,** 149–154.

Kreig, T., Lissner, R., Bolsen, K., Goetz, G., and Ulrich, V. (1977). *O*-Dealkylation activity in rat liver following application of hexachlorobenzene. *Arch. Dermatol. Res.* **258,** 93.

Krijnen, C. J. and Boyd, E. M. (1970). Susceptibility to captan pesticide of albino rats fed from weaning on diets containing various levels of protein. *Food Cosmet. Toxicol.* **8,** 35–42.

Krolikowska-Prasal, I. (1973). The influence of captan on the metabolism of liver cells in cytochemical studies. *Ann. Univ. Mariae Curie-Sklodowska, Sect. D* **28,** 81–90 (in Polish).

Krolikowska-Prasal, I. (1974). Histochemical studies on the gastric epithelium and glands in guinea pigs subjected to the action of a fungicide (captan). *Folia Morphol. (Warsaw)* **33,** 427–435.

Krupa, A., Pienkowska, H. and Tarka, Z. (1971). Acute poisoning with "thiram." *Med. Wiejsk.* **6,** 29–31 (in Polish).

Krupka, R. M. (1974). On the anti-cholinesterase activity of benomyl. *Pestic. Sci.* **5,** 211–216.

Kuchar, E. J., Geenty, F. O., Griffith, W. P., and Thomas, R. J. (1969). Analytical studies of metabolism of Terraclor in beagle dogs, rats and plants. *J. Agric. Food Chem.* **17,** 1237–1240.

Kuiper-Goodman, T., Grant, D., Korsrud, G., Moodie, C. A., and Munro, I. C. (1974). Toxic effects of hexachlorobenzene in the rat: Correlations of electron microscopy with other toxic parameters. *Toxicol. Appl. Pharmacol.* **29,** 101.

Kuiper-Goodman, T., Grant, D. L., Moodie, C. A., Korsrud, G., and Munro, I. C. (1975). Subacute toxicity of hexachlorobenzene in the rat. *Toxicol. Appl. Pharmacol.,* **33,** 157.

Kuiper-Goodman, T., Grant, D. L., Moodie, C. A., Korsrud, G. O., and Munro, I. C. (1977). Subacute toxicity of hexachlorobenzene in the rat. *Toxicol. Appl. Pharmacol.* **40,** 529–549.

Kumar, S. S., Sikka, H. C., Saxena, J., and Zweig, G. (1975). Membrane damage in human erythrocytes caused by captan and captafol. *Pestic. Biochem. Physiol.* **5,** 338–347.

Kusevitskiy, I. A., Kirlich, A. Ye., and Khovayeva, L. A. (1970). The action of maneb and Sevin on the thyroid gland. *Veterinariya (Moscow)* **46,** 73–74 (in Russian).

Kvitnitskaya, V. A., and Kolesnichenko, T. X. (1971). The transplacental blastomogenic action of zineb on mouse progeny. *Vopr. Pitan.* **30,** 49–50 (in Russian).

Laborie, F., Laborie, R., and Dedieu, E. H. (1964). Allergy to the fungicides maneb and zineb. Prophylaxis preliminary research. *Arch. Mal. Prof. Med. Trav. Secur. Soc.* **25,** 419–424 (in French).

Laisi, A., Tuominen, R., Mannisto, P., Savolainen, K., and Mattila, J. (1985). The effect of maneb, zineb and ethylenethiourea on the humoral activity of the pituitary–thyroid axis in rat. *Arch. Toxicol., Suppl.* **8,** 253–258.

Larsson, K. S., Armander, C., Cekanova, E., and Kjellberg, M. (1976). Studies of teratogenic effects of the dithiocarbamates maneb, mancozeb, and propineb. *Teratology* **14,** 171–184.

Lee, C. C., and Peters, P. J. (1976). Neurotoxicity and behavioral effects of thiram in rats. *Environ. Health Perspect.* **17,** 35–43.

Lee, C. C., Russell, J. Q., and Minor, J. L. (1978). Oral toxicity of ferric dimethyldithiocarbamate (ferbam) and tetramethylthiuram disulfide (thiram) in rodents. *J. Toxicol. Environ. Health* **4,** 93–106.

Legator, M., and Zimmering, S. (1975). Genetic toxicology. *Annu. Rev. Pharmacol. Toxicol.* **15,** 387–408.

Legator, M. S., Kelly, F. J., Green, S., and Oswald, E. (1969). Mutagenic effects of captan. *Ann. N.Y. Acad. Sci.* **160,** 44–351.

Lehman, A. J. (1951). Chemicals in foods: A report to the Association of Food and Drug officials on current developments. II. Pesticides. Section I: Introduction. *Q. Bull.—Assoc. Food Drug Off.* **15,** (I), 122–133.

Lehman, A. J. (1952). Chemicals in foods: A report to the Association of Food and Drug Officials on current developments. II. Pesticides. Section II. Dermal toxicity. Section III. Subacute and chronic toxicity. Section IV. Biochemistry. Section V. Pathology. *Q. Bull.—Assoc. Food Drug Off.* **16** (II), 3–9; (III), 47–53; (IV), 85–91; (V) 126–132.

Lehman, A. J. (1965). "Summaries of Pesticide Toxicity." Association of Food and Drug Officials of the United States, Topeka, Kansas.

Lippmann, W., and Lloyd, K. (1971). Effects of tetramethylthiuram disulfide and structurally-related compounds on the dopamine-hydroxylase activity in the rat and hamster. *Arch. Intern. Pharmacodyn. Ther.* **189,** 348–357.

Lisi, P., and Caraffini, S. (1985). Pellagroid dermatitis from mancozeb with vitiligo. *Contact Dermatitis* **13,** 124–125.

Lissner, R., Goerz, G., Eichenauer, M. G., and Ippen, H. (1975). Hexachlorobenzene-induced porphyria in rats—relationship between porphyrin excretion and induction of drug metabolizing liver enzymes. *Biochem. Pharmacol.* **24,** 1729–1731.

Loose, L. D., Pittman, K. A., Benitz, K. F., and Silkworth, J. B. (1977). Polychlorinated biphenyl and hexachlorobenzene induced humoral immunosuppression. *J. Reticuloendothel. Soc.* **22,** 253–271.

Loose, L. D., Silkworth, J. B., Pittman, K. A., Benitz, K. F., and Mueller, W. (1978a). Impaired host resistance to endotoxin and malaria in polychlorinated biphenyl- and hexachlorobenzene treated mice. *Infect. Immun.* **20,** 30–35.

Loose, L. D., Pittman, K. A., Benitz, K. F., Silkworth, J. B., Mueller, W., and Coulston, F. (1978b). Environmental chemical-induced immune dysfunction. *Ecotoxicol. Environ. Saf.* **2,** 173–198.

Louw, M., Neethling, A. C., Percy, V. A., Carstens, M., and Shanley, B. C. (1977). Effects of hexachlorobenzene feeding and iron overload on enzymes of haem biosynthesis and cytochrome P 450 in rat liver. *Clin. Sci. Mol. Med.* **53,** 111–115.

Lowy, R., Albrecht, R., Pelissier, M. A., and Manchon, P. (1977). Determination of the "no-effect levels" of two pesticides, lindane and zineb, on the microsomal enzyme activities of rat liver. *Toxicol. Appl. Pharmacol.* **42,** 329–338.

Lu, M.-H., and Kennedy, G. L. (1986). Teratogenic evaluation of mancozeb in the rat following inhalation exposure. *Toxicol. Appl. Pharmacol.* **84,** 355–368.

Lui, H., and Sweeney, G. D. (1975). Hepatic metabolism of hexachlorobenzene in rats. *FEBS Lett.* **51,** 225–226.

Lukens, R. J. (1971). "Chemistry of Fungicidal Action," Molecular Biol., Biochem. Biophys., No. 10. Springer-Verlag, New York.

Lyubchenko, P. N., Chemnyy, A. B., Boyarchuk, Z. I., Ginzburg, D. A., and Sukova, V. M. (1973). Effects of a BHC–thiram combination in humans. *Gig. Tr. Prof. Zabol.* **17,** 50–52 (in Russian).

Makita, T., Hashimoto, Y., and Noguchi, T. (1973). Mutagenic, cytogenetic and teratogenic studies on thiophanate-methyl. *Toxicol. Appl. Pharmacol.* **24,** 206–215.

Malling, H. V., and DeSerres, F. J. (1970). Captan—a potent fungicide with mutagenic activity. *Newsl. Environ. Mutagen. Soc.* **3,** 37.

Marcinkowski, T., and Manikowski, W. (1973). Fatal case of intoxication with "Seed Dressing T." *Med. Pr.* **24,** 91–95 (in Polish).

Martson', L. V. (1969). The effects of maneb on embryonic development and the generative function of rats. *Farmakol. Toksikol. (Moscow)* **32,** 731–732 (in Russian).

Martson', L. V., and Pilinskaya, M. A. (1971). Hygienic characteristics of working conditions in production of ziram. *Gig. Sanit.* **36,** 107–108 (in Russian).

Maté, C., Ryan, A. J., and Wright, S. E. (1967). Metabolism of some 4-nitroaniline derivatives in the rat. *Food Cosmet. Toxicol.* **5,** 657–663.

Matokhnyuk, L. A. (1971). Maneb toxicity following inhalational exposure. *Gig. Sanit.* **36,** 22–26 (in Russian).

Matsushita, T., Arimatsu, T., and Nomura, S. (1977). Contact allergy due to two fungicides, benomyl and thiophanate methyl. *Jpn. J. Ind. Health* **19,** 354 (in Japanese).

Matsushita, T., Nomura, S., Wakatsuki, A., Matsushima, S., and Sugaya, H. (1979). Actual state of occurrence of skin impairment due to agricultural chemicals in Japan. *J. Jpn. Soc. Rural Med.* **28,** 454–455 (in Japanese).

Matthiaschk, G. (1973). The influence of L-cystein on the teratogenicity caused by thiram (TMTD) in MMRI mice. *Arch. Toxicol.* **30,** 251, 262 (in German).

Mazzei, E. S., and Mazzei, C. M. (1972). Porphyria from hexachlorobenzene. *Prensa Med. Argent.* **59,** 1205–1211.

Mazzei, E. S., and Mazzei, C. M. (1973). Poisoning by the fungicide hexachlorobenzene through contamination of wheat grains. *Sem. Hop.* **49,** 63–67 (in French).

McLaughlin, J., Jr., Reynaldo, E. F., Lamar, J. K., and Marliac, J. P. (1969). Teratology studies in rabbits with captan, folpet and thalidomide. *Toxicol. Appl. Pharmacol.* **14,** 641.

McPherson, F. J., Bridges, J. W., and Parke, D. V. (1975). The enhancement of biphenyl 2-hydroxylation by carcinogens *in vitro*. *Biochem. Soc. Trans.* **2,** 618–619.

Medline, A., Bain, E., Menon, A. I., and Haberman, H. F. (1973). Hexachlorobenzene and rat liver. *Arch. Pathol.* **96,** 61–65.

Mehendale, H. M., Fields, M., and Matthews, H. B. (1975). Metabolism and effects of hexachlorobenzene on hepatic microsomal enzymes in the rat. *J. Agric. Food Chem.* **23,** 261–263.

Melson, F., and Weigelt, H. (1967). The influence of tetramethyl thiuram and carbon disulphide on the enzymes monoaminoxidase and alcoholdehydrogenase. *In* "Toxicology of Carbon Disulphide" (H.Brieger and J.Teisinger, eds.). Excerpta Med. Found., Amsterdam.

Mendoza, C. E., Grant, D. L., and Shields, J. B. (1975). Body burden of hexachlorobenzene in suckling rats and its effects on various organs and on liver porphyrin accumulation. *Environ. Physiol. Biochem.* **5**, 460–464.

Mendoza, C. E., Shields, J. B., and Laver, G. W. (1976). Body burden of hexachlorobenzene and its effects on some esterases in tissues of young male rats. *Toxicol. Appl. Pharmacol.* **38**, 499–506.

Mendoza, C. E., Collins, B., Shields, J. B., and Laver, G. W. (1977). Hexachlorobenzene residues and effects of esterase activities in pre-weanling rats after a reciprocal transfer between HCB-treated and control dams. *Arch. Toxicol.* **38**, 191–199.

Mendoza, C. E., Collins, B., Shields, J. B., and Laver, G. W. (1978). Effects of hexachlorobenzene on body and organ weights of preweanling rats after a reciprocal transfer between the treated and control dams. *J. Agric. Food Chem.* **26**, 941–945.

Merlevede, E., and Casier, H. (1961). Carbon disulphide in expired air of alcoholic patients treated with Antabuse (disulfiram), and sodium diethyldithiocarbamate. *Arch. Int. Pharmacodyn. Ther.* **132**, 427–453 (in French).

Meyer, T., Aarbakke, J., and Scheline, R. R. (1976). The metabolism of biphenyl. I. Metabolic disposition of ^{14}C biphenyl in the rat. *Acta Pharmacol. Toxicol.* **39**, 412–418.

Mihail, G., Bodnar, J., Zlavog, A., Branisteanu, D., Mihaila, D., and Ambrono, V. (1970). Researches concerning the exposure risk and the toxicology of one dithiocarbamic fungicide. *J. Jpn. Assoc. Rural Med.* **63**.

Mollet, P. (1973). Mutagenicity and toxicity testing of captan in *Drosophila*. *Mutat. Res.* **21**, 137–148 (in German).

Mollet, P., and Wurgler, F. E. (1974). Detection of somatic recombination and mutation in *Drosophila*. A method for testing genetic activity of chemical compounds. *Mutat. Res.* **25**, 421–424.

Moriya, M., Kato, K., Shirasu, Y., and Kada, T. (1976). Mutagenicity screening of pesticides in microbial systems. III. Fate of mutagenicity. *Mutat. Res.* **38**, 342.

Moriya, M., Kato, K., Shirasu, Y., and Kada, T. (1978a). Mutagenicity screening of pesticides in microbial systems. IV. Mutagenicity of dimethyldithiocarbamates and related fungicides. *Mutat. Res.* **54**, 221.

Moriya, M., Kato, K., and Shirasu, Y. (1978b). Effects of cysteine and a liver metabolic activation system on the activities of mutagenic pesticides. *Mutat. Res.* **57**, 259–263.

Mueller, W. F., Hobson, W., Fuller, G. B., Knauf, W., Coulston, F., and Korte, F. (1978a). Endocrine effects of chlorinated hydrocarbons in rhesus monkeys. *Ecotoxicol. Environ. Saf.* **2**, 161–172.

Mueller, W. F., Iatropoulos, M. J., Rozman, K., Korte, F., and Coulston, F. (1978b). Comparative kinetic, metabolic, and histopathologic effects of chlorinated hydrocarbon pesticides in rhesus monkeys. *Toxicol. Appl. Pharmacol.* **45**, 283–284.

Mull, R. L., Winterlin, W. L., Peoples, S. A., Giri, S. N., and Ocampo, L. (1978). Hexachlorobenzene. II. Effects on growing lambs of prolonged low-level oral exposure to hexachlorobenzene (HCB). *J. Environ. Pathol. Toxicol.* **1**, 927–937.

Nadzhimutdinov, K. N., Kamilov, I. K., and Muzrabekov, Sh.M. (1974). Influence of pesticides on the duration of hexobarbital-induced sleep. *Farmakol. Toksikol. (Moscow)* **37**, 533–537 (in Russian).

Nakamura, I., Kudo, Y., Horrie, Y., and Nishida, N. (1977). Change of erythrocytic cells in peripheral blood of rabbit by several pesticides for agriculture. *Jpn. J. Ind. Health* **19**, 354–355 (in Japanese).

Nater, J. P., Terpstra, H., and Bleumink, E. (1979). Allergic contact sensitization to the fungicide maneb. *Contact Dermatitis* **5**, 24–26.

National Cancer Institute (NCI) (1977). Bioassay of captan for possible carcinogenicity. *U.S. NTIS, PB Rep.* **PB-273**, 475.

Nelson, B. D. (1971a). Action of the fungicides captan and folpet on rat liver mitochondria. *Biochem. Pharmacol.* **20**, 737–748.

Nelson, B. D. (1971b). Induction of mitochondrial swelling by the fungicide captan. *Biochem. Pharmacol.* **20**, 749–758.

Newton, K. G., and Greene, N. C. (1972). Organochlorine pesticide residue levels in human milk—Victoria, Australia—1970. *Pestic. Monit. J.* **6**, 4–8.

Neyko, E. M., Drin, M. M., Lanoviy, I. D., and Yurkevich, S. T. (1974). Certain parameters of peripheral blood, enzyme activity, and reproductive function in women working in zineb manufacturing plants. *Pediatr., Akush. Ginekol.* **36**, 56–59 (in Ukrainian).

Nishiyama, K. (1974). Studies on the prevention of pesticidal hazards: Part 1. On the aerial concentration of pesticides applied in a vinyl greenhouse and the acute effects of applied pesticides on living organisms. *J. Jpn. Assoc. Rural Med.* **23**, 1–7 (in Japanese).

Noguchi, T. (1972). Environmental evaluation of systemic fungicides. *In* "Environmental Toxicology of Pesticides" (F. Matsumura, G. M. Bousch, and T. Misato, eds.), Academic Press, New York.

Nomura, K., and Wakatsuki, S. (1976). Studies on the effects of pesticides on living organisms. 7. Results of examinations for dermatergosis among fruit tree cultivators. *J. Jpn. Assoc. Rural Med.* **25**, 46–47 (in Japanese).

Nomura, S., Matsushita, T., Arimatsu, T., and Tomio, T. (1976). Results of health examination on persons applying organosulfur fungicides. *J. Jpn. Soc. Rural Med.* **1–2**, 36–42 (in Japanese).

Novak, L., Djuric, D., and Fridman, V. (1969). Specificity of the iodine-azide test for carbon disulfide exposure. *Arch. Environ. Health* **19**, 473–477.

Ockner, R. K., and Schmid, R. (1961). Acquired porphyria in man and rat due to hexachlorobenzene intoxication. *Nature (London)* **189**, 499.

Palmer, J. S. (1963a). Tolerance of sheep to captan. *J. Am. Vet. Med. Assoc.* **143**, 513–514.

Palmer, J. S. (1963b). Tolerance of sheep to the organic-zine fungicide, zineb. *J. Am. Vet. Med. Assoc.* **143**, 994–995.

Palmer, J. S., and Radeleff, R. D. (1964). The toxicologic effects of certain fungicides and herbicides in sheep and cattle. *Ann. N.Y. Acad. Sci.* **111**, 729–736.

Pearson, R. W., and Malkinson, F. D. (1965). Some observations on hexachlorobenzene induced experimental porphyria. *J. Invest. Dermatol.* **44**, 420–432.

Pedersen, L. G., and Carlson, G. L. (1975). The planarity of hexachlorobenzene: An *ab initio* investigation. *J. Chem. Phys.* **62**, 2009–2010.

Pelissier, M. A., Atteba, S., Manchon, P., and Albrecht, R. (1976). Diminution of activity of microsomal oxygenases of the liver of rats fed a supplement of zineb. *Ann. Nutr. Aliment.* **30**, 45–54 (in French).

Percival, G. H. (1942). Cure of scabies and new remedy. *Br. Med. J.* **2**, 451–452.

Perelygin, V. M., Shpirt, M. B., Aripov, O. A., and Ershova, V. I. (1971). Effects of some pesticides on immunological reactivity. *Gig. Sanit.* **36**, 29–33 (in Russian).

Pergal, M., Vukojevic, N., Cirin-Popov, N., Djuric, D., and Bojovic, T. (1972a). Carbon disulfide metabolites excreted in the urine of exposed workers. II. Isolation and identification of 2-mercapto-2-thiazolinone-5. *Arch. Environ. Health* **25**, 38–41.

Pergal, M., Vukojevic, N., and Djuric, D. (1972b). Carbon disulfide metabolites excreted in the urine of exposed workers. II. Isolation and identification of thiocarbamide. *Arch. Environ. Health* **25**, 42–44.

Peters, H. A., Johnson, S. A. M., Cam, S., Oral, S., Muftu, Y., and Ergene, T. (1966). Hexachlorobenzene-induced porphyria: Effect of chelation on the disease, porphyrin and metal metabolism. *Am. J. Med. Sci.* **251**, 314–322.

Petrova-Vergieva, T., and Ivanova-Tchemishanska, L. (1971). Teratogenicity of zinc ethylenebisdithiocarbamate (zineb) in rats. *Eksp. Med. Morfol.* **10**, 226–230 (in Bulgarian).

Petrova-Vergieva, T., and Ivanova-Tchemishanska, L. (1973). Assessment of the teratogenic activity of dithiocarbamate fungicides. *Food Cosmet. Toxicol.* **11**, 239–244.

Pilinskaya, M. A. (1970). Chromosome aberrations in individuals coming in contact with ziram under industrial conditions. *Genetika (Moscow)* **6**, 157–163 (in Russian).

Pilinskaya, M. A. (1971). Cytogenetic effects of the fungicide ziram on cultured human lymphocytes *in vitro*. *Genetika (Moscow)* **7**, 138–143 (in Russian).

Pilinskaya, M. A. (1974). Results of cytogenetic examination of persons occupationally exposed to the fungicide zineb. *Genetika (Moscow)* **10**, 140–146 (in Russian).

Pilinskaya, M. A. (1976). Genetic hazards of the fungicide zineb during manufacture. *Gig. Tr. Prof. Zabol.* **12**, 26–29 (in Russian).

Pinkhas, J., Djaldetti, M., Joshua, H., Resnick, C., and DeVries, A. (1963). Sulfhemoglobinemia and acute hemolytic anemia with Heinz bodies following contact with a fungicide—zinc ethylene bisdithiocarbamate—in a subject with glucose-6-phosphate dehydrogenase deficiency and hypocatalasemia. *Blood* **21**, 484–494.

Popov, T. A. (1977). Significance of hepatic mixed-function oxidases for the solution of some problems of current interest in hygienic toxicology. *Gig. Sanit.* **10**, 23–27 (in Russian).

Pozo Lora, R., Herrera Marteache, A., Polo Villar, L. M., Jodral Villarejo, M., Mallol Escobar, J., and Polo Villar, G. (1978). Presence of the synthetic fungicide, hexachlorobenzene, in human fatty tissues in Spain. Part I. *Rev. Sanid. Hig. Publica* **52**, 1145–1150 (in Spanish).

Propping, P., Buselmaier, W., and Roehrborn, G. (1973). A critical examination of a mutagenicity assay for chemicals in cultured animal micro-organisms. *Arzneim.-Forsch.* **23**, 746–749 (in German).

Rainey, J. M., Jr., and Neal, R. A. (1975). Disulfiram, carbon disulphide, and atherosclerosis. *Lancet* **1**, 284–285.

Raizada, R. B., Datta, K. K., and Dikshith, T. S. S. (1979). Effect of zineb on male rats. *Bull. Environ. Contam. Toxicol.* **22**, 208–213.

Ranek, L., and Andreasen, P. B. (1977). Disulfam hepatotoxicity. *Br. Med. J.* **2**, 94–96.

Rannug, A., and Rannug, U. (1984). Enzyme inhibition as a possible mechanism of the mutagenicity of dithiocarbamic acid derivates in *Salmonella typhimurium*. *Chem.-Biol. Interact.* **49**, 329–340.

Reinl, W. (1966). Hypersensitivity to alcohol after exposure to the fungicide tetramethylthiuram disulfide (TMTD). *Arch. Toxikol.* **22**, 12–15 (in German).

Renner, G., and Schuster, K. P. (1977). 2,4,5-Trichlorophenol, a new urinary metabolite of hexachlorobenzene. *Toxicol. Appl. Pharmacol.* **39**, 355–356.

Renner, G., and Schuster, K. P. (1978a). N-Acetyl-S-(pentachlorophenyl)cysteine, a new urinary metabolite of hexachlorobenzene. *Chemosphere* **7**, 663–668.

Renner, G., and Schuster, K. P. (1978b). Synthesis of hexachlorobenzene metabolites. *Chemosphere* **7**, 669–674.

Reynolds, W. A., and Lowe, F. H. (1965). Mushrooms and a toxic reaction to alcohol. *N. Engl. J. Med.* **272**, 630–631.

Richter, E., and Schmid, A. (1976). Hexachlorobenzene blood concentrations in children. *Arch. Toxicol.* **35**, 141–147.

Richter, E., Lay, J. P., Klein, W., and Korte, F. (1977). Enhanced elimination of hexachlorobenzene in rats by light paraffin. *Chemosphere* **6**, 357–369.

Rios de Molina, M. C., de Calmanovici, R. W., Tomio, J. M., and San Martin de Viale, L. C. (1975). HCB-induced porphyria in rats. Effect of the drug on the porphyrin content and uroporphyrinogen decarboxylase activity in various organs. *An. Asoc. Quim. Argent.* **63**, 313–332 (in Spanish).

Robens, J. F. (1969). Teratologic studies of carbaryl, diazinon, norea, disulfiram and thiram in small laboratory animals. *Toxicol. Appl. Pharmacol.* **15**, 152–163.

Robens, J. F. (1970). Teratogenic activity of several phthalimide derivatives in the golden hamster. *Toxicol. Appl. Pharmacol.* **16**, 24–34.

Robinson, H. J., Phares, H. F., and Graessle, O. E. (1964). Antimycotic properties of thiabendazole. *J. Invest. Dermatol.* **42**, 479–482.

Robinson, H. J., Graessle, O. E., Lehman, E. G., Kelley, K. L., Geoffrey, R. F., and Rosenblum, C. (1966). Ocular absorption of thiabendazole-¹⁴C by the rabbit. *Am. J. Ophthalmol.* **62**, 710–715.

Roll, R. (1971). Teratogenic studies of thiram in two mice strains. *Arch. Toxikol.* **27**, 137–186 (in German).

Rosenstein, L., Lowder, J., Deskin, R., Roger, N., Jenkins, K., and Westbrook, B. (1978). Toxicity of maneb as a function of age and sex with special emphasis on the peripheral nervous system. *Toxicol. Appl. Pharmacol.* **45**, 233.

Rozman, K., Mueller, W., Iatropoulos, M., Coulston, F., and Korte, F. (1975). Separation, excretion, and metabolism of hexachlorobenzene after single oral doses in rats and rhesus monkeys. *Chemosphere* **4**, 289–298.

Rozman, K., Mueller, W. F., Coulston, F., and Korte, F. (1977). Long-term feeding study of hexachlorobenzene in rhesus monkeys. *Chemosphere* **6**, 81–84.

Rozman, K., Mueller, W. F., Coulston, F., and Korte, F. (1978). Chronic low dose exposure of rhesus monkeys to hexachlorobenzene (HCB). *Chemosphere* **7**, 177–184.

Rozman, K., Mueller, W. F., Coulston, F., and Korte, F. (1979a). The involvement of the lymphatic system in the absorption, transport, and excretion of hexachlorobenzene in rats and rhesus monkeys. *Toxicol. Appl. Pharmacol.* **48**, A93.

Rozman, K., Williams, J., Mueller, W. F., Coulston, F., and Korte, F. (1979b). Metabolism and pharmacokinetics of pentachlorobenzene in the rhesus monkey. *Bull. Environ. Contam. Toxicol.* **22**, 190–195.

Rudner, E. J. (1977). North American group results. *Contact Dermatitis* **3**, 208–209.

Ruzicska, P., Sandor, P., Jozsef, L., and Endre, C. (1976). Study on the chromosomal mutagenicity of Fundazol 50 WP. *Egeszsegtudomany* **20**, 74–83 (in Hungarian).

Ryazanova, R. A. (1967a). On the toxic properties of zineb pesticide. *Gig. Sanit.* **31**, 25–29 (in Russian).

Ryazanova, R. A. (1967b). Effects of ziram and zineb fungicides on the regenerative functions of experimental animals. *Gig. Sanit.* **32**, 26–30 (in Russian).

San Martin de Viale, L. C., Viale, A. A., Nacht, S., and Grinstein, M. (1970). Experimental porphyria induced in rats by hexachlorobenzene: A study of the porphyrins excreted by urine. *Clin. Chim. Acta* **28**, 13–23.

San Martin de Viale, L. C., Rios de Molina, M. del C., Wainstok de Calmanovici, R., and Tomio, J. M. (1977). Porphyrins and porphyrinogen carboxylase in hexachlorobenzene-induced porphyria. *Biochem. J.* **168**, 393–400.

Savitakii, J. V. (1964). The basis for determining safe permissible concentrations of hexachlorobenzene and pentachloronitrobenzene in the air. *Vopr. Prom.-Toksikol.*, pp. 158–173 (in Russian).

Savitt, L. E. (1972). Contact dermatitis due to benomyl insecticide. *Arch. Dermatol.* **105**, 926–927.

Schmid, R. (1960). Medical intelligence. Cutaneous porphyria in Turkey. *N. Engl. J. Med.* **263**, 397–398.

Schubel, F., and Linss, G. (1971). Respiratory allergy caused by zineb 80. *Dtsch. Gesundheitswes.* **26**, 1187–1189.

Schumann, A. M., and Borzelleca, J. F. (1978). The potential methemoglobin and Heinz body inducing capacity of pentachloronitrobenzene (PCNB) in the cat. *Toxicol. Appl. Pharmacol.* **44**, 523–529.

Schwartz, L., and Tulipan, L. (1933). Outbreak of dermatitis among workers in a rubber manufacturing plant. *Public Health Rep.* **48**, 809–814.

Searle, C. E. (1966). Tumor initiatory activity of some chloromononitrobenzenes and other compounds. *Cancer Res.* **26**, 12–17.

Sedokur, L. K. (1971). Rat liver nucleic acids as affected by dithiocarbamic acid derivatives. *Ukr. Biokhim. Zh.* **43**, 511–514 (in Ukranian).

Sedokur, L. K., and Lukyanchuk, V. D. (1976). Xanthurenic aciduria as a specific test for dithiocarbamate intoxication. *Gig. Tr. Prof. Zabol.* **2**, 55–56 (in Russian).

Seidler, H., Haertig, M., Schnaak, W., and Engst, R. (1970). Studies on the metabolism of some insecticides and fungicides in the rat. 2. The distribution of ¹⁴C maneb. *Nahrung* **14**, 363–373 (in German).

Seidler, H., Haertig, M., Schnaak, W., and Engst, R. (1971). Studies on the metabolism of some insecticides and fungicides in the rat. 3. Excretion, distribution and metabolism of ³⁵S captan. *Nahrung* **15**, 177–185 (in German).

Seidler, H., Haertig, M., and Lewerenz, H. J. (1975). A controlled study on the function of the thyroid using radioactive iodine for toxicological investigation. *Nahrung* **19**, 715–726 (in German).

Seiler, J. P. (1973). A survey on the mutagenicity of various pesticides. *Experientia* **29**, 622–623.

Seiler, J. P. (1976). The mutagenicity of benzimidazole and benzimidazole derivatives. IV. Cytogenic effects of benzimidazole derivatives in the bone marrow of the mouse and the Chinese hamster. *Mutat. Res.* **40**, 339–348.

Selling, H. A., Vouk, J. M., and Sijpesteijn, A. K. (1970). Transformation of the systemic fungicide methyl thiophanate into 2-benzimidazole carbamic acid methyl ester. *Chem. Ind. (London)*, pp. 1625–1626.

Seppalainen, A. M., and Hakkinen, I. (1975). Electrophysiological findings in diphenyl poisoning. *J. Neurol., Neurosurg. Psychiatry* **38**, 248–252.

Serrone, D. M., Pakdman, P., Stein, A. A., and Coulston, F. (1967). Comparative toxicology of 2,6-dichloro-4-nitroaniline in rats and monkeys. *Toxicol. Appl. Pharmacol.* **10**, 404.

Shanley, B. C., Taljaard, J. J. F., Deppe, W. M., and Joubert, S. M. (1972). Haem biosynthesis in "experimental porphyria." *S. Afr. J. Lab. Clin. Med.* **18**, 118.

Shelley, W. B. (1964). Golf-course dermatitis due to thiram fungicide. Cross-hazards of alcohol, disulfiram, and rubber. *JAMA J. Am. Med. Assoc.* **188**, 415–417.

Sherman, H., Culik, R., and Jackson, R. A. (1975). Reproduction, teratogenic, and mutagenic studies with benomyl. *Toxicol. Appl. Pharmacol.* **32**, 305–315.

Shiaku, K., Torii, M., and Hirai, K. (1979). Results of survey on health impairment due to application of pesticides in citrus culturing district in Ehime Prefecture. *J. Jpn. Soc. Rural Med.* **28**, 456–457 (in Japanese).

Shirai, T., Miyata, Y., Nakanishi, K., Murasaki, G., and Ito, N. (1978). Hepatocarcinogenicity of polychlorinated terphenyl (PCT) in ICR mice and its enhancement by hexachlorobenzene (HCB). *Cancer Lett.* **4**, 299–303.

Shirasu, Y., Tezuka, H., Henmi, R., Teramoto, S., Shingu, A., and Kaneda, M. (1978). Cytogenic and dominant-lethal studies on captan. *Mutat. Res.* **54**, 227–228.

Short, R. D., Jr., Russel, J. Q., Minor, J. L., and Lee, C. C. (1976). Developmental toxicity of ferric dimethyldithiocarbamate and bis(dimethylthiocarbamoyl) disulfide in rats and mice. *Toxicol. Appl. Pharmacol.* **35**, 83–94.

Shpirt, M. B. (1973). Toxicological assessment of DDT, BHC, TMTD, Sevin, and zineb acting on human cell cultures. *Gig. Tr. Prof. Zabol.* **17**, 32–35 (in Russian).

Shtenberg, A. I., and Torchinskiy, A. M. (1972). Relationships between general toxic, embryotoxic, and teratogenic effects of exogenous chemicals and the possibility of predicting their influence on antenatal ontogenesis. *Vestn. Akad. Med. Nauk SSSR* **27**, 39–46 (in Russian).

Shtenberg, A. I., Kirlich, A. E., and Orlova, N. V. (1969). The toxicological characteristics of maneb used for treating food crops. *Vopr. Pitan.* **28**, 66–72 (in Russian).

Shtenberg, A. I., Ashemnskas, Yu. I., and Kusevitskiy, I. A. (1972). Immunobiological reactivity changes under the influence of some pesticides belonging to the groups of carbamate and dithiocarbamate compounds. *Vopr. Pitan.* **31**, 58–63 (in Russian).

Siebert, D., Zimmermann, F. K., and Lemperle, E. (1970). Genetic effects of fungicides. *Mutat. Res.* **10**, 533–543.

Silkworth, J. B., and Loose, L. D. (1978). Cell-mediated immunity in mice fed either Aroclor 1016 or hexachlorobenzene. *Toxicol. Appl. Pharmacol.* **45**, 326–327.

Simeray, A. (1966). The use of an agricultural fungicide (orthicide) in 250 cases of pityriasis versicolor. *Bull. Soc. Fr. Dermatol. Syphiligr.* **73**, 337–338 (in French).

Simon, G. S., Kipps, B. R., Tardiff, R. G., and Borzelleca, J. F. (1978). Failure of Kepone and hexachlorobenzene to induce dominant lethal mutations in the rat. *Toxicol. Appl. Pharmacol.* **45**, 330–331.

Simon, N., Siklosi, Cs., and Koszo, F. (1978). The influence of environmental factors on porphyrin metabolism. *Therapiewoche* **28**, 8452, 8454, 8457–8458 (in German).

Sivitskaya, I. I. (1974). State of the organ of vision in persons working in contact with tetramethylthiuram disulfide (TMTD). *Oftal'mol. Zh.* **28**, 286 (in Russian).

Siyali, D. S. (1972). Hexachlorobenzene and other organochloride pesticides in human blood. *Med. J. Aust.* **2**, 1063–1066.

Siyali, D. S. (1973). Polychlorinated biphenyls, hexachlorobenzene and other organochloride pesticides in human milk. *Med. J. Aust.* **2**, 815–818.

Siyali, D. S., and Ouw, K. H. (1973). Chlorinated hydrocarbon pesticides in human blood—Wee Waa survey. *Med. J. Aust.* **2**, 908–909.

Smith, R. B., Jr., Finnegan, J. K., Larson, P. S., Sahyoun, P. F., Dreyfuss, M. L., and Haag, H. B. (1953). Toxicological studies of zinc and disodium ethylene bisdithiocarbamates. *J. Pharmacol. Exp. Ther.* **109**, 159–166.

Smyth, H. F., Jr., Carpenter, C. P., Weil, C. S., Pozzani, U. C., and Striegel, J. A. (1962). Range-finding toxicity data: List VI. *Am. Ind. Hyg. Assoc. J.* **23**, 95–107.

Sobotka, T. (1971). Comparative effects of 60-day feeding of maneb and of ethylenethiourea on thyroid electrophoretic patterns of rats. *Food Cosmet. Toxicol.* **9**, 537–540.

Spencer, F. (1984). Structural and reproductive modifications in rats following a post-implantation exposure to captan. *Bull. Environ. Contam. Toxicol.* **33**, 84–91.

Spindeldreir, A., and Deichmann, B. (1980). Contact dermatitis caused by a wood preservative containing a new fungicide. *Dermatosen Beruf Umwelt* **28**, 88–90 (in German).

Steckerl, F., and Turner, M. L. (1965). The effect of "Captan" on the mouse ascites tumour of Ehrlich. *Nature (London)* **206**, 839.

Steinwandter, H., and Bruene, J. (1977). No natural occurrence of hexachlorobenzene in the ecosphere. *Chemosphere* **6**, 77–80.

Stevens, J. T., Farmer, J. D., and Dipasquale, L. C. (1978). The acute inhalation toxicity of technical captan and folpet. *Toxicol. Appl. Pharmacol.* **45**, 320.

Stiller, R. L., and Stevens, D. A. (1986). Studies with a plant fungicide, imazalil, with vapor-phase activity, in the therapy of human alternariosis. *Mycopathologia* **93**, 169–172.

Stonard, M. D. (1974). Experimental hepatic porphyria induced by hexachlorobenzene as a model for human symptomatic porphyria. *Br. J. Haematol.* **27**, 617–626.

Stonard, M. D. (1975). Mixed type hepatic microsomal enzyme induction by hexachlorobenzene. *Biochem. Pharmacol.* **24**, 1959–1963.

Stonard, M. D., and Greig, J. B. (1976). Different patterns of hepatic microsomal enzyme activity produced by administration of pure hexachlorobiphenyl isomers and hexachlorobenzene. *Chem.-Biol. Interact.* **15**, 365–379.

Stonard, M. D., and Nonov, P. Z. (1974). Effect of hexachlorobenzene on hepatic microsomal enzymes in the rat. *Biochem. Pharmacol.* **23**, 2175–2183.

Strohmayer, A., Desi, I., Erdos, G., Dura, G., Gonczi, C., and Kneffel, Z. (1975). Complex toxicological investigation of Fundazol 50 WP (benomyl) fungicide in animal experiments. *Egeszsegtudomany* **19**, 168–181 (in Hungarian).

Strömme, J. H. (1965). Metabolism of disulfiram and diethyldithiocarbamate in rats with demonstration of an *in vivo* ethanol-induced inhibition of the glucuronic acid conjugation of the thiol. *Biochem. Pharmacol.* **14**, 393–410.

Stoud, S. W. (1940). The metabolism of the parent compounds of some simple synthetic oestrogenic phenol. *J. Endocrinol.* **2**, 55–62.

Styles, J. A., and Garner, R. (1974). Benzimidazolecarbamate methyl ester—evaluation of its effects *in vivo* and *in vitro*. *Mutat. Res.* **26**, 177–187.

Sutou, S., and Tokuyama, F. (1974). Induction of endoreduplication in cultured mammalian cells by some chemical mutagens. *Cancer Res.* **34**, 2615–2623.

Sweeney, G. D., and Jones, K. G. (1976). Hexachlorobenzene (HCB) porphyria in rats: Difference between sexes. *Pharmacologist* **18**, 245.

Szabo, E., Berko, G., Husz, S., and Simon, M. (1973a). Demonstration of tissue porphyrins in hexachlorobenzene model experiment by the fluorescence technique. *Acta Morphol. Acad. Sci. Hung.* **21**, 155–163.

Szabo, E., Husz, S., Berko, G., and Simon, M. (1973b). Immunofluorescence studies in hexachlorobenzene model experiments. *Acta Morphol. Acad. Sci. Hung.* **21**, 165–174.

Sziza, M., and Magos, L. (1959). Toxicological examination of some aromatic nitrogen compounds encountered in Hungarian industry. *Munkavedelem* **5**, 45–58.

Takamatsu, M., Futatsuka, M., Arimatsu, Y., Maeda, H., Inuzuka, T., and Takamatsu, S. (1968). Epidemiologic survey on dermatitis from a new fungicide used in tangerine orchards in Kimamoto Prefecture. *J. Kumamoto Med. Soc.* **42**, 854–859 (in Japanese).

Taljaard, J. J. F., Shanley, B. C., and Joubert, S. M. (1971). Decreased uroporphyrinogen decarboxylase activity in "experimental symptomatic porphyria." *Life Sci.* **10**, (Part 2), 887–893.

Taljaard, J. J. F., Shanley, B. C., Deppie, W. M., and Joubert, S. M. (1972). Porphyrin metabolism in experimental hepatic siderosis in the rat. II. Combined effect of iron overload and hexachlorobenzene. *Br. J. Haematol.* **23**, 513–519.

Texas Reports on Biology and Medicine (1969). "Thiabendazole Symposium." *Tex. Rep. Biol. Med.* **27**, Suppl. 2, 533–708.

Tezuka, H., Teramoto, S., Kaneda, M., Henmi, R., Murakami, N., and Shirasu, Y. (1978). Cytogenic and dominant lethal studies on captan. *Mutat. Res.* **57**, 201–207.

Thienpont, D., Van Cutsem, J., Van Cauteren, H., and Marsboom, R. (1981). The biological and toxicological properties of imazalil. *Arzneim.-Forsch.* **31**, 309–315 (in German).

Thorn, G. D., and Ludwig, R. A. (1962). "The Dithiocarbamates and Related Compounds." Elsevier, Amsterdam.

Tocco, D. J., Rosenblum, C., Martin, C. M., and Robinson, H. J. (1966). Absorption, metabolism and excretion of thiabendazole in man and laboratory animals. *Toxicol. Appl. Pharmacol.* **9**, 31–39.

Tomashivskiy, D. I. (1975). Occupational dermatoses in workers dealing with fungicides. *Vestn. Dermatol. Venerol.* **4**, 59–62 (in Russian).

Torchinskiy, A. M. (1973). Significance of diets with different protein content in manifestations of teratogenic and embryotoxic action of some pesticides. *Vopr. Pitan.* **3**, 76–80 (in Russian).

Torgeson, D. C., ed. (1967). "Fungicides: An Advanced Treatise," Vol. 1. Academic Press, New York.

Torgeson, D. C., ed. (1969). "Fungicides: An Advanced Treatise," Vol. 2. Academic Press, New York.

Torracca, A. M., Cardamone, G. C., Ortali, V., Carere, A., Raschetti, R., and Ricciardi, G. (1976). Mutagenicity of pesticides as pure compounds and after metabolic activation with rat liver microsomes. *Atti Assoc. Genet. Ital.* **21**, 28–29 (in Italian).

Truhaut, R. F., Fujita, M., Lich, N. P., and Chaigneau, M. (1973). Study of the metabolic changes of zineb (ethylenebisdithiocarbamate) in the rat. *C.R. Hebd. Seances Acad. Sci., Ser. D* **276**, 229–233 (in French).

Tschudy, D. P., and Bonkowsky, H. L. (1972). Experimental porphyria. *Fed. Proc., Fed. Am. Soc. Exp. Biol.* **31**, 147–159.

Turner, J. C., and Green, R. S. (1974). Effect of hexachlorobenzene on microsomal enzyme systems. *Biochem. Pharmacol.* **23**, 2387–2390.

Urbanek-Karlowska, B. (1975). The effect of protein deficiency in rats on captan toxicity. I. Acute toxicity of captan. *Rocz. Panstw. Zakl. Hig.* **26**, 137–144 (in Polish).

Van Etten, C. H., and Wolff, I. A. (1973). Natural sulfur compounds. *In* "Toxicants Occurring Naturally in Foods" (Committee on Food Protection, Food and Nutrition Board, National Research Council, ed.), 2nd ed., National Academy of Sciences, Washington, D.C.

Van Haver, W., Vandezande, A., and Gordts, L. (1978). Organochlorine pesticides in human fatty tissues. *Arch. Belg. Med. Soc., Hyg., Med. Trav. Med. Leg.* **36**, 147–155 (in Flemish).

van Hecke, E., and De Vos, L. (1983). Contact sensitivity to enilconazole. *Contact Dermatitis* **9**, 144.

van Joost, T., Naafs, B., and van Ketel, W. G. (1983). Sensitization to benomyl and related pesticides. *Contact Dermatitis* **9**, 153–154.

van Ketel, W. G. (1977). Sensitivity to the pesticide benomyl. *Contact Dermatitis* **2**, 290–291.

van Ketel, W. G. (1984). Contact urticaria from rubber gloves after dermatitis from thiurams. *Contact Dermatitis* **11**, 323–324.

van Ketel, W. G., and van den Berg, W. H. H. W. (1984). The problem of the sensitization to dithiocarbamates in thiuram-allergic patients. *Dermatologica* **169**, 70–75.

Vargas, M. I., Lamas, J. M., and Alvarenga, V. (1983). Tibial dyschondroplasia in growing chickens experimentally intoxicated with tetramethylthiuram disulfide. *Poult. Sci.* **62**, 1195–1200.

Vashakidze, V. I., Mandzhgaladze, R. N., and Zhorzholiani, V. S. (1973). The toxicity of captan and its hygienic standardization in food products. *Gig. Sanit.* **38**, 24–27 (in Russian).

Vasilos, A. F., Anisimova, L. A., Todorova, E. A., and Dmitrienko, V. D. (1978). The reproductive function of rats in acute and chronic intoxication with thiram. *Gig. Sanit.* **43**, 37–40 (in Russian).

Vekshtein, M.Sh., and Khitsenko, I. I. (1971). The metabolism of ziram in warm-blooded animals. *Gig. Sanit.* **36**, 23–27 (in Russian).

Veltmann, J. R., and Linton, S. S. (1986). Influence of dietary tetramethylthiuram disulfide (a fungicide) on growth and incidence of tibial dys-

chondroplasia in single-comb white leghorn chicks. *Poult. Sci.* **65**, 1205–1207.

Veltmann, J. R., Rowland, G. N., and Linton, S. S. (1985). Tibial dyschondroplasia in single-comb white leghorn chicks fed tetramethylthiuram disulfide (a fungicide). *Avian Dis.* **29**, 1269–1200.

Verhagen, A. R. H. B. (1974). Contact dermatitis in Kenya. *Trans. St. John's Hosp. Dermatol. Soc.* **60**, 86–90.

Vettorazzi, G. (1977). State of the art of toxicological evaluation carried out by the Joint FAO/WHO Expert Committee on Pesticide Residues. III. Miscellaneous pesticides used in agriculture and public health. *Residue Rev.* **66**, 137–184.

Villanueva, E. C., Jennings, R. W., Burse, V. W., and Kimbrough, R. D. (1974). Evidence of chlordibenzo-*p*-dioxin and chlorodibenzofuran in hexachlorobenzene. *J. Agric. Food Chem.* **22**, 916–917.

Villeneuve, D. C., and Khera, K. S. (1975). Placental transfer of halogenated benzenes (pentachloro-, pentachloronitro-, and hexabromo-) in rats. *Environ. Physiol. Biochem.* **5**, 328–331.

Villeneuve, D. C., and Newsome, W. H. (1975). Toxicity and tissue levels in the rat and guinea pig following acute hexachlorobenzene administration. *Bull. Environ. Contam. Toxicol.* **14**, 297–300.

Villeneuve, D. C., Phillips, W. E., Panopio, L. G., Mendoza, C. E., Hatina, G. V., and Grant, D. L. (1974a). The effects of phenobarbital and carbon tetrachloride on the rate of decline of body burdens of hexachlorobenzene in the rat. *Arch. Environ. Contam. Toxicol.* **2**, 243–252.

Villeneuve, D. C., Panopio, L. G., and Grant, D. L. (1974b). Placental transfer of hexachlorobenzene in the rabbit. *Toxicol. Appl. Pharmacol.* **29**, 108.

Villeneuve, D. C., Panopio, L. G., and Grant, D. L. (1974c). Placental transfer of hexachlorobenzene in the rabbit. *Environ. Physiol. Biochem.* **4**, 112–115.

Villeneuve, D. C., Van Logten, M. J., Vox, J. G., Den Tonkelaar, E. M., Greve, P. A., Speijers, G. J. A., and van Esch, G. J. (1977). Effect of food deprivation on low level hexachlorobenzene exposure in rats. *Sci. Total Environ.* **8**, 179–186.

Vizethum, W., Dahlmann, D., Bolsen, K., and Goerz, G. (1979). Influence of chloroquine (Resochin) on hexachlorobenzene (HCB) induced porphyria of the rat. *Arch. Dermatol. Res.* **264**, 125.

Vondruska, J. F., Fancher, O. E., and Calandra, J. C. (1971). An investigation into the teratogenic potential of captan, folpet and Difolatan in nonhuman primates. *Toxicol. Appl. Pharmacol.* **18**, 619–624.

Vonk, J. W., and Sijpesteijn, A. K. (1971). Methylbenzimidazol-2-ylcarbamate, the fungitoxic principal of thiophanate-methyl. *Pestic. Sci.* **2**, 160–164.

Vos, J. G., and Krajne, E. I. (1983). Immunotoxicity of pesticides. *In* "Developments in the Science and Practice of Toxicology" (A. W. Hayes, R. C. Schnell, and T. S. Miya, eds.). Am. Elsevier, New York.

Vos, J. G., VanLogten, M. J., Kreeftenberg, J. G., and Kruizinga, W. (1979). Hexachlorobenzene-induced stimulation of the humoral immune response in rats. *Ann. N.Y. Acad. Sci.* **320**, 535–550.

Waldenström, J., and Haeger-Aronsen, B. (1963). Different patterns of human porphyria. *Br. Med. J.* **2**, 272–273.

Watanabe, S. (1971). Medical observation on pesticide poisonings with dermatitis as the chief complaint. *J. Jpn. Assoc. Rural Med.* **19**, 371 (in Japanese).

Watson, C. J. (1960). Problem of porphyria. Some facts and questions. *N. Engl. J. Med.* **263**, 1025–1215.

Wattenberg, L. W., Lam, L. K. T., Fladmoe, A. V., and Borchert, P. (1977). Inhibitors of colon carcinogenesis. *Cancer (Philadelphia)* **40**, 2432–2435.

Weil, E., Kusterer, L., and Brogard, M.-H. (1965). Reaction to an antifungal citrus fruit agent. *Arch. Mal. Prof. Med. Trav. Secur. Soc.* **26**, 405–408.

West, H. D. (1940). Evidence for the detoxication of diphenyl through a sulfur mechanism. *Proc. Soc. Exp. Biol. Med.* **43**, 373–375.

West, H. D., and Jefferson, N. C. (1942). The effect of aromatic hydrocarbons on the growth of young rats. *J. Nutr.* **23**, 425–430.

West, H. D., Lawson, J. R., Miller, I. H., and Mathura, G. R. (1956). The fate of diphenyl in the rat. *Arch. Biochem. Biophys.* **60**, 14–20.

World Health Organization (WHO) (1974). World Health Organization International Agency for Research on Cancer. Some anti-thyroid and related substances, nitrofurans and industrial chemicals. *IARC Monogr. Eval. Carcinog. Risk. Chem. Man* **7.**

World Health Organization (WHO) (1975). Chlorothalonil. *WHO Pestic. Residues Ser.* **4,** 101–148.

World Health Organization (WHO) (1976). World Health Organization International Agency for Research on Cancer. Some carbamates, thiocarbamates, and carbazides. *IARC Monogr. Eval. Carcinog. Risk Chem. Man* **12.**

Worthing, C. R., and Walker, B. (1983). "The Pesticide Manual." Br. Crop Prot. Counc. Croydon, U.K.

Wray, J. E., Muftu, Y., and Dogramace, I. (1962). Hexachlorobenzene as a cause of porphyria turcica. *Turk. J. Pediatr.* **4,** 132–137.

Yang, R. S. H. (1975). Species-specific binding of ^{14}C-hexachlorobenzene to animal blood cells. *Toxicol. Appl. Pharmacol.* **33,** 147–148.

Yang, R. S. H., and Pittman, K. A. (1975). Fate of (^{14}C)hexachlorobenzene in the rhesus monkey and the rat. *Toxicol. Appl. Pharmacol.* **33,** 147.

Yang, R. S. H., Pittman, K. A., Rourke, D. R., and Stein, V. B. (1978). Pharmacokinetics and metabolism of hexachlorobenzene in the rat and the rhesus monkey. *J. Agric. Food Chem.* **26,** 1076–1083.

Yurchenko, I. V., Kazakevich, R. L., and Sasinovich, L. M. (1976). Neurosomatic disorders due to prolonged effect of tetramethylthiuram disulfide. *Vrach. Delo* **4,** 135–138 (in Russian).

Zawirska, B., and Dzik, D. (1977). Experimental hepatic synporphyringenesis.

Patol. Pol. **28,** 349–354 (in Polish).

Zdzienicka, M., Zielenska, M., Tudek, B., and Seymezyk, T. (1979). Mutagenic activity of thiram in Ames tester strains of *Salmonella typhimurium. Mutat. Res.* **68,** 9–13.

Zemaitas, M. A., and Greene, F. E. (1979). *In vivo* and *in vitro* effects of thiuram disulfides and dithiocarbamates on hepatic microsomal drug metabolism in the rat. *Toxicol. Appl. Pharmacol.* **48,** 343–350.

Zeman, A., Wolfram, G., and Zollner, N. (1971). Serum, hexachlorobenzene levels in humans. *Naturwissenschaften* **58,** 276 (in German).

Zeman, F. J., Hoogenboom, E. R., Kavlock, R. J., and Semple, J. L. (1986). Effects on the fetus of maternal benomyl exposure in the protein-deprived rat. *J. Toxicol. Environ. Health* **17,** 405–417.

Zhorzholiani, V. S. (1971). Effect of prolonged injection of captan on the function of gonads. *Soobshch. Akad. Nauk Gruz. SSR* **64,** 749–751 (in Russian).

Zhorzholiani, V. S. (1972). Materials on the cumulation of captan in experimental animals. *Soobshch. Akad. Nauk Gruz. SSR* **65,** 225–227 (in Russian).

Zorin, P. M. (1970). Allergic dermatitis from zineb. *Vestn. Dermatol. Venerol.* **44,** 65–68 (in Russian).

Zweig, G., Gao, R.-Y., and Popendorf, W. (1983). Simultaneous dermal exposure to captan and benomyl by strawberry harvesters. *J. Agric. Food Chem.* **31,** 1109–1113.

Miscellaneous Pesticides

Charles O. Knowles
University of Missouri–Columbia

22.1 INTRODUCTION

There are many compounds that are active against a variety of invertebrate and vertebrate pests of agriculture, domestic animals, and humans and whose chemical configuration precludes their assignment to any of the traditional major groups of pesticides. Included among these materials are some of the insecticides, acaricides, and molluscicides as well as the chemosterilants, repellents, and synergists. These miscellaneous compounds are not necessarily minor pesticides in terms of their benefit to humans. However, as a result of their rather high degree of specificity, they might be regarded by some as less important than many of the more broad-spectrum chemicals that are in such wide use.

22.2 SYNTHETIC ACARICIDES

Acaricides can be divided into the insecticides/acaricides and the specific acaricides. Insecticides/acaricides are compounds that are active in laboratory tests against insects, mites, and ticks. In practice, very few of these compounds are used against all three groups; individual compounds in this category usually are used for some insects and mites or for some insects and ticks. Insecticides/acaricides include some of the organophosphates (e.g., demeton, dimethoate, parathion, chlorpyrifos, diazinon, and azinphos-methyl), carbamates (e.g., formetanate, aldicarb, methomyl, and oxamyl), organochlorines (e.g., endosulfan and toxaphene), pyrethroids (e.g., fluvalinate, fenpropathrin, and bifenthrin), and formamidines (e.g., chlordimeform and amitraz). The specific acaricides are not lethal to insects at practical doses but are lethal to mites and/or ticks. In practice, however, specific acaricides have been used mainly for mite control. Specific acaricides include some of the diphenyl aliphatics (e.g., dicofol, chlorobenzilate, chloropropylate, and bromopropylate), organotins (e.g., cyhexatin, azocyclotin, and fenbutatin oxide), sulfur-bridged compounds (e.g., chlorfenson, tetradifon, tetrasul, PPPS, and propargite), dinitrophenol derivatives (e.g., dinocap, dinobuton, and binapacryl), and other structurally unrelated compounds (e.g., dienochlor, azoxybenzene, clofentezene, hexythiazox, flubenzimine, and oxythioquinox). The insecticides/acaricides, except for the formamidines and some of the specific acaricides (e.g., diphenyl aliphatics, organotins, dinitrophenol derivatives, and dienochlor), are more appropriately addressed in other chapters. Discussed here are two sulfur-bridged compounds (chlorfenson and propargite), two formamidines (chlordimeform and amitraz), and azoxybenzene. The structures of these and related compounds are given in Figs. 22.1 and 22.2.

22.2.1 CHLORFENSON

22.2.1.1 Identity, Properties, and Uses

Chemical Name Chlorfenson is 4-chlorophenyl 4-chlorobenzenesulfonate.

Structure See Fig. 22.1.

Synonyms Chlorfenson is the common name approved by BSI and ISO. The compound also is known as chlorofénizon (France), difenson (Denmark), CPCBS (JMAF, Japan), ephirsulphonate (USSR), ovatran (Argentina), ovex (ANSI, United States and Canada), and PCPCBS. Trade names have included Estonmite®, Genite 883®, Trichlorfenson®, Lethalaire G-58®, Mitran®, Orthotran®, Ovochlor®, Ovitox®, Ovotran®, Sappiran®, Erysit Super®, and Fac Super®. Code designations have included C-854, K-6,451, and C-1,006. The CAS registry number is 80-33-1.

Physical and Chemical Properties Chlorfenson has the empirical formula $C_{12}H_8Cl_2O_3S$ and a molecule weight of 303.2. It is a white crystalline solid with a characteristic odor. Technical chlorfenson is a colorless to tan flaky solid with a melting point of about 80°C. The vapor pressure of the compound at 25°C is negligible. Chlorfenson is practically insoluble in water, moderately soluble in ethyl alcohol and petroleum oils, and readily soluble in acetone and aromatic solvents. It is hydrolyzed by alkali but is compatible with most pesticides.

History, Formulations, and Uses Chlorfenson was introduced in 1949. It is a miticide active mainly against eggs but with some toxicity to motile forms. Chlorfenson has been formulated as a wettable powder either alone (500 gm/kg) or in

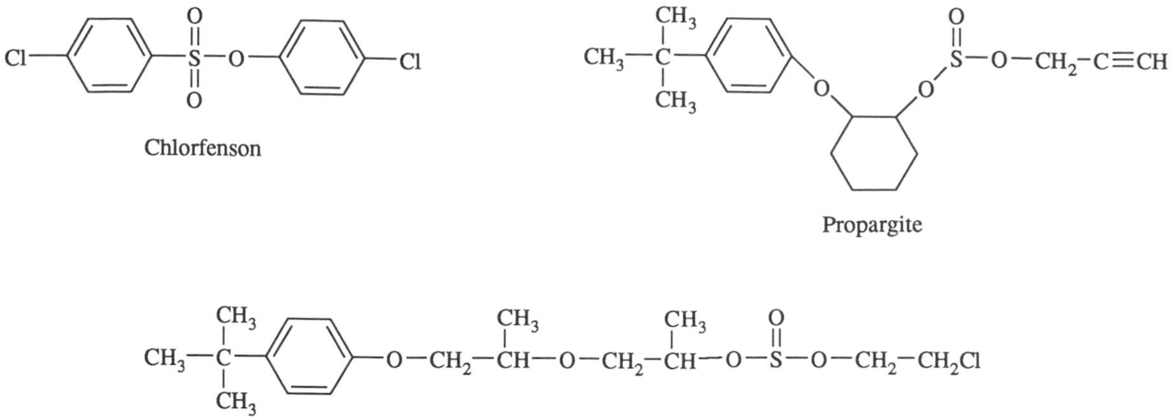

Chlorfenson

Propargite

PPPS

Figure 22.1 Three organosulfur acaricides.

combination with other compounds such as prothoate, chlorfenethol, or carbaryl.

22.2.1.2 Toxicity to Laboratory Animals

Basic Findings The acute oral LD 50 of chlorfenson to rats was found to be about 2000 mg/kg, while the dermal LD 50 was greater than 10,000 mg/kg (Worthing and Walker, 1983). Chlorfenson may cause skin irritation (Worthing and Walker, 1983). In the mouse, the acute oral LD 50 of chlorfenson was greater than 4000 mg/kg in both males and females. Definite toxic effects consisting of respiratory difficulty and spasms were evident at 2000 mg/kg (Taniguchi et al., 1978).

When fed to rats for 90 days at a dietary level of 3000 ppm, chlorfenson caused significant retardation of growth, increase in liver size, increase in thyroid size, and characteristic histological changes in the liver and thyroid, all in both males and females. Except for body growth in males, similar but lesser changes were produced by 1000 ppm. At 200 ppm, only the changes in liver and thyroid weights and in the induction of liver microsomal enzymes and the corresponding morphological changes were statistically significant. Even at 50 ppm, there was a trend to enzyme induction and corresponding histological change, but statistical significance was not established. The study was made with a diet very low in iodine, and this may have conditioned the thyroid response (Verschuuren et al., 1973).

In a 2-year study in rats, a minimal effect was produced by chlorfenson at a dietary level of 50 ppm, and 25 ppm was a no-effect level (Weil and McCollister, 1963).

Biochemical Effects Chlorfenson was a potent inhibitor of the oxidative deamination of 5-hydroxytryptamine and dopamine but not of 2-phenylethylamine, octopamine, and tryptamine by preparations of rat brain (Kadir and Knowles, 1981).

Effects on Organs and Tissues Chlorfenson was not mutagenic in bacterial assay systems involving strains of *Salmonella typhimurium* (Shirasu et al., 1976; Quinto et al., 1981; Moriya et al., 1983), *Escherichia coli* (Shirasu et al., 1976; Moriya et

al., 1983), and *Bacillus subtilis* (Shirasu et al., 1976). However, when chlorfenson was administered orally to rats daily for 6 days at 7.0% of the LD 50, an increase in the number of bone marrow cells with chromosomal aberrations was observed (Kiryushin, 1977).

Innes et al. (1969) treated 7-day-old male and female mice with daily oral dosages of chlorfenson (464 mg/kg) for 21 days until the mice were weaned, after which time they received the compound in the feed at 1019 ppm. No evidence of tumorigenic activity was found upon necropsy of mice at 18 months of age (Innes et al., 1969).

Chlorfenson provided *ad libitum* in the diet of male weanling rats for 3 weeks at concentrations of 2500, 250, or 25 ppm produced no apparent adverse effects on several immune parameters including number of lymphocytes and monocytes; levels of serum immunoglobulins IgM and IgG; and weight and histopathology of thymus, spleen, and mesenteric and popliteal lymph nodes. However, some liver effects, which included increased weight and histopathology, were found (Vos and Krajnc, 1983; Vos et al., 1983).

Factors Influencing Toxicity No studies of factors influencing chlorfenson toxicity to laboratory animals were found in the literature. However, chlorfenson does have a moderating effect on the toxicity of some insecticides that is probably due to its activity as an enzyme inducer. Treatment of rats with chlorfenson (100 mg/kg, oral) provided protection from a lethal dose of parathion (100 mg/kg, oral) and paraoxon (50 mg/kg, oral); the duration of protection was longer for parathion than for paraoxon. Chlorfenson caused a significant reduction in the concentrations of organophosphate in the livers of parathion- and paraoxon-exposed rats. Moreover, chlorfenson was shown to increase the rate of parathion metabolism by whole liver homogenates but had only a marginal effect on the rate of paraoxon metabolism. Chlorfenson also increased liver weight/body weight ratios (Black et al., 1973, 1975).

Pathology Induction of microsomal enzymes in rats is reflected by an increase in liver weight and by the formation of whorls of smooth endoplasmic reticulum in the hepatocytes. The lowest dietary level producing whorls within 90 days was 1000 ppm, but less striking changes in hepatocytes were produced by 50 ppm (Verschuuren *et al.*, 1973). In some acutely poisoned mice, the only change noted was hemorrhage of the spleen (Taniguchi *et al.*, 1978).

22.2.1.3 Toxicity to Humans

Accidents and Use Experience Apparently, the only report of human injury that may have been related to chlorfenson is that of Platonova (1970), who found a tendency to gastritis in 84 of 533 outpatients and in 86 of 104 inpatients, all of whom worked in the production of DDT, BHC, and chlorfenson. In the absence of reports of similar effects in exposed persons or in animals (including those receiving repeated doses at toxic levels), the cause of the gastritis remains unclear. Highly positive reactions to patch tests with chlorfenson among farmers, greenhouse workers, and others with dermatitis attributed to pesticides have been reported. A number of other compounds also gave positive reactions (Horiuchi and Ando, 1980; Horiuchi *et al.*, 1976, 1980).

Treatment of Poisoning Treatment is symptomatic.

22.2.2 PROPARGITE

22.2.2.1 Identity, Properties, and Uses

Chemical Name Propargite is 2-[4-(1,1-dimethylethyl)phenoxy]cyclohexyl 2-propynyl sulfite.

Structure See Fig. 22.1.

Synonyms Propargite is the common name approved by ANSI, BSI, and ISO. It also is known as BPPS (JMAF). Trade names have included Omite® and Comite®. Code designations have included DO-14 and ENT-27,226. The CAS registry number is 2312-35-8.

Physical and Chemical Properties Propargite has the empirical formula $C_{19}H_{26}O_4S$ and a molecular weight of 350.5. Technical propargite is 85% pure and forms a dark brown, viscous liquid with a vapor pressure of 3 mm Hg at 20°C. It is practically insoluble in water but is soluble in most organic solvents.

History, Formulations, and Uses Propargite was introduced in 1967 by the Uniroyal Chemical Company. It is an acaricide with activity mainly against motile stages of mites. It is formulated as emulsifiable concentrates (570, 680, or 750 gm/liter), wettable powders (300 gm/kg), and dusts (40 gm/kg).

22.2.2.2 Toxicity to Laboratory Animals

Basic Findings Propargite is a compound of low toxicity. Gaines (1969) reported an oral LD 50 value of 1480 mg/kg in both male and female rats but dermal values of 250 and 680 mg/kg in males and females, respectively. The time to death after an oral dose ranged from 43 hr to 16 days. The interval was similar after dermal exposure. Wiswesser (1976) quoted an oral LD 50 value of 2200 mg/kg in the rat and a dermal LD 50 value of over 10,000 mg/kg in the rabbit. A dermal LD 50 value of about 3200 mg/kg in the rabbit also has been reported [Food and Agriculture Organization/World Health Organization (FAO/WHO), 1978a]. No reason is apparent for the marked species difference in dermal toxicity. The relationship between oral and dermal toxicity in the rat suggests the presence of rapid effective detoxification of the compound in the liver of that species.

Ninety-day feeding studies with propargite have been conducted in rats and dogs. Groups of male and female rats were fed propargite in their diet at 4000, 2000, 800, 400, and 200 ppm, which corresponded in adult animals to 200, 100, 40, 20, and 10 mg/kg, respectively. Growth retardation and reduction of food intake were observed at the two highest levels. Hematological examinations and clinical chemistry tests revealed no abnormalities. At 200 and 100 mg/kg, the relative liver weights were increased; relative kidney weights were increased only in the 200 mg/kg group. In groups of male and female dogs provided a diet containing propargite at 2000 ppm (increased to 2500 ppm after 3 weeks), no effects on appearance or behavior were observed, and results of hematological and clinical chemistry tests were normal. However, in most propargite-treated dogs, reduced food consumption, reduced body weight, and increased relative liver and kidney weights were evident (FAO/WHO, 1978a).

Two-year feeding studies with rats and dogs also have been conducted with propargite. For 104 weeks, groups of male and female rats were fed propargite at 900, 300, and 100 ppm, which corresponded to 45, 15, and 5 mg/kg, respectively. No propargite-related effects were evident after 26 weeks; therefore, another study with propargite at 2000 ppm, which corresponded to 100 mg/kg, was initiated and continued for 78 weeks. Rats sacrificed at the end of 104 weeks and 78 weeks, along with those that died, were examined. At 100 mg/kg, reductions in food consumption and body weight gains were observed; mortality of male rats was 32%, compared to 7% in the control. No effects on appearance, behavior, growth rate, and survival were observed at levels up to and including 45 mg/kg. Hematological examinations and clinical laboratory studies revealed no propargite-related effects. Reductions in absolute and relative weights of liver and kidney were found in animals treated at levels of 45, 15, and 5 mg/kg which died or were sacrificed, but dose–response relationships could not be established. In animals treated at 100 mg/kg, an increase in relative liver and kidney weights of about 30% was found. In groups of dogs fed propargite at dietary levels of 900, 300, and 100 ppm for 2 years, no treatment-related effects were observed on growth rate and organ weights. Results of clinical laboratory studies and urinalyses were normal (FAO/WHO, 1978a).

Absorption, Distribution, Metabolism, and Excretion When rats were treated orally with a single dose of radiolabeled propargite (271 mg/kg), it was absorbed from the gastrointestinal tract and rapidly metabolized, mainly to polar compounds that were eliminated in the urine (47%) and feces (32%). Levels of radiocarbon remaining in the total carcass were low (about 9%).

Propargite metabolism *in vivo* and *in vitro* has been examined using several animal species. Propargite was hydrolyzed at the sulfite ester linkage to propargyl alcohol and to 2-*p-tert*-butylphenoxycyclohexanol, which was subsequently cleaved at the ether moiety to *tert*-butylphenol and cyclohexandiol. Other polar metabolites including *tert*-butylpyrocatechol and conjugates also were formed (FAO/WHO, 1978a,b, 1981b).

Biochemical Effects   Propargite was a weak inhibitor of the oxidative deamination of dopamine, octopamine, 2-phenylethylamine, and tryptamine by rat brain homogenates (Kadir and Knowles, 1981).

Effects on Organs and Tissues   Propargite was not mutagenic in several assays with strains of *S. typhimurium* (TA1535, TA1536, TA1537, TA1538), *E. coli* (WP2 strains), and *B. subtilis* (H17 Rec$^+$, M45 Rec$^-$) (Shirasu *et al.*, 1976). In other studies, propargite at concentrations ranging from 0.001 to 5.0 mg/plate was examined for mutagenic potential using *Salmonella* spp. and *Saccharomyces* spp. in the presence and absence of liver microsomal preparation from Aroclor 1254-induced rats (S9 activation). Although the higher concentrations caused some cellular toxicity, propargite did not induce mutagenic activity (FAO/WHO, 1981a).

To evaluate the carcinogenic potential, groups of male and female mice (Charles River, CD-1) were fed propargite in the diet at dosage levels of 1000, 500, 160, and 50 mg/kg for 18 months. There was no excessive mortality during the study as a consequence of the propargite. Further, there was no effect of propargite on food consumption, growth, appearance, or behavior. Hematological values were not affected by propargite at any dosage level. A slight reduction in kidney weight and enlarged uterus in the animals fed at the highest dosage were noted. However, no additional adverse effects were revealed on gross and histological examinations, and it was concluded that propargite was not tumorigenic or carcinogenic in these studies (FAO/WHO, 1981a).

Effects on Reproduction   Groups of female rats were treated with propargite at levels ranging from 450 to 6 mg/kg/day on days 6–15 of gestation. Animals were sacrificed on day 20 of gestation, and fetuses were removed and examined. Maternal mortality at 450 mg/kg was high, and this dose level was discontinued. Females at 105 mg/kg showed signs of acute poisoning including bloody nasal discharge, alopecia, urinary incontinence, and bloody vaginal discharge, but only occasional toxic signs of poisoning were observed at levels of 25 and 6 mg/kg. There were no differences in any of the treatment groups with respect to the maintenance of pregnancy, implantation sites, numbers of live and dead fetuses, or resorption sites. There was an increased number of smaller pups and an in-

creased incidence of hemorrhagic abdomen in more litters at 105 and 25 mg/kg than in those at 6 mg/kg or in the controls. No differences with respect to the average weight of live fetuses in any of the groups were noted. It was concluded that propargite was not teratogenic in these studies (FAO/WHO, 1981a, 1982).

Pathology   No propargite-related lesions were found upon gross and microscopic examination of tissues from rats in the 90-day feeding trial or dogs in the 2-year feeding study. However, in the 2-year feeding study with rats, some animals in the 100 mg/kg group and in the control had enlarged and/or dark red lymph nodes that were involved in abdominal masses in some cases. In the 90-day feeding study with dogs, tissues were normal upon gross examination, but histopathological examination showed an increased amount of pigment in the liver reticuloendothelial cells and increased hemosiderosis of the spleen (FAO/WHO, 1978a). In the rat teratology study, missing sternebrae and missing or reduced hyoid were significantly increased at 105 and 25 mg/kg, and an increased incidence of incomplete closure of the skull also was observed at 105 mg/kg. It was suggested that these abnormalities were indicative of retarded development and were probably reflective of the toxic maternal effects observed at higher dosage levels (FAO/WHO, 1981a, 1982).

22.2.2.3   Toxicity to Humans

Use Experience   Propargite has been involved in numerous cases of dermatitis in the United States and elsewhere (Nagai, 1976; Churchill *et al.*, 1986). For example, during the 12-year period from 1974 through 1985, 506 cases of dermatitis associated with exposure to propargite among agricultural workers were reported in California. This number was second only to sulfur, with 677 recorded cases. Two occurrences in California, one in 1974 and one in 1986, are noteworthy. In 1974 there were 36 recorded complaints of dermatitis and eye irritation caused by propargite associated with the application of 358,477 kg of the compound on 179,160 ha. During the investigation in 1975, many complaints that had not been officially reported were found by questioning workers. Most complaints were associated with a single water-wettable powder, which was very dusty, and most of the difficulty was associated with mixing and loading. Following a meeting called by the State Department of Food and Agriculture, the manufacturers cooperated fully and rapidly. The offending formulation was withdrawn from sale in California and a newly developed wettable powder with negligible dustiness was substituted, which essentially solved the problem (K. T. Maddy, personal communication to W. J. Hayes, Jr., 1976). In May 1986 another outbreak of dermatitis occurred involving 114 of 198 orange pickers working for a packer. Interviews revealed that the dermatitis occurred commonly in the exposed areas of the neck (81%) and chest (42%). The dermatitis started with burning, redness, and itching and in many instances progressed to small papules, vesicles with weeping and crusting, exfoliation, and hyperpigmentation. One-third of the interviewed workers reported exfoliation, and

34% reported eye irritation, for which 8% received medical treatment. On-site observations revealed that the pickers frequently leaned into dense foliage to harvest oranges and that this direct contact with the treated foliage probably resulted in exposure to pesticide residues. Additional interviews and leaf residue sampling indicated that propargite (Omite-CR) was the causative agent. The California registration for Omite-CR was subsequently withdrawn by the manufacturer (Churchill *et al.*, 1986).

Treatment of Poisoning Treatment of poisoning by propargite is symptomatic.

22.2.3 CHLORDIMEFORM

22.2.3.1 Identity, Properties, and Uses

Chemical Name Chlordimeform is *N'*-(4-chloro-*o*-tolyl)-*N*,*N*-dimethylformamidine; it is marketed as the base and as the hydrochloride salt.

Structure See Fig. 22.2.

Synonyms The common name chlordimeform is approved by ANSI, BSI, and E-ISO; other common names have included chlordiméforme (F-ISO), chlorophenamidine (JMAF), chlorodimeform, and chlorophedine. Trade names have included Fundal®, Galecron®, Bermat®. Fundex®, and Spanone®. Code designations have included Ciba-8,514, OMS-1,209, and ENT-27,335 for the base and EP-333, ENT-27,567, and Schering-36,268 for the salt. The CAS registry numbers are 6164-98-3 and 19750-95-9 for the base and salt forms, respectively.

Physical and Chemical Properties Chlordimeform has the empirical formula $C_{10}H_{13}ClN_2$ and a molecular weight of 196.7. The pure material forms colorless crystals with a boiling point of 163–165°C at 14 mm Hg and a melting point of 32°C. The vapor pressure at 20°C is 3.5×10^{-4} mm Hg. The compound is only slightly soluble in water but readily soluble in organic solvents. The hydrochloride, which melts at 225–227°C with decomposition, is quite soluble in water. Although the hydrochloride is stable in aqueous solution for several days under acidic conditions, the base is hydrolyzed under neutral and acidic conditions.

History, Formulations, and Uses Chlordimeform was introduced in 1966 by Schering A.G. It is active mainly against eggs and motile forms of mites and ticks and against eggs and early instars of some Lepidoptera. The base is formulated as emulsifiable concentrates (500 gm/liter), and the hydrochloride is formulated as soluble powders (800 gm/kg).

22.2.3.2 Toxicity to Laboratory Animals

Basic Findings Chlordimeform is a compound of moderate acute toxicity (see Table 22.1). The base, but not the hydrochloride, is readily absorbed by the skin. The compound is not irritating to animals. Rats killed by oral treatment with chlordimeform displayed hyperactivity, tremors, convulsions, and respiratory arrest.

In studies of the toxicity to mice of chlordimeform and its mammalian metabolites, acute oral LD 50 values were found to be 267 mg/kg for chlordimeform, 163 mg/kg for demethylchlordimeform, 78 mg/kg for didemethylchlordimeform, 750 mg/kg for *N*-formyl-4-chloro-*o*-toluidine, between 500 and 1000 mg/kg for 3-(4-chloro-*o*-toly)urea, and greater than 1000 mg/kg for 4-chloro-*o*-toluidine, 1,1-dimethyl-3-(4-chloro-*o*-tolyl)urea, and 1-methyl-3-(4-chloro-*o*-tolyl)urea. Symptoms manifested by mice treated with lethal doses of the three formamidines generally were similar but some differences were noted. Symptoms included restlessness, hyperreflexia, and tremors, particularly of the head and forelimbs, that developed to one or more episodes of clonic convulsions. Death usually occurred within the first hour during one of the convulsive episodes. Tremors were not observed in mice poisoned with demethylchlordimeform and didemethylchlordimeform, and the convulsive stage was longer than that with chlordimeform. The

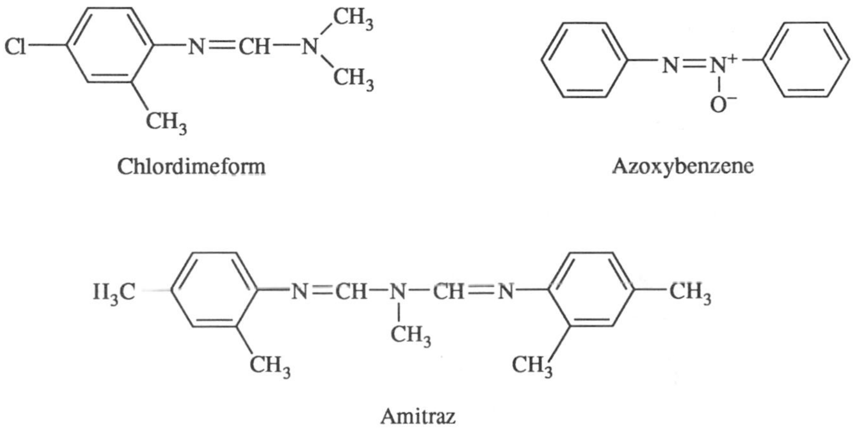

Figure 22.2 Three organonitrogen acaricides.

Table 22.1
Single-Dose LD 50 Values of Chlordimeform

Species	Route	LD 50 (mg/kg)	Reference
Rat	oral	250	Haddow and Shankland (1969)
Rat	oral	340[a]	Worthing and Walker (1983)
Rat	oral	170–220[a]	Larson et al. (1985)
Rat	oral	225–330[b]	Larson et al. (1985)
Rat	oral	335[b]	Worthing and Walker (1983)
Rat, M	oral	123	Robinson et al. (1975)
Rat, M	oral	178–220	FAO/WHO (1972)
Rat, F	oral	170–460	FAO/WHO (1972)
Rat	dermal	640	FAO/WHO (1972)
Mouse	oral	290	Haddow and Shankland (1969)
Mouse, M	oral	267	Ghali and Hollingworth (1985)
Mouse	oral	160[a]	Larson et al. (1985)
Mouse	dermal	225[a]	Larson et al. (1985)
Mouse	intraperitoneal	110	FAO/WHO (1972)
Rabbit	oral	625	Haddow and Shankland (1969)
Rabbit	oral	625	Worthing and Walker (1983)
Rabbit	dermal	>4000[b]	Worthing and Walker (1983)
Dog, M	oral	~150	FAO/WHO (1972)
Dog, F	oral	~100	FAO/WHO (1972)

[a]Chlordimeform base.
[b]Chlordimeform hydrochloride.

locomotor difficulty usually observed in chlordimeform-treated mice was absent from those treated with the two N-demethylated metabolites. N-Formyl-4-chloro-o-toluidine, 4-chloro-o-toluidine, and the three substituted urea metabolites were depressants; death of mice with these compounds frequently occurred many hours following treatment (Ghali and Hollingworth, 1985).

The toxicity to rats of chlordimeform and four of its mammalian metabolites following intraperitoneal, subcutaneous, and intracerebroventricular injection was investigated. Chlordimeform and its two formamidine metabolites, N'-(4-chloro-o-tolyl)-N-methylformamidine (demethylchlordimeform) and N'-(4-chloro-o-tolyl)formamidine (didemethylchlordimeform), were more toxic by intraperitoneal treatment than by subcutaneous treatment. Chlordimeform also was more toxic by intraperitoneal injection than by intracerebroventricular injection. However, demethylchlordimeform and especially didemethylchlordimeform were much more toxic when injected directly into the brain than when injected intraperitoneally and subcutaneously. With the three formamidines, toxicity decreased in the order didemethylchlordimeform > demethylchlordimeform > chlordimeform for each of the three modes of

treatment. N-Formyl-4-chloro-o-toluidine and 4-chloro-o-toluidine were of low acute toxicity upon injection. Symptoms manifested by rats poisoned with chlordimeform following intraperitoneal and subcutaneous injection were similar. A marked hyperexcitability, which increased in intensity with time, with a sensitivity to external stimuli ensued about 20 min following subcutaneous injection of a lethal dose (200 mg/kg). Running and intense escape behavior also were evident. Prostration with hyperextension of hind legs occurred at later stages of poisoning, and death occurred between 50 and 143 min postinjection. Following subcutaneous injection of rats with a lethal dose of demethylchlordimeform (150 mg/kg), symptoms elicited were qualitatively similar to those with chlordimeform but were more intense. Hyperexcitation began about 5 min after treatment and death occurred between 17 and 50 min postinjection. When rats were injected with a lethal dose of didemethylchlordimeform (35 mg/kg), hyperexcitability began within 3–4 min posttreatment, and by 5–6 min convulsions were evident. Rats died between 9 and 10 min postinjection. Symptoms from intracerebroventricular treatment of rats with the three formamidines were similar to those from subcutaneous treatment. However, symptoms following intracerebroventricular injection of didemethylchlordimeform began immediately after treatment, whereas those from chlordimeform and demethylchlordimeform occurred after a latent period. Rats treated with N-formyl-4-chloro-o-toluidine were asymptomatic following subcutaneous (400 mg/kg) and intracerebroventricular (67 mg/kg) treatment at the highest dosages tested. However, when administered intraperitoneally (400 mg/kg), a sedative action was apparent followed in about 15 min by a condition in which rats failed to respond to external stimuli. A similar depressant effect that ensued about 1 min after treatment was observed when rats were treated intraperitoneally with 4-chloro-o-toluidine (500 mg/kg) (Benezet et al., 1978).

Several short-term and long-term feeding studies of chlordimeform have been conducted with groups of male and female rats and mice. Rats fed chlordimeform at the rate of 100 mg/kg/day for 28 days showed retarded growth without morphological change; 80 mg/kg/day produced no toxic effect (Haddow and Shankland, 1969). In other studies, male and female rats and mice were fed chlordimeform in their diet for 60 days at concentrations of 6000, 3000, 1500, and 750 ppm, which corresponded to average dosages of 463, 227, 129, and 78 mg/kg body weight for rats and 1522, 643, 197, and 113 mg/kg for mice. There was slight mortality in rats at the highest dosage (463 mg/kg) and some mortality in mice at the two highest dosages (1522 and 643 mg/kg). Food consumption and growth rate were reduced in both rats and mice (females only) at all levels. No clinical signs of toxicity were noted. Changes in hematological parameters were found in both species but were more dramatic in mice. In rats, levels of methemoglobin were increased at all levels in a dose-related manner, and Heinz bodies were observed at dosages of 129 mg/kg and above. In mice, a toxic hemolytic anemia was found in both sexes in all treated groups. It was characterized by reduced hemoglobin concentration, red blood cell count, and packed cell volume;

these reductions were associated with increased methemoglobin levels and Heinz body formation. Mice of both sexes treated at 643 mg/kg showed slight reticulocytosis that was accompanied in females by a shift in the differential leukocyte count due to an increase in the percentage of polymorphonuclear neutrophils and a decrease in the percentage of lymphocytes. Small changes in several clinical chemistry parameters were noted in both species. Reduction in relative weights of many organs was observed in rats of both sexes (FAO/WHO, 1981a).

In long-term studies, male and female rats were fed chlordimeform for 24 months in the diet at levels of 500, 100, 20, and 2 ppm, which corresponded to average dosages of 26, 5.5, 1.1, and 0.1 mg/kg body weight, and mice were fed chlordimeform hydrochloride at dietary levels of 500, 100, and 20 ppm. Excessive mortality was not observed in rats, but mortality in mice was significantly increased at 500 and 100 ppm in females after 60 and 90 weeks, respectively, and in males after 70 and 110 weeks, respectively. In rats, growth rate was reduced at 500 ppm (26 mg/kg) in both sexes, but no effects on growth were found in mice. No clinical signs of poisoning or abnormal behavior were observed in rats or mice. Analyses of blood and urine of rats revealed slight changes in several parameters at higher dosages, including increased formation of methemoglobin and Heinz bodies. There were no chlordimeform-related changes in organ weights in rats. Results of blood and urine analyses and organ weights were not provided for mice (FAO/WHO, 1979a, 1981a).

In another 2-year feeding study of chlordimeform in rats, a dietary level of 1000 ppm (approaching 50 mg/kg/day) caused severe inhibition of growth within 3 months. Even at 500 ppm, food intake and growth were reduced in both sexes. Red cell count, hematocrit, and hemoglobin were decreased in females during the first year, but during the second year only the hematocrit was consistently depressed. Changes in the ratio of organ to body weights were not dosage-related (FAO/WHO, 1972).

In a 2-year feeding study with dogs, body weight, red cell count, hematocrit, and hemoglobin were reduced at a dietary level of 1000 ppm. Leukocyte count and serum albumin were decreased sporadically. The relative weights of the spleen and kidneys were increased in one or both sexes at 1000 ppm (FAO/WHO, 1972).

Additional short-term and long-term feeding studies have been carried out with groups of male and female rats and mice with two chlordimeform metabolites, N-formyl-4-chloro-o-toluidine (FAO/WHO, 1979a, 1981a) and 4-chloro-o-toluidine [FAO/WHO, 1979a, 1981a; National Cancer Institute (NCI), 1979a; Weisburger et al., 1978]. The results of these studies will not be discussed, except for associated histopathology (see Pathology below).

Absorption, Distribution, Metabolism, and Excretion When radioactive chlordimeform was administered as a single oral dose to rats (Knowles and Sen Gupta, 1970; Morikawa et al., 1975; Knowles and Benezet, 1977), mice (FAO/WHO, 1980; Ghali and Hollingworth, 1985), dogs (Sen Gupta and Knowles, 1970), or goats (Sen Gupta and Knowles, 1970), it

was rapidly absorbed, distributed, metabolized, and eliminated. The majority of the radiocarbon was present in the urine during the initial 24 hr posttreatment. Some radioactivity was found in dog bile and in the feces of the four animal species. A similar pattern of fast absorption, distribution, metabolism, and elimination was observed when female mice were treated with multiple daily doses of chlordimeform; excretion was largely complete within 24 hr after the last treatment (FAO/WHO, 1980). Tissue residues generally were low, and no evidence was found for any selective tissue storage of chlordimeform or its metabolites with single or multiple oral dosing regimes. Moreover, chlordimeform was not secreted in goat milk to any appreciable extent (Sen Gupta and Knowles, 1970). Chlordimeform also was degraded by mice treated intraperitoneally (Kimmel et al., 1986) and in vitro by rat and mouse liver preparations (Ahmad and Knowles, 1971a; Morikawa et al., 1975; Ghali and Hollingworth, 1985; Kimmel et al., 1986).

Products of chlordimeform metabolism in vivo or in vitro or both included demethylchlordimeform, didemethylchlordimeform, N-formyl-4-chloro-o-toluidine, 4-chloro-o-toluidine, N-formyl-5-chloroanthranilic acid, 5-chloroanthranilic acid, 1,1-dimethyl-3-(4-chloro-o-tolyl)urea, 1-methyl-3-(4-chloro-o-tolyl)urea, 3-(4-chloro-o-tolyl)urea, 4-chloro-2-methylnitrosobenzene, and unidentified compounds including sulfate and glucuronide conjugates. Metabolic paths for the formation of these compounds and discussions of associated mechanisms have been presented (Knowles, 1970, 1974, 1982; Ahmad and Knowles, 1971a,b; Benezet and Knowles, 1976a; Knowles and Benezet, 1977; Kimmel et al., 1986).

Pharmacological and Biochemical Effects Chlordimeform elicits a variety of pharmacological and biochemical effects when administered to laboratory animals. Considerable effort has been devoted in an attempt to describe these actions and to explain their significance. Chlordimeform is rapidly metabolized by laboratory animals, and several of its metabolites are biologically active, even more so than the parent compound in some instances. Thus, any attempt to understand the actions of chlordimeform must include consideration of its metabolites.

The observation that chlordimeform administered intraperitoneally to rabbits at 200 mg/kg caused a marked decrease in mean arterial blood pressure of almost 50% within 30 min of treatment focused attention on the cardiovascular system as a potential target (Matsumura and Beeman, 1976). In subsequent work it was found that chlordimeform induced marked cardiovascular changes in the dog (Lund et al., 1978a,b; Rieger et al., 1981). Chlordimeform administered intravenously to pentobarbital-anesthetized dogs at dosages from 1 to 30 mg/kg caused a biphasic effect on blood pressure consisting of an initial depressor response and a secondary pressor response. The depressor and pressor responses were associated with decreased and increased cardiac contractility, respectively. Another experiment with the dog perfused hind-limb preparation indicated that the chlordimeform-mediated depressor and pressor responses also were associated with decreased and increased vascular resistance, respectively. It was concluded that decreased cardiac contractility and vascular resistance accounted for the initial depressor response, whereas the increased cardiac contractility and vascular resistance accounted for the secondary pressor response. Other research indicated that the initial depressor response was the result of a nonspecific direct action on the cardiac and vascular smooth muscle and was independent of the autonomic nervous system, since blockade of the parasympathetic nervous system or histaminergic receptors had no effect on the response, nor did chlordimeform have any blocking effect on the sympathetic nervous system. The secondary pressor response was the result of action on the autonomic system inasmuch as interference with the function of the sympathetic nervous system at the level of the brain, sympathetic ganglia, or neuroeffector junction blocked the response. Chlordimeform administered intravenously to dogs at lethal dosages (50 mg/kg) caused a rapid, irreversible hypotension that resulted from severe depression of heart and peripheral vasculature. The cardiovascular collapse was followed quickly by respiratory arrest. Since artificial respiration would not afford protection against hypotension and death, it was concluded that cardiovascular collapse was a primary cause of death (Lund *et al.*, 1978a,b). These and other actions of chlordimeform on the cardiovascular and central nervous systems of dogs, mice, and rats are similar in many respects to those of local anesthetics, such as procaine and lidocaine (Chinn *et al.*, 1976, 1977; Lund *et al.*, 1978a,b, 1979; Pfister *et al.*, 1978b).

Watkinson (1985a,b, 1986a,b) examined the effects of chlordimeform on cardiovascular functional parameters in postweanling (22–30-day-old) and geriatric (2-year-old) rats. For intravenous treatment, postweanling rats were sequentially dosed with 5, 10, 30, 60, and 120 mg/kg and geriatric rats were sequentially dosed with 5, 20, 30, and 60 mg/kg; the injection period lasted about 1 min per dose, and 10–15 min were allowed between doses. For intraperitoneal treatment, postweanling rats received a single injection of 60, 30, or 10 mg/kg. Chlordimeform administered intravenously produced profound and abrupt decreases in heart rate and blood pressure within 0–3 min. Multiple arrhythmias and alterations in electrocardiogram waveforms and intervals also were observed. After the initial acute stage there was a transient recovery followed by a persistent delayed depression of heart rate and blood pressure. These effects were more severe in geriatric rats than in postweanling rats. In rats treated intraperitoneally, decreased heart rate also was observed and was comparable to the delayed heart rate effect seen in rats treated intravenously. Interestingly, bradycardia was not found in rats treated intraperitoneally with chlordimeform at 50–100 mg/kg (Beeman and Matsumura, 1973) or intravenously at 0.03–10 mg/kg (Hsu and Kakuk, 1984).

Numerous studies of the inhibition of monoamine oxidase *in vivo* by chlordimeform have been conducted mainly in rats and occasionally in mice. Chlordimeform was administered orally, intraperitoneally, and subcutaneously, and the dosage was varied from single lethal doses to single, sublethal, behaviorly active doses; multiple doses also were used. At various post-treatment intervals, radiometric, fluorometric, or colorimetric methods using 5-hydroxytryptamine, tryptamine, tyramine, dopamine, 2-phenylethylamine, benzylamine, and kynuramine as substrates were used to assay monoamine oxidase activity in brain, liver, and occasionally intestine. As would be expected, the results were variable, but chlordimeform clearly inhibited monoamine oxidase *in vivo*, although it was less potent than classical monoamine oxidase inhibitors such as tranylcypromine and pargyline (Beeman and Matsumura, 1973; Benezet *et al.*, 1978; Maitre *et al.*, 1978; Kaloyanova *et al.*, 1978, 1979, 1981; Pfister *et al.*, 1978a; Bainova *et al.*, 1979; Hollingworth *et al.*, 1979; MacPhail and Leander, 1980, 1981; Bailey *et al.*, 1982; Witkin and Leander, 1982; Boyes *et al.*, 1985c). Chlordimeform, demethylchlordimeform, didemethylchlordimeform, and *N*-formyl-4-chloro-*o*-toluidine, but not 4-chloro-*o*-toluidine, *N*-formyl-5-chloroanthranilic acid, and 5-chloroanthranilic acid, were *in vitro* inhibitors of brain and liver monoamine oxidase (Aziz and Knowles, 1973; Beeman and Matsumura, 1973; Knowles and Aziz, 1974; Benezet and Knowles, 1976b; Knowles, 1976; Neumann and Voss, 1977; Benezet *et al.*, 1978; Hollingworth *et al.*, 1979; Urbaneja and Knowles, 197; Rieger *et al.*, 1980; Kadir and Knowles, 1981). *N*-Formyl-4-chloro-*o*-toluidine was more potent than chlordimeform and its two *N*-demethyl metabolites as an *in vitro* inhibitor of rat and mouse brain monoamine oxidase (Benezet *et al.*, 1978; Hollingworth *et al.*, 1979). Chlordimeform, demethylchlordimeform, didemethylchlordimeform, and *N*-formyl-4-chloro-*o*-toluidine were reversible fully competitive inhibitors of monoamine oxidase (Benezet *et al.*, 1978; Hollingworth *et al.*, 1979), and they inhibited both monoamine oxidase types A and B *in vitro* (Benezet *et al.*, 1978; Hollingworth *et al.*, 1979). Inhibition of both types A and B was observed when rats were treated with chlordimeform (Maitre *et al.*, 1978; Kaloyanova *et al.*, 1981; Bailey *et al.*, 1982; Boyes *et al.*, 1985c), and there was variation among the studies as to which type, if either, was preferentially inhibited. This apparent disparity can be resolved when one keeps in mind the fact that chlordimeform and three of its metabolites inhibit both types of monoamine oxidase *in vitro* with slightly different preferences and that in the assays from chlordimeform treatment *in vivo* one is measuring the net contribution of the four compounds, which will vary depending on rate of metabolism and other related pharmacokinetic factors. Although it seemed certain that monoamine oxidase inhibition was not the major lesion in laboratory animals killed by chlordimeform (Neumann and Voss, 1977; Robinson and Smith, 1977; Hollingworth *et al.*, 1979), it may be involved in some of the sublethal actions (Boyes *et al.*, 1985c). In this connection, Boyes *et al.* (1985c) reported that since chlordimeform is a reversible inhibitor and since earlier *in vivo* studies used heavily diluted fractions, the amount of monoamine oxidase inhibition was underestimated. They reported that in rats intraperitoneal dosages of 30 and 8 mg/kg were sufficient to give 50% inhibition of brain monoamine oxidase types A and B, respectively, after 2 hr (Boyes *et al.*, 1985c).

Chlordimeform treatment of rats has been shown to alter levels of biogenic amines in brain and plasma. Maitre *et al.* (1978) monitored amine levels in rat brain at 1, 2, 4, and 6 hr following oral treatment with 200 mg/kg; 5-hydroxytryptamine, norepinephrine, and dopamine peak levels were 21% (2 hr), 21% (6 hr), and 26% (2 hr) higher than controls, respectively. When rats were injected intraperitoneally with chlordimeform at 200 mg/kg, 5-hydroxytryptamine and norepinephrine levels in brain were 70 and 22% higher, respectively, than control levels at 1 hr (Beeman and Matsumura, 1973); however, it should be mentioned that differences between norepinephrine levels in the treatment (0.22 ± 0.01 $\mu g/gm$) and control (0.18 ± 0.02 $\mu g/gm$) rats probably were not statistically significant. However, when Johnson and Knowles (1983) treated rats subcutaneously with chlordimeform at 200 mg/kg, at 1 hr brain levels of 5-hydroxytryptamine, norepinephrine, dopamine, and 2-phenylethylamine did not differ significantly from controls, but levels of tyramine were 62% less than controls. Benezet et al. (1978) found that the level of 5-hydroxytryptamine in rat brain 1 hr following subcutaneous treatment with chlordimeform at 150 mg/kg was 58% higher than the control level. When rats were injected intraperitoneally with chlordimeform at the low dosage of 25 mg/kg, brain levels of norepinephrine and dopamine were increased by 52 and 70%, respectively, within 14 hr of treatment (Bailey et al., 1982). Plasma levels of 5-hydroxytryptamine, norepinephrine, and 2-phenylethylamine were 64, 38, and 83% less than controls, respectively, and the tyramine level was the same as control 1 hr following subcutaneous treatment of rats with chlordimeform at 200 mg/kg (Johnson and Knowles, 1983). Several chlordimeform metabolites also elicited changes in levels of some biogenic amines in brain and plasma when administered to rats. When demethylchlordimeform was administered subcutaneously to rats at 100 mg/kg, levels of 5-hydroxytryptamine and dopamine were 38 and 26% higher than controls, respectively, at 1 hr and reached peak values of 62 and 47%, respectively, at 4 hr (Benezet et al., 1978). In rats treated similarly with demethylchlordimeform, Johnson and Knowles (1983) found that at 1 hr brain levels of 5-hydroxytryptamine, dopamine, and 2-phenylethylamine were not significantly different from controls, but levels of norepinephrine and tyramine were decreased 12 and 66%, respectively; however, norepinephrine levels peaked at 22% higher than controls at 12 hr and dopamine levels peaked at 13% higher than controls. Levels in plasma of rats injected subcutaneously with demethylchlordimeform at 100 mg/kg at 1 hr were 83, 63, and 86% lower than controls for 5-hydroxytryptamine, norepinephrine, and 2-phenylethylamine, respectively, but tyramine levels were unchanged (Johnson and Knowles, 1983). Didemethylchlordimeform injected subcutaneously into rats at 25 mg/kg resulted in brain levels of norepinephrine and tyramine at 1 hr that were 23 and 59% lower than controls, respectively, but levels of 5-hydroxytryptamine, dopamine, and 2-phenylethylamine were not significantly different from controls (Johnson and Knowles, 1983). In plasma 1 hr after rats received didemethylchlordimeform subcutaneously at 25 mg/kg, levels of 5-hydroxytryptamine, norepinephrine, and 2-phenylethylamine were lower than controls by 78, 69, and 72%, respectively, while the level of tyramine was 98% higher than the control (Johnson and

Knowles, 1983). Rats treated subcutaneously with N-formyl-4-chloro-o-toluidine at 175 mg/kg had brain levels of 5-hydroxytryptamine and dopamine that were 56 and 35% higher than controls at 8 and 2 hr posttreatment, respectively (Benezet et al., 1978). The toxicological significance of these effects on biogenic amine levels by chlordimeform and its metabolites is difficult to assess. They probably are due, at least in part, to inhibition of monoamine oxidase, but other factors, including stimulation of amine release, also may be involved. In any event, the changes in amine levels were not as great as those induced by classical monoamine oxidase inhibitors, and Robinson et al. (1975) found that neither blockade of serotonergic or α-adrenergic receptors or both nor depletion of tissue stores of these amines reduced the lethality in rats of chlordimeform, and they concluded that it was improbable that death resulted from stimulation of α-adrenergic or excitatory serotonergic receptors.

Chlordimeform and certain metabolites have been shown to affect platelet function (Knowles and Johnson, 1984a). Uptake of radioactive 5-hydroxytryptamine by platelets from rats treated intraperitoneally with chlordimeform (25 mg/kg) was not significantly influenced at 1 hr; however, uptake of this amine by platelets from rats treated with demethylchlordimeform (25 mg/kg) was significantly inhibited. At 1 and/or 24 hr posttreatment, chlordimeform effected significant decreases in platelet levels of 5-hydroxytryptamine, norepinephrine, and dopamine and plasma levels of 5-hydroxytryptamine, whereas demethylchlordimeform caused significant decreases in both platelet and plasma levels of 5-hydroxytryptamine (Knowles and Johnson, 1984b). On direct treatment of isolated rat platelets, formamidines inhibited uptake of 5-hydroxytryptamine and induced release of endogenous stores of this amine in a concentration-dependent manner; potency decreased in the order didemethylchlordimeform > demethylchlordimeform > chlordimeform (Johnson and Knowles, 1981, 1982). Aggregation of rat platelets induced by ADP, collagen, and arachidonic acid was inhibited by chlordimeform (1×10^{-5} M) and N-formyl-4-chloro-o-toluidine (arachidonic acid only). Chlordimeform (1×10^{-5} M), demethylchlordimeform, and didemethylchlordimeform also increased cyclic AMP levels in platelet-rich plasma (Johnson and Knowles, 1985).

Chlordimeform induces hypothermia in rats (Yim et al., 1978a; Boyes and Dyer, 1984c; Boyes et al., 1985b) and mice (Gordon and Long, 1985; Gordon et al., 1985) under normothermic conditions. It was suggested that this action of chlordimeform in mice was likely of central neural origin (Gordon et al., 1985). Moreover, there is some evidence to suggest that in rats the severity of some of the cardiotoxic effects of chlordimeform mentioned earlier (e.g., decreased heart rate) may be causally related to the concomitant decrease in body temperature (Watkinson and Gordon, 1987).

Chlordimeform also has antipyretic and anti-inflammatory actions. When injected intraperitoneally into rats at dosages from 5 to 80 mg/kg, chlordimeform reduced yeast-induced fever with a potency intermediate between those of indomethacin and aspirin (Pfister and Yim, 1977; Yim et al., 1978a). The compound also was shown to antagonize both early (5-hydroxytryptamine and histamine-mediated) and late (prostaglandin-mediated) phases of carrageenan-induced hind-paw edema, albumin-induced hind-paw edema, and edema induced upon direct injection of 5-hydroxytryptamine and histamine (Yim *et al.*, 1978a; Holsapple *et al.*, 1980). Chlordimeform injected intraperitoneally into rats (80, 40, 20 mg/kg) induced mild gastric ulcers, while oral treatment (140, 80, 40 mg/kg) did not elicit gastric ulceration. Aspirin, however, induced moderate gastric ulcers when injected (240, 140, 80 mg/kg) and severe ulcers when administered orally (240, 140, 80 mg/kg). Neither chlordimeform nor aspirin induced intestinal ulceration when administered orally to rats (Holsapple and Yim, 1979, 1981). Some of these actions doubtless are related to the ability of chlordimeform to inhibit prostaglandin biosynthesis (Yin *et al.*, 1978a; Holsapple and Yim, 1979). Chlordimeform inhibited the synthesis of prostaglandin E_2 from arachidonic acid by bovine seminal vesicle microsomes (Holsapple *et al.*, 1977; Yim *et al.*, 1978a).

Chlordimeform at 40 mg/kg facilitated electrical kindling of the amygdala and hippocampus of rats; no effect on after-discharge thresholds was found. It was suggested that this chlordimeform-mediated enhanced susceptibility to kindling might have resulted from a depletion of brain levels of norepinephrine by the formamidine (Gilbert, 1987).

The effects of chlordimeform on mammalian visual function have been examined. Intraperitoneal treatment of male rats with acute dosages (40, 15, 5 mg/kg) of chlordimeform 30 min prior to testing revealed a temporary increase in both the amplitude and latency of pattern reversal-evoked potentials and an increase only in the latency of flash-evoked potentials (Dyer and Boyes, 1983; Boyes and Dyer, 1984a,b,c). In a subsequent study, it was found that the action of chlordimeform on visual evoked potentials was dependent on the amount of contrast in the stimulus pattern, and it was suggested that the formamidine altered the encoding of visual contrast (Boyes *et al.*, 1985a). Boyes *et al.* (1985b) observed that peak latencies of flash-evoked potentials were prolonged by chlordimeform at 22°C but not at 30°C. Moreover, the rate of axonal transport was slowed in chlordimeform-treated hypothermic rats but not in chlordimeform-treated warmed rats. In contrast, chlordimeform increased pattern reversal-evoked potential peak latencies and peak-to-peak amplitudes independent of body temperature. Thus, the flash-evoked potential and axonal transport changes produced by chlordimeform were an indirect consequence of the hypothermia (Boyes *et al.*, 1985b). In a related study, it was found that inhibition of monoamine oxidase by chlordimeform was not directly responsible for the visual evoked changes, since rats injected with pargyline (0.4 or 20 mg/kg) responded similarly to untreated controls (Boyes *et al.*, 1985c). It was mentioned that the chlordimeform effects on the pattern reversal-evoked potentials might be mediated by α_2-adrenergic receptors, known to be present along the primary visual pathway (Boyes *et al.*, 1985c). In a subsequent study of pattern reversal visual evoked potentials, it was found that injection of rats with clonidine (0.05–0.5 mg/kg), an α_2-agonist, enhanced the P1N3 component and suppressed the N2P2 component in a manner similar to

that of chlordimeform. In contrast, the N2P2 component was enhanced by injection of rats with yohimbine (0.5–2.0 mg/kg), an α_2-antagonist. Pretreatment of rats with yohimbine (2 mg/kg) diminished the effects of both clonidine and chlordimeform, providing support for the hypothesis of an α_2-adrenergic receptor action for chlordimeform on rat visual function (Boyes and Moser, 1985). Subsequent research has revealed that intraperitoneal treatment of rats with chlordimeform at 40 mg/kg augmented the visual evoked potential component at peak N2, which is thought to be due to a response of a sustained visual subsystem (pattern detection), but not that at P1, which is thought to be due to a response of a transient visual subsystem (motion detection) (Boyes and Hudnell, 1987).

The auditory system also is affected by chlordimeform. Janssen *et al.* (1983), using the brain stem auditory evoked response, which allows separation of central from peripheral effects, injected rats with chlordimeform (40 mg/kg) or pargyline (0.4 or 20 mg/kg). Two hours after treatment evoked responses were measured. Peak I latency was not affected by chlordimeform, but the interpeak latency between peaks I and IV was lengthened, indicating that alterations were central in origin. Although pargyline also produced auditory dysfunction, the pattern was different from that induced by chlordimeform, and it was concluded that monoamine oxidase inhibition could not account fully for the action of this formamidine.

The nature of the interaction of chlordimeform with vascular muscle tissue has been investigated. Robinson *et al.* (1976) and Zelenski *et al.* (1978) examined the effects of chlordimeform on agonist-induced contractions of rabbit aortic strips and on calcium flux in deadventitiated strips. Chlordimeform relaxed contractions induced by potassium, histamine, 5-hydroxytryptamine, and norepinephrine and decreased the rate of contraction of strips exposed to each of the four agonists. Chlordimeform increased the rate of washout of ^{45}Ca from the media-intimal layer of aorta in most cases, but it did not affect ^{45}Ca uptake by media-intimal strips. In a subsequent study of the effects of chlordimeform on rabbit aortic strips, Robinson (1982) concluded that chlordimeform relaxes vascular smooth muscle by interference with calcium utilization and not by antagonism at the usual vascular relaxant receptors. Using a preparation from rabbit central ear artery, Robinson and Bittle (1979) reported that demethylchlordimeform antagonized contractions induced by vasoactive agents and contracted vascular tissue as a partial α-adrenergic receptor agonist. However, demethylchlordimeform did not alter ^{45}Ca uptake into deadventitiated rabbit aorta strips or norepinephrine-stimulated efflux from ^{45}Ca-loaded, superfused aorta strips (Robinson and Pento, 1980).

In light of the effects of chlordimeform on rabbit aorta *in vitro*, Pento *et al.* (1979) examined the effects of single and repeated administration of the formamidine on calcium and glucose homeostasis in the rat. A single intraperitoneal injection of chlordimeform at 100 mg/kg produced a rapid 15% decrease in plasma calcium and a 64% increase in plasma glucose. Intraperitoneal treatment at 75 mg/kg twice daily for 7 days resulted in an 8% reduction in plasma calcium, a 50% decrease in duodenal calcium transport, and a 20% decrease in body weight.

Emran *et al.* (1980) found that chlordimeform and its metabolites at $3 \times 10^{-4} M$ inhibited the acetylcholine-mediated catecholamine release from isolated bovine adrenals; potency decreased in the order didemethylchlordimeform > demethylchlordimeform > chlordimeform > N-formyl-4-chloro-o-toluidine. Demethylchlordimeform also strongly inhibited calcium-evoked secretion from adrenals, suggesting that blockade of calcium influx might be important.

Demethylchlordimeform is a potent agonist of octopamine-sensitive adenylate cyclase in insects. Moreover, perturbation of octopaminergic transmission by this metabolite probably is responsible for many of the sublethal effects of chlordimeform in insects (Hollingworth and Lund, 1982). Chlordimeform itself is only weakly active in this connection. Demethylchlordimeform stimulated rat caudate nucleus dopamine-sensitive adenylate cyclase, rat heart ventricle β_1-adrenergic-sensitive adenylate cyclase, and rat liver β_2-adrenergic-sensitive adenylate cyclase, but high concentrations were required, and in no case was the formamidine more active than the endogenous agonist. Chlordimeform was a weak inhibitor of basal and isoproterenol-stimulated adenylate cyclase activities in rat liver and of basal and dopamine-stimulated adenylate cyclase activities in rat caudate nucleus (Nathanson and Hunnicutt, 1981). Demethylchlordimeform did not inhibit the binding of norepinephrine to rat cardiac microsomes, a preparation that contained putative β-adrenergic receptors (Knowles and Aziz, 1974).

At a concentration of $1 \times 10^{-4} M$, chlordimeform suppressed the amplitude of miniature end-plate potentials with significant change in their frequency on frog sciatic nerve–sartorius muscle preparations. At $1 \times 10^{-4} M$ it completely blocked these potentials without affecting the resting membrane potential. The end-plate potential evoked by nerve stimulation also was blocked, even though the action potential from the nerve terminal was not impaired. Sensitivity of the end plate to acetylcholine was decreased, even though release of this neurohormone was not affected. This change in sensitivity of the end plate is consistent with the observed paralysis of animals poisoned by chlordimeform (Wang et al., 1975; Watanabe et al., 1975). Demethylchlordimeform, N-formyl-4-chloro-o-toluidine, and 4-chloro-o-toluidine also induced contractions at 1×10^{-4} to $1 \times 10^{-3} M$. Demethylchlordimeform strongly inhibited the acetylcholine-induced contraction, but N-formyl-4-chloro-o-toluidine and 4-chloro-o-toluidine were inactive at $1 \times 10^{-3} M$ (Watanabe et al., 1976).

Chlordimeform is an uncoupler of oxidative phosphorylation, about as active as the classical inhibitor 2,4-dinitrophenol. The addition of chlordimeform to rat liver mitochondria at the concentration of 0.01 μmol/mg protein caused a 34.3% decrease in oxidative phosphorylation, a 71.0% decrease in respiratory control, and a 73.5% increase in state-4 respiration. It also stimulated ATPase activity (Abo-Khatwa and Hollingworth, 1973).

Effects on Organs and Tissues Chlordimeform and several of its metabolites have been tested for mutagenic activity in a number of bacteria. Chlordimeform was negative in the recassay with two strains of *Bacillus subtillis* (H17 rec$^+$ and M45

rec$^-$) without S9 activation (Shirasu et al., 1976; Waters et al., 1982). It also was without mutagenic activity when incubated with histidine-dependent strains of *S. typhimurium* (TA98, TA100, TA1535, TA1537, TA1538) (Shirasu et al., 1976; FAO/WHO, 1979a; Waters et al., 1982; Rashid et al., 1984; Kimmel et al., 1986), tryptophan-dependent strains of *Escherichia coli* (WP$_2$, WP$_2$uvrA, WP67, CM611, CM571) (Waters et al., 1982; Rashid et al., 1984), and a streptomycin-dependent strain of *E. coli* (FAO/WHO, 1979a), in the presence and absence of S9 activation. Chlordimeform was negative in studies with *S. cerevisiae* (D3) (Waters et al., 1982). Demethylchlordimeform, however, was slightly mutagenic when assayed with *S. typhimurium* TA1535 but not with the other four strains (FAO/WHO, 1979a). N-Formyl-4-chloro-o-toluidine was not mutagenic when assayed with the five strains of *S. typhimurium* or *E. coli* WP$_2$ (FAO/WHO, 1979a; Rashid et al., 1984). However, 4-chloro-o-toluidine was weakly mutagenic in *S. typhimurium* strain TA1535 without S9 activation (FAO/WHO, 1979a; Rashid et al., 1984) and was strongly mutagenic in strain TA100 with S9 activation (Zimmer et al., 1980; Kimmel et al., 1986). The chlordimeform metabolite 4-chloro-2-methylnitrosobenzene also was mutagenic with TA100 in presence of S9 activation (Kimmel et al., 1986).

N-Formyl-4-chloro-o-toluidine and 4-chloro-o-toluidine, but not chlordimeform, were active in inducing damage in some tests using *S. typhimurium* and *E. coli* multirepair-deficient systems (Rashid et al., 1984).

Chlordimeform, N-formyl-4-chloro-o-toluidine, and 4-chloro-o-toluidine were examined for mutagenic activity in the mouse dominant lethal test. Male mice were treated orally with a single dose of chlordimeform (66 and 22 mg/kg), N-formyl-4-chloro-o-toluidine (315 and 105 mg/kg), and 4-chloro-o-toluidine (330 and 110 mg/kg). The mice were mated with untreated females weekly for 6 consecutive weeks. No evidence for any dominant lethal effects was observed in the progeny of male mice treated with these three compounds (FAO/WHO, 1979a, 1980).

Lang and Adler (1982) examined the mutagenic potential of chlordimeform and two metabolites in the mouse heritable translocation assay. Male mice were given single daily oral doses of chlordimeform (120 mg/kg), N-formyl-4-chloro-o-toluidine (100 mg/kg), or 4-chloro-o-toluidine (200 mg/kg) for 49 days. F$_1$ male offspring were tested for their reproductive performance by a sequential decision procedure on litter sizes to select males with translocation heterozygosity. Partially sterile, sterile, and nonclassifiable F$_1$ males were examined cytogenetically by scoring meiotic chromosomes for translocation multivalents or analyzing mitotic divisions for marker chromosomes. No induction of translocation heterozygosity by chlordimeform or the two metabolites was found (Lang and Adler, 1982).

Lang (1984) examined the mutagenic potential of chlordimeform, N-formyl-4-chloro-o-toluidine, and 4-chloro-o-toluidine using a mammalian spot test. Pregnant mice were treated orally with chlordimeform (160 mg/kg), N-formyl-4-chloro-o-toluidine (100 mg/kg), and 4-chloro-o-toluidine (100 mg/kg) on days 8, 9, and 10 of gestation. Mutation induction was monitored postnatally by checking the fur of the offspring for color spots that resulted from expression of a recessive gene involved in the coat-color determination. 4-Chloro-o-toluidine, but not chlordimeform and its N-formyl metabolite, was mutagenic (Lang, 1984).

In an *in vivo* mutagenesis assay evaluating chromatid-type and chromosome-type aberrations in bone marrow cells, groups of male and female Chinese hamsters were given two consecutive daily oral doses of chlordimeform (240, 120, and 60 mg/kg), N-formyl-4-chloro-o-toluidine (1200, 600, and 300 mg/kg), and 4-chloro-o-toluidine (400, 200, and 100 mg/kg). There was no evidence for mutagenic activity of chlordimeform or of the two metabolites in these tests (FAO/WHO, 1980).

Chlordimeform, N-formyl-4-chloro-o-toluidine, and 4-chloro-o-toluidine were not carcinogenic in rats in long-term feeding trials (FAO/WHO, 1981a). However, they were carcinogenic in similar studies with mice (FAO/WHO, 1979a,b, 1980, 1981a,b; Feng *et al.*, 1985; Weisburger *et al.*, 1978; NCI, 1979a). The major neoplasm was of vascular origin and was histologically characterized as hemangioendothelioma (FAO/WHO, 1979a, 1981a) or hemangiosarcoma (Weisburger *et al.*, 1978; NCI, 1979a).

The effect of chlordimeform at either 148 mg/kg (LD 50) or 14.8 mg/kg (0.1 LD 50) on the subsequent immune response of mice to sheep erythrocytes was investigated. Chlordimeform given in a single oral dose of 148 mg/kg administered 2 days after immunization or on the day of immunization resulted in significant suppression of humoral immune response. However, when mice were treated orally with either 8 or 28 consecutive daily doses of the compound, no significant change in numbers of plaque-forming cells was found (Wiltrout *et al.*, 1978; Ceglowski *et al.*, 1979).

In another study, mice were treated intraperitoneally with chlordimeform daily for 14 days at 30 and 10 mg/kg. The numbers of IgM antibody-forming cells per spleen were decreased by 72 and 22% in the high- and low-dose groups, respectively. The suppression of antibody-forming cells occurred in the absence of any effects on body and spleen weights, spleen cell number, or leukocyte differential. Two models of a delayed hypersensitivity response were not affected at either dosage. It was suggested that these effects were not attributable to general systemic toxicity but resulted from a relatively specific suppression of B-lymphocyte activity (Holsapple *et al.*, 1983).

Effects on Reproduction In a three-generation study, rats received dietary levels of 500, 250, and 100 ppm. Food consumption and body weight prior to mating tended to be low, especially at 500 ppm. At 500 ppm, the lactation index was reduced in F_{1a}, and F_{1b}, and F_{3a} litters, and the weight of pups in all litters was low. Fertility index, gestation index, live birth index, sex ratio, mean litter size, and birth weight were normal. Dietary levels of 250 and 100 ppm were no-effect levels. No dietary level produced any teratologic change (FAO/WHO, 1972).

Groups of female rats were given chlordimeform orally at dosages of 50, 25, and 10 mg/kg/day from day 6 to day 15 of pregnancy. Examination of fetuses taken on day 21 revealed a slight delay in growth at the two highest levels. However, this effect was likely due to maternal toxicity, since reduced body weight gain, reduced food intake, and somnolence were observed on days 6–18 of pregnancy. No teratogenic events were observed in progeny, but an increased incidence of sternal ossification defects occurred at 25 mg/kg (FAO/WHO, 1979a).

Rabbits intubated with chlordimeform on days 8–16 of gestation at rates of 30 and 7.5 mg/kg/day were killed on day 28 or permitted to bear their young. Parental mortality, abortion rate, ratio of implantations to corpora lutea, litter size, incidence of resorption, fetal weight, fetal length, and incidence of skeletal and soft tissue anomalies were not affected. In rabbits that gave birth, the length of gestation and the size and weight of litters were normal (FAO/WHO, 19720.

In another study, groups of female rabbits were administered chlordimeform orally from day 6 to day 18 of pregnancy at levels of 100, 30, and 10 mg/kg. The high dosage produced some adverse effects in the first 4 days of treatment. In fetuses removed on day 28 of pregnancy, there was a slight increase over controls in the number of incompletely ossified sternebrae in the high-dose group. However, there was no evidence of teratogenic effects in fetuses from the low-dose group (FAO/WHO, 1979a).

Behavioral Effects Laboratory animals treated with chlordimeform manifest a number of behavioral aberrations.

Chlordimeform at low dosages has been shown to be an appetite stimulant in rats (Pfister *et al.*, 1978a; Yim *et al.*, 1978b; Witkin and Leander, 1982). Pfister *et al.* (1978a) treated rats with chlordimeform intraperitoneally at 6 mg/kg for 5 days, followed by 60 mg/kg daily for an additional 4 days. Marked hyperphagia began shortly after the first treatment and continued until the initial injection at 60 mg/kg, after which time anorexia was induced. Hyperphagia and anorexia were accompanied by increases and decreases in body weight, respectively. Hyperphagia was especially pronounced when non-food-deprived rats were injected intraperitoneally with chlordimeform at 10 mg/kg; food intakes were 5 times control levels after 3 hr and 1.1 times control levels after 24 hr. Demethylchlordimeform also was an appetite stimulant in rats, but it was not as potent as chlordimeform (Pfister *et al.*, 1978a). Witkin and Leander (1982) administered chlordimeform or chlordiazepoxide intraperitoneally to non-food-deprived rats at dosages ranging from 1.25 to 40 mg/kg 30 min before a 1-hr period of access to food and water. Both compounds (2.5–10 mg/kg) increased food intake, and chlordiazepoxide, but not chlordimeform, also increased water consumption of 23-hr water-deprived rats. Chlordimeform produced dose-related decreases in water consumption.

Chlordimeform also induces flavor aversions in rats (MacPhail and Leander, 1980) and mice (Landauer *et al.*, 1984). Rats were adapted to a daily 30-min period of water availability. After stabilization of intake, they were allowed access to water and to a saccharin solution (0.1%) for 15 min, and then they were treated intraperitoneally with chlordimeform (10, 5,

2.5 mg/kg). Three days later rats were given access to both water and saccharin. Rats treated with chlordimeform showed an aversion to saccharin that was proportional to dosage (MacPhail and Leander, 1980). Mice treated with chlordimeform and tested under a slightly different protocol also displayed a dose-related aversion to saccharin (Landauer et al., 1984).

Chlordimeform produced dosage-related decreases in overall rates of responding of rats and mice under fixed-ratio and fixed-interval scales of reinforcement (MacPhail and Leander, 1981; Peele et al., 1984; MacPhail, 1985; Glowa, 1986; Moser and MacPhail, 1986). Aberrant behavior also was observed in pigeons and bobwhite chicks treated with chlordimeform (Leander and MacPhail, 1980; Fleming et al., 1985).

Rats were fed chlordimeform in such a way that they received 0.1 mg/kg/day, beginning on the fifth day of gestation, and the pups received the same diet after they were weaned. Under these circumstances, treated pups showed significantly slower overall development of the ability to swim. No significant differences appeared in maze or motivation tests (Olson et al., 1978).

In addition, chlordimeform has been shown to increase tail-flick latencies and raise thresholds for vocalization induced by electrical stimulation of the tail in rats (Pfister and Yim, 1977) and to decrease time spent investigating a female conspecific and to decrease rearing proportionately greater than ambulation in mice (Landauer et al., 1984).

Moser et al. (1987), using a functional observational battery including home-cage and open-field observations, neuromuscular and sensorimotor tests, and physiological measures, found that the profiles of the effects elicited by intraperitoneal treatment of rats with chlordimeform (56, 25, 1 mg/kg) and carbaryl (30, 10, 3 mg/kg) were clearly different.

Factors Influencing Toxicity Ghali and Hollingworth (1985) studied the effects of various inhibitors and inducers of metabolism on chlordimeform toxicity to mice. Potential modifiers of toxicity included SKF 525A and pipcronyl butoxide administered intraperitoneally at 50 and 400 mg/kg, respectively, 2 hr prior to subsequent treatment; phenobarbital administered intraperitoneally at 50 mg/kg daily for 4 days prior to subsequent treatment; Aroclor 1254 administered intraperitoneally at 500 mg/kg in one dose 5 days prior to subsequent treatment; and 3-methylcholanthrene administered intraperitoneally at 40 mg/kg in two successive daily doses with the second dose 2 days prior to subsequent treatment. SKF 525A, piperonyl butoxide, and phenobarbital had no significant effect on the toxicity of chlordimeform to mice, whereas 3-methylcholanthrene and Aroclor 1254 slightly decreased toxicity. In the case of the toxicity to mice of demethylchlordimeform and didemethylchlordimeform, 3-methylcholanthrene and Aroclor 1254 had a protective action, but piperonyl butoxide was without effect. Pretreatment of mice with these inhibitors and inducers appreciably affected chlordimeform metabolism in vitro and in vivo even though they were without significant effect on toxicity. For example, treatment of mice as described above with SKF 525A or piperonyl butoxide decreased the degradation of chlordimeform in vitro

by liver preparations, whereas phenobarbital, Aroclor 1254, and 3-methylcholanthrene caused rapid degradation of chlordimeform. Chlordimeform was administered orally to mice at 40 mg/kg following pretreatment with piperonyl butoxide, phenobarbital, or 3-methylcholanthrene as described above. Mice were killed 40 min following chlordimeform treatment, and blood, liver, and brain were analyzed. Pretreatment of mice with phenobarbital or 3-methylcholanthrene had no significant effect on total levels of radioactivity in tissues; however, piperonyl butoxide reduced the radiocarbon content of the tissues by about 50%. Treatment with each of the three compounds resulted in changes in the ratios of chlordimeform and its metabolites in tissues that were quite pronounced in some cases (Ghali and Hollingworth, 1985).

Durations of zoxazolamine-induced paralysis and of pentobarbital-induced hypnosis were increased significantly after intraperitoneal treatment of rats with a single dose of chlordimeform (100 mg/kg); however, following repeated administration (75 mg/kg) for 4 days, a decrease was observed in zoxazolamine-induced paralysis time, but pentobarbital-induced hypnosis was not altered (Raupp et al., 1980; Budris et al., 1983). Intraperitoneal treatment of mice with a single dose of chlordimeform (50 mg/kg), demethylchlordimeform (50 mg/kg), or N-formyl-4-chloro-o-toluidine significantly extended ethyl alcohol-induced sleep time in mice (Benezet et al., 1978; Knowles and Benezet, 1979).

Sixty minutes following intraperitoneal treatment of rats with chlordimeform at 100 mg/kg, ethylmorphine N-demethylase activity, cytochrome P-450 content, NADPH–cytochrome-c reductase activity, and the spectral binding of hexobarbital and aniline were decreased, whereas aniline hydroxylase and p-nitroanisole-O-demethylase activities were unchanged. Following four daily intraperitoneal injections of chlordimeform (75 mg/kg), male rats showed decreased ethylmorphine N-demethylase and aniline hydroxylase activities and spectral binding of hexobarbital, but no differences were observed in p-nitroanisole-O-demethylase activity, cytochrome P-450 levels, and spectral binding of aniline. In female rats similarly treated, aniline hydroxylase activity was decreased, but no changes in ethylmorphine N-demethylase or p-nitroanisole-O-demethylase activities were observed (Raupp et al., 1980; Budris et al., 1983). However, when Bentley et al. (1985) treated rats and mice orally at 150, 100, or 50 mg/kg daily for 7 days, induction of various hepatic drug-metabolizing enzymes was apparent. Microsomal cytochrome P-450 content was elevated in both male and female rats and mice. Ethoxycoumarin O-deethylase activity was induced in male and female rats but not in mice, whereas ethylmorphine N-demethylase activity was elevated in mice but not in rats. Benzo[a]pyrene hydroxylase activity was increased in female rats and mice but not in males. UDP-glucuronyl transferase, glutathione S-transferase, and microsomal epoxide hydrolase were induced in a dose-dependent manner in male rats and female rats and mice, but not in male mice.

Crowder and Whitson (1980) treated mice orally with radioactive chlordimeform alone (3.25 mg/kg), in binary mixtures with toxaphene (25 mg/kg) or methyl parathion (12.5 mg/kg), or in a tertiary mixture with toxaphene and methyl parathion and measured the rates of elimination of radiocarbon in urine and feces for 8 days posttreatment, as well as levels of radiocarbon in selected tissues at 8 days. Toxaphene and/or methyl parathion had no significant effect on the elimination of chlordimeform equivalents. At least 83% of the initial dose was accounted for in the urine and feces by 8 days in all cases. However, combinations of toxaphene and/or methyl parathion with chlordimeform resulted in lower radiocarbon levels in some tissues compared to tissue levels in mice receiving chlordimeform alone. The combination of methyl parathion and chlordimeform yielded lower radiocarbon levels in the liver, whereas combinations of methyl parathion, toxaphene, or both gave lower radiocarbon levels in lipid, muscle, and testes.

Kaloyanova *et al.* (1979, 1981) treated rats with chlordimeform alone and in combination with nialamide or analgin (methylamine sulfomethane), using several different regimes. Chlordimeform in combination with nialamide or analgin yielded greater inhibition of monoamine oxidase in brain and liver as assayed with several different substrates than did treatment with chlordimeform or either drug alone.

Pathology In 60-day feeding studies of chlordimeform in rats, hemosiderosis of spleen, focal hyperplasia of small biliary ducts and of the transitional epithelium of liver, increased vascularization in the mucous membranes of the bladder, atrophy of thymus, and reduced spermatogenesis were observed at one or both of the highest concentrations (3000 and 6000 ppm); no chlordimeform-related histopathological changes were found at levels of 1500 ppm or lower (FAO/WHO, 1981a). The short-term study in mice also revealed hemosiderosis of spleen and atrophy of thymus at high chlordimeform concentrations, but no other pathology was observed (FAO/WHO, 1981a). The long-term study in rats indicated no significant pathological changes that were attributed to chlordimeform (FAO/WHO, 1981a). However, mice fed chlordimeform at levels of 100 ppm and above had an increased incidence of hemorrhagic tissue masses in subcutaneous tissues, retroperitoneum, and in some internal organs including kidney, liver, and spleen. These masses, which were classified as malignant hemangioendotheliomas, were reported to occur rarely in controls and were found mainly in the 500 and 100 ppm groups. In some animals, the tumors were of multiple origin, and metastases to lungs were observed. No other chlordimeform-related neoplasms were found (FAO/WHO, 1979a).

In short-term feeding studies of *N*-formyl-4-chloro-*o*-toluidine in rats, atrophy of spleen and thymus was noted during the initial 3 weeks at 6000 ppm. Liver changes consisting of hyperplasia of the bile duct epithelium and changes in the distribution of lipid were found at all treatment levels (6000, 3000, 1500, 750 ppm); in addition, hyperplasia of bladder epithelium and testes and increased mitotic incidence in hepatocytes were observed at the highest dietary level (FAO/WHO, 1981a). In mice, pathological changes included congestion of organs, especially liver, thymic atrophy, and increased hemosiderosis of spleen (FAO/WHO, 1981a). The long-term study of *N*-formyl-4-chloro-*o*-toluidine in rats revealed no significant pathology (FAO/WHO, 1981a). In mice, however, an increase in number of malignant hemangioendotheliomas was found in some internal organs at all treatment levels (500, 100, 20 ppm). Moreover, the time-to-tumor relationship was decreased as dietary level of compound was increased (FAO/WHO, 1979a).

The short-term study with 4-chloro-*o*-toluidine in rats revealed enlarged and congested spleen with hemorrhage, hypertrophy of hepatocytes, and moderate proliferation of transitional cell epithelium in bladder, all occurring at the highest dietary levels (6000 and/or 3000 ppm) (FAO/WHO, 1979a). In mice, slight to moderate vascular changes of hepatocytes which were pronounced at 3000 ppm or greater were observed. Urinary bladder changes included hyperemia, dilation of capillaries in mucosal layer, edema, and multiple intraepithelial hemorrhage and focal proliferation of transitional cell epithelium; those changes sometimes occurred at the lowest dietary levels (FAO/WHO, 1979a). Long-term studies of 4-chloro-*o*-toluidine in rats revealed a slight but significant increase in incidence of multilocular cholangiogenic cysts in liver at the highest dietary level (500 ppm); incidence of cysts at lower levels was similar to that in controls. No evidence of carcinogenesis was found in rats (FAO/WHO, 1981a). In mice fed levels of 20 ppm or higher, an increased incidence of malignant hemangioendotheliomas was found in subcutaneous tissue, in the retroperitoneum, and in some internal organs. Metastases were observed in some cases. There was a significant dose-dependent increase in the total incidence of tumors, and tumors occurred in animals at the higher concentrations at an earlier date than those at lower concentrations. A benign variant of the neoplasm was found in all groups (FAO/WHO, 1979a).

In the long-term feeding study of 4-chloro-*o*-toluidine conducted by Weisburger *et al.* (1978), there was no significant increase in the incidence of tumors in rats, but mice had hemangiosarcomas or hemangiomas mainly in the spleen and the subcutaneous and retroperitoneal adipose tissue.

In the National Cancer Institute Study (NCI, 1979a), rats fed 4-chloro-*o*-toluidine had an increased incidence of chromophobe adenomas of the pituitary; however, this finding may be of questionable significance, in view of the reduced survival among controls and the unusually low incidence of chromophobe adenomas among matched controls compared with that in historical controls [International Agency for Research on Cancer (IARC), 1983a]. In the study with 4-chloro-*o*-toluidine-fed mice, hemangiosarcomas occurred in both males and females, mainly in the fatty tissue adjacent to the genital organs (NCI, 1979a).

Long-term feeding of chlordimeform to dogs produced congestion of liver, kidneys, and lungs as well as edema and hemorrhage of the lungs. Bile duct hyperplasia, pericholangitis, and nodular hyperplasia and hypertrophy of hepatocytes in both sexes were observed at 1000 ppm. The kidneys showed increased pigmentation. These changes were less or absent at a dietary level of 500 ppm (FAO/WHO, 1972).

In other studies, cats were injected subcutaneously with five daily doses of chlordimeform or 4-chloro-*o*-toluidine at 50 mg/kg. Cats were killed 4 days after the last dose except for two cats treated with chlordimeform that died 5 days after dosing was begun. The livers of cats treated with chlordimeform had a yellowish-green tinge. The bladder mucosa was edematous and congested in cats treated with both compounds; the bladder of one cat treated with chlordimeform was filled with bloody urine. Microscopic examination of liver showed bile pigment in hepatocytes, Kupffer cells, and macrophages of chlordimeform-treated cats, and hepatocytes of cats given chlordimeform and one cat given 4-chloro-*o*-toluidine were vacuolated. The bladder mucosa was congested, and the transitional epithelium was degenerated or lost completely. However, it is noteworthy that none of the cats treated with chlordimeform or 4-chloro-*o*-toluidine displayed the severe acute hemorrhagic cystitis observed in humans that is discussed in the following section (Folland *et al.,* 1978; Kimbrough, 1980).

22.2.3.3 Toxicity to Humans

Biochemical Effects   When chlordimeform was incubated with cultured human embryonic lung cells, it was taken up (Murakami and Fukami, 1976) and degraded to *N*-formyl-4-chloro-*o*-toluidine (81.9%) and 4-chloro-*o*-toluidine (2.3%); minor metabolites included chlordimeform and two unknowns (Lin *et al.,* 1975).

Monolayer cultures of HeLa cells were exposed to chlordimeform, and its effects on nucleic acid and protein synthesis were examined. No influence on macromolecule synthesis was found at $1 \times 10^{-5} M$. At a chlordimeform concentration of $1 \times 10^{-4} M$, the synthesis of RNA was slightly inhibited; however, synthesis of DNA and protein was unaffected. At $1 \times 10^{-3} M$, RNA synthesis was reduced to 30% of the control, and DNA and protein synthesis were reduced to 50–60% of the control. Chlordimeform, demethylchlordimeform, *N*-formyl-4-chloro-*o*-toluidine, and 4-chloro-*o*-toluidine at a concentration of $1 \times 10^{-3} M$ were incubated with HeLa cells for 5 days, after which time total protein content of the cultures was measured. Values for 50% inhibition of cell growth were $7.6 \times 10^{-5} M$ for chlordimeform, $6.7 \times 10^{-5} M$ for demethylchlordimeform, $6.4 \times 10^{-5} M$ for *N*-formyl-4-chloro-*o*-toluidine, and $10.1 \times 10^{-5} M$ for 4-chloro-*o*-toluidine (Murakami *et al.,* 1972; Murakami and Fukami, 1974).

Effects on Organs and Tissues   Chlordimeform was not mutagenic when tested in a human lung fibroblast unscheduled DNA synthesis assay with or without S9 activation (Waters *et al.,* 1982).

Accidental and Intentional Poisoning   A woman intentionally ingested 30 ml of a 50% formulation of chlordimeform (about 214 mg/kg). No respiration or heartbeat was detectable when she was admitted to the hospital. This patient died within 24 hr, even though heart action was restored and a machine was used to maintain respiration. Apparently, no autopsy was done (FAO/WHO, 1972).

An unsuccessful suicide attempt involved a 76-year-old male who arrived at the hospital in acute distress within 50 min after ingesting 100 gm of chlordimeform. He had vomited several times while en route to the emergency room. He was lethargic, and generalized muscular weakness was present. His peripheral pulse was moderately weak, and an unusual brownish-purple cyanosis was associated with the lips, nails, and skin. The methemoglobin concentration in the blood was 17% of the total hemoglobin at 5 hr after admission but was in the normal range in the next 2 days. In addition to the methemoglobinemia, moderate neutrophilic leukocytosis and minimum microhematuria with moderate proteinuria also were found. He had regained complete consciousness by about 50 hr after admission, but complained of headache and blurred vision. His urine became normal on the fifth day. The only intervention reported was gastric lavage, which was performed shortly after his arrival at the hospital (Arima *et al.,* 1976).

Tao *et al.* (1985) cited a report of the ingestion of chlordimeform (100–200 ml) by two individuals; unconsciousness resulted, and no monoamine oxidase activity was detectable in either case on the day of ingestion.

Use Experience   Chlordimeform concentrations were measured in an agrochemical factory in China. The levels of airborne chlordimeform varied, depending on the working area, but a mean value of <0.16 mg/m^3 was reported. Skin contamination was highest in workers in the packaging area, where the average contamination was 0.993 mg/cm^2 or 2.988 mg/day. Chlordimeform residues in the urine of workers in the packaging area were about 0.513 mg/liter. Major symptoms of chlordimeform-exposed workers included lack of appetite, fatigue, dizziness, swollen liver, and dermatitis. Some abnormalities were found in electrocardiograms and in liver function tests of some of the exposed workers, but monoamine oxidase activity was not significantly different from that of controls (Tao *et al.,* 1985).

In another instance, 9 of 22 men who had worked between 20 and 23 May 1975 in a separate shed where chlordimeform was packaged developed dysuria (9), urgency to void (7), increased frequency (7), nocturia (6), urethral discharge (6), gross hematuria (6), abdominal pains (7), back pain (4), feeling hot (6), sleepiness (9), sweet taste (4), and skin rash (5). The skin rash, which was on the face and arms, began as a fine papular eruption 2–3 days after exposure and then, within 2 or 3 days, desquamated and itched. There were no signs or symptoms of photosensitivity or anticholinesterase effects. Four other workers exposed at different times also had urinary symptoms. No cases were found among family contacts or others in the community (see apparent exception mentioned below under Atypical Cases).

Hematuria was documented in all 10 affected persons who saw physicians, and 7 of them had proteinuria. The three most seriously affected workers were hospitalized on June 6, 2 weeks after onset of symptoms, for complete urological examination. Intravenous urograms revealed small bladder capacity (75, 150, and 200 ml) in all three, and two had urethral reflux. All had hemorrhagic cystitis as determined by cystoscopy. One patient had mild elevations of SGOT and alkaline phosphatase, but all renal function tests were normal.

The urinary illness lasted 2–14 days in most patients, but 2 months in those who were hospitalized. When reexamined a little over 2 months after admission, the three patients were asymptomatic and their bladder capacities had returned to normal (Folland *et al.,* 1978; Kimbrough, 1980).

This outbreak of urinary disease was detected by a physician who, within a matter of days, saw four patients with hematuria, an unusual condition. Three of the patients not only worked in the same plant but also began work just 2 days before developing hematuria; the severity of their conditions eventually led to their hospitalization. The results of the subsequent investigation raised a question of why the illnesses had occurred, although chlordimeform had been packaged at the same plant in earlier years without recognized harm. During the previous year, the plant had packaged some 136,000 kg of a 95% chlordimeform formulation. The explanation was completely clear for the three men most severely affected and probably satisfactory for the other workers. The three workers had been assigned to the night shift without adequate instruction or supervision. They had operated the equipment improperly and produced more dust than usual and thus exposed themselves and others to excessive respiratory and dermal intake. The apparent lack of cases in earlier years almost certainly depended on the fact that the processing of chlordimeform had been transferred to a hotter, more poorly ventilated building, which was part of the same plant (Armstrong *et al.,* 1975; Folland *et al.,* 1978; Kimbrough, 1980).

Urine from some of the ill workers was analyzed for total amines, with the highest concentrations being found in samples from those who packaged chlordimeform. Analyses of urine samples collected from the three patients hospitalized 3 days after exposure revealed the following concentrations (ppm) of total amines, chlordimeform, 4-chloro-*o*-toluidine, and conjugates, respectively: for patient A, 11.0, 1.10, 3.75, and 6.25; for patient B, 15.2, 2.16, 4.16, and 8.67; and for patient C, 2.6, 0.04, 1.25, and 1.17 (Folland *et al.,* 1978).

A survey was made of 10 farmers who used chlordimeform. None had experienced gross hematuria, but one had experienced dysuria. Microscopic hematuria was found in only one of six farmers tested. Although levels of amines were higher in urine of farmers after they had used chlordimeform, they were lower than in all but one symptomatic employee from the packaging plant (Folland *et al.,* 1978).

An occupational exposure surveillance program associated with the aerial application of chlordimeform to cotton was conducted in 1979 and involved workers from nine countries, including Australia and some in Africa and the Americas. Over 28,000 urine samples were analyzed. Only 1.0% of the assays showed substantial chlordimeform urinary residues, and over 75% of the samples were at or below the level of detectability. No cases of hematuria were reported (FAO/WHO, 1981a).

A field exposure monitoring program also in association with the application of chlordimeform to cotton has been in use in California since 1982 (Coye *et al.,* 1986; Maddy *et al.,* 1986). At one point in the program 130 workers had been monitored, and 1000 urine samples were analyzed. No chlordimeform metabolites were detected in about two-thirds of all samples (limit of detection, 0.05 ppm). Of all samples, 97% had less than 0.5 ppm, and average levels ranged from 0.10 to 0.12 ppm; six mixer/loader/applicators had levels exceeding 1.0 ppm (Coye *et al.,* 1986). Thus, chlordimeform residues can be found in the urine of workers who handle or who are involved in application of the product, even when they are wearing special protective clothing and respirators (Maddy *et al.,* 1986). In these reports, there was no mention of any cystitis, although it was indicated that bladder cancer was detected in one pilot who had had at least seven seasons of exposure (Maddy *et al.,* 1986).

It is probable that the hemorrhagic cystitis that has been observed in some workers exposed to high levels of chlordimeform is caused mainly by the 4-chloro-*o*-toluidine metabolite (sometimes reported in early literature under a different nomenclature as "5-chloro-2-toluidine" or "5-chloro-*o*-toluidine"). 4-Chloro-*o*-toluidine-induced hemorrhagic cystitis has been reported previously in humans (Currie, 1933; Lehmann, 1933).

Atypical Cases of Various Origins   Hemorrhagic cystitis developed in a young woman who was a romantic contact of one of the affected new employees in the outbreak discussed above. She never entered the plant building, but she did ride home in the same car with the workers, whose body and clothes, particularly trouser cuffs, were contaminated with chlordimeform. The precise nature of the woman's physical exposure to her friend was not established; however, it seemed highly probable that her illness was a result of secondary exposure to the chlordimeform (Folland *et al.,* 1978).

Pathology   Bladder biopsy specimens of hospitalized workers revealed changes of acute hemorrhagic cystitis including local ulceration of epithelium with some areas of complete slough, moderate submucosal chronic inflammation, and conspicuous congestion and dilation of submucosal blood vessels. Calcium concrements also were occasionally present. No cytologically atypical epithelial cells were observed (Folland *et al.,* 1978; Kimbrough, 1980).

Treatment of Poisoning   Treatment of poisoning by chlordimeform is symptomatic; there is no specific antidote. Sympathomimetic drugs should be avoided.

22.2.4 AMITRAZ

22.2.4.1 Identity, Properties, and Uses

Chemical Name   Amitraz is *N'*-(2,4-dimethylphenyl)-*N*-[[(2,4-dimethylphenyl)imino]methyl]-*N*-methylmethanimidamide.

Structure   See Fig. 22.2.

Synonyms The common name amitraz is approved by ANSI, BSI, E-ISO, BPC, and JMAF; it also has been called amitraze (F-ISO), triazid, and azaform. Trade names have included BAAM®, Ectodex®, Mitac®, Triatox®, and Taktic®. Code designations have included U-36,059, BTS-27,419, JA-119, and ENT-27,967. The CAS registry number is 33089-61-1.

Physical and Chemical Properties Amitraz has the empirical formula $C_{19}H_{23}N_3$ and a molecular weight of 293.4. The pure material forms colorless needles with a melting point of 86–87°C. The vapor pressure at 20°C is 3.8×10^{-7} mm Hg. The compound is soluble in most organic solvents and sparingly soluble in water. Amitraz is unstable under acidic conditions.

History, Formulations, and Uses Amitraz was introduced by The Boots Company Limited (now Schering A.G.) to control eggs and motile forms of mites and ticks on crops and domestic animals. It also is active against eggs and early instars of some Lepidoptera and against several other insects including scale insects, mealy bugs, and aphids. It is formulated as an emulsifiable concentrate (200 gm/liter) and a wettable powder (500 gm/kg) for crop use, as an emulsifiable concentrate (125 gm/liter) for farm animal use, and as an emulsifiable concentrate (50 gm/liter) and dispersal powder (250 or 500 gm/kg) dog shampoo.

22.2.4.2 Toxicity to Laboratory Animals

Basic Findings Amitraz possesses moderate acute toxicity to laboratory animals (see Table 22.2). Turnbull treated rats orally with a commercial formulation containing amitraz (20%) and xylene (75%) and with amitraz and xylene alone. When the formulation was administered undiluted to males at a dosage of 2050 mg/kg (440 mg/kg amitraz) and to females at 1700 mg/kg (365 mg/kg amitraz) (approximately LD 80 rate for both sexes), toxic signs included coolness to touch, reduced spontaneous activity, episodes of increased induced activity such as aggres-

Table 22.2
Single-Dose LD 50 Values for Amitraz

Species	Route	LD 50 (mg/kg)[a]
Rat, M	oral	800
Rat	oral	600[b]
Rat, M	dermal	>1600
Rat, M	intraperitoneal	~800
Mouse, M	oral	>1600
Mouse	intraperitoneal	>100[c]
Guinea pig, F	oral	400–800
Rabbit, F	oral	>100
Rabbit	dermal	>200
Dog	oral	~100
Baboon	oral	100–250

[a]From FAO/WHO (1981a) unless indicated otherwise.
[b]Hollingworth (1976).
[c]Benezet et al. (1978).

sion in response to handling, and signs of general debilitation including exophthalmos, facial staining, hunched posture, and piloerection. Amitraz alone at 600 mg/kg caused hypothermia, reduced spontaneous activity, episodes of increased induced activity, and similar signs of general debilitation. In addition, amitraz produced a slowly reversed emaciation in survivors that was not seen in rats treated with the formulation. Xylene alone at 3225 mg/kg caused reduced spontaneous activity, facial soiling, and, unlike amitraz, reduced muscle tone and ataxia (Turnbull, 1983). Other adverse reactions to amitraz in animals have included mydriasis, bradycardia, hypotension, sedation, bloat, polyuria, vomiting, and hyperglycemia (Dobozy, 1982; Hsu and Kakuk, 1984; Hsu and McNeel, 1985).

N'-(2,4-Xylyl)-N-methylformamidine (U-40481 or BTS-27271), a mammalian metabolite of amitraz, was found to have acute oral LD 50 values of 200 mg/kg in rats, 100–200 mg/kg in mice, 200 mg/kg in guinea pigs, >25 mg/kg in rabbits, and >20 mg/kg in dogs (FAO/WHO, 1981a). Ravikumar and Rieger (1983) determined a subcutaneous LD 50 for U-40481 in mice of 107 mg/kg; signs of acute toxicity included abnormal gait, hind-limb hyperextension, transient hyperactivity followed by a protracted phase of hypoactivity, ataxia, progressive respiratory difficulty, cyanosis, loss of righting reflex, and death.

Amitraz was not an irritant when applied to the rabbit eye. Neither amitraz nor U-40481 showed sensitization activity in guinea pigs (FAO/WHO, 1981a).

When rabbits were treated dermally with amitraz in acetone solution in 15 doses of 200 or 50 mg/kg over a 21-day period, sedation was observed in both sexes at 200 mg/kg and only in males at 50 mg/kg. In males at both dosages, slight to moderate erythema, desquamation of skin, and subcutaneous hemorrhage were evident (FAO/WHO, 1981a).

Groups of male and female rats were exposed daily for 6 hr to amitraz at concentrations in the air of 1.0, 0.1, and 0.01 mg/liter for 14 days over a 3-week period. At 1.0 mg/liter, ataxia, increased nasal secretion, polyuria, body tremors, and slight coma were observed. Eye irritation and hyposensitivity to noise were found at 0.1 mg/liter. Body weight gains were reduced in both sexes at the two highest levels. Hematological analyses revealed a decreased packed cell volume, hemoglobin, and red blood cell count and increased numbers of neutrophils in males and females and a decreased mean corpuscular hemoglobin concentration and number of lymphocytes in males of the highest dose group. Relative weights of liver, heart, and pituitary in males and of liver in females were increased at 1.0 mg/liter (FAO/WHO, 1981a).

In short-term feeding studies, groups of male and female rats and mice were fed amitraz in the diet for 90 days at 50, 12, and 3 mg/kg/day, assuming daily food intakes of 20 gm and 5 gm for rats and mice, respectively. Survival of rats apparently was unaffected, but six male mice died; the deaths probably were not related to amitraz. Decreases in body weight gains were found in female rats and male and female mice at 50 and 12 mg/kg and in male rats at 50 mg/kg. Food and water consumption were decreased in rats in all cases; they were slightly decreased in mice at 50 and 12 mg/kg, and the effect was more pronounced in males than in females. In rats, relative weights of brain, heart, lung, liver, kidney, spleen, and uterus or testes were increased in both sexes at 50 mg/kg, while thymus and adrenals in males at 50 mg/kg increased and decreased in weight, respectively. In mice, increases in brain (50 mg/kg) and heart (50 and 12 mg/kg) weights were observed in males, whereas kidney weight was decreased in females at 50 mg/kg. Hematological analyses of rats revealed a dose-related decrease in numbers of platelets in males at 50 and 12 mg/kg and a significant increase in eosinophils in females at 50 mg/kg. Serum of male rats at 50 mg/kg had decreased alkaline phosphatase activity and blood sugar concentration and increased potassium concentration. Serum of mice had decreased alkaline phosphatase and SGPT activities. In addition, mice serum had increased albumin–globulin ratios at 50 and 12 (males only) mg/kg. Urinalysis revealed several rats with proteinurea and decreased potassium concentration at 50 and 12 mg/kg (FAO/WHO, 1981a).

Male and female dogs received amitraz in capsules at 4, 1, or 0.25 mg/kg once daily for 90 days. Central nervous system depression, ataxia, and vomiting were observed during the initial 3–6 hr after treatment for the first few days, and dogs were subdued throughout the experiment. Temperature and pulse rate were decreased slightly after treatment but returned to normal within 24 hr. Hyperglycemia was observed in some cases. An increase in relative liver weights was found in both sexes at 4 mg/kg (FAO/WHO, 1981a).

In long-term studies, amitraz was administered in the diet at 200, 50, or 15 ppm for 2 years to groups of male and female rats. Rats at the highest dose were aggressive, nervous, and excitable, and growth rate and food intake were decreased during the first weeks of the experiment. No dose-related anomalies were found in organ weights or in hematological and biochemical analyses. Male and female mice were fed amitraz in the diet at 400, 100, or 25 mg/kg for 80 weeks. Food consumption was increased in male mice at 400 and 100 mg/kg and was decreased at 100 and 25 mg/kg and increased at 400 mg/kg in female mice (FAO/WHO, 1981a).

Absorption, Distribution, Metabolism, and Excretion
Amitraz administered orally to rats, mice, or dogs was rapidly absorbed, distributed, metabolized, and eliminated mainly in the urine but also in the feces (FAO/WHO, 1981a; Knowles and Benezet, 1981). For example, in rats treated orally with amitraz at 5 mg/kg, 78 and 9% of the administered radiocarbon were found in the urine and feces, respectively, by 96 hr (Knowles and Benezet, 1981). Ninety-six hours after treating dogs with a single oral dose of amitraz, 57% of the radiocarbon had been eliminated in the urine and 24% in the feces (FAO/WHO, 1981a). Amitraz was eliminated from most tissues of rats within a few days following single or multiple dosing (FAO/WHO, 1981a; Knowles and Benezet, 1981).

Amitraz degradation products found in urine or feces or both included U-40481, 2,4-dimethylformanilide, 2,4-dimethylaniline, 4-formamido-3-methylbenzoic acid, 4-amino-3-methylbenzoic acid, conjugates, and several unknowns (FAO/WHO,

1981a; Knowles and Benezet, 1981). Kimmel *et al.* (1986) reported that amitraz was metabolized upon intraperitoneal treatment of rats and *in vitro* by rat liver preparations to 2,4-dimethylaniline, which was subsequently converted to 2,4-dimethylnitrosobenzene.

Pharmacological and Biochemical Effects Hsu and Kakuk (1984) treated anesthetized rats intravenously with amitraz at dosages ranging from 0.03 to 1 mg/kg. Amitraz induced mydriasis and bradycardia, both of which were blocked by the α_2-adrenoreceptor antagonists yohimbine and phentolamine but not by prazosin, an α_1-adrenoreceptor antagonist. Also, it was suggested that the amitraz-induced mydriasis was mediated by postsynaptic α_2-adrenoreceptors, while the amitraz-induced bradycardia was mediated by presynpatic α_2-adrenoreceptors. In subsequent studies, amitraz was shown to induce bradycardia and hypertension when administered to conscious dogs. Intravenous injection of amitraz (1 mg/kg) caused a decrease in heart rate, which was accompanied by sinus arrhythmia for at least 60 min, and an increase in mean aortic blood pressure. Atropine sulfate (0.045 mg/kg, intravenous) increased heart rate and prevented the bradycardia, but potentiated the hypertension. Tolazoline (5 mg/kg, intravenous), a nonselective α-adrenoreceptor antagonist, reduced the bradycardia and sinus arrhythmia but did not affect hypertension. Prazosin (1 mg/kg, intravenous) did not affect the cardiovascular actions of amitraz. However, yohimbine (0.1 mg/kg, intravenous) prevented the amitraz-induced hypertension, bradycardia, and sinus arrhythmia (Hsu *et al.*, 1986).

Pascoe and Reynoldson (1986) found that amitraz induced hypotension and bradycardia in pentobarbital-anesthetized guinea pigs. When tested on isolated guinea pig atria, amitraz did not significantly affect the response curve to isoprenaline or acetylcholine, but it antagonized the histamine-induced response competitively in the presence of propranolol. Amitraz increased the atrial force of contraction in the absence of propranolol and depressed the atrial rate directly to a minor degree. It was suggested that the cardiovascular depression observed in the guinea pig was caused by an alteration in autonomic drive rather than a significant direct effect on the heart.

Amitraz induces intestinal stasis in some animals. For example, in horses amitraz has been found to induce stasis of the large intestine that has resulted in severe colic and even death in some cases (Pass and Seawright, 1982). Sellers *et al.* (1985) observed that injection of amitraz into the horse ileocolic artery produced a fall in colon blood flow, an effect that was prevented by yohimbine. Amitraz also produced intestinal stasis in dogs and mice (Hsu and Lu, 1984; Hsu and McNeel, 1985). Amitraz treatment of dogs (1 mg/kg, intravenous) prolonged the time for barium sulfate to move from the stomach to the duodenojejunal junction from 6 to 251 min, and there were no vigorous gastric contractions for at least 180 min. Yohimbine (0.1 mg/kg, intravenous) reversed the intestinal stasis in dogs when administered 20 min after amitraz (Hsu and McNeel, 1985); yohimbine also countered this effect of amitraz in mice

(Hsu and Lu, 1984). Pass and Seawright (1982) examined the effects of amitraz on the motility of isolated pieces of guinea pig ileum. Amitraz inhibited contractions induced by histamine and the histamine H_1 agonists 2-methylhistamine and 2-pyridylethylamine, but not those induced by acetylcholine, methacholine, or dimethylphenylpiperazinium. Amitraz also stimulated contractions directly.

U-40481, an amitraz metabolite, caused contractions of the rabbit central ear artery, an action that was antagonized by phentolamine. It also reversibly antagonized contractions induced by 5-hydroxytryptamine, norepinephrine, histamine, and to some extent potassium. U-40481 did not change the resting rate of washout of radioactivity from radioactive norepinephrine-preloaded strips, but it reduced electrically induced release of this amine. It was concluded that U-40481 was a partial α-adrenoreceptor agonist (Robinson, 1979). U-40481 also reduced the rate of both ^{45}Ca uptake and norepinephrine-stimulated ^{45}Ca uptake into deadventitiated rabbit aorta strips and reduced norepinephrine-stimulated efflux from ^{45}Ca-loaded, superfused aorta strips. It seemed possible that the action of this amitraz metabolite on unstimulated ^{45}Ca uptake may have resulted from uncoupling oxidative phosphorylation, and the reduction in norepinephrine-induced ^{45}Ca flux may have resulted from antagonism of norepinephrine receptors (Robinson and Pento, 1980).

Amitraz, U-40481, and 2,4-dimethylformanilide, but not 2,4-dimethylaniline, were inhibitors of rat and mouse monoamine oxidase *in vitro* (Aziz and Knowles, 1973; Knowles and Aziz, 1974; Benezet and Knowles, 1976b; Benezet *et al.*, 1978; Urbaneja and Knowles, 1979; Rieger *et al.*, 1980; Kadir and Knowles, 1981; Moser and MacPhail, 1984b). However, neither amitraz nor U-40481 appeared to have significant central or peripheral monoamine oxidase-inhibiting activity in rats *in vivo* (Bonsall and Turnbull, 1983; Moser and MacPhail, 1984b).

Amitraz was a weak inhibitor of 5-hydroxytryptamine uptake by isolated rat blood platelets; U-40481 was considerably more active than amitraz (Johnson and Knowles, 1982; Knowles and Johnson, 1984a). Amitraz also inhibited arachidonic acid-induced aggregation of rat platelets but was without effect on that induced by collagen or ADP. Amitraz did not significantly elevate cyclic AMP levels in platelet-rich plasma (Johnson and Knowles, 1985).

Amitraz also affects visual evoked potentials in rats. Specifically, amitraz (50 or 100 mg/kg, intraperitoneal) caused a significant increase in pattern reversal-evoked potential and flash-evoked potential latencies and in the pattern reversal-evoked potential but not the flash-evoked potential amplitude (Boyes and Dyer, 1984c).

Amitraz has antipyretic and anti-inflammatory activity. When injected into rats (5–80 mg/kg, intraperitoneal), it reduced the yeast induced fever and antagonized the carrageenan-induced swelling of the hind paw (Yim *et al.*, 1978a). Also, amitraz inhibited the synthesis of prostaglandin E_2 from arachidonic acid by bovine seminal vesicle microsomes (Yim *et al.*, 1978a).

U-40481 has been found to reduce isometric contractions of the isolated rat hemidiaphragm induced by electrical stimulation of either the phrenic nerve or the diaphragm itself (Ravikumar and Rieger, 1983).

Gilbert (1987) found that amitraz at 50 mg/kg facilitated electrical kindling of the amygdala but not the hippocampus in rats and suggested that the enhanced susceptibility to kindling might have resulted from depletion of norepinephrine by the formamidine.

Effects on Organs and Tissues Amitraz was not mutagenic when assayed with *S. typhimurium* (TA98, TA100, TA1535, TA1537, TA1538) and *E. coli* (WP$_2$, WP$_2$uvrA) in the presence or absence of S9 activation (FAO/WHO, 1981a; Ghali, 1981; Kimmel *et al.*, 1986). Also, amitraz showed no increase in point mutational activity against *S. typhimurium* (G46, TA1532, TA1964) when tested in the mouse perivisceral host-mediated assay at single oral doses up to 400 mg/kg with or without S9 activation (FAO/WHO, 1981a). However, the amitraz metabolite U-40481 showed weak but consistent mutagenic activity with *S. typhimurium* TA100 (FAO/WHO, 1981a). In the presence of S9 activation, 2,4-dimethylaniline also was mutagenic with stains TA98 and TA100 (Zimmer *et al.*, 1980; FAO/WHO, 1981a; Ghali, 1981; Kimmel *et al.*, 1986).

Female mice were treated orally for 5 consecutive days with amitraz at 50 or 12 mg/kg, and subgroups were mated with untreated males on day 3, 9, 14, or 19 posttreatment. A slight increase in mean postimplantation loss and decrease in mean viable litter size at 50 mg/kg was observed (FAO/WHO, 1981a). In another study, male mice were treated orally with amitraz for 5 consecutive days at 50 or 12 mg/kg and mated with untreated females for 6 weeks. A significantly lower implantation rate was found at 50 mg/kg at the first mating and a higher implantation rate at 12 mg/kg at the fifth mating. No treatment-related changes with regard to number of embryonic deaths and postimplantation losses were found (FAO/WHO, 1981a).

In the Chinese hamster lung fibroblast assay, there was no evidence of induction of DNA damage by amitraz, U-40481, or 2,4-dimethylaniline (FAO/WHO, 1981a).

Amitraz was not carcinogenic in long-term feeding studies with rats. However, in mice, an increased incidence of lymphoreticular tumors was observed in females as compared to controls (FAO/WHO, 1981a). On the basis of long-term feeding studies, it was concluded that 2,4-dimethylaniline was not carcinogenic in rats or male mice, but pulmonary tumors were significantly increased in female mice at the highest dosage (Weisburger *et al.*, 1978; FAO/WHO, 1981a). However, additional research is required before a definitive statement can be made about the carcinogenic activity of amitraz and its metabolites in laboratory animals (FAO/WHO, 1981a,b).

Using an in-depth tumor data evaluation system, Wang (1984a,b) classified amitraz in category IV, which included compounds that were "noncarcinogenic to no more than of borderline significance."

Effects on Reproduction Groups of male and female rats were fed amitraz in the diet at 200, 50, or 15 mg/kg. The animals were mated after 10 weeks. After the F_1 generation was weaned, males and females from each group were kept for breeding and maintained on the amitraz-treated diet, a procedure that was continued until the F_3 generation was weaned. Amitraz at 200 mg/kg caused decreased growth and food consumption in the F_0 generation. A decrease in fertility and viability also was observed. The 200 mg/kg dose group was discontinued when the F_1 generation was weaned due to low survival. At 50 mg/kg no effect was found on the number of litters and mean litter size, but a decrease in number of young alive at 21 days in all generations was found (FAO/WHO, 1981a).

When female mice were fed amitraz in the diet at 400 mg/kg for up to 33 weeks, a reduction in body weight and an increase in food consumption were observed. Analysis of vaginal smears indicated that the mean duration of estrus and the incidence of prolonged estrus were significantly increased. β-Estradiol levels in plasma were normal (FAO/WHO, 1981a). Female rats fed amitraz at 200 mg/kg for 18 weeks had longer estrous cycles than controls (FAO/WHO, 1981a).

Amitraz was administered to rats in doses of 12, 3, or 1 mg/kg from day 1 of pregnancy until the young were weaned at 21 days old. Weight gains of dams and mean number of young born and alive at day 4 were reduced at 12 mg/kg. No treatment-related effects were observed in the other groups (FAO/WHO, 1981a).

Rats were treated with amitraz at 12, 3, or 1 mg/kg/day from day 8 to day 20 of pregnancy. Rats were killed on day 21. Average litter size, fetal viability, and implantation index were not affected. In the 12 mg/kg group, fetal weight loss was less than in the controls, and calcification of sternebrae was less advanced (FAO/WHO, 1981a).

Rabbits received amitraz at 25, 5, or 1 mg/kg from day 6 to day 18 of pregnancy. When rabbits were killed on day 30, number of litters and mean litter size were decreased at 25 mg/kg. No increase in congenital abnormalities was observed (FAO/WHO, 1981a).

Behavioral Effects In rats, amitraz induced hyperphagia (Pfister *et al.*, 1978a), decreased ambulation and rearing (Moser and MacPhail, 1984b), and decreased fixed-interval schedule-controlled responding (Moser and MacPhail, 1984a,b, 1986). In dogs, amitraz suppressed open-field activity, an index of central nervous system depression; this and other behavior indicative of depression were prevented by yohimbine (Schaffer *et al.*, 1985; Hsu and Hopper, 1986).

Relatively low doses of U-40481 (1–20 mg/kg, subcutaneous) markedly impaired the ability of trained mice to ride a rotating rod (Ravikumar and Rieger, 1983).

In another study, Crofton *et al.* (1987) found that oral treatment of rats with amitraz at 25–200 mg/kg decreased motor activity and acoustic startle response. Significant behavioral effects were observed at otherwise asymptomatic dosages (25–50 mg/kg).

Factors Influencing Toxicity Moser and MacPhail (1985) found that amitraz induced delayed lethality in mice and that yohimbine (10 mg/kg, intraperitoneal) immediately before an injection of amitraz (600 mg/kg) and twice daily thereafter for 8 days protected mice from the lethal action of this formamidine.

Pathology Microscopic examination of rats fed 12 or 3 mg/kg of amitraz for 90 days showed some liver pathology, manifested as a slight increase in lymphoid infiltration with some leukocytosis and a loss of glycogen (FAO/WHO, 1981a). In the similar study with mice, the liver had a slight black discoloration mainly in the 12 mg/kg group; a slight centrilobular degeneration in the liver at all dose groups was the only histopathology found (FAO/WHO, 1981a). In the 90-day study with dogs, livers showed enlargement of the central and midzonal hepatocytes. Hyperplasia of the small periportal hepatocytes and increase in binucleate cells were evident in the 12 mg/kg group. Thinning of the zonae fasciculata and reticularis, sometimes associated with slight hyperplasia of the zona glomerulosa, was observed in the adrenals at all dose levels (FAO/WHO, 1981a).

Treatment of Poisoning in Animals Some domestic and farm animals are intentionally exposed to formulations containing amitraz to control mites and ticks. Although occasional side effects such as depression, anorexia, and sometimes vomiting have been reported, the compound has been found to be quite safe to these animals.

Roberts and Seawright (1979) reported that horses sprayed with 0.025% amitraz showed somnolence and reduced intestinal activity for 12–24 hr. Treatment with 0.1% amitraz produced somnolence, reduced intestinal activity, severe abdominal discomfort after 48 hr, and progressive impaction of the large intestine. Suggested treatment included cold water wash to remove the compound from the coat, lubricants by stomach tube, enemas, chloral hydrate/magnesium sulfate mixture, pentazocine or xylazine to relieve pain, oral fluids containing electrolytes by stomach tube, and large volumes of fluids intravenously.

No specific antidote presently exists for amitraz, although results from some of the pharmacological studies suggest that yohimbine might function in this capacity.

22.2.4.3 Toxicity to Humans

Experimental Exposure No reports of oral treatment of humans with amitraz were found. However, 2 mg of the amitraz metabolite U-40481 were administered in a single oral dose to six volunteers. Differences in blood pressure, pulse rate, temperature, and mental alertness were observed between those receiving the formamidine and those receiving the placebo (FAO/WHO, 1981a).

About 10 mg of amitraz in 0.02 ml of a 50% acetone solution were applied to the arms of nine volunteers; after 6 hr the arms were cleaned. One, who had previously reacted to the compound, had a slight erythema localized to the patch area. Three other volunteers who had previously reacted to the compound were administered a paraffin-based ointment containing 5% amitraz. One individual reported a delayed reaction that occurred 14 hr after treatment and consisted of a reddening in the area of his earlier reaction (FAO/WHO, 1981a).

In 1977, a program was conducted with amitraz to determine the dermal and respiratory exposure of sprayers and the potential dermal exposure of workers in a pear orchard at various times after spraying. Three different spray concentrations of BAAM® were applied by airblast sprayers: "semi-concentrated," containing 6.4–10 pints of BAAM/100 gallons of tank mix; "normal," containing 3 pints/100 gallons; and "dilute," containing 1.5 pints/100 gallons. Sprayers had α-cellulose pads on shoulders, upper back, upper chest, and forearms, and the exposed body area was calculated to be 1730 cm^2. Little difference in exposure was found with pad location or spray concentration, although a trend toward an inverse relationship between tank mix concentration and dermal exposure was suggested. Taking into account a 60% loss of amitraz by volatilization from the pads during storage prior to analysis, it was concluded that the dermal exposure would have ranged from less than 0.175 to 250 mg/person/hr with a mean of 31.8 mg/person/hr. Respiratory exposure, also corrected for the 60% loss, ranged from less than 0.075 to 86.5 μg/person/hr with a mean exposure for all tank mixes of 75.5 μg/person/hr. Analyses of alcohol hand rinses of sprayers, air samples, and pear foliage yielded unsatisfactory results [U.S. Department of Agriculture (USDA), 1978].

Accidents and Use Experience Bonsall and Turnbull (1983) summarized four cases of amitraz poisoning in humans. In 1977, a 74-year-old diabetic male suffering from confusion due to cerebral atherosclerosis drank a product containing amitraz and an organic solvent. Less than 30 ml of the product containing 6 gm of amitraz probably was ingested. At the hospital an hour later he was conscious, unstable, and smelled of xylene. Upon gastric lavage, his stomach contained food and an oily aromatic liquid. His level of consciousness decreased, and he was admitted to the hospital. His blood pressure was 200/100 mm Hg; he had moderate glycosuria and a trace of ketones in the urine. He was treated with antibiotics, insulin, and "cardiokinetic therapy." He was unconscious for 24 hr. SGOT, SGPT, alkaline phosphatase, and acid phosphatase activities were increased. Neutrophilic leukocytosis also was present. After 48 hr he was still confused but otherwise normal. He was discharged after 14 days. He subsequently developed a urinary tract infection, septicemia, and died 30 days after discharge. In 1978, a 29-year-old man fell into a cattle dip and was immersed to shoulder level for only a few seconds. He quickly washed in a nearby stream. He probably was in contact with the diluted amitraz formulation for about 3 min; washing and decontamination probably were not thorough. After 36 hr, he had a generalized throbbing headache and vomiting; no other specific symptoms were present. He was symptomatic for 3 days, except for the vomiting, which had stopped 24 hr earlier. It was not

determined whether the symptoms were a result of amitraz exposure or of a coincidental viral infection. In 1979, a successful suicide with amitraz occurred. The patient apparently survived for 6 days prior to death. In 1980 a 3-year-old child ingested a small quantity of an amitraz formulation. He was drowsy for several hours but was well the next day.

Some people involved in the development of amitraz have occasionally noticed a flushing of the skin. Interviews by medical staff led to the conclusions that the phenomenon was due to capillary dilation caused by amitraz or U-40481 or both and was the result of systemic absorption. The condition, which appeared to be temporary and disappeared soon after contact was discontinued, was more likely to occur when large quantities of the offending materials were processed (FAO/WHO, 1981a).

Laboratory Findings The amitraz metabolite 4-amino-3-methylbenzoic acid has been detected in the urine of production workers and volunteers (FAO/WHO, 1981a).

Treatment of Poisoning Impaired consciousness, hypotension, bradycardia, hypothermia, and possibly hypoglycemia may occur in severe cases of poisoning by some products containing amitraz. A typical product contains 75% xylene, which can cause a burning sensation in the mouth and throat with substernal and abdominal pain upon ingestion. Nausea, vomiting, diarrhea, headache, dizziness, and incoordination also may occur. Skin contact with amitraz alone is without toxic effect; however, skin contact with xylene may cause irritation, erythema, and dermatitis. Management of poisoning due to an amitraz formulation containing xylene should include gastric lavage (with precautions to avoid aspiration) along with symptomatic and supportive therapy directed especially at the respiratory and cardiovascular systems. No specific antidote for amitraz currently is known (Bonsall and Turnbull, 1982, 1983; Turnbull, 1983).

22.2.5 AZOXYBENZENE

22.2.5.1 Identity, Properties, and Uses

Chemical Name Azoxybenzene is diphenyldiazene 1-oxide.

Structure See Fig. 22.2.

Synonyms Other names for azoxybenzene include azobenzene oxide, azossibenzene, azoxybenzeen, azoxybenzol, azoxybenzide, and azoxydibenzene. The CAS registry number is 495-48-7.

Physical and Chemical Properties Azoxybenzene has the empirical formula $C_{12}H_{10}N_2O$ and a molecular weight of 198.2. It forms pale yellow orthorhombic needles melting at 36°C. Azoxybenzene is insoluble in water but soluble in alcohol and ether. It is slightly volatile in steam and easily volatile in superheated steam (140–150°C).

Use   Azoxybenzene is a component in some acaricides.

22.2.5.2 Toxicity to Laboratory Animals

Basic Findings   The following LD 50 values have been reported for azoxybenzene: rat oral, 620 and 700 mg/kg; rat intraperitoneal (male), 115 mg/kg; mouse oral, 500, 515, and 2760 mg/kg; mouse intraperitoneal, 500 mg/kg; rabbit dermal, 1090 mg/kg; and rabbit subcutaneous, 250 mg/kg (Smyth *et al.,* 1954; Nakamura *et al.,* 1977; Tsunenari, 1973; Salamone, 1981).

Absorption, Distribution, Metabolism, and Excretion
Pregnant rats were treated intragastrically with azoxybenzene at 50 mg/kg/day on day 18 of gestation; on days 15, 16, and 17 of gestation; or on days 12, 13, and 14 of gestation. Rats were sacrificed 24 hr after the last treatment, and levels of azoxybenzene and two of its metabolites were measured in the maternal liver, the placenta, and the fetuses. Livers from the three treatments contained mainly the metabolite 2-hydroxy-azobenzene, although small amounts of the parent compound also were present. Placentas and fetuses of the group receiving the single dose contained only 2-hydroxyazobenzene, whereas those of the two groups receiving multiple doses also contained some azoxybenzene. In addition, fetuses in the multiple-dosed groups also contained small amounts of azobenzene. 2-Hydroxyazobenzene levels in liver were lower than those in fetuses and placentas (Kujawa *et al.,* 1985).

Effects on Organs and Tissues   Azoxybenzene was one of 42 chemicals selected for extensive mutagenicity evaluation in five groups of assays. They included bacterial mutation, bacterial repair, lower eukaryotes, higher eukaryotes *in vitro,* and higher eukaryotes *in vivo.* A total of 42 separate tests were conducted with azoxybenzene; 16 tests gave a negative response, 25 were positive, and one was questionable. Azoxybenzene was a bacterial mutagen and gave a positive result in a number of repair assays in the presence of S9 activation. It apparently was inactive in tests with lower eukaryotes, but there were insufficient data for evaluation in tests with higher eukaryotes. Azoxybenzene probably was negative in both the *in vivo* micronucleus tests (Ashby, 1981).

Pathology   Icteritious skin, methemoglobinemia, swelling of spleen and liver, and atrophy of testes and epididymis were observed in laboratory animals treated orally with azoxybenzene (Nakamura *et al.,* 1977).

22.2.5.3 Toxicity to Humans

A 19-year-old youth attempted suicide by drinking about 50 ml of an acaricide consisting of 38% azoxybenzene, 22% PPPS (see Fig. 22.2), and 40% xylene. No symptoms appeared within 19 hr, but jaundice and sporadic unconsciousness were observed at 72 hr. He lapsed into hepatic coma within 96 hr and died of cardiac insufficiency at 140 hr after ingestion. Autopsy was refused (Tsunenari *et al.,* 1972; Tsunenari, 1973). The esti-

mated dosages for the three ingredients were: azoxybenzene, 380 mg/kg; PPPS, 220 mg/kg; and xylene, 400 mg/kg. All of these compounds are toxic to the liver, but azoxybenzene is the most toxic in this regard and probably accounted for much of the injury. The delayed onset and protracted course were reminiscent of the picture seen in rats poisoned by azoxybenzene. The contribution of PPPS probably was minor, inasmuch as Tsunenari (1973) found that the oral LD 50 of PPPS in mice is 5624 mg/kg. Mice that died slowly after receiving the mixture showed reduced movement, clonic convulsions, ataxia, and irregular respiration. Autopsy demonstrated degeneration of the renal tubular epithelium, pulmonary edema, hemorrhagic pneumonia, and congestion of the liver and necrosis of liver cells.

Treatment of poisoning by azoxybenzene is symptomatic.

22.3 SYNTHETIC MOLLUSCICIDES

Snails and slugs are relatively minor pests in agriculture. They usually thrive best under greenhouse conditions. Partly for this reason and partly because only crops of high unit value are raised in greenhouses, much of the agricultural use of molluscicides is in greenhouses.

On the contrary, schistosomiasis, one of the great endemic diseases of humankind, depends on certain snails for its continued existence. It has been estimated that more than 200 million people in 73 countries are infected. The prevalence of the disease has declined in a few places, including Japan, but the disease is uncontrolled in some endemic areas, and in several places it is spreading or increasing in importance as a result of population movements or the exploitation of water resources and the creation of artificial lakes.

Schistosomiasis, or bilharziasis as it is called, is really a constellation of three major diseases caused by *Schistosoma haematobium, S. mansoni,* and *S. japonicum* and one minor disease caused by *S. intercalatum.* All these blood flukes are obligate parasites. The adults inhabit specific veins of mammals; parts of the immature stages develop in aquatic or amphibious snails, while other immature stages are free swimming. The life-cycle details differ with the species of worm. Only certain snails are capable of serving as intermediate hosts. In Egypt, where both *S. haematobium* and *S. mansoni* occur, each requires a different species of snail.

Even though infected snails may be present, transmission of the disease to humans may be limited by hygienic measures, such as filtration and other appropriate processing of water used for household purposes. In addition to the personal benefit, treatment of human cases may help to limit transmission. However, the value of such measures is severely limited where the raising of important crops, especially rice, requires workers to wade in water. In most situations, control of the disease requires control of the snail host, and different species of snails are important in different parts of the world. In certain situations, biological control of the snail host has been possible. The most fascinating biological method involved the introduction of new snails that were incapable of being hosts of the developmental

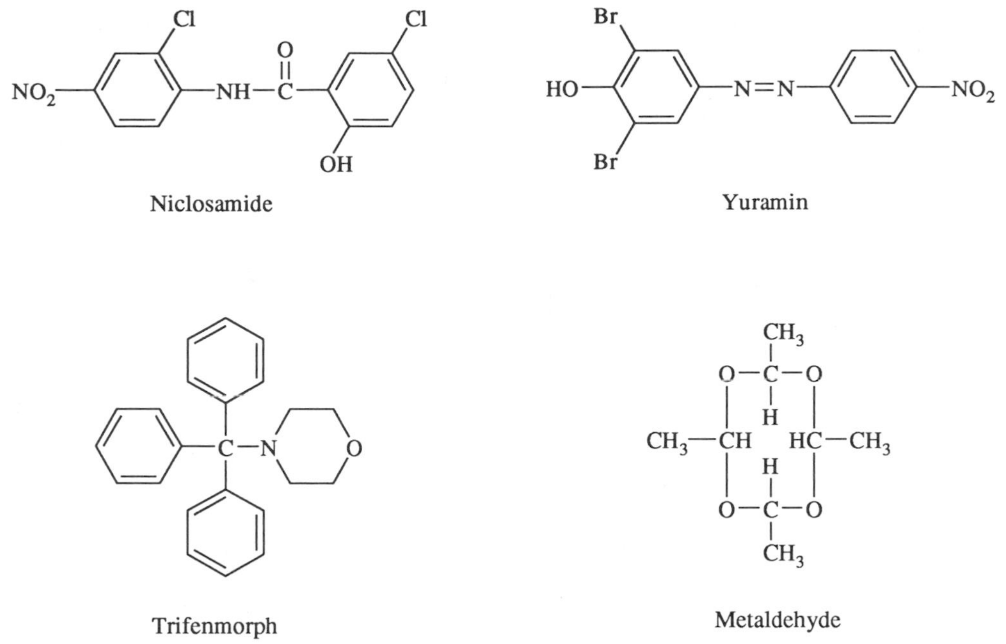

Figure 22.3 Some synthetic molluscicides.

stages of the parasite but were so competitive that the host snail was reduced significantly or even eliminated (Ferguson, 1975).

Although more extensive use of biological control may be possible for the snail hosts of schistosomiasis and thus for the human disease, a need for chemical control of the snails likely will continue.

Compounds that have proved useful for snail control do not constitute one or even a few chemical groups clearly set apart from other pesticides. In fact, copper sulfate and sodium pentachlorophenate have been used extensively for control of aquatic snails, but they are better known as fungicides. Some carbamate insecticides also are used in agriculture for control of snails and slugs. These compounds include methiocarb (see Section 17.3.13) and mexacarbate (see Section 17.3.15). Other synthetic organic molluscicides have included Yurimin, trifenmorph, metaldehyde, and niclosamide. The structures for some molluscicides are given in Fig. 22.3. Much more information than can be presented here on schistosomiasis and on some molluscicides may be found in a book entitled "Toxicology of Molluscicides" (Webbe, 1987).

22.3.1 METALDEHYDE

22.3.1.1 Identity, Properties, and Uses

Chemical Name Metaldehyde is metaacctaldehyde, a tetramer of acetaldehyde.

Structure See Fig. 22.3.

Synonyms Metaldehyde is accepted in lieu of a common name by BSI, ISO, and JMAF. Trade names have included Antimilace®, Ariotox®, Meta®, Slug Death®, Antimitace®, Cekumeta®, Halizan®, Metason®, Namekil®, Slugit Pellets®, Slug Pellets®, and Mini Slug Pellets®. The CAS registry numbers are 108-62-3 for the tetramer and 9002-91-9 for the homopolymer.

Physical and Chemical Properties Metaldehyde has the empirical formula $C_8H_{16}O_4$ and a molecular weight of 176.2. It is a flammable, colorless, crystalline solid that burns with a nonsmoky flame. The pure tetramer melts (in a sealed tube) at 246°C and sublimes at 110–120°C. It is subject to depolymerization, but the polymer itself does not respond to tests for the aldehyde group. The polymer is so flammable that it is used as a fuel. At 17°C the solubility in water of metaldehyde is only 200 ppm. In benzene and chloroform the compound is fully soluble, but in ethyl alcohol and diethyl ether it is only slightly soluble.

History, Formulations, and Uses For control of slugs and snails, metaldehyde is used in the form of granules, sprays, and dusts (Verschuuren *et al.*, 1975). Although sometimes used with bran as a bait, the compound alone is attractive to snails. It is interesting that neither acetaldehyde nor paraldehyde (a trimer) is an effective molluscicide.

22.3.1.2 Toxicity to Laboratory Animals

Basic Findings Metaldehyde is a compound of moderate oral toxicity. Acute oral LD 50 values of 227–690, 200, 175–700, 290–1250, and 100–1000 mg/kg were reported for rats, mice, guinea pigs, rabbits, and dogs, respectively (Booze and Oehme, 1985). Dosages that are nontoxic when given singly show little tendency to cause illness when repeated (Dobryanskiy, 1972).

Mice treated orally with metaldehyde at 1000 mg/kg showed

signs of toxicity within 10 min including sedation and shivering followed by whole body tremors, and tonic-clonic convulsions; death occurred within 2 hr of exposure (Homeida and Cooke, 1982b). In dogs, initial signs of metaldehyde poisoning may appear any time during the first 3 hr after exposure. Signs of metaldehyde toxicity include increased heart rate, anxiety, nystagmus, mydriasis, hyperpnea, panting, hypersalivation, ataxia (due to stiff legs), muscle tremors, vomiting, hyperesthesia, continuous convulsions, cyanosis, acidosis, diarrhea, depression, and narcosis. Death is usually due to respiratory failure and occurs between 4 and 24 hr postexposure (Boswood, 1962; Turner, 1962; Bishop, 1975; Maddy, 1975; Hatch, 1982; Booze and Oehme, 1985, 1986). A dog that survived poisoning by metaldehyde was totally blind initially but gradually regained normal vision within a period of 3 weeks (Bishop, 1975). Signs of metaldehyde toxicity in cats are similar to those in dogs (Booze and Oehme, 1985).

A dietary level of 10,000 ppm metaldehyde led to paralysis of the hindquarters of some rats after 126 days.

A 2-year study in rats fed metaldehyde at a level of 5000 ppm showed that growth was not significantly affected, but intermittent reduction of food intake by females occurred. Posterior paralysis was observed in 5 of 25 females (but not in males), and this was the cause of increased mortality in the females. The latency period prior to onset of paresis was more than 550 days, except in one instance, where it was less than 1 month. A significant increase in the relative weights of livers (in males) and ovaries was evident. At a dietary level of 1000 ppm, growth and survival were normal. Posterior paralysis was observed in one male and one female. An increase in liver size also was evident, but it was less striking than at the higher dosage. The only effects of a dietary level of 200 ppm for 2 years were posterior paresis in one male rat (latency period, 569 days) and increased relative weights of ovaries (Verschuuren *et al.*, 1975).

Absorption, Distribution, Metabolism, and Excretion Metaldehyde was found in the plasma and urine of dogs given a single oral dose of 600 mg/kg. The urinary excretion of metaldehyde was less than 1% of the dose (Booze and Oehme, 1986). It was of interest that acetaldehyde was not found in plasma or urine of metaldehyde-treated dogs (Booze and Oehme, 1986), since the prevailing view is that acetaldehyde formed by gastric hydrolysis of metaldehyde is responsible for the toxicity (Beran *et al.*, 1982; Dreisbach, 1983).

Biochemical Effects Mice treated orally with metaldehyde showed a significant decrease in brain levels of γ-aminobutyric acid, norepinephrine, 5-hydroxytryptamine, and 5-hydroxyindoleacetic acid and a significant increase in monoamine oxidase activity (Homeida and Cook, 1982a,b).

Effects on Organs and Tissues There was no evidence of mutagenicity when metaldehyde was evaluated with five strains of *Salmonella* in the presence and absence of S9 activation (Quinto *et al.*, 1981).

The incidence of tumors in male and female rats was not increased by dietary levels of metaldehyde as high as 5000 ppm for 2 years (Verschuuren *et al.*, 1975).

Effects on Reproduction Dietary levels of 1000 and 5000 ppm metaldehyde, which were toxic to female rats, also interfered with their reproduction in a three-generation, 2-year test. A dietary level of 200 ppm did not affect reproduction. Although none of the levels evaluated were teratogenic, increases in relative liver weights were observed in some offspring (Verschuuren *et al.*, 1975).

Pathology The most interesting pathology associated with metaldehyde was fracture or dislocation of vertebrae and subsequent compression of the spinal cord in rats. The condition was seen more often in females on 5000 ppm, and its frequency was increased by pregnancy, the incidence reaching more than 50%. Histological study excluded the possibility of osteomalacia or muscular dystrophy but failed to establish a cause. It seemed possible that the kink of the vertebral column was caused by uncontrolled body movements and subsequent mechanical damage, but this was not proved. Whatever its cause, the lesion usually occurred in the thoracic cord but was seen in the neck and lumbar region also (Verschuuren *et al.*, 1975).

Postmortem examinations of dogs poisoned with metaldehyde have revealed hepatic, renal, and pulmonary congestion usually with hyperemia and interstitial hemorrhages. Petechial and ecchymotic hemorrhages have been found in the gastrointestinal mucosa, and massive subendocardial and subepicardial hemorrhages also have been observed (Booze and Oehme, 1985).

Treatment of Poisoning in Animals In small animals, apomorphine is generally recommended as the emetic; in large animals, mineral oil has been used as a laxative. In dogs, the use of an emetic should be followed with light anesthesia or tranquilization to control convulsions and to facilitate gastric lavage if required. Diazepam and triflupromazine are among those that have been suggested. Lactated Ringer solution can be given to combat acidosis and dehydration, and parenteral administration of dextrose, saline, or calcium borogluconate solution has been suggested to prevent liver damage (Booze and Oehme, 1986).

22.3.1.3 Toxicity to Humans

Accidental and Intentional Poisoning Metaldehyde-induced poisoning of humans in Europe is caused by tablets intended for use as a fuel in lamps and in small stoves as well as by the molluscicide. Metaldehyde poisoning in the United States is due exclusively to the molluscicide, since meta-fuel is not available. Several detailed accounts of metaldehyde poisoning in children and adults occur in the literature.

In one well-described case, a 2.5-year-old boy was thought to have eaten only one tablet and that at about 1715 hr. The mother gave the child a large dose of castor oil. About 20 min later he fell asleep but awoke about an hour later crying, retching, and complaining of abdominal pain. At 1845 hr, the boy was seen by a physician, who recovered some of the poison in vomitus and some in stomach washings. The child seemed relieved and in about 15 min fell asleep. Later he had a few attacks of retching, but he seemed better when seen again by a physician at 2030 hr. At 2200 hr the child awoke from a short sleep, complained of a return of abdominal pain, and had a convulsion lasting about 3 min. For about an hour before midnight, convulsions recurred about every 10 min. At about midnight the child lost consciousness completely, and convulsions became more frequent. Chloral and potassium bromide were used but without noticeable improvement. At 0145 hr next morning the boy became much worse. Convulsions were almost continuous. Risus sardonicus and opisthotonos were present. The temperature rose to 40°C and the pulse to 140. Death occurred within 33 hr of ingestion (Lewis *et al.*, 1939). Autopsy findings are mentioned below.

Greater delay in onset and a milder course are characteristic of nonfatal cases. A boy of 16 years who mistook a metaldehyde tablet for candy remained well for 7 hr and without convulsions for an additional 3 hr. He had only six episodes of convulsions within a period of 14 hr; he never became fully unconscious, and his temperature rose only to 38.3°C. A striking feature of the case was loss of memory for the illness and other recent events; even 3 months after the episode, memory remained poor for a holiday 2 months after the ingestion (Miller, 1928).

Longstreth and Pierson (1982) described the attempted suicide of a 32-year-old woman who ingested about 470 ml of a commercial slug bait that contained 4% metaldehyde; the dosage was about 330 mg of metaldehyde per kilogram of body weight. Soon after ingestion nausea and vomiting occurred, followed in 2 hr by the first of many generalized convulsions. She was treated initially with gastric lavage, activated charcoal, and diazepam; convulsions continued accompanied by decreased mental status, muscle spasms, and coma. Her blood pressure was 130/90 mm Hg, temperature 38.1°C, and respirations 20/min. She was unresponsive to voice or painful stimuli. Her pupils were reactive; she turned her eyes and head toward sounds; and corneal reflexes were present. Chvostek's sign also was present. Clinical laboratory tests revealed a high anion gap (23 mEq/ml) and a urine pH of 5.5 with ketones indicating metabolic acidosis. Respiratory alkalosis was present (arterial blood gas pH, 7.57; pCO_2 21 mm Hg), as were elevated serum transaminase and creatine kinase levels. Pneumonia and increased oral and tracheobronchial secretions also were found. Muscle spasms and generalized convulsions continued despite therapy with phenytoin, phenobarbital, and diazepam. Convulsions and coma lasted for 3 and 7 days, respectively. Her strength improved and anticonvulsant drug therapy was discontinued. When communication was possible, she was found to have pronounced memory deficits including adaptive problem-solving impairment and severe impairment of memory in both verbal and visual–spatial areas. She was discharged after 51 days. Her memory almost completely returned to normal by 1 year following ingestion of metaldehyde (Longstreth and Pierson, 1982).

Other signs and symptoms in addition to those mentioned

above that have been associated with metaldehyde toxicosis in humans have included blurred vision, dilated pupils, conjunctival irritation, dermatitis, pruritis, edema, erythema, confusion, agitation, depression, general apathy, drowsiness, fainting, salivation, frontal lobe damage, and regression to infant-like reflexes [Borbely, 1970; Environmental Protection Agency (EPA), 1980; Booze and Oehme, 1985].

Although most poisoning by metaldehyde has been the result of accidental ingestion by children or suicide by adults, at least two murders have involved this compound (Lüden, 1958).

Dosage Response In cases of poisoning by "meta-fuel," many authors apparently have failed to report the weight of the tablets their patients had swallowed, and it is unlikely that the tablets were all of the same size and weight. Belfrage (1927) equated half a tablet with about 2000 mg. This dose was ingested by a 2.8-year-old child who survived the dosage, which in view of his weight was 136 mg/kg. However, a 2.5-year-old boy died after eating one tablet measuring "two inches long by half an inch thick," even though part of the poison was recovered in vomitus and stomach washings (Lewis *et al.*, 1939).

A 53-year-old man with a history of chronic cardiopulmonary disease and alcoholism died about 38 hr after ingesting six tablets, presumably a total of 24,000 mg (Vischer, 1935). On the contrary, a woman who swallowed six tablets vomited immediately and made a complete recovery (Lewis *et al.*, 1939). Several other adults survived following attempted suicide by ingesting one to three tablets (Vischer, 1935).

Borbely (1970) reviewed 213 cases of metaldehyde poisoning from 1966 to 1969 in the records of the Swiss Toxicological Information Center. In the case of children, all instances were accidental and were divided equally between meta-fuel tablets and molluscicides. None of the children died. In adults 20 of 24 cases were intentional and all involved tablets; two of the adults died. Borbely (1970) suggested the following relationships between clinical effects and ingested dose: salivation, facial flushing, fever, abdominal cramps, nausea, and vomiting from a "few" mg/kg; drowsiness, tachycardia, spasms, irritability, salivation, abdominal cramps, facial flushing, and nausea from up to 50 mg/kg; ataxia and increased muscle tone from 50–100 mg/kg; convulsions, tremor, and hyperreflexia from 100–200 mg/kg; and coma and death from about 400 mg/kg (Borbely, 1970; Longstreth and Pierson, 1982).

Laboratory Findings The urine may be very acid in spite of extensive alkali therapy. Casts and albumin may occur in the urine and may persist for several days after symptomatic recovery. Elevated serum transaminase and creatine kinase levels also have been reported.

Pathology At autopsy of a 2.5-year-old boy who lived 33 hr after ingesting metaldehyde, the lungs showed areas of collapse and congestion, the right ventricle and auricle of the heart were dilated, the liver was pale and yellow, and other organs were grossly normal, except for petechial hemorrhages in the brain, endocardium, stomach mucosa, and liver. Microscopic examination revealed intense fatty degeneration with zonal necrosis of the liver and swelling and desquamation of the renal tubular epithelium (Lewis *et al.*, 1939).

Treatment of Poisoning To remove metaldehyde from the digestive tract and to prevent additional absorption, emesis or gastric lavage or both followed by administration of activated charcoal has been used. Administration of barbiturates during the early stages of metaldehyde poisoning in adults may be contraindicated, since respiratory and cardiovascular systems may be depressed. Antibiotics, chlorpromazine, and additional supportive therapy for coma, hypoxia, and/or pulmonary edema may be required (Arenz, 1983; Booze and Oehme, 1985). Depending on the severity of the poisoning, many patients appear to recover fully in 2–5 days except for loss of memory, which may last several months (Booze and Oehme, 1985).

22.3.2 NICLOSAMIDE

22.3.2.1 Identity, Properties, and Uses

Chemical Name Niclosamide is 5-chloro-*N*-(2-chloro-4-nitrophenyl)-2-hydroxybenzamide. In addition to the free base, it is marketed as the ethanolamine salt, piperazine salt, and monohydrate.

Structure See Fig. 22.3.

Synonyms Niclosamide is the common name accepted by BSI, ISO, and BPC. Clonitralide also has been used as a common name. Trade names for the base or various other forms have included Bayluscide®, Bayluscit®, Mollutox®, Mansonil®, Taenifugin®, Lintex®, Cestocide®, Atenase®, Aten®, Copharten®, Fenasal®, Grandal®, Helmiantin®, Iometan®, Kontal®, Mato®, Niclocide®, Sagimid®, Teniamida®, Vermitin®, Yomesan®, Zemun®, and Zestocarp®. Code designations have included Bayer-2,353, Bayer-6,076, Bayer-9,045, Bayer-73, G-501, HL-2,448, and SR-73. The CAS registry numbers are 50-65-7 for the base and 1420-04-8 for the ethanolamine salt.

Physical and Chemical Properties Niclosamide is a yellowish gray crystalline solid with an empirical formula of $C_{13}H_8O_4N_2Cl_2$ and a molecular weight of 327.1. Its melting point is 222–224°C, and its vapor pressure at 20°C is less than 7.5×10^{-6} mm Hg. Its solubility in water at room temperature ranges from 5 to 8 mg/liter. The ethanolamine salt is a yellow solid with a melting point of 216°C. Its solubility in water at room temperature is 180–280 mg/liter. The ethanolamine salt is stable to heat and is hydrolyzed by concentrated acid or base.

History, Formulations, and Uses The molluscicidal properties of niclosamide were first described by Gönnert and Schraufstätter (1959) of Bayer AG. The compound is toxic to a variety of species of aquatic snails, with those that serve as intermediate hosts of trematodes, especially the schistosomes,

attracting most attention. In addition to killing the snails, niclosamide is lethal to miracidia and cercariae, larval stages of trematodes that are infective for either the intermediate or final hosts. Niclosamide also is used in human and veterinary medicine as a cestocide and trematocide. For molluscicidal use, the base is formulated as an emulsifiable concentrate (250 gm/liter), and the ethanolamine salt is formulated as a wettable powder (700 or 600 gm/kg). Granule, sand, and gelatin formulations also have been used. For human medicine, niclosamide free base is used, and for veterinary medicine, various preparations of niclosamide free base, piperazine salt, and monohydrate are used.

22.3.2.2 Toxicity to Laboratory Animals

Basic Findings Niclosamide, its ethanolamine salt, and the monohydrate have low acute oral and subcutaneous toxicity to laboratory animals (Table 22.3). The compounds were of higher toxicity following intraperitoneal and intravenous administration (Andrews *et al.*, 1983).

Symptoms of acute niclosamide poisoning included disturbances in behavior, hypopnea, convulsions, and sedation. Vomiting was observed in dogs and cats (Andrews *et al.*, 1983).

Groups of male and female rats were treated orally with 24 daily doses of niclosamide ethanolamine salt at 5000, 2000, 800, or 320 mg/kg body weight or with 30 daily doses at 250 mg/kg body weight. Rats treated at 5000 mg/kg had marginal decreases in hemoglobin and erythrocyte values, but rats at 2000 mg/kg and lower were without symptoms and showed no evidence of damage based on clinical chemistry tests and histopathological examination. Groups of male and female rats treated dermally with 15 daily doses at 200 mg/kg body weight also tolerated the chemical without any evidence of damage (Gönnert and Schraufstätter, 1959; Andrews *et al.*, 1983).

Mice were treated with six daily subcutaneous injections of niclosamide ethanolamine salt at 2500 and 1000 mg/kg body weight. The high dosage level was lethal, but the lower level was tolerated without clinical symptoms (Gönnert and Schraufstätter, 1959).

Groups of male and female rabbits were treated orally with 24 daily doses of niclosamide ethanolamine salt at 900, 300, or 100 mg/kg body weight. Doses of 900 mg/kg resulted in slight decreases in hemoglobin and plasma urea values. The weights of the adrenals and thyroids were slightly increased in males that received 900 and 300 mg/kg. Doses of 100 mg/kg or less were tolerated without apparent damage. It may be noteworthy that the rabbits in these tests were infected inadvertently with coccidia (Andrews *et al.*, 1983). In another study, rabbits received 11 daily doses of 100 mg/kg body weight without clinical or hematological symptoms (Hecht and Gloxhuber, 1960).

Groups of male and female dogs were treated only with 24 daily doses of niclosamide ethanolamine salt at 4500, 1500, and 500 mg/animal (increased to 6000 mg/animal after 8 days), and groups of male and female cats were treated with 24 daily doses at 900, 300, and 100 mg/kg body weight. Except for the cats, which experienced slight but quickly reversible weight loss,

Table 22.3
Single-Dose LD 50 Values for Niclosamide, Niclosamide Ethanolamine
Salt, and Niclosamide Monohydrate[a]

Substance and species	Route	LD 50 (mg/kg)
Niclosamide		
Rat	oral	>5,000
Rat, M	oral	>3,710
Rat, F	oral	3,710
Rat	subcutaneous	>10,200
Rat	intraperitoneal	750[b]
Rat, M	intraperitoneal	610
Rat, F	intraperitoneal	740
Rat, F	intravenous	6
Mouse, F	oral	1,500
Mouse, F	subcutaneous	>20,000
Mouse, F	intraperitoneal	210
Mouse	intravenous	8[b]
Rabbit	oral	>5,000[b]
Dog	oral	>250[b]
Cat	oral	>1,000[b]
Cat	intravenous	>5
Niclosamide ethanolamine salt		
Rat	oral	>10,000[c]
Rat, M	oral	>5,000
Rat	intraperitoneal	250[c]
Rat, M	intraperitoneal	44–110
Rat, M	intravenous	7
Mouse	intravenous	9–15[c]
Guinea pig, M	intraperitoneal	31
Guinea pig, M	intravenous	3
Rabbit	oral	>4,000[c]
Cat	oral	>500[c]
Niclosamide monohydrate		
Rat, M	oral	>5,000
Mouse, M	oral	>10,000

[a]Table modified from Andrews et al. (1983). Data from unpublished Bayer documents
unless indicated otherwise.
[b]From Hecht and Gloxhuber (1960).
[c]From Hecht and Gloxhuber (1962).

there was no evidence of damage (Hecht and Gloxhuber, 1960;
Andrews et al., 1983).

In longer-term toxicity tests, groups of male and female rats
were given niclosamide ethanolamine salt in the feed at levels of
15 or 5 ppm for 90 days or 25,000 ppm (about 1250 mg/kg body
weight) and 10,000 ppm for 319 and 326 days, respectively.
The two highest concentrations caused a reduction of body
weight in male rats, but no other treatment-related effects were
found (Hecht and Gloxhuber, 1962; Andrews et al., 1983).
Groups of male and female dogs were fed niclosamide ethanolamine salt in gelatin capsules at 100 mg/kg body weight per
day for 252 days over a 1-year period with no evidence of any
treatment-related effects based on symptoms, clinical chemistry
tests, and dissection (Hecht and Gloxhuber, 1962).

Several long-term studies also have been conducted with
niclosamide. Groups of male and female rats were given the
compound in the feed at levels of 20,000 (about 1610 mg/kg
body weight), 8000, 4000, and 2000 ppm for 14 weeks without
evidence of any treatment-related effects (Andrews et al.,
1983). In another study, male rats were given niclosamide at
2500 mg/kg body weight oral daily for 65 days and thereafter
25,000 ppm in the feed for 381 days or 1000 mg/kg oral daily
for 55 days and thereafter 10,000 ppm in the feed for 365 days.
Rats in the high-dose group experienced reduced weight gains.
Some mortality of unknown etiology also occurred. However, it
was concluded that based on symptoms, hematology, urinalysis, dissection, and histopathology, the level of 25,000 ppm
was tolerated without damage (Hecht and Gloxhuber, 1962).
Male and female dogs also tolerated niclosamide given orally in
capsules at 100 mg/kg body weight for over 1 year without
damage (Hecht and Gloxhuber, 1962).

In rabbits, niclosamide ethanolamine salt and two of its formulations, a wettable powder (700 gm/kg) and an emulsifiable
concentrate (250 gm/liter), had a strong irritating effect on the
mucosal membranes of the eye and were locally corrosive to the
cornea. The two formulations also elicited skin reactions in
rabbits, but high concentrations (>10%) or repeated applications of lower concentrations were required (Andrews et al.,
1983).

Absorption, Distribution, Metabolism, and Excretion
When radiolabeled niclosamide ethanolamine salt was administered orally to male rats at 50 mg/kg, about one-third of the dose
was absorbed from the gastrointestinal tract and eliminated in
the urine within 24 hr; the remainder of the dose was eliminated
in the feces. Similar absorption and excretion patterns were
found when rats were given seven oral doses of 50 mg/kg
(Duhm et al., 1961). The major excretory product was 2,5'-
dichloro-4'-aminosalicylanilide, which was formed by reduction of the 4'-nitro moiety of the parent compound (Duhm et al.,
1961).

Pregnant rats were treated orally with niclosamide at
1000 mg/kg on day 13, 19, or 20 of gestation, and rats were
sacrificed at 4, 8, 16, or 24 hr posttreatment. Highest concentrations of niclosamide and 2,5'-dichloro-4'-aminosalicylanilide
were detected in liver and kidney 8 hr after treatment. Niclosamide, but not its amino metabolite, was present in fetuses
from rats treated on day 13, whereas both compounds were
found in fetuses from rats treated on day 19 or 20. It was
suggested that 19- and 20-day-old fetuses, but not 13-day-old
fetuses, were able to metabolize niclosamide (Andrews et al.,
1983).

Absorption of niclosamide and its piperazine salt by dogs
receiving a single oral dose of 125 mg/kg also was examined.
Maximum concentrations of 1.6 ppm were found in plasma at
1–24 hr posttreatment. No differences in absorption between
niclosamide and its piperazine salt were observed (Andrews et
al., 1983).

Biochemical Effects   Niclosamide given orally to cats at 100
or 30 mg/kg body weight resulted in increased methemoglobi-

nemia; an intravenous dose of 5 mg/kg had no effect on blood pressure (Andrews *et al.*, 1983).

Using rat liver mitochondrial preparations, Pütter (1970) examined the effects of niclosamide on the activity of acetylase, catalase, peroxidase, succinate dehydrogenase, and ATPase, and on the formation of ATP and methemoglobin. Niclosamide in low concentrations activated ATPase activity and inhibited the formation of ATP but was without appreciable influence on the other processes (Pütter, 1970).

Effects on Organs and Tissues The dominant lethal test was used to evaluate the mutagenic potential of niclosamide ethanolamine salt. Male mice were treated orally with the compound at 500 mg/kg body weight and mated to untreated females. Although the treated males showed some acute effects of the chemical (light somnolence), no evidence for any mutagenic activity was observed in the progeny (Andrews *et al.*, 1983). No evidence of mutagenic activity was found when niclosamide ethanolamine salt or its wettable powder formulation (700 gm/kg) was incubated with *S. typhimurium* in the absence of S9 activation; however, the ethanolamine salt yielded a slight mutagenic effect in the presence of induced microsomes (Lemma and Ames, 1975; Andrews *et al.*, 1983).

Groups of male and female rats (Osborne–Mendel) were given niclosamide ethanolamine salt in the feed at time-weighted average levels of 28,433 and 14,216 ppm and groups of male and female mice (B6C3F1) were given 549 and 274 ppm in the feed for 78 weeks followed by observation periods of 33 and 14 weeks for rats and mice, respectively. There was no convincing evidence of carcinogenic activity in rats or female mice; poor survival of male mice precluded evaluation (NCI, 1978).

Effects on Reproduction Female rats were treated orally with niclosamide at a daily rate of 1000 mg/kg body weight for 3–4 consecutive days on days 4–6, 7–9, or 10–12 of pregnancy, and female rabbits were similarly treated on days 7–10, 10–12, or 13–16 of pregnancy. None of the progeny showed any embryotoxic or teratogenic effects (Andrews *et al.*, 1983).

Factors Influencing Toxicity When ethyl alcohol and niclosamide (2000 mg/kg) were administered concurrently to male mice, enhancement of toxicity was observed (Airaksinen *et al.*, 1967).

22.3.2.3 Toxicity to Humans

Experimental Exposure No signs of intoxication were observed when adult males and females were treated once or twice orally with niclosamide at 1000 mg per person (Hecht and Gloxhuber, 1960). Children aged 6–15 years showed no signs of niclosamide intoxication when treated at dosages ranging from 1000 to 750 mg per person (Andrews *et al.*, 1983).

Humans have been exposed experimentally to niclosamide and its ethanolamine salt. A transient erythema was the only reaction in 4 of 7 persons when niclosamide was applied to their forearms for 24 hr; 2 of 6 reacted similarly to the ethanolamine

salt (Gönnert, 1961). In other experiments, niclosamide ethanolamine salt caused no skin irritation in adults over a 24-hr exposure period (Hecht and Gloxhuber, 1962; Andrews *et al.*, 1983), and cutaneous application of niclosamide had no sensitizing effect in humans suffering from a photoallergy to tribromosalicylanilide (Osmundsen, 1971).

Therapeutic Use Niclosamide in the free-base form only is used primarily as a cestocide and to a lesser extent as a trematocide. The drug is formulated as a chewable tablet containing 500 mg of niclosamide. It is very effective against tapeworm infections caused by *Taenia saginata*, *T. solium*, and *Diphyllobothrium latum;* tapeworms such as *Hymenolepis diminuta*, *H. nana*, and *Dipylidium caninum* are somewhat more recalcitrant. For infections of *T. saginata*, *T. solium*, and *D. latum*, single oral dosages of 2 gm (adult), 1.5 gm (child > 34 kg), and 1.0 gm (child 11–34 kg) are recommended. Other tapeworms may require repeated treatment—for example, 2 gm/day in single daily doses for 7 days (adults), 1.5 gm given in a single dose on the first day followed by 1 gm/day for the next 6 days (child > 34 kg), and 1 gm given in a single dose on the first day followed by 500 mg/day for next 6 days (child 11–34 kg). Safety for use in children under 2 years of age has not been established. Since niclosamide is active only against intestinal cestodes, it is not effective for treatment of cysticercosis (Compendium of Drug Therapy, 1986). As a trematocide, niclosamide is active mainly against flukes such as *Fasciolopsis buski* in the intestines (Idris *et al.*, 1980).

Signs and symptoms associated with niclosamide therapy, though infrequent, include nausea and vomiting, abdominal discomfort including anorexia, diarrhea, drowsiness, and dizziness; those of lesser frequency include constipation, headache, irritability, rash including pruritus ani, alopecia, oral irritation, fever, rectal bleeding, bad taste in mouth, sweating, palpitations, edema of an arm, and backache.

Accidents and Use Experience Even though niclosamide has been widely used as a molluscicide to control snails and as a cestocide in human and veterinary medicine, no cases of accidental or intentional poisoning were found.

Skin reactions have been reported occasionally following field application of niclosamide emulsifiable concentrate (250 gm/liter) (Andrews *et al.*, 1983). In one incident, a 20-year-old sprayman in good health and with no known allergies developed an itching papular eruption on the fingers of both hands following application of the material for snail control. The condition was relieved by topical treatment with hydrocortisone cream. A year later, during a period of intensive application of the molluscicide, the same man developed a pruritic vesicular cutaneous eruption on an indurated erythematous base where clothing, drenched with spray from dense vegetation in the habitat under treatment, touched his legs. Patch testing on his back for 24 hr with the niclosamide formulation gave sloughing with formation of vesicles and papules. The lesions responded to hydrocortisone cream. He was able to continue work without difficulty by avoiding prolonged contact with the formulation. Additional tests were conducted without positive results on three other spraymen, two of whom had complained of minor itching and skin eruptions at various times. Tests were repeated using the formulation and the active ingredient. Neither sprayman gave any reactions. It was suggested that the sprayman in question was allergic to components in the formulation other than the active ingredient (Cook *et al.*, 1972).

Niclosamide has been used in over 40 pilot and expanded control projects in Brazil, Puerto Rico, Egypt, Iran, Liberia, Indonesia, Saint Lucia, and other countries for control of snails transmitting schistosomiasis. In most instances chemotherapy of target human populations with drugs such as praziquantel, niridazole, and metrifonate has been combined with application of niclosamide molluscicide (Jobin, 1979; Putrali *et al.*, 1980; Barnish *et al.*, 1982; Saladin *et al.*, 1983). Niclosamide is active against some intestinal trematodes in humans but apparently is ineffective against blood flukes such as the schistosomes. Thus niclosamide has not been used as a chemotherapeutic agent in these control projects.

In Bangladesh, niclosamide was used to treat 20 children, up to the age of 14 years, parasitized with the trematode *Fasciolopsis buski*. Three doses, 150, 110, and 70 mg/kg, were used, and the compound was administered to the children in the morning following a light supper. In some cases, the drug was readministered about 7–10 days after the initial treatment. Egg reduction was 60.0, 47.9, and 39.9% for the high, medium, and low dosages, respectively. Patients tolerated the niclosamide well, and none of the subjects complained of any adverse effects attributable to the compound (Idris *et al.*, 1980).

Laboratory Findings   When male and female volunteers each were treated orally with 2000 mg of radiocarbon-labeled niclosamide, between 2 and 25% of the dose was eliminated in the urine over a 4-day period; the remainder was found in the feces. Elimination of niclosamide equivalents was essentially complete after 1–2 days. Glucuronides of the following were eliminated: niclosamide, 2′,5-dichloro-4′-aminosalicylanide, and 2′,5-dichloro-4′-acetaminosalicylanilide. Maximal niclosamide equivalents in serum ranged from 0.25 to 6.0 ppm; the variation associated with this parameter was attributed to differential rates of absorption among the individuals (Andrews *et al.*, 1983).

In children aged 6–15 years given oral doses of niclosamide ranging from 1000 to 750 mg/kg, the results of analyses of urine and blood and of liver and kidney function tests were normal. No methemoglobinemia was observed in males treated orally with niclosamide at 30 mg/kg (Andrews *et al.*, 1983).

The genotoxic effects to peripheral lymphocytes from five patients before and after treatment with niclosamide for *H. nana* parasitism were examined; the treatment regimen was 1–2 gm of niclosamide orally the first day followed by 0.5 gm in a daily oral dose for the next 6 days. Lymphocytes from three of the five patients showed an increase in chromosomal aberrations following niclosamide therapy; breaks were the aberration observed most frequently. In none of the five was an increase in sister chromatid exchanges observed. In *in vitro* studies, niclosamide added in 2-hr pulses to lymphocyte cultures induced a small clastogenic effect in blood from one donor and inhibited mitosis in blood from two other donors. A dose-related increase in clastogenicity was found in two of four blood samples in the presence of S9 activation, and a weak dose-related increase in sister chromotid exchange was observed in one sample (Ostrosky-Wegman *et al.*, 1986).

Pathology   No niclosamide-induced pathology in humans has been reported.

Treatment of Poisoning   Treatment of an overdose includes a fast-acting laxative and enema; use of an emetic is contraindicated (Compendium of Drug Therapy, 1986).

22.4 REPELLENTS

Repellents prevent pests from approaching a treated area or cause them to leave promptly if they do approach. The best-known examples are insect repellents for application to human skin or clothing. Such preparations greatly increase the comfort of people exposed to mosquitoes or other biting species. If the insect or tick is capable of transmitting a disease either directly by biting or by a more indirect means, the use of a repellent will minimize disease transmission.

Repellents effective against field rodents may be used to protect forest tree seeds sown by aircraft until the seeds have time to germinate. Those effective against birds, dogs, and cats can contribute to convenience.

Apparently, little attention has been given to the possibility of protecting field crops from insect pests by means of repellents, and no practical method has been developed along this line. However, some of the insecticides have been reported to have repellent-like activity, and this action may contribute to their overall efficacy. That such an approach to crop protection might hold promise is indicated by the fact that certain vegetables are relatively immune to insect attack. A difficulty that appears likely on *a priori* grounds is that most, if not all, repellents—including those in insect-resistant plants—are volatile. If an effective, safe repellent were available for crops, it might have to be applied so often as to be impractical. There might be no good way to simulate the constant production and availability of repellent accomplished by certain species of plants. In spite of this evident difficulty, the problem deserves more attention. The naturally occurring, effective compounds apparently are of low toxicity, being constituents of wholesome vegetables.

The insect repellents for human use generally have little irritancy. However, exceptions do exist, and some examples with deet will be discussed under Section 22.4.1. It is of some interest that deet, which previously was known only as a synthetic compound, was found to occur naturally in adult female pink bollworm moths in amounts ranging from 0.075 to 0.604 mg/insect; its function is unknown (Jones and Jacobson, 1968).

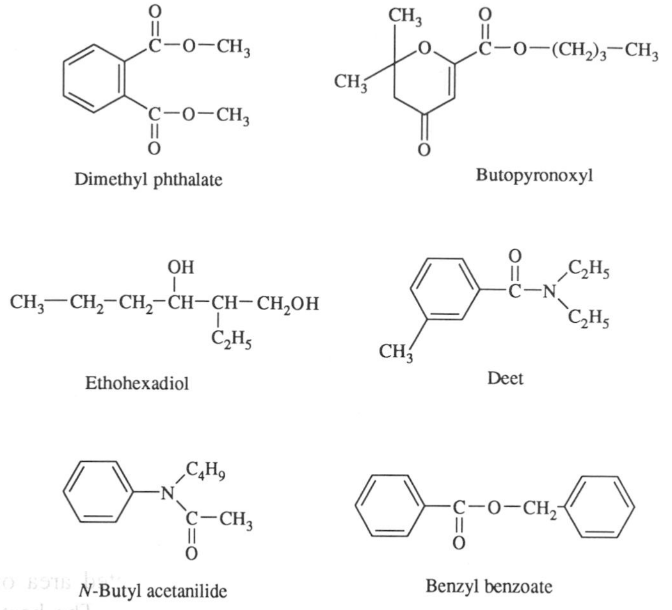

Figure 22.4 Some repellents.

Some repellents are shown in Fig. 22.4; the four at the top are used mainly against insects and the two at the bottom mainly against ticks and chiggers. Ethoxadiol is called Rutgers 6–12, and butopyronoxyl generally is known by a trade name, Indolone®.

22.4.1 DEET

22.4.1.1 Identity, Properties, and Uses

Chemical Name Deet is *N*,*N*-diethyl-3-methylbenzamide or *N*,*N*-diethyl-*m*-toluamide.

Structure See Fig. 22.4.

Synonyms Deet is the common name accepted by ANSI, ESA, and NTMA; diethyltoluamide is accepted in lieu of a common name by BSI and E-ISO. The compound also is known as detamide, *m*-delphene, and metadelphene and by the acronyms DET, DETA, and M-DET. Trade names for some products containing deet include Autan®, Black Flag®, Tabard®, Delphene®, Detamide®, Dieltamide®, Flypel®, *m*-Delphene®, Meta-Delphene®, Muskol®, Naugatuck Det®, Off®, 612 Plus®, Jungle Plus®, and Pellit®. Code designation include ENT 20,218. The CAS registry number is 134-62-3.

Physical and Chemical Properties Deet has the empirical formula $C_{12}H_{17}NO$ and a molecular weight of 191.3. It is a colorless to amber liquid with a boiling point of 111°C at 1 mm Hg. It is practically insoluble in water but miscible with ethyl alcohol, isopropyl alcohol, propylene glycol, and cottonseed oil.

History, Formulations, and Uses Deet was introduced in 1955 by Hercules Incorporated. As an insect repellent, deet is especially effective against mosquitoes. It is usually supplied in an ethyl alcohol or isopropyl alcohol base in concentrations ranging from about 11 to 95%; end-use products are formulated as solutions, lotions, gels, aerosol sprays, sticks, and impregnated towelettes (Robbins and Cherniack, 1986). Technical deet is 95% *m* isomer. The *o* and *p* isomers, which are highly repellent but less effective than the *m* isomer, are contaminants of technical grade deet.

22.4.1.2 Toxicity to Laboratory Animals

Basic Findings The acute oral LD 50 values were about 3000 mg/kg in male rats and about 2000 mg/kg in females (Ambrose *et al.*, 1959; Carpenter *et al.*, 1974; Macko and Weeks, 1980). Rats killed by dosages in the LD 50 range showed lacrimation, chromodacryorrhea, depression, prostration, tremors, and asphyxial convulsions; respiratory failure usually preceded cardiac failure (Ambrose *et al.*, 1959).

In rabbits, an intravenous dosage of 75 mg/kg was rapidly fatal, but 50 mg/kg was not. Five doses at the rate of 25 mg/kg/day produced no cumulative effect, except for injury of the intima of some veins used for injection (Ambrose *et al.*, 1959).

The acute dermal LD 50 of deet to rabbits was about 3180 mg/kg (Carpenter *et al.*, 1974). Ambrose *et al.* (1959) found that single dermal applications to rabbits at rates of about 2000 or 4000 mg/kg produced no systemic effect but did produce mild to moderate erythema. Repeated dermal application of 50% solutions for 13 weeks at the rate of about 200 mg/kg/day produced no evidence of systemic toxicity but did produce desquamation, coriaceousness, dryness, and fissuring in the same species. Except for some scarring, these lesions cleared within 3 weeks. Instillation of deet into the eyes of rabbits produced mild to moderate edema of the nictitating membrane, lacrimation, conjunctivitis, and some corneal injury, as revealed by fluorescein staining. After 5 days all eyes appeared normal (Ambrose *et al.*, 1959). The irritating effects of deet at the dermal application site and to the eye have been corroborated by others (Carpenter *et al.*, 1974; Wong and Yew, 1978; Macko and Weeks, 1980). No sensitization was seen in guinea pigs (Ambrose *et al.*, 1959).

Repeated dermal application to horses produced hypersteatosis, an overactivity of the sebaceous glands, when the solution of deet was 15% or higher (Palmer, 1969). Apparently, this particular form of dermatitis has not been described in other species.

No systematic toxicity was observed in rats exposed 8 hr/day, 5 days/week, for 7 weeks to air saturated with deet. No toxic effects were observed in rats exposed for 6 hr to an aerosol of deet. No gross or significant histological changes were seen (Ambrose *et al.*, 1959). An exudate from the nose and eyes of rats and nausea and vomiting in dogs were seen when these animals were exposed for 13 weeks to deet at 1500 mg/m³ and 750–1500 mg/m³, respectively (Macko and Bergman, 1979).

When rats were fed deet at a dietary level of 10,000 ppm for about 200 days, their growth was decreased without a decrease in food intake. There was a significant increase in the relative weight of the testes and liver in males, of the liver and spleen in females, and of the kidneys in both males and females. Some of these changes were seen in lesser degree at a dietary level of 1000 ppm. No gross or significant histological changes were seen at any dietary level, and no changes of any kind were observed at 100 or 500 ppm (about 25 mg/kg/day) (Ambrose *et al.*, 1959).

Similar results were found in other subacute dermal and feeding studies with deet in rats, rabbits, and dogs. In these oral studies, 2000 ppm proved to be a no-effect level. Oral administration of deet to dogs at rates of 100 and 300 mg/kg/day caused tremor and hyperactivity and occasional vomiting, but no other effects. Blood studies (hemoglobin, hematocrit, sedimentation rate, platelet counts, total and differential white cell counts) on dogs receiving 300 mg/kg orally or dermally or on rabbits receiving 300 mg/kg dermally revealed no effect on the hematopoetic system (Keplinger *et al.*, 1961).

Rabbits receiving 528 mg/kg of deet for 15 days had a progressive decrease in body weight. Serum calcium levels were decreased, and cholesterol and triglyceride levels were increased. No other signs of toxicity were apparent (Haight *et al.*, 1979).

Either *o*-DET or *p*-DET or both occur as impurities in commercial *m*-DET (deet). A thorough study of the *o* and *p* isomers showed that the *o* isomer is slightly more toxic than the others (oral LD 50 1210 mg/kg in rats). However, no alarming difference was found, and it was concluded that the presence of 5% of *o*-DET or *p*-DET as impurities in the insect repellent is not a serious health problem (Ambrose and Yost, 1965).

Absorption, Distribution, Metabolism, and Excretion There have been numerous studies both *in vivo* and *in vitro* of the penetration of topically applied deet into and through the skin of mice, rats, dogs, pigs, guinea pigs, and rabbits (Schmidt *et al.*, 1959; Gleiberman and Voronkina, 1972; Gleiberman *et al.*, 1975; Blomquist and Thorsell, 1977; Lurie *et al.*, 1978; Reifenrath *et al.*, 1980, 1981, 1984; Snodgrass *et al.*, 1982; Hawkins and Reifenrath, 1986). Following movement through the skin, deet is absorbed and distributed rather rapidly. For example, topically applied radioactive deet reached a maximum concentration in the blood by 1 hr postapplication; it was almost completely eliminated from the blood within 1–3 days (Lurie *et al.*, 1978). Deet is rapidly eliminated mainly in the urine and to a lesser extent in the feces (Lurie *et al.*, 1978; Snodgrass *et al.*, 1982). Although the metabolites of deet have yet to be completely characterized, Christensen *et al.* (1969) found *m*-toluric, hippuric, and benzoic acids in urine of rats and rabbits exposed to deet in aerosol form; no unchanged deet was detected. By use of autoradiography following intravenous injection of radiocarbon-labeled deet into mice, high tissue levels were found initially in the liver, kidney, lacrimal gland, and nasal mucosa. Very soon, concentrations higher than that in blood were found

in the thyroid and brown fat. Concentrations were highest and most persistent in the lacrimal gland. Concentrations in the fetus remained lower than those in the mother. By 4 hr after injection, very little radioactivity remained in any tissue, except the lacrimal gland (Blomquist *et al.*, 1975). Deet does cross the placenta (Blomquist *et al.*, 1975; Gleiberman *et al.*, 1976; Snodgrass *et al.*, 1982); however, pregnant rabbits receiving repeated dermal applications of deet throughout gestation showed no evidence of bioaccumulation in maternal tissue or individual fetuses (Snodgrass *et al.*, 1982).

Pharmacological Effects At an *in vitro* concentration of 200 ppm, deet decreased the amplitude of rhythmic contraction of rat uterus, and at 10 ppm it had a similar effect on the ileum. Contractions were restored by washing, and the responses to acetylcholine and barium chloride were not altered (Ambrose *et al.*, 1959).

The intravenous injection of anesthetized rabbits with deet at a rate of 5 mg/kg produced a slight, evanescent fall in blood pressure. Larger dosages produced a more pronounced and sustained effect (Ambrose *et al.*, 1959).

Leach *et al.*, (1987) examined the cardiovascular effects of deet in rats and dogs. When anesthetized rats were treated intraperitoneally with 75% deet in ethyl alcohol at dosages of 225, 125, and 63 mg/kg, a dose-related drop in mean blood pressure was observed within 30 min; heart rate also was reduced at 225 mg/kg. Dogs similarly treated at 225 mg/kg had decreased blood pressure, heart rate, and cardiac output, along with minor changes in the electrocardiogram. Deet at 225 mg/kg also reduced the responsiveness of anesthetized rats to exogenous acetylcholine, indicating that the hypotensive effects of the repellent might be due partly to an interaction with cholinergic systems.

Effects on Organs and Tissues Stenbäck (1977) treated mice and rabbits cutaneously on their back and ear, respectively, with 20, 10, and 2 mg of deet twice a week for their lifetime. No deet-related tumors were found.

Swentzel (1977), in a dominant lethal study, treated male mice orally with deet at 600 mg/kg. No evidence of mutagenicity was observed during an 8-week mating period. Further, there was no evidence of mutagenicity of deet in a bacterial plate assay (Ficsor and Nii Lo Piccolo, 1972).

Effects on Reproduction When deet was applied to the skin of rats at 1000 mg/kg/day throughout pregnancy, implantation was reduced significantly. Prenatal mortality was 34.1%, compared with 20.9% in the control. No teratogenic effect was detected. Mortality between birth and weaning was 44%, compared to 15.7% in the control. Injury was less, but probably significant, at a dosage of 100 mg/kg/day throughout pregnancy (Gleiberman *et al.*, 1975). In a subsequent study, Gleiberman *et al.* (1976) applied deet topically to the skin of male and female rats at 1000 or 100 mg/kg/day for periods of 1–6 months. Residues of deet were detected in brain, adrenals, and adipose tissue and in the placenta and embryos even when its administration to females was discontinued prior to pregnancy. Deet residues in offspring persisted throughout the 4-month observation period following termination of treatment. Dose- and time-related effects included decreased motility of spermatozoa, increased proportion of abnormal spermatozoa, decreased number of corpora lutea, increased embryonic and postnatal mortality, decreased weight of offspring, and retarded development of offspring. Lebowitz *et al.* (1981, 1983) administered deet dermally at 1000, 300, and 100 mg/kg/day to male rats 5days/week for 9 weeks. Evaluation of sperm at 35, 65, and 95 days revealed no toxicity or sperm head abnormalities, perhaps because of the relatively short period of dosing. Although weight changes were observed in livers and kidneys, no changes in weight of testes or testicular histopathology were found. Testicular hypertrophy in rats, however, was found in long-term feeding studies with deet (Ambrose *et al.*, 1959).

Angerhofer and Weeks (1981) treated pregnant rabbits from day 1 through day 29 of gestation with daily dermal doses of deet in ethyl alcohol at 1000, 500, 100, and 50 mg/kg/day. All maternal and fetal indices were within normal limits.

Kuhlman *et al.* (1981) injected fertilized white leghorn chicken eggs with about 243 μg of deet in mineral oil at various times during the second incubation day. Forty-one percent of the embryos survived to day 15 of incubation; 33% of them had gross malformations including ventricular septal defects, abnormal aortic arch patterns, rumplessness, malrotated limbs, absence of limbs, and some defects of the central nervous system. The mineral oil carrier also induced mortality.

Some, but not all, of the studies mentioned above would indicate that deet has appreciable reproductive and teratologic toxicity. Although a conclusion regarding these points must await additional research, results of some of the ongoing and/or unpublished studies cited by Robbins and Cherniack (1986) provide a basis for suggesting that deet may have little, if any, reproductive toxicity and teratogenic activity in laboratory animals.

Behavioral Effects   Groups of male and female rats were exposed to deet aerosols at concentrations of 4100, 2900, or 2300 mg/m³ for 4 hr or at concentrations of 1500, 750, or 250 mg/m³ for 6 hr/day, 5 days/week, for 13 weeks. A battery of behavioral tests measuring balance, endurance, activity, tactile sensitivity, learning and recall was administered immediately upon termination of exposure. Concentration-dependent behavioral changes were observed (Sherman, 1979a,b; Sherman *et al.*, 1980).

Factors Influencing Toxicity   Liu *et al.* (1984) found that pretreatment of rats with deet had a biphasic effect on the hypnotic activity of pentobarbital. When administered orally to rats at 400 mg/kg 1, 2, or 6 hr prior to intraperitoneal injection of pentobarbital at 25 mg/kg, sleeping time was prolonged by 2- to 6- fold. However, when administered 0.5, 1, 2, 3, or 6 days before pentobarbital, sleeping time was shortened markedly. The increase in sleeping time was associated with increased brain and plasma levels of pentobarbital and, according to the

authors, an increase in pentobarbital hydroxylase activity. The decrease in sleeping time was associated with decreased brain and plasma levels and a decrease in liver pentobarbital hydroxylase activity.

Pathology   In the studies of Ambrose *et al.* (1959) with rats and rabbits, no significant deet-related gross or histopathological lesions were found; a few rats that died following lethal doses of deet in propylene glycol or neat showed varying degrees of hyperemia of the gastrointestinal tract. Gross and microscopic examination of organs from dogs, rats, and rabbits treated with deet revealed slight damage to rabbit kidneys typical of that associated with burns of the skin, but no effects were observed on 13 other organs including liver, spleen, and bone marrow (Keplinger *et al.*, 1961).

22.4.1.3 Toxicity to Humans

Experimental Exposure   Application of deet to the face and arms of five volunteers daily for 5 consecutive days produced only slight irritation of the face and nose and some desquamation about the nose. Similar changes, plus dryness of the face and a slight tingling sensation, occurred among those who received applications for 3 consecutive days/week for 6 weeks, but all symptoms disappeared during each 4-day period of rest (Ambrose *et al.*, 1959). Phillips *et al.* (1972), in their study of the irritancy of 12 compounds topically applied to the ventral aspects of the forearms or to the backs of male volunteers, found that deet did not have significant irritancy potential when tested by several different protocols.

In studies of the penetration of deet, Smith *et al.* (1963) found that from 7 to 13% of a topical treatment of about 1 mg/cm² and from 9% of a dose of 1.86 mg/cm² to 56% of a dose of 0.077 mg/cm² penetrated the skin of volunteers. Feldmann and Maibach (1970) observed that only 16% of a topical application to the forearm at 4 μg/cm² penetrated during a 96-hr interval. In their *in vitro* study, Reifenrath and Robinson (1982) found that the penetration of deet into and through human abdominal skin was 29.8% (29.6% remained in skin, 0.2% penetrated) at 1 hr after application of the lower concentration and 36.3% (29.7% remained in skin, 6.6% penetrated) at 12 hrs following application of the higher concentration.

Blomquist and Thorsell (1977) applied 250 μCi of radiocarbon-labeled deet in 0.030 ml of 25% absolute ethyl alcohol on a 9-cm² area of the forearm of a male volunteer and monitored the total radioactivity in the urine for 48 hr; the experiment was repeated in the same volunteer. Eight hours following each application, the treated area was washed with 10 ml of absolute ethyl alcohol, recovering 8 and 15%, respectively, of the applied radioactivity. During the two 48-hr experiments, 5.5 and 3.8% of the applied radioactivity were recovered in the urine. The nature of the urinary radioactivity was not reported. In other experiments, deet was detected in the urine of some (Wu *et al.*, 1979) but not all (Christensen *et al.*, 1969) volunteers following topical application. Wu *et al.* (1979) estimated that from 10 to 14% of a topical dose of deet was eliminated in the urine as the parent compound during the first hour after treatment. In addition to deet, two metabolites were identified in the urine. One, m-carboxyl-N,N-diethylbenzoylamide, was formed by oxidation of the tolyl methyl moiety. The other, N-hydroxyethyl-N-ethyl-m-toluamide glucuronide, was formed by N-ethyl hydroxylation and subsequent conjugation with glucuronic acid.

Accidents and Use Experience   Use experience with deet has been excellent, from the standpoints of both effectiveness and safety. However, deleterious side effects have been reported in a few cases following the use of deet as recommended in addition to those resulting from chronic overdosage and accidental ingestions of the repellent.

Four cases of side effects, including contact dermatitis, conjunctivitis, and exacerbation of seborrhea and acne vulgaris, were observed in a study of 85 persons who used between 4 and 6 ml of a 40% alcoholic solution of deet once or twice daily for prolonged periods. The preparation also was capable of causing local eye irritation (Rabinovich, 1966). Fifty-eight workers engaged in the manufacture of deet lotion (DETA-20) were examined for occupational exposure; 14 developed severe skin disease. It was indicated that direct contact with deet causes disturbances of the local thermoregulation reaction, not only in the skin damage area but also in intact areas (Prishchepov et al., 1981).

More serious dermatological manifestations associated with the use of deet have been described. A bullous eruption was observed in the antecubital fossae of some military personnel in South Vietnam. In every instance the first indication of the eruption was noticed in the morning on awakening from sleep in the field. At first the cause was thought to be a vesicating insect of the genus *Paederus*. Eventually it was realized that the eruption occurred only in those who had used deet. The repellent issued to the military is 75% deet in 25% ethyl alcohol or dichlorodifluoromethane, depending on whether it is used as a liquid or as a spray under pressure. It was concluded that the restricted distribution of the dermatitis (mainly antecubital fossae, occasionally popliteal fossae) was due at least in part to occlusion and sweating of the affected parts. When first seen in the morning in the field, one or sometimes both antecubital fossae were red and tender. Within the next hours, blisters developed on the tender base. The blisters remained intact for 1–3 days and then broke down, leaving an area that remained eroded and purulent for 2–3 weeks. During this period, the dermatitis was disabling; the arm could not be extended because of pain. The degree of skin necrosis was sufficient that permanent scarring remained in most cases. The condition was reproduced using 75% deet in some of 63 volunteer military personnel in DaNang and 14 in Oakland, California. Further testing of some of those with positive reactions with 5% deet in petrolatum or with ethyl alcohol alone yielded no dermatitis, even in the antecubital fossae. It was suggested that deet not be applied to regions of skin flexion such as the antecubital and popliteal areas (Lamberg and Mulrennan, 1969). Reuveni and Yagupsky (1982) reported a similar bullous eruption in ten 18–20-year-old soldiers with a history of local use of 50% deet 18–24 hr earlier.

The repellent had been applied to the uncovered skin of the face, neck, upper part of the trunk, and legs before sleep. In each case, there was sudden onset of a burning sensation and erythema of the antecubital fossa of one or both arms that progressed to hemorrhagic blisters which drained spontaneously after 1–2 days, and in some cases deep ulcerations and scarring remained.

Maibach and Johnson (1975) reported the results of an investigation of a 35-year-old woman for presumed allergy to insect repellents. She had used several repellents on frequent camping trips and noticed that a "red, raised lesion" appeared about 30 min after application. Open patch testing on the forearm with "pure" deet revealed, within 20 min, a macular erythema that evolved into a wheal-and-flare response. Similar tests with dimethyl phthalate and butopyronoxyl were negative. The response was passively transferred, suggesting a possible immunologic mechanism. It was indicated that this particular case of contact urticaria was of immediate-type hypersensitivity (stage 1). An immunological mechanism also was shown in a 4-year-old boy who developed contact urticaria following application of deet (von Mayenburg and Rakoski, 1983). A case of anaphylactic hypersensitivity associated with deet was described by Miller (1982). A 42-year-old woman with no prior atopic history touched a companion who had just sprayed himself with repellent containing 52% deet. Generalized pruritus rapidly developed and progressed to generalized angioedema. The woman became nauseated and unconscious en route to hospital, where her blood pressure was found to be 70/40 mm Hg. She responded to treatment with epinephrine, diphenhydramine, and corticosteroids. Periorbital edema developed after another exposure to deet 1 week later. In a controlled setting, a small amount of deet in isopropyl alcohol was applied to the patient's forearm. Pruritus occurred in the treated area within 15 sec and progressed to localized urticaria despite immediate washing of the arm. The patient was treated with epinephrine and diphenhydramine when she reported pruritis of lips and the contralateral arm. She responded to therapy, but the localized urticaria lasted for over 1 hr. Isopropyl alcohol alone elicited no response.

Several cases of a deet-associated toxic encephalopathy have been reported in young females. A 3.5-year-old girl suffered a bizarre illness after all of a 180 ml aerosol can of deet (Off®) had been used each evening for 2 weeks to spray her and her nightclothes and bedding. Because of this exposure and because careful medical examination failed to suggest any other cause, the possibility was considered that deet was the cause. However, it was pointed out that, even if the child had absorbed all of the deet discharged from the aerosol can, the dosage of active ingredient would have been only 0.14 ml/kg/day, a level tolerated by animals. The signs were disorientation, staggering gait, slurred speech, and episodes consisting of stiffening into a sitting position, crying out, extending the extremities, flexing the fingers, and dorsiflexing the toes. Therapy, which began 1 day after onset, was symptomatic. Recovery was complete in 4 days (Gryboski et al., 1961). Zadikoff (1979) described two cases. One involved a 5-year-old girl who had been sprayed with 10%

deet (Mylol®) nightly for almost 3 months. She was referred to the hospital following 10 days of progressively worsening headaches; prior to admission she was unduly agitated and mildly disoriented. On the day of her admission, she had slurred speech, severe confusion, ataxia, and a generalized convulsion. She had constant involuntary movements involving the head, trunk, and limbs. Athetosis and wild thrashing movements alternating with short periods of quiet and episodes of marked shaking and crying or screaming were present. She was treated for meningitis, but there was no improvement in her condition. She continued to have convulsions, developed pneumonia which cleared, deteriorated steadily, and died 24 hr after admission. The second case involved a 1.5-year-old girl who was admitted to the hospital following ingestion of an unknown, but probably small, amount of Mylol® the previous day. She also was extremely irritable and lay in an opisthotonic posture. She displayed bizarre movements with periods of shaking and crying. On examination, no localizing neurologic deficit was found; however, muscle stretch reflexes were depressed. She improved slowly over a 6-week period and was discharged, although her head control was not yet normal and her tendon reflexes remained depressed (Zadikoff, 1979). Heick *et al.* (1980) described the case of a 6-year-old girl who had used a spray containing 15% deet on at least 10 occasions on extensive areas of the skin. She presented with a 4-day history of lethargy, mood changes, and nightmares. Many of her subsequent signs and symptoms were similar to those above. Her condition steadily deteriorated and required assisted ventilation and peritoneal dialysis. Electroencephalograms on hospital days 7 and 8 were flat and supportive therapy discontinued on day 8. A different diagnosis of Reye's syndrome or ornithine carbamoyltransferase deficiency was made based on laboratory findings and previous history. The mother also had low hepatic levels of this enzyme (Heick *et al.*, 1980). Pronczuk de Garbino and Laborde (1983) reported the case of a 17-month-old girl admitted to hospital with acute encephalopathy of unknown etiology. However, for 3 weeks prior to admission she had received frequent skin applications of a deet-containing lotion. Deterioration was rapid and death ensued. Another case of toxic encephalopathy, described by Roland *et al.* (1985), involved an 8-year-old girl who was hospitalized for recurrent seizures and behavior change. Four days prior to admission she had begun to apply copious amounts of 15% deet (Off®), and 2 days later a raised, erythematous, pruritic rash developed mainly on the face and extremities; altered behavior also was noted. The next day she applied "100%" deet (Muskol®). During the night she had a brief convulsion with clonic movements of all limbs; about 5 hr later she had a second seizure and was taken to the hospital, where she had a third seizure. The child received phenytoin therapy. The restlessness settled, the rash faded, and she apparently recovered completely. At least three other cases of encephalopathy in individuals of unspecified sex and age following ingestion of deet have been reported. The onset, signs, and symptoms were similar to those mentioned above. Following treatment, recovery was complete (Tenebein, 1981). The fact that most, if not all, of these deet-related toxic encephalopathies

involved only young females is both intriguing and surprising, since one would expect repellent use to be at least as great and probably greater among males. Heick *et al.* (1980) had good reason to suspect that their patient was heterozygous for ornithine carbamoyltransferase activity. Further, they conjectured that it was possible the other young females also had a similar deficiency. This condition is sex-linked and is fatal in males during the neonatal period but of variable severity in females. It was suggested that drugs that are considered safe in the normal population may produce catastrophic effects in patients with an unrecognized genetic susceptibility (Heick *et al.*, 1980).

A rather bizarre case of acute manic psychosis occurred in a 30-year-old man following self-medication with 75% deet for a papular, truncal, erythematous rash that was later diagnosed as pityriasis rosea. It was his recollection that he had used deet successfully to treat a similar condition 4 years previously. Beginning 2 weeks prior to admission to the hospital, he daily applied deet on one side of his body and entered a homemade sauna for 60–90 min; he emerged from the sauna, treated the other side of his body, and reentered the sauna for another 60–90 min. This procedure was continued for 1 week. He was occasionally lethargic and incoherent following the deet-sauna treatment. Four days prior to admission, he developed marked personality changes that included delusions of grandeur and verbal aggressivity. He became more irritable and belligerent and was admitted to the hospital, where he required seclusion because of his violent behavior. His condition worsened and was diagnosed as acute manic psychosis. By the sixth hospital day, he was more calm, more cooperative, and accepted haloperidol medication. He had previously refused haloperidol and lithium carbonate. He continued to improve, the medication was discontinued on day 8, and he was discharged on day 10. No recurrence of dermatologic or psychiatric symptoms was reported on follow-up 3 months later. Analysis of urine collected on hospital day 8 revealed the presence of free deet at a concentration of 0.18 ppm; gas chromatographic–mass spectrometric (GC–MS) analyses revealed the presence of ions with molecular weights of 163, 191, 207, 235, 221, and 249, and it was suggested that they possibly represented *N*-ethyl-*m*-toluamide, deet, and hydroxylated, methylated, and oxidized metabolites, respectively. Since resolution of the patient's symptoms began within 72 hr of hospitalization and was complete within 6 days, the clinical course was atypical for classic endogenous mania. Other than the exposure to deet, there was nothing in the results of tests made during hospitalization or in the patient's family history that provided insight into the etiology of the illness (Snyder *et al.*, 1986).

Atypical Cases of Various Origins An 18-year-old man was admitted to hospital because of jaundice 1 day in duration. For 24 or 36 hr he had noted dark urine, clay-colored stools, and itching, but felt well. Past history indicated celiac disease as an infant and an undiagnosed febrile illness that began 2 weeks before onset of the jaundice and that lasted only 1 day. Except for jaundice and associated findings, the results of examination on admission were normal; specifically, the red cell count, hemoglobin, white cell count, and percentages of polymorphonuclear lymphocytes were normal. A few purpuric areas in the skin were considered to be associated with the jaundice. During the next day or two, several new purpuric or ecchymotic areas appeared, and the patient began bleeding from the gums and the postnasal area. The red cell count had fallen to 4,500,000, the hemoglobin to 13.5 gm %, the white cell count to 3600, the polymorphonuclear lymphocytes to 29%, and the platelet count to 88,000. Bleeding continued, and the blood picture worsened. Several bone marrow studies revealed aplasia. The patient did not respond to treatment with prednisone, antibiotics, and transfusions. Bleeding increased, both externally and into the tissues. During the last few days, the temperature rose as high as 40.56°C and remained elevated for about 48 hr. The patient died following a generalized convulsive seizure, less than a month after onset. Recognized exposures included one 4-mg chlorpheniramine tablet 2 or 3 months before onset, one aspirin tablet 2 weeks before onset, two vaccines (DPT and poliomyelitis) administered separately 1 day or less before onset, and deet applied as an aerosol for "several weeks" before onset (Beckerman, 1960).

Two sisters exposed to large amounts of deet, piperonyl butoxide, *N*-octylbicycloheptene dicarboximide (MGK 264®), allethrin, and dichlorvos, during their first trimester of pregnancy each gave birth to a male with coarctation of the aorta (Hall *et al.*, 1975).

Laboratory Findings An 18-year-old woman, who was killed by an oncoming train, was found to have ingested deet. Analysis of postmortem specimens revealed levels of deet (corrected for recovery) of 767 mg in stomach and contents, 51 ppm in liver, 6.4 ppm in blood, and 0.4 ppm in urine; the identity of deet in these four extracts was confirmed by mass spectrometry (Crowley *et al.*, 1986).

Pathology The brain of the 5-year-old girl showed generalized edema with intense congestion of brain and meninges. Cerebral vessels showed swelling of endothelial cells; there was no perivenous or other demyelination and no perivascular infiltrate. No evidence of meningitis was found (Zadikoff, 1979). In the other reported fatality (Heick *et al.*, 1980), the brain, which weighed 1460 gm, also was edematous and soft. The cerebellar tonsils were necrotic and portions of necrotic cerebellum had herniated down around the spinal cord. Alzheimer type II astrocytes were present in the putamen. The liver was enlarged (642 gm) but otherwise normal in appearance. However, most liver parenchymal cells were foamy and contained abundant glycogen. Centrilobular liver cells were vacuolated and contained fat dispersed in fine droplets. Liver biopsy taken just prior to death showed mild mitochondrial pleomorphism, possible loss of dense bodies, and minor abnormalities of cristae. The smooth endoplasmic reticulum was distended and contained an unidentified material (Heick *et al.*, 1980).

Treatment of Poisoning Treatment is symptomatic.

22.4.2 BENZYL BENZOATE

22.4.2.1 Identity, Properties, and Uses

Chemical Name Benzyl benzoate is benzoic acid phenylmethyl ester.

Structure See Fig. 22.4.

Synonyms Trade names for some products containing benzyl benzoate include Ascarbin®, Ascabiol®, Benylate®, Scabanca®, Tenutex®, Vanzoate®, and Venzoate®. The CAS registry number is 120-51-4.

Physical and Chemical Properties Benzyl benzoate has the empirical formula $C_{14}H_{12}O_2$ and a molecular weight of 212.2. It exists as leaflets with a melting point of 21°C or as an oily liquid with a boiling point of 323–324°C and a specific gravity of 1.1210 at 16.5°C. It has a faint, pleasant, aromatic odor and a sharp, burning taste. Benzyl benzoate is insoluble in water or glycerol but miscible with alcohol, chloroform, ether, oils, acetone, and benzene. It is hydrolyzed to benzoic acid and benzyl alcohol in the presence of alkali.

History, Formulation, and Uses In addition to being prepared synthetically, benzyl benzoate occurs naturally in balsams of Peru and Tolu and certain other essential oils. In liquid formulation (300 gm/liter), it is used on humans as a repellent for chiggers, ticks, and mosquitoes. Formulated in emulsions or lotions (200–350 gm/liter) it is used on humans as an acaricide (scabicide). For veterinary application, benzyl benzoate is used as a scabicide and pediculicide; however, its use on cats is contraindicated. Other nonpesticidal uses for benzyl benzoate include solvent, camphor substitute, and perfume fixative; it also can be found in some confectionery and chewing gum flavors.

22.4.2.2 Toxicity to Laboratory Animals

Basic Findings Benzyl benzoate is of low toxicity to laboratory animals. The following acute oral LD 50 values have been reported: 2800 mg/kg (Graham and Kuizenga, 1945) and 1906 mg/kg (Draize *et al.*, 1948) for rats; 1569 mg/kg for mice (Draize *et al.*, 1948); 1121 mg/kg for guinea pigs (Draize *et al.*, 1948); 2018 mg/kg (Draize *et al.*, 1948) and 1680 mg/kg (Graham and Kuizenga, 1945) for rabbits; >22,440 mg/kg for dogs (Graham and Kuizenga, 1945); and 2240 mg/kg for cats (Graham and Kuizenga, 1945). A dog also was reported to have survived a single oral dose of 7847 mg without harmful effects (Macht, 1918). Thus, dogs can tolerate oral doses of benzyl benzoate of about 10 times the quantity that is lethal to rats, rabbits, and cats. The acute dermal LD 50 to rats is 4484 mg/kg, and the 90-day subacute dermal LD 50 to rabbits is 2242 mg/kg (Draize *et al.*, 1948). Dogs have survived six local applications on their backs of 112 or 224 gm each without toxic symptoms (Graham and Kuizenga, 1945). However, one local application of 22,420 mg and two local applications of 8408 mg each were lethal to cats; cats receiving the single and multiple doses survived for 22 and about 48 hr, respectively (Graham and Kuizenga, 1945). Cats receiving 33% benzyl benzoate in isopropyl alcohol (two doses of 22,420 mg each), ethyl alcohol (two doses of 22,420 mg each), or water (three doses of 22,420 mg each) locally died at 43, 46, and 69 hr after treatment, respectively (Graham and Kuizenga, 1945). Upon subcutaneous and/or intramuscular injection, the minimum lethal dosage was 2242–3363 mg/kg for rats, 561 mg/kg for mice, 1121 mg/kg for guinea pigs, about 2242 mg/kg for rabbits, and 1212–1686 mg/kg for cats (Macht, 1918). A dosage of 2242 mg/kg administered subcutaneously or intraperitoneally was not fatal to dogs, but about 1682 mg/kg administered intravenously was lethal (Macht, 1918).

Signs of poisoning manifested by animals receiving toxic oral doses of benzyl benzoate included salivation, piloerection, muscular incoordination, tremors, progressive paralysis of hind limbs, prostration, violent convulsions, dyspnea, and death, which usually was preceded by respiratory paralysis (Graham and Kuizenga, 1945). Death of rabbits treated with a large single dermal dose of benzyl benzoate was delayed, and the animals died without exhibiting prior symptoms of systemic effects (Draize et al., 1948). Cats receiving a lethal dermal dose of benzyl benzoate exhibited excessive salivation and twitching of the treated areas of their backs. Generalized tremors, muscular incoordination, paralysis of hind limbs, convulsions, respiratory failure, and death followed. In some instances, the cats remained prostrate following the convulsive seizures for many hours prior to death. All of the cats that died lost from 200 to 400 gm in weight, probably as a result of decreased intakes of food and water (Macht, 1918). In rabbits, benzyl benzoate was reported to cause very mild gross skin irritation (Draize et al., 1948).

Absorption, Distribution, Metabolism, and Excretion
Benzyl benzoate is rapidly absorbed and hydrolyzed to benzoic acid and benzyl alcohol. The benzyl alcohol is subsequently oxidized to benzoic acid (Williams, 1959). The metabolism of benzoic acid does not differ significantly whether the compound is administered as such or produced metabolically (Testa and Jenner, 1976). Benzoic acid is conjugated with glycine to yield benzoylglycine (hippuric acid) and with glucuronic acid to yield benzoylglucuronic acid. These conjugates are eliminated in the urine in varying ratios depending on species and dose. Herbivorous animals excrete benzoic acid almost entirely as hippuric acid, whereas carnivores and omnivores usually excrete moderate to high levels of the glucuronide (Williams, 1959).

Pharmacological and Biochemical Effects The initial pharmacological studies of benzyl benzoate were conducted by Macht (1918). Using chiefly rabbits, dogs, and cats, he found that the compound had actions on smooth muscle and on the respiratory, circulatory, and central nervous systems. Effects of benzyl benzoate on smooth muscle organs, including the intestine, urinary bladder, gallbladder, and uterus, consisted of inhibition of contractions, lowering of tonicity, and relaxation of

spasm. Although large oral doses and small injected doses resulted in no appreciable change in respiration, very large doses, especially when administered intravenously, tended to depress respiration, and death after lethal doses occurred from paralysis of the respiratory center. In small animals, such as mice, rats, and guinea pigs, effects on respiration were seen even after subcutaneous treatment. Following injection of benzyl benzoate, a fall in blood pressure was observed which was due to peripheral vasodilation resulting from the action of the compound on the smooth muscle of the arterial walls. This depressor effect was found when benzyl benzoate was injected intramuscularly, subcutaneously, intraperitoneally, and intravenously, but was most pronounced following the latter route. Actions on the vasomotor center and the heart were deemed insignificant. Oral doses of benzyl benzoate were without striking effect on the central nervous system; however, spastic convulsions were present following injection of large doses. In mice, guinea pigs, and cats following paralysis of the respiratory center, death was preceded by convulsions (Macht, 1918).

These actions of benzyl benzoate on laboratory animals generally were corroborated and extended by Mason and Pieck (1920), Nielsen and Higgins (1920, 1921), and Gruber (1923a,b). In their study of the effects of benzyl benzoate administered intravenously to anesthetized dogs, Nielsen and Higgins (1920, 1921) noted a marked relaxation of intestinal muscles, a diminution of barium chloride-induced intestinal contractions, a lowering of blood pressure, and a decrease in respiration. Gruber (1923a), working with anesthetized and unanesthetized dogs, found that orally administered benzyl benzoate produced no change in blood pressure, a result that differed from those of Macht (1918), Mason and Pieck (1920), and Nielsen and Higgins (1921) in which the drug was injected. When given orally, benzyl benzoate did not alter the pulse rate (Gruber, 1923a). Moderately large doses of benzyl benzoate accelerated respiration but decreased the depth, whereas large doses paralyzed the respiratory center. Repeated injections caused edema of the lungs, fluid in the bronchioles, and marked passive congestion of the lower and middle lobes due probably to emboli (Gruber, 1923b). Gruber (1923b) also observed that repeated intravenous injections of benzyl benzoate into dogs, cats, or rabbits caused a permanent increase in the pressure of the superior vena cava and lowered arterial pressure. Moreover, one moderate dose temporarily increased the pressure in the superior vena cava. Comparatively large doses lowered blood pressure; moderate doses increased pressure on some occasions and were without effect on others. Benzyl benzoate was more toxic to the auricles than to the ventricles, and it was observed that the compound may paralyze heart muscle before the respiratory center. Other effects on the heart included increased volume in most cases and paroxysmal flutter approaching fibrillation, pulsus alternans, and trigeminal pulse following large doses. Benzyl benzoate had the same action on blood vessels in the perfused kidney and limb (vasodilation) as it had on vessels of the intact intestine (Gruber, 1923b).

Benzyl benzoate also has emetic, cathartic, narcotic, antipyretic, and diuretic actions in laboratory animals. In some cases, oral treatment of animals produced emesis. It was concluded that this was due to local irritation of the alimentary canal and not to excitation of the vomiting center, since subcutaneous and intramuscular injections of the same dosage did not induce vomiting (Gruber, 1923a). The cathartic activity observed in some animals receiving moderate doses of benzyl benzoate also was thought to result from local irritation (Gruber, 1923a). A slight narcosis was observed in dogs given huge dosages (1021 mg/kg) of benzyl benzoate (Gruber, 1923a). Oral administration of benzyl benzoate also was effective in reducing hyperpyrexia in rabbits induced by some but not all methods. This action was thought to be due almost entirely to a greater dissipation of heat through dilation of blood vessels (Macht and Leach, 1929). A diuretic effect was observed when dogs or rabbits were administered benzyl benzoate intravenously, intramuscularly, or intraperitoneally. The latent period between intraperitoneal injection and the beginning of increased urine secretion was 19 min; a 215% increase in urine flow was found. Diuresis occurred even after pyloric sphincter ligation; thus it was not due to relaxation of smooth muscles permitting rapid emptying of fluid contents of the stomach into the intestine (Gruber, 1924).

Effects on Reproduction Pregnant rats were fed benzyl benzoate in their diet at 10,000 ppm from the beginning of gestation to 21 days postparturition. No external, skeletal, or visceral abnormalities in the fetuses were observed (Morita et al., 1981).

Pathology Inanition was present in rabbits treated dermally with benzyl benzoate daily for 90 days. Survivors at the two highest levels (dosages not specified) had atrophy of testes and possibly increased incidence of focal nephritis and encephalitis (Draize et al., 1948).

Treatment of Poisoning Treatment of benzyl benzoate poisoning in animals would be symptomatic.

22.4.2.3 Toxicity to Humans

Therapeutic Use Products containing benzyl benzoate are used as a scabicide in some countries; however, since commercial formulations containing this compound are not available in the United States, benzyl benzoate is only rarely used for scabies in this country. For treatment of scabies, benzyl benzoate emulsions or lotions (200–350 gm/liter) are applied nightly or every other night for a total of three applications (Orkin et al., 1976; Gurevitch, 1985).

From the earlier literature, one finds that benzyl benzoate was efficacious in the treatment of a number of conditions including excessive peristalsis of the intestine as in diarrhea and dysentery, intestinal colic and enterospasm, pylorospasm, spastic constipation in which there was a tonic spastic condition of the intestine, biliary colic, ureteral or renal colic, spasm of the urinary bladder, spasms associated with contraction of seminal vesicles, uterine colic as in spastic dysmenorrhea, arterial spasm including hypertension, and bronchial spasms as in asthma and pertussis (Macht, 1918; 1919a;b; 1920). The use of benzyl benzoate in the treatment of these conditions has been superseded by the use of other more effective drugs.

Effects on Organs and Tissues Benzyl benzoate at a concentration of 1×10^{-5} M was without significant effect on human lymphocyte mitogenic response to phytohemagglutinin and neutrophil chemotaxis (Lee et al., 1979).

Accidents and Use Experience In 1929, Macht and Leach reported that the most remarkable feature of benzyl benzoate therapy in humans was the low toxicity of the drug, which was due to its being converted into and excreted as hippuric acid. They were unaware of any serious cases of poisoning following its use in "thousands upon thousands" of cases.

Following oral administration of therapeutic doses, one of the first symptoms was a sensation of warmth and slight flushing of the skin due to peripheral vasodilation (Macht and Leach, 1929). Macht (1918) also observed occasional gastric irritation following oral administration of benzyl benzoate.

Benzyl benzoate solutions are irritating to the eyes and can cause stinging and conjunctivitis (Orkin et al., 1976). Although it is not highly irritating to the skin, sensitivity to benzyl benzoate does occur (Meynadier et al., 1982).

There have been a number of incidents or accidents associated with the use of benzyl benzoate as a scabicide (Castot et al., 1980; Lanfranchi and Bavoux, 1982). Three will be described. A 2-month-old boy weighing 4.2 kg, who was hospitalized for scabies, was bathed over the body, except for the face, with a solution containing benzyl benzoate (43%), soap (20%), ethyl alcohol (20%), and distilled water (17%). Convulsions appeared 2.5 hr later and were controlled with diazepam. About 1.5 hr later, convulsions recurred requiring even stronger doses of diazepam. There was no hyperthermia, hypocalcemia, or hypoglycemia. The cerebrospinal fluid was normal, as were X rays of the head. All organic causes and subdural hematoma were eliminated. It was highly probable that the condition was iatrogenic and that the etiological agent was the benzyl benzoate. However, this could not be proved, since benzyl benzoate was not found in the urine and since the quantity of urine was too small for analysis of metabolites such as hippuric acid. The boy apparently fully recovered and was in good health when last examined at 6 months of age (Lanfranchi and Bavoux, 1982). In another case, a 7-year-old boy died following a transplant for aplastic bone marrow. The etiology of his condition was not established with certainty. However, the month preceding diagnosis he was bathed over the body every other day with Ascabiol®, a scabicide which contained benzyl benzoate (10%) and disulfiram (2%) in addition to ethyl alcohol, water, and polysorbate. It seemed likely that the condition resulted from chronic overdosage with the scabicide (Lanfranchi and Bavoux, 1982). A 24-year-old inmate of a penal institution, who was suffering from scabies, was painted on the body below the neck with an emulsion of benzyl benzoate of unspecified concentration. After treatment, the brush was steeped in 80% phenol antiseptic. The next day the brush was taken from the phenol solution and washed under running water, and the inmate was again treated with benzyl benzoate. This time the man complained of stinging during treatment. Ten or so minutes following treatment he became unsteady, collapsed on the floor, and appeared to be suffering an epileptic fit. His eyes were open, pupils were dilated, face was blue, fists were clenched tight, and he was gasping and frothing at the mouth. He stopped breathing and failed to respond to resuscitation efforts and cardiac massage. Phenol was detected in the liver (3.3 ppm unhydrolyzed, 7.1 ppm hydrolyzed) and blood (4.7 ppm) but not in lung, stomach contents, or urine. Moreover, the plastic bag containing the paint brush had an odor of phenol. It was concluded that the phenol, which was absorbed through the skin, was the cause of death (Lewin and Cleary, 1982). Although no mention was made of the potential role of benzyl benzoate in this poisoning, it may have been a contributory factor, since the compound has been shown to induce convulsions in laboratory animals and humans (Graham and Kuizenga, 1945; Lanfranchi and Bavoux, 1982).

Treatment of Poisoning   Treatment of benzyl benzoate poisoning in humans is symptomatic.

22.5 SYNERGISTS

The possibility that synergists might assist in the control of pests is an attractive one that has been widely considered and selectively explored. Certain compounds increase the toxicity of pyrethrins to insects by as much as 100 times. Consequently, unsynergized formulations of them are used only rarely. Synergists also are used with some of the other pyrethroids, although the performance of these compounds usually is improved to a lesser degree. Synergists for certain carbamates, organophosphates, chlorinated hydrocarbons, and other insecticides and acaricides also are known. In fact, representatives of almost all types of organic insecticides and acaricides can be synergized, at least in the laboratory. However, relatively few combinations of insecticides and acaricides with synergists lend themselves to practical use, either because the degree of improved performance is small or because too much of the expensive synergist is required, or both (Casida, 1970). By the same token, although synergism of inherently toxic compounds such as organophosphates against laboratory animals has been observed (see, e.g., Robbins *et al.*, 1959), no example of increased toxicity to humans or useful animals under practical conditions has been reported.

Synergistic activity is found among methylenedioxyphenolic compounds (see Table 22.4), 2-propynyl esters and esters, *N*-alkyl compounds (e.g., SKF 525A, MGK 264, WARF antiresistant for DDT, and *N*-isobutylundecylenamide used in MYL antilouse powder), thiocyanates (e.g., Thanite®) and related benzothiadiazoles, and even some organophosphate (e.g., TOCP and DEF), carbamate, formamidine, and other compounds. However, the methylenedioxyphenolic compounds are of greatest importance as synergists from the standpoint of historical development, current use, and number of active compounds (Casida, 1970). Thus, the remainder of this section will be concerned with these compounds in general and with piperonyl butoxide in particular.

The chemistry of synergists for pyrethrins and other insecticides and their mode of action in insects have been reviewed thoroughly by Metcalf (1955, 1967) and by Casida (1970). Insects receive a higher dosage of an aerosol while in flight than while at rest. Thus, anything about an aerosol that excites insects to fly or prolongs their flight will increase the effectiveness of the aerosol. Synergists are known that have these actions and whose effectiveness, therefore, must depend partly on them. These and some other mechanisms that may influence synergistic action in insects would have no bearing on their action in mammals. However, Metcalf (1955) concluded that the major cause of synergistic effects of the compounds that increased the action of insecticides was their physiological and biochemical activity in increasing the toxic response to a given dosage and, more specifically, was interference with the detoxification of these insecticides by insects (Metcalf, 1967). Most evidence bearing on the exact nature of the action indicated that it consists in inhibition of microsomal enzymes by the methylenedioxyphenyl compounds (Metcalf, 1967; Casida, 1970).

The methylenedioxyphenyl synergists are substrates for the microsomal enzyme–NADPH$_2$ system, which also metabolizes many drugs and insecticides. By serving as alternative substrates (and, therefore, as competitive inhibitors) for this system, these compounds prolong the persistence of the drug or insecticide so that a lower initial dose is effective (Casida *et al.*, 1966; Kamienski and Casida, 1970; Casida, 1970).

Although insecticide synergists inhibit mixed-function oxidases in mammals as well as in insects, there is a marked difference in susceptibility. Compounds studied so far are active in mammals only at high dosages and for brief periods (Casida, 1970). It is true that for periods of 4 days or less piperonyl butoxide (500 mg/kg) can block the inductive action of phenobarbital (75 mg/kg) (Friedman and Couch, 1974). However, although the initial action is inhibition of microsomal enzymes and reduction of the apparent level of P-450, after 24–72 hr synergists induce increased enzyme activity and P-450 content (Skrinjaric-Spoljar *et al.*, 1971; Bick and Fishbein, 1972; Mirer *et al.*, 1975; Friedman *et al.*, 1975). Both purified and technical grade piperonyl butoxide are equally effective in inducing microsomal enzymes and cytochrome P-450 and the proliferation of smooth endoplasmic reticulum. The induction of different enzymes reached a maximum in 1–8 weeks, but liver weight, cellular hypertrophy, and proliferation of smooth endoplasmic reticulum appeared greater after 8 weeks of dietary intake at the rate of 10,000 ppm than after 1 week (Goldstein *et al.*, 1973).

Black pepper, which contains methylenedioxyphenyl compounds, was used as an insecticide many years ago. However, it was the discovery (patented in 1940) that oil from sesame seed activates pyrethrins that motivated extensive research on the constituents of this oil and on their analogs. One active material, sesamin, was isolated and identified by Haller *et al.* (1942), and another even more active one, sesamolin, was isolated and identified by Beroza (1954).

Table 22.4
Chemical Structure of Naturally Occurring and Synthetic Synergists of the General Form

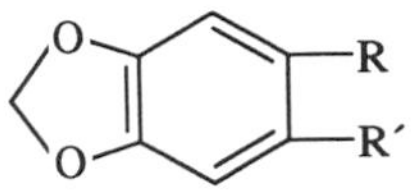

R and R′	R and R′
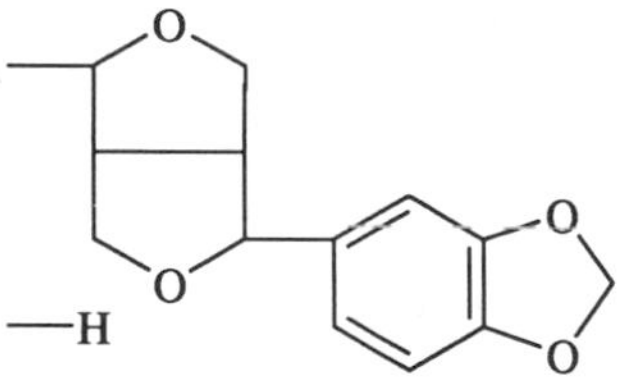 —H Sesamin	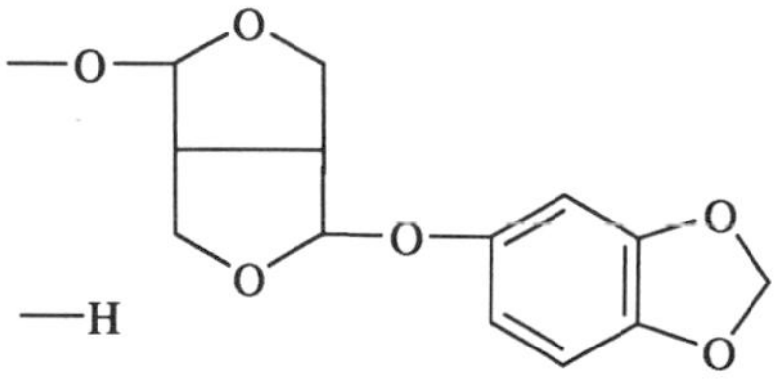 —H Sesamolin
$—CH_2—(O—CH_2—CH_2)_2—O—(CH_2)_3—CH_3$ $—CH_2—CH_2—CH_3$ Piperonyl butoxide	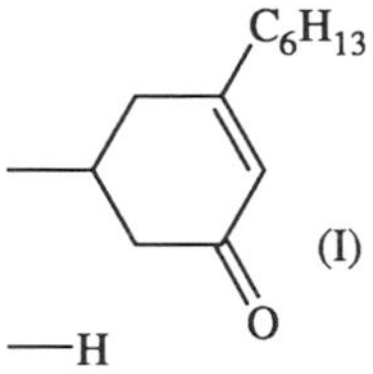 (I) —H 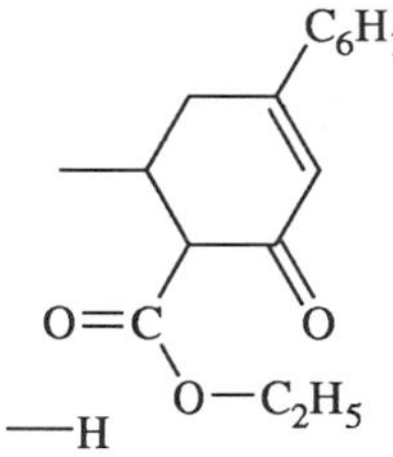 (II) —H Piperonyl cyclonone
$—CH\langle^{O—(CH_2—CH_2—O)_2—(CH_2)_3—CH_3}_{O—(CH_2—CH_2—O)_2—(CH_2)_3—CH_3}$ —H Piprotal	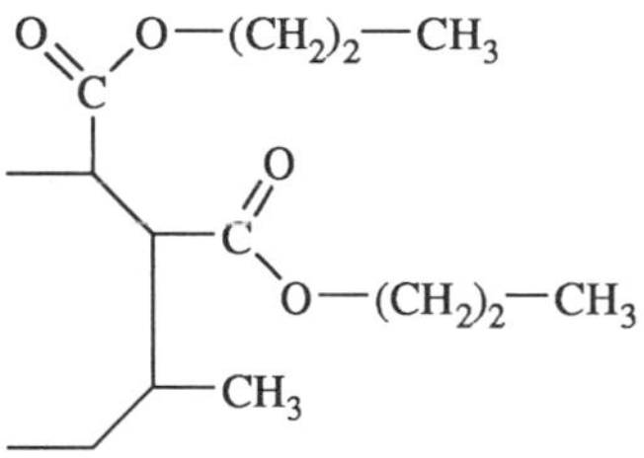 Propyl isome
$—O—CH(CH_3)—(O—CH_2—CH_2)_2—O—CH_2—CH_3$ —H Sesamex	$—CH_2—CH(CH_3)—S(=O)—(CH_2)_7—CH_3$ —H Sulfoxide

The methylenedioxyphenyl synergists are chemically related to sesamol and safrole, although these compounds have little or no synergistic action. Sesamol is an antioxidant found in processed sesame oil. Its side chains (see Table 22.4) are —OHand —H, respectively. Although dietary levels as high as 10,000 ppm for 400 days or more have no effect on mortality or growth of rats, levels of 300 ppm or greater produce benign and malignant tumors not observed in controls or in rats fed levels of 80–160 ppm (Ambrose *et al.*, 1958). The side chains of safrole are $—CH_2—CH{=}CH_2$ and —H, respectively. Safrole is a recognized cause of liver dysplasia (Homburger *et al.*, 1962) and a variety of benign and malignant tumors of the liver in rats (Long *et al.*, 1963). Safrole does not cause esophageal tumors in rats, but high dietary levels of the flavoring agent dihydrosafrole (side chains $—CH_2—CH_2—CH_3$ and —H) do cause such tumors but not liver tumors (Long and Jenner, 1963). Because piperonyl butoxide and sulfoxide inhibit the metabolism of benzpyrene and because of their close chemical similarity to sesamol and safrole, all methylenedioxyphenyl synergists are suspect as liver tumorigens. Because methylenedioxyphenyl synergists are inducers of microsomal enzymes and because some features of the tumors described by Long *et al.* (1963) are similar to those induced in mice by some chlorinated hydrocarbon insecticides, there is reason to think that the safrole tumors may be peculiar to rodents. However, the synergists initially inhibit microsomal enzymes in a way that the chlorinated hydrocarbons do not, and the pathology is not identical (e.g., safrole caused proliferation of bile ducts).

22.5.1 PIPERONYL BUTOXIDE

22.5.1.1 Identity, Properties, and Uses

Chemical Name Piperonyl butoxide is 5-[[2-(2-butoxy ethoxy)ethoxy]methyl]-6-propyl-1,3-benzodioxole.

Structure See Table 22.4. The names piperonyl butoxide (BSI, E-ISO, BPC, ESA) and piperonyl butoxyde (F-ISO) are accepted in lieu of a common name. Trade names have included Butoxide®, Butacide®, Butocide®, and Pyrenone® (mixture with allethrin). Code designations have included FAC-5,273, NIA-5,273, and ENT 14,250. The CAS registry number is 51-03-6.

Physical and Chemical Properties Piperonyl butoxide has the empirical formula $C_{19}H_{30}O_5$ and a molecular weight of 338.4. The technical material can range from 71.6 to 90.1% piperonyl butoxide with the remainder consisting of a number of chemically related compounds. Much of the toxicological research has used the technical material. It is a pale yellow oil with a faint bitter taste. It has a density of 1.07, a boiling point of 180°C at 1 mm Hg, and a flash point of 171.1°C. Piperonyl butoxide is miscible with benzene, dichlorofluoromethane, methyl alcohol, ethyl alcohol, Freons, Geons, petroleum oils, and other organic solvents. It is noncorrosive and resistant to hydrolysis.

History, Formulations, and Uses Developed in 1947, piperonyl butoxide is an insecticide synergist for pyrethroids and rotenone. It is used with these insecticides in ratios of 5 : 1 to 20 : 1 by weight in the form of aerosols, dusts, emulsions, and solutions. In concentrations of less than 5% it is a component in some insect repellents.

22.5.1.2 Toxicity to Laboratory Animals

Basic Findings A single large oral dose of piperonyl butoxide produces anorexia, unsteadiness, rough coat, watering eyes, irritability, prostration, coma, and death. Onset may be as early as 20 min after dosing. Illness may last several days, and death may be delayed by as much as 1 week (Lehman, 1951, 1952). The signs are similar but are delayed following a small number of repeated doses sufficient to produce death. Repeated doses that kill rats only after several or many weeks produce anorexia,

stunting, and cachexia. Dogs react in a similar way but also vomit (Sarles and Vandegrift, 1952).

Undiluted piperonyl butoxide is mildly irritating to rabbit skin on repeated application, but it is not sensitizing (Sarles *et al.*, 1949).

The acute oral toxicity of piperonyl butoxide is low. See Table 22.5. The compound is even less toxic to rats when injected subcutaneously, presumably because of poor absorption. A spray concentrate containing unusually high proportions of piperonyl butoxide (20%) and pyrethrins (2.5%) was found to be little, if any, more toxic for rats than the petroleum oil solvent alone (Sarles *et al.*, 1949).

Rabbits generally survive a single dermal application at the rate of 1880 mg/kg in the form of a 20% solution in dimethyl phthalate; it causes no skin irritation but does cause hyperexcitability and convulsions (Lehman, 1951, 1952).

A dietary level of 25,000 ppm caused rats to eat only about one-third as much food as controls; the dosage was about 780 mg/kg/day (see results for dosages of 8.4 and 84 mg/kg/day below). These rats gained very little weight. About half of them died within 26 weeks, all of them within 78 weeks. They showed a very marked increase in the relative weight of the liver (relative weight of the kidney also in some experiments), decrease in relative weight of the testes, definite morphological changes in the liver, and no reproduction (Sarles and Vandegrift, 1952). Judging from these results, the chronicity index at 90 days must be near 10 but is not truly representative because the animals continued to die. The 90-dose dermal LD 50 in rabbits is 200 mg/kg/day (Lehman, 1951, 1952), indicating a chronicity index under these conditions of about 15.

A dietary level of 10,000 ppm, which produced about 22% food refusal compared with that of controls and therefore a dosage of only about 650 mg/kg/day, led to moderate reduction of weight gain, increased relative weight of the kidneys in some experiments, increased relative weight of the liver in all experiments, and decreased reproduction (average delay of over 23 days to first litter, reduced average number of litters per female,

Table 22.5
Single-Dose LD 50 Values for Piperonyl Butoxide

Species	Route	LD 50 (mg/kg)	Reference
Rat	oral	7,500–10,000	Sarles *et al.* (1949)
Rat	oral	11,500	Lehman (1951, 1952)
Rat	oral	8,000	Adolphi (1958)
Rat, M	oral	7,500	Gaines (1969)
Rat, F	oral	6,150	Gaines (1969)
Rat, M	dermal	>7,950	Gaines (1969)
Rat, F	dermal	>7,950	Gaines (1969)
Mouse	oral	8,000	Adolphi (1958)
Mouse	intraperitoneal	3,800	Adolphi (1958)
Rabbit	oral	2,500–5,000	Sarles *et al.* (1949)
Dog	oral	>7,500	Sarles *et al.* (1949)
Cat	oral	>7,500	Sarles *et al.* (1949)

reduced average weight of young per litter at 4 weeks of age, and trend to a smaller number of young per litter). Mortality was not clearly increased within 52 weeks, but it increased above that of controls within 104 weeks (Sarles and Vendegrift, 1952).

Lehman (1952, 1952) reported that even a dietary level of 5000 ppm (about 250 mg/kg/day) produced illness and tissue change.

Rats tolerated dietary levels of 100 and 1000 ppm (approximately 8.4 and 84 mg/kg/day) with little or no effect on weight gain, relative weights of organs, survival during the first 52 weeks of feeding, reproductive ability through two complete generations, and organ morphology. There may have been a trend to greater mortality during the second year, but the difference from that of controls was not significant. Feeding of pyrethrins at 14 mg/kg/day, in addition to piperonyl butoxide at 84 mg/kg/day, for 2 years had no greater effect than piperonyl butoxide alone at 84 mg/kg/day (Sarles and Vandegrift, 1952).

Dogs showed a progressive increase in liver weight associated with dosage rates of 3, 31, 105, and 315 mg/kg/day. Dosages of 105 and 315 mg/kg/day produced weight loss; morphological changes in the liver, kidney, and adrenal gland; and, at the higher level, death of all animals in 4–15 weeks attributed to liver injury (Sarles and Vandegrift, 1952). The death of one dog that received 31 mg/kg/day was attributed to natural causes but involved severe, unexplained liver injury. Dogs tolerated piperonyl butoxide administered in capsules at rates of 3 mg/kg/day, and most of them tolerated 31 mg/kg/day, although the relative weight of the liver was slightly but not statistically increased, even at the lower dosage.

A goat tolerated about 66 mg/kg/day for a year without clinical effect. During that period, she successfully nursed a kid. At autopsy the liver of the mother showed minimal change, but that of the kid was normal (Sarles and Vandegrift, 1952).

African green monkeys tolerated piperonyl butoxide better than dogs at doses as high as 105 mg/kg/day, but the monkeys received only 24 doses rather than a year of treatment.

Absorption, Distribution, Metabolism, and Excretion
Piperonyl butoxide is poorly absorbed from the gastrointestinal tract. In two experiments, 78 and 87%, respectively, of the dose administered orally to dogs were recovered in the feces (Sarles and Vandegrift, 1952). The small proportion that was absorbed from the gastrointestinal tract was rapidly excreted in the urine. Intratracheal administration led to a more prolonged excretion of metabolites in the bile and urine, but even in this instance residues in lung tissue were less than they were following intravenous administration (Fishbein *et al.*, 1972).

The metabolism of methylenedioxyphenyl compounds has been studied by Casida *et al.* (1966), Fishbein *et al.* (1967), and Kamienski and Casida (1970). Briefly, it was found that the [^{14}C]methylene group of piperonyl butoxide was hydroxylated by liver microsomal enzymes, yielding [^{14}C]formate by a route that did not involve formaldehyde but eventually did yield $^{14}CO_2$ in living mice and house flies. Within 48 hr after oral administration to mice, 61–76% of the radioactive methylene carbon was expired as $^{14}CO_2$ hr. The percentage of radioactive methylene carbon excreted in the urine within 48 hr was lower for compounds with long apolar side chains (e.g., sulfoxide, piperonyl butoxide) than for others (e.g., safrole). The amount of radioactive methylene carbon excreted in the feces (3–6%) or remaining in the body as a residue (9–14%) 48 hr after oral administration of these synergists was similar to that found after the administration of [^{14}C]formate.

Thus the major metabolic pathway for piperonyl butoxide and certain other methylenedioxyphenyl synergists in mice involves cleavage of the methylenedioxyphenyl moiety and expiration of the methylene carbon as carbon dioxide. By contrast, the methylenedioxyphenyl moiety of piprotal and related materials generally remains intact, and the major metabolic pathway involves oxidation or conjugation, or both, of the side chain (Kamienski and Casida, 1970).

Following a single intravenous injection of piperonyl butoxide in rats, the number of radioactive metabolites recovered in the bile and urine were 13 and 11, respectively, when tagging was on the methylenedioxy group, and 24 and 26, respectively, when tagging involved the α-carbon of the propyl side chain. There were, in addition, eight nonradioactive biliary metabolites. In spite of this extensive fragmentation of the molecule, an unexpectedly large percentage of total radioactivity in the form of unchanged piperonyl butoxide was retained in the lung and fat (Fishbein *et al.*, 1969).

Pharmacological and Biochemical Effects From the toxicological viewpoint, the most significant action of piperonyl butoxide in laboratory animals is its effect on enzymes, chiefly mixed-function oxidases. As mentioned earlier, this action can be biphasic and can consist of inhibition and induction, depending on time and dose. Either inhibition or induction of microsomal mixed-function oxidases can have a profound influence on the toxicities of xenobiotics that are metabolized by this system. Thus, piperonyl butoxide has been widely used by pharmacologists and toxicologists as a research tool to probe mechanisms associated with the toxic actions of a variety of pesticides and drugs. The results of some of these studies are mentioned under Factors Influencing Toxicity.

Treatment of rats orally with piperonyl butoxide at 750 mg/kg resulted in inhibition of the activity of several serum enzymes including glutamate-oxaloacetic transaminase, glutamic-pyruvic transaminase, glutamyltransferase, and lactate dehydrogenase (Enan *et al.*, 1982). The compound inhibited state 3 respiration and uncoupled oxidative phosphorylation in isolated rat liver mitochondria (Nelson *et al.*, 1971). Piperonyl butoxide also caused a transient decrease in glomerular filtration rate (Davis, 1984).

Piperonyl butoxide treatment of mice induced hypothermia (Massey *et al.*, 1982), depleted hepatic levels of glutathione (James and Harbison, 1982), and increased δ-aminolevulinic acid synthetase activity (Yoshida *et al.*, 1976).

Piperonyl butoxide also was shown to have anticonvulsant activity when administered to mice in both the electroshock seizure test and the pentylenetetrazole test. In the maximal electroshock seizure test, which measures the ability of an anticonvulsant drug to abolish the hind limb tonic–extensor component of maximal seizures, piperonyl butoxide had an intraperitoneal ED 50 value of 457 mg/kg, a dosage that was higher than that for valproate (272 mg/kg), clonazepam (92.7 mg/kg), phenobarbital (21.8 mg/kg), phenytoin (9.5 mg/kg), and carbamazepine (8.81 mg/kg) but lower than that for ethosuximide (>1000 mg/kg). Piperonyl butoxide had low neurotoxicity with a median neurotoxic dose or TD 50 of 1690 mg/kg as measured by the rotorod test. In the maximal electroshock seizure test, piperonyl butoxide yielded a protective index (TD 50/ED 50) of 3.69, which was greater than those for phenobarbital (3.17), valproate (1.57), ethosuximide (<0.44), and clonazepam (0.002) but lower than those for carbamazepine (8.12) and phenytoin (6.89). Piperonyl butoxide had a safety ratio (TD 3/ED 97) of <1 in both the maximal electroshock seizure and pentylenetetrazole tests; therefore, anticonvulsant activity can be achieved with a minimally neurotoxic dose (Ater *et al.*, 1984).

Effects on Organs and Tissues   Piperonyl butoxide was not mutagenic with *S. typhimurium* (TA98, TA100, TA1537) with or without S9 activation (White *et al.*, 1978; Kawachi *et al.*, 1980), with *E. coli* WP2 (trp) without activation (Ashwood-Smith *et al.*, 1972), or with *B. subtilis* (H17 rec$^+$, M45 rec$^-$) Kawachi *et al.*, 1980). It also was inactive in tests for chromosomal aberrations in cultured Chinese hamster cells and rat bone marrow (Kawachi *et al.*, 1980). When injected intraperitoneally into mice at 1000 or 200 mg/kg, no dominant lethal mutations were observed (Epstein *et al.*, 1972).

In long-term feeding studies, the occurrence and types of benign tumors in rats fed piperonyl butoxide were similar to those in the controls, except that rats receiving 10,000 and 20,000 ppm showed a marked increase in liver nodules. Three hepatomas were observed. A carcinoma with metastasis to lymph nodes, lungs, and mediastinum was seen in a rat that had received 25,000 ppm for 64 weeks (Sarles and Vandegrift, 1952). In a subsequent study, groups of male and female rats (Fischer 344) were fed piperonyl butoxide (technical grade, 90.1%) at concentrations of 10,000 or 5000 ppm for 107 weeks. Mean body weights of both sexes were lower than those of corresponding controls. Survival was not affected by treatment. A statistically significant dose-related increase in the incidence of lymphoreticular neoplasia (lymphomas and leukemias) was found in females; however, the incidence of these neoplasms was higher in control males than in treated males (Cardy *et al.*, 1979; NCI, 1979b). It should be kept in mind that hematopoietic neoplasms are among the most frequently occurring spontaneous neoplasms in F344 rats (Cardy *et al.*, 1979). In a more recent study, Maekawa *et al.* (1985) fed piperonyl butoxide (technical grade) at dietary levels of 10,000 and 5000 ppm to F344 rats for 2 years and found no significant dose-related increase of any tumor. Thus, piperonyl butoxide was not carcinogenic in F344 rats (NCI, 1979b; Maekawa *et al.*, 1985).

Innes *et al.* (1969) evaluated piperonyl butoxide (technical

grade, 80%) for possible tumorigenicity in two strains of mice. Groups of male and female mice received piperonyl butoxide by stomach tube at 464 or 100 mg/kg at 7 days of age, followed by the same amount daily up to 4 weeks of age; subsequently, the mice were fed 1112 ppm or 300 ppm in the diet up to 70 weeks of age. No significant difference was found in the incidence of tumors between treated and control mice (Innes *et al.*, 1969; IARC, 1983b). In another study, groups of male and female mice (B6C3F1) were fed piperonyl butoxide (technical grade, 90.1%) at concentrations of 5000 or 2500 ppm up to week 30 and thereafter at 500 or 2000 ppm for 82 weeks, yielding time-weighted average doses of 1036 or 2804 ppm. Dose-related decreases in mean body weights were observed; however, survival was unaffected. No statistically significant dose-related neoplasms were found (NCI, 1979b).

Groups of male and female mice were injected subcutaneously with piperonyl butoxide at 1000 or 100 mg/kg on day 28 of life and were observed until they were 78 weeks of age. No significant increase in tumor incidence was observed (NTIS [National Technical Information Service, 1968]).

Piperonyl butoxide in combination with either Freon 112 or Freon 113 increased the appearance of hepatomas when injected subcutaneously into mice. Piperonyl butoxide alone was not tumorigenic. The compounds were given in four doses at intervals of 1 week, beginning the date after birth; the initial dosage rate was about 2625 mg/kg for piperonyl butoxide and twice that for the Freon. The other three doses were about 1050, 1050, and 700 mg/kg, respectively. This total dosage (piperonyl butoxide plus Freon) was sufficient to produce a mortality of 46–55% before weaning, chiefly during the first week, compared with 2–11, 15, and 14% in the Freon, piperonyl butoxide, and control treatments, respectively. After weaning, mortality was much greater in males, which were genetically subject to obstructive uropathy. Hepatomas were found only in the males, including some hepatomas in control males. Malignant lymphomas were found in females of different groups, including the controls (Epstein *et al.*, 1967a).

Especially during the first week of life, the same dosage of piperonyl butoxide increased the mortality produced by Freon 112, Freon 113, griseofulvin, and benzo[*a*]pyrene. Survivors of these tests grew faster than controls (Epstein *et al.*, 1967b), perhaps because there were fewer left to suckle each mother.

Effects on Reproduction   Rats tolerated dietary levels as high as 1000 ppm or 84 mg/kg/day with little or no effect on reproduction through two complete generations (Sarles and Vandegrift, 1952).

Rats were treated by gavage with piperonyl butoxide at rates of 300 or 1000 mg/kg/day on days 6–15 of gestation. Maternal growth during gestation was slightly reduced, but no dams died. The numbers of corpora lutea, implantations, resorptions, and viable fetuses per female were not altered, compared to those of controls. No anomalies that could be related to the synergist were revealed by external inspection or study of the soft tissues or skeleton (Kennedy *et al.*, 1977). Khera *et al.* (1979) found no adverse effect on fetal development when female rats were treated orally with piperonyl butoxide (technical grade) at dosages ranging from 500 to 62.5 mg/kg on days 6–15 of gestation.

Factors Influencing Toxicity Piperonyl butoxide is of low toxicity to laboratory animals, and little, if any, information is currently available on factors that influence its toxicity. However, the literature is replete with references to the influence of piperonyl butoxide on pesticide and drug toxicity, pharmacokinetics, and pharmacodynamics in laboratory animals (see review by Haley, 1978). Piperonyl butoxide afforded protection against the acutely toxic effects of the insecticides methyl parathion, azinphos-methyl, and dimethoate (Kamienski and Murphy, 1971). The compound has been shown to increase barbiturate sleeping time (Anders, 1968; Fujii et al., 1970; Jaffe and Neumeyer, 1970; Lush, 1976) and to enhance zoxazolamine-induced paralysis in some (Fujii et al., 1970; Jaffe and Neumeyer, 1970) but not all cases (Lush, 1976). It also enhanced the neurotoxicity induced by TOCP (Veronesi, 1984) and methyl mercury (Friedman and Eaton, 1978). Piperonyl butoxide increased the hepatotoxicity of 4-acetylaminobiphenyl, N-hydroxy-4-acetylaminobiphenyl, 2-acetylaminofluorene, N-hydroxy-2-acetylaminofluorene, and 7,12-dimethylbenz[a] anthracene (Fujii and Epstein, 1979). It prevented bromobenzene-induced hepatotoxicity (Reid et al., 1971) and bromobenzene- and chlorobenzene-induced nephrotoxicity (Reid, 1973). With regard to cephalosporin-mediated nephrotoxicity, piperonyl butoxide protected against that induced by cephaloridine but not that induced by cephaloglycin (Tune et al., 1983). Piperonyl butoxide enhanced methylcyclopentadienylmanganese-induced pulmonary toxicity (Haschek et al., 1982) but decreased that induced by naphthalene (Warren et al., 1982). Piperonyl butoxide decreased overall alveolar cell proliferation mediated by urethane and butylated hydroxytoluene when administered after urethane and before butylated hydroxytoluene; however, it did not completely suppress type II alveolar cell proliferation (Witschi, 1986). It potentiated the genotoxicity of 1,2-dichloroethane (Storer and Conolly, 1985). The compound reduced some of the toxic effects of acetaminophen (Mitchell et al., 1973; Harman and Fischer, 1983) but enhanced acetaminophen-induced hypothermia (Massey et al., 1982).

Piperonyl butoxide decreased the incidence of o-bromophenol-induced elevated levels of blood urea nitrogen (Lau et al., 1984). When administered prior to benzene, it reduced the urinary excretion of benzene metabolites at 24 hr but increased overall urinary excretion and expiration of benzene (Timbrell and Mitchell, 1977). Piperonyl butoxide increased brain levels of Δ^1-tetrahydrocannabinol (Gill and Jones, 1972). It also increased the inhibition of acetylcholinesterase in animals treated with coumaphos (Robbins et al., 1959).

Many of these interactions are due to inhibition of the metabolism of the xenobiotic by piperonyl butoxide. In studies in vivo or in vitro or both, piperonyl butoxide has been shown to inhibit mainly certain of the oxidative metabolic paths of some organophosphate (Dahm et al., 1962; Normal and Neal, 1976) carbamate (Hodgson and Casida, 1961; Casida, 1970), pyrethroid (Jao and Casida, 1974), and formamidine (Ghali and Hollingworth, 1985) insecticides and acaricides as well as those of hexobarbital (Jaffe et al., 1968a,b; Jaffe and Neumeyer, 1970), aniline (Anders, 1968; Friedman et al., 1972), dimethylaminopyrine (Jaffe et al., 1968a,b), aminopyrine (Poland and Kappas, 1971; Friedman et al., 1972), ethylmorphine (Anders, 1968), p-nitroanisole (Anders, 1968), biphenyl (Jaffe et al., 1969; Jaffe and Neumeyer, 1970), aminophenazone (Jaffe and Neumeyer, 1970), bromobenzene (Reid et al., 1971), p-chloroacetanilide (Hinson et al., 1975), N-2-fluorenylacetamide (Levine, 1971), 3-methylcholanthrene (Levine, 1972), 7,12-dimethylbenz[a]anthracene (Levine, 1974), dimethylnitrosoamine (Friedman et al., 1975; Friedman and Sanders, 1976), 1-naphthol (Lucier et al., 1971), and testosterone (Lucier et al., 1971). Cholesterol biosynthesis also was inhibited by piperonyl butoxide (Mitoma et al., 1968).

Piperonyl butoxide has been found to enhance the metabolism of a number of xenobiotics including biphenyl (Jaffe et al., 1969; Jaffe and Neumeyer, 1970), dimethylnitrosamine (Friedman et al., 1975; Friedman and Sanders, 1976), p-nitroanisole (Wagstaff and Short, 1971; Goldstein et al., 1973), EPN (Wagstaff and Short, 1971), hexobarbital (Wagstaff and Short, 1971; Goldstein et al., 1973), aniline (Goldstein et al., 1973), and benzpyrene (Lake et al., 1973).

Piperonyl butoxide inhibited the induction by phenobarbital of microsomal enzymes (Friedman and Couch, 1974).

Pathology Rats killed by a single large dose of piperonyl butoxide showed liver damage, including fatty change, vacuolation of the cytoplasm, and hydropic swelling of the nucleus and nucleolus. Those dying within the first 4 days also showed damage to ganglion cells of the brain stem (Sarles and Vandegrift, 1952).

Following repeated intake at dietary levels of 5000 ppm or more, rats showed enlargement of the liver, periportal hepatic cell hypertrophy, and slight fatty change (Lehman, 1951, 1952). Induction of ileocecal ulcers also has been found in rats following repeated intake at levels of 10,000 and 5000 ppm (Maekawa et al., 1985).

At a dosage of 780 mg/kg/day and in the presence of marked inanition, some rats showed dystrophy, dysplasia, slight to moderate focal necrosis, cystic bile ducts, diffuse lobular cirrhosis, and toxic pigmentation of the liver. Changes similar to those in the liver, but less severe, were found in the fascicular and glomerular zone of the adrenal gland and in the proximal convoluted tubules of the kidneys (Sarles and Vandegrift, 1952). At a dosage of 650 mg/kg/day for 2 years, Sarles and Vandegrift, 1952) found no pathology distinctly different from that of controls. However, Kimbrough et al. (1968), being more alert to the liver changes associated with induction of microsomal enzymes, found increased hypertrophy, margination, and inclusion bodies in rats that had received only 500 mg/kg/day.

Dogs given piperonyl butoxide at rates of 105 and 315

mg/kg/day showed changes similar to those in rats, but with rather less injury to the liver and more to the kidneys and adrenals. Nodules, hepatomas, and carcinomas have not been observed in dogs (Sarles and Vandegrift, 1952).

22.5.1.3 Toxicity to Humans

Effects on Organs and Tissues   Lee *et al.* (1979) examined the effects of piperonyl butoxide on human leukocyte functions. When a diluted whole blood culture was incubated with piperonyl butoxide at a concentration of 1×10^{-5} *M* for 24 hr, 26% inhibition of lymphocyte mitogenic response to phytohemagglutinin was obtained; however, no significant effect on this process was observed when the phytohemagglutinin was incubated with the blood cells for 24 hr prior to adding the piperonyl butoxide. This indicated that the action of piperonyl butoxide was involved with early biochemical events associated with cellular activation and might be due to the inhibition of microsomal protein synthesis in the activated lymphocytes. Piperonyl butoxide was without significant effect on neutrophil chemotaxis (Lee *et al.*, 1979).

Experimental Exposure   Eight male volunteers ranging in age from 22 to 57 years old were given a single oral dose of 50 mg of piperonyl butoxide which corresponded to an average dosage of 0.71 mg/kg; no toxic signs were recorded. This level of piperonyl butoxide, which is 50 times greater than the daily exposure of individuals using sprays extensively in enclosed areas, did not affect the metabolism of antipyrine, and it was concluded that it was unlikely that environmental exposure to this chemical would result in inhibition of microsomal enzyme function in humans (Conney *et al.*, 1972).

Therapeutic Use   Piperonyl butoxide itself has no known therapeutic use. However, formulations of pyrethrins containing piperonyl butoxide are used as a pediculicide to control the body louse *Pediculus humanus humanus,* the head louse *P. humanus capitis,* and the crab louse *Pthirus pubis* (Smith, 1973; Compendium of Drug Therapy, 1986).

Accidents and Use Experience   A 66-year-old man, who for the previous 15 years had worked in a small, unventilated store where he regularly used generous amounts of an aerosol mixture containing lindane, piperonyl butoxide, and pyrethrum dissolved in xylene, toluene, and kerosene, was hospitalized for pneumonia. Results of bone marrow aspiration and trephine bone biopsy were indicative of hypoplastic anemia even though his peripheral blood count including platelets was normal 1 year prior to admission. The urine contained traces of toluene and xylene. He was treated with antibiotics and leukocyte transfusions, and his condition gradually improved over a 3-month period except for a drop in hemoglobin which necessitated several blood transfusions. Results of a subsequent bone marrow test were compatible with aplastic anemia. He continued to use the insecticide and died from septicemia 1 month following the diagnosis of acute myeloblastic leukemia (Sidi *et al.,* 1983). In another instance, each of two sisters, who were exposed during the first trimester of pregnancy to large amounts of piperonyl butoxide, N-octylbicycloheptene dicarboximide (MGK® 264), allethrin, pyrethrins, diethyl-*m*-toluamide, and dichlorvos, gave birth to a male infant with coarctation of the aorta (Hall *et al.,* 1975). Although Sidi *et al.* (1983) thought it probable that the evolution of the leukemic process was related to exposure to the insecticide, it is impossible to discern the role, if any, played by piperonyl butoxide in either of these instances.

Laboratory Findings   According to Arena (1974), exposure to piperonyl butoxide can result in blood disorders including pancytopenia, thrombocytopenia, leukopenia, polycythemia, and unspecified anemias.

Treatment of Poisoning   Treatment of poisoning by piperonyl butoxide would be entirely symptomatic.

22.6 CHEMOSTERILANTS

Chemosterilants are chemicals that induce sterilization in one or both sexes of a pest organism. The basic concepts underlying this particular form of control were reviewed by Hayes (1982) and in far greater detail by Knipling (1979). Briefly, there are two main approaches that exploit the ability of certain chemicals to induce sterility. The biological and operational distinctions between the two methods were made very early by Knipling, but only in a descriptive way, and no distinct names were assigned to them. In the first method, insects are mass-produced and sterilized by a chemical under essentially factory conditions and subsequently released in the field. Biologically, there is no limit on the number of individuals that can be processed; specifically, it is possible to release as many—or even more—individuals in succeeding generations. Operationally, extremely dangerous chemicals can be used because the critical process can be confined to a closed system within the factory analogous to the closed system that was used to sterilize screwworm flies by radiation. This method was referred to by Hayes (1982) as the "factory method"; it is now called the sterile insect release method (SIRM) (Borkovec, 1985). In the second method, some individuals of a natural population of pests are sterilized by a chemical placed in their environment. Biologically, if the method is successful at all, the number of individuals in succeeding generations must decrease because the population is decreased. Operationally, only chemicals that are safe enough for humans and the environment may be used. This method was referred to by Hayes (1975) as the "field method"; unfortunately, the corresponding term now in use—that is, field sterilization method or FSM (Borkovec, 1985)—has been interpreted so generally that it is not limited to the action of chemosterilants but may include the action of juvenoids, chitin synthesis inhibitors, and possibly other classes of chemicals.

True chemosterilants (see Fig. 22.5) include some of the alkylating agents (e.g., busulfan, chlorambucil, tepa, and thiotepa), analogs of alkylating agents (e.g., hexamethylmela-

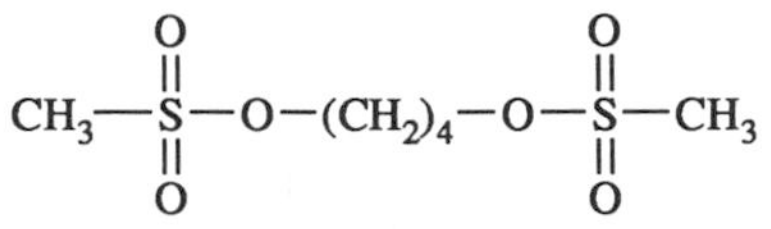

Busulfan

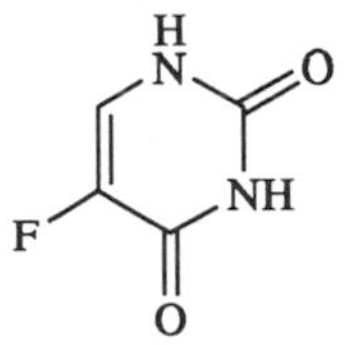

Fluorouracil

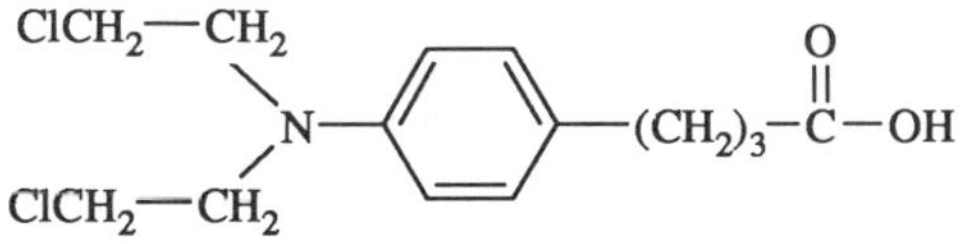

Chlorambucil

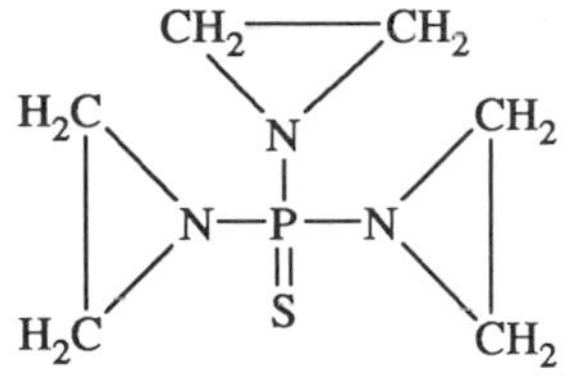

Thiotepa

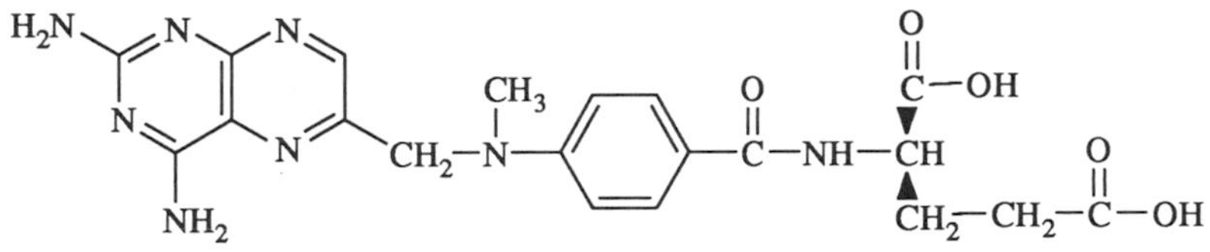

Methotrexate

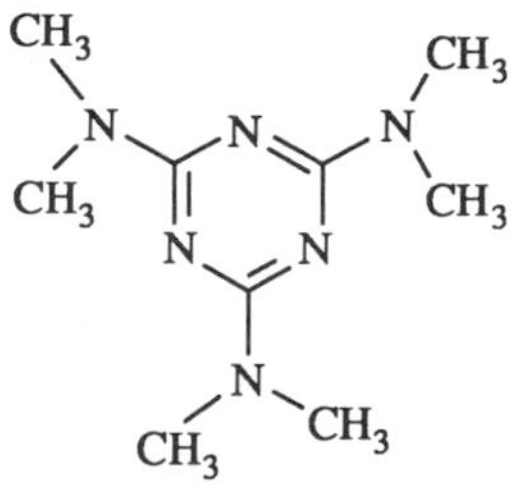

Hexamethylmelamine

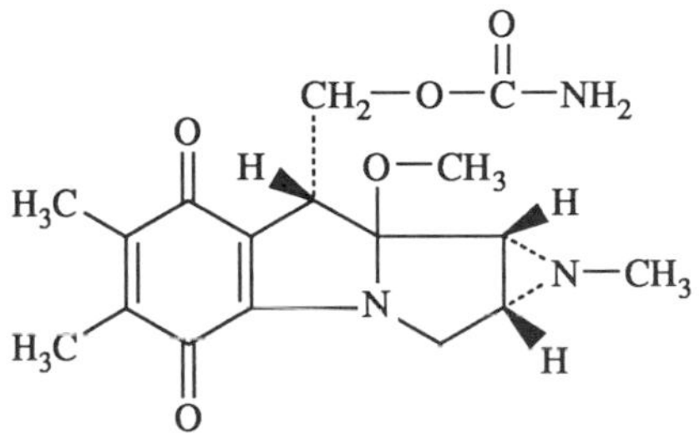

Porfirmycin

Figure 22.5 Examples of insect chemosterilants.

mine), antimetabolites (e.g., 5-fluorouracil and methotrexate), and certain antibiotics (e.g., porfirmycin). They must be used for practical pest control under very strict security in a factory setting. No chemosterilant safe enough for unrestricted field use is known, although some of them have received very limited field tests, mainly by combining them with baits to minimize the total amount released.

As for each compound that happens to have some sterilizing action in one or more species in addition to some other more prominent mode of action, its toxicity must be judged on its own merits.

22.6.1 BUSULFAN

The most common side effect of the use of this aklylating agent for treatment of chronic myclocytic leukemia or polycythemia vera is depression of the bone marrow, but testicular atrophy, renal failure, an Addison-like syndrome, or other injuries may occur. Although a cause-and-effect relationship had not been proved, cases suggest that busulfan is teratogenic and carcinogenic in people, as has been proved in animals [Hayes, 1982; American Medical Association (AMA), 1986].

22.6.2 CHLORAMBUCIL

This alkylating agent has been used in the palliative treatment of several neoplastic diseases. Treatment may cause depression of the bone marrow or hyperuricemia. Leukemia, lymphosarcoma, and other cases of neoplasia associated with chlorambucil have been reported. Teratogenesis, apparently related to the compound, has been recorded also (Hayes, 1982; AMA, 1986).

22.6.3 THIOTEPA

Thiotepa is quite useful in the palliative treatment of carcinoma of the ovary and breast and is of some use for lymphomas and a few other neoplastic diseases. It can cause bone marrow depression, sometimes delayed. In several instances patients have developed new neoplastic conditions during or following treatment with thiotepa (Hayes, 1982; AMA, 1986).

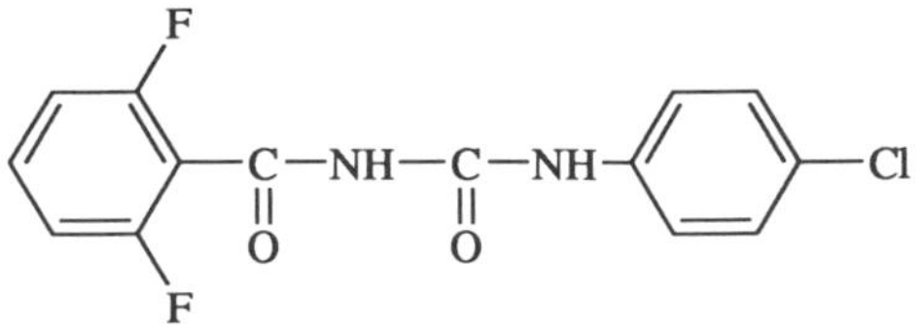

22.6.4 HEXAMETHYLMELAMINE

This analog of an alkylating agent is used for treating several carcinomas; it has caused thrombocytopenia and peripheral neuropathy as well as less serious side effects (Hayes, 1982; AMA, 1986).

22.6.5 5-FLUOROURACIL

This antimetabolite has been used for treating several carcinomas, especially those of the gastrointestinal tract. Leukopenia usually is the first adverse effect, but many other less serious side effects can occur (Hayes, 1982; AMA, 1986).

22.6.6 METHOTREXATE

This antimetabolite leads to long-term survival of some patients with trophoblastic tumors, and it (often in combination with other drugs) is useful in some leukemias, lymphomas, carcinomas, and sarcomas. It may produce ulcerative lesions of the gastrointestinal tract, serious kidney injury, cirrhosis of the liver, pulmonary infiltrations, and severe bone marrow depression. Methotrexate produced teratogenesis when ingested with the hope of producing an abortion (Hayes, 1982; AMA, 1986).

22.6.7 PORFIRMYCIN

This antibiotic has been used in treating cervical, ovarian, hepatocellular, and gastrointestinal neoplasms. Toxic effects include leukopenia and thrombocytopenia (Hayes, 1982).

22.7 INHIBITORS OF CHITIN SYNTHESIS

The target for most of the conventional insecticides is the nervous system. However, a recently discovered novel class of insecticides, the benzoylphenylureas, interfere with the formation of chitin. Chitin, a polysaccharide, is a major constituent of the exoskeleton of insects. This skeleton supports the organism. Without a rigid skeleton, effective movement of the legs and wings would be impossible. The tracheae through which most insects breathe are held open by rings of chitin. Finally, the exoskeleton and its waxy covering are of great importance in preventing loss of water. Therefore, it seems likely that anything that effectively interferes with the formation of chitin by

Figure 22.6 Diflubenzuron.

insects would be useful in their control. Furthermore, because vertebrates and most plants do not form chitin, a compound that inhibits its formation but lacks other pharmacological or toxic effects at the required dosage should be safe for humans, domestic animals, wildlife, and plants. Such a compound might, however, be dangerous to other arthropods, including beneficial insects and edible crustaceans. This is because arthropods form chitin and depend on it to a greater or lesser degree. Chitin also is formed by many fungi; therefore, an inhibitor of chitin synthesis might injure some of these organisms.

Diflubenzuron or Dimlin® is the forerunner of the benzoylphenylurea insecticides (Fig. 22.6). It appears that the major action of diflubenzuron in insects is inhibition of the synthesis of chitin, although it can inhibit other enzymes and interfere with other processes. The final stage in the formation of chitin is the polymerization of uridine-diphospho-N-acetyl-glucosamine units, a reaction catalyzed by chitin synthase. Diflubenzuron exerts its action on chitin synthesis by inhibiting the proteolytic activation of the chitin synthase zymogen (Marks et al., 1982). Other promising benzoylphenylurea insecticides include 2-chloro-[[[4-(trifluoromethoxy)phenyl]amino]-carbonyl]benzamide (triflumuron or Alsystin®) and N-[4-(3-chloro-5-(trifluoromethyl)-2-pyridinyloxy)-3,5-dichloro-phenylaminocarbonyl]-2,6-difluorobenzamide (Aim®). Interestingly, these three compounds apparently possess little, if any, activity against mites. However, certain of the nucleoside antibiotic nikkomycins, whose actions include competitive inhibition of chitin synthase, appear to be more active against mites than insects (Mothes, 1981; Mothes-Wagner, 1984a,b; Zebitz et al., 1981; Mothes and Seitz, 1982; Zoebelein and Kniehase, 1985). No studies of the benzoylphenylureas or nikkomycins in humans were found.

REFERENCES

Abo-Khatwa, N., and Hollingworth, R. M. (1973). Chlordimeform: Uncoupling activity against rat liver mitochondria. *Pestic. Biochem. Physiol.* **3**, 358–369.

Adolphi, Dr. (1958). Examination of a pyrethrum synergist: Preliminary information. *Pyrethrum Post* **4**, 3–5.

Ahmad, S., and Knowles, C. O. (1971a). Metabolism of N'-(4-chloro-o-tolyl)-N,N-dimethylformamidine (chlorphenamidine) and 4-chloro-o-formoto-luidide by rat hepatic microsomal and soluble enzymes. *Gen. Pharmacol.* **2**, 189–197.

Ahmad, S., and Knowles, C. O. (1971b). Formamidase involvement in the metabolism of chlorphenamidine and formetanate acaricides. *J. Econ. Entomol.* **64**, 792–795.

Airaksinen, M. M., Mattila, M. J., and Takki, S. (1967). The oral toxicity in mice and the uptake by *Diphyllobothrium latum* and the host gut of some anthelmintics *in vitro*. *Acta Pharmacol. Toxicol.* **25**, 33–40.

Ambrose, A. M., and Yost, D. H. (1965). Pharmacologic and toxicologic studies of *N,N*-diethyltoluamide. II. *N,N*-Diethyl-*p*-toluamide. *Toxicol. Appl. Pharmacol.* **7**, 772–780.

Ambrose, A. M., Cox, A. J., Jr., and DeEds, F. (1958). Toxicological studies on sesamol. *J. Agric. Food Chem.* **6**, 600–604.

Ambrose, A. M., Huffman, D. K., and Salamone, R. T. (1959). Pharmacologic and toxicologic studies of *N,N*-diethyl-*m*-toluamide. *Toxicol. Appl. Pharmacol.* **1**, 97–115.

American Medical Association (AMA) (1986). "AMA Drug Evaluations", 4th ed. Am. Med. Assoc., Chicago, Illinois.

Anders, M. W. (1968). Inhibition of microsomal drug metabolism by methylenedioxybenzenes. *Biochem. Pharmacol.* **17**, 2367–2370.

Andrews, P., Thyssen, J., and Lorke, D. (1983). The biology and toxicology of molluscicides, Bayluscide®. *Pharmacol. Ther.* **19**, 245–295.

Angerhofer, R. A., and Weeks, M. H. (1981). "Phase 7, Effect of Dermal Applications of *N,N*-Diethyl-*m*-toluamide (*m*-DET) on the Embryonic Development of Rabbits." Study 75-51-0034-80, March 1979-July 1980. U.S. Army Environ. Hyg. Agency, Aberdeen Proving Ground, Maryland.

Arena, J. M. (1974). "Poisoning," 3rd ed., p. 13. Thomas, Springfield, Illinois.

Arena, J. M. (1983). Acute miscellaneous poisoning. *In* "Current Therapy" (H. F. Conn, ed.), pp. 931–949. Saunders, Philadelphia, Pennsylvania.

Arima, T., Morooka, H., Tanigawa, T., Imal, M., Tsunashima, T., and Kita, S. (1976). Methemoglobinemia induced by chlorphenamidine. *Acta Med. Okayama* **30**, 57–60.

Armstrong, J., Somerville, O. G., Lovejoy, G., Swiggart, R., and Hutcheson, R. H., Jr. (1975). Insecticide-induced acute hemorrhagic cystitis—Tennessee. *Morbid. Mortal. Wkly. Rep.* **24**, 374.

Ashby, J. (1981). Overview of study and test chemical activities. Prog. Mutat. Res. **1**, 112–171.

Ashwood-Smith, M. J., Trevino, J., and Ring, R. (1972). Mutagenicity of dichlorvos. *Nature (London)* **240**, 418–420.

Ater, S. B., Swinyard, E. A., Tolman, K. G., and Franklin, M. R. (1984). Anticonvulsant activity and neurotoxicity of piperonyl butoxide in mice. *Epilepsia* **25**, 551–555.

Aziz, S. A., and Knowles, C. O. (1973). Inhibition of monoamine oxidase by the pesticide chlordimeform and related compounds. *Nature (London)* **242**, 417–418.

Bailey, B. A., Martin, R. J., and Downer, R. G. H. (1982). Monoamine oxidase inhibition and brain catecholamine levels in the rat following treatment with chlordimeform. *Pestic. Biochem. Physiol.* **17**, 293–300.

Bainova, A. I., Zaprianov, Z., and Kaloyanova-Simeonova, F. (1979). Effect of pesticides on the activity of monoamine oxidase (MAO) in rats. *Arch. Hig. Rada Toksikol.* **30**, Suppl., 531–535.

Barnish, G., Jordan, P., Bartholomew, R. K., and Grist, E. (1982). Routine focal mollusciciding after chemotherapy to control *Schistosoma mansoni* in Cul de Sac Valley, Saint Lucia. *Trans. R. Soc. Trop. Med. Hyg.* **76**, 602–609.

Beckerman, S. C. (1960). An unusual case of aplastic anemia. *J. Maine Med. Assoc.* **51**, 53, 54, 60.

Beeman, R. W., and Matsumura, F. (1973). Chlordimeform: A pesticide acting upon amine regulatory mechanisms. *Nature (London)* **242**, 273–274.

Belfrage, H. (1927). Poisoning through metaldehyde. *Acta Paediatr. (Stockholm)* **6**, 481–483 (in German).

Benezet, H. J., and Knowles, C. O. (1976a). *N'*-(4-Chloro-*o*-tolyl)-*N*-methylformamidine (demethylchlordimeform) metabolism in the rat. *J. Agric. Food Chem.* **24**, 152–154.

Benezet, H. J., and Knowles, C. O. (1976b). Inhibition of rat brain monoamine oxidase by formamidines and related compounds. *Neuropharmacology* **15**, 369–373.

Benezet, H. J., Chang, K.-M., and Knowles, C. O. (1978). Formamidine pesticides—metabolic aspects of neurotoxicity. *In* "Pesticide and Venom Neurotoxicity" (D. L. Shankland, R. M. Hollingworth, and T. Smyth, Jr., eds.), pp. 189–206. Plenum, New York.

Bentley, P., Stäubli, W., Bieri, F., Muecke, W., and Waechter, F. (1985).

Induction of hepatic drug-metabolising enzymes following treatment of rats and mice with chlordimeform. *Toxicol. Lett.* **28**, 143–149.

Beran, F., Kahle, E., and Klimmer, O. R. (1982). Metaldehyde. *In* "Compendium of Plant-Protection Agents and Guidelines for the Management of Plant-Protection Agents," pp. 347–348. Literature Research, Annandale, Virginia.

Beroza, M. (1954). Pyrethrum synergists in sesame oil. Sesamolin, a potent synergist. *J. Am. Oil Chem. Soc.* **31**, 302–305.

Bick, M., and Fishbein, L. (1972). The inductive effect of piperonyl butoxide on microsomal demethylase activity. *Sci. Total Environ.* **1**, 197–203.

Bishop, C. H. G. (1975). Blindness associated with metaldehyde poisoning. *Vet. Rec.* **96**, 438.

Black, W. D., Wade, A. E., and Talbot, R. B. (1973). A study of the effect of ovex on parathion toxicity in rats. *Can. J. Physiol. Pharmacol.* **51**, 682–685.

Black, W. D., Talbot, R. B., and Wade, A. E. (1975). A study of the effect of ovex on parathion and paraoxon toxicity in rats. *Toxicol. Appl. Pharmacol.* **33**, 393–400.

Blomquist, L., and Thorsell, W. (1977). Distribution and fate of the insect repellent ^{14}C-*N,N*-diethyl-*m*-toluamide in the animal body. II. Distribution and excretion after cutaneous application. *Acta Pharmacol. Toxicol.* **41**, 235–243.

Blomquist, L., Stroman, L., and Thorsell, W. (1975). Distribution and fate of the insect repellent ^{14}C-*N,N*-diethyl-*m*-toluamide in the animal body. I. Distribution and excretion after injection into mice. *Acta Pharmacol. Toxicol.* **37**, 121–133.

Borbely, A. (1970). Contribution to the question of metaldehyde poisoning. Dissertation, University of Zurich. Juris Druck and Verlag, Zurich. (in German).

Bonsall, J. L., and Turnball, G. J. (1982). Extrapolation from safety data to management of poisoning with reference to amitraz (a formamidine pesticide) and xylene. *Hum. Toxicol.* **2**, 416.

Bonsall, J. L., and Turnbull, G. J. (1983). Extrapolation from safety data to management of poisoning with reference to amitraz (a formamidine pesticide) and xylene. *Hum. Toxicol.* **2**, 587–592.

Booze, T. F., and Oehme, F. W. (1985). Metaldehyde toxicity: A review. *Vet. Hum. Toxicol.* **27**, 11–19.

Booze, T. F., and Oehme, F. W. (1986). An investigation of metaldehyde and acetaldehyde toxicities in dogs. *Fundam. Appl. Toxicol.* **6**, 440–446.

Borkovec, A. B. (1985). Chemicals for the control of insect reproduction. *Beltsville Symp. Agric. Res.* **8**.

Boswood, B. (1962). Metaldehyde poisoning. *Vet Rec.* **74**, 517–518.

Boyes, W. K., and Dyer, R. S. (1984a). Pattern evoked potential changes at high but not low contrast produced by chlordimeform insecticide *Soc. Neurosci. Abstr.* **10**, 115.

Boyes, W. K., and Dyer, R. S. (1984b). Chlordimeform produces profound, selective and transient changes in visual evoked potentials of hooded rats. *Exp. Neurol.* **86**, 434–447.

Boyes, W. K., and Dyer, R. S. (1984c). Comparison of amitraz and chlordimeform effects on hooded rat visual evoked potentials. *Neurotoxicology* **5**, 76.

Boyes, W. K., and Hudnell, H. K. (1987). Chlordimeform action on the sustained and transient components of rat pattern evoked potentials. *Toxicologist* **7**, 97.

Boyes, W. K., and Moser, V. C. (1985). A possible α2-adrenergic mode of chlordimeform action on rat visual function. *Toxicologist* **5**, 82.

Boyes, W. K., Jenkins, D. E., and Dyer, R. S. (1985a). Chlordimeform produces contrast-dependent changes in visual evoked potentials of hooded rats. *Exp. Neurol.* **89**, 391–407.

Boyes, W. K., Padilla, S., and Dyer, R. S. (1985b). Body temperature-dependent and independent actions of chlordimeform on visual evoked potentials and axonal transport in optic system of rat. *Neuropharmacology* **24**, 743–749.

Boyes, W. K., Moser, V. C., MacPhail, R. C., and Dyer, R. S. (1985c). Monoamine oxidase inhibition cannot account for changes in visual evoked potentials produced by chlordimeform. *Neuropharmacology* **24**, 853–860.

Budris, D. M., Yim, G. K. W., Carlson, G. P., and Schnell, R. C. (1983).

Effect of acute and repeated chlordimeform treatment on rat hepatic microsomal drug metabolizing enzymes. *Toxicol. Lett.* **18**, 63–71.

Cardy, R. H., Renne, R. A., Warner, J. W., and Cypher, R. L. (1979). Carcinogenesis bioassay of technical-grade piperonyl butoxide in F344 rats. *JNCI, J. Natl. Cancer Inst.* **62**, 569–576.

Carpenter, C. P., Weil, C. S., and Smyth, H. F., Jr. (1974). Range-finding toxicity data: List VIII. *Toxicol. Appl. Pharmacol.* **28**, 313–319.

Casida, J. E. (1970). Mixed-function oxidase involvement in the biochemistry of insecticide synergists. *J. Agric. Food Chem.* **18**, 753–772.

Casida, J. E., Engle, J. L., Essac, E. G., Kamienski, F. X., and Kuwatsuka, S. (1966). Methylene-C^{14} dioxyphenyl compounds: Metabolism in relation to their synergistic action. *Science* **153**, 1130–1132.

Castot, A., Garnier, R., Lanfranchi, C., and Bavoux, F. (1980). Systemic side effects of drugs applied cutaneously. *Therapie* **35**, 423–432 (in French).

Ceglowski, W. S., Ercegovich, C. D., and Pearson, N. S. (1979). Effects of pesticides on the reticuloendothelial system. *Adv. Exp. Med. Biol.* **121A**, 569–576.

Chinn, C., Pfister, W. R., and Yim, G. K. W. (1976). Local anesthetic-like actions of the pesticide, chlordimeform (CDM). *Fed. Proc., Fed. Am. Soc. Exp. Biol.* **35**, 729.

Chinn, C., Lund, A. E., and Yim, G. K. W. (1977). The central actions of lidocaine and a pesticide, chlordimeform. *Neuropharmacology* **16**, 867–871.

Christensen, H. E., Zaratzian, V. L., and Poczenik, A. (1969). "Parameters of the Use of *N,N*-Diethyl-*m*-toluamide as Pressurized Spray to Prevent Transmission of Communicable Disease from Arthropod Vectors," Final Rep., Proj. RP004T1-64/69, March 1964–May 1969. U.S. Army Environ. Hyg. Agency, Edgewood Arsenal, Maryland.

Churchill, C., Pendleton, J., Maddy, K., Ames, R. G., Knaak, J. B., Jackson, R., and Kizer, K. W. (1986). Outbreak of severe dermatitis among orange pickers—California. *Morbid. Mortal. Wkly. Rep.* **35**, 465–467.

Compendium of Drug Therapy (1986). Biomedical Information Corporation, New York.

Conney, A. H., Chang, R., Levin, W. M., Garbut, A., Munro-Faure, A. D., Peck, A. W., and Bye, A. (1972). Effects of piperonyl butoxide on drug metabolism in rodents and man. *Arch. Environ. Health* **24**, 97–106.

Cook, J. A., Sturrock, R. F., and Barnish, G. (1972). An allergic skin reaction to a new formulation of the molluscicide clonitralide (Bayluscide). *Trans. R. Soc. Trop. Med. Hyg.* **66**, 954–955.

Coye, M. J., Lowe, J. A., and Maddy, K. J. (1986). Biological monitoring of agricultural workers exposed to pesticides: II. Monitoring of intact pesticides and their metabolites. *J. Occup. Med.* **28**, 628–636.

Crofton, K. M., Boncek, V. M., and Reiter, L. M. (1987). The effects of amitraz (AMZ) administration on locomotor activity and the acoustic startle response: Dosage and time dependent effects in the rat. *Toxicologist* **7**, 254.

Crowder, L. A., and Whitson, R. S. (1980). Fate of toxaphene, methyl parathion, and chlordimeform combinations in the mouse. *Bull. Environ. Contam. Toxicol.* **24**, 444–451.

Crowley, R. J., Geyer, R., and Muir, S. G. (1986). Analysis of *N,N*-diethyl-*m*-toluamide (DEET) in human postmortem specimens. *J. Forensic Sci.* **31**, 280–282.

Currie, A. N. (1933). Chemical haematuria from handling 5-chloro-*ortho*-toluidine. *J. Ind. Hyg.* **15**, 205–213.

Dahm, P. A., Kopecky, B. E., and Walker, C. B. (1962). Activation of organophosphorus insecticides by rat liver microsomes. *Toxicol. Appl. Pharmacol.* **4**, 683–696.

Davis, M. F. (1984). Changes of hexachlorobutadiene nephrotoxicity after piperonyl butoxide treatment. *Toxicology* **30**, 217–225.

Dobozy, V. S. (1982). Mitaban safety. *DVM* **13**, 54–55.

Dobryanskiy, V. M. (1972). Toxicologic characteristics of the molluscicide metaldehyde. *Zdravookhranenie* **18**(3), 13–16 (in Russian).

Draize, J. H., Alvarez, E., Whitesell, M. F., Woodard, G., Hagan, E. C., and Nelson, A. A. (1948). Toxicological investigations of compounds proposed for use as insect repellents. A. Local and systemic effects following topical skin application. B. Acute oral toxicity. C. Pathological examination. *J. Pharmacol. Exp. Ther.* **93**, 26–39.

Dreisbach, R. H. (1983). "Handbook of Poisoning Diagnosis and Treatment," 11th ed., pp. 202–205. Lange Med. Publ., Los Altos, California.

Duhm, von B., Maul, W., Medenwald, H., Patzschke, K., and Wegner, L.-A. (1961). Radioactive investigations with a new molluscicide. *Z. Naturforsch., B: Anorg. Chem., Org. Chem., Biochem., Biophys., Biol.* **16B**, 509–515 (in German).

Dyer, R. S., and Boyes, W. K. (1983). Chlordimeform differentially affects pattern reversal-evoked and flash-evoked potentials in rats. *Toxicologist* **3**, 13.

Emran, A., Shanbaky, N. M., and Borowitz, J. L. (1980). Blockade of adrenal catecholamine release by chlordimeform and its metabolites. *Bull. Environ. Contam. Toxicol.* **25**, 197–202.

Enan, E. E., El-Sebae, A. H., Enan, O. H., and El-Fiki, S. (1982). *In vitro* interaction of some organophosphorus insecticides with different biochemical targets in white rats. *J. Environ. Sci. Health, Part B* **B17**, 549–570.

Environmental Protection Agency (EPA) (1980). "Summary of Reported Pesticide Incidents Involving Metaldehyde-pesticide," Incident Monit. Rep. No. 285, March 1980. Health Eff. Branch, Hazard Eval. Div. Off. Pestic. Programs, Environ. Prot. Agency, Washington, D.C.

Epstein, S. S., Joshi, S., Andrea, J., Clapp, P., Falk, H., and Mantel, N. (1967a). Synergistic toxicity and carcinogenicity of "Freons" and piperonyl butoxide. *Nature (London)* **214**, 526–528.

Epstein, S. S., Andrea, J., Clapp, P., and MacKintosh, D. (1967b). Enhancement by piperonyl butoxide of acute toxicity due to Freons, benzo[α]pyrene, and griseofulvin. *Toxicol. Appl. Pharmacol.* **11**, 442–448.

Epstein, S. S., Arnold, E., Andrea, J., Bass, W., and Bishop, Y. (1972). Detection of chemical mutagens by the dominant lethal assay in the mouse. *Toxicol. Appl. Pharmacol.* **23**, 288–325.

Feldmann, R. J., and Maibach, H. I. (1970). Absorption of some organic compounds through skin in man. *J. Invest. Dermatol.* **54**, 399–404.

Feng, L., Ching, Z. S., Kwang, H. T., Ah, C. S., and Fong, W. Y. (1985). Carcinogenic effects of chlordimeform in mice from lifetime oral dosing experiment. *J. Chin. Prev. Med.* **19**, 154–156 (in Chinese).

Ferguson, F. F. (1975). "The Role of Biological Agents in the Control of Schistosome-Bearing Snails." U.S. Department of Health, Education, and Welfare, Public Health Service, Centers for Disease Control, Atlanta, Georgia.

Ficsor, G., and Nii Lo Piccolo, G. (1972). Survey of pesticides for mutagenicity by the bacterial-plate assay method. *Environ. Mutagen. Soc. Newsl.* **6**, 6–8.

Fishbein, L., Fawkes, J., Falk, H. L., and Thompson, S. (1967). Thin-layer chromatography of rat bile and urine following intravenous administration of pesticidal synergists. *J. Chromatogr.* **27**, 153–166.

Fishbein, L., Falk, H. L., Fawkes, J., Jordan, S., and Corbett, B. (1969). The metabolism of piperonyl butoxide in the rat with 14-C in the methylenedioxy or alpha-methylene group. *J. Chromatogr.* **41**, 61–79.

Fishbein, L., Falk, H. L., Fawkes, J., and Jordan, S. (1972). The metabolism of ^{14}C-piperonyl butoxide in the rat. *In* "Fate of Pesticides in Environment," pp. 503–519. Gordon & Breach, London.

Fleming, W. J., Heinz, G. H., and Schuler, C. A. (1985). Lethal and behavioral effects of chlordimeform in bobwhite. *Toxicology* **36**, 37–47.

Folland, D. S., Kimbrough, R. D., Cline, R. E., Swiggart, R. C., and Schaffner, W. (1978). Acute hemorrhagic cystitis: Industrial exposure to the pesticide chlordimeform. *JAMA, J. Am. Med. Assoc.* **239**, 1052–1055.

Food and Agriculture Organization/World Health Organization (FAO/WHO) (1972). "1971 Evaluations of Some Pesticide Residues in Food." Report of 1971 Joint Meeting of the FAO Working Party of Experts on Pesticide Residues and the WHO Expert Committee on Pesticide Residues. (WHO Pestic. Residues Ser., No. 1). World Health Organ., Geneva.

Food and Agriculture Organization/World Health Organization (FAO/WHO) (1978a). "1977 Evaluations of Some Pesticide Residues in Food," FAO Plant Prod. Prot. Pap. No. 10, Suppl. Food Agric. Organ./World Health Organ., United Nations, Rome.

Food and Agriculture Organization/World Health Organization (FAO/WHO) (1978b). "Pesticide Residues in Food." Report of the 1977 Joint Meeting of the FAO Panel of Experts on Pesticide Residues and the Environment and the

WHO Expert Committee on Pesticide Residues (WHO Pestic. Residues Ser. No. 10, Rev.). Food Agric. Organ./World Health Organ., Rome.

Food and Agriculture Organization/World Health Organization (FAO/WHO) (1979a). "1978 Evaluations of some Pesticide Residues in Food," FAO Plant Prod. Prot. Pap. No. 15, Suppl. Food Agric. Organ./World Health Organ., United Nations, Rome.

Food and Agriculture Organization/World Health Organization (FAO/WHO) (1979b). "Pesticide Residues in Food." Report of the 1977 Joint Meeting of the FAO Panel of Experts on Pesticide Residues and the Environment and the WHO Expert Group of Pesticide Residues (WHO Pestic. Residues Ser., No. 15). Food Agric. Organ./World Health Organ. Rome.

Food and Agriculture Organization/World Health Organization (FAO/WHO) (1980). "1979 Evaluations of Some Pesticide Residues in Food," FAO Plant Prod. Prot. Pap. No. 20, Suppl. Food Agric. Organ./World Health Organ. United Nations, Rome.

Food and Agriculture Organization/World Health Organization (FAO/WHO) (1981a). "1980 Evaluations of Some Pesticide Residues in Food," FAO Plant Prod. Prot. Pap. No. 26, Suppl. Food Agric. Organ./World Health Organ., United Nations, Rome.

Food and Agriculture Organization/World Health Organization (FAO/WHO) (1981b). Pesticide Residues in Food." Report of the 1980 Joint Meeting of the FAO Panel of Experts on Pesticide Residues in Food and the Environment and the WHO Expert Group on Pesticide Residues (WHO Pestic. Residues Ser. No. 26.) Food Agric. Organ./World Health Organ., Rome.

Food and Agriculture Organization/World Health Organization (FAO/WHO) (1982). "1982 Evaluations of Some Pesticide Residues in Food," FAO Plant Prod. Prot. Pap. no. 49. Food Agric. Organ./World Health Organ., United Nations, Rome.

Friedman, M. A., and Couch, D. B. (1974). Inhibition by piperonyl butoxide of phenobarbital mediated induction of mouse liver microsomal enzyme activity. *Res. Commun. Chem. Pathol. Pharmacol.* **8**, 515–526.

Friedman, M. A., and Eaton, L. R. (1978). Potentiation of methylmercury toxicity by piperonyl butoxide. *Bull. Environ. Contam. Toxicol.* **20**, 9–16.

Friedman, M. A., and Sanders, V. (1976). Effects of piperonyl butoxide on dimethylnitrosamine metabolism and toxicity in Swiss mice. *J. Toxicol. Environ. Health* **2**, 67–75.

Friedman, M. A., Greene, E. J., Csillag, R., and Epstein, S. S. (1972). Paradoxical effects of piperonyl butoxide on the kinetics of mouse liver microsomal enzyme activity. *Toxicol. Appl. Pharmacol.* **21**, 419–427.

Friedman, M. A., Woods, S., Sanders, V., and Couch, D. B. (1975). Effects of piperonyl butoxide on dimethylnitrosamine metabolism and toxicity in Swiss mice. *Proc. Am. Assoc. Cancer Res. Am. Soc. Clin. Oncol.* **16**, 160.

Fujii, K., and Epstein, S. S. (1979). Effects of piperonyl butoxide on the toxicity and hepatocarcinogenicity of 2-acetylaminofluorene and 4-acetylaminobiphenyl, and their N-hydroxylated derivatives, following administration to newborn mice. *Oncology* **36**, 105–112.

Fujii, K., Jaffe, H., Bishop, Y., Arnold, E., Mackintosh, D., and Epstein, S. S. (1970). Structure activity relations for methylenedioxyphenyl and related compounds on hepatic microsomal enzyme function, as measured by prolongation of hexobarbital narcosis and zoxazolamine paralysis in mice. *Toxicol. Appl. Pharmacol.* **16**, 482–494.

Gaines, T. B. (1969). Acute toxicity of pesticides. *Toxicol. Appl. Pharmacol.* **14**, 515–534.

Ghali, G. Z. (1981). The metabolic basis for the acute and chronic toxicity of formamidine pesticides. *Diss. Abstr. Int B* **42**, 57.

Ghali, G. Z., and Hollingworth, R. M. (1985). Influence of mixed function oxygenase metabolism on the acute neurotoxicity of the pesticide chlordimeform in mice. *Neurotoxicology* **6**, 215–238.

Gilbert, M. E. (1987). Enhanced susceptibility to amygdaloid kindling following treatment with formamidine pesticides amitraz and chlordimeform. *Toxicologist* **7**, 98.

Gill, E. W., and Jones, G. (1972). Brain levels of Δ^1-tetrahydrocannabinol and its metabolites in mice. Correlation with behavior, and the effect of the metabolic inhibitors SKF 525A and piperonyl butoxide. *Biochem. Pharmacol.* **21**, 2237–2248.

Gleiberman, S. E., and Voronkina, T. M. (1972). Study into the resorption of the repellent diethyltoluamide. *Med. Parazitol. Parazit. Bolezni* **41**, 189–197 (in Russian).

Gleiberman, S. E., Volkova, A. P., Nikolaev, G. M., and Zhukova, E. V. (1975). A study on embryotoxic properties of the repellent diethyltoluamide. *Farmakol. Toksikol. (Moscow)* **2**, 202–205 (in Russian).

Gleiberman, S. E., Volkova, A. P., Nikolaev, G. M., and Zhukova, E. V. (1976). Study of the long-range consequences of using repellents. I. Experimental study of the consequences of the long-term effect of the repellent diethyltoluamide (DETA). *Med. Parazitol. Parazit. Bolezni* **45**, 65–69 (in Russian).

Glowa, J. R. (1986). Acute and sub-acute effects of deltamethrin and chlordimeform on schedule-controlled responding in the mouse. *Neurobehav. Toxicol. Teratol.* **8**, 97–102.

Goldstein, J. A., Hickman, P., and Kimbrough, R. D. (1973). Effects of purified and technical piperonyl butoxide on drug-metabolizing enzymes and ultrastructure of rat liver. *Toxicol. Appl. Pharmacol.* **26**, 444–458.

Gönnert, R. (1961). Results with laboratory and field trials with the molluscicide Bayer 73. *Bull. W. H. O.* **25**, 483–501.

Gönnert, R., and Schraufstätter, E. (1959). A new molluscicide: Molluscicide Bayer 73. *Proc. Int. Congr. Trop. Med. Malaria, 6th, 1958*, vol. **2**, pp. 197–202.

Gordon, C. J., and Long, M. D. (1985). Effect of chlordimeform on behavioral and autonomic thermoregulation in mice. *Toxicologist* **5**, 25.

Gordon, C. J., Long, M. D., and Stead, A. G. (1985). Thermoregulation in mice following acute chlordimeform administration. *Toxicol. Lett.* **28**, 9–15.

Graham, B. E., and Kuizenga, M. H. (1945). Toxicity studies on benzyl benzoate and related benzyl compounds. *J. Pharmacol. Exp. Ther.* **84**, 358–362.

Gruber, C. M. (1923a). The pharmacology of benzyl alcohol and its esters. I. The effect of benzyl alcohol, benzyl acetate, and benzyl benzoate when given by mouth upon the blood pressure, pulse and alimentary canal. *J. Lab. Clin. Med.* **9**, 15–33.

Gruber, C. M. (1923b). The pharmacology of benzyl alcohol and its esters. II. Some of the effects of benzyl alcohol, benzyl benzoate and benzyl acetate when injected intravenously upon the respiratory and circulatory systems. *J. Lab. Clin. Med.* **9**, 92–112.

Gruber, C. M. (1924). The pharmacology of benzyl alcohol and its esters. IV. The diuretic effect of benzyl alcohol, benzyl-acetate and benzyl-benzoate. *J. Lab. Clin. Med.* **10**, 284–294.

Gryboski, J., Weinstein, D., and Ordway, N. K. (1961). Toxic encephalopathy apparently related to the use of an insect repellent. *N. Engl. J. Med.* **264**, 289–291.

Gurevitch, A. W. (1985). Scabies and lice. *Pediatr. Clin. North Am.* **32**, 987–1018.

Haddow, B. C., and Shankland, G. R. (1969). C 8514, N-(2-methyl-4-chlorophenyl)-N',N'-dimethylformamidine, a promising new acaricide. *Proc. Br. Insectic. Fungic. Conf.* **2**, 538–545.

Haight, E. A., Harvey, J. G., Singer, A. W., and Pope, C. R. (1979). "Phase 5, Subchronic Oral Toxicity Study of the Insect Repellent N,N-Diethyl-m-toluamide (m-DET)." Study 75-51-0034-80, September 1978–May 1979. U.S. Army Environ. Hyg. Agency, Aberdeen Proving Ground, Maryland.

Haley, T. J. (1978). Piperonyl butoxide, α[2-(2-butoxyethoxy)ethoxy]-4,5-methylenedioxy-2-propyltoluene: A review of the literature. *Ecotoxicol. Environ. Saf.* **2**, 9–31.

Hall, J. G., McLaughlin, J. F., and Stamm, S. (1975). Coarctation of the aorta in male cousins with similar maternal environmental exposure to insect repellent and insecticides. *Pediatrics* **55**, 425–427.

Haller, H. L., Laforge, F. B., and Sullivan, W. N. (1942). Effect of sesamin and related compounds in the insecticidal action of pyrethrum in houseflies. *J. Econ. Entomol.* **35**, 247–248.

Harman, A. W., and Fischer, L. J. (1983). Hamster hepatocytes in culture as a model for acetaminophen toxicity: Studies with inhibitors of drug metabolism. *Toxicol. Appl. Pharmacol.* **71**, 330–341.

Haschek, W. M., Hakkinen, P. J., Witschi, H. P., Hanzlik, R. P., and Traiger, G. J. (1982). Nonciliated bronchiolar epithelial (Clara) cell necrosis induced by organometallic carbonyl compounds *Toxicol. Lett.* **14**, 85–92.

Hatch, R. C. (1982). Metaldehyde. *In* "Veterinary Pharmacology and Therapeutics" (N. H. Booth and L. E. McDonald, eds.), pp. 1012–1014. Iowa State Univ. Press, Ames.

Hawkins, G. S., and Reifenrath, W. G. (1986). Influence of skin source, penetration cell fluid, and partition coefficient on *in vitro* skin penetration. *J. Pharm. Sci.* **75,** 378–381.

Hayes, W. J., Jr. (1975). "Toxicology of Pesticides." Williams & Wilkins, Baltimore, Maryland.

Hayes, W. J., Jr. (1982). "Pesticides Studied in Man." Williams & Wilkins, Baltimore, Maryland.

Hecht, G., and Gloxhuber, C. (1960). Experimental investigations with *N'*-(2'-chloro-4'-nitrophenyl)-5-chlorosalicylamide, a new tapeworm remedy. 2. Communication: Toxicological investigations. *Arzneim.-Forsch.* **10,** 884–885 (in German).

Hecht, G., and Gloxhuber, C. (1962). Tolerance to 2',5-dichloro-4-nitrosalicylanilide ethanolamine salt. *Z. Tropenmed. Parasitol.* **13,** 1–8 (in German).

Heick, H. M., Shipman, R. T., Norman, M. G., and James, W. (1980). Reye-like syndrome associated with use of insect repellent in a presumed heterozygote for ornithine carbamoyl transferase deficiency. *J. Pediatr.* **97,** 471–473.

Hinson, J. A., Mitchell, J. R., and Jallow, D. J. (1975). Microsomal *N*-hydroxylations of *p*-chloroacetanilide. *Mol. Pharmacol.* **11,** 462–469.

Hodgson, E., and Casida, J. E. (1961). Metabolism of *N,N*-dialkylcarbamates and related compounds by rat liver. *Biochem. Pharmacol.* **8,** 179–191.

Hollingworth, R. M. (1976). Chemistry, biological activity, and uses of formamidine pesticides. *Environ. Health Perspect.* **14,** 57–69.

Hollingworth, R. M., and Lund, A. E. (1982). Biological and neurotoxic effects of amidine pesticides. *In* "Insecticide Mode of Action" (J. R. Coats, ed.), pp. 189–277. Academic Press, New York.

Hollingworth, R. M., Leister, J., and Ghali, G. (1979). Mode of action of formamidine pesticides: An evaluation of monoamine oxidase as the target. *Chem.-Biol. Interact.* **24,** 35–49.

Holsapple, M. P., and Yim, G. K. W. (1979). Anti-inflammatory and ulcerogenic actions of chlordimeform, an alkaline PGBS inhibitor. *Fed. Proc., Fed. Am. Soc. Exp. Biol.* **38,** 440.

Holsapple, M. P., and Yim, G. K. W. (1981). Decreased gastrointestinal ulcerogenicity of chlordimeform, a basic anti-inflammatory agent. *Toxicol. Appl. Pharmacol.* **59,** 107–110.

Holsapple, M. P., Blake, D. E., Hollingworth, R. M., and Yim, G. K. W. (1977). Prostaglandin synthetase inhibited by a formamidine pesticide. *Pharmacologist* **19,** 147.

Holsapple, M. P., Schnur, M., and Yim, G. K. W. (1980). Pharmacological modulation of edema mediated by prostaglandin, serotonin and histamine. *Agents Actions* **10,** 368–373.

Holsapple, M. P., Shopp, G. R., Munson, J. A., and Tucker, A. (1983). Selective immunosuppression by a formamidine pesticide. *Toxicologist* **3,** 59.

Homburger, F., Kelly, T., Jr., Baker, T. R., and Russfield, A. B. (1962). Sex effect on hepatic pathology from deficient diet and safrole in rats. *Arch. Pathol.* **73,** 118–125.

Homeida, A. M., and Cooke, R. G. (1982a). Pharmacological aspects of metaldehyde poisoning in mice. *J. Vet. Pharmacol. Ther.* **5,** 77–81.

Homeida, A. M., and Cooke, R. G. (1982b). Anti-convulsant activity of diazepam and clonidine on metaldehyde-induced seizures in mice: Effects on brain gamma-aminobutyric acid concentrations and monoamine oxidase activity. *J. Vet Pharmacol. Ther.* **5,** 187–190.

Horiuchi, N., and Ando, S. (1980). Contact dermatitis due to pesticides for agricultural use. *Jpn. J. Dermatol.* **90,** 289 (in Japanese).

Horiuchi, N., Kambe, Y., Kato, E., and Ando, S. (1976). Studies on the criteria of diagnosis in dermatitis due to pesticides. Part 3. Results of patch tests on pesticide-dermatitis patients engaged in lettuce cultivation and irradiation. *J. Jpn. Assoc. Rural Med.* **25,** 340–341 (in Japanese).

Horiuchi, N., Ando, S., and Kambe, Y. (1980). Dermatitis due to pesticides for agricultural use. *Jpn. J. Dermatol.* **90,** 277 (in Japanese).

Hsu, W. H., and Hopper, D. L. (1986). Effect of yohimbine on amitraz-induced CNS depression and bradycardia in dogs. *J. Toxicol. Environ. Health* **18,** 423–429.

Hsu, W. H., and Kakuk, T. J. (1984). Effect of amitraz and chlordimeform on

heart rate and pupil diameter in rats: Mediated by alpha-2-adrenoreceptors. *Toxicol. Appl. Pharmacol.* **73,** 411–415.

Hsu, W. H., and Lu, Z. (1984). Amitraz-induced delay of gastrointestinal transit in mice: Mediated by alpha 2-adrenergic receptors. *Drug Rev. Res.* **4,** 655–660.

Hsu, W. H., and McNeel, S. V. (1985). Amitraz-induced prolongation of gastrointestinal transit and bradycardia in dogs and then antagonism by yohimbine: Preliminary study. *Drug Chem. Toxicol.* **8,** 239–253.

Hsu, W. H., Lu, Z. X., and Hembrough, F. B. (1986). Effect of amitraz on heart rate and aortic blood pressure in conscious dogs: Influence of atropine, prazosin, tolazoline, and yohimbine. *Toxicol. Appl. Pharmacol.* **84,** 418–422.

Idris, M., Rahman, K. M., Muttalib, M. A., and Azad Khan, A. K. (1980). The treatment of fasciolopsiasis with niclosamide and dichlorophen. *J. Trop. Med. Hyg.* **83,** 71–74.

Innes, J. R. M., Ulland, B. M., Valerio, M. G., Petrucelli, L., Fishbein, L., Hart, E. R., Pallotta, A. J., Bates, R. R., Falk, H. L., Gart, J. J., Klein, G. M., Mitchell, I., and Peters, J. (1969). Bioassay of pesticides and industrial chemicals for tumorigenicity in mice: A preliminary note. *J. Natl. Cancer Inst. (U.S.)* **42,** 1101–1114.

International Agency for Research on Cancer (IARC) (1983a). Chlordimeform. *IARC Monogr. Eval. Carcinog. Risk Chem. Hum.* **30,** 61–72.

International Agency for Research on Cancer (IARC) (1983b). Piperonyl butoxide. *IARC Monogr. Eval. Carcinog. Risk Chem. Hum.* **30,** 183–195.

Jaffe, H., and Neumeyer, J. L. (1970). Comparative effects of piperonyl butoxide and *N*-(4-pentynyl)phthalimide on mammalian microsomal enzyme functions. *J. Med. Chem.* **13,** 901–903.

Jaffe, H., Fujii, K., and Epstein, S. S. (1968a). In vivo inhibition of mouse liver microsomal hydroxylating systems by methylenedioxyphenyl insecticidal synergists and related compounds. *Fed. Proc. Fed. Am. Soc. Exp. Biol.* **27,** 721.

Jaffe, H., Fujii, K., Sengupta, M., Guérin, H., and Epstein, S. S. (1968b). *In vivo* inhibition of mouse liver microsomal hydroxylating systems by methylene dioxyphenyl insecticidal synergists and related compounds. *Life Sci.* **7** (Part 1), 1051–1062.

Jaffe, H., Fujii, K., Guérin, H., Sengupta, M., and Epstein, S. S. (1969). Bimodal effect of piperonyl butoxide on the *o*- and *p*-hydroxylations of biphenyl by mouse liver microsomes. *Biochem. Pharmacol.* **18,** 1045–1051.

James, R. C., and Harbison, R. D. (1982). Hepatic glutathione and hepatotoxicity: Effects of cytochrome P-450 complexing compounds SKF 525-A, *L*-alpha-acetylmethadol (LAAM), norLAAM, and piperonyl butoxide. *Biochem. Pharmacol.* **31,** 1829–1835.

Janssen, R., Boyes, W. K., and Dyer, R. S. (1983). Effects of chlordimeform on the brainstem auditory evoked response in rats. *In* "Developments in the Science and Practice of Toxicology" (A. W. Hayes, R. C. Schnell, and T. S. Miya, eds.), pp. 533–536, Am. Elsevier, New York.

Jao, L. T., and Casida, J. E. (1974). Esterase inhibitors as synergists for (+)-transchrysanthemate insecticide chemicals. *Pestic. Biochem. Physiol.* **4,** 456–464.

Jobin, W. R. (1979). Cost of snail control. *Am. J. Trop. Med. Hyg.* **28,** 142–154.

Johnson, T. L., and Knowles, C. O. (1981). Inhibition of rat platelet 5-hydroxytryptamine uptake by chlordimeform. *Toxicol. Lett.* **9,** 1–4.

Johnson, T. L., and Knowles, C. O. (1982). Interaction of formamidines with the rat platelet 5-hydroxytryptamine uptake system. *Gen. Pharmacol.* **13,** 299–307.

Johnson, T. L., and Knowles, C. O. (1983). Influence of formamidines on biogenic amine levels in rat brain and plasma. *Gen. Pharmacol.* **14,** 591–596.

Johnson, T. L., and Knowles, C. O. (1985). Formamidine-mediated inhibition of rat platelet aggregation. *Gen. Pharmacol.* **16,** 321–325.

Jones, W. A., and Jacobson, M. (1968). Isolation of *N,N*-diethyl-*m*-toluamid (deet) from female pink bollworm moths. *Science* **159,** 99–100.

Kadir, H., and Knowles, C. O. (1981). Inhibition of rat brain monoamine oxidase by insecticides, acaricides, and related compounds. *Gen. Pharmacol.* **12,** 239–247.

Kaloyanova, F. P., Zaprianov, Z., and Bainova, A. I. (1978). Influence of the insecticide chlorodimeform of the activity of the monoamine oxidase (MAO) of albino rats. *Dokl. Bolg.. Akad. Nauk* **31**, 491–493.

Kaloyanova, F. P., Zaprianov, Z., and Bainova, A. I. (1979). Inhibition of the monoamine oxidase (MAO) after the combined action of the insecticide chlordimeform with analgin. *Dokl. Bolg. Akad. Nauk* **32**, 1153–1155.

Kaloyanova, F., Bainova, A., and Zaprianov, Z. (1981). Inhibition of monoamine oxidase activity after combined action of chlordimeform with the antidepressant nialamide. *Arch. Environ. Contam. Toxicol.* **10**, 1–8.

Kamienski, F. X., and Casida, J. E. (1970). Importance of demethylenation in the metabolism *in vivo* and *in vitro* of methylenedioxyphenyl synergists and related compounds in mammals. *Biochem. Pharmacol.* **19**, 91–112.

Kamienski, F. X., and Murphy, S. D. (1971). Biphasic effects of methylenedioxyphenyl synergists on the action of hexabarbital and organophosphate insecticides in mice. *Toxicol. Appl. Pharmacol.* **18**, 883–894.

Kawachi, T., Yahagi, T., Kada, T., Ishidate, M., Sasaki, M., and Sugiyama, T. (1980). Cooperative programme on short-term assays for carcinogenicity in Japan. *IARC Sci. Publ.* **27**, 323–330.

Kennedy, G. L., Jr., Smith, S. H., Kinoshita, F. K., Keplinger, M. L., and Calandra, J. C. (1977). Teratogenic evaluation of piperonyl butoxide in the rat. *Food Cosmet. Toxicol.* **15**, 337–339.

Keplinger, M. L., Frawley, J. P., Tusing, T. W., Woodard, G., and Dardin, V. J. (1961). Subacute oral and dermal toxicity of deet (*N,N*-diethyl-*m*-toluamide). *Fed. Proc., Fed. Am. Soc. Exp. Biol.* **20**, 432.

Khera, K. S., Whalen, C., Angers, G., and Trivett, G. (1979). Assessment of the teratogenic potential of piperonyl butoxide, biphenyl, and phosalone in the rat. *Toxicol. Appl. Pharmacol.* **47**, 353–358.

Kimbrough, R. D. (1980). Human health effects of selected pesticides, chloroaniline derivatives. *J. Environ. Sci. Health, Part B* **B15**, 977–992.

Kimbrough, R. D., Gaines, T. B., and Hayes, W. J., Jr. (1968). Combined effect of DDT, pyrethrins and piperonyl butoxide on rat liver. *Arch. Environ. Health* **16**, 333–341.

Kimmel, E. C., Casida, J. E., and Ruzo, L. O. (1986). Formamidine insecticides and chloroacetanilide herbicides: Disubstituted anilines and nitrosobenzenes as mammalian metabolites and bacterial mutagens. *J. Agric. Food Chem.* **34**, 157–161.

Kiryushin, V. A. (1977). Mutagenic effect of pesticides of different chemical structure during isolated intake by white rats. *Gig. Aspekty Okhr. Zdorov'ya Naseleniya*, p. 196 (in Russian).

Knipling, E. F. (1979). The basic principles of insect population suppression and management. *U.S., Dep. Agric, Agric. Handb.* **512.**

Knowles, C. O. (1970). Metabolism of two acaricidal chemicals, *N'*-(4-chloro-*o*-tolyl)-*N,N*-dimethylformamidine (chlorphenamidine) and *m*{[(dimethylamino)methylene]amino}phenyl methylcarbamate hydrochloride (formetanate). *J. Agric. Food Chem.* **18**, 1038–1047.

Knowles, C. O. (1974). Detoxication of acaricides by animals. *In* "Survival in Toxic Environments" (M. A. Q. Khan and J. P. Bederka, Jr., eds.), pp. 155–176. Academic Press, New York.

Knowles, C. O. (1976). Chemistry and toxicology of quinoxaline, organotin, organofluorine, and formamidine acaricides. *Environ. Health Perspect.* **14**, 93–102.

Knowles, C. O. (1982). Structure–activity relationships among amidine acaricides and insecticides. *In* "Insecticide Mode of Action" (J. R. Coats, ed.), pp. 243–277. Academic Press, New York.

Knowles, C. O., and Aziz, S. A. (1974). Interaction of formamidines with components of the biogenic amine system. *ACS Symp. Ser.* **2**, 92–99.

Knowles, C. O., and Benezet, H. J. (1977). Mammalian metabolism of chlordimeform. Formation of metabolites containing the urea moiety. *J. Agric. Food Chem.* **25**, 1022–1026.

Knowles, C. O., and Benezet, H. J. (1979). Inhibition of ethanol and acetate metabolism in mice by chlordimeform and related compounds *Gen. Pharmacol.* **10**, 499–503.

Knowles, C. O., and Benezet, H. J. (1981). Excretion balance, metabolic fate and tissue residues following treatment of rats with amitraz and *N'*-(2,4-dimethylphenyl)-*N*-methylformamidine. *J. Environ. Sci. Health, Part B* **B16**, 547–556.

Knowles, C. O., and Johnson, T. L. (1984a). Formamidine interactions with rat platelet biogenic amine regulatory mechanisms. *Neurotoxicology* **5**, 78–79.

Knowles, C. O., and Johnson, T. L. (1984b). Effect of formamidines on 5-hydroxytryptamine uptake and biogenic amine levels in rat platelets. *Toxicology* **31**, 91–98.

Knowles, C. O., and Sen Gupta, A. K. (1970). *N'*-(4-Chloro-*o*-tolyl)-*N,N*-dimethylformamidine-C^{14} (Galecron) and 4-chloro-*o*-toluidine-C^{14} metabolism in the white rat. *J. Econ. Entomol.* **63**, 856–859.

Kuhlman, R. S., Cameron, R. H., Kolesari, G. L., and Wu, A. (1981). *N,N*-Diethyl-*meta*-toluamide: Embryonic sensitivity. *Teratology* **23**, 48A.

Kujawa, M., Macholz, R., Bleyl, D., Nickel, B., and Seidler, H. (1985). Analysis of azobenzene and its metabolites as well as the placental transfer of azoxybenzene. *Z. Gesamte Hyg. Ihre Grenzgeb.* **31**, 464–465 (in Japanese).

Lake, B. G., Hopkins, R., Chakraborty, J., Bridges, J. W., and Parke, D. V. W. (1973). Influence of some hepatic enzyme inducers and inhibitors on extrahepatic drug metabolism. *Drug Metab. Dispos.* **1**, 342–349.

Lamberg, S. I., and Mulrennan, J. A., Jr. (1969). Bullous reaction to diethyl toluamide (deet) resembling a blistering insect eruption. *Arch. Dermatol.* **100**, 582–586.

Landauer, M. R., Tomlinson, W. T., Balster, R. L., and MacPhail, R. C. (1984). Some effects of the formamidine pesticide chlordimeform on the behavior of mice. *Neurotoxicology* **5**, 91–100.

Lanfranchi, C., and Bavoux, F. (1982). Difficulties in the treatment of scabies in infants. *Arch. Fr. Pediatr.* **39**, 845–849 (in French).

Lang, R. (1984). The mammalian spot test and its use for testing of mutagenic and carcinogenic potential: Experience with the pesticide chlordimeform, its principal metabolites and the drug lisuride hydrogen maleate. *Mutat. Res.* **135**, 219–224.

Lang, R., and Adler, I.-D. (1982). Studies on the mutagenic potential of the pesticide chlordimeform and its principal metabolites in the mouse heritable translocation assay. *Mutat. Res.* **92**, 243–248.

Larson, L. L., Kenaga, E. E., and Morgan, R. W. (1985). "Commercial and Experimental Organic Insecticides." Entomol. Soc. Am., College Part, Maryland.

Lau, S. S., Monks, T. J., Greene, K. E., and Gillette, J. R. (1984). The role of *ortho*-bromophenol in the nephrotoxicity of bromobenzene in rats. *Toxicol. Appl. Pharmacol.* **72**, 539–549.

Leach, G. J., Russell, R. D., and Houpt, J. T. (1987). Cardiovascular effects of *N,N*-diethyl-*m*-toluamide. *Toxicologist* **7**, 91.

Leander, J. D., and MacPhail, R. C. (1980). Effect of chlordimeform (a formamidine pesticide) on schedule-controlled responding of pigeons. *Neurobehav. Toxicol. Teratol.* **2**, 315–321.

Lebowitz, H., Young, R., Galloway, S., and Brusick, D. (1981). The effect of *N,N*-diethyltoluamide (deet) on sperm number, viability and head morphology in male rats treated dermally. *Environ. Mutagen.* **3**, 370.

Lebowitz, H., Young, R., Kidwell, J., McGowan, J., Langloss, J., and Brusick, D. (1983). Deet (*N,N*-diethyltoluamide) does not affect sperm number, viability and head morphology in male rats treated dermally. *Drug Chem. Toxicol.* **6**, 379–395.

Lee, T.-P., Moscati, R., and Park, B. H. (1979). Effects of pesticides on human leukocyte functions. *Res. Commun. Chem. Pathol. Pharmacol.* **23**, 597–609.

Lehman, H. J. (1951). Chemicals in foods: A report to the Association of Food and Drug Officials on current developments. Part II. Pesticides. Section I. Introduction. *Q. Bull.—Assoc. Food Drug Off.* **15** (I), 122–133.

Lehman, H. J. (1952). Chemicals in foods: A report to the Association of Food and Drug Officials in current developments. Part II. Pesticides. Section II. Dermal toxicity. Section III. Subacute and chronic toxicity. Section IV. Biochemistry. Section V. Pathology. *Q. Bull.—Assoc. Food Drug Off.* **16** (II), 3–9; (III), 47–53; (IV), 85–91; (V), 126–132.

Lehmann, K. B. (1933). Studies on the action of chloroaniline and chlorotoluidine and the hydrochloride of 5-chloro-2-toluidine. *Arch. Hyg. Bakteriol.* **110**, 12–32 (in German).

Lemma, A., and Ames, B. N. (1975). Screening for mutagenic activity of some molluscicides. *Trans. R. Soc. Trop. Med. Hyg.* **69**, 167–168.

Levine, W. G. (1971). Metabolism and biliary excretion of *N*-2-fluorenylacetamide and *N*-hydroxy-2-fluorenylacetamide. *Life Sci.* **10**, 727–735.

Levine, W. G. (1972). Biliary excretion of 3-methylcholanthrene as controlled by its metabolism. *J. Pharmacol. Exp. Ther.* **183**, 420–426.

Levine, W. G. (1974). Hepatic uptake, metabolism and biliary excretion of 7,12-dimethylbenzanthracene in the rat. *Drug Metab. Dispos.* **2**, 169–177.

Lewin, J. F., and Cleary, W. T. (1982). An accidental death caused by the absorption of phenol through skin. A case report. *Forensic Sci. Int.* **19**, 177–179.

Lewis, D. R., Madel, G. A., and Drury, J. (1939). Fatal poisoning by "Meta Fuel" tablets. *Br. Med. J.* **1**, 1283–1284.

Lin, T. H., North, H. H., and Menzer, R. E. (1975). The metabolic fate of chlordimeform [*N*-(4-chloro-*o*-tolyl)-*N'*,*N'*-dimethylformamidine] in human embryonic lung cell cultures. *J. Agric. Food Chem.* **23**, 257–258.

Liu, S., Wu, A., and Wang, R. I. H. (1984). Biphasic effect of *N*,*N*-diethyl-*m*-toluamide (deet) on the hypnotic activity and metabolism of pentobarbital in rats. *Fed. Proc., Fed. Am. Soc. Exp. Biol.* **43**, 762.

Long, E. L., and Jenner, P. M. (1963). Esophageal tumors produced in rats by the feeding of dihydrosafrole. *Fed. Proc., Fed. Am. Soc. Exp. Biol.* **22**, 275.

Long, E. L., Nelson, A. A., Fitzhugh, O. G., and Hansen, W. H. (1963). Liver tumors produced in rats by feeding safrole. *Arch. Pathol.* **75**, 595–604.

Longstreth, W. T., Jr., and Pierson, D. J. (1982). Metaldehyde poisoning from slug bait ingestion. *West. J. Med.* **137**, 134–137.

Lucier, G. W., McDaniel, O. S., and Matthews, H. B. (1971). Microsomal rat liver UDP glucuronyltransferase: Effects of piperonyl butoxide and other factors on enzyme activity. *Arch. Biochem. Biophys.* **145**, 520–530.

Lüdin, M. (1958). Murder with meta? *Schweiz. Med. Wochenschr.* **88**, 381–384 (in German).

Lund, A. E., Yim, G. K. W., and Shankland, D. L. (1978a). The cardiovascular toxicity of chlordimeform: A local anesthetic-like action. *In* "Pesticide and Venom Neurotoxicity" (D. L. Shankland, R. M. Hollingworth, and T. Smyth, Jr., eds.), pp. 171–177. Plenum, New York.

Lund, A. E., Shankland, D. L., Chinn, C., and Yim, G. K. W. (1978b). Similar cardiovascular toxicity of the pesticide chlordimeform and lidocaine. *Toxicol. Appl. Pharmacol.* **44**, 357–365.

Lund, A. E., Hollingworth, R. M., and Yim, G. K. W. (1979). The comparative neurotoxicity of formamidine pesticides *In* "Neurotoxicology of Insecticides and Pheromones" (T. Narahashi, ed.), pp. 119–137. Plenum, New York.

Lurie, A. A., Gleiberman, S. E., and Tsizin, Y. S. (1978). Pharmacokinetics of the repellent *N*,*N*-diethyl-3-methylbenzamide. *Med. Parazitol. Parazit. Bolezni* **47**, 72–77 (in Russian).

Lush, I. E. (1976). A survey of the response of different strains of mice to substances metabolized by microsomal oxidation; hexobarbitone, zoxazolamine and warfarin. *Chem.-Biol. Interact.* **12**, 363–373.

Macht, D. I. (1918). On the relation between the chemical structure of the opium alkaloids and their physiological action on smooth muscle with a pharmacological and therapeutic study of some benzyl esters. II. A pharmacological and therapeutic study of some benzyl esters. *J. Pharmacol. Exp. Ther.* **11**, 419–446.

Macht, D. I. (1919a). A therapeutic study, pharacologic and clinical, of benzyl benzoate. *JAMA, J. Am. Med. Assoc.* **73**, 599–601.

Macht, D. I. (1919b). A therapeutic study of benzyl benzoate in bronchial spasm or asthma. *South. Med. J.* **12**, 367–371.

Macht, D. I. (1920). On the use of benzyl benzoate in some circulatory conditions. *N. Y. Med. J.* **112**, 269–271.

Macht, D. I., and Leach, H. P. (1929). Concerning the antipyretic properties of benzyl benzoate. *J. Pharmacol. Exp. Ther.* **35**, 281–296.

Macko, J. A., Jr., and Bergman, J. D. (1979). "Phase 4, Inhalation Toxicities of *N*,*N*-Diethyl-*meta*-toluamide (*m*-DET)." Study 75-51-0034-80, January–May 1979. U.S. Army Environ. Hyg. Agency, Aberdeen Proving Ground, Maryland.

Macko, J. A., Jr., and Weeks, M. H. (1980). "Phase 6, Acute Toxicity Evaluation of *N*,*N*-Diethyl-*meta*-toluamide (*m*-DET). Animal Studies." Study 75-51-0034-81, March 1977–January 1980, 39 pp. U.S. Army Environ. Hyg. Agency, Aberdeen Proving Ground, Maryland.

MacPhail, R. C. (1985). Effects of pesticides on schedule-controlled behavior. *In* "Behavioral Pharmacology: The Current Status" (L. S. Seiden and R. L. Balster, eds.), pp. 519–535. Alan R. Liss, New York.

MacPhail, R. C., and Leander, J. D. (1980). Flavor aversions induced by chlordimeform. *Neurobehav. Toxicol. Teratol.* **2**, 363–365.

MacPhail, R. C., and Leander, J. D. (1981). Chlordimeform effects on schedule-controlled behavior in rats. *Neurobehav. Toxicol. Teratol.* **3**, 19–26.

Maddy, K. T. (1975). Poisoning of dogs with metaldehyde in snail and slug poison bait—conclusion. *Calif. Vet.* **29**, 24–25.

Maddy, K. T., Knaak, J. B., and Gibbons, D. B. (1986). Monitoring the urine of pesticide applicators in California for residues of chlordimeform and its metabolites 1982–1985. *Toxicol. Lett.* **33**, 37–44.

Maekawa, A., Onodera, H., Furuta, K., Tanigawa, H., Ogiu, T., and Hayashi, Y. (1985). Lack of evidence of carcinogenicity of technical-grade piperonyl butoxide in F344 rats: Selective induction of ileocaecal ulcers. *Food Chem. Toxicol.* **23**, 675–682.

Maibach, H. I., and Johnson, H. L. (1975). Contact urticaria syncrome. Contact urticaria to diethyltoluamide (immediate-type hypersensitivity). *Arch. Dermatol.* **111**, 726–730.

Maitre, A. F., Waldmeier, P., and Kehr, W. (1978). Monoamine oxidase inhibition in brain and liver of rats treated with chlordimeform. *J. Agric. Food Chem.* **26**, 442–446.

Marks, E. P., Leighton, T., and Leighton, F. (1982). Modes of action of chitin synthesis inhibitors. *In* "Insecticide Mode of Action" (J. R. Coats, ed.), pp. 281–313. Academic Press, New York.

Mason, E. C., and Pieck, C. E. (1920). A pharmacological study of benzyl benzoate. *J. Lab. Clin. Med.* **6**, 62–77.

Massey, T. E., Walker, R. M., McElligott, T. F., and Racz, W. J. (1982). Acetaminophen-induced hypothermia in mice: Evidence for a central action of the parent compound. *Toxicology* **25**, 187–200.

Matsumura, F., and Beeman, R. W. (1976). Biochemical and physiological effects of chlordimeform. *Environ. Health Perspect.* **14**, 71–82.

Metcalf, R. L. (1955). "Organic Insecticides—Their Chemistry and Mode of Action." (Wiley Interscience), New York.

Metcalf, R. L. (1967). Mode of action of insecticide synergists. *Annu. Rev. Entomol.* **12**, 229–256.

Meynadier, J. M., Meynadier, J., Colmas, A., Castelain, P. Y., Ducombs, G., Chabeau, G., Lacroix, M., Martin, P., and Ngangu, Z. (1982). Allergy to preservatives. *Ann. Dermatol. Venereol.* **109**, 1017–1023 (in French).

Miller, J. D. (1982). Anaphylaxis associated with insect repellent (letter). *N. Engl. J. Med.* **307**, 1341–1342.

Miller, R. (1928). Poisoning by "Meta Fuel" tablets (metacetaldehyde). *Arch. Dis. Child.* **3**, 292–295.

Mirer, F. E., Cheever, K. L., and Murphy, S. D. (1975). A comparison of gas chromatographic and anti-cholinesterase methods for measuring parathion metabolism in vitro. *Bull. Environ. Contam. Toxicol.* **13**, 745–750.

Mitchell, J. R., Jollow, D. J., Potter, W. Z., Davis, D. C., Gillette, J. R., and Brodie, B. B. (1973). Acetaminophen-induced hepatic necrosis. I. Role of drug metabolism *J. Pharmacol. Exp. Ther.* **187**, 185–194.

Mitoma, C., Yasuda, D., Yagg, J. S., Neubauer, S. E., Calderoni, F. J., and Tanabe, M. (1968). Effects of various chemical agents on drug metabolism and cholesterol biosynthesis. *Biochem. Pharmacol.* **17**, 1377–1383.

Morikawa, M., Yokoyama, S., and Fukami, J. (1975). Comparative metabolism of chlordimeform on rat and rice stem borer. *Botyu-Kagaku* **40**, 162–184.

Morita, S., Yamada, A., Ohgaki, S., Noda, T., and Taniguchi, S. (1981). Safety evaluation of chemicals for use in household products. II. Teratological studies on benzyl benzoate and 2-(morpholinothio)benzothiazole in rats. *Annu. Rep. Osaka City Inst. Public Health Environ. Sci.* **43**, 90–97 (in Japanese).

Moriya, M., Ohta, T., Watanabe, K., Miyazawa, T., Kato, K., and Shirabu, Y. (1983). Further mutagenicity studies on pesticides in bacterial reversion assay systems. *Mutat. Res.* **116**, 185–216.

Moser, V. C., and MacPhail, R. C. (1984a). Differential effects of formamidine pesticides on multiple fixed-interval responding in rats. *Neurosci. Abstr.* **10**, 1071.

Moser, V. C., and MacPhail, R. C. (1984b). Some neurobehavioral effects of amitraz in rats. *Neurotoxicology* **5**, 75–76.

Moser, V. C., and MacPhail, R. C. (1985). Yohimbine attenuates the delayed lethality induced in mice by amitraz, a formamidine pesticide. *Toxicol Lett.* **28**, 99–104.

Moser, V. C., and MacPhail, R. C. (1986). Differential effects of formamidine pesticides on fixed-interval behavior in rats. *Toxicol. Appl. Pharmacol.* **84**, 315–324.

Moser, V. C., McCormick, J. P., and MacPhail, R. C. (1987). Comparison of chlordimeform and carbaryl using a functional observational battery. *Toxicologist* **7**, 251.

Mothes, U. (1981). Electron microscopial changes of the cuticle of *Tetranychus urticae* Koch (Acari, Tetranychidae) after treatment with nikkomycin (AMS 0896 Bayer Leverkusen). *Mitt. Dtsch. Ges. Allg. Angew. Entomol.* **2**, 172–179 (in German).

Mothes, U., and Seitz, K.-A. (1982). Action of the microbial metabolite and chitin synthesis inhibitor nikkomycin on the mite *Tetranychus urticae;* an electron microscope study. *Pestic. Sci.* **13**, 426–441.

Mothes-Wagner, U. (1984a). Fine structure of the cuticle and structural changes occurring during moulting in the mite *Tetranychus urticae*. II. Moulting process (Chelicerata, Acarina). *Zoomorphology* **104**, 105–110.

Mothes-Wagner, U. (1984b). Effects of the chitin synthesis inhibitor complex nikkomycin on oogenesis in the mite *Tetranychus urticae*. *Pestic. Sci.* **15**, 455–461.

Murakami, M., and Fukami, J. (1974). Effects of chlorphenamidine and its metabolites on HeLa cells. *Bull. Environ. Contam. Toxicol.* **11**, 184–188.

Murakami, M., and Fukami, J. (1976). Uptake and persistence of pesticides in cultured human cells. *Bull. Environ. Contam. Toxicol.* **15**, 425–428.

Murakami, M., Fukami, J., and Fukunaga, K. (1972). Effects of chlorphenamidine on cultured cells. *Seikagaku* **44**, 496 (in Japanese).

Nagai, R. (1976). Occupational and allergic dermatitis in Japan. *Clin. Dermatol.* **18**, 601–610.

Nakamura, E., Kimura, M., Kato, R., and Noda, F. (1977). The toxicity of azoxybenzene. *Kyoritsu Yakka Daigaku Kenkyu Nempo* **21**, 25–47 (in Japanese).

Nathanson, J. A., and Hunnicutt, E. J. (1981). *N*-Demethylchlordimeform, a potent partial agonist of octopamine-sensitive adenylate cyclase. *Mol. Pharmacol* **20**, 68–75.

National Cancer Institute (NCI) (1978). "Bioassay of Clonitralid for Possible Carcinogenicity." Carcinogenesis Tech. Rep. Series No. 91, DHEW Publ. No. (NIH) 78–1341. U.S. Gov. Printing Office, Washington, D.C.

National Cancer Institute (NCI) (1979a). "Bioassay of 4-Chloro-*o*-toluidine Hydrochloride for Possible Carcinogenicity," Carcinogenesis Tech. Rep. Ser. No. 165, DHEW Publ. No. (NIH) 79–1721. U.S. Gov. Printing Office, Washington, D.C.

National Cancer Institute (NCI) (1979b). "Bioassay of Piperonyl Butoxide for Possible Carcinogenicity," Carcinogenesis Tech. Rep. Ser. No. 120, DHEW Publ. No. (NIH) 79–1375. U.S. Gov. Printing Office, Washington, D.C.

National Technical Information Service (NTIS) (1968). "Evaluation of Carcinogenic, Teratogenic and Mutagenic Activities of Selected Pesticides and Industrial Chemicals," Vol. **1**, Carcinogenic Study (PB-223159). U.S. Govt. Printing Office, Washington, D.C.

Nelson, B. D., Drake, R., and McDaniel, O. (1971). Effects *in vitro* and *in vivo* of methylenedioxyphenyl compounds on oxidative phosphorylation in rat liver mitochondria. *Biochem. Pharmacol.* **20**, 1139–1149.

Neumann, R., and Voss, G. (1977). MAO inhibition, an unlikely mode of action for chlordimeform. *Experientia* **33**, 23–24.

Nielsen, C., and Higgins, J. A. (1920). Observations on the pharmacology of some benzyl esters. *J. Lab. Clin. Med.* **6**, 388–392.

Nielsen, C., and Higgins, J. A. (1921). Further observations on the pharmacology of benzyl compounds. *J. Lab. Clin. Med.* **7**, 69–83.

Norman, B. J., and Neal, R. A. (1976). Examination of the metabolism *in vitro* of parathion (diethyl *p*-nitrophenyl phosphorothioate) by rat lung and brain. *Biochem. Pharmacol.* **25**, 37–45.

Olson, K. L., Boush, G. M., and Matsumura, F. (1978). Behavioral effects of

perinatal exposure of chlordimeform in rats. *Bull. Environ. Contam. Toxicol.* **20**, 760–768.

Orkin, M., Epstein, E., and Maibach, H. I. (1976). Treatment of today's scabies and pediculosis *JAMA, J. Am. Med. Assoc.* **236**, 1136–1139.

Osmundsen, P. E. (1971). Contact photo-allergy to tribromosalicylanilide. *Boll. Chim.-Farm.* **110**, 590–594.

Ostrosky-Wegman, P., Garcia, G., Montero, R., Pérez Romero, B., Alvarez Chácon, R., and Cortinas de Nava, C. (1986). Susceptibility to genotoxic effects of niclosamide in human peripheral lymphocytes exposed *in vitro* and *in vivo*. *Mutat. Res.* **173**, 81–87.

Palmer, J. S. (1969). Toxicologic effects of aerosols of *N,N*-diethyl-*m*-toluene (deet) applied on skin of horses. *Am. J. Vet. Res.* **30**, 1929–1932.

Pascoe, A. L., and Reynoldson, J. A. (1986). The cardiac effects of amitraz in the guinea pig *in vivo* and *in vitro*. *Comp. Biochem. Physiol. C* **83C**, 413–417.

Pass, M. A., and Seawright, A. A. (1982). Effect of amitraz on contractions of the guinea-pig ileum *in vitro*. *Comp. Biochem. Physiol. C* **73C**, 419–422.

Peele, D. P., MacPhail, R. C., and Cannon, S. E. (1984). Comparison of the effects of environmental challenges and chlordimeform on the schedule-controlled performance of young-adult and senescent rats. *Fed. Proc., Fed. Am. Soc. Exp. Biol.* **43**, 1018.

Pento, J. T., Robinson, C. P., Rieger, J. A., and Horton, P. A. (1979). The influence of chlordimeform on calcium and glucose homeostasis in the rat. *Res. Commun. Chem. Pathol. Pharmacol.* **24**, 127–142.

Pfister, W. R., and Yim, G. K. W. (1977). Antipyretic–analgesic actions of the formamidine pesticide, chlordimeform. *Pharmacologist* **19**, 216.

Pfister, W. R., Hollingworth, R. M., and Yim, G. K. W. (1978a). Increased feeding in rats treated with chlordimeform and related formamidines: A new class of appetite stimulants. *Psychopharmacology* **60**, 47–51.

Pfister, W., Chinn, C., Noland, V., and Yim, G. K. W. (1978b). Similar pharmacological actions of chlordimeform and local anesthetics. *Pestic. Biochem. Physiol.* **9**, 148–156.

Phillips, L., II, Steinberg, M., Maibach, H. I., and Akers, W. A. (1972). A comparison of rabbit and human skin response to certain irritants. *Toxicol. Appl. Pharmacol.* **21**, 369–382.

Platonova, V. I. (1970). Disturbances in the functional condition of the stomach with the prolonged effect on the body of some organochlorine pesticides. *Gig. Tr.* **6**, 142–147 (in Russian).

Poland, A., and Kappas, A. (1971). The metabolism of aminopyrine in chick embryo hepatic cell culture: Effects of competitive substrates and carbon monoxide. *Mol. Pharmacol.* **7**, 697–706.

Prishchepov, V. F., Mikhailuts, A. P., Ostapenko, I. T., Urbanskii, A. S., and Gubin, V. I. (1981). Occupational skin disease of workers in the production of diethyltoluamide-20 repellent lotion. *Gig. Tr. Prof. Zabol.* **10**, 11–13 (in Russian); *Chem. Abstr.* 9673940Y.

Pronczuk de Garbino, J., and Laborde, A. (1983). Toxicity of an insect repellent: *N,N*-Diethyltoluamide. *Vet. Hum. Toxicol.* **25**, 422–423.

Putrali, J., Dazo, B. C., Hardjawidjaja, L., Sudomo, M., and Barodji, A. (1980). A schistosomiasis pilot control project in Lindu Valley, Central Sulawesi, Indonesia. *Southeast Asian J. Trop. Med. Public Health* **11**, 480–486.

Pütter, von J. (1970). On the biological and chemical actions of the tapeworm remedy *N*-(2'-chloro-4'-nitrophenyl)-5-chlorosalicylamide. 1. Communication: Action on enzyme systems. *Arzneim.-Forsch.* **20**, 203–205 (in German).

Quinto, I., Martire, G., Vricella, G., Riccardi, F., Perfumo, A., Giulivo, R., and Delorenzo, F. (1981). Screening of 24 pesticides by *Salmonella* microsome assay, mutagenicity of benazolin, etoxuron, and paraoxon. *Mutat. Res.* **85**, 165.

Rabinovich, M. V. (1966). On the effect of diethyltoluamide on the skin and mucous membranes of the human eye. *Zh. Mikrobiol., Epidemiol. Immunol.* **43**, 109–112 (in Russian).

Rashid, K. A., Ercegovich, C. D., and Mumma, R. O. (1984). Evaluation of chlordimeform and degradation products for mutagenic and DNA-damaging activity in *Salmonella Typhimurium* and *Escherichia coli*. *J. Environ. Sci. Health, Part B* **19**, 95–110.

Raupp, D. R., Yim, G. K. W., and Schnell, R. C. (1980). Effect of acute and chronic chlordimeform treatment on rat hepatic microsomal drug metabolizing enzymes. *Abstr. Pap., 19th Annu. Meet. Soc. Toxicol.,* p. A82.

Ravikumar, V. C., and Rieger, J. A. (1983). Potential neuromuscular toxicity of *N'*-(2,4-xylyl)-*N*-methylformamidine HC1 in rodents. *Toxicology* **27,** 71–80.

Reid, W. D. (1973). Mechanism of renal necrosis induced by bromobenzene and chlorobenzene. *Exp. Mol. Pathol.* **19,** 197–214.

Reid, W. D., Christie, B., Krishna, G., Mitchell, J. R., Moskowitz, J., and Brodie, B. B. (1971). Bromobenzene metabolism and hepatic necrosis. *Pharmacology* **6,** 41–55.

Reifenrath, W. G., and Robinson, P. B. (1982). *In vitro* skin evaporation and penetration characteristics of mosquito repellents. *J. Pharm. Sci.* **71,** 1014–1018.

Reifenrath, W. G., Hill, J. A., Robinson, P. B., McVey, D. L., Akers, W. A., Anjo, D. M., and Maibach, H. I. (1980). Percutaneous absorption of carbon 14 labeled insect repellents in hairless dogs. *J. Environ. Pathol. Toxicol.* **4,** 249–256.

Reifenrath, W. G., Robinson, P. B., Bolton, V. D., and Aliff, R. E. (1981). Percutaneous penetration of mosquito repellents in the hairless dog—effect of dose on percentage penetration. *Food Cosmet. Toxicol.* **19,** 195–199.

Reifenrath, W. G., Chellquist, E. M., Shipwash, E. A. Jederberg, W. W., and Krueger, G. G. (1984). Percutaneous penetration in the hairless dog, weanling pig and grafted nude mouse: Evaluation of models for predicting skin penetration in man. *Br. J. Dermatol., Suppl.* **111,** 123–135.

Reuveni, H., and Yagupsky, P. (1982). Diethyltoluamide-containing insect repellent: Adverse effects in worldwide use. *Arch. Dermatol.* **118,** 582–583.

Rieger, J. A., Robinson, C. P., Gherezghiher, T., and Leung, T. (1980). Inhibition of mammalian monoamine oxidase by two formamidine pesticides *Pharmacologist* **22,** 172.

Rieger, J. A., Robinson, C. P., Cox, P., and Horst, M. A. (1981). Cardiovascular actions and interactions of chlordimeform in the dog. *Bull. Environ. Contam. Toxicol.* **27,** 707–715.

Robbins, P. J., and Chernaick, M. G. (1986). Review of the biodistribution and toxicity of the insect repellent *N,N*-diethyl-*m*-toluamide (deet). *J. Toxicol. Environ. Health* **18,** 503–525.

Robbins, W. E., Hopkins, T. L., and Darrow, D. I. (1959). Synergistic action of piperonyl butoxide with Bayer 21/199 and its corresponding phosphate in mice. *J. Econ. Entomol.* **52,** 660–663.

Roberts, M. C., and Seawright, A. A. (1979). Amitraz induced large intestinal impaction in the horse. *Aust. Vet. J.* **55,** 553–554.

Robinson, C. P. (1979). Effects of U-40481 and formetanate on the isolated rabbit central ear artery. *Pestic. Biochem. Physiol.* **12,** 109–116.

Robinson, C. P. (1982). The mechanism of relaxation of rabbit aorta by chlordimeform. *Toxicologist* **2,** 145.

Robinson, C. P., and Bittle, I. (1979). Vascular effects of demethylchlordimeform, a metabolite of chlordimeform *Pestic. Biochem. Physiol.* **11,** 46–55.

Robinson, C. P., and Pento, J. T. (1980). The effects of U-40481, demethylchlordimeform, and formetanate on calcium flux in the isolated rabbit aorta. *Res. Commun. Chem. Pathol. Pharmacol.* **28,** 215–228.

Robinson, C. P., and Smith, P. W. (1977). Lack of involvement of monoamine oxidase in the lethality of acute poisoning by chlordimeform. *J. Toxicol. Environ. Health* **3,** 565–568.

Robinson, C. P., Smith, P. W., Zelenski, J. D., and Endecott, B. R. (1975). Lack of an effect of interference with amine mechanisms on the lethality of chlordimeform in the rat. *Toxicol. Appl. Pharmacol.* **33,** 380–383.

Robinson, C. P., Zelenski, J. D., and Pento, J. T. (1976). The effects of chlordimeform on agonist-induced contractions of vascular smooth muscle. *Pharmacologist* **18,** 141.

Roland, E. H., Jan, J. E., and Rigg, J. M. (1985). Toxic encephalopathy in a child after brief exposure to insect repellents *Can. Med. Assoc. J.,* **132,** 155–156.

Saladin, B., Saldin, K., Holzer, B., Dennis, E., Hanson, A., and Degrémont, A. (1983). A pilot control trial of schistomiasis in central Liberia by mass chemotherapy of target populations, combined with focal application of molluscicide. *Acta Trop.* **40,** 271–295.

Salamone, M. F. (1981). Toxicity of 41 carcinogens and noncarcinogenic analogs. *Prog. Mutat. Res.* **1,** 682–685.

Sarles, M. P., and Vandegrift, W. B. (1952). Chronic oral toxicity and related studies on animals with the insecticide and pyrethrum synergist, piperonyl butoxide. *Am. J. Trop. Med.* **1,** 862–883.

Sarles, M. P., Dove, W. E., and Moore, D. H. (1949). Acute toxicity and irritation tests on animals with the new insecticide, piperonyl butoxide. *Am. J. Trop. Med.* **29,** 151–162.

Schaffer, D. D., Hsu, W. H., and Hopper, D. L. (1985). The effects of yohimbine, tolazoline, atropine, prazosin, and naloxone on amitraz-induced depression of shuttle-avoidance response in dogs. *Abstr. Conf. Res. Workers Anim. Dis., 66th,* Chicago, p. 14.

Schmidt, C. H., Acree, F., Jr., and Bowman, M. C. (1959). Fate of C^{14}-diethyltoluamide applied to guinea pigs. *J. Econ. Entomol.* **52,** 928–930.

Sellers, A. F., Lowe, J. E., and Cummings, J. F. (1985). Trials of serotonin, substance P and α_2-adrenergic receptor effects on the equine large colon. *Cornell Vet.* **75,** 319–323.

Sen Gupta, A. K., and Knowles, C. O. (1970). Galecron-C^{14}, *N'*-(4-chloro-*o*-tolyl)-*N,N*-dimethylformamidine, metabolism in the dog and goat. *J. Econ. Entomol.* **63,** 951–956.

Sherman, R. A. (1979a). "Phase 2, Behavioral Effects of Acute Aerosol Exposure to *N,N*-Diethyl-*meta*-toluamide (*m*-DET)." Study 75-51-0034-80, January–February 1979. 28 pp. U.S. Army Environ. Hyg. Agency, Aberdeen Proving Ground, Maryland.

Sherman, R. A. (1979b). "Phase 3, Behavioral Effects of Subchronic Aerosol Exposure to *N,N*-Diethyl-*meta*-toluamide (*m*-DET)." Study 75-51-0034-80, February–May 1979. U.S. Army Environ. Hyg. Agency, Aberdeen Proving Ground, Maryland.

Sherman, R. A., Weeks, M. H., Asaki, A., Kerby, W., Bergmann, J., and Macko, J. (1980). Behavioral effects of acute and subchronic aerosol exposure of rats to *m*-DET. *Abstr. Pap., 19th Annu. Meet. Soc. Toxicol.,* p. A28.

Shirasu, Y., Moriya, M., Kato, K., Furuhashi, A., and Kada, T. (1976). Mutagenicity screening of pesticides in the microbial system. *Mutat. Res.* **40,** 19–30.

Sidi, Y., Kiltchevsky, E., Shaklai, M., and Pinkhas, J. (1983). Acute myeloblastic leukemia and insecticide. *N. Y. State J. Med.* **83,** 161.

Skrinjaric-Spoljar, M., Matthews, H. B., Engel, J. L., and Casida, J. E. (1971). Response of hepatic microsomal mixed function oxidases to various types of insecticide chemical synergists administered to mice. *Biochem. Pharmacol.* **20,** 1607–1618.

Smith, C. N. (1973). Pyrethrum for control of insects affecting man and animals. *In* "Pyrethrum: The Natural Insecticide" (J. E. Casida, ed.), pp. 225–241. Academic Press, New York.

Smith, C. N., Gilbert, I. H., Gouck, H. C., Bowman, M. C., Acree, F., Jr., and Schmidt, C. H. (1963). Factors affecting the protection period of mosquito repellents. *U.S., Dep. Agric., Tech. Bull.* **1285,** 1–36.

Smyth, H. F., Jr., Carpenter, C. P., Weil, S. C., and Pozzani, U. C. (1954). Range-finding and toxicity data. *AMA Arch. Ind. Health* **10,** 61–68.

Snodgrass, H. L., Nelson, D. C., and Weeks, M. H. (1982). Dermal penetration and potential for placental transfer of the insect repellent, *N,N*-diethyl-*m*-toluamide. *Am. Ind. Hyg. Assoc. J.* **43,** 747–753.

Snyder, J. W., Poe, R. O., Stubbins, J. F., and Garrettson, L. K. (1986). Acute manic psychosis following dermal application of *N,N*-diethyl-*m*-toluamide (deet) in an adult. *J. Toxicol. Clin. Toxicol.* **24,** 429–439.

Stenbäck, F. (1977). Local and systemic effects of commonly used cutaneous agents: Lifetime studies of 16 compounds in mice and rabbits *Acta Pharmacol. Toxicol.* **41,** 417–431.

Storer, R. D., and Conolly, R. B. (1985). An investigation of the role of microsomal oxidative metabolism in the *in vitro* genotoxicity of 1,2-dichloroethane. *Toxicol. Appl. Pharmacol.* **77,** 36–46.

Swentzel, K. C. (1977). Investigation of *N,N*-Diethyl-*m*-toluamide (*m*-DET) for Dominant Lethal Effects in the Mouse. Study 51-0034-78, September–November 1977, 12 pp. U.S. Army Environ. Hyg. Agency, Aberdeen Proving Ground, Maryland.

Taniguchi, Y., Nishibe, T., and Tsubura, Y. (1978). Toxicity test of *p*-chlorophenyl *p*-chlorobenzene sulfonate. Part I. Acute oral toxicity in BDF mice. *J. Nara Med. Assoc.* **29**, 534–538 (in Japanese).

Tao, X. M., Sun, R., and Wang, M. (1985). Health survey of workers in Cuiqiao agrochemical factory manufacturing chlordimeform hydrochloride. *Zhonghua Laodong Weisheng Zhiyebing Zazhi* **3**, 272–274 (in Chinese).

Tenebein, M. (1981). Toxic encephalopathy due to insect repellent ingestion. *Vet. Hum. Toxicol.* **23**, 363.

Testa, B., and Jenner, P. (1976). "Drug Metabolism: Chemical and Biochemical Aspects." Dekker, New York.

Timbrell, J. A., and Mitchell, J. R. (1977). Toxicity-related changes in benzene metabolism *in vivo*. *Xenobiotica* **7**, 415–423.

Tsunenari, S. (1973). Studies on an organic miticide, Azomite, from forensic toxicological aspects. *Jpn. J. Leg. Med.* **27**, 123–133 (in Japanese).

Tsunenari, S., Ogata, Y., Matsumoto, S., Abe, Y., and Yanda, M. (1972). A death by intoxication due to Azomite, an acaricide, and experimental studies on the acaricide. *Jpn. J. Leg. Med.* **26**, 381 (in Japanese).

Tune, B. M., Kuo, C. H., Hook, J. B., Hsu, C. Y., and Fravert, D. (1983). Effects of piperonyl butoxide on cephalosporin nephrotoxicity in the rabbit. An effect on cephaloridine. *J. Pharmacol. Exp. Ther.* **224**, 520–524.

Turnbull, G. J. (1983). Animal studies on the treatment of poisoning by amitraz (a formamidine pesticide) and xylene. *Hum. Toxicol.* **2**, 579–586.

Turner, T. (1962). Metaldehyde poisoning in the dog. *Vet Rec.* **74**, 592–593.

Urbaneja, M., and Knowles, C. O. (1979). Formanilide inhibition of rat brain monoamine oxidase. *Gen. Pharmacol.* **10**, 309–314.

U.S. Department of Agriculture (USDA) (1978). "The biologic and economic assessment of amitraz. A report of the amitraz assessment team to the rebuttable presumption against registration of amitraz submitted to EPA. *U.S., Dep. Agric., Tech. Bull.* **1637**, 1–82.

Veronesi, B. (1984). Effect of metabolic inhibition with piperonyl butoxide on rodent sensitivity to tri-*ortho*-cresyl phosphate. *Exp. Neurol.* **85**, 651–660.

Verschuuren, H. G., Kroes, R., and Den Tonkelaar, E. M. (1973). Toxicity studies on tetrasul. III. Short-term comparative studies in rats with tetrasul and structurally related acaricides. *Toxicology* **1**, 113–123.

Verschuuren, H. G., Kroes, R., Den Tonkelaar, E. M., Berkvens, J. M., and Van Esch, G. J. (1975). Long-term toxicity and reproduction studies with metaldehyde in rats. *Toxicology* **4**, 97–115.

Vischer, A. (1935). Contribution to the symptoms of metaldehyde poisoning. *Schweiz. Med. Wochenschr.* **65**, 827–829 (in German).

von Mayenburg, J., and Rakoski, J. (1983). Contact urticaria to diethyltoluamide. *Contact Dermatitis* **9**, 171.

Vos, J. G., and Krajnc, E. I. (1983). Immunotoxicity of pesticides. *Dev. Toxicol. Environ. Sci.* **11**, 229–240.

Vos, J. G., Krajnc, E. I., Beekhof, P. K., and Van Logten, M. J. (1983). Methods of testing immune effects of toxic chemicals: Evaluation of the immunotoxicity of various pesticides in the rat. *Proc. Int. Congr. Pestic. Chem., 5th* Vol. 3, pp. 497–504.

Wagstaff, D. J., and Short, C. R. (1971). Induction of hepatic microsomal hydroxylating enzymes by technical piperonyl butoxide and some of its analogs. *Toxicol. Appl. Pharmacol.* **19**, 54–61.

Wang, C. M., Narahashi, T., and Fukami, J. (1975). Mechanism of neuromuscular block by chlordimeform. *Pestic. Biochem. Physiol* **5**, 119–125.

Wang, G. M. (1984a). Evaluation of pesticides which pose carcinogenicity potential in animal testing. I. Developing a tumor data evaluation system. *Regul. Toxicol. Pharmacol.* **4**, 355–360.

Wang, G. M. (1984b). Evaluation of pesticides which pose carcinogenicity potential in animal testing. II. Consideration of human exposure conditions for regulatory decision making. *Regul. Toxicol. Pharmacol.* **4**, 361–367.

Warren, D. L., Brown, D. L., Jr., and Buckpitt, A. R. (1982). Evidence for cytochrome P-450 mediated metabolism in the bronchiolar damage by naphthalene. *Chem.-Biol. Interact.* **40**, 287–303.

Watanabe, H., Tsuda, S., and Fukami, J. (1975). Effects of chlordimeform on recuts abdominis muscle of frog. *Pestic. Biochem. Physiol.* **5**, 150–154.

Watanabe, H., Ishibashi, S., and Fukami, J. (1976). Chlordimeform and its metabolites: Toxicity and inhibition of acetylcholine-induced contraction of frog muscle. *J. Pestic. Sci.* **1**, 301–305.

Waters, M. D., Sandhu, S. S., Simmon, V. F., Mortelmans, K. E., Mitchell, A.

D., Jorgenson, T. A., Jones, D. C. L., Valencia, R., and Garrett, N. E. (1982). Study of pesticide genotoxicity. *In* "Genetic Toxicology: An Agricultural Perspective" (R. Fleck and A. Hollaender, eds.), pp. 275–326. Plenum, New York.

Watkinson, W. P. (1985a). Effects of chlordimeform on cardiovascular functional parameters in the postweanling rat. *Toxicologist* **5**, 95.

Watkinson, W. P. (1985b). Effects of chlordimeform on cardiovascular functional parameters: Part 1. Lethality and arrhythmogenicity in the geriatric rat. *J. Toxicol. Environ. Health* **15**, 729–744.

Watkinson, W. P. (1986a). Effects of chlordimeform on cardiovascular functional parameters: Part 2. Acute and delayed effects following intravenous administrations in the postweanling rat. *J. Toxicol. Environ. Health* **19**, 195–206.

Watkinson, W. P. (1986b). Effects of chlordimeform on cardiovascular functional parameters: Part 3. Comparison of different routes of administration in the postweanling rat. *J. Toxicol. Environ. Health* **19**, 207–218.

Watkinson, W. P., and Gordon, C. J. (1987). Effects of chlordimeform on heart rate and body temperature of unanesthetized, unrestrained rats. *Toxicol. Lett.* **35**, 209–216.

Webbe, G., ed. (1987). "Toxicology of Molluscicides," Int. Encycl. Pharmacol. Ther., Sect. 125. Pergamon, Oxford.

Weil, C. S., and McCollister, D. D. (1963). Relationship between short- and long-term feeding studies in designing an effective toxicity test. *J. Agric. Food Chem.* **11**, 486–491.

Weisburger, E. K., Russfield, A. B., Homburger, F., Weisburger, J. H., Boger, E., Van Dongen, G., and Chu, K. C. (1978). Testing of twenty-one environmental aromatic amines or derivatives for long-term toxicity or carcinogenicity. *J. Environ. Pathol. Toxicol.* **2**, 325–356.

White, T. J., Goodman, D., Shulgin, A. T., Castagnoli, N., Jr., Lee, R., and Petrakis, N. L. (1978). Mutagenic activity of some centrally active aromatic amines in *Salmonella typhimurium*. *Mutat. Res.* **56**, 199–202.

Williams, R. T. (1959). "Detoxication Mechanisms." Wiley, New York.

Wiltrout, R. W., Ercegovich, C. D., and Ceglowski, W. S. (1978). Humoral immunity in mice following oral administration of selected pesticides. *Bull. Environ. Contam. Toxicol.* **20**, 423–431.

Wiswesser, W. J., ed. (1976). "Pesticide Index," 5th ed. Entomol Soc. Am., College Part, Maryland.

Witkin, J. M., and Leander, J. D. (1982). Effects of the appetite stimulant chlordimeform on food and water consumption of rats: Comparison with chlordiazepoxide. *J. Pharmacol. Exp. Ther.* **223**, 130–134.

Witschi, H. P. (1986). Separation of early diffuse alveolar cell proliferation from enhanced tumor development in mouse lung. *Cancer Res.* **46**, 2675–2679.

Wong, M. H., and Yew, D. T. (1978). Dermotoxicity of the mosquito repellent related to rabbit ears. *Acta Anat.* **100**, 129–131.

Worthing, C. R., and Walker, S. B., eds. (1983). "The Pesticide Manual," 7th ed. Br. Crop Prot. Counc., Lavenham Press Ltd., Lavenham, Suffolk, U.K.

Wu, A., Pearson, M. L., Shekoski, D. L., Soto, R. J., and Stewart, R. D. (1979). High resolution gas chromatography/mass spectrometric characterization of urinary metabolites of *N,N*-diethyl-*m*-toluamide (deet) in man *HRC CC, J. High Resolut. Chromatogr. Chromatogr. Commun.* **2**, 558–562.

Yim, G. K. W., Holsapple, M. P., Pfister, W. R., and Hollingworth, R. M. (1978a). Prostaglandin synthesis inhibited by formamidine pesticides. *Life Sci.* **23**, 2509–2516.

Yim, G. K. W., Pfister, W. R., Yau, E. T., and Mennear, J. H. (1978b). Comparison of appetite stimulation by chlordiazepoxide, chlordimeform, clonidine, and cyproheptadine in rats *Fed. Proc., Fed. Am. Soc. Exp. Biol.* **37**, 860.

Yoshida, T., Suzuki, Y., and Uchiyama, M. (1976). Effect of piperonyl butoxide on hepatic delta-aminolevulinic acid synthetase activity in mice. *Biochem. Pharmacol.* **25**, 2418–2420.

Zadikoff, C. M. (1979). Toxic encephalopathy associated with use of insect repellent. *J. Pediatr.* **95**, 140–142.

Zebitz, C. P. W., Holst, H., and Schmutterer, H. (1981). Effect of nikkomycin (GT 25/76, AMS 0896) on the predaceous mite *Phytoseiulus persimilis*

Athias-Henriot (Acari, Phytoseiidae). *Mitt. Dtsch. Ges. Allg. Angew, Entomol.* **2,** 180–185 (in German).

Zelenski, J. D., Robinson, C. P., and Pento, J. T. (1978). Effects of chlordimeform on vascular smooth muscle. *Pestic. Biochem. Physiol.* **11,** 278–286.

Zimmer, D., Mazurek, J., Petzold, G., and Bhuyan, B. K. (1980). Bacterial mutagenicity and mammalian cell DNA damage by several substituted anilines. *Mutat. Res.* **77,** 317–326.

Zoebelein, G., and Kniehase, U. (1985). Laboratory, greenhouse and field trials on the effect of nikkomycins on insects and mites. *Pflanzenschutz-Nachr.* **38,** 203–304.

Cumulative Index

This index covers all three volumes, but the volumes are treated differently. Important subheadings are shown for each compound discussed in Volume 1 but, with certain exceptions, only the range of pages is recorded for its discussion in Volumes 2 and 3. Volume 1 is concerned mainly with *concepts* so that mention of any particular compound there would be lost if it were not indexed; on the contrary, Volumes 2 and 3 are concerned largely with *compounds*, and details about each one are presented in an orderly way under three numbered subheadings: *Identity, Properties, and Uses; Toxicity to Laboratory Animals;* and *Toxicity to Humans.* Each of these headings is further subdivided by several paragraph headings, depending on the amount of information available for presentation on each particular compound. This arrangement should make it easy for the reader to find any particular information presented within the range of pages devoted to each compound in Volumes 2 and 3, and duplication of the subdivisions in the index would make the index much longer without being more helpful. Exceptions concern (*a*) the heading *Studies in Humans*, which is subdivided in the index to indicate individual compounds that have caused illness, that have been studied in workers, that have been studied in volunteers, or that have been used theraputically and (*b*) introductory material in Volumes 2 and 3, which generally concerns a group of compounds and not any one compound to which a separate numbered section is devoted.